CT and MRI in Congenital Heart Diseases

Ramiah Rajeshkannan
Vimal Raj • Sanjaya Viswamitra
Editors

CT and MRI in Congenital Heart Diseases

Springer

Editors
Ramiah Rajeshkannan
Department of Radiology
Amrita School of Medicine, Amrita
Institute of Medical Sciences
and Research Centre
Amrita Vishwa Vidyapeetham
Kochi
Kerala
India

Vimal Raj
Department of Cardiothoracic imaging
Narayana Hrudayalaya
Bangalore
Karnataka
India

Sanjaya Viswamitra
Department of Radiology
Sri Sathya Sai Institute of Higher
Medical Sciences
Bengaluru
Karnataka
India

ISBN 978-981-15-6754-4 ISBN 978-981-15-6755-1 (eBook)
https://doi.org/10.1007/978-981-15-6755-1

This Springer imprint is published by the registered company Springer Nature Singapore Pte Ltd.
The registered company address is: 152 Beach Road, #21-01/04 Gateway East, Singapore 189721, Singapore

Foreword

At the outset, let me congratulate Dr. Rajeshkannan, the Editor-in-Chief of this book, for the stupendous effort that has gone into putting it together. As someone who has gone through the pain associated with writing books, I can only empathize with Rajesh for the time, energy, and effort that he and his coeditors, Dr. Vimal Raj and Dr. Sanjaya Viswamitra, have put into the whole process, from picking out the topics, allotting authors, chasing them, and editing the articles and images to giving all of them a coherent flow. And in a country like India, where deadlines often have no meaning and authors do not deliver their book chapters for sometimes up to a year after the deadline is past, I can tell you that this is no easy task.

The book comprehensively covers the techniques, the embryology, anatomy, and then the individual diseases. Both intra-cardiac and extra-cardiac anomalies are dealt with in detail by authors who are experts in the field of cardiac imaging and have an in-depth knowledge of their individual subjects.

The images are of high quality, along with the videos. In many chapters, especially embryology, aortic anomalies, and vascular rings, the colored diagrams go a long way in making these complex anomalies seem simple.

The book ends with a section discussing alternate topics such as the role of echocardiography, the use of CT versus MRI in different forms of congenital heart disease (CHD), 3D printing, which many surgeons and cardiologists find useful, and radiation issues.

The book is a must-read for those who perform scans in patients with CHD, and even if you do not go through it at one go, it would be a good reference book to have by your side if you ever get stuck with a case or want to know what points to cover, both when these patients are being scanned and when you are generating the report.

As with all multi-author books, the language varies from chapter to chapter…this only brings out the heterogeneity of our country and its different voices that this book captures well.

I wish the authors and editors all success and again…congrats to everyone involved for a job well done.

Bhavin Jankharia
Radiology Education Foundation
Mumbai, Maharashtra, India

Preface

This book fills the growing need for a comprehensive resource in the imaging of congenital heart disease (CHD). We started this off as a modest effort to explain the complexities of imaging in CHD. We soon realized that we needed to expand the text for such a resource to be beneficial. Dr. R. Rajeshkannan has worked tirelessly to put together a veritable who's who of Indian authors with years of experience in imaging of CHD. He has been the conductor of this orchestra of professional imagers. This book's success owes as much to his successful efforts in creating a symphony as it does to the knowledge of the individual contributors. We are grateful to all the authors for their time and energy in creating this tome.

The book's 25 chapters cover everything from the aorta to vascular rings, embryology to postsurgical evaluation, and the simplest to the most complex congenital heart disease. The book begins with "Basics of imaging" in CT and MRI and then progresses to the core topics on congenital heart disease. It ends with a unique section on advanced topics such as 3D printing. There is even a chapter on the physics of CT and MRI, and a chapter on radiation—issues relevant to those who "image gently!"

Keeping in track with the changing world where books are being supplemented by digital reading materials, we have created a repository of nearly 300 videos. These videos fit in very well and will help you to get a holistic approach.

We hope that there is something for everyone in this book. The novice will welcome the liberal use of tables and figures used to emphasize and to add clarity. The book's images and illustrations reflect the experience and enthusiasm of all the authors. We hope that the experienced imager finds the writing lucid and engaging and, perhaps, even new gems within the chapters.

We trust that this book finds a special place in your office, reporting room, and at your scanner and, finally, that you enjoy this book as much as we have enjoyed bringing it to you.

Kochi, India — Ramiah Rajeshkannan
Bangalore, India — Vimal Raj
Bengaluru, India — Sanjaya Viswamitra

Contents

About the Editors and Contributors

About the Editors

Ramiah Rajeshkannan, MD, DNB, PDCC graduated from JIPMER, Puducherry University, India. He works as clinical professor at the Department of Radiology, Amrita Institute of Medical Sciences, Kochi. He holds fellowship in cardiovascular and neuro-interventional radiology from Sree Chitra Tirunal Institute of Medical Sciences, Trivandrum. He is the general secretary and founder member of Indian Association of Cardiac Imaging (IACI). The global academy of MRI has awarded him the title "ESMRMB and ISMRM certified teacher in Clinical MRI." He has many peer-reviewed national and international publications.

Vimal Raj, FRCR, CCT, EDM, PGDMLS is a renowned specialist in the field of cardiothoracic imaging. He currently heads the Department of Radiology in Narayana Hrudayalaya, Bangalore. He has worked in three of the leading cardiothoracic centers of the world, i.e., Cambridge (Papworth Hospital), London (Royal Brompton Hospital), and Leicester (Glenfield Hospital). He has also worked with the British Army and was deployed in the war zone in Afghanistan. He has teaching interests and has published two books and multiple book chapters for radiologists and clinicians. He has published several articles in peer-reviewed journals. He also holds a patent in catheter design for performing postmortem CT coronary angiography. He has the distinction of conducting the only Cardiac MR fellowship program in India, under the aegis of the European Society of Cardiology in India. He also holds the distinction of training more than 2000 imagers in the last 3 years on cardiothoracic imaging across the Indian subcontinent, the Middle East, South Asia, Africa, and Europe.

Sanjaya Viswamitra graduated from the Jawaharlal Institute of Medical Education and Research, Puducherry University, Puducherry, India, in 1991. He completed a Body Imaging Fellowship from Thomas Jefferson University Hospital and a Nuclear Medicine Fellowship from the Hospital of the University of Pennsylvania, Philadelphia, PA. He is heading the Department of Radiology, Sri Sathya Sai Institute of Higher Medical Sciences, Bangalore. He is also a faculty at the University of Arkansas for Medical Sciences, Little Rock, AR, USA, and specializes in radiology and nuclear medicine. He is the past president of the Indian Association of Cardiac Imaging and one of its founder members. He holds many Editor's Recognition Awards from AJR (ARRS) and Radiology (RSNA). He has been practicing cardiac imaging since 2003 and is passionate about teaching cardiac imaging.

Contributors

Onkar B. Auti Ruby Hall Clinic, Pune, Maharashtra, India

Ashita Barthur Department of Radiology, Sri Jayadeva Institute of Cardiovascular Sciences and Research, Bangalore, India

Alpa Bharati BJ Wadia Hospital for Children, Holy Family Hospital, Mumbai, India

Salil Bhargava Department of Radiology, Sir Ganga Ram Hospital, New Delhi, India

Binita Chacko Department of Radiology, Christian Medical College and Hospital, Vellore, Tamil Nadu, India

Johann Christopher CARE Hospitals, Hyderabad, India

Subhajit Das Rabindranath Tagore International Institute of Cardiac Sciences, Kolkata, India

Amit Ajit Deshpande Department of Cardiovascular Radiology & Endovascular Interventions, All India Institute of Medical Sciences, New Delhi, India

Amol Dikshit Infinity Medical Centre, Parel, Mumbai, India

Jahnavi Gaduputi Department of Radiology, Sri Sathya Sai Institute of Higher Medical Sciences, Whitefield, Bengaluru, Karnataka, India

Archita Goel Department of Radiology, Sri Sathya Sai Institute of Higher Medical Sciences, Whitefield, Bengaluru, Karnataka, India

Gurpreet Gulati Department of Cardiovascular Radiology & Endovascular Interventions, All India Institute of Medical Sciences, New Delhi, India

Aparna Irodi Department of Radiology, Christian Medical College and Hospital, Vellore, Tamil Nadu, India

Shaik Ismail Department of Radiology, Sri Sathya Sai Institute of Higher Medical Sciences, Whitefield, Bengaluru, Karnataka, India

Priya Jagia Department of Cardiovascular Radiology and Endovascular Interventions, All India Institute of Medical Sciences, New Delhi, India

Elizabeth Joseph Department of Radiology, Christian Medical College and Hospital, Vellore, Tamil Nadu, India

Shruthi Kalyan Star Hospitals, Hyderabad, India

T. R. Kapilamoorthy Department of Imaging Sciences and Interventional Radiology, Sree Chitra Tirunal Institute for Medical Sciences and Technology, Trivandrum, Kerala, India

Mahesh Kappanayil Department of Pediatric Cardiology, Amrita School of Medicine, Amrita Institute of Medical Sciences and Research Centre, Amrita Vishwa Vidyapeetham, Kochi, Kerala, India

Rishabh Khurana Department of Cardiovascular Radiology & Endovascular Interventions, All India Institute of Medical Sciences, New Delhi, India

R. Krishna Kumar Department of Pediatric Cardiology, Amrita School of Medicine, Amrita Institute of Medical Sciences and Research Centre, Amrita Vishwa Vidyapeetham, Kochi, Kerala, India

Linu Kuruvilla Department of Radiology, Christian Medical College and Hospital, Vellore, Tamil Nadu, India

Srikanth Moorthy Amrita School of Medicine, Amrita Institute of Medical Sciences and Research Centre, Amrita Vishwa Vidyapeetham, Kochi, Kerala, India

Ashirwad Pasumarthy AIG Hospitals, Hyderabad, Telangana, India

Ramiah Rajeshkannan Department of Radiology, Amrita School of Medicine, Amrita Institute of Medical Sciences and Research Centre, Amrita Vishwa Vidyapeetham, Kochi, Kerala, India

Vimal Raj Department of Cardiothoracic Imaging, Narayana Hrudayalaya, Bangalore, Karnataka, India

Yashpal Rana U.N. Mehta Institute of Cardiology and Research Centre, Ahmedabad, Gujarat, India

Radiscan Diagnostics, Ahmedabad, Gujarat, India

Bhavana Nagabhushana Reddy Department of Radiology, Sri Sathya Sai Institute of Higher Medical Sciences, Whitefield, Bengaluru, Karnataka, India

D. Prashanth Reddy Department of Radiology, Sri Sathya Sai Institute of Higher Medical Sciences, Whitefield, Bengaluru, Karnataka, India

Megha M. Sheth U. N. Mehta Institute of Cardiology and Research Centre, Ahmedabad, Gujarat, India

Mumun Sinha Department of Cardiovascular Radiology and Endovascular Interventions, All India Institute of Medical Sciences, New Delhi, India

Hemant B. Telkar Infinity Medical Centre, Next to Gandhi (MGM) hospital, Parel, Mumbai, India

Sudeep Verma CARE Hospitals, Hyderabad, India

Sanjaya Viswamitra Department of Radiology, Sri Sathya Sai Institute of Higher Medical Sciences, Whitefield, Bengaluru, Karnataka, India

Part I

The Basics of CHD imaging

CMR Physics

1

Amit Ajit Deshpande, Rishabh Khurana, and Gurpreet Gulati

1.1 Introduction

The importance of magnetic resonance imaging (MRI) in the field of cardiovascular radiology is growing day by day. As it offers several advantages compared to computed tomography (superior contrast and temporal resolution, no exposure to radiation or iodinated contrast and multiparametric imaging), MRI is being utilized more often in the management of congenital heart diseases. It is important to understand the physics behind the MRI for its optimum utilization. This chapter will focus on the basic principles and working of the MRI.

1.2 Hardware

MRI has three main components, i.e., magnets, coils, and computer systems. Magnet is the heart of the scanner and coils are the main workhorse. Magnets provide the constant magnetic field (B_0), while the coils generate magnetic field gradients, transmit and receive the signals. The signals received are fed into the computer system to generate the images.

A. A. Deshpande · R. Khurana · G. Gulati (✉)
Department of Cardiovascular Radiology & Endovascular Interventions, All India Institute of Medical Sciences, New Delhi, India

1.2.1 Magnets

- Magnets can be of three types: (1) Permanent, (2) Resistive, and (3) Super-conducting electromagnet.
- Permanent magnets are generally a part of an open bore type of system. It consists of two opposing flat magnetized poles fixed to an iron frame. This system gives low strength (up to 0.3 T) and a vertical magnetic field.
- Resistive electromagnets have a set of DC coils and require a continuous supply of around 50–100 kW of power [1]. The magnetic field generated by this magnet is limited to 0.5 T due to heat production.
- The superconducting electromagnet has niobium-titanium (Nb-Ti) alloy wires in a copper matrix. This metal, when kept at a very low temperature (below 9.4 °K), loses the electric resistance so that the flow of current increases and so does the magnetic field strength. Once the electric resistance is eliminated, higher magnetic field strength can be achieved by a continuous flow of current in a loop. There is no loss of power, so it does not require a continuous power supply as long as the wires are maintained below the critical temperature. The critical temperature is maintained by the liquid helium (4 °K) surrounding the coil, known as a cryostat. Cryostat is a multi-compartmental structure containing various insulating and vacuum layers. It is further

R. Rajeshkannan et al. (eds.), *CT and MRI in Congenital Heart Diseases*,
https://doi.org/10.1007/978-981-15-6755-1_1

encased by the external casing made of non-ferromagnetic materials (mostly stainless steel) (Fig. 1.1). These insulating layers shield the coils from the external environment. Now, with the "*Zero boil off*" technique, it is possible to run the system without the need for a helium refill [2].

1.2.2 Coils

- These are of three types, i.e., (1) outermost shim coil, (2) middle gradient coils, and (3) innermost radio-frequency (RF) coils (Fig. 1.2).
- Shim coils make the magnetic field as homogenous as possible throughout the volume of interest. The inhomogeneity in the main magnetic field (B_0) is nullified by the shim coil. This is important to generate good quality images. Homogeneity is expressed as parts per million (ppm). For the optimum quality of images, 10 ppm is required for spin-echo sequences whereas spectroscopy requires homogeneity of <1 ppm [3].
- Three sets of gradient coils produce magnetic field gradients along *x*, *y*, and *z*-axis. The current in these coils must be switched on and off rapidly. This results in the formation of eddy currents, which degrades the magnetic field homogeneity. It also produces heat, which results in the boiling of the helium (cryogen). These gradients are perpendicular to each other and used for slice selection, phase encoding, and frequency encoding.
- Radio-frequency coils transmit the RF pulses and receive the signal from the patient. These coils produce the magnetic field (B_1) perpendicular to the main magnetic field. Depending on the type of surface to be imaged, RF coils can be of various types, i.e., body coil, surface coil, and phased array coil.

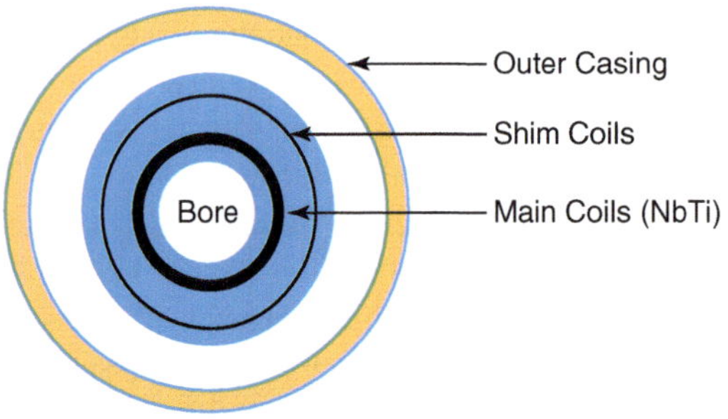

Fig. 1.1 Superconducting electromagnet, showing the main coil and shim coil immersed in liquid helium (blue) maintained at 4 °K. It is encased by the outer casing insulating the coils from external heat

1.3 Principle

- MRI works on the principle of nuclear magnetic resonance (NMR). Purcell and Bloch first described this in 1946. NMR is the physical process to record the absorption and emission of the energy from the nuclei in the magnetic field. It basically deals with the behavior of an atom when subjected to the magnetic field. This behavior depends on the property of "nuclear spin (*I*)." Nuclear spin is the property of the atomic nucleus, i.e., protons and neutrons. Both protons and neutrons have a net spin of the half. Calculating the nuclear spin of a particular atom can be a complex process that is beyond the scope of this chapter. Generally, nuclei with an odd mass

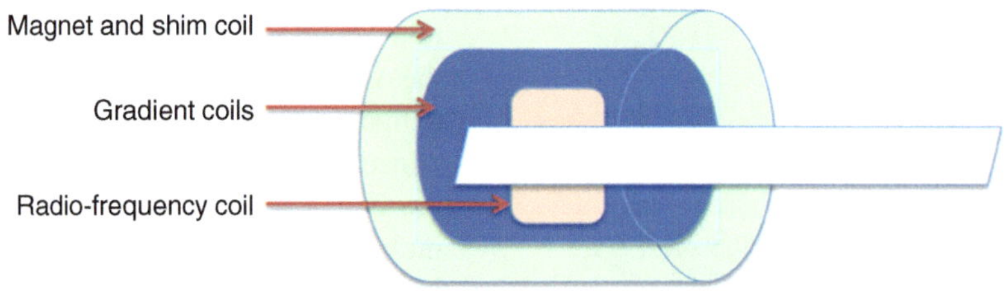

Fig. 1.2 Arrangement of coils. Gradient coils (blue) produce magnetic gradients along *x*, *y*, and *z*-axis. RF coils (orange) generate the signal while the shim coil (green) maintains the homogeneity of the volume

number (e.g., ^{1}H, ^{19}F, ^{31}P, ^{13}C) have spun with half-integral ($I = ½$) [4]. When these nuclei are subjected to magnetic fields, they can have two orientations, which can be either parallel (+½) or antiparallel (−½) to the magnetic fields.

- The human body has a very high concentration of ^{1}H protons in mainly water and fat. Since ^{1}H has a "spin," it can be imaged with MRI. Each of these positively charged protons rotates around an axis resulting in the formation of a small magnetic field. Generally, these protons are arranged randomly with the net magnetization of zero. When subjected to the magnetic field, these protons align themselves either parallel or antiparallel to the magnetic field as explained previously (Fig. 1.3a, b). The protons with the higher energy levels align antiparallel to the magnetic field and vice versa. Once these protons are aligned, they "precess" (spin) along B_0 in addition to their native spin around themselves (Fig. 1.3c). This precession frequency is also called Larmor frequency and is defined by the equation:

$$\nu = Y / 2\pi \times B_0,$$

where ν = Precession frequency (Hertz or cycles/min), Y = gyromagnetic ratio, B_0 = magnetic field strength. Y is specific for specific proton. Thus, the precession frequency of a water proton is roughly twice in a 3 T scanner as compared to a 1.5 T scanner. For example, the precession frequency of a water proton at 1.5 T is around 64 and 127 MHz in a 3 T scanner [5].

1.4 MR Signal Formation

1.4.1 Radio-frequency Excitation

- When the patient is placed in the magnetic bore, the protons spin along the direction of the main magnetic field (B_0), i.e., along the *z*-axis. The resultant net magnetization will be along the *z*-axis (also called equilibrium magnetization M_0), with no net magnetization in $x - y$ (transverse) plane (M_{xy}). MR image is formed by the net magnetization in the $x - y$ plane, while the *z*-axis magnetization is not enough for image formation (Fig. 1.4a).
- When an external radio-frequency (RF) pulse (B_1) is applied, the protons absorb this energy and move to a state of higher energy. This is called radio-frequency excitation. The frequency of the applied RF pulse should match the Larmor frequency of the protons. This phenomenon is called *resonance.*

1.4.2 180° and 90° Pulse

- A pulse having the energy to flip the protons through 180° and resulting in a reversal of the

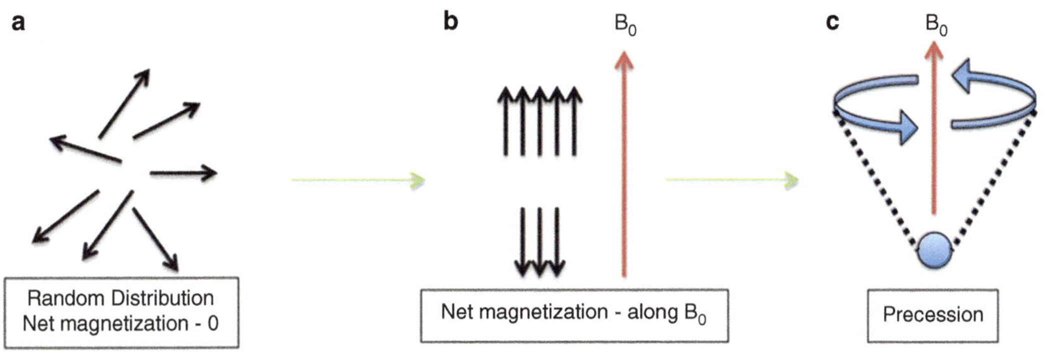

Fig. 1.3 Protons in the body are oriented randomly along all the axes of the body (**a**) with the resultant net magnetization of zero. When subjected to B_0, these protons get aligned either parallel or antiparallel to the magnetic field producing net magnetization (**b**). Each proton spins (precess) around the B_0 in conical fashion in addition to its native spin around itself (**c**). This precession frequency is given by the Larmor equation

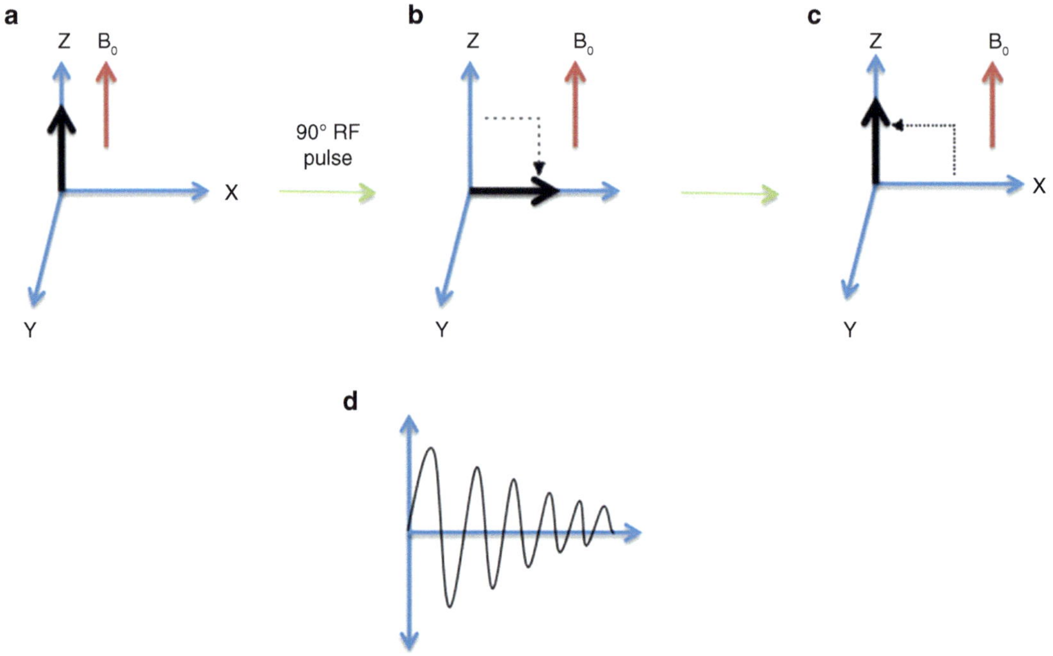

Fig. 1.4 Net magnetization (black arrow) along the Z-axis or the direction of B_0 (M_0). No net magnetization in the $x-y$ plane (M_{xy}), which is essential for the formation of image (**a**). After the application of 90° pulse, the net magnetization flips in the $x-y$ plane (**b**) with the formation of the signal. After the RF pulse is stopped, the net magnetization again spirals to its original orientation (**c**). The strength of M_{xy} and the MR signal is strongest when the RF pulse is stopped. The decay of M_{xy} and the MR signal is called free induction decay (**d**)

magnetic field is called 180° pulse or an inversion pulse. When a pulse with half the energy is applied, it results in the 90° flip of the protons with resultant net magnetization in the $x-y$ plane, also called transverse magnetization (M_{xy}) (Fig. 1.4b). Thus, it is called a 90° pulse or saturation pulse. In reality, it is possible to flip the magnetization to anywhere between 0° and 180°, depending on the energy of the applied pulse. The frequency of these pulses should also match the Larmor frequency of protons.

- The RF pulse is applied transiently to shift the net magnetization in the $x-y$ plane. The oscillating M_{xy} forms a current, which is picked up by the receiver coil. This process occurs due to the "relaxation" of the protons. Once the RF pulse is switched off, the M_{xy} and the MR signal is the highest. As the B_0 is the only magnetic field acting on the protons, protons in the transverse plane return to their original orientation (Fig. 1.4c), some before the other (depending on their energies and type of interactions, i.e., spin–spin or spin–lattice relaxation). As a result, longitudinal magnetization (M_z) regrows and M_{xy} decays. Thus, the MR signal strength also decreases. This phenomenon is called *Free induction decay* (Fig. 1.4d). This occurs by two different mechanisms called T1 relaxation and T2 decay.

1.4.3 T1 Relaxation/Spin: Lattice Relaxation

- T1 relaxation is the recovery of the M_0, by releasing the energy to the surrounding or the lattice. The time required to recover 63% of the M_0 is called T1 [5] (Fig. 1.5). It depends on the lattice in which the proton is oscillating and the strength of the magnetic field. Thus,

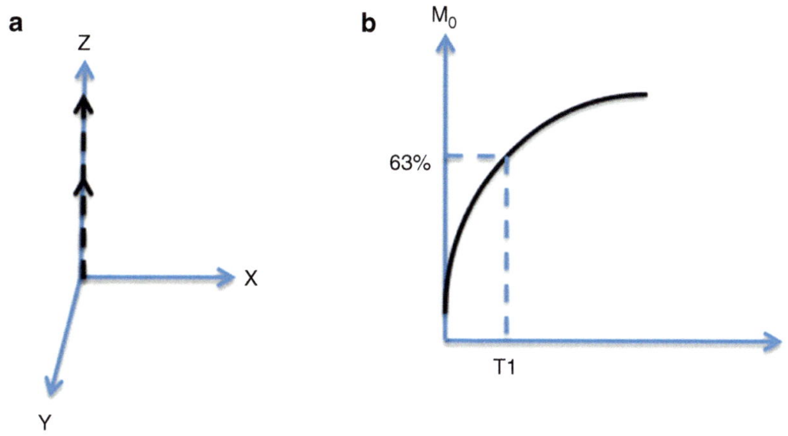

Fig. 1.5 Black dashed lines in (**a**) denote the growth of M_z. The time required for M_z to grow to 63% of M_0 is called T1 (**b**)

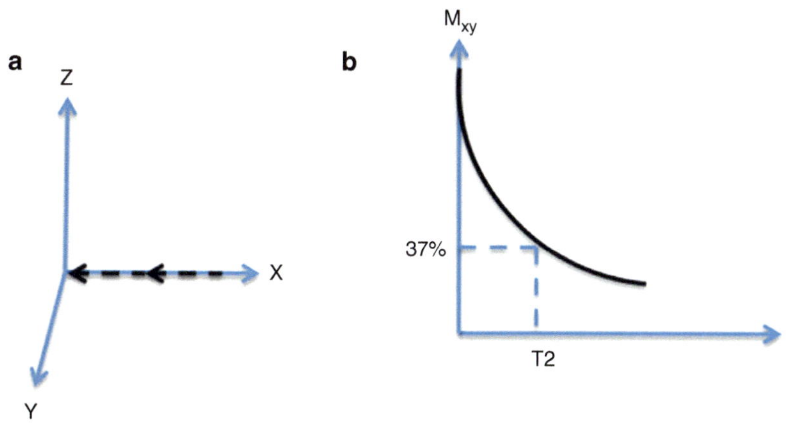

Fig. 1.6 The black dashed line in (**a**) denotes the decay of M_{xy}. The time required for M_{xy} to reduce to 37% of its maximum value is called T2 (**b**)

T1 is a constant for a particular tissue at a particular magnetic field strength. The transfer of energy to the surrounding is faster if the protons in the surrounding matter resonate at Larmor frequency. This is the case in fat, so it has short T1. Water, on the other hand, has the protons, which are moving too rapidly with different frequencies, resulting in a longer time to transfer the energy. So, water has a long T1 value.

- After the 90° pulse, M_z is zero, but it regrows with the constant T1 to achieve the equilibrium state (M_0). The value M_z at a particular time (t) after the 90° pulse is given by the formula:

$$M_z(t) = M_0\left(1 - e^{-t/T1}\right).$$

1.4.4 T2 Decay or Spin: Spin Relaxation

- The time required for the M_{xy} to fall to 37% of its maximum value is called T2 [6] (Fig. 1.6). Similar to T1, it depends on the tissue composition and the magnetic field strength. And thus, T2 is a constant for a particular tissue at a particular magnetic field strength.
- T2 decay is the reduction of M_{xy}, by interacting with other nuclei in the vicinity. Each proton in tissue has its tiny magnetic field (around 1 μT). It results in a change in B_0 from place to place on a submicroscopic scale. It alters the precessional frequency of protons (also known as dephasing) due to variations in the magnetic field. This variation is greatest in solids as the atoms are relatively fixed and close to

each other. Therefore, solid tissues have short T2 and produce a weaker signal. On the other hand, liquids like water have their atoms in random motion and loosely spaced. As a result, water has a long T2 and stronger signals as well.

- After the 90° pulse, M_{xy} is maximum (M_{xy0}). It decays with the constant T2. The value of M_{xy} after the time (t) of 90° pulse can be given by the formula:

$$M_{xy}(t) = M_{xy0}\left(e^{-t/T2}\right).$$

1.4.5 T2* Relaxation

- In addition to the inhomogeneity intrinsic to tissues, the external magnetic field is inhomogeneous as well. T2* relaxation occurs as a combination of spin–spin in relaxation and external magnetic field inhomogeneity. While this inhomogeneity in the external magnetic field is eliminated in spin-echo (SE) sequences (as will be discussed in Sect. 1.6), it persists in the gradient-echo (GRE) sequences. So T2* can only be seen in GRE sequences and not in SE sequences. Transverse relaxation in GRE sequences is given by T2* rather than T2. Since T2* is a combination of T2 and magnetic field inhomogeneity, it is shorter than T2 (Fig. 1.7). The relationship can be given as:

$$1/T2^{*} = 1/T2 + Y \cdot \Delta B_{\text{in homo}},$$

where Y = gyromagnetic ratio and ΔB_{inhomo} = magnetic field inhomogeneity.

- Normal T1, T2, and T2* values are given in Table 1.1. Since these values depend on the tissue characteristics as well as the magnetic field strength, the values are altered in altered tissue morphology (diseased state) [7]. T1, T2, and T2* values are the basis of the generation of the image contrast in an MR image. In addition, the exogenous intravenously administered contrast agent, i.e., gadolinium shortens T1, T2, and T2* values of a tissue in which it accumulates. It is possible to image these signals with the help of specific sequences and thus add to the diagnostic ability of the image.

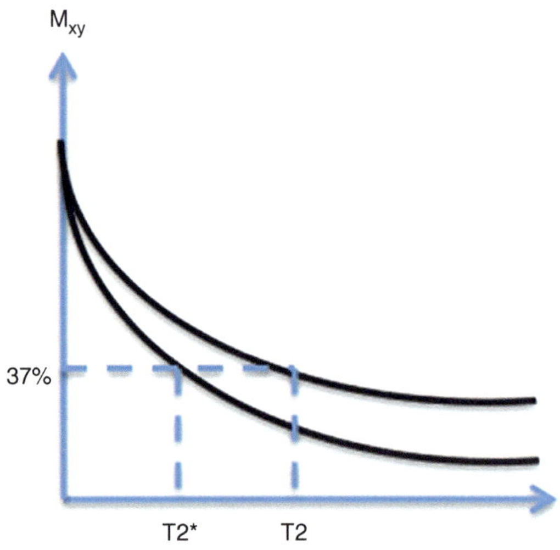

Fig. 1.7 T2* relaxation curve. T2* is shorter than T2 due to inhomogeneity in the external magnetic field in addition to spin–spin in relaxation

1.5 MR Signal Localization

We have seen how the signal is generated from a particular tissue by the use of three constants T1, T2, and T2*. However, it is important to localize the signal in three dimensions, i.e., x, y, and z to form the image. It is generally done in three steps: (1) Slice selection, (2) Phase encoding, and (3) Frequency encoding or readout step. Each of these steps can be rotated in any plane, i.e., x, y, and z as required. The localization is done by three magnetic fields superimposed on the B_0. These magnetic fields are produced by gradient coils and are also referred to as gradient fields.

1.5.1 Slice Selection

- Slice selection is the first step in the image localization. In this step, the gradient is applied along the direction of B_0 (usually along the z-axis). The slice selection gradient is applied along with the 90° RF pulse (Fig. 1.9). This produces a steady gradient in the magnetic field along the Z-axis. The pro-

Table 1.1 Normal T1 and T2 values at 1.5 T and 3 T

	T1 value (ms)		T2 values (ms)		T2* values (ms)	
Tissue	1.5 T	3 T	1.5 T	3 T	1.5 T	3 T
Myocardium	950 ± 21 [8]	1052 ± 23 [8]	55.8 ± 2.8 [9]	51.6 ± 3 [9]	36 ± 5 [10]	24 ± 5 [11]
Skeletal muscle	1130 ± 91.7 [12]	1420 ± 38.1 [12]	35.3 ± 3.85 [12]	31.7 ± 1.9 [12]	–	–
Blood	1441 ± 120 [13]	1932 ± 85 [13]	290 ± 30 [13]	275 ± 50 [13]	–	–

Note that T1 value increases and T2 value decreases with an increase in the magnetic field strength. Also, change in the T1 value is much more significant as compared to change in the T2 value

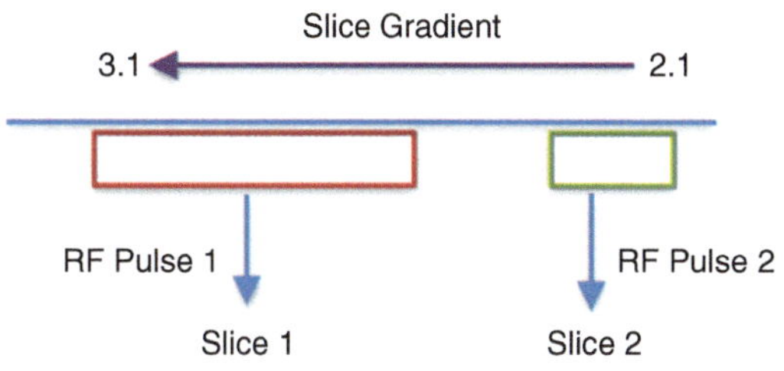

Fig. 1.8 After the slice selection gradient is applied, the RF pulse of a particular bandwidth is applied to select the slice thickness. RF pulse with a particular bandwidth (range of frequencies) will excite all the portions with the matching Larmor frequencies. RF pulse 1 (red rectangle) with broader bandwidth will produce a thicker slice as compared to RF pulse 2 (green rectangle) with a narrower bandwidth

tons at one end will precess faster and those at the other end will precess slower after the gradient pulse is applied. Now, the RF pulse having a particular bandwidth of frequency is applied using a gradient coil. Only the protons precessing with the frequency lying within the bandwidth of applied RF pulse will be excited and produce an MR signal (Fig. 1.8).

- The thickness of the slice is also determined at this step (Fig. 1.8). The thickness can be decreased by increasing the gradient across the field or narrowing the bandwidth of the applied RF pulse. Thinner the slice, better is the resolution due to a reduction in the partial volume effect.

1.5.2 Phase Encoding

- Once the location of the signal along one axis is determined, the next step is to determine the location along the rest of the axes. Every pixel of the image has a particular phase-frequency combination and it is not possible to decode the phase shift of every pixel from a single pulse by Fourier Transformation. Thus, each pixel row requires a separate phase encoding gradient pulse, e.g., 256 steps for an image size of 256 × 256. As a result, it requires multiple measurements from multiple phase encoding steps to accurately identify the location of a proton, unlike frequency encoding.

1.5.3 Frequency Encoding

- For frequency encoding, the gradient pulse is applied perpendicular to the slice selection and phase encoding gradients. When this gradient pulse is on, different protons along with this particular axis experience slightly different magnetic fields. Subsequently, the signal received from each of the protons will be different depending on the individual precessional frequency. By measuring these frequencies, the location of each proton is determined by Fourier Transformation. The gradient is applied during the time at which the MR signal is measured. Thus, it is also called the readout phase (Fig. 1.9).

1.5.4 *k*-Space

- The data from the frequency and phase encoding step is combined to form *k*-space. Each *k*-space point corresponds to phase and frequency information about every pixel in the image. This information is converted into the final image using a mathematical software called Fourier Transformation.

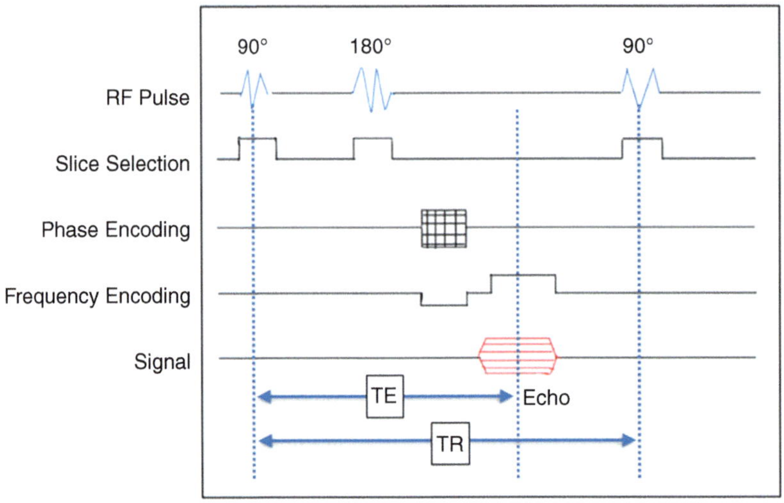

Fig. 1.9 Spin-echo sequence. 90° and 180° pulses are applied in series. The slice selection gradient is applied at the time of the RF pulse. Multiple phase encoding gradients are applied before the frequency encoding gradient, which should be on during the time echo is generated (also called readout gradient). The time from 90° pulse to the echo is called Time-to-Echo (TE) and time from one 90° pulse to the next 90° pulse is called Time-to-repetition (TR)

1.5.5 Scan Time

- Scan time or time of acquisition of a sequence depends on the TR, number of phase encoding steps, and number of excitations (Nex) or number of images averaged. The formula is given as:

$$\text{Scan time} = \text{TR} \times \text{phase encoding steps} \times \text{Nex}.$$

- The signal-to-noise ratio (SNR) is proportional to the square root of Nex and thus can be improved with increasing Nex, at the cost of increased scan time.
- Scan time can be significantly reduced by reducing the number of phase encoding steps, which is the principle of Parallel imaging (will be discussed in Sect. 1.6.3).

1.6 Sequences

These are specialized software programs that define the type, magnitude, and timing of the RF pulses. Depending on these factors, sequences can be of several types. Broadly, pulse sequences are divided into spin-echo and gradient-echo sequences.

1.6.1 Spin-Echo (SE) Imaging

- SE sequences involve sending two RF pulses (Fig. 1.9) and measuring the echo generated. As described earlier, transverse relaxation (decay) of the protons after the RF pulse is a measurement of T2*, rather than "true T2" due to the inhomogeneity in the magnetic field along with the spin–spin dephasing. This can be avoided using the SE sequence. The 180° pulse (following the first 90° pulse) eliminates the effects of inhomogeneity in the magnetic field. The signal generated at the time of echo decays by T2.
- The factors influencing the contrast in the MR signal are Time-to-Echo (TE) and Time-to-Repetition (TR) (Fig. 1.9). TE and TR determine whether the image is T1, T2, or proton density (PD) weighted. If the TR is kept short, the M_z will not have recover fully by the time the next 90° pulse is applied. This causes a

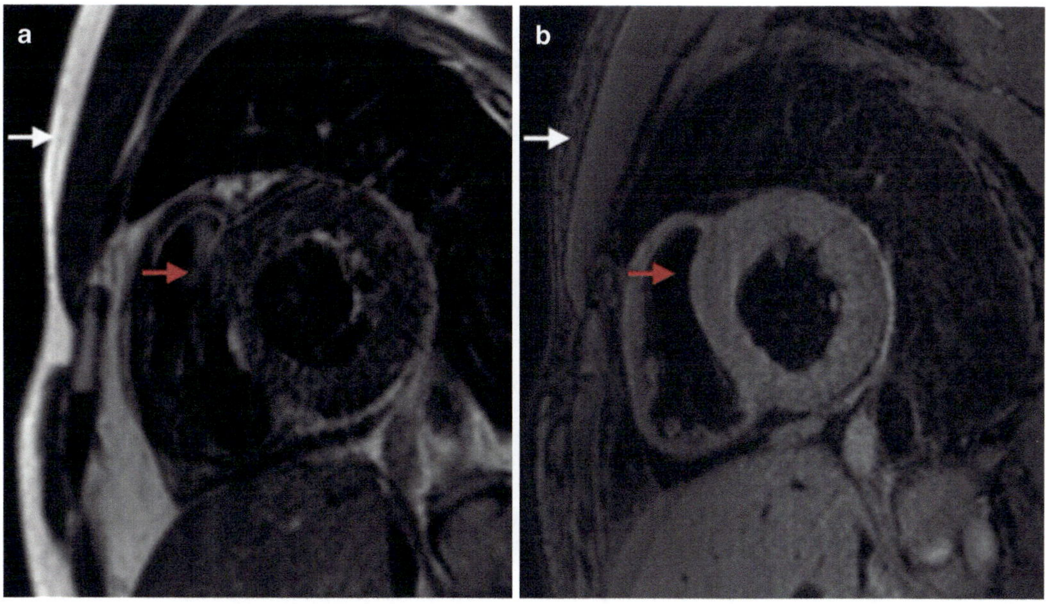

Fig. 1.10 Comparison of T2 TSE (**a**) and triple IR black blood T2 short axis (**b**) sequence. Note the suppression of fat signal (white arrow) as well as homogenous suppression of blood (red arrow) in triple IR black blood T2 sequence (**b**)

reduction in the MR signal which is dependent on the T1 value of the sample as well as TR. Thus, T1 weighted image can be achieved by short TR with short TE (to minimize T2 weighting). On the other hand, T2 weighted image is obtained by long TR and a long TE. PD weighted image is obtained by using short TE and long TR [5].

- *Dark blood imaging* used in CMR is based on SE imaging and is a double inversion recovery sequence (DIR-SE). Two preparatory 180° RF inversion pulses are used to highlight the signal from the myocardium. First is a nonselective pulse inverting the magnetization of the entire volume of the coil. Second is a selective pulse restoring magnetization of the particular area of interest, i.e., both blood and myocardium. However, the magnetization of blood outside this area remains inverted and it starts to undergo T1 recovery moving from the zero, attempting to realign with B_0. This blood enters the area of interest. The imaging time is chosen such that the magnetization of inflowing blood is zero, highlighting the signal from the myocardium. The third RF inversion pulse may be added to suppress the fat signals (*dark blood dark fat*) (Fig. 1.10). Modifications of SE sequence, i.e., Fast SE or Turbo SE are used for dark blood imaging [14]. In FSE, multiple 180° pulses are used after 90° pulse with phase encoding gradients applied after each 180° pulse. It can be a T1 or T2 weighted (Fig. 1.11). Continuously flowing blood appears dark; however, slow-moving blood may appear bright, resulting in artifacts. It is done for the anatomic assessment of the cardiac chambers, major vessels, and cardiac masses. T2 weighted dark blood image is also used to identify edematous myocardial tissue secondary to acute infarct, cardiomyopathy, or myocarditis.

1.6.2 Gradient-Echo (GRE) Imaging

- GRE is the most commonly used sequence in the CMR. It uses a very short TR along with shorter flip angles. These modifications allow the sequence time to be as short as milliseconds. Hence, they can be used to eliminate

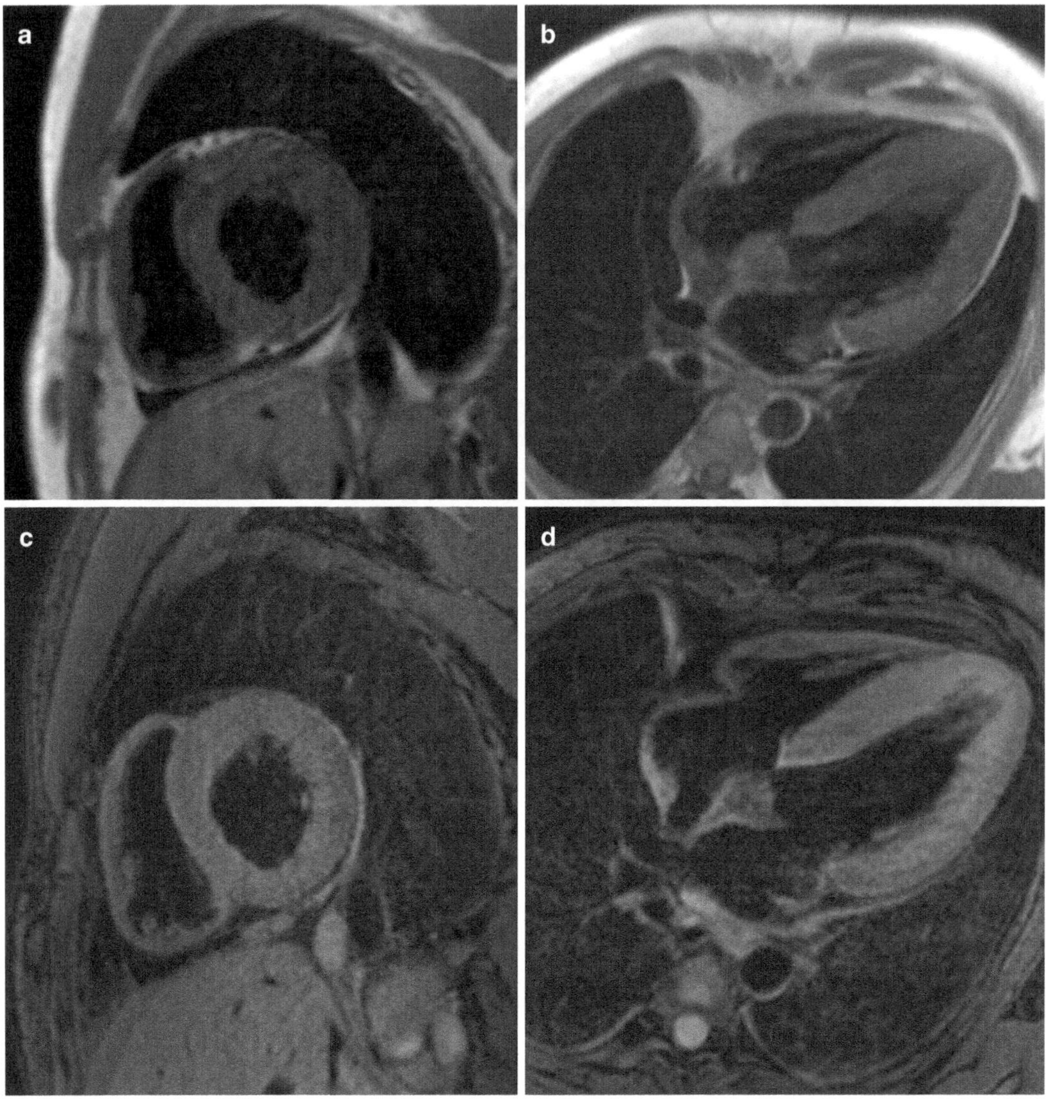

Fig. 1.11 Double IR black blood T1 (**a**, **b**) and triple IR black blood T2 (**c**, **d**) short axis and axial sequences. Note the additional suppression of fat signals in triple IR T2 images (**c**, **d**)

motion artifacts of moving heart along with ECG gating. The 180° pulse used in the SE image is omitted in GRE. Thus, the transverse magnetization now decays with the T2*, instead of T2 (as magnetic field inhomogeneity is not eliminated).

- *Bright blood imaging* (Fig. 1.12) used in CMR is based on GRE imaging. Various modifications of GRE, i.e., steady-state free precession (SSFP), echo-planar imaging (EPI), TRUFI are used more commonly for various assessments. These are used for ventricular function assessment (cine imaging), perfusion imaging, and phase-contrast imaging (flow quantifications). SSFP sequence is based on the principle of "steady magnetization" which is achieved after multiple RF pulses. It results in excellent T1/T2 contrast and thus used for the cine imaging (as discussed in the next paragraph). On the other hand, EPI is an ultrafast technique that fills the entire *k*-space in one shot. It is relatively insensitive to motion and

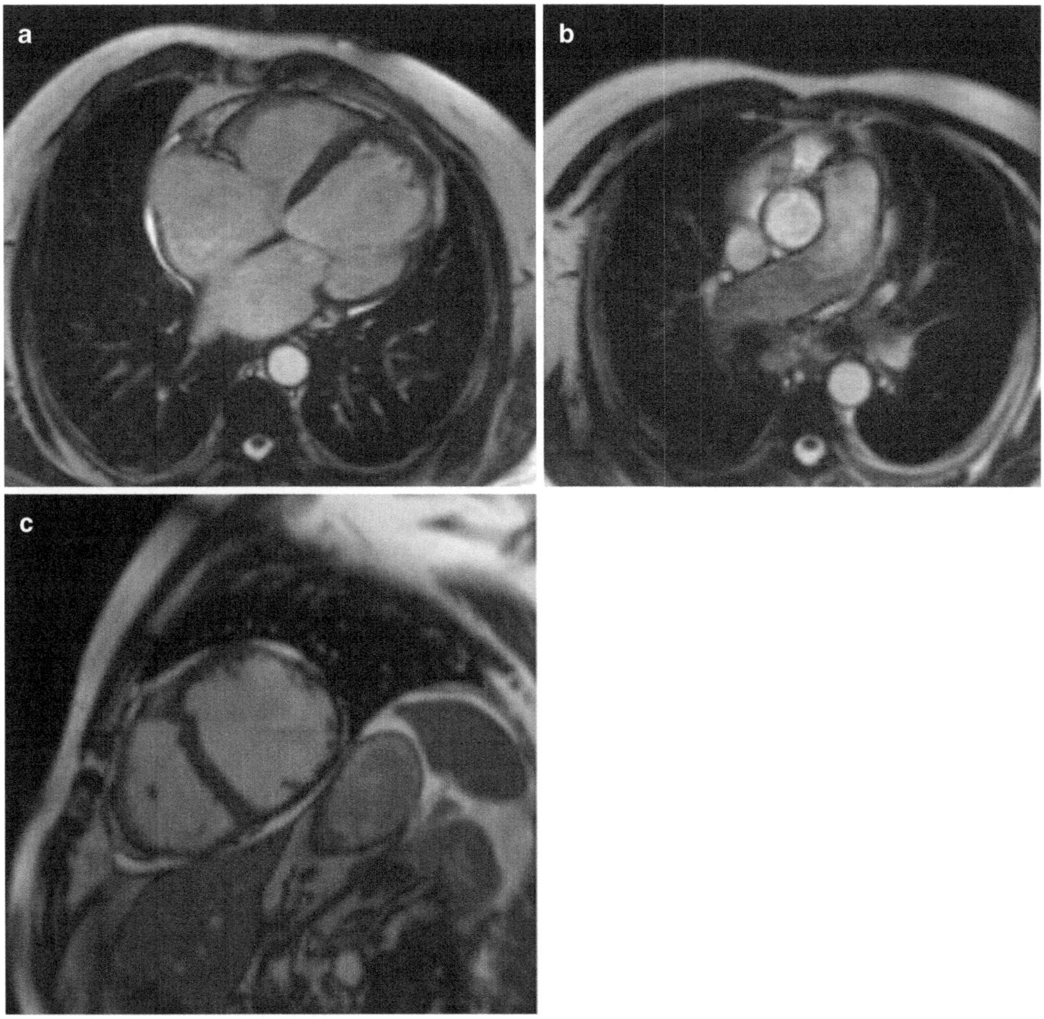

Fig. 1.12 White blood (GRE sequence) axial (**a**, **b**), short-axis (**c**) SSFP images. These are used for cine imaging. Note the excellent T2/T1 contrast with resultant high contrast between myocardium and moving blood

the *k*-space is filled with *long echo train*. EPI is the basis of myocardial tagging and perfusion imaging (will be discussed in Sects. 1.6.4 and 1.6.5, respectively) due to its ultrafast nature.

- *Cine imaging* is primarily based on a balanced steady-state free precession (bSSFP) technique along with retrospective ECG gating (will be discussed in Sect. 1.7). Due to its ultra-fast nature and excellent T1/T2 contrast, it gives high contrast between myocardium and moving blood. This is used for the assessment of regional wall motion abnormalities of the ventricular wall, flow of blood, and assessment of the movement of cardiac tumors.
- *Phase-contrast imaging* is a velocity encoded sequence based on GRE imaging. It is used to calculate systemic (Qs) and pulmonary (Qp) blood flow. The ratio of Qp/Qs is essential in the treatment planning of congenital heart disease. The value of ratio > 1.5 is indicative of significant left-to-right shunt, indicating that it may require correction [13]. It is also used to estimate regurgitation fraction of blood or flow across a stenotic segment of a vessel or a graft. These measurements indicate the severity of the regurgitation or stenosis, respectively.

1.6.3 Parallel Imaging

- Long scan acquisition time is one of the major limitations of CMR. The data acquisition window is constrained by the physiologic motion of the heart as well as the blood flow. The conventional method of spatial encoding, i.e., slice selection, phase encoding, and frequency encoding, requires rapid switching of gradient coils and application of various RF pulses. In spite of various newer pulse sequences and data acquisition methods, there is a limit up to which the scan time can be minimized.
- The concept of parallel imaging helps to circumvent these issues. It utilizes the known position and sensitivity of the coil for spatial localization of the signal. This allows a reduction in the phase encoding steps and a resultant decrease in the imaging time. In routine imaging, the signals from the multiple coils are combined, digitized, and converted into an image. However, in parallel imaging, the signal from each coil is processed separately. To reduce the time of acquisition to half, each coil acquires only half of the k-lines which would result in reduced FOV and wrap-around or aliasing artifacts. SMASH (Spatial Acquisition of Spatial Harmonics) and GRAPPA (GeneRalized Autocalibrating Partially Parallel Acquisition) generate the missing harmonics before the image formation and thus eliminate the artifact. GRAPPA algorithm provides a better signal-to-noise ratio (SNR) than SMASH. These are known as *k*-space based parallel imaging techniques [15].
- Another image-based technique to eliminate the wrap-around or aliasing artifact is known as SENSE (SENSitivity Encoding). It reconstructs the partial images from each coil and then combines all the images [15].
- Parallel imaging is used for "*rapid MRI,*" i.e., to minimize the scan time in cine imaging, phase-contrast imaging, coronary evaluation, perfusion imaging as well as viability imaging.
- Parallel imaging, when used with *k-t techniques* such as TSENSE, k-t BLAST, k-t SENSE, k-t GRAPPA, FOCUS [16] can reduce the scan time further, e.g., time required to acquire each slice of 2D cine image using balanced steady-state free precision (b-SSFP) sequence is around 10 s. This can be reduced to 4–5 s per slice using parallel imaging and can be reduced further to 2–3 s per slice using k-t methods.

1.6.4 Myocardial Tagging

- The functional evaluation of the heart using cine imaging is based on the ejection fraction, myocardial thickness, and end-diastolic/systolic volume. However, regional myocardial functions (such as strain and torsion) are important for the early identification of an at-risk individual. The cardiac pathologies do not affect the myocardium uniformly, e.g., a small infarct can cause the regional myocardial wall abnormality but the ejection fraction could be normal. Thus, the important underlying pathology can be missed if only the global chamber function is considered.
- Myocardial tagging (Fig. 1.13) deals with the regional myocardium function evaluation. Earlier it used to be done by implanting radio-opaque markers within the myocardium and tracking their movements by imaging [17]. CMR allows noninvasive measurement of the regional myocardial function or strain. The latest sequence for the myocardial tagging offered a better spatial and temporal resolution. These include SPAMM (spatial modulation of magnetization), HARP (harmonic phase), and strain ending (SENC). Each of these sequences offers some advantages over the other [17]. Myocardial tagging is used to assess regional myocardial dysfunctions in cardiomyopathies (dilated cardiomyopathy, hypertrophic cardiomyopathy, muscular dystrophies) in addition to ischemic cardiomyopathy [18].

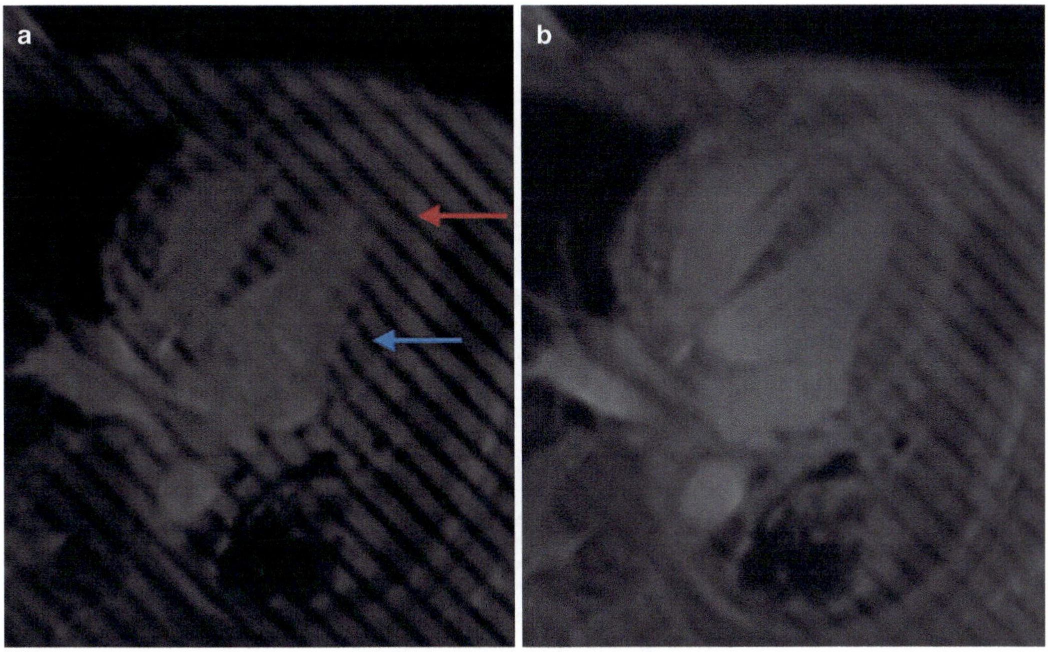

Fig. 1.13 (**a**, **b**) Myocardial tagging in a case of constrictive pericarditis. The adhesions between the pericardial layers prevent the normal shearing (red arrow in **a**) of the tagged stripes. Normal shearing of the tagged stripes is also seen as denoted by the blue arrow in (**a**)

1.6.5 Contrast-Enhanced (CE) Imaging

- Gadolinium (Gd)-based water soluble is the most commonly used contrast agent in MRI. It has primarily intravascular distribution and also permeates into the interstitial space. However, it does not enter the intracellular space, nor does it cross the blood–brain barrier [19]. Thus, contrast imaging depends on the differential distribution of the gadolinium. It shortens both T1 and T2 values of tissue; however, T1 shortening is much more significant than T2 shortening.
- The infarcted or fibrosed myocardium has much higher interstitial space than normal myocardium. The Gd permeates into these spaces and delayed imaging (~10 min) will show increased MR signal from these tissues (due to T1 shortening). This is the basis of *late gadolinium-enhanced (LGE) imaging.* It utilizes a T1-based GRE sequence. The signal from the myocardium needs to be nulled using an inversion recovery (IR) sequence before the delayed imaging. Thus, accurate inversion time (TI) is essential to detect subtle LGE (Fig. 1.14). However, the Gd washes out from the myocardium with time, that result in increase in the TI of the myocardium (Figs. 1.15 and 1.16). Thus, TI can change many times after Gd administration and thus needs to be adjusted every time [19]. LGE is also important in the diagnosis of cardiomyopathies such as amyloidosis, sarcoidosis, hypertrophic cardiomyopathy, Fabry's disease as well as myocarditis. It is the basis for viability imaging before revascularization (Fig. 1.17).
- *First-pass contrast-enhanced MRI* also uses a T1-based GRE sequence. It is specifically done to assess the passage of Gd through the heart, vessels, and myocardium (Fig. 1.18). As the Gd passes through, normal myocardium enhances whereas the ischemic myocardium

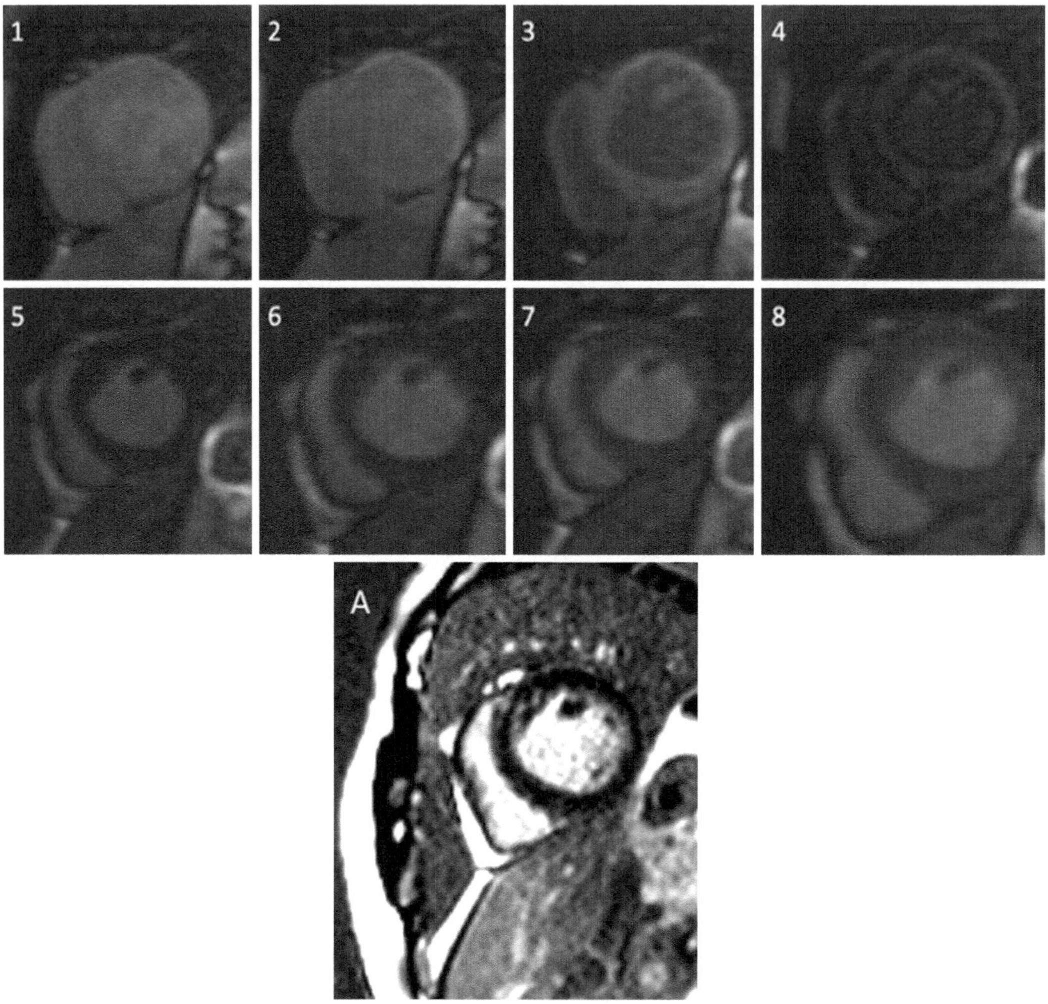

Fig. 1.14 TI scout images used to find the accurate inversion time of myocardium. Image 5 with TI of 260 ms nulls the myocardium effectively. LGE scan is done using a TI value of 260 ms (**a**)

enhances at a slower rate highlighting the perfusion deficits. Combined with pharmacological stress, first-pass imaging forms the basis for the evaluation of ischemic myocardium in coronary artery disease.

- *Contrast-Enhanced MR angiography (CE-MRA)* is used to image the vessels efficiently (Fig. 1.19). Arteries and veins can be imaged by adjusting the timing of the sequence. With the use of parallel imaging, it is possible to image larger areas with good signal-to-noise ratio (SNR). Thus, it can be used to assess aortic pathologies, pulmonary thromboembolism, peripheral vascular diseases.

1.6.6 Mapping Sequences

- In addition to the usual sequences, mapping sequences are used for the objective assessment of the pathology. These pathologies alter the T1, T2, and T2* values of the myocardium. Specialized pulse sequences are used to quantify these values and create color-coded anatomic maps.
- *T1 mapping* (Fig. 1.20a) is used to objectively assess the myocardial pathologies. It is done by using modified Look–Locker Inversion Recovery sequences (MOLLI). T1 quantification is done using the map gener-

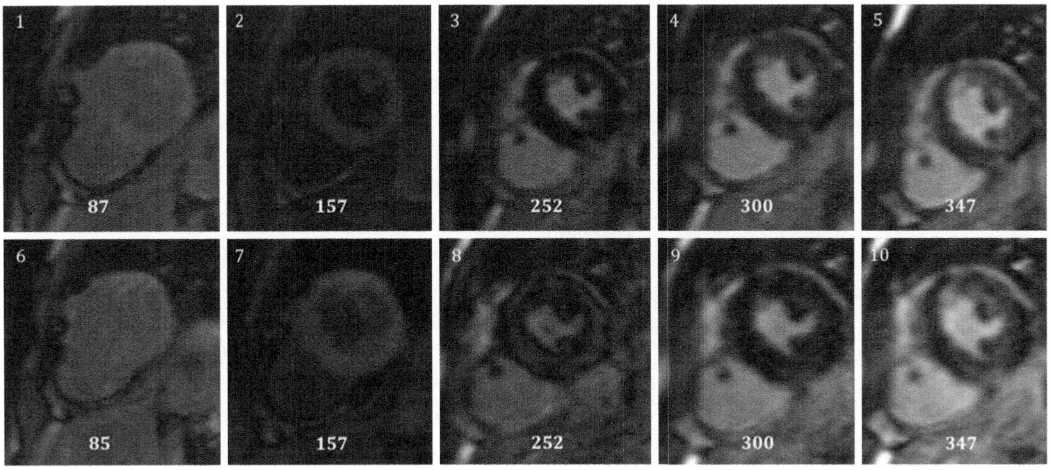

Fig. 1.15 TI scout images of a normal myocardium, 5 min (1–5) and 10 min (6–10) post-Gd administration with corresponding TIs. The time of nulling of myocardium increased from 252 to 300 ms in 5 and 10 min post-Gd images, respectively

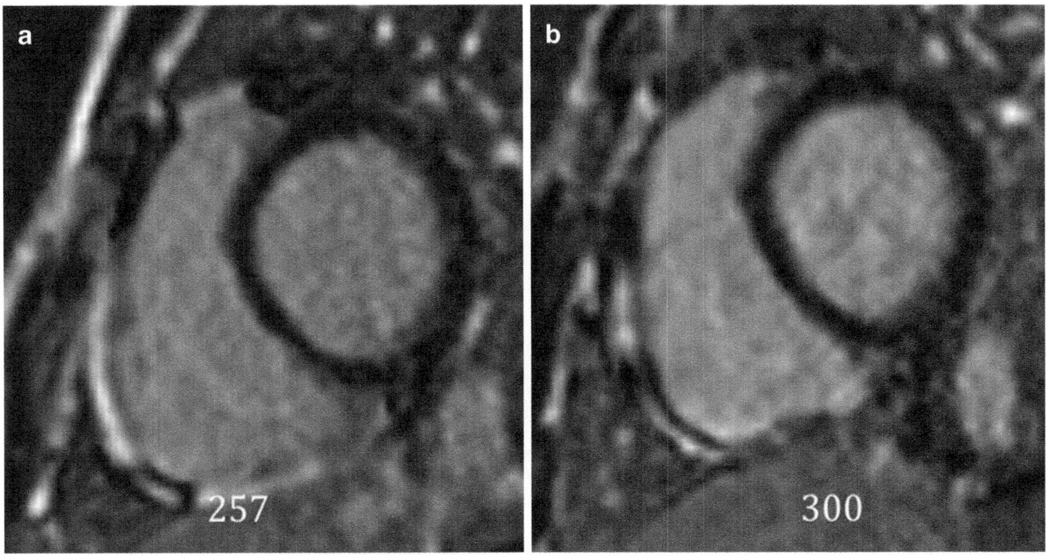

Fig. 1.16 Short axis PSIR (phase-contrast inversion recovery) sequence shows increased nulling time of myocardium from 257 to 300 ms in 5 and 10 min post-Gd images, respectively

ated by the MOLLI sequence. Non-contrast T1 mapping is useful in cardiomyopathies and iron-overload scenarios as these conditions lead to a significant alteration in the T1 values of the myocardium which can be objectively assessed. Diffuse or subtle fibrosis that may be missed on LGE can be picked on the T1 map. Pre- and post-contrast T1 mapping is used to calculate Extra-cellular volume (ECV) [20]. Diffuse or focal fibrosis and edema disturb the ECV values of the myocardium [21]. Diffuse changes are difficult to assess or quantify using LGE, pre- and post-contrast T1 mapping alone. ECV maps generated using pre- and post-T1 maps and hematocrit levels of the patient correlates well with the degree of myocardial fibrosis [20].

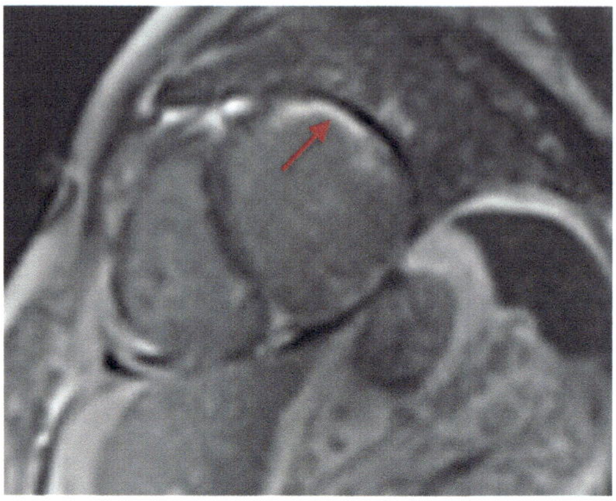

Fig. 1.17 Late gadolinium enhancement (LGE). The red arrow shows the subendocardial LGE. The location, extent, and transmurality of the LGE are important to establish a particular diagnosis

- Similarly, *T2 mapping* (Fig. 1.20b) *and T2* mapping* (Fig. 1.20c) can be done. T2 mapping is especially useful for the assessment of water accumulation in the myocardium in cases with acute infarction, transplant rejection, and myocarditis. T2* mapping is very sensitive to assess the iron accumulation in the myocardium in patients receiving frequent blood transfusions such as thalassemia major [22].

1.7 ECG Gating

- The majority of the CMR sequences are based on ECG gating. The ECG gated imaging generally depends on the structure evaluated. Static structure evaluation is done by the *prospective gating.*
- The scan is usually acquired in the mid-diastole or *diastasis* which is the most quiescent phase in the cardiac cycle to avoid the motion artifacts (Fig. 1.21). R wave marks the start of the sequence in prospective gating and is completed before the next R wave. This interval is called *the R–R interval*. This is divided into trigger delay, acquisition window, and trigger window (Fig. 1.22). The trigger delay is the interval between the R wave and the start of acquisition. It is kept around 0–50 ms for systolic and 150–250 ms for the diastolic phase. Trigger window is buffer period, including the final 10–15% of R–R interval. It allows a slight variation in the heart rate. Any R wave falling outside the trigger window is rejected [23]. It causes partial *k*-space-filling spanning over several cardiac cycles and averaging these signals. This is known as multi-segmental reconstruction. The data is acquired during successive trigger windows and the final image is reconstructed averaging all these signals. Any ectopic R wave due to premature ventricular contractions or arrhythmias is rejected and no data is acquired during that period.
- On the other hand, in *retrospective gating,* the signal and the ECG are acquired continuously over many cardiac cycles, regardless of the cardiac cycle phase (Fig. 1.20). The signal grouping is done according to the specific cardiac cycle retrospectively using the ECG data. This is especially used in dynamic imaging to assess the perfusion and the flow.

1.8 MR Artifacts

- Having studied the principles of magnetic resonance imaging acquisition and image formation, it is essential to learn about the various challenges in acquisition of high-quality diagnostic images. All MRI images have artifacts to some degree. These may render images nondiagnostic and various measurements as non-reliable. Moreover, cardiac and respiratory motion along with fast-flowing blood and the presence of implants add to the problem. Hence, it is important to understand the causes of these artifacts and compensate for them, if possible. A few of these artifacts are irreversible and can only be reduced rather than being completely eliminated. Others can be completely avoided. In subsequent sections, the various types of artifacts will be discussed along with illustrations, their cause, and remedial measures to minimize/eliminate them.
- Most of the artifacts can be corrected during scan acquisition itself. Hence, it is essential

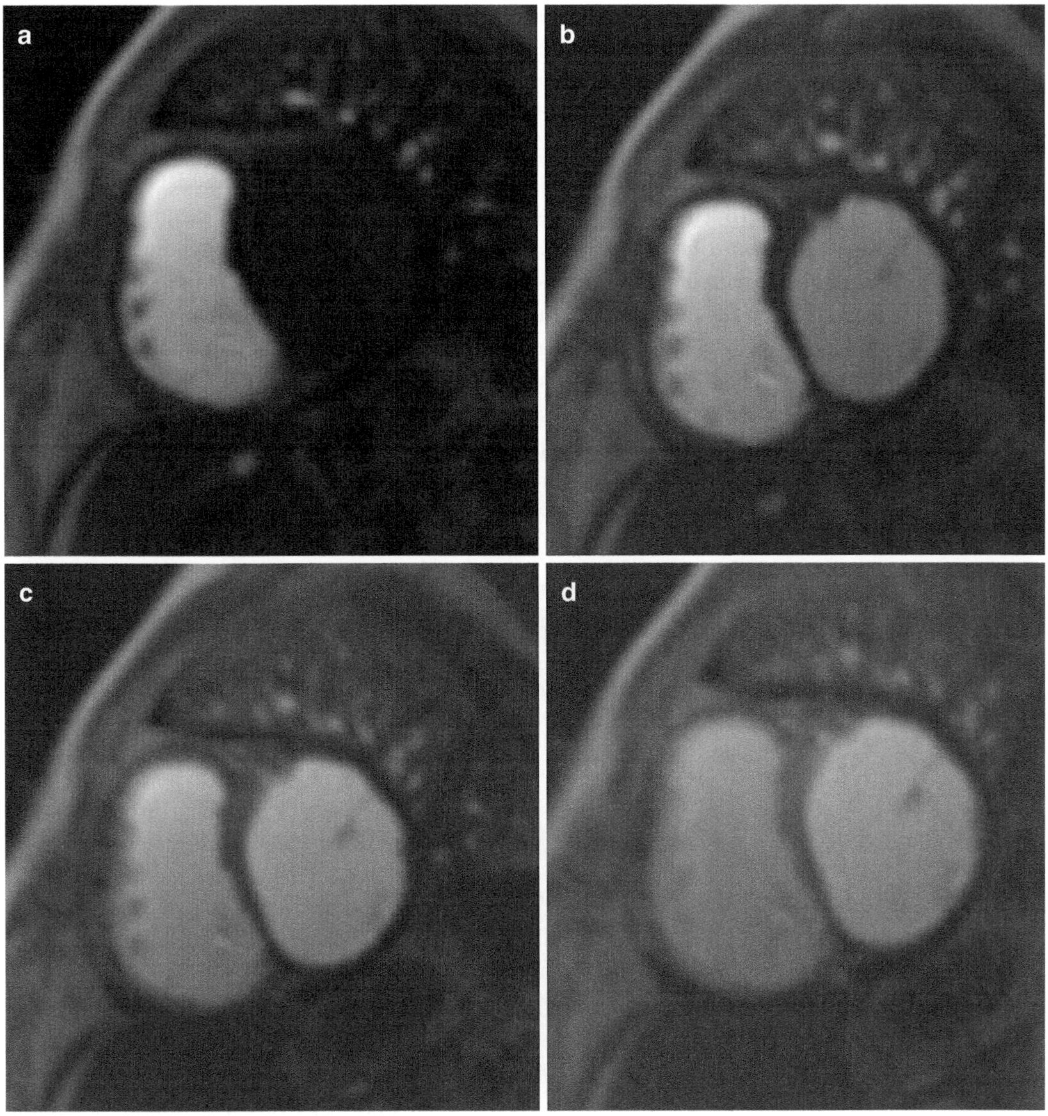

Fig. 1.18 First passed contrast-enhanced MRI, showing normal opacification of the right ventricle (**a**) followed by the left ventricle (**b**, **c**) and enhancement of myocardium (**d**) sequentially. Any myocardial perfusion defect can be identified in this image

to recognize the type during the procedure itself so that remedial measures can be carried out.

1.8.1 Equipment-Related Artifacts

1. Radio-frequency/Zipper artifact:
   - It is a common artifact that is seen as the presence of regular stripes across all the images. These are seen irrespective of the MR sequence used. It extends in the frequency encoding direction.
   - It occurs due to external RF source leakage into the magnet room which distorts the magnetic field. This may occur if any electronic device has been carried in the MR room or if the door of the MR room is not properly closed or there has been damage to the Faraday cage (loss of shielding). If

the problem persists even after the removal or electrical disconnection of all electronic equipment in the MR room, this may indicate a compromise of the RF shield.

2. Motion-related artifacts

It is a commonly seen artifact that occurs due to patient motion during image acquisition. This can be seen as blurring of the image or presence of parallel lines or double contours in the image (referred to as ghosting). In general, nonperiodic movements cause a smearing of the image (Fig. 1.23a) whereas periodic movements cause coherent ghosts (Fig. 1.23b, c). It originates from the part that moves periodically throughout the scan, for example, breathing movements, vessel pulsations [24]. It is seen along the phase encoding direction. This is because the time difference in acquiring adjacent points along the frequency encoding direction is shorter (~microseconds). It depends upon the sampling frequency or bandwidth used. On the contrary, the time difference in acquiring adjacent points along the phase encoding direction is relatively longer (equal to repetition time of the sequence). This positional difference due to motion introduces a phase difference between the views in *k*-space and appears as a ghost on the image. On looking at an image, the direction of phase encoding can always be determined by the direction of the phase mismapping or ghosting artifact.

There are various ways to reduce the phase mismapping or ghosting:

(a) Controlled breathing during MR acquisition and coaching the patients with breathing instructions before starting the acquisition. When a patient is unable to hold the breath in expiration, a breath-hold in inspiration can also be used. Acquisition speed can be increased (and hence reducing the breath-hold duration) using single-shot imaging sequences or reducing the spatial resolution and use of parallel imaging.
(b) In faster sequences, breath-hold instructions can suffice. However, in longer sequences, a method known as respiratory compensation or respiratory ordered phase encoding (ROPE) can greatly reduce ghosting from breathing movements. Respiratory gating or

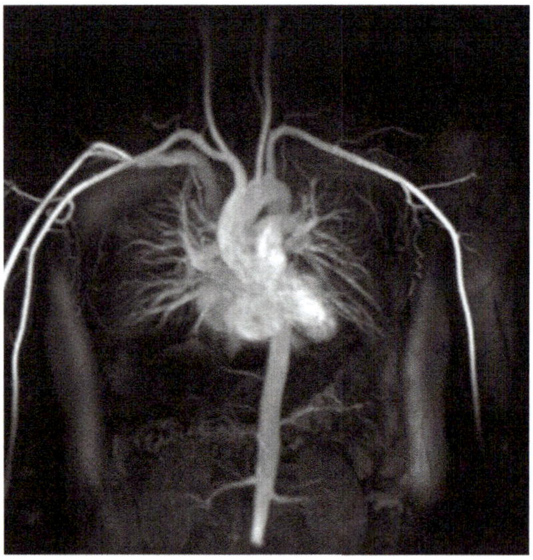

Fig. 1.19 CE-MRA of the thoracoabdominal aorta and bilateral upper limbs

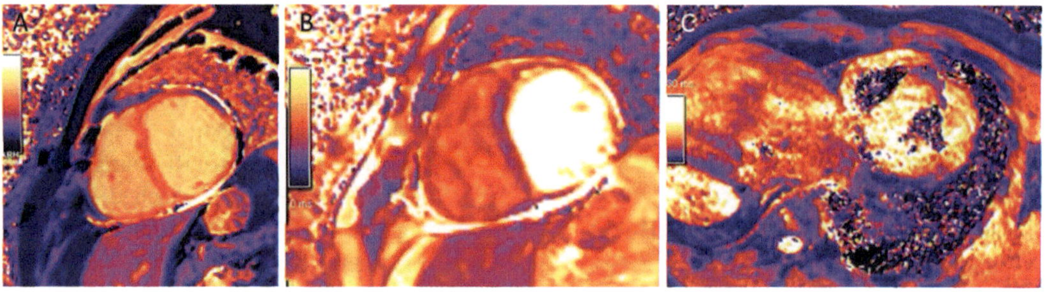

Fig. 1.20 T1 (**a**), T2 (**b**), and T2* (**c**) mapping sequences. The color-coded maps are used to objectively define the diseased myocardial tissue. The actual T1, T2, and T2* value can be calculated by drawing an ROI

triggering method can also be used. It times the RF excitation with a certain phase of respiration. Each slice of the acquisition is therefore obtained at the same phase of respiration. Respiratory navigator echoes can also be used to reduce phase mismapping caused by respiratory motion. In this technique, a region of interest (ROI) is placed across the diaphragm in either coronal or sagittal localizers. Image acquisition is synchronized to the diaphragmatic excursions. The system monitors the signal intensity within this ROI and throws out data acquired outside prescribed boundaries [25]. Alternatively, in patients who have difficulty in performing breath-holds or in arrhythmia cases, real-time imaging can be used. These sequences do not require breath-holds and are not ECG triggered. However, the drawback is that the scan acquisition time will increase and there is a marked reduction in the image quality. We can invert the signal from the abdominal wall by applying a saturation band.

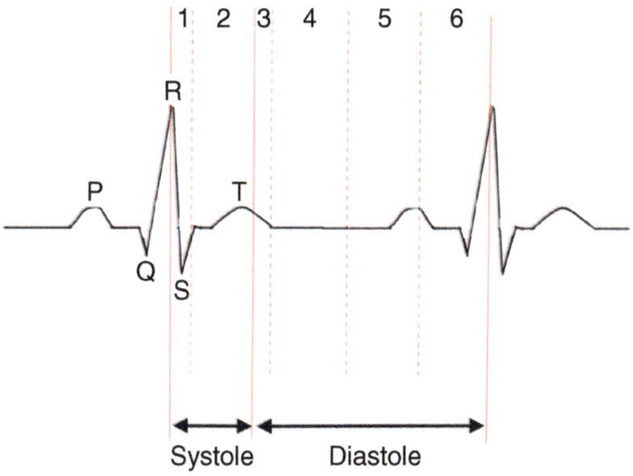

Fig. 1.21 ECG with various phases in the cardiac cycle. R wave denotes the start of ventricular systole. Various phases of the cardiac cycle are marked. 1. Isovolumetric contraction (AV and semilunar valve closed), 2. Ejection of blood (opening of semilunar valves), 3. Isovolumetric relaxation (AV and semilunar valve closed), 4. Rapid LV inflow (AV valve open), 5. Diastasis, 6. Atrial systole

(c) ECG gating: Just as respiratory gating monitors respiration, cardiac gating monitors cardiac motion by coordinating the excitation pulse with the R wave of systole.
(d) Swapping phase and frequency: As ghosting is seen only along the phase axis, the direction of phase encoding can be changed, so that the artifact does not interfere with the area of interest.
(e) Using pre-saturation pulses: Pre-saturation can null the signal from specified areas. Placing the pre-saturation volumes over the area producing artifact will null the signal and reduces the artifact. Also, pre-saturation reduces artifacts from flowing nuclei in blood vessels. Pre-saturation produces a low signal from these nuclei and is most effective when placed between the origin of the flow and the FOV.
(f) Voluntary motion can be reduced by making the patient as comfortable as possible, using

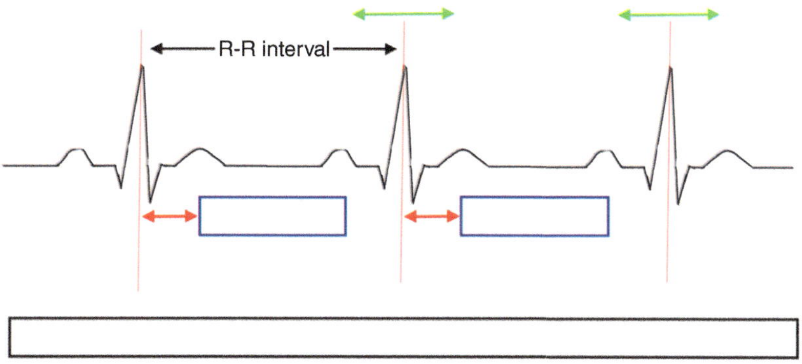

Fig. 1.22 Prospective and retrospective gating. In prospective gating, the scan is acquired (blue rectangle) in the R–R interval after the trigger delay (red double arrow). Trigger window (green double arrow) allows a slight variation in the heart rate. R wave falling outside the trigger delay is rejected. In retrospective gating, the scan is acquired continuously irrespective of the cardiac phase (black rectangle)

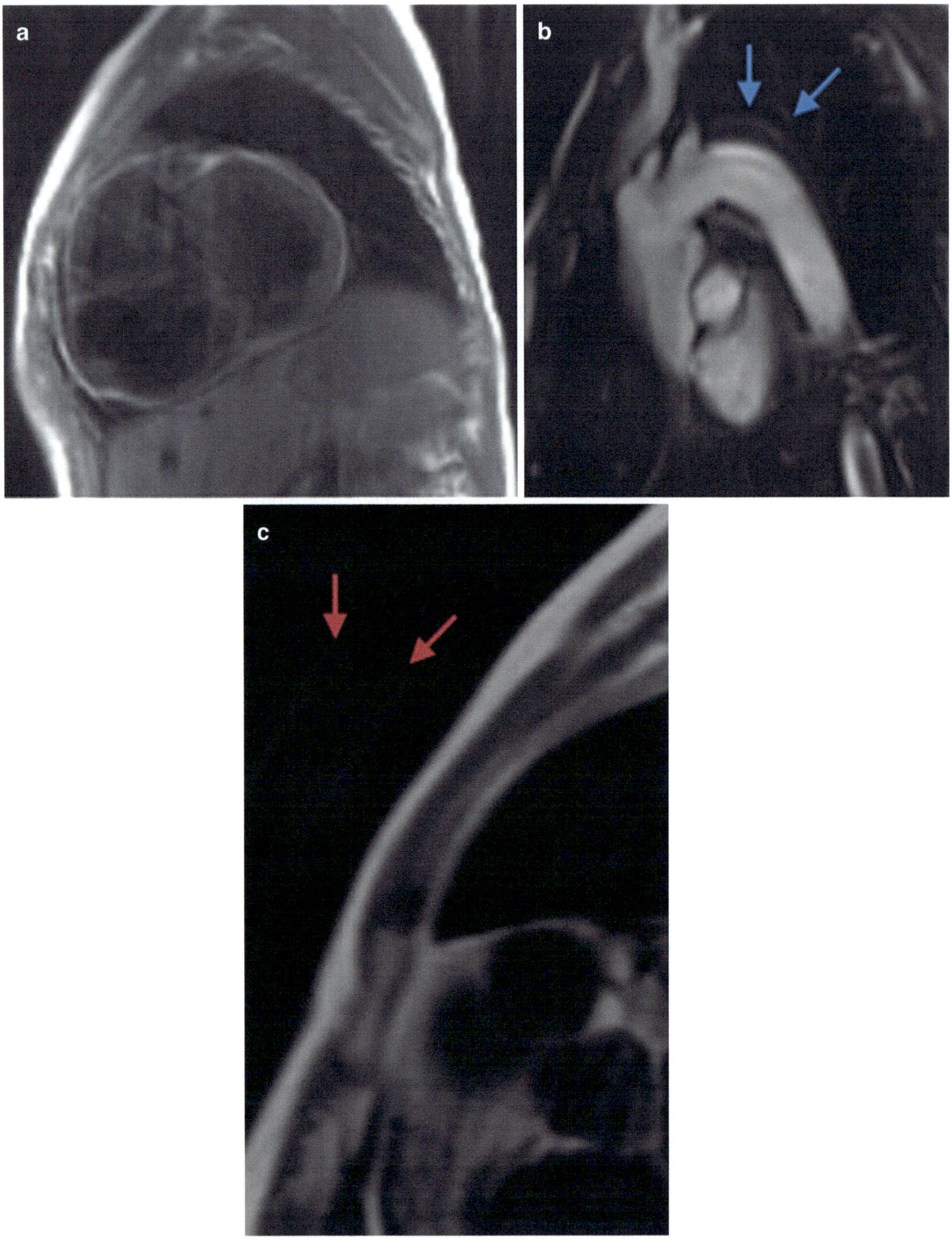

Fig. 1.23 Motion-related artifacts. Smearing (**a**) occurs due to incoherent motion during the scanning. Ghosting (parallel lines) occurs due to periodic motion such as pulsations (blue lines in **b**) and breathing (red lines in **c**)

pads and straps for immobilization. Sedation of the patient may be required in extreme cases.

1.8.2 Aliasing or Wrap-Around Artifact

- When anatomy present outside the FOV is folded onto the top of anatomy inside the FOV (and overlaps the area of interest), it is referred to as aliasing or wrap-around artifact [26]. If an anatomical structure is in close proximity to the receiver coil, it can still produce a signal even if it is outside the FOV. Data from this signal must be allocated a pixel position, thus causing the artifacts (Fig. 1.24).
- To compensate for aliasing, we can enlarge the FOV so that all anatomy producing signal is incorporated within the FOV. But this will also result in a loss of spatial resolution. Also, we can increase the number of phase encoding steps (oversampling). Alternatively, the frequency and phase encoding direction in the acquisition process can be swapped. Regarding the asymmetry of the torso, the number of phase-encoding steps may be adequate for acquisition in the opposite direction. Moreover, saturation bands can be used which inverts the signal from the body part outside the FOV so that it cannot cause aliasing.

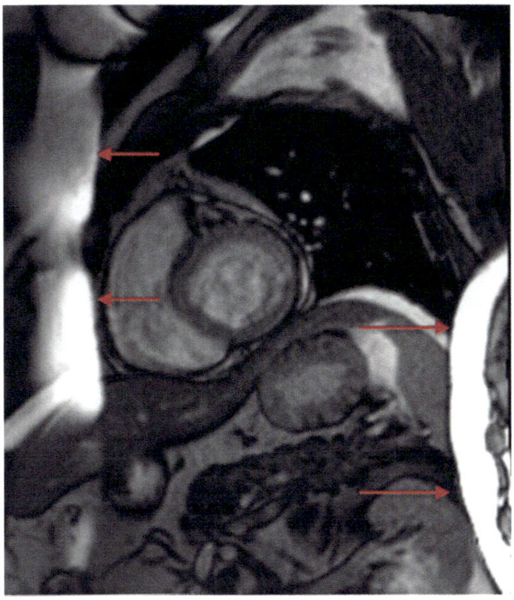

Fig. 1.24 Wrap-around artifact. Overlapping of different anatomic structures (red arrows) is seen. This can be corrected by increasing the FOV

1.8.3 Aliasing During Flow Analysis

- In flow analysis, an aliasing phenomenon is used to estimate the velocity of protons in a vessel or across a valve as well as to estimate the pressure gradient across a stenotic lesion. This is based on the fact that there is a phase shift of moving protons in flow sequences, which is proportional to their velocity. Encoded velocity (VENC) refers to the maximum velocity present in an imaging volume. Any velocity which is lesser than VENC value (depending on the direction of blood flow) will produce aliasing (Fig. 1.25a) (and appear as black holes) [27]. The recognition of this artifact becomes essential in flow sequences as it will lead to under- or overestimation of the true velocity. These values can be manually adjusted until the velocity encoded on the scanner is slightly more than the velocity in the body of the patient. The artifact will be eliminated using the correct adjustment of the VENC (Fig. 1.25b).

1.8.4 Chemical Shift Artifact

- It is seen as a dark edge at the interface of water and fat [28]. These occur due to the different chemical environments of fat and water. Fat processes at a lower frequency than water. Due to a misregistration of the signal from water and fat present in the same voxel along the frequency encoding direction, the difference in resonance frequency between fat and

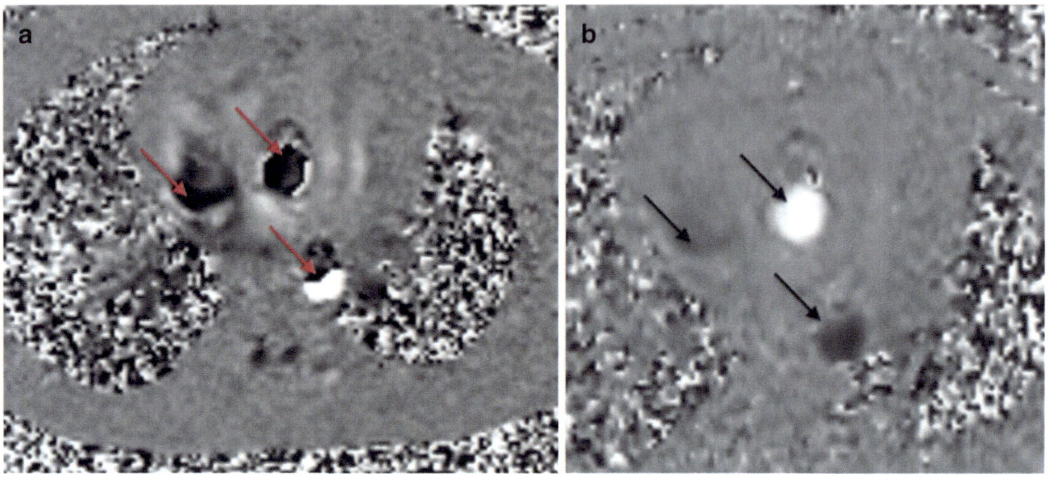

Fig. 1.25 Aliasing artifacts in phase-contrast imaging. If the maximum velocity in the imaging volume is greater than the VENC, it produces artifact in the form of dark circles (**a**). This is eliminated by raising the VENC till the dark circles disappear (**b**)

water causes a separation (pixel shift) in the reconstructed images producing the artifact.

- To reduce chemical shift artifact, always use the widest receive bandwidth in keeping with good signal-to-noise ratio. If the bandwidth is reduced to increase the SNR, use chemical saturation to saturate out the signal from either fat or water. By doing so, as either fat or water is nulled, there is nothing for one tissue to shift against and therefore, chemical shift artifact will be eliminated.

1.8.5 Truncation or Gibbs Artifact or Dark Rim Artifact

- This refers to the presence of a band at the interfaces of high and low signals. In CMR, these can be observed in any image at the intersection of bright blood and darker myocardium [29]. These may mimic subendocardial perfusion defects (Fig. 1.26). It occurs due to data under-sampling (i.e., too few *k*-space lines filled) so that interfaces of high and low signals are incorrectly represented on the image, resulting in a dark band. Truncation artifact occurs in the phase direction only and produces a low-intensity band running through a high-intensity area.

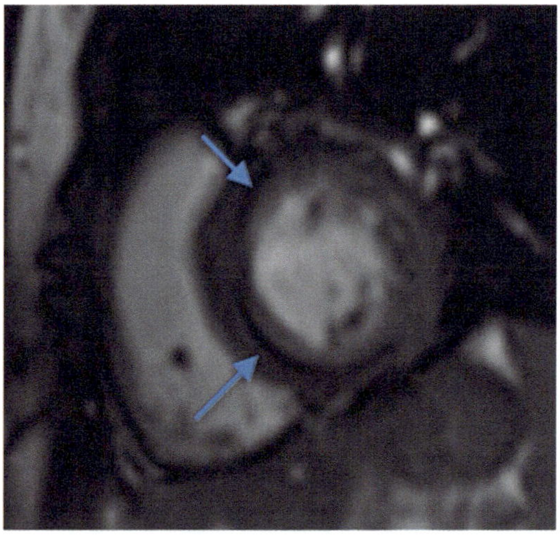

Fig. 1.26 Truncation artifact. The black lines (blue arrows) are seen at the junction of high-intensity blood and low-intensity myocardium. This can mimic the subendocardial perfusion defect

- To prevent these, avoid data under-sampling by increasing the number of phase-encoding steps. For example, use a 256 × 256 matrix instead of 256 × 128. Increasing the spatial resolution can reduce this artifact. However, the presence of dark rim artifact does not prohibit image analysis for cardiac imagers. A true perfusion defect can be discriminated, even in the presence of a dark rim artifact.

This artifact usually lasts for only a few heartbeats, whereas a real perfusion defect tends to be more persistent.

1.8.6 Magnetic Susceptibility Artifact

- This artifact produces image distortion together with large signal voids. Magnetic susceptibility is the ability of a substance to become magnetized. Different tissues magnetize to different degrees, which results in a difference in precessional frequency and phase. This leads to dephasing at the interface of these tissues and a signal alteration. In practice, the main causes of this artifact are metal (e.g., sternal wires, pacemakers) within the imaging volume, although it can also be seen from naturally occurring iron content of hemorrhage, as these magnetize to a much greater degree than the surrounding tissue. Ferromagnetic objects have a very high magnetic susceptibility and cause distortion of the image. Magnetic susceptibility artifact is more prominent in gradient-echo sequences as the gradient reversal cannot compensate for the phase difference at the interface.
- This artifact can, under some circumstances, be used to aid in diagnosis, e.g., for detecting hemorrhage, hemosiderin deposition, and calcification. It also forms the basis of post-contrast T2*-weighted MR perfusion studies and sequences to quantify myocardial and liver iron load.

1.8.7 Trigger Artifact

- It is seen as blurring (or become less well-defined) of myocardial borders leading to image degradation which renders them nondiagnostic. Moreover, the subsequent measurements or calculations performed will be unreliable.
- As we have studied previously that the cardiac scan data acquisition is synchronized to the R wave in the QRS complex. Normally, data is acquired during the complete heart cycle. It is then retrospectively assigned to specific phases of the cardiac cycle, referred to as retrospective triggering. If the ECG signal is poor or in cases of arrhythmias, data acquisition becomes a challenging task.
- This can be taken care of by using arrhythmia rejection software in patients having an irregular heartbeat. All the images which are obtained during irregular RR intervals are rejected. Another remedial measure is by using prospective triggering in which data is acquired during a predefined cardiac cycle phase. However, an important limitation of the prospective triggering approach is that the image acquisition does not cover the complete RR interval. Therefore, this results in an underestimation of stroke volume in the volume analysis.

1.8.8 Blood Flow Artifact

- This is seen as due to disturbance of the homogeneous steady-state magnetization by protons flowing at a high velocity near or in the selected imaging slice [30]. It is usually seen when the area of interest is near to outflow tracts or large arteries.
- To overcome this: improve main magnetic field homogeneity (shimming), reduce TR or TE (this results in a sequence less susceptible for turbulent flow artifacts), apply saturation band across the outflow tract or large arteries, swap phase and frequency encoding direction.

1.9 Conclusion

To conclude, it is important to be aware of basic physics behind CMR to be able to correctly plan the scan. The basic understanding of each of the sequences allows the radiologist to tailor the scan to answer specific questions asked by the physician. It is also important to know about different artifacts, why they occur, and ways to eliminate them, to improve the quality of the scan.

References

1. Allisy-Roberts P, Williams J. Chapter 10 - Magnetic resonance imaging. In: Farr's physics for medical imaging. 2nd ed. Philadelphia: W.B. Saunders; 2008. p. 169–95.
2. Winkler SA, Schmitt F, Landes H, de Bever J, Wade T, Alejski A, Rutt BK. Gradient and shim technologies for ultra high field MRI. NeuroImage. 2018;168:59–70. https://doi.org/10.1016/j.neuroimage.2016.11.033.
3. Juchem C, de Graaf RA. B0 magnetic field homogeneity and shimming for in vivo magnetic resonance spectroscopy. Anal Biochem. 2017;529:17.
4. Tognarelli JM, et al. Magnetic resonance spectroscopy: principles and techniques: lessons for clinicians. J Clin Exp Hepatol. 2015;5(4):320–8. https://doi.org/10.1016/j.jceh.2015.10.006.
5. Manning WJ, Pennell DJ. Cardiovascular magnetic resonance: a companion to Braunwald's heart disease. New York: Elsevier; 2019.
6. Plewes DB, Kucharczyk W. Physics of MRI: a primer. J Magn Reson Imaging. 2012;35(5):1038–54. https://doi.org/10.1002/jmri.23642.
7. Spieker M, Katsianos E, Gastl M, Behm P, Horn P, Jacoby C, et al. T2 mapping cardiovascular magnetic resonance identifies the presence of myocardial inflammation in patients with dilated cardiomyopathy as compared to endomyocardial biopsy. Eur Heart J Cardiovasc Imaging. 2018;19(5):574–82. https://doi.org/10.1093/ehjci/jex230.
8. Dabir D, et al. Reference values for healthy human myocardium using a T1 mapping methodology: results from the International T1 Multicenter cardiovascular magnetic resonance study. J Cardiovasc Magn Reson. 2014;16(1):69. https://doi.org/10.1186/s12968-014-0069-x.
9. Granitz M, Motloch LJ, Granitz C, Meissnitzer M, Hitzl W, Hergan K, et al. Comparison of native myocardial T1 and T2 mapping at 1.5T and 3T in healthy volunteers: reference values and clinical implications. Wien Klin Wochenschr. 2019;131(7–8):143–55. https://doi.org/10.1007/s00508-018-1411-3.
10. Ramazzotti A, Pepe A, Positano V, Rossi G, De Marchi D, Brizi MG, et al. Multicenter validation of the magnetic resonance T2* technique for segmental and global quantification of myocardial iron. J Magn Reson Imaging JMRI. 2009;30(1):62–8. https://doi.org/10.1002/jmri.21781.
11. Roy C, Slimani A, de Meester C, Amzulescu M, Pasquet A, Vancraeynest D, et al. Age and sex corrected normal reference values of T1, T2 T2* and ECV in healthy subjects at 3T CMR. J Cardiovasc Magn Reson. 2017;19(1):72. https://doi.org/10.1186/s12968-017-0371-5.
12. Gold GE, Han E, Stainsby J, Wright G, Brittain J, Beaulieu C. Musculoskeletal MRI at 3.0 T: relaxation times and image contrast. AJR Am J Roentgenol. 2004;183(2):343–51. https://doi.org/10.2214/ajr.183.2.1830343.
13. Stanisz GJ, Odrobina EE, Pun J, Escaravage M, Graham SJ, Bronskill MJ, Henkelman RM. T1, T2 relaxation and magnetization transfer in tissue at 3T. Magn Reson Med. 2005;54(3):507–12. https://doi.org/10.1002/mrm.20605.
14. Ginat DT, Fong MW, Tuttle DJ, Hobbs SK, Vyas RC. Cardiac imaging: part 1, MR pulse sequences, imaging planes, and basic anatomy. Am J Roentgenol. 2011;197(4):808–15. https://doi.org/10.2214/AJR.10.7231.
15. Glockner JF, Hu HH, Stanley DW, Angelos L, King K. Parallel MR imaging: a user's guide. Radiographics. 2005;25(5):1279–97. https://doi.org/10.1148/rg.255045202.
16. Kozerke S, Plein S. Accelerated CMR using zonal, parallel and prior knowledge driven imaging methods. J Cardiovasc Magn Reson. 2008;10(1):29. https://doi.org/10.1186/1532-429X-10-29.
17. Ibrahim E-SH. Myocardial tagging by cardiovascular magnetic resonance: evolution of techniques—pulse sequences, analysis algorithms, and applications. J Cardiovasc Magn Reson. 2011;13(1):36. https://doi.org/10.1186/1532-429X-13-36.
18. Shehata ML, Cheng S, Osman NF, Bluemke DA, Lima JAC. Myocardial tissue tagging with cardiovascular magnetic resonance. J Cardiovasc Magn Reson. 2009;11(1):55. https://doi.org/10.1186/1532-429X-11-55.
19. Tseng W-YI, Su M-YM, Tseng Y-HE. Introduction to cardiovascular magnetic resonance: technical principles and clinical applications. Acta Cardiol Sin. 2016;32(2):129–44. https://doi.org/10.6515/ACS20150616A.
20. Kellman P, Wilson JR, Xue H, Ugander M, Arai AE. Extracellular volume fraction mapping in the myocardium, part 1: evaluation of an automated method. J Cardiovasc Magn Reson. 2012;14:63. https://doi.org/10.1186/1532-429X-14-63.
21. Flett AS, Hayward MP, Ashworth MT, Hansen MS, Taylor AM, Elliott PM, et al. Equilibrium contrast cardiovascular magnetic resonance for the measurement of diffuse myocardial fibrosis: preliminary validation in humans. Circulation. 2010;122(2):138–44. https://doi.org/10.1161/CIRCULATIONAHA.109.930636.
22. Pennell DJ. T2* magnetic resonance and myocardial iron in thalassemia. Ann N Y Acad Sci. 2005;1054:373–8. https://doi.org/10.1196/annals.1345.045.
23. Nacif MS, Zavodni A, Kawel N, Choi EY, Lima JA, Bluemke DA. Cardiac magnetic resonance imaging and its electrocardiographs (ECG): tips and tricks. Int J Cardiovasc Imaging. 2012;28(6):1465–75. https://doi.org/10.1007/s10554-011-9957-4.
24. Niendorf T, Winter L, Frauenrath T. Electrocardiogram in an MRI environment: clinical needs, practical considerations, safety implications, technical solutions, and future directions. In: Mills RM, editor. Advances

in electrocardiograms - methods and analysis. InTech Open Access Publishing, London, 2012.
25. Barish MA, Jara H. Motion artifact control in body MR imaging. Magn Reson Imaging Clin N Am. 1999;7(2):289–301.
26. Matsumoto H, Matsuda T, Miyamoto K, Nakatsuma K, Sugahara M, Shimada T. Feasibility of free-breathing late gadolinium-enhanced cardiovascular MRI for assessment of myocardial infarction: navigator-gated versus single-shot imaging. Int J Cardiol. 2013;20(1):94–9.
27. Pusey E, Yoon C, Anselmo ML, Lufkin RB. Aliasing artifacts in MR imaging. Comput Med Imaging Graph. 1988;12(4):219–24.
28. Henk CB, Grampp S, Koller J, et al. Elimination of errors caused by first-order aliasing in velocity encoded cine-MR measurements of postoperative jets after aortic coarctation: in vitro and in vivo validation. Eur Radiol. 2002;12(6):1523–31.
29. Graves MJ, Mitchell DG. Body MRI artifacts in clinical practice: a physicist's and radiologist's perspective. J Magn Reson Imaging. 2013;38(2):269–87.
30. Gerber BL, Raman SV, Nayak K, et al. Myocardial first-pass perfusion cardiovascular magnetic resonance: history, theory, and current state of the art. J Cardiovasc Magn Reson. 2008;28(10):1–18.

Cardiac Embryology

2

D. Prashanth Reddy and Sanjaya Viswamitra

2.1 Introduction

The cardiac imager needs to understand the embryology and development of the heart to predict the combinations of associated congenital anomalies and make developmentally plausible diagnoses. Cardiac development is a complex process involving contributions from all three germ layers. Congenital heart defects (CHD) arise due to an arrest in development at a particular stage or as a result of inappropriate growth or involution. This occurs either due to inherited or de novo genetic defects or due to external precipitating events such as teratogenic drugs, radiation, infections, or metabolic disorders. The molecular biology and genetics which drive these changes are still poorly understood. Most congenital heart diseases are not associated with mutations in a specific gene, rather they are multifactorial in etiology. Less than 20% of CHD can be explained by a chromosomal abnormality or a single gene defect [1]. There are a few well-known genetic associations which will be discussed later in the chapter [2]. The stages in development up to the 3-week stage will be discussed in brief, followed by a more detailed description of the development of the heart, the venous, and arterial systems. The developmental basis for common CHD will be discussed. The purpose of this chapter is to shed light and understanding on the various CHD chapters that follow, rather than to suggest a definitive nomenclature for cardiac embryology.

D. P. Reddy · S. Viswamitra (✉)
Department of Radiology, Sri Sathya Sai Institute of Higher Medical Sciences,
Whitefield, Bengaluru, Karnataka, India

2.2 Early Embryonic Development

Fertilization occurs in the fallopian tube. This results in the restoration of a diploid number of chromosomes and the formation of a zygote. The zygote undergoes multiple cell divisions forming a mass of cells called the morula. A series of changes occur within the morula which forms the blastocyst. Within the blastocyst, cells are arraigned as an inner cell mass which forms the embryo and the outer cell mass which forms the placenta. The blastocyst undergoes the process of implantation following which the inner cell mass is rearranged to form the epiblast and hypoblast cell layers. This is called the two-layered disc. At this stage, the primitive streak, primitive node, and primitive pit form and divide the embryo into a cranial and caudal pole [3] (Figs. 2.1 and 2.2).

Epiblast cells migrate through the primitive pit to form the mesoderm and endoderm in a process called gastrulation. The result is a three-layered disc composed of the ectoderm, mesoderm, and endoderm cell layers. The mesoderm further differentiates into three parts. The somatic meso-

R. Rajeshkannan et al. (eds.), *CT and MRI in Congenital Heart Diseases*,
https://doi.org/10.1007/978-981-15-6755-1_2

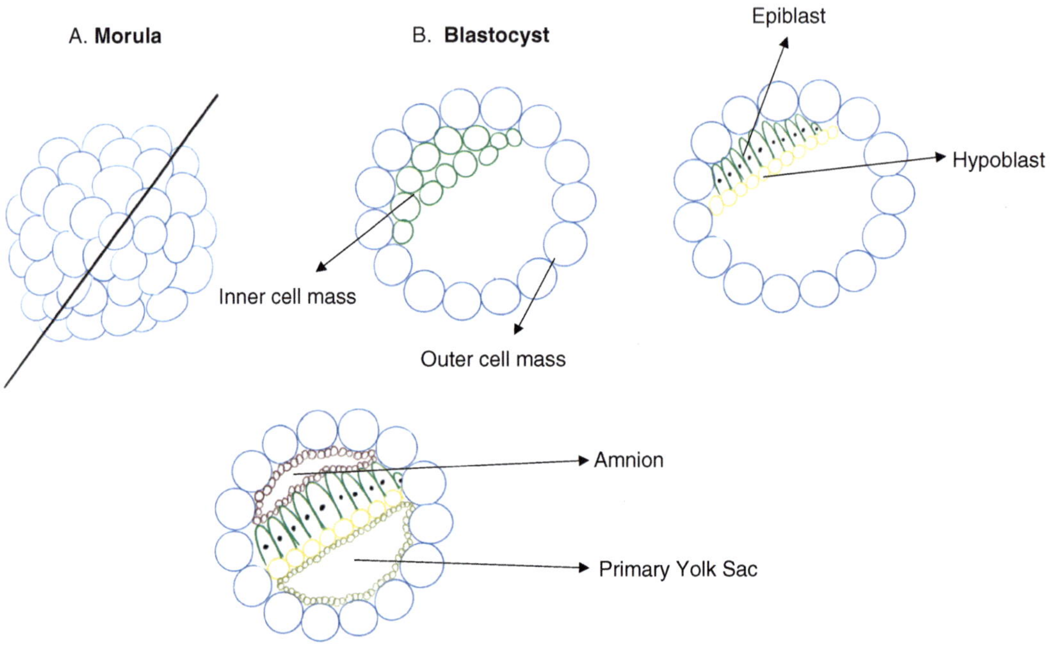

Fig. 2.1 Development of the embryo up to the blastocyst stage

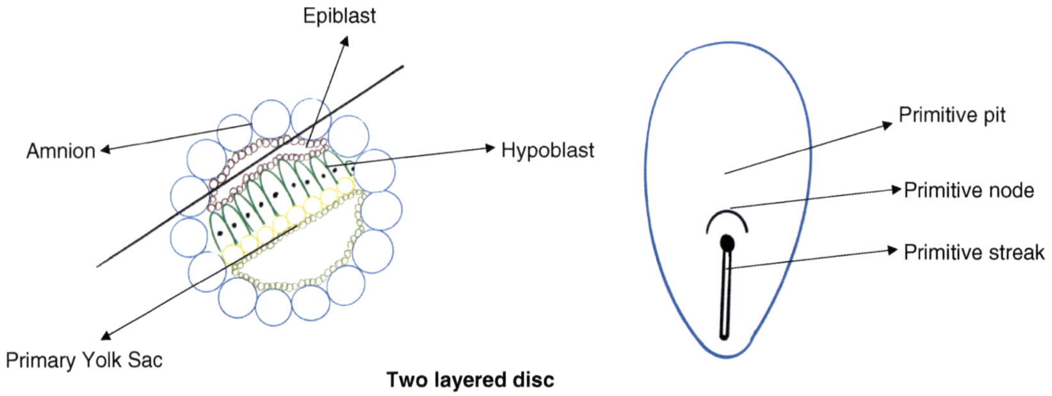

Fig. 2.2 Formation of the primitive streak

derm forms the somites, intermediate mesoderm, and the lateral plate mesoderm. The lateral plate mesoderm further divides into the somatic layer which is related to the ectoderm layer and the visceral mesoderm which is related to the endoderm. The intraembryonic coelom forms between the two layers of the lateral plate mesoderm. The formation of the gut tube and body wall causes the intraembryonic coelom to be encased between the somatic and visceral layers of the lateral plate mesoderm. The intraembryonic coelom contributes to the development of the pericardial and pleural cavities as discussed later.

Cardiac development begins in the visceral layer of the mesoderm within two crescent-shaped zones termed the primary and secondary heart fields which are located around the developing pharynx [4] (Fig. 2.3).

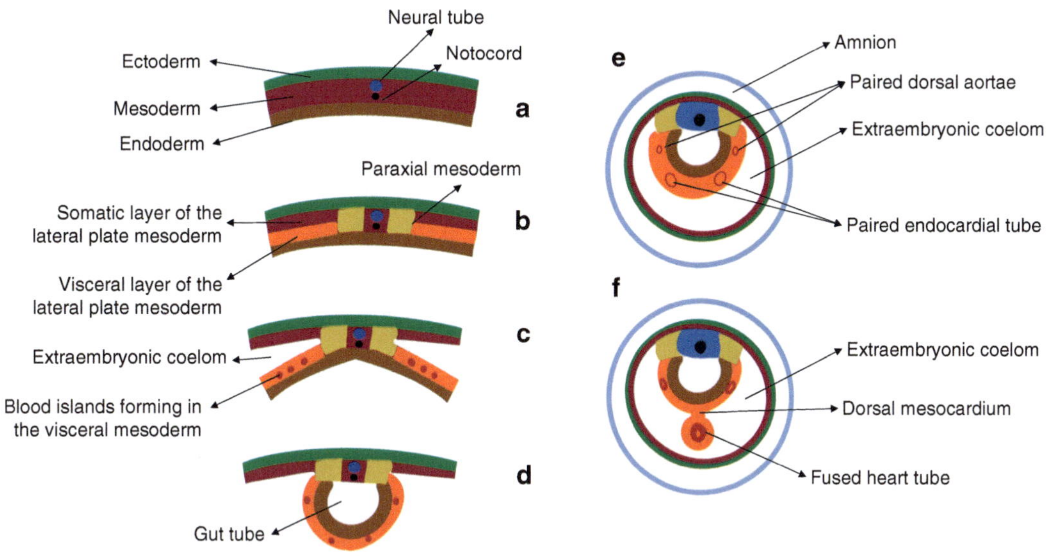

Fig. 2.3 (**a**) Development of the three germ layers. (**b**) Division of the mesoderm into the somatic mesoderm, intermediate mesoderm, and the lateral plate mesoderm. (**c**) Separation of the two layers of the lateral plate mesoderm by the extraembryonic coelom and formation of blood islands in the visceral mesoderm. (**d**) Formation of the gut tube. (**e**) Formation of the body wall. (**f**) Fusion of the paired endocardial tubes to form a single heart tube

2.3 Cardiac Development

2.3.1 Formation of the Endocardial Tube

Nutrition is initially supplied by diffusion. Circulation must replace diffusion for the embryo to develop. Hence, the cardiovascular system is the first to develop. The pregnant woman is often unaware of her pregnancy at this stage and may be exposed to external teratogenic insults. Heart development is complete by 10 weeks. Most teratogenic insults occur during the first 8 weeks of gestation. This is the reason that heart defects are one of the more common congenital defects [5].

Blood islands develop in the cardiogenic areas within the visceral layer of the lateral plate mesoderm which differentiates into the endothelial lining of primitive blood vessels as well as the primitive erythrocytes. The primitive blood vessels coalesce to form the paired endocardial tubes ventral to the developing gut tube and the paired dorsal aorta dorsal to the gut tube. The paired endocardial tubes fuse around day 22 to form a single tube which is connected to the developing body wall by the dorsal mesocardium [6]. The heart tube connects with the paired dorsal aortae through the aortic arches. The paired dorsal aorta fuse to form a signal aorta toward the caudal end of the embryo. There is now a directionality to blood flow in the embryo. Blood flows into the endocardial tube through the early cardiac veins (common cardinal veins) and out through the aortic archs and dorsal aortae to the rest of the embryo and back to the placenta. Further development of the heart tube involves the formation of loose mesenchymal tissue around the heart tube called cardiac jelly. The cardiac jelly separates the endocardial tube from the foregut. The heart tube begins pumping at around day 23 due to the formation of a layer of myocardium external to the cardiac jelly [6]. The cardiac jelly eventually regresses with the inward development of the myocardium. The dorsal mesocardium which connects the heart tube to the foregut also disappears allowing the heart tube to move into the pericardial cavity. The developing heart is cranial to the neural tube in the early embryo. Enlargement of the central nervous system and folding of the embryo push the developing heart tube caudally and into the extraembryonic coelom (Fig. 2.4).

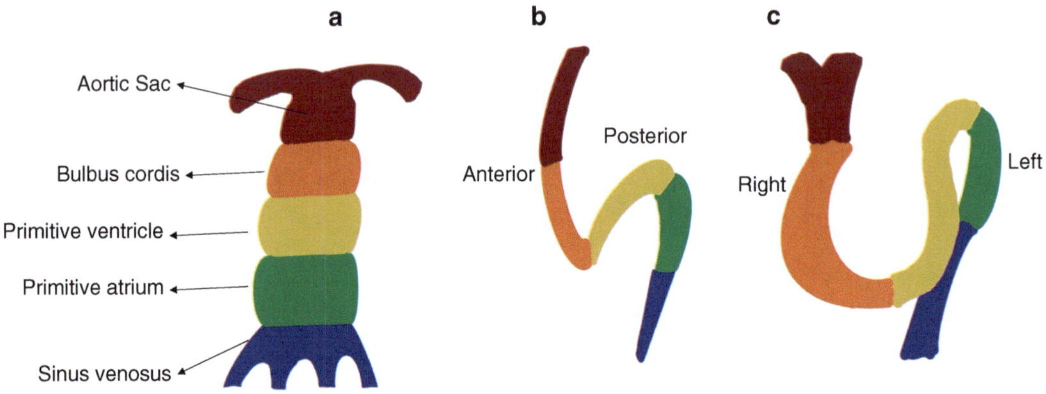

Fig. 2.4 (**a**) Parts of the heart tube. (**b**) Elongation of the heart tube causes it to fold anteriorly and cranially. (**c**) Further growth pushes the bulbus cordis to the right and the primitive ventricle to the left. The primitive atrium is now posterior to the primitive ventricle

The enlarging heart tube pushes itself into the back of the extraembryonic coelom which forms the visceral layer of the pericardium. Thus, the heart tube is surrounded by the extraembryonic coelom from the pericardial cavity. Further growth of the heart tube subdivides it into the various regions which are separated by myocardial constrictions. The portion of the embryonic heart which is receiving blood is called the sinus venosus. The sinus venosus has two horns: the right and the left horn. Blood flows from the sinus venosus into the primitive atrium, primitive ventricle, bulbus cordis, and the aortic sac. The sinus venosus forms the right atrium, vena cava junction, and the coronary sinus. The primitive atrium forms parts of the right atrium and the left atrium. The primitive ventricle forms the left ventricle. Elongation of the bulbus cordis divides it into three regions. The proximal third of the bulbus cordis forms the muscular right ventricle. The mid-third called the conus cordis forms the smooth outflow portions of the right and left ventricles. The distal third called the Truncus arteriosus forms the proximal aorta and the pulmonary trunk. The aortic sac forms portions of the aorta and the pulmonary artery. The endocardial tube folds craniocaudally to bring the sinus venosus and the primitive atrium posterior to the primitive ventricle. At the same time, the tube loops so that the bulbus cordis moves toward the right side of the body and the primitive ventricle moves toward the left side of the body. At this stage, the primitive atria are posterior to the ventricles. The bulbus cordis which forms the right ventricle is more to the right side of the body and the primitive ventricle which forms the left ventricle is to the left side of the body. The embryonic circulation forms a single circuit. The formation of septations between the different primitive chambers converts the single circuit into two parallel circuits for the systemic and pulmonary circulations. Table 2.1 describes the relation of the primitive chamber and its equivalent derivation in the adult.

Table 2.1 Adult derivatives of the primitive heart tube

Primitive chamber	Adult derivative
Sinus venosus	Smooth part of the right atrium Coronary sinus Oblique vein of the left atrium
Primitive atrium	Trabeculated parts of the right and left atria
Primitive ventricle	Trabeculated parts of the right and left ventricles
Bulbus cordis	Smooth outflow regions of the right and left ventricles
Truncus arteriosis	Ascending aorta and pulmonary trunk

2.3.1.1 Clinical Correlate

D—looping: Refers to normal looping of the cardiac chambers cephalocaudally, anteriorly, and to the right (Fig. 2.4c). At this stage, the primitive atrium still lies on top of the primitive ventricle and the bulbus cordis gives rise to the Truncus arteriosus. *An arrest in development at this age would result in a double inlet left ventricle which is the most common type of single ventricle* [7].

L—looping: Refers to looping of the cardiac chambers cephalocaudally, anteriorly, however, to the left. The bulbus cordis which forms the right ventricle is more to the left side of the body and the primitive ventricle which forms the left ventricle is to the right side of the body. *This causes L-TGA or physiologically corrected transposition* [8]. This is quite rare.

2.4 Determination of Right-Left Symmetry

How does the embryo know left from right? This process begins in the region of the embryo known as the node. Ciliated cells in this region create a left-ward flow of extraembryonic fluid which is thought to be responsible for the establishment of left-right symmetry [9]. Mouse models in which the cilia fail to beat have demonstrated the formation of organs on the wrong side of the body [10].

2.4.1 Clinical Correlate

Heterotaxy syndromes occur when this process is disrupted. Two groups of heterotaxy syndromes have been identified:

- Left isomerism with polysplenia and bilateral left lungs and right isomerism with asplenia and bilateral right lungs.
- Right isomerism is commonly associated with more severe congenital heart defects [11].

2.5 Formation of the Myocardium

Blebs develop in the endocardial tube which carves out the cardiac jelly and forms scaffolds for the structures of the mature heart such as the papillary muscles, chordae tendineae, and the valves. The myocardium grows into these spaces [4].

2.5.1 Clinical Correlate

The myocardium initially forms as a compact outer layer and a trabeculated, spongy inner layer. The compact layer provides most of the contractile force. The trabecular layer aids in nutrient exchange especially before the establishment of the coronary circulation. The trabecular myocardium undergoes a process of compaction that begins from the base of the heart and proceeds toward apex. *Failure of this process leads to LV non-compaction cardiomyopathy* [12]. In this condition, the trabeculated myocardium persists and predisposes the patient to arrhythmias and thromboembolic phenomena. The compact layers in the region of non-compaction is thin and has poor contractility. *For a diagnosis of LV non-compaction trabeculated myocardium must be present in the apex as it is the last to undergo the compaction process* [13].

2.6 Formation of the Four-Chambered Heart

Septations form at the level of the common atrioventricular canal, the interventricular foramen, and in the primitive atrium. Endocardial cushions anterior, posterior, right, and left aid in the separation of the atria from the ventricles and in the formation of the right and left atrioventricular canals. The interventricular foramen (also called the bulboventricular foramen) is located between the primitive ventricle and the bulbus cordis. An outgrowth at this location forms the muscular interventricular septum which grows upward toward the bulboventricular flange as well as the central area of the common atrioventricular canal. The separation of the right and left atrium involves the formation of primary and secondary septae and is discussed in the coming sections. The formation of the four-chambered heart can be summarized into the following four stages which occur simultaneously over the course of about 10 days during normal development [14]:

1. Formation of the right and left atrioventricular canals

2. Separation of the primitive ventricle from the bulbus cordis to form the left and right ventricles
3. Separation of the sinus venosus and primitive atrium into the right and left atria
4. Separation of the conus cordis and truncus arteriosus to become the proximal aorta and the pulmonary trunk (Fig. 2.5)

2.7 Formation of the Right and Left Atrioventricular Canals

Endocardial cushions are derived from neural crest cells. Four endocardial cushions from anterior, posterior, right, and left to the atrioventricular canal. They grow and squeeze the atrioventricular canal into a separate right and left canal [15] (Fig. 2.6).

2.7.1 Clinical Correlate

Persistent atrioventricular canal:

- Persistent atrioventricular canal occurs due to the underdevelopment of the endocardial cushions. There is a *lack of division of the atrioventricular canal into right and left canals. This defect is commonly associated with large atrial and ventricular septal defects* [16].

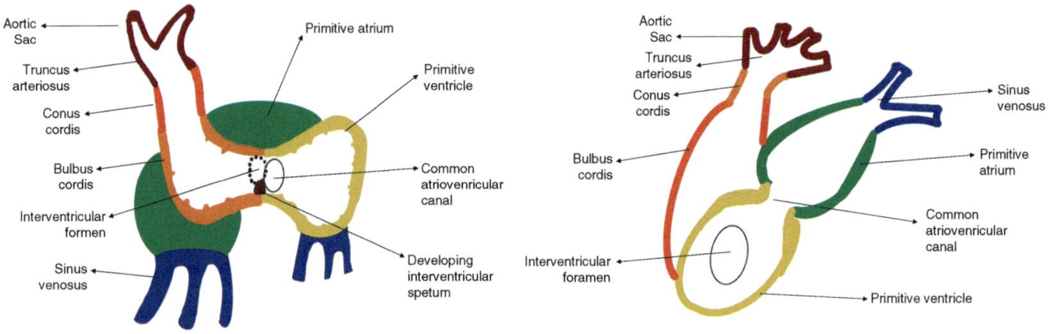

Fig. 2.5 Configuration of the heart tube before the formation of septations. The bulbus cordis which forms the right ventricle is to the right side of the body. The primitive ventricle which forms the left ventricle is to the left side of the body and the primitive atrium is posterior to the ventricle. There are pinch points for the flow of blood at the common atrioventricular canal and the interventricular foramen

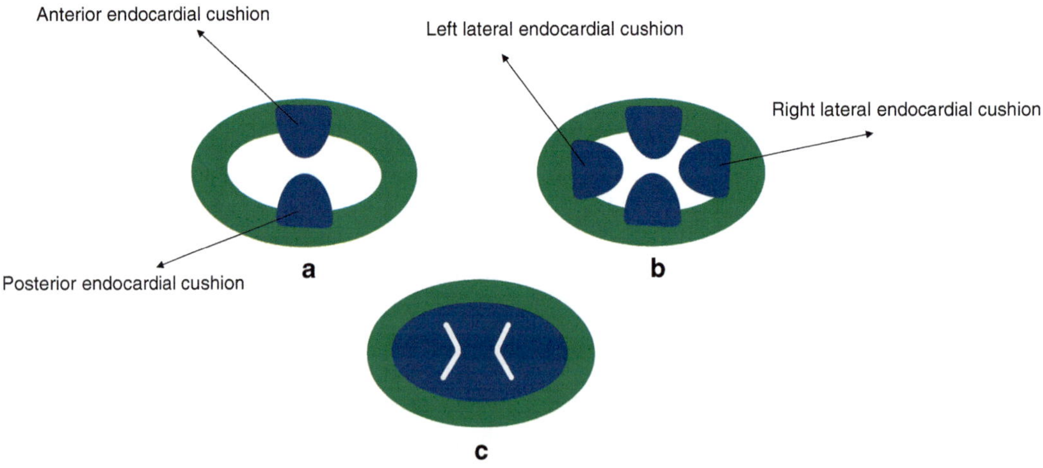

Fig. 2.6 Formation of separate right and left atrioventricular canals by the growth of the endocardial cushions. (**a**) Formation of the anterior and posterior endocardial cushions. (**b**) Formation of the right and left lateral endocardial cushions. (**c**) Progressive growth and fusion of the endocardial cushions and formation of the atrioventricular valves to form separate right and left atrioventricular canals

- There is an association of facial anomalies and atrioventricular canal defects due to common neural crest origin [17].

Tricuspid and mitral atresia:

- The normal communication between the right atrium and the right ventricle is occluded. Blood cannot enter the lungs through the right ventricle and pulmonary circulation must be satisfied through a secondary lesion which is necessary for survival. The right ventricle is severely hypoplastic. An ASD must shunt blood from the right atrium into the left atrium [18]. Blood can gain access to the pulmonary circulation either through a VSD or a PDA.
- "No flow no grow" is a common theme in congenital heart disease embryology. Cardiac chambers that do not receive blood fail to develop. Another example is the early closure of the patent foramen ovale in-utero which reduces the blood flow across the mitral valve. *This is hypothesized to cause mitral atresia and hypoplastic left heart syndrome* [19].
- Mitral or tricuspid stenosis may also occur with varying degrees of functional impairment due to hypoplastic ventricles.
- The atrioventricular valves form through erosion of the endocardial cushions. Partial erosion or the valves causes foreshortened, tethered chordae with single or bifid papillary muscles.

2.8 Formation of the Interventricular Septum (IVS)

The ventricles enlarge by pushing outward toward apex of the bulbus cordis and the primitive ventricle. The muscular septum enlarges toward the endocardial cushions. A down growth from the endocardial cushions completes the interventricular septum. This portion is called the membranous part of the interventricular septum [20] (Fig. 2.7).

2.8.1 Clinical Correlate

Interventricular septal defects are the most common congenital heart defects in infants. In adults, atrial septal defects are more common. This is

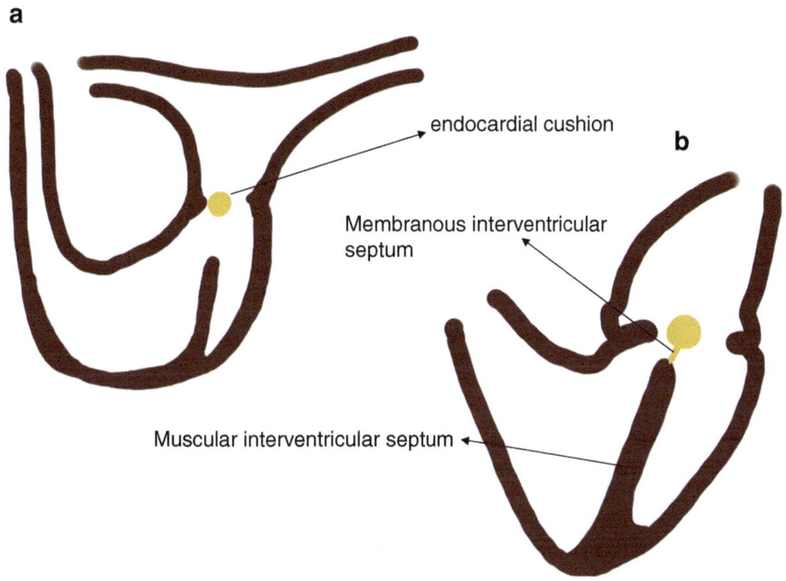

Fig. 2.7 Formation of the muscular and membranous parts of the interventricular septum. (**a**, **b**) A down growth from the endocardial cushion contributes to the formation of the membranous portion of the interventricular septum

because many VSDs close before the age of 10 years. *About 70% of VSDs occur in the membranous part of the septum. The truncal septum, inlet septum from the AV canal, and the native IVS all attach at a single point to form the membranous septum.* This is the most common location for VSDs due to the convergence of several embryonic structures.

Conoventricular VSDs occur due to incomplete formation of the inferior truncal spiral septum which is derived from neural crest migration. These defects never close spontaneously.

Inlet VSDs occur due to incomplete formation of the superior endocardial cushion which forms the inlet part of the interventricular septum.

Muscular VSDs have a different etiology and occur due to cell death in the trabecular septum [21].

2.9 Formation of the Interatrial Septum

There are two openings in the primitive atrium. On the right side is the opening of the sinus venosus and on the left side is the opening of the common pulmonary vein. The septum primum grows downward from the midline of the primitive atrium as the atrium enlarges. The septum primum separates the common atrium into the left and the right atria (Fig. 2.8).

The right and left atria communicate with each other through the ostium primum. Blood can enter either the right or the left ventricle through the ostium primum. The ostium primum closes and simultaneous apoptosis in the superior part of the septum primum forms the ostium secundum. Oxygenated blood can still reach the left ventricle through the ostium secundum (Fig. 2.9).

This configuration is compatible with intrauterine life but is not ideal after birth as it would result in the mixing of oxygenated blood coming from the pulmonary veins with deoxygenated blood coming from the vena cavae. An ingenious mechanism now develops which permits uninterrupted blood flow through the ostium secundum during fetal life and will interrupt blood flow after birth. The way this happens is through the formation of a second septum parallel to the septum primum called the septum secundum. The right atrium enlarges by incorporation of the

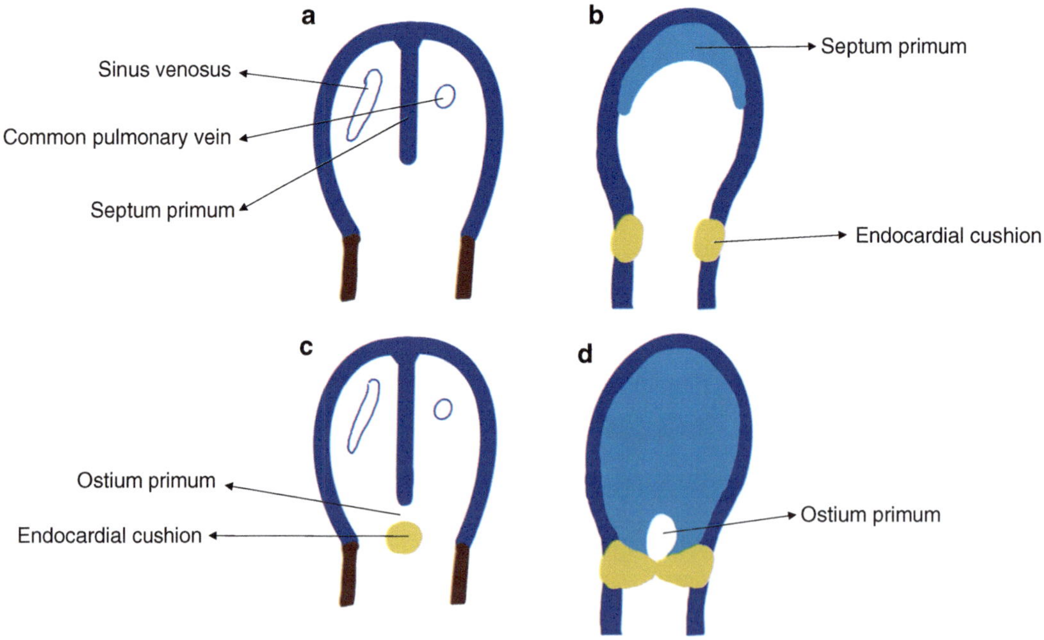

Fig. 2.8 Formation of the ostium primum. (**a**, **b**) End on views of the interatrial septum (**c**) are views of the interatrial septum looking in from the right side

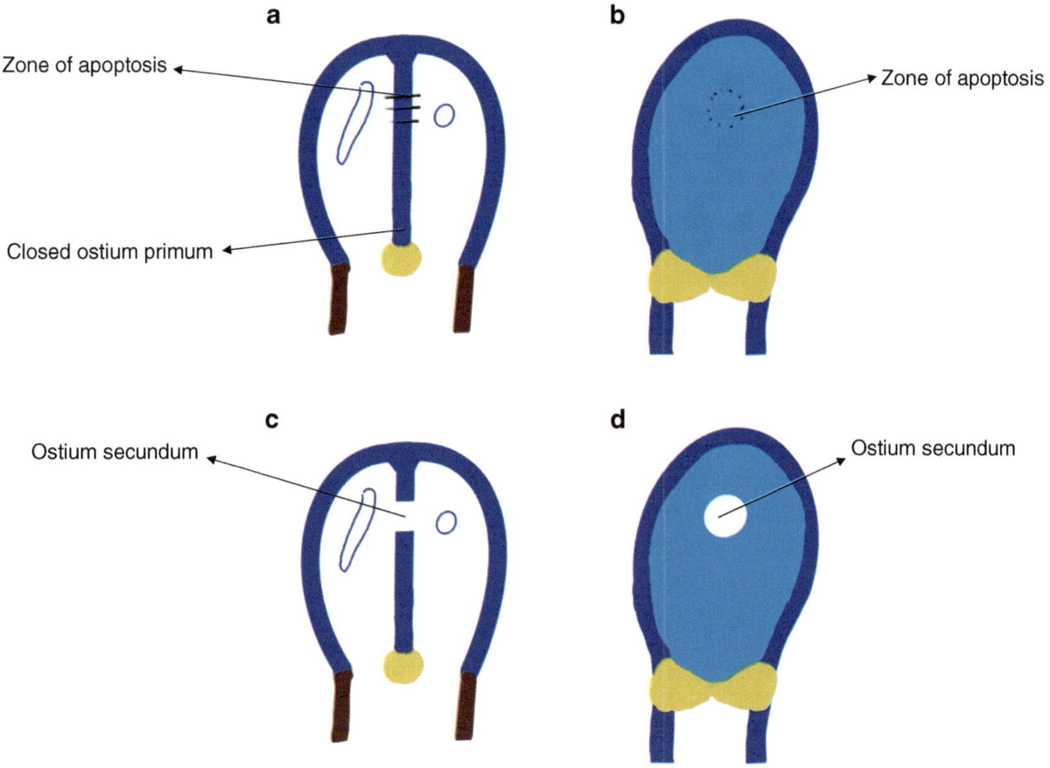

Fig. 2.9 Closure of the ostium primum and formation of the ostium secundum. (**a**, **b**) End on and lateral views of the zone of apoptosis in the septum primum. (**c**, **d**) End on and lateral views showing interatrial communication through the completed ostium secundum

sinus venosus into the wall of the right atrium. As the sinus venosus is pulled into the right atrium, it forms the septum secundum. The septum secundum has a gap called the foramen ovale. The foramen ovale overlaps a portion of the septum primum. Oxygenated blood flowing in through the inferior vena cava is directed in such a way that it flows directly toward the foramen ovale. The blood then hits the septum primum. The septum primum is actually a very thin structure compared to the septum secundum and is easily displaced by the inflow blood. The region of the septum primum which is displaced is called the valve of the foramen ovale. Oxygenated blood is thus shunted from right to left and to the rest of the body.

The left atrium enlarges by incorporation of the pulmonary veins. This pulls the tributaries of the pulmonary veins into the left atrium resulting in the usual configuration of four pulmonary vein ostia in the left atrium [22] (Fig. 2.10).

2.9.1 Clinical Correlates

Atrial septal defects (ASD):

- Atrial septal defect is the third most common congenital heart defect. Atrial septal defects are classified based on location into patent foramen ovale, ostium primum defect, ostium secundum defect, sinus venosus defect, coronary sinus defect, and common atrium [22].
- The leading part of the septum primum contains a mesenchymal cap. The dorsal mesenchymal protrusion which is derived from the dorsal mesocardium grows along with the septum primum. The ostium primum normally closes by the fusion of the mesenchymal cap with the atrioventricular endocardial cushions and the dorsal mesenchymal protrusion. *Defects in the formation of the dorsal mesenchymal protrusion have been implicated in the formation of ostium primum and atrioventric-*

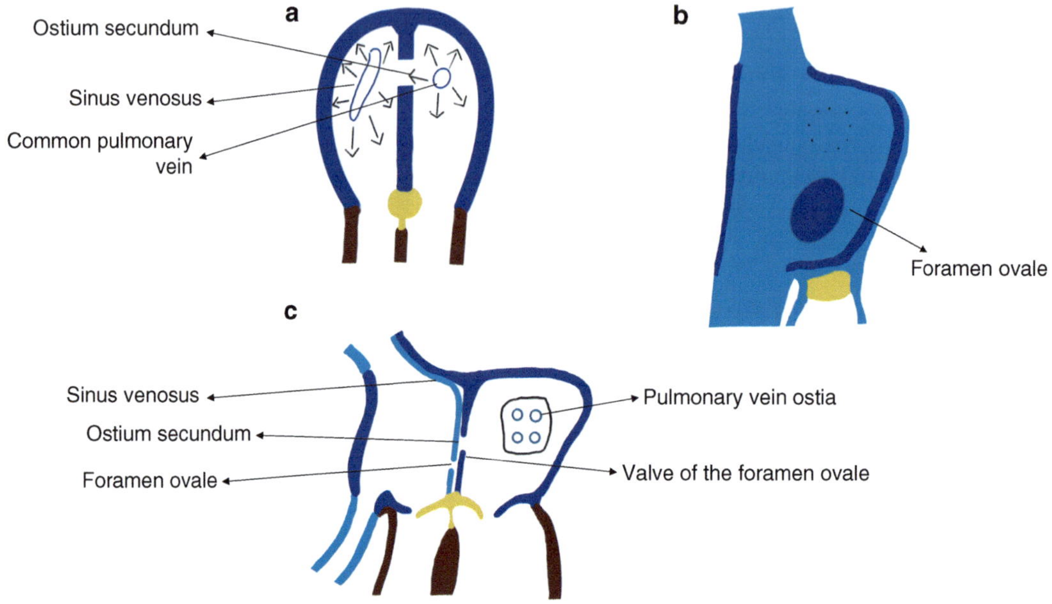

Fig. 2.10 (**a**) Formation of the septum secundum and the foramen ovale. (**b**) Viewing the interatrial septum from the right side, we see part of the septum primum (valve of the foramen ovale) through the foramen ovale. (**c**) Most of the right atrium including the septum secundum is formed by ingrowth of the sinus venosus

ular canal defects [23]. If the defect is the result of a deficiency of the atrioventricular valve tissue associated defects of the atrioventricular valves can complicate the lesion [24].

- Common atrium is the result of a complete lack of septation of the primitive atrium and is usually associated with other congenital heart diseases [25].
- The cause for sinus venosus ASDs is controversial. They are thought to arise due to a lack of separation between the pulmonary veins and the superior vena cava (SVC) or right atrium [26].
- The unroofed coronary sinus is the least common type of ASD. In this condition there is a lack of septation between the left atrium and the roof of the coronary sinus, allowing communication between the left atrium and the right atrium. It is commonly associated with a left-sided SVC [27].
- Individuals with Down's syndrome have a high incidence of atrial and ventricular septal defects. Another condition that is strongly associated with ASDs is Holt–Oram syndrome which is associated with upper limb anomalies [2].

Anomalous pulmonary venous return:

- The pulmonary veins are endodermal in origin. Normal development of the pulmonary venous system involves the creation of a connection between the mesodermal common atrium and the endodermal pulmonary venous plexus. Once this happens, other pulmonary–systemic connections involute. Disruption of this process can result in anomalous pulmonary venous drainage. Communication with the common pulmonary vein and other endodermal venous structures such as the SVC, Brachiocephalic veins, IVC, and Portal vein causes total anomalous pulmonary venous return [28]. Atresia of one side of the splanchnic vitelline system causes partial anomalous pulmonary venous return [28].
- Incomplete incorporation of the CPV into the LV causes Cor Triatriatum Sinister. These

come from the Latin terms for right and left—Sinister in Latin means left while Dexter is right. This results in a membrane in the left atrium which separates the atrium into two chambers. A proximal chamber which contains the ostia of the pulmonary veins and a distal chamber which contains the atrioventricular valve. The presence, size, and number of openings in the membrane determine the degree of obstruction to flow across the membrane [29].

2.10 Separation of the Outflow Tracts

The outflow tracts must permit blood leaving the right ventricle to enter the pulmonary circulation and blood leaving the left ventricle to enter the systemic circulation. They do this by shifting toward and straddling the common atrioventricular canal. A septum forms which splits the conus cordis and the Truncus arteriosus into an anterior and posterior tubes. The septum is formed by the fusion of the right and left conotruncal swellings (right superior truncus swelling, right dorsal conus swelling, left inferior truncus swelling, and left ventral conus swelling) [15] (Fig. 2.11).

The inferior part of the conotruncal septum is formed by cells from the endocardial cushion. This is why conotruncal anomalies can be associated with midline defects such as spina bifida as the neural arch is also a neural crest derivative. The septum spirals due to a surge of growth below the pulmonary artery. The aorta exits from the left ventricle and to the right of the pulmonary artery. The aorta then arches to the left. The pulmonary artery exits from the right ventricle anterior and to the left of the aorta [30] (Figs. 2.12 and 2.13).

2.10.1 Clinical Correlate

2.10.1.1 Conotruncal Anomalies

Malformation of the outflow tract is responsible for 20–30% of all cases of congenital heart disease.

2.10.1.2 Truncus Arteriosus

Failure of formation of the conotruncal septum causes persistent truncus arteriosus. This defect is commonly associated with a ventricular septal defect because the ventricular septum is formed in part by contributions from the conotruncal ridges. A common outflow vessel overrides the ventricular septum and receives blood from both ventricles. This results in severe cyanosis [31].

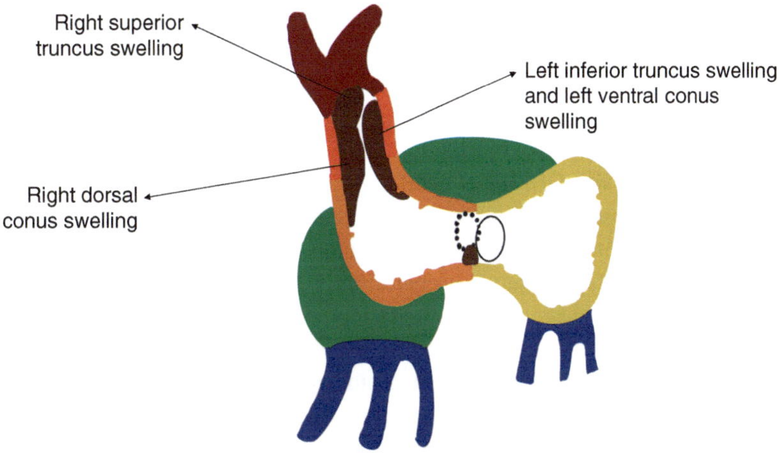

Fig. 2.11 Formation of conotruncal swellings dividing the outflow track into anterior and posterior channels

Fig. 2.12 Contribution of the endocardial cushion to the inferior conotruncal septum

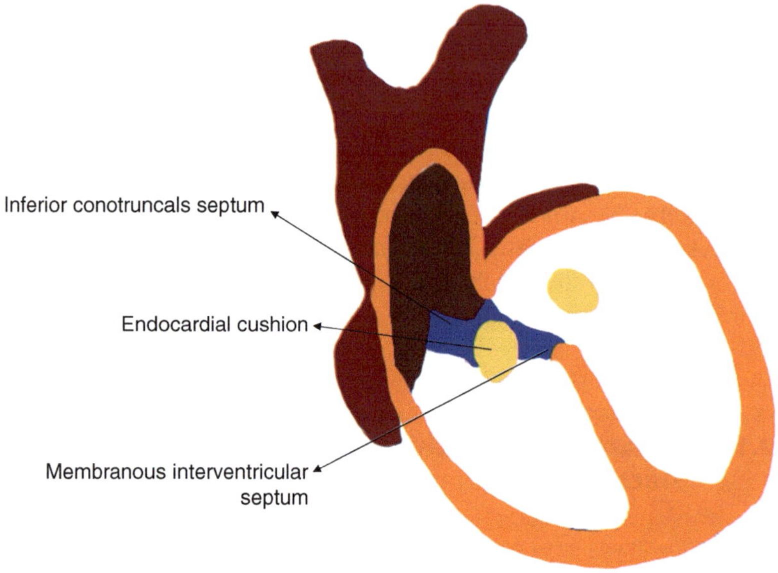

Fig. 2.13 Spiraling of the conotruncal septum allows blood from the mitral valve and left ventricle to flow posteriorly into the aorta and blood from the tricuspid valve and right ventricle to flow anteriorly into the pulmonary artery

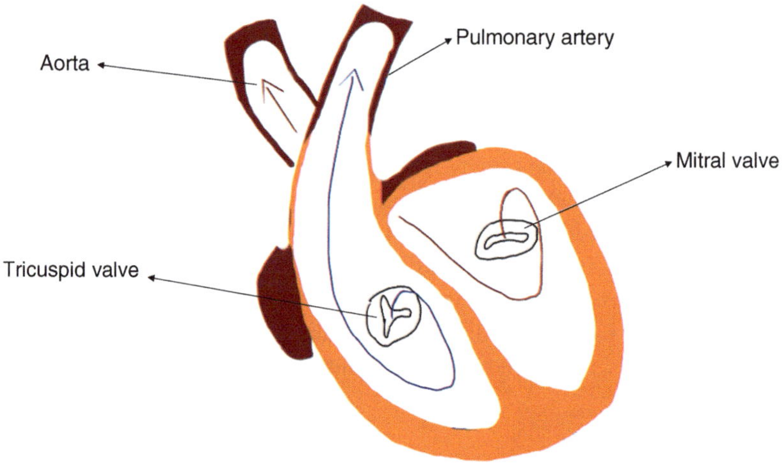

2.10.1.3 D: Transposition of the Great Arteries

Failure of spiraling of the conotruncal septum results in the transposition of the great arteries. This defect results in complete separation of the pulmonary and systemic circulations. The right ventricle empties into the aorta and the left ventricle into the pulmonary artery. This lesion is the most common cause of cyanosis in newborns. It is only compatible with life if there is an associated ASD, VSD, or PDA present [32].

2.10.1.4 Tetralogy of Fallot (TOF)

Deviation of the conotruncal septum to the one side results in asymmetry and narrowing of the aorta or pulmonary artery. Deviation of the conotruncal septum anteriorly and to the right results in TOF. This causes varying degrees of pulmonary stenosis, a membranous VSD, a large aorta overriding the right ventricle and right ventricular hypertrophy due to pulmonary stenosis [33].

2.10.1.5 Double Outlet Right Ventricle (DORV)

Normal development of the outflow tract involves a leftwards shift of the conus to straddle the common atrioventricular canal. In DORV this shift fails to occur. The arterial trunk stays over the RV but septates. This causes DORV where the aorta and pulmonary artery arise from the right ventricle. Pulmonary stenosis is commonly present due to the associated right deviation of the conotruncal septum. In the primitive heart of DORV, the most common relation of the great arteries is D-malposed. The aorta is anterior and to the right of the pulmonary artery. Other combinations are possible depending on the stage of the arrest of development which determines the degree of spiraling of the conotruncal septum [34].

2.11 Development of the Aortic Arches and the Great Vessels

Early in development blood flows from the primitive heart into the truncus arteriosus, the aortic sac, and through the aortic arches into the paired dorsal aortae which then fuse to form a single aorta caudally. This configuration resembles the gill arch structures which form in fish. These structures still form in humans but undergo extensive morphological changes to form the mature arterial system. The truncus arteriosus forms the proximal part of the ascending aorta and the pulmonary trunk. The aortic sac forms the ascending aorta and the right brachiocephalic trunk. The first and second arches form small arteries in the middle ear, head, and neck. The third arch forms the left and right common and internal carotid arteries. The fourth arch forms part of the right subclavian artery and part of the aortic arch. The fifth arch is nonexistent in humans. The sixth arch forms the right and left pulmonary arteries. The dorsal aorta forms part of the right subclavian artery, the arch of the aorta, and the descending aorta.

As development progresses, the number of arches increases. The dorsal aorta gives rise to branches called intersegmental arteries. The first and second arches start to degenerate. The third and fourth arches develop and carry most of the blood to the dorsal aorta. A bridging artery forms between the first to the seventh intersegmental arteries and starts growing cranially. The aortic arches grow adjacent to the developing pharynx and are associated with pharyngeal pouches. The dorsal aorta

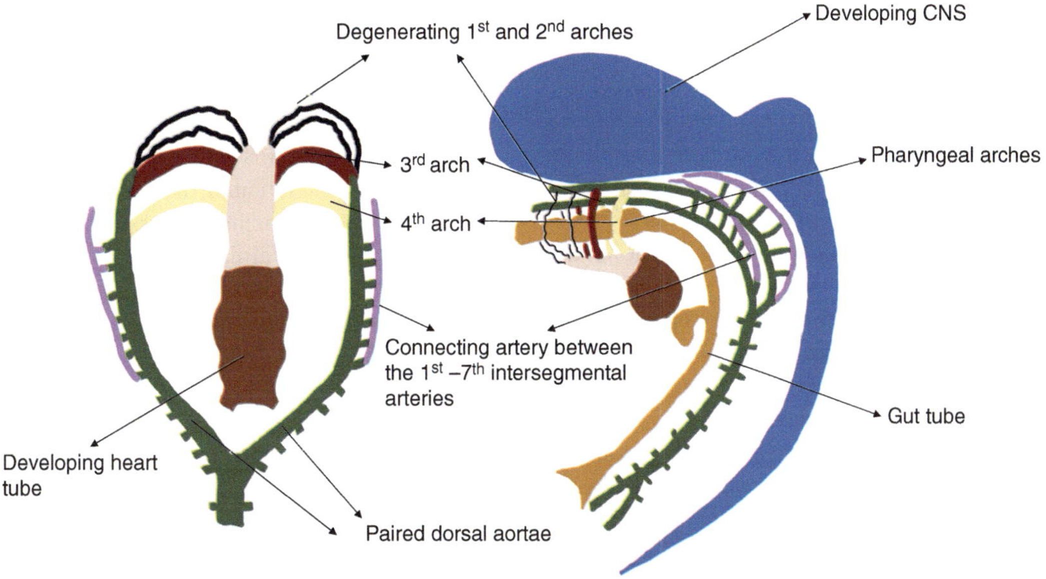

Fig. 2.14 Formation of the third and fourth aortic arches. Note the relationship of the aortic arches to the developing foregut and central nervous system

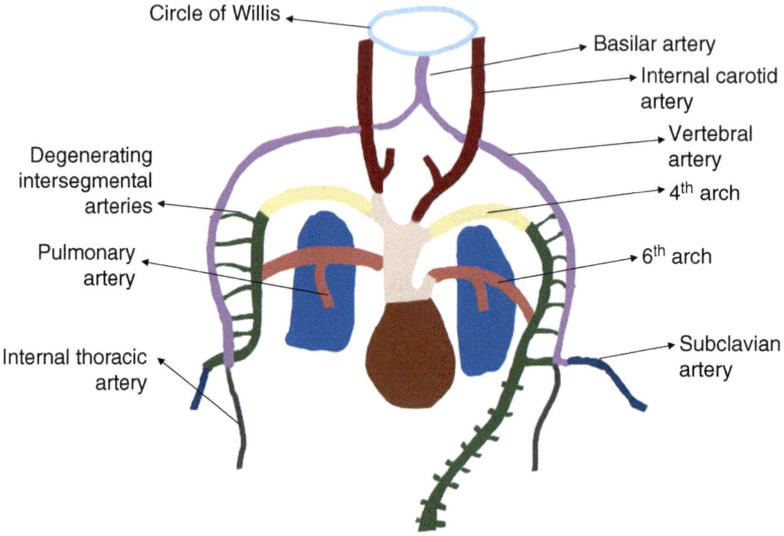

Fig. 2.15 Formation of the vertebral artery, internal carotid artery, and the circle of Willis. The seventh intersegmental artery forms the subclavian artery

between the third and fourth arches degenerates separating the third and fourth arches (Fig. 2.14).

The seventh intersegmental artery elongates and supplies the limb bud. The third arch along with the bridging artery grows cranially toward a plexus of vessels at the base of the brain. The first to sixth intersegmental arteries degenerate. Blood flows through the seventh intersegmental artery to the upper limb and through the bridging artery toward the brain. Another inferior branch develops from the seventh intersegmental artery which forms the internal mammary artery. The third arch forms the internal carotid arteries, the bridging arteries form the vertebral arteries which fuse to form the basilar artery and these vessels anastomose with vessels at the base of the brain to form the circle of Willis (Fig. 2.15).

The sixth arch develops as a plexus of vessels associated with the lung bud but is shown as a separate vessel for ease of representation. Branches form the sixth arch from the right and left pulmonary arteries and the ductus arteriosus (Fig. 2.16).

The right dorsal aorta degenerates associating the right dorsal aorta with the right subclavian artery. At this stage, the aorta and pulmonary artery are coming into existence through the formation of the conotruncal septum. The left dorsal aorta remains intact and forms the descending aorta. The lower intersegmental arteries form the intercostal arteries and the abdominopelvic arteries [35] (Fig. 2.17 and Table 2.2). Table 2.2 gives a summary of the derivatives of the aortic arches.

2.11.1 Clinical Correlate

2.11.1.1 Double Aortic Arch

The segment of the right dorsal aorta between the origin of the left subclavian artery and its point joining the left subclavian artery persists instead of regressing forming a vascular loop around the esophagus and the trachea. This condition may cause symptoms due to tracheal or esophageal compression [36].

2.11.1.2 Right Aortic Arch

A right arch arises due to the persistence of the left dorsal aorta and involution of the left dorsal aorta caudal to the origin of the left subclavian artery. The aortic arch is to the right and is the mirror image of the left arch. This condition can occur as an isolated anomaly or associated with other congenital heart diseases [37]. It is usually asymptomatic unless associated with an anomalous left subclavian artery running posterior to the esophagus.

2.11.1.3 Aberrant Right Subclavian Artery

The right subclavian artery is normally formed by the right fourth arch. Degeneration of the right fourth arch between the common carotid artery and the exit of the right seventh intersegmental artery and persistence of the segment between the origin of the right subclavian artery and the more distal right aortic arch causes the right subclavian

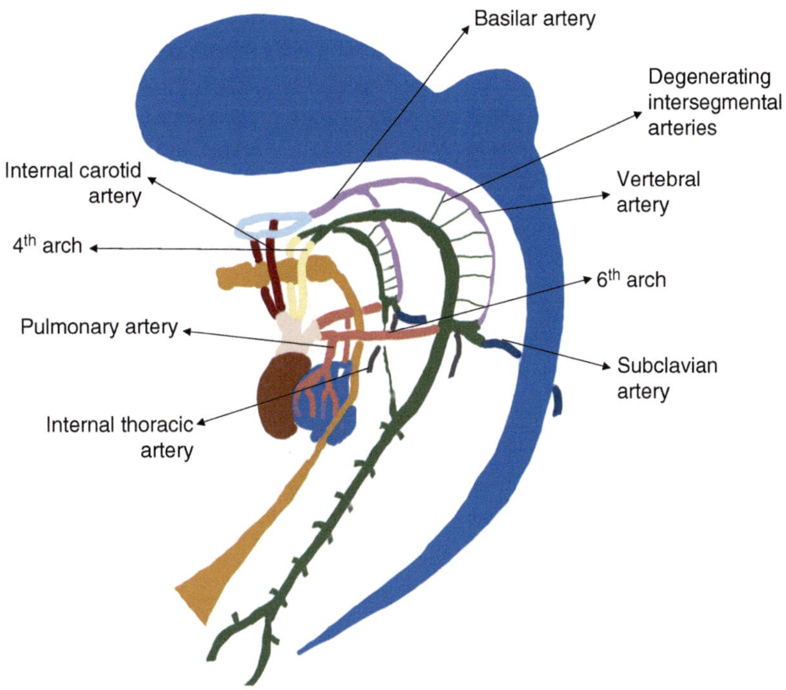

Fig. 2.16 The pulmonary arteries from the sixth arch and supply the lung buds. The distal part of the right dorsal aorta degenerates associating the remnant of the right dorsal aorta with the subclavian artery

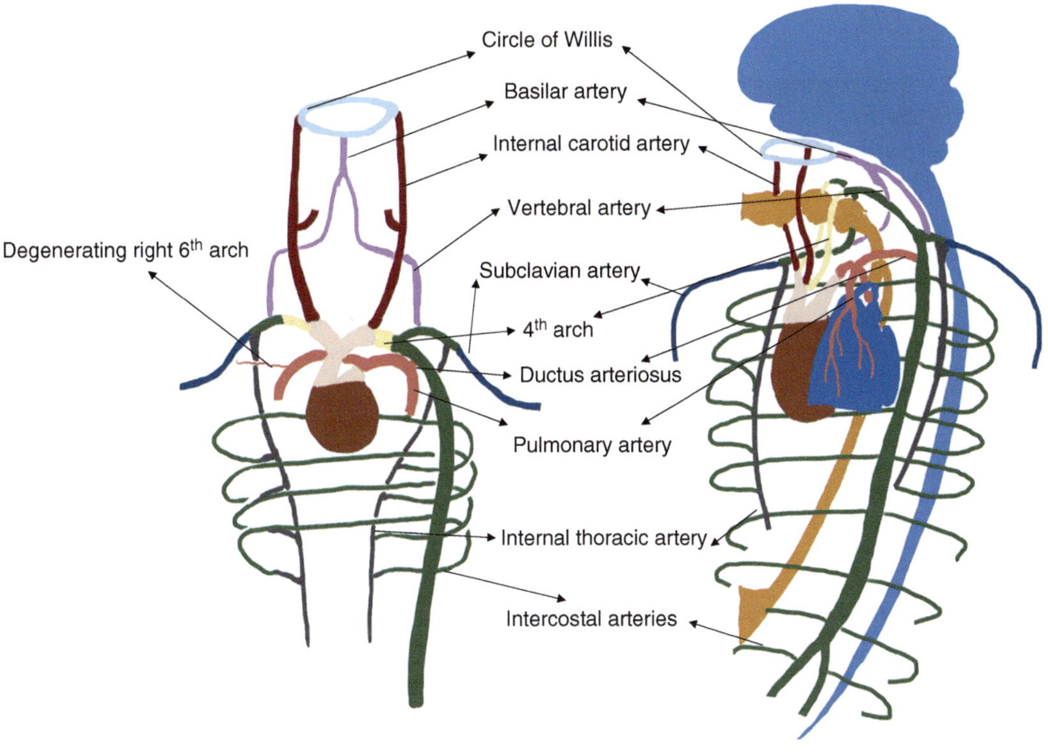

Fig. 2.17 Near mature circulation. Separate aortic and pulmonary circulations have been established. The right sixth arch degenerates. The ductus venous drains blood from the pulmonary artery into the aorta. The intersegmental arteries form the intercostal arteries as well as the abdominopelvic arteries

Table 2.2 Aortic arches and their adult derivatives

Aortic arch derivatives		
Vessel	Left	Right
First arch	Maxillary artery	
Second arch	Stapedial and hyoid arteries	
Third arch	Common carotid, internal and external carotid arteries	
Fourth arch	Part of aortic arch	Part of the right subclavian artery
Sixth arch	Left pulmonary artery and ductus arteriosus	Right pulmonary artery
Seventh intersegmental artery	Left subclavian artery	Part of the right subclavian artery
Dorsal aorta	Descending thoracic aorta	Part of right subclavian artery
Aortic sac	Part of aortic arch	Brachiocephalic trunk

artery to arise from the left aortic arch and pass posterior to the esophagus and trachea to supply the right arm [38].

2.11.1.4 Interruption of the Aortic Arch

A break in the aortic arch usually distal to the origin of the left subclavian artery is termed interruption of the aortic arch. It is due to the failure of the development of the left fourth arch segment which contributes to part of the aortic arch. The descending aorta and lower limbs are supplied by a patent ductus arteriosus. Arch interruption is further defined by the site of interruption. In type A, interruption is distal to the left subclavian artery; in type B, interruption is between the left carotid and left subclavian arteries; and in type C, interruption occurs between the innominate and left carotid arteries [37].

2.11.1.5 Patent Ductus Arteriosus (PDA)

This condition is due to the failure of closure of the ductus arteriosus after birth. Several chromosomal anomalies have been implicated [39]. Congenital rubella syndrome and fetal alcohol syndrome are associated with PDA. It is more common in preterm neonates due to lung immaturity, reduction oxygen saturation, and inadequate clearance of prostaglandins [40].

2.11.1.6 Coarctation of the Aorta

The embryogenesis of coarctation is unclear. One theory is that cells from the ductus arteriosus move into the aorta and constrict in response to increasing oxygen saturation after birth. Another theory proposes that reduced blood flow in the aorta at the level of the isthmus as the cause for hypoplasia of this segment. Coarctation of the aorta is more common in Down's syndrome and Turner's syndrome [37].

2.12 Formation of the Venous System

The venous inflow into the developing heart tube is through the sinus venosus. The sinus venosus receives blood through the common cardinal veins, the umbilical veins, and the vitelline veins which go on to form different components of the adult venous system.

The anterior cranial veins drain the cranial end of the embryo, the posterior cardinal veins drain the caudal end of the embryo and converge to the form the paired common cardinal veins. Umbilical veins come from the placenta. The vitelline veins drain the yolk sac and form an anastomosis around the gut tube. The vitelline veins are important in forming tributaries of the hepato-portal system (Fig. 2.18).

We will first discuss the formation of the hepato-portal system followed by the formation of the systemic veins. It should be kept in mind that both systems develop simultaneously (Fig. 2.19).

The umbilical veins lose their communication with the sinus venosus. They instead drain into the right and left hepatocardiac channels with a drain into the sinus venosus. The hepatocardiac channels form from the vitelline anastomosis within the developing liver. The right umbilical vein involves. The left umbilical vein enlarges and communicates with the left hepatocardiac channel (Fig. 2.20).

The ductus venosus develops from the left hepatocardiac channel in the liver which bypasses the liver sinusoids and drains into the hepatic seg-

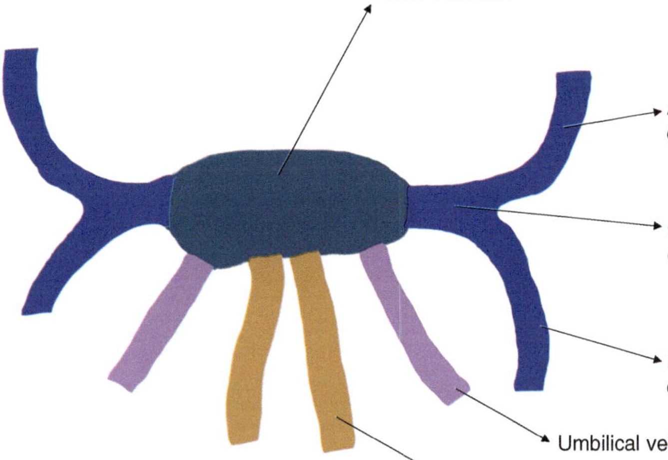

Fig. 2.18 Venous structures of the early embryo

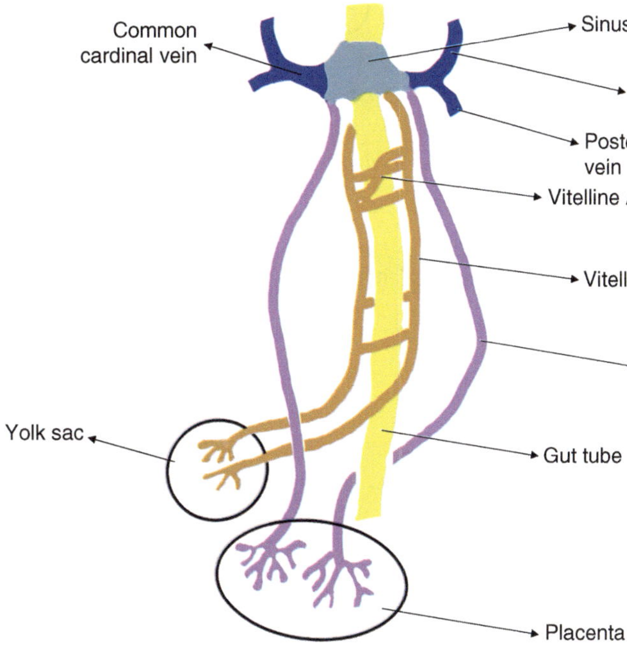

Fig. 2.19 The vitelline veins are associated with the yolk sac and the gut tube. The umbilical veins initially drain directly into the sinus venosus. Later on, this communication is lost

ment of the inferior vena cava which is also derived from the vitelline veins. The right hepatocardiac channel disappears (Fig. 2.21).

The vitelline veins form the portal venous system. Blood from the gut tube drains into the portal venous system and accesses the hepatic sinusoids. The hepatic sinusoids drain into the central veins of the hepatic lobules and thence into larger and larger hepatic veins which eventually drain into the IVC. Blood from the umbilical vein bypasses the portal circulation and directly enters the IVC through the ductus venosus (Fig. 2.22).

Changes in the cardinal veins are occurring simultaneously. Subcardinal veins develop toward the dorsal surface of the embryo. They form a subcardinal anastomosis and communicate with the posterior cardinal veins through several channels. The posterior cardinal veins supply the mesonephric kidney. The mesonephric

Fig. 2.20 Formation of hepatocardiac channels and loss of communication of the umbilical veins with the sinus venosus

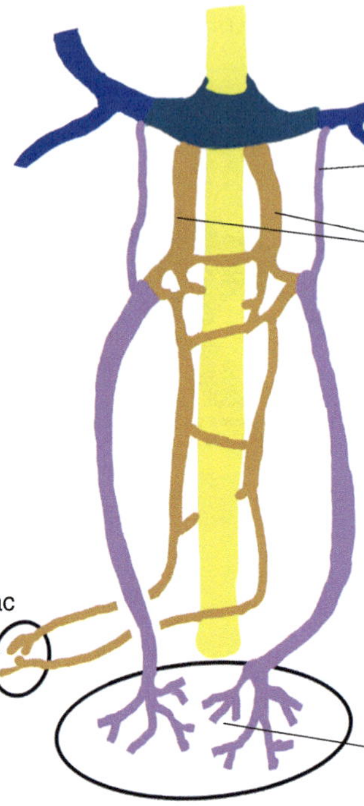

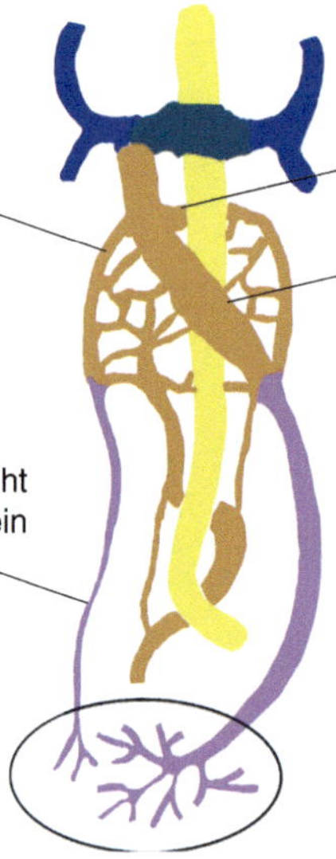

Fig. 2.21 Formation of the ductus venosus and involution of the right umbilical vein. The yolk sac has also disappeared

kidney is transiently present and regresses with the development of the metanephric kidney. The posterior cardinal veins regress along with it (Fig. 2.23).

Another set of veins develops toward the back of the embryo called the supracardinal veins. These veins connect with the posterior cardinal veins and also with the subcardinal veins. The anastomosis between the supracardinal veins and the subcardinal veins is called the subsupracardinal anastomosis (Figs. 2.24 and 2.25).

The subcardinal veins and the supracardinal veins take on a more prominent role with the disappearance of the posterior cardinal veins. Simultaneously anastomotic channels develop between the right and left superior cardinal veins and supracardinal veins. A communication develops between the subcardinal veins and the hepatic segment of the inferior vena cava. The metanephric kidney develops in association with the subsupracardinal anastomoses which eventually form the renal veins. The gonads are drained through the subcardinal veins (Figs. 2.26 and 2.27).

The proximal portion of the left anterior cardinal vein, the connection between the subcardinal veins and the posterior cardinal vein, the cranial portion of the left supracardinal vein constrict. The connection between the supracardinal veins

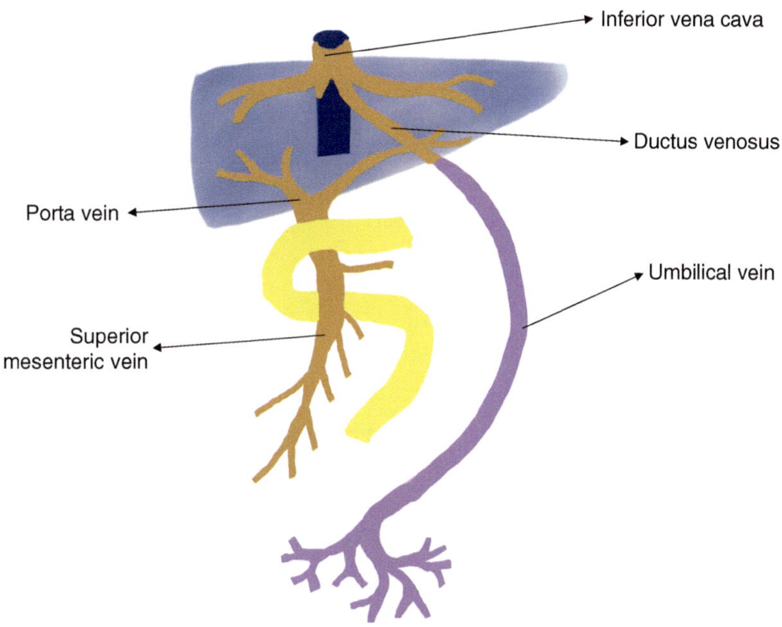

Fig. 2.22 Formation of the mature portal system from the vitelline veins. The ductus venosus closes after birth to form the ligamentum venosum of the liver. The umbilical vein forms the ligamentum teres

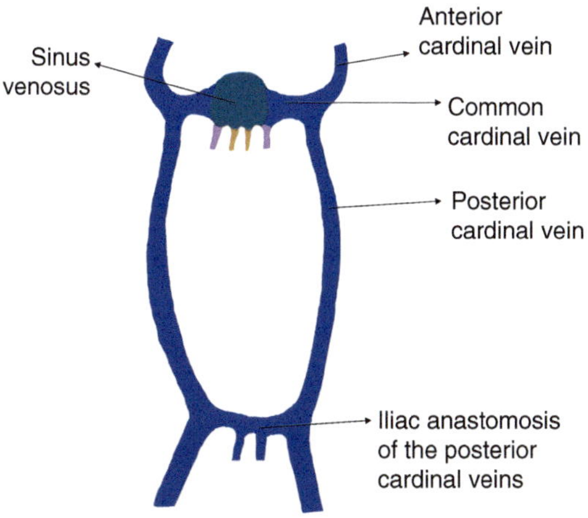

Fig. 2.23 The anterior and posterior cardinal veins drain into the sinus venosus through the common cardinal veins

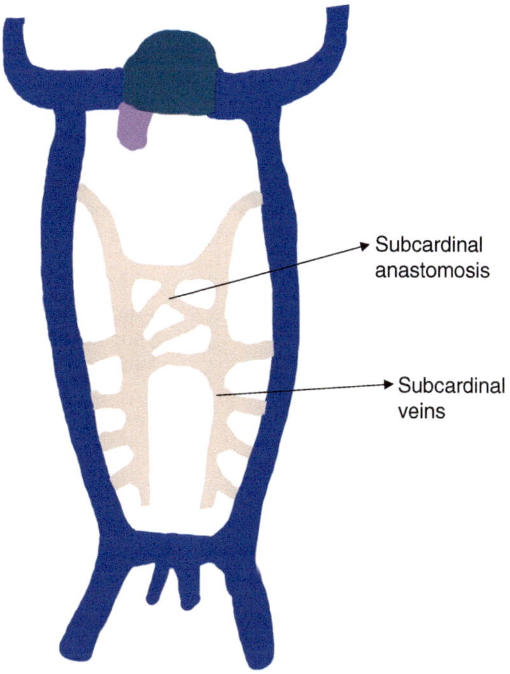

Fig. 2.24 Formation of the subcardial veins and subcardinal anastomosis

and the subsupracardinal anastomosis degenerates (Fig. 2.28).

Constriction of these vessels results in a pattern of vessels that resembles the adult venous system. The right and left brachiocephalic veins are derived from the anterior cardinal vein. The coronary sinus is formed from the left common cardinal vein. The azygous, hemiazygous, and accessory hemiazygous veins are derived from the supracardinal veins. The right and left renal veins form the subsupracardinal anastomosis. The right and left gonadal and suprarenal veins form the subcardinal veins. The IVC forms from a combination of several veins. The left and right iliac veins form from the anastomosis

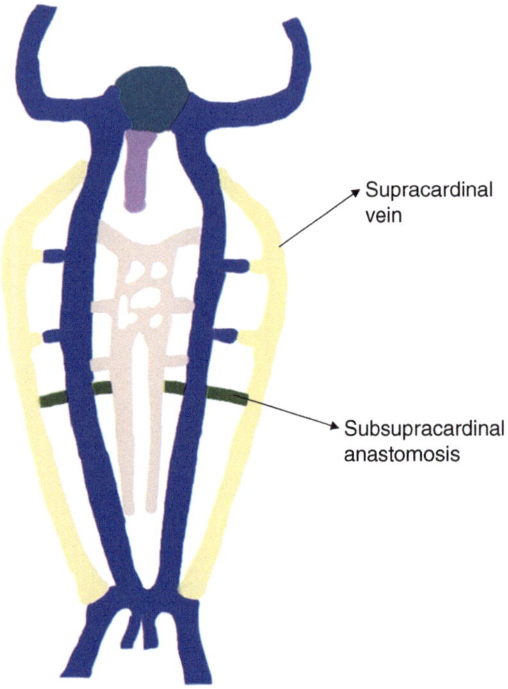

Fig. 2.25 Formation of the supracardinal veins and the subsupracardinal anastomosis

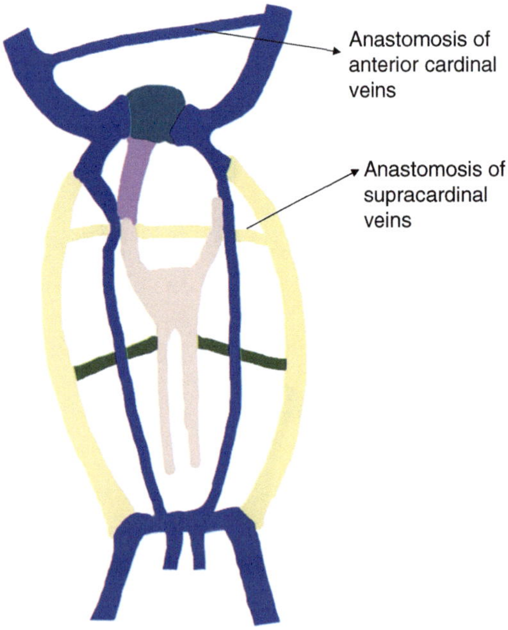

Fig. 2.26 Formation of the anastomosis between the supracradinal veins, anterior cardinal veins. The subcardinal veins form a communication with the hepatic segment of the inferior vena cava

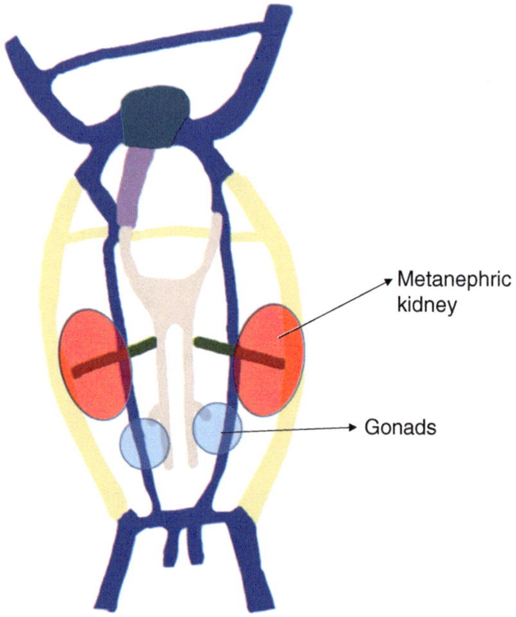

Fig. 2.27 Relationship of the subsupracardinal veins to the metanephric kidney and the subcardinal veins to the gonads

between the posterior cardinal veins [41] (Fig. 2.29).

2.12.1 Clinical Correlate

2.12.1.1 Persistent Left Superior Vena Cava

Degeneration of the intercardinal vein anastomosis results in the preservation of the left anterior supracardinal veins. Blood from the left upper limb and head and neck flows through the left anterior cardinal vein into the coronary sinus and then the right atrium. This results in the formation of a persistent left superior vena cava [42] (Fig. 2.30).

2.12.1.2 Isolated Left Superior Vena Cava

Constriction of the right common cardinal vein causes the right SVC not to develop. All the blood from the upper limbs now travels through the left superior vena and drains into the right atrium through the coronary sinus [42] (Fig. 2.31).

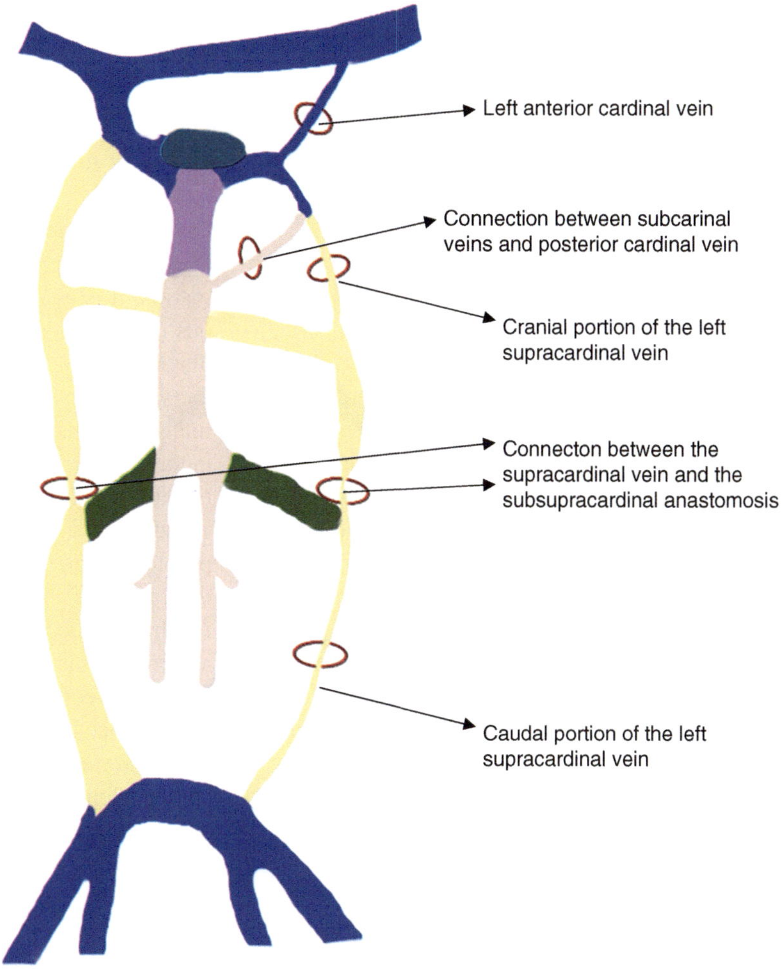

Fig. 2.28 Constriction and involution of several embryonic venous structures on the left side and one structure on the right side

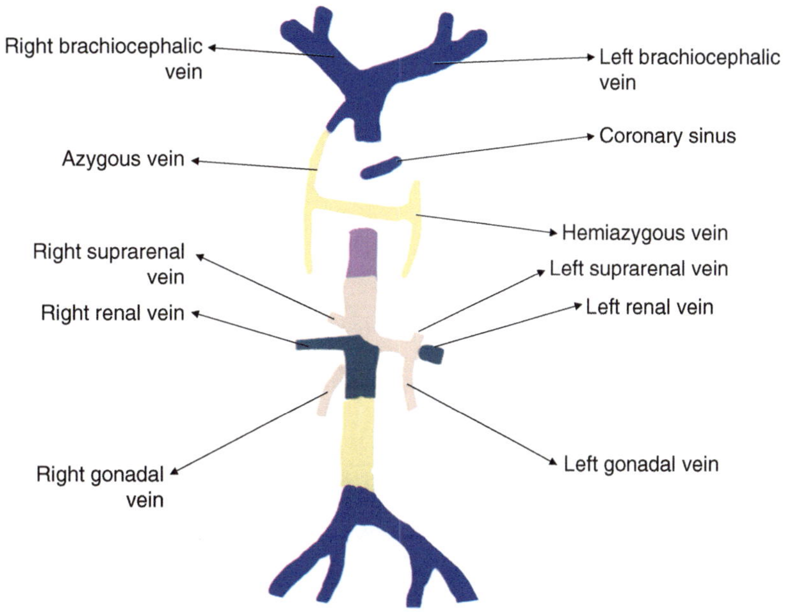

Fig. 2.29 Mature systemic venous system. The IVC is derived from several embryonic veins

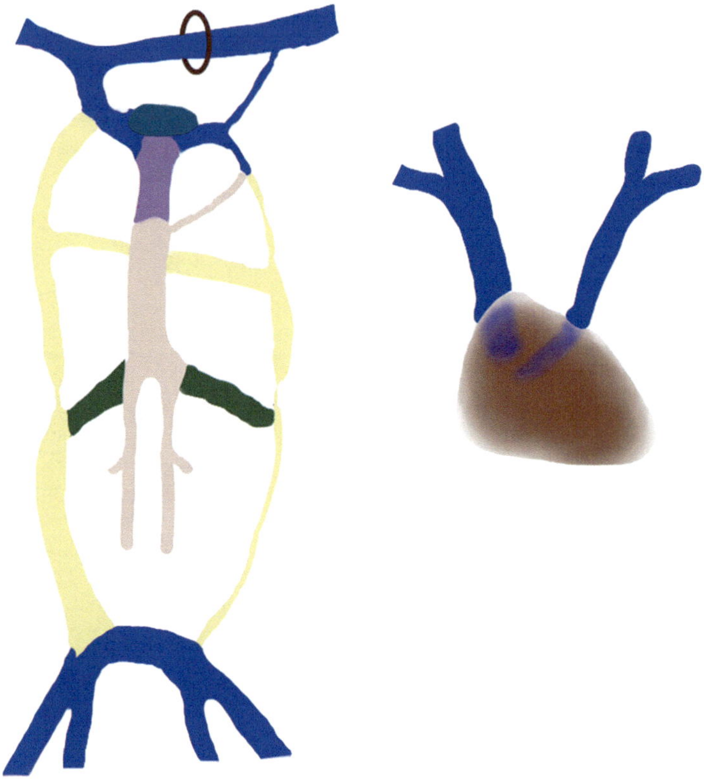

Fig. 2.30 Constriction of the anterior intercardinal vein anastomosis causes the development of a persistent left SVC

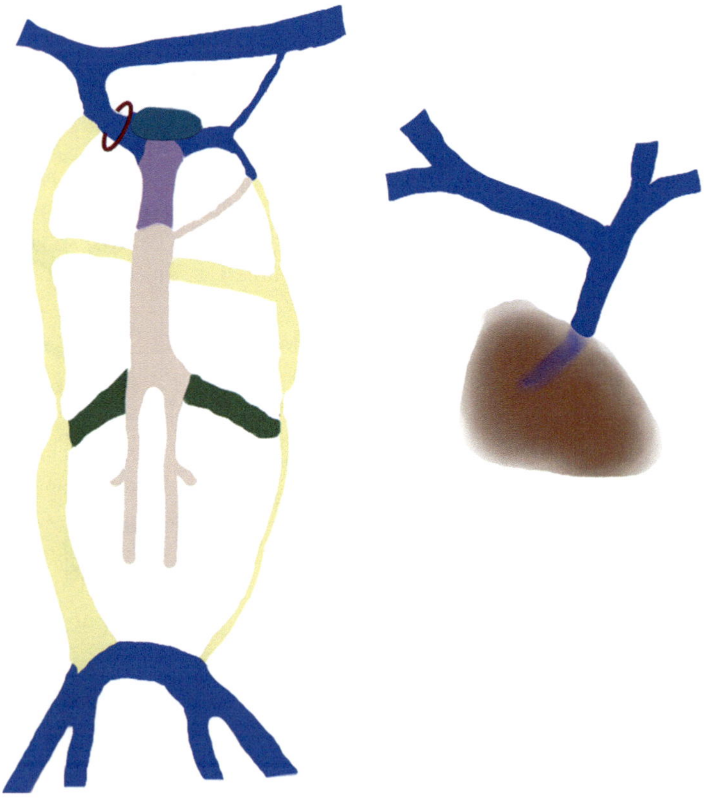

Fig. 2.31 Isolated left superior vena cava due to constriction of the right common cardinal vein

2.12.1.3 Azygous Continuation of the Inferior Vena Cava

Lack of formation of the anastomosis between the hepatic segment of the IVC derived from the vitelline veins and the segment derived from the subcardinal veins results in azygous continuation of the IVC. Blood from the lower limbs and abdominal organs now drains into the azygous vein with drains into the superior vena cava. The portal venous system drains normally into the liver. The hepatic veins and hepatic segment of the IVC drain into the right atrium [43] (Fig. 2.32).

2.12.1.4 Double Interior Vena Cavae

This condition is caused by involution of the inter posterior cardinal vein iliac anastomosis. In such cases, the caudal portion of the left supracardinal vein remains open and drains blood from the left lower limb and pelvic organs into the left renal vein (Fig. 2.33).

2.13 Fetal Circulation

Blood flows from the placenta to the umbilical veins. The ductus venosus shunts oxygenated blood from the umbilical vein to the inferior vena cava where it mixes with deoxygenated blood from the abdominopelvic organs and the lower limbs and enters the right atrium. From the right atrium blood from the IVC is preferentially shunted to the left atrium through the foramen ovale. Blood from the left atrium is pumped into the left ventricle, the preductal aorta, and the head and upper limbs. Deoxygenated blood from the SVC tends to flow to the right ventricle, pulmonary trunk, and the lungs. High vascular resistance in the pulmonary circulation causes shunting of blood through the ductus arteriosus into the postductal aorta. Only about 10% of the right ventricular output passes through the pulmonary circulation. The remaining is shunted into the aorta through the ductus arteriosus. Hence, blood with a

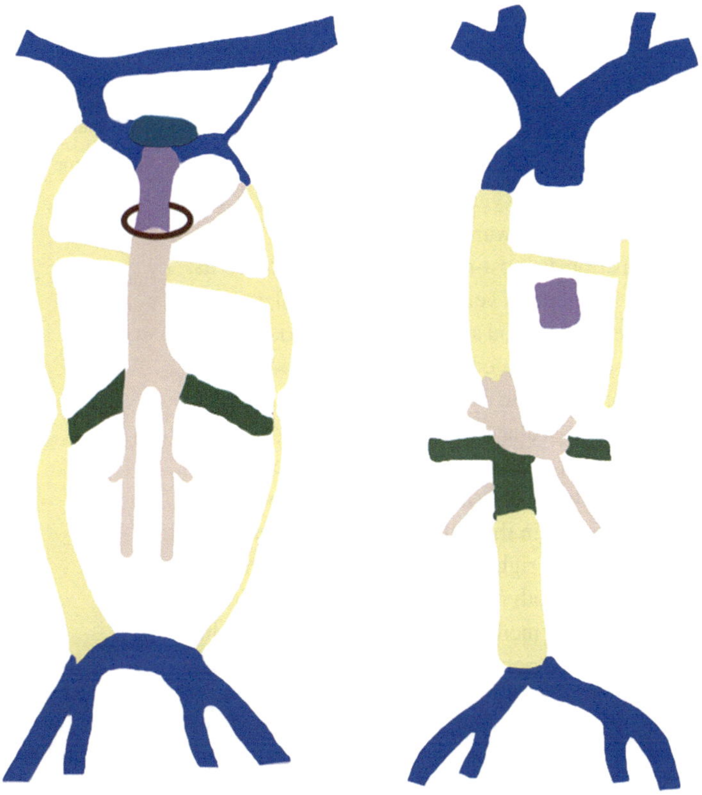

Fig. 2.32 Lack of communication between the subcardial veins and the intrahepatic segment of the IVC cause azygous continuation of the IVC. This condition is associated with the left isomerism polysplenia syndrome

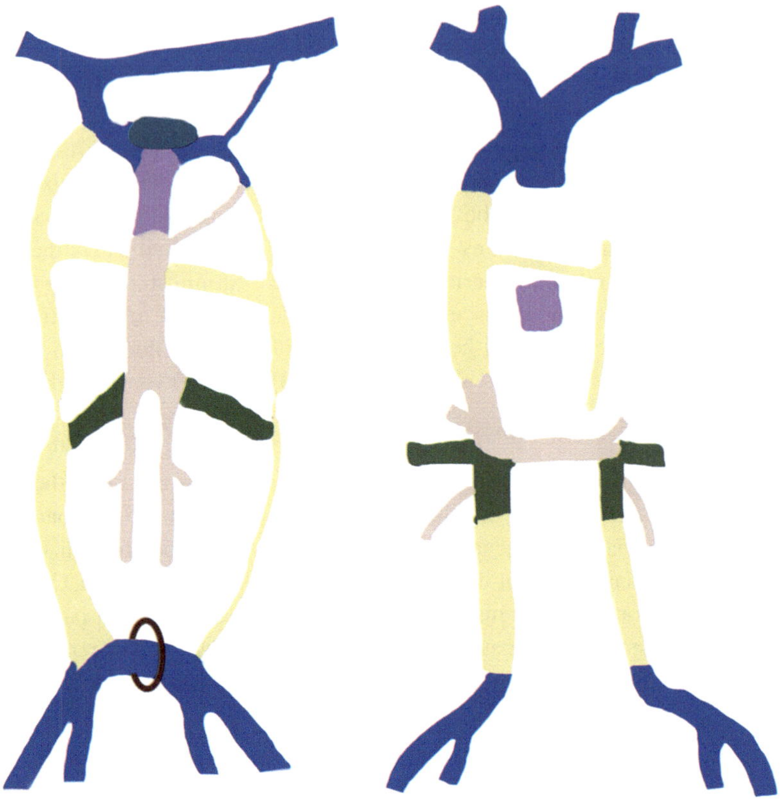

Fig. 2.33 Involution of the inter posterior cardinal vein iliac anastomosis causes double SVC

higher oxygen saturation is reaching the developing brain whereas relatively deoxygenated blood is reaching the abdominopelvic organs and the lower limbs. Deoxygenated blood flows via the umbilical artery toward the placenta.

Transition to post-natal blood flow occurs as follows. The ductus venosus and umbilical arteries no longer carry blood and close. The IVC is receiving poorly oxygenated blood from the abdominopelvic organs. The lungs fill with air and the pulmonary vascular resistance decreases, increasing left atrial pressure. The increased left atrial pressure is due to increased blood flow through the lungs. Pressure in the left atrium now exceeds the pressure in the right atrium closing the foramen ovale. The smooth muscle of the ductus arteriosus responds to the increased oxygen saturation in the blood and constricts closing the ductus arteriosus. The systemic and pulmonary circuits are now separate and the circulation is mature [3] (Table 2.3).

Table 2.3 Chronology of developmental events and malformations

Time frame	Developmental event	Malformation
20–24 days	• Determination of left and right sidedness	• Heterotaxy syndromes
End of fourth week	• Incorporation of sinus venosus into the right atrium • Appearance of endocardial cushions • Formation of the septum primum • Formation of the muscular interventricular septum • Formation of conotruncal ridges • Formation of the fourth aortic arch	• Abnormalities of systemic venous return • Persistent atrioventricular canal • Common atrium • Common ventricle • Persistent Truncus arteriosus • Interrupted aortic arch

Table 2.3 (continued)

Time frame	Developmental event	Malformation
Start of fifth week	• Growth of endocardial cushions forming right and left AV canals • Further growth of the muscular IVS • Spiraling of the conotruncal septum • Incorporation of pulmonary veins into the LA	• Atrioventricular canal defects • Muscular VSDs • Transposition of the great arteries • Anomalous pulmonary venous connections
End of fifth week to early sixth week	• Closure of the ostium primum • Formation of the membranous interventricular septum • Formation of the semilunar valves	• Ostium primum ASDs • Membranous VSDs • Aortic and pulmonary valvar stenosis
Late sixth week	• Ostium secundum forms • Atrioventricular valves and papillary muscles form • Membranous septum continues to form	• Ostium secundum ASDs • Tricuspid and mitral valvar stenosis/atresia • Membranous VSDs
Eighth to ninth week	• Membranous septum is completed	• Membranous VSDs

References

1. Hoffman JIE, Kaplan S. The incidence of congenital heart disease. J Am Coll Cardiol. 2002 Jun 19;39(12):1890–900.
2. Gelb BD, Chung WK. Complex genetics and the etiology of human congenital heart disease. Cold Spring Harb Perspect Med. 2014; https://doi.org/10.1101/cshperspect.a013953.
3. Sadler TW. Langman's medical embryology. Philadelphia: Lippincott Williams & Wilkins; 2011. p. 387.
4. Kelly RG, Buckingham ME, Moorman AF. Heart fields and cardiac morphogenesis. Cold Spring Harb Perspect Med. 2014 Oct;4(10):a015750.
5. Anderson RH, Webb S, Brown NA, Lamers W, Moorman A. Development of the heart: (2) Septation of the atriums and ventricles. Heart. 2003 Aug;89(8):949–58.
6. Gittenberger-de Groot AC, Bartelings MM, Deruiter MC, Poelmann RE. Basics of cardiac development for the understanding of congenital heart malformations. Pediatr Res. 2005 Feb;57(2):169–76.
7. van Praagh R, Plett JA, van Praagh S. Single ventricle. Pathology, embryology, terminology and classification. Herz. 1979 Apr;4(2):113–50.
8. de la Cruz MV, Arteaga M, Espino-Vela J, Quero-Jiménez M, Anderson RH, Díaz GF. Complete transposition of the great arteries: types and morphogenesis of ventriculoarterial discordance. Am Heart J. 1981 Aug;102(2):271–81.
9. Hirokawa N, Tanaka Y, Okada Y, Takeda S. Nodal flow and the generation of left-right asymmetry. Cell. 2006 Apr 7;125(1):33–45.
10. Shiraishi I, Ichikawa H. Human heterotaxy syndrome – from molecular genetics to clinical features, management, and prognosis. Circ J Off J Jpn Circ Soc. 2012;76(9):2066–75.
11. Jacobs JP, Anderson RH, Weinberg PM, Walters HL, Tchervenkov CI, Del Duca D, et al. The nomenclature, definition and classification of cardiac structures in the setting of heterotaxy. Cardiol Young. 2007 Sep;17(Suppl 2):1–28.
12. Left ventricular non-compaction: genetics and embryology - Oxford Medicine. Available from https://oxfordmedicine.com/view/10.1093/med/9780198784906.001.0001/med-9780198784906-chapter-362
13. Zuccarino F, Vollmer I, Sanchez G, Navallas M, Pugliese F, Gayete A. Left ventricular noncompaction: imaging findings and diagnostic criteria. Am J Roentgenol. 2015;204(5):W519–30.
14. Anderson RH, Brown NA, Mohun TJ, Moorman AFM. Insights from cardiac development relevant to congenital defects and adult clinical anatomy. J Cardiovasc Transl Res. 2013 Apr;6(2):107–17.
15. Lin C-J, Lin C-Y, Chen C-H, Zhou B, Chang C-P. Partitioning the heart: mechanisms of cardiac septation and valve development. Dev Camb Engl. 2012 Sep 15;139(18):3277–99.
16. Anatomical-embryological correlates in atrioventricular septal defect. Available from https://www.ncbi.nlm.nih.gov/pmc/articles/PMC481158/
17. Keyte A, Hutson MR. The neural crest in cardiac congenital anomalies. Differ Res Biol Divers. 2012 Jul;84(1):25–40.
18. Rossignol AM, Delisle G, Guay JM. Tricuspid atresia: anatomo-embryological and clinical study of 11 cases. Union Med Can. 1974 May;103(5):833–8.
19. Barron DJ, Kilby MD, Davies B, Wright JGC, Jones TJ, Brawn WJ. Hypoplastic left heart syndrome. Lancet Lond Engl. 2009 Aug 15;374(9689):551–64.
20. Goor DA, Edwards JE, Lillehei CW. The development of the interventricular septum of the human heart; Correlative Morphogenetic Study. Chest. 1970 Nov 1;58(5):453–67.

21. Minette MS, Sahn DJ. Ventricular septal defects. Circulation. 2006 Nov 14;114(20):2190–7.
22. Geva T, Martins JD, Wald RM. Atrial septal defects. Lancet Lond Engl. 2014 May 31;383(9932):1921–32.
23. Snarr BS, Wirrig EE, Phelps AL, Trusk TC, Wessels A. A spatiotemporal evaluation of the contribution of the dorsal mesenchymal protrusion to cardiac development. Dev Dyn Off Publ Am Assoc Anat. 2007 May;236(5):1287–94.
24. Briggs LE, Kakarla J, Wessels A. The pathogenesis of atrial and atrioventricular septal defects with special emphasis on the role of the dorsal mesenchymal protrusion. Differ Res Biol Divers. 2012 Jul;84(1):117–30.
25. Musuku SR, Cagino J. Congenital common atrium. Turk J Anaesthesiol Reanim. 2018 Aug;46(4):335–6.
26. Oliver JM, Gallego P, Gonzalez A, Dominguez FJ, Aroca A, Mesa JM. Sinus venosus syndrome: atrial septal defect or anomalous venous connection? A multiplane transoesophageal approach. Heart. 2002 Dec;88(6):634–8.
27. Shah SS, Teague SD, Lu JC, Dorfman AL, Kazerooni EA, Agarwal PP. Imaging of the coronary sinus: normal anatomy and congenital abnormalities. Radiographics. 2012 Jun 27;32(4):991–1008.
28. Douglas YL, Jongbloed MRM, DeRuiter MC, Groot ACG. Normal and abnormal development of pulmonary veins: state of the art and correlation with clinical entities. Int J Cardiol. 2011 Feb 17;147(1):13–24.
29. Bharucha T, Spicer DE, Mohun TJ, Black D, Henry GW, Anderson RH. Cor triatriatum or divided atriums: which approach provides the better understanding? Cardiol Young. 2015 Feb;25(2):193–207.
30. Neeb Z, Lajiness JD, Bolanis E, Conway SJ. Cardiac outflow tract anomalies. Wiley Interdiscip Rev Dev Biol. 2013 Jul;2(4):499–530.
31. de la Cruz MV, Sánchez Gómez C, Arteaga MM, Argüello C. Experimental study of the development of the truncus and the conus in the chick embryo. J Anat. 1977 Jul;123(Pt 3):661–86.
32. Unolt M, Putotto C, Silvestri LM, Marino D, Scarabotti A, Massaccesi V, et al. Transposition of great arteries: new insights into the pathogenesis. Front Pediatr. 2013 Jun 6;1:11.
33. Apitz C, Webb GD, Redington AN. Tetralogy of Fallot. Lancet Lond Engl. 2009 Oct 24;374(9699):1462–71.
34. Obler D, Juraszek AL, Smoot LB, Natowicz MR. Double outlet right ventricle: aetiologies and associations. J Med Genet. 2008 Aug;45(8):481–97.
35. Aorta and Great Vessels: Aortic Development and Anomalies. Available from https://www.ncbi.nlm.nih.gov/pmc/articles/PMC3036416/
36. "Double Aortic Arch" embryological basis and its surgical implications. Available from https://www.researchgate.net/publication
37. Hanneman K, Newman B, Chan F. Congenital variants and anomalies of the aortic arch. Radiographics. 2017 Jan;37(1):32–51.
38. The Aberrant Right Subclavian Artery (Arteria Lusoria): the morphological and clinical aspects of one of the most important variations—a systematic study of 141 reports. Available from https://www.hindawi.com/journals/tswj/2014/292734/
39. Bökenkamp R, DeRuiter MC, van Munsteren C, Gittenberger-de Groot AC. Insights into the pathogenesis and genetic background of patency of the ductus arteriosus. Neonatology. 2010 Jun;98(1):6–17.
40. Coceani F, Baragatti B. Mechanisms for ductus arteriosus closure. Semin Perinatol. 2012 Apr;36(2):92–7.
41. Yagel S, Kivilevitch Z, Cohen SM, Valsky DV, Messing B, Shen O, et al. The fetal venous system, part I: normal embryology, anatomy, hemodynamics, ultrasound evaluation and Doppler investigation. Ultrasound Obstet Gynecol. 2010;35(6):741–50.
42. Saha S, Paoletti D, Robertson M. Persistent left superior vena cava – considerations in fetal, pediatric and adult populations. Australas J Ultrasound Med. 2012 May;15(2):61–6.
43. Radiological features of azygos and hemiazygos continuation of inferior vena cava. Available from https://www.ncbi.nlm.nih.gov/pmc/articles/PMC5944491/

Cross-Sectional Imaging Atlas 3

Yashpal Rana, Megha M. Sheth,
and Ramiah Rajeshkannan

Figure Labels Part 1: CT Anatomy

1. Right brachiocephalic trunk
2. Left common carotid artery
3. Left subclavian artery
4. Trachea, 4B. Carina, 4C. Right main bronchus 4D. Left main bronchus
5. Oesophagus
6. SVC, 6A—azygos vein
7. Lung apices
8. Left innominate vein
9. Common trunk of right brachiocephalic trunk and left common carotid artery
10. A—Ascending aorta, 10B—Left aortic arch, 10C—Descending thoracic aorta 10D—Abdominal Aorta
11. Right internal mammary artery (RIMA)
12. Left internal mammary artery (LIMA)
13. A—Main pulmonary trunk, 13B—Right pulmonary artery, 13C—Left pulmonary artery, 13D—Right descending pulmonary artery, 13E—Left descending pulmonary artery
14. A—Right superior pulmonary vein, 14B—Left superior pulmonary vein, 14C—Right inferior pulmonary vein, 14D—Left inferior pulmonary vein
15. A. Right atrial appendage
16. A. Left atrial appendage
17. Left main coronary artery (LMCA)
18. Left atrium
19. Aortic valve, 19A—Aorto-mitral fibrous continuity
20. Right ventricular outflow tract (RVOT)
21. Right atrium
22. Right ventricle
23. Left ventricle
24. Mitral valve
25. Right coronary artery (RCA)
26. Tricuspid valve
27. Coronary sinus
28. IVC
29. Liver
30. Spleen
31. Stomach
32. Pancreas
33. Right kidney
34. Left kidney
35. Sternum
36. Pulmonary valve

Y. Rana (✉)
U.N. Mehta Institute of Cardiology and Research Centre, Ahmedabad, Gujarat, India

Radiscan Diagnostics, Ahmedabad, Gujarat, India

M. M. Sheth
U.N. Mehta Institute of Cardiology and Research Centre, Ahmedabad, Gujarat, India

R. Rajeshkannan
Department of Radiology, Amrita School of Medicine, Amrita Institute of Medical Sciences and Research Centre, Amrita Vishwa Vidyapeetham, Kochi, Kerala, India

R. Rajeshkannan et al. (eds.), *CT and MRI in Congenital Heart Diseases*,
https://doi.org/10.1007/978-981-15-6755-1_3

37. Gall bladder
38. Celiac Trunk
39. Left ventricular outflow tract (LVOT)

- Figs. 3.1–3.23: Axial CT anatomy
- Figs. 3.24–3.34: Coronal CT anatomy
- Figs. 3.35–3.42: Sagittal CT anatomy

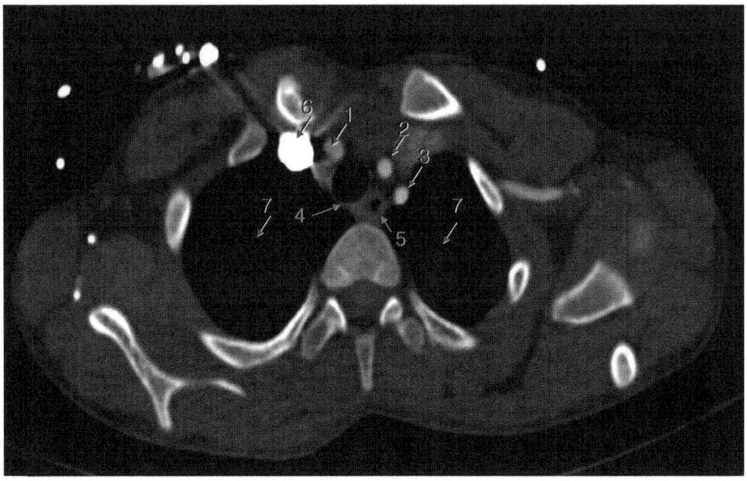

Fig. 3.1 1. Right brachiocephalic trunk; 2. Left common carotid artery; 3. Left subclavian artery; 4. Trachea; 5. Oesophagus; 6. SVC; 7. Lung apices

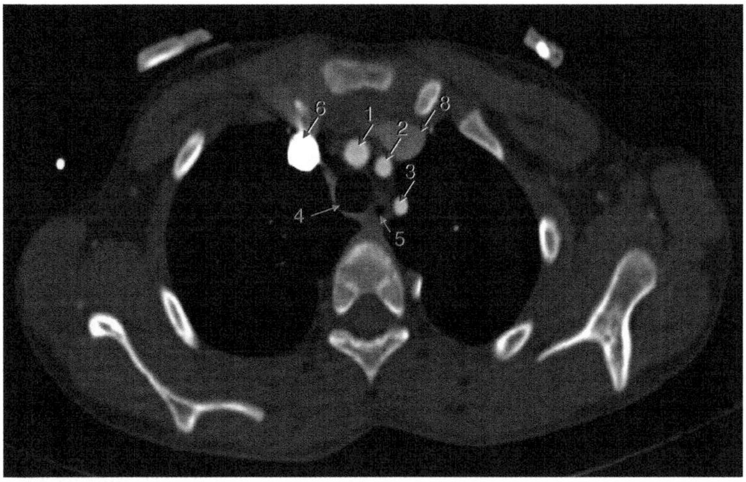

Fig. 3.2 1. Right brachiocephalic trunk; 2. Left common carotid artery; 3. Left subclavian artery; 4. Trachea; 5. Oesophagus; 6. SVC; 8. Left innominate vein

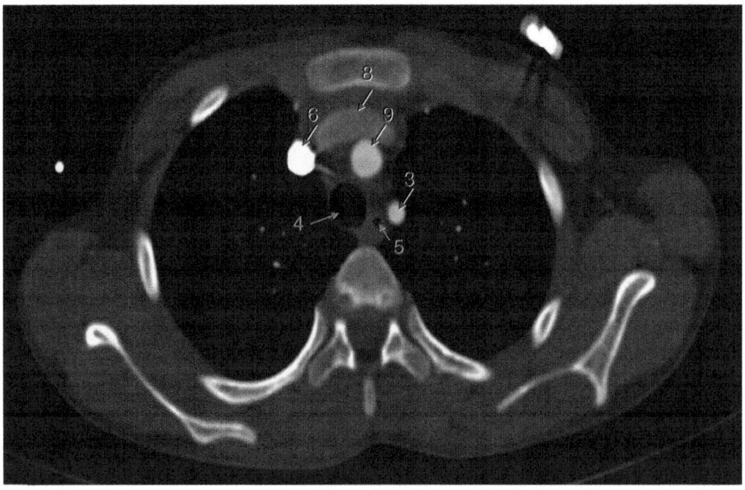

Fig. 3.3 3. Left subclavian artery; 4. Trachea; 5. Oesophagus; 6. SVC; 8. Left innominate vein; 9. Common trunk of right brachiocephalic trunk and left common carotid artery

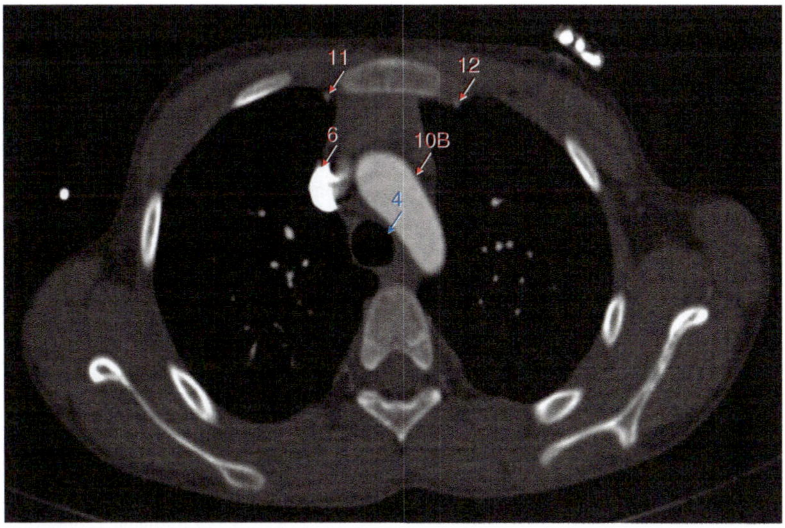

Fig. 3.4 4. Trachea; 6. SVC; 10B—Left aortic arch; 11. Right internal mammary artery (RIMA); 12. Left internal mammary artery (LIMA)

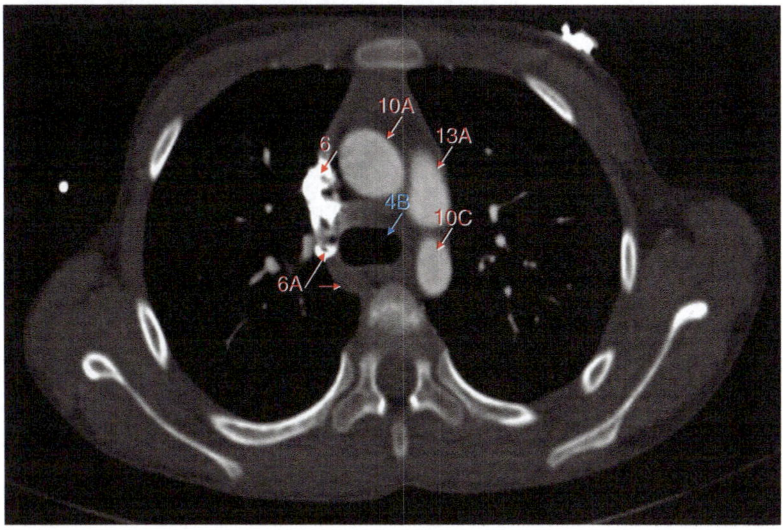

Fig. 3.5 4B. Carina; 6. SVC; 6A Azygos vein 10A—Ascending aorta, 10C—Descending thoracic aorta; 13A—Main pulmonary trunk

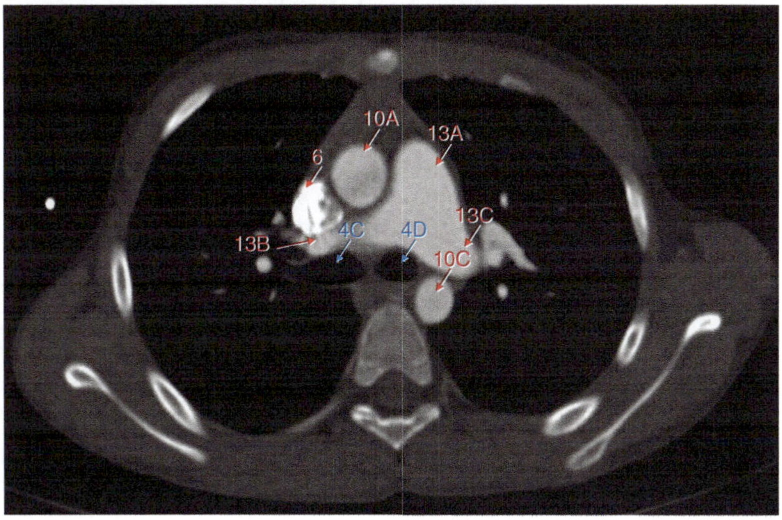

Fig. 3.6 4C. Right main bronchus 4D. Left main bronchus; 6. SVC; 10A—Ascending aorta, 10C—Descending thoracic aorta; 13A—Main pulmonary trunk, 13B—Right pulmonary artery, 13C—Left pulmonary artery

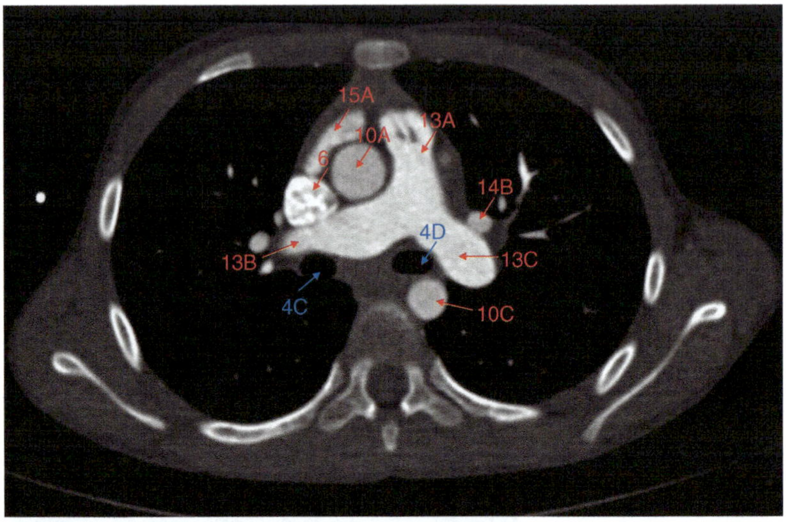

Fig. 3.7 4C. Right main bronchus 4D. Left main bronchus; 6. SVC; 10A—Ascending aorta, 10C—Descending thoracic aorta; 13A—Main pulmonary trunk, 13B—Right pulmonary artery, 13C—Left pulmonary artery; 14B—Left superior pulmonary vein; 15A—Right atrial appendage

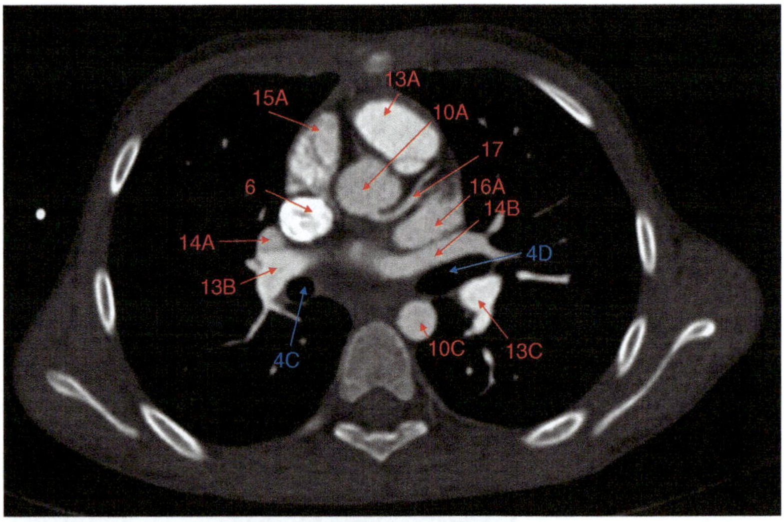

Fig. 3.8 4C. Right main bronchus 4D. Left main bronchus; 6. SVC; 10A—Ascending aorta, 10C—Descending thoracic aorta; 13A—Main pulmonary trunk, 13B—Right pulmonary artery, 13C—Left pulmonary artery; 14A—Right superior pulmonary vein, 14B—Left superior pulmonary vein; 15A. Right atrial appendage; 16A. Left atrial appendage; 17. Left main coronary artery (LMCA)

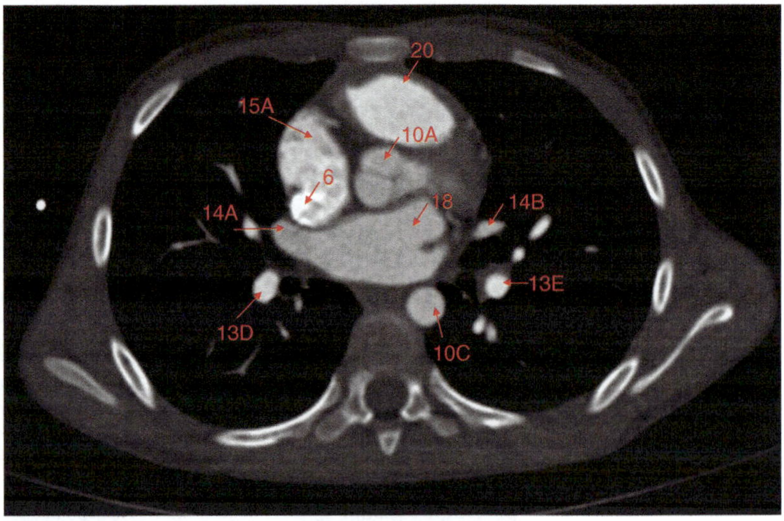

Fig. 3.9 6. SVC; 10A—Ascending aorta, 10C—Descending thoracic aorta; 13D—Right descending pulmonary artery, 13E—Left descending pulmonary artery, 14A—Right superior pulmonary vein, 14B—Left superior pulmonary vein; 15A. Right atrial appendage; 18. Left atrium, 20—RVOT

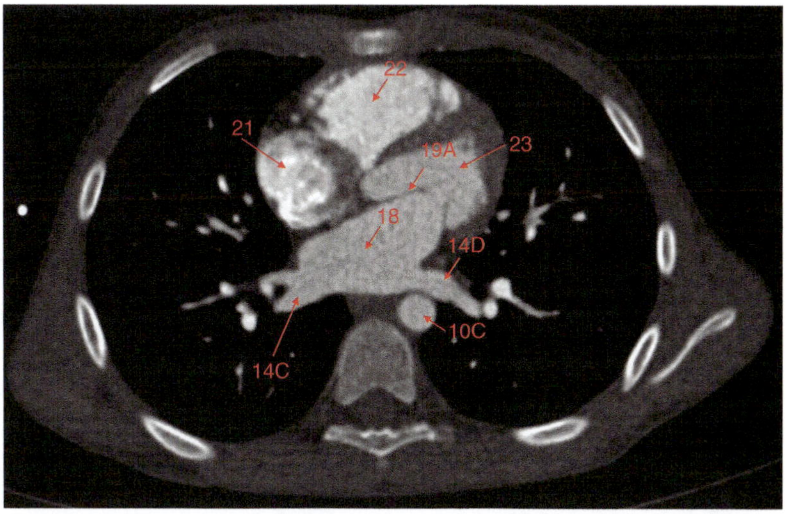

Fig. 3.10 10C—Descending thoracic aorta; 14C—Right inferior pulmonary vein; 14D—Left inferior pulmonary vein; 18. Left atrium; 19A—Aorto-mitral fibrous continuity; 21. Right atrium; 22. Right ventricle; 23. Left ventricle

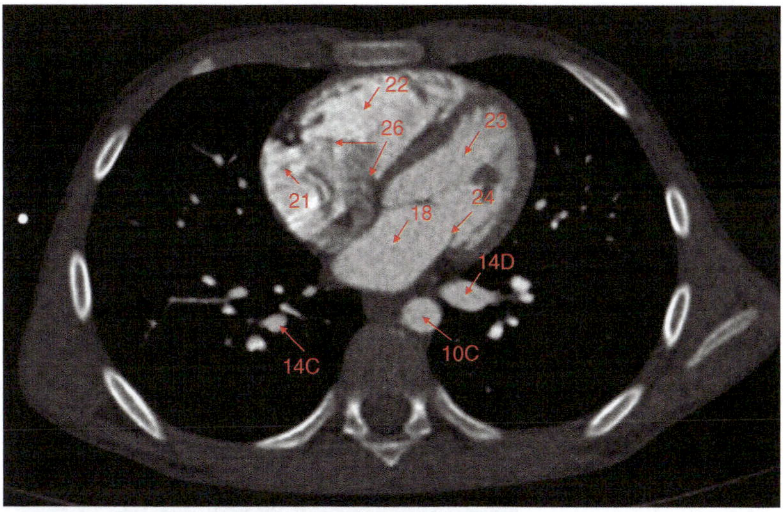

Fig. 3.11 10C—Descending thoracic aorta; 14C—Right inferior pulmonary vein; 14D—Left inferior pulmonary vein; 18. Left atrium; 21. Right atrium; 22. Right ventricle; 23. Left ventricle; 24. Mitral valve; 26. Tricuspid valve

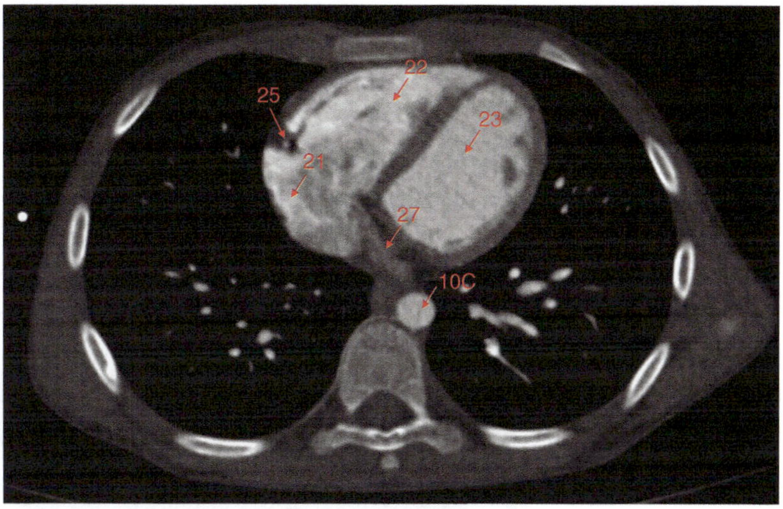

Fig. 3.12 10C—Descending thoracic aorta; 21. Right atrium; 22. Right ventricle; 23. Left ventricle; 25. Right coronary artery (RCA); 27. Coronary sinus

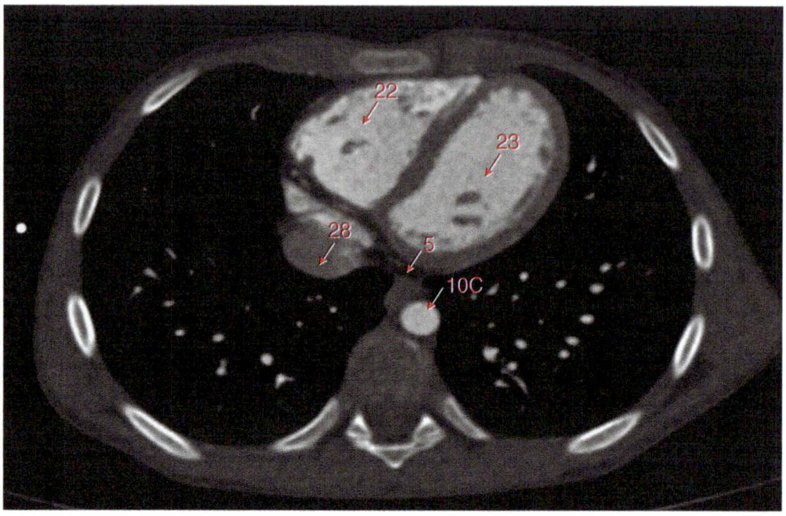

Fig. 3.13 5. Oesophagus; 10C—Descending thoracic aorta; 22. Right ventricle; 23. Left ventricle; 28. IVC

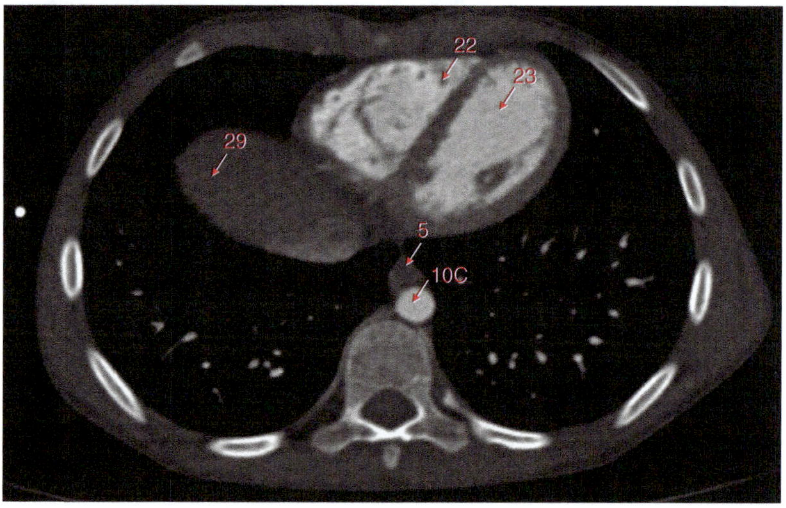

Fig. 3.14 5. Oesophagus; 10C—Descending thoracic aorta; 22. Right ventricle; 23. Left ventricle; 29. Liver

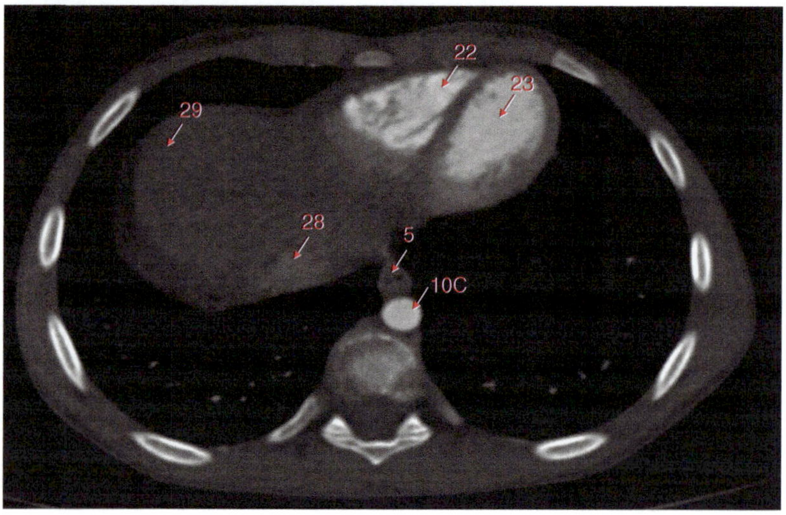

Fig. 3.15 5. Oesophagus; 10C—Descending thoracic aorta; 22. Right ventricle; 23. Left ventricle, 28. IVC; 29. Liver

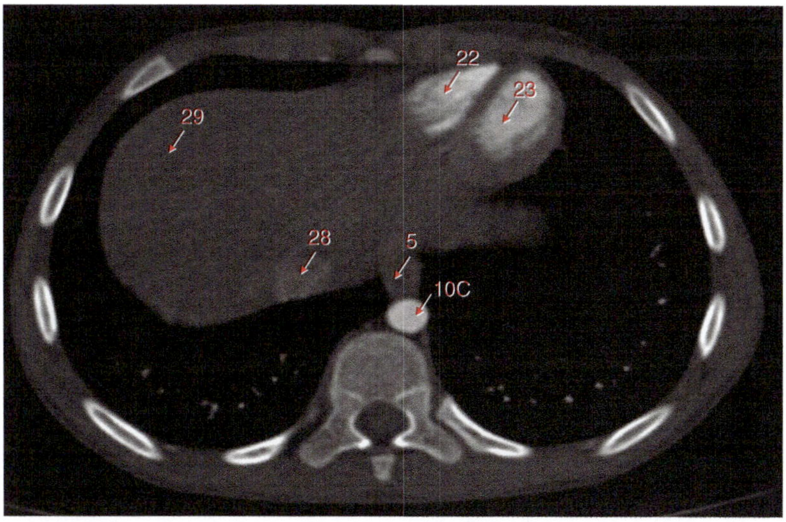

Fig. 3.16 5. Oesophagus; 10C—Descending thoracic aorta; 22. Right ventricle; 23. Left ventricle, 28. IVC; 29. Liver

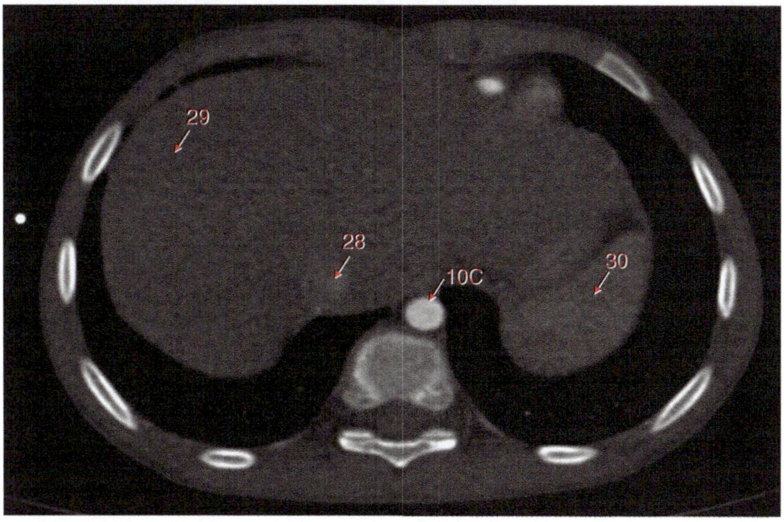

Fig. 3.17 10C—Descending thoracic aorta; 28. IVC, 29. Liver; 30. Spleen

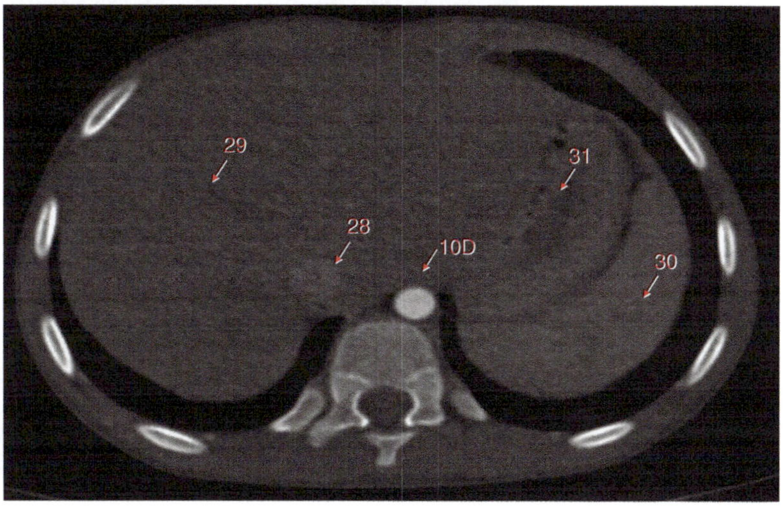

Fig. 3.18 10D—Abdominal aorta; 28-IVC; 29. Liver; 30. Spleen; 31. Stomach

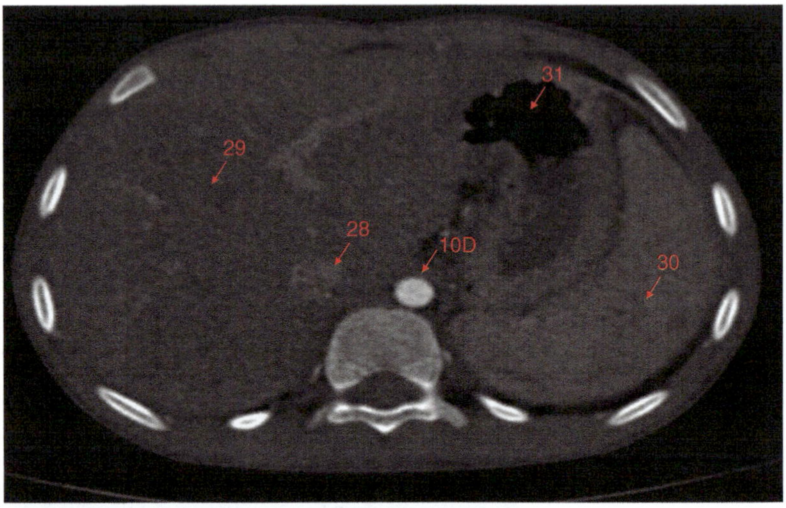

Fig. 3.19 10D—Abdominal aorta; 28 IVC; 29. Liver; 30. Spleen; 31. Stomach

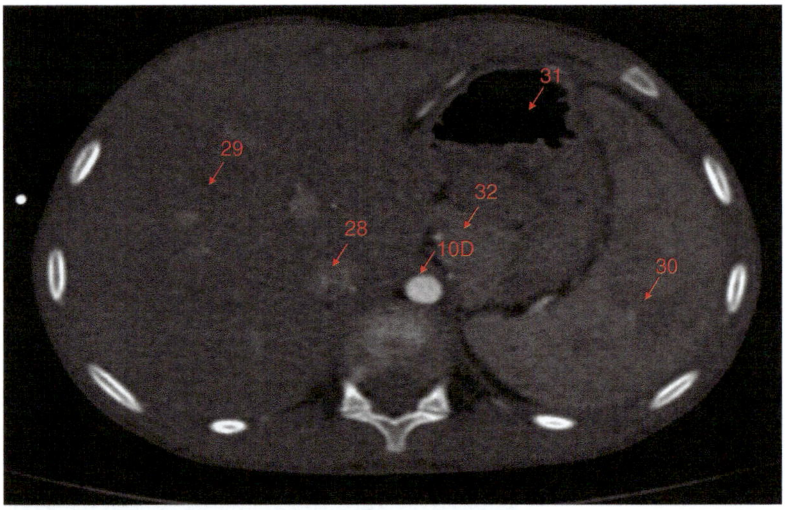

Fig. 3.20 10D—Abdominal aorta; 28 IVC; 29. Liver; 30. Spleen; 31. Stomach; 32. Pancreas

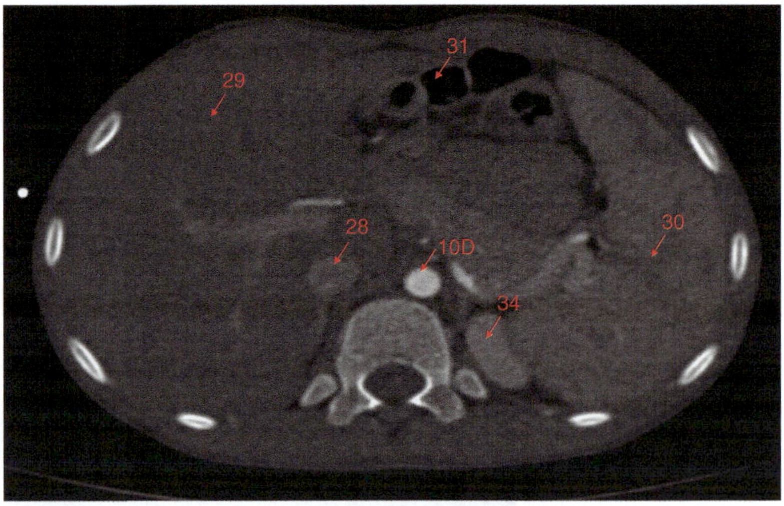

Fig. 3.21 10D—Abdominal aorta; 28-IVC; 29. Liver; 30. Spleen; 31. Stomach; 34. Left kidney

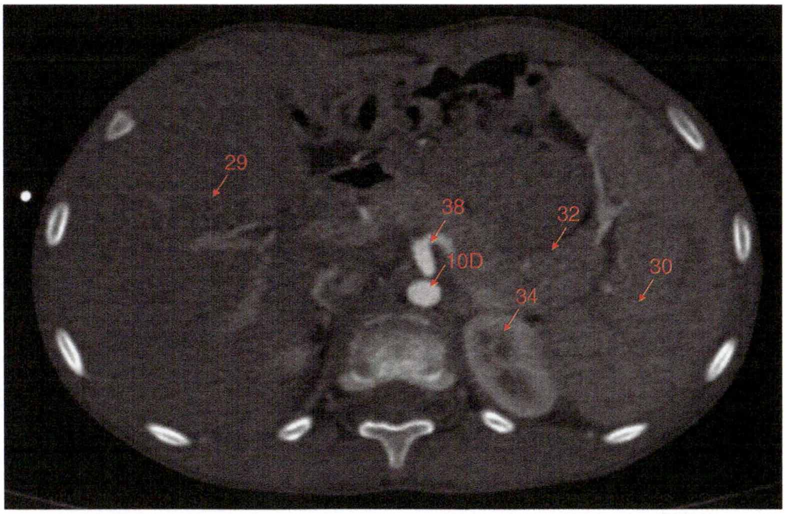

Fig. 3.22 10D—Abdominal aorta; 29. Liver; 30. Spleen; 32. Pancreas; 34. Left kidney; 38. Celiac trunk

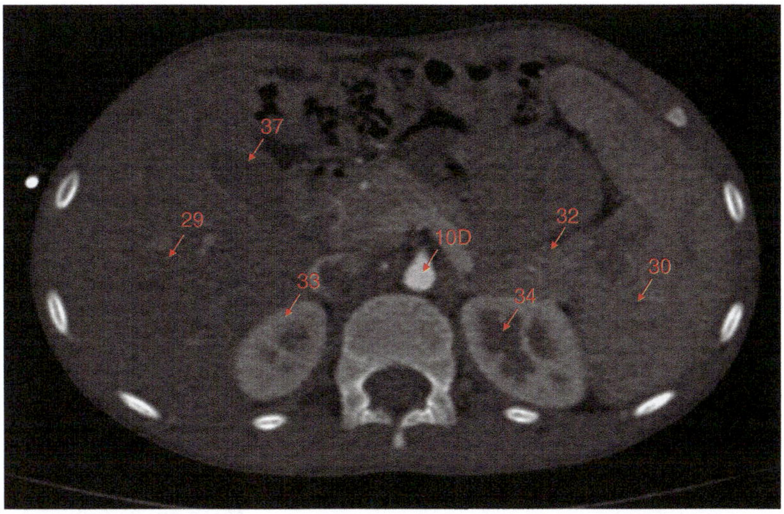

Fig. 3.23 10D—Abdominal aorta; 29. Liver; 30. Spleen; 32. Pancreas; 33. Right kidney; 34. Left kidney; 37. Gall bladder

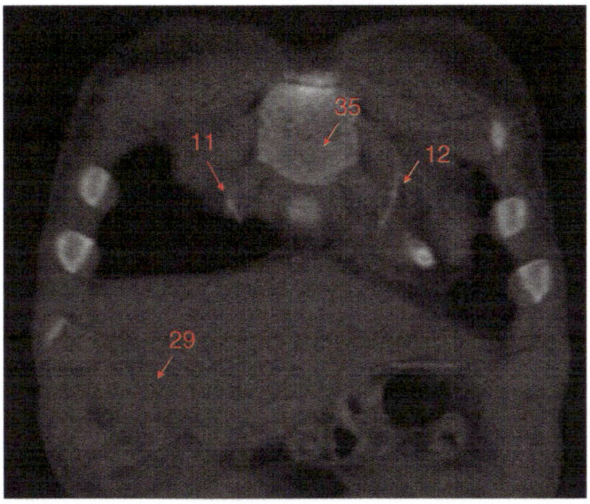

Fig. 3.24 11. Right internal mammary artery (RIMA); 12. Left internal mammary artery (LIMA); 29. Liver; 35. Sternum

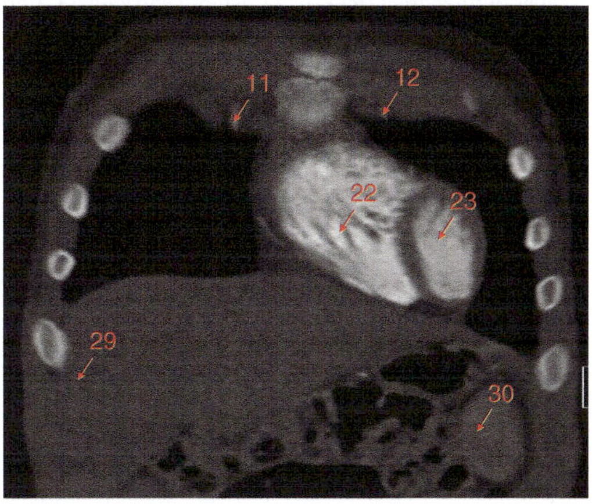

Fig. 3.25 11. Right internal mammary artery (RIMA); 12. Left internal mammary artery (LIMA) 22. Right ventricle; 23. Left ventricle 29. Liver; 30. Spleen

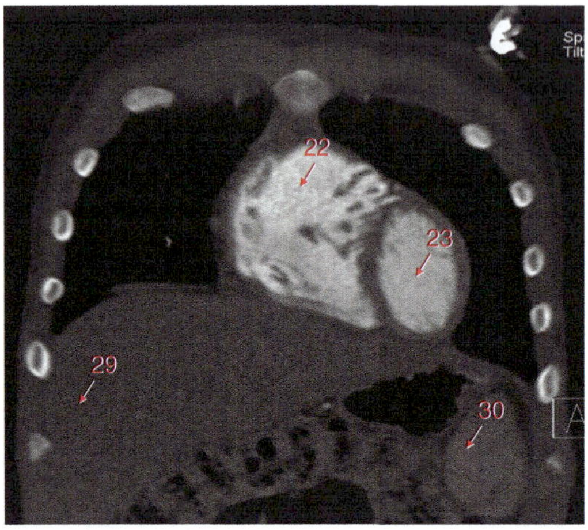

Fig. 3.26 22. Right ventricle; 23. Left ventricle 29. Liver; 30. Spleen

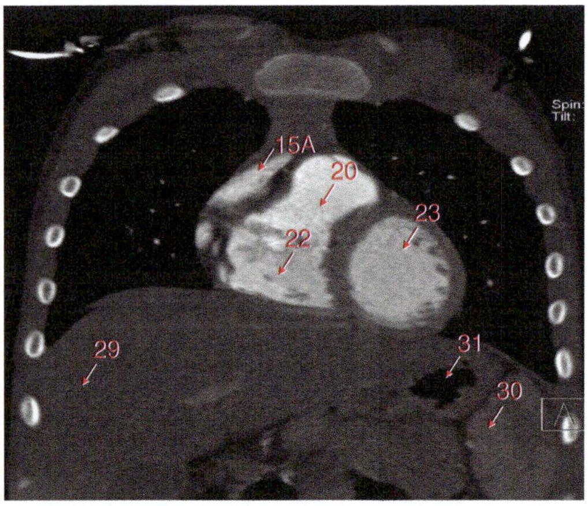

Fig. 3.27 15A. Right atrial appendage; 20. Right ventricular outflow tract (RVOT) 22. Right ventricle; 23. Left ventricle; 29. Liver; 30. Spleen; 31. Stomach

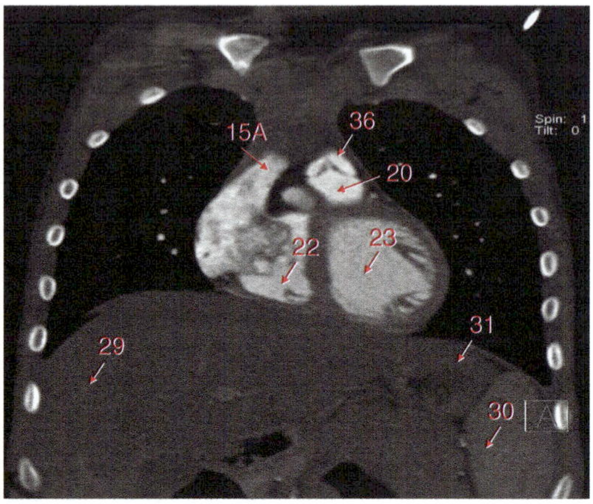

Fig. 3.28 15A. Right atrial appendage; 20. Right ventricular outflow tract (RVOT); 22. Right ventricle; 23. Left ventricle; 29. Liver; 30. Spleen; 31. Stomach; 36. Pulmonary valve

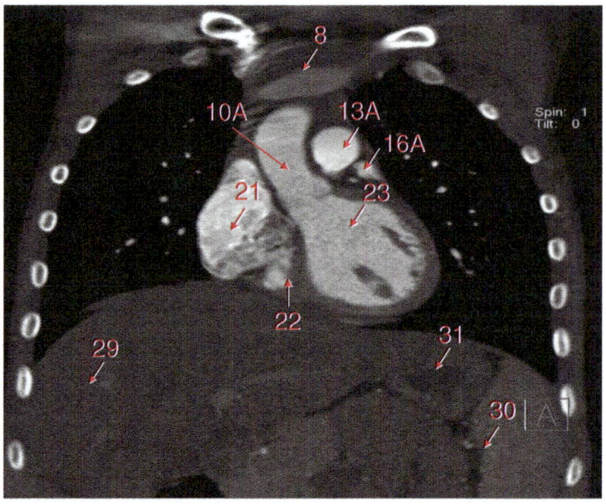

Fig. 3.29 8. Left innominate vein; 10A—Ascending aorta; 13A—Main pulmonary trunk; 16A. Left atrial appendage; 21. Right atrium; 22. Right ventricle; 23. Left ventricle; 29. Liver; 30. Spleen; 31. Stomach

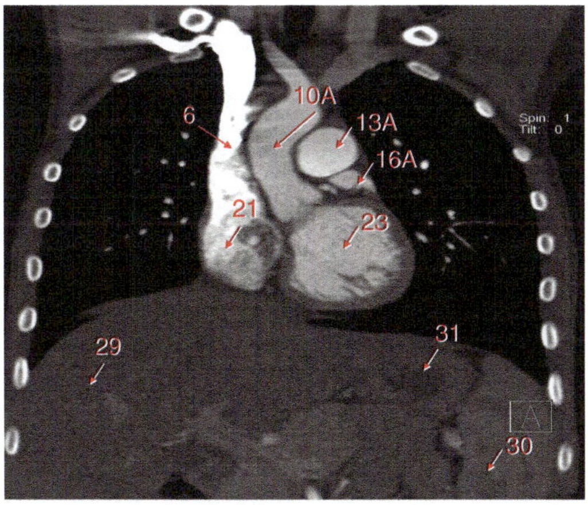

Fig. 3.30 6. SVC; 10A—Ascending aorta; 13A—Main pulmonary trunk; 16A. Left atrial appendage; 21. Right atrium; 23. Left ventricle; 29. Liver; 30. Spleen; 31. Stomach

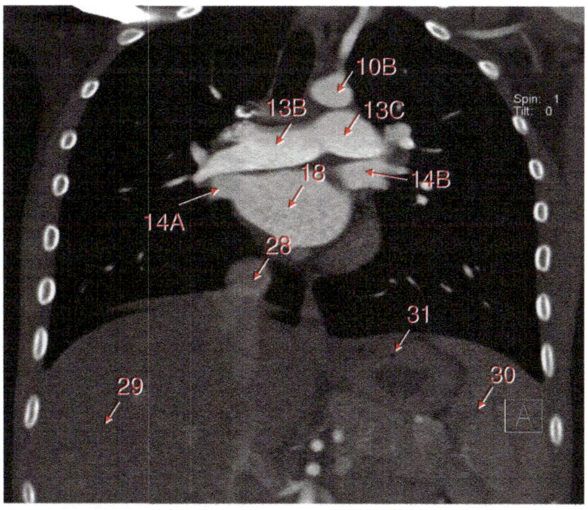

Fig. 3.32 10B—Left aortic arch; 13B—Right pulmonary artery, 13C—Left pulmonary artery; 14A—Right superior pulmonary vein 14B—Left superior pulmonary vein; 18 Left atrium; 28. IVC; 29. Liver; 30. Spleen; 31. Stomach

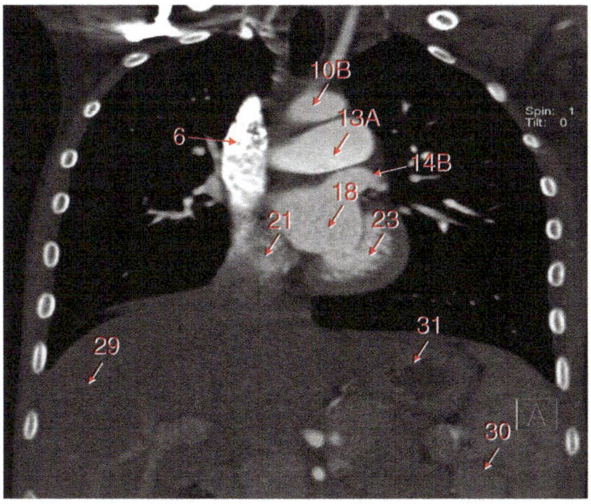

Fig. 3.31 6. SVC; 10B—Left aortic arch; 13A—Main pulmonary trunk, 14B—Left superior pulmonary vein; 18 Left atrium; 21. Right atrium; 23. Left ventricle; 29. Liver; 30. Spleen; 31. Stomach

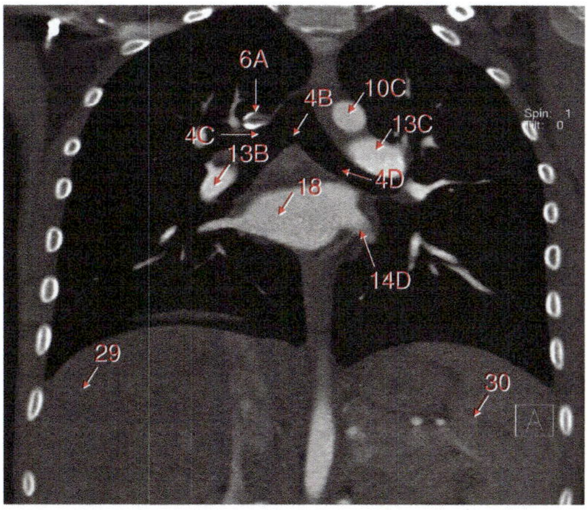

Fig. 3.33 4B. Carina, 4C. Right main bronchus 4D. Left main bronchus, 6A—azygos vein; 10C—Descending thoracic aorta; 13B—Right pulmonary artery, 13C—Left pulmonary artery; 14D—Left inferior pulmonary vein; 18 Left atrium; 29. Liver; 30. Spleen

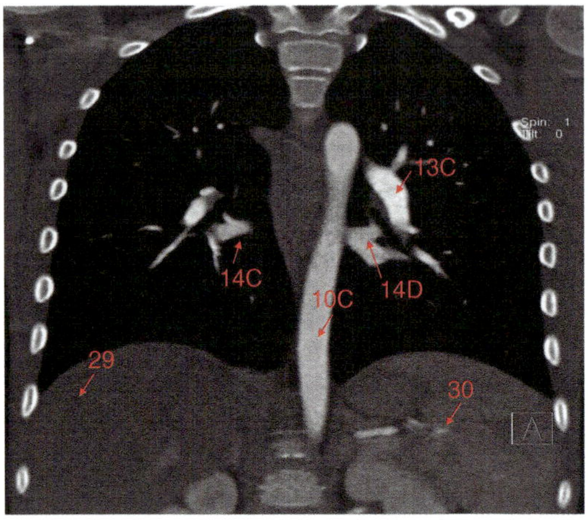

Fig. 3.34 10C—Descending thoracic aorta; 13C—Left pulmonary artery; 14C—Right inferior pulmonary vein, 14D—Left inferior pulmonary vein; 29. Liver; 30. Spleen

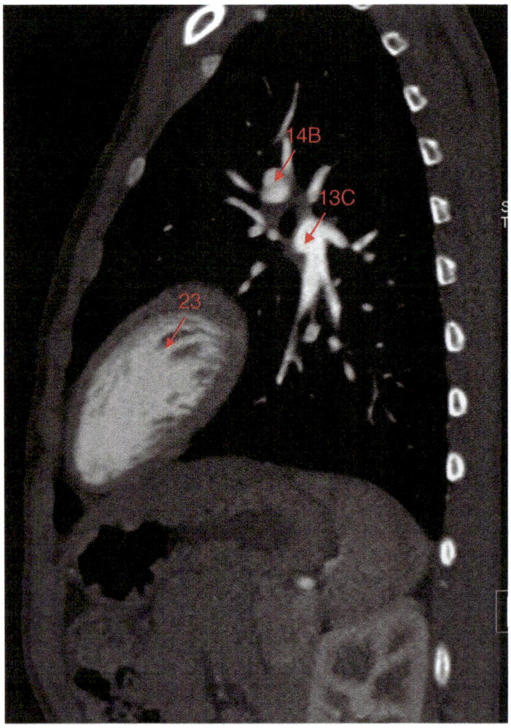

Fig. 3.35 13C—Left pulmonary artery; 14B—Left superior pulmonary vein; 23. Left ventricle

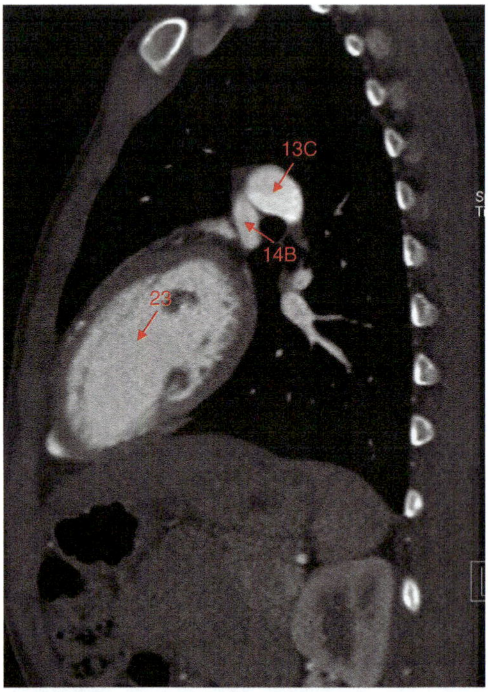

Fig. 3.36 13C—Left pulmonary artery; 14B—Left superior pulmonary vein; 23. Left ventricle

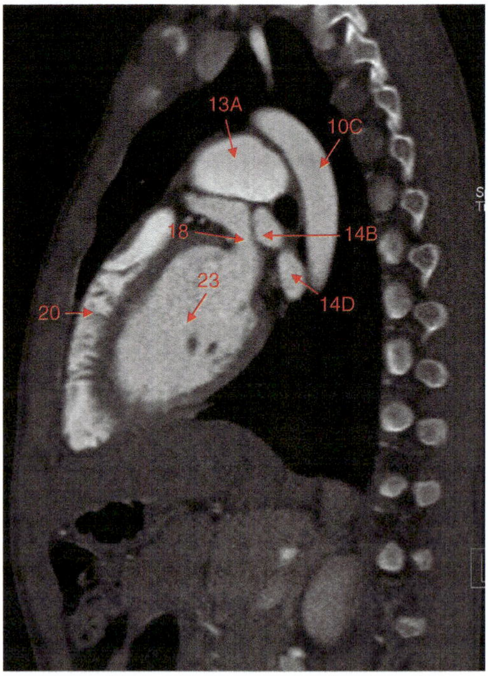

Fig. 3.37 10C—Descending thoracic aorta; 13A—Main pulmonary trunk; 14B—Left superior pulmonary vein; 14D—Left inferior pulmonary vein; 18. Left atrium; 22. Right ventricle; 23. Left ventricle

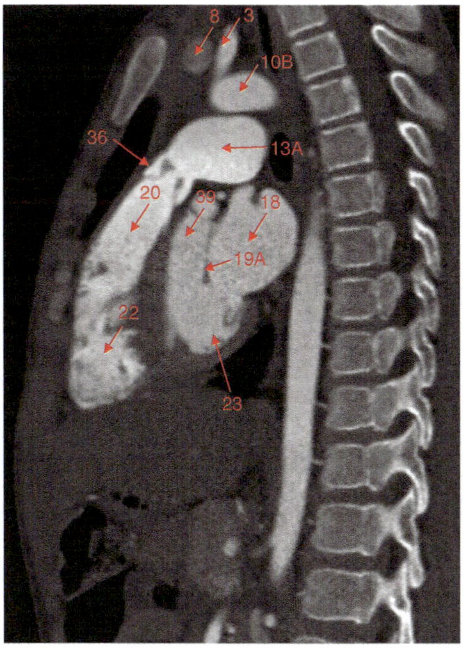

Fig. 3.38 3. Left subclavian artery; 8. Left innominate vein; 10B—Left aortic arch; 13A—Main pulmonary trunk; 18. Left atrium; 19A—Aorto-mitral fibrous continuity; 20. Right ventricular outflow tract (RVOT); 22. Right ventricle; 23. Left ventricle; 36. Pulmonary valve; 39. Left ventricular outflow tract (LVOT)

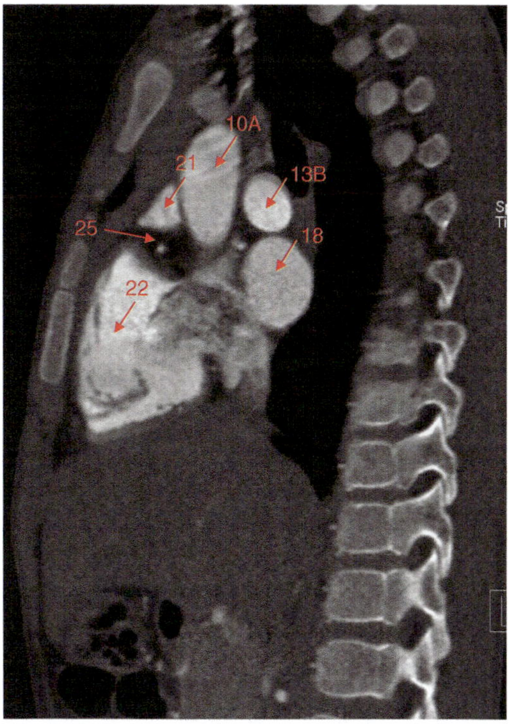

Fig. 3.40 10A—Ascending aorta; 13B—Right pulmonary artery; 18. Left atrium; 21. Right atrium; 22. Right ventricle; 25. Right coronary artery (RCA)

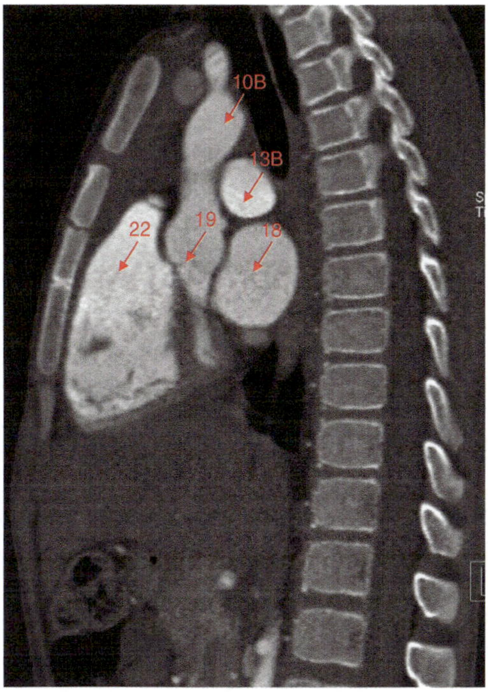

Fig. 3.39 10B—Left aortic arch; 13B—Right pulmonary artery; 18. Left atrium; 19 Aortic valve; 22. Right ventricle

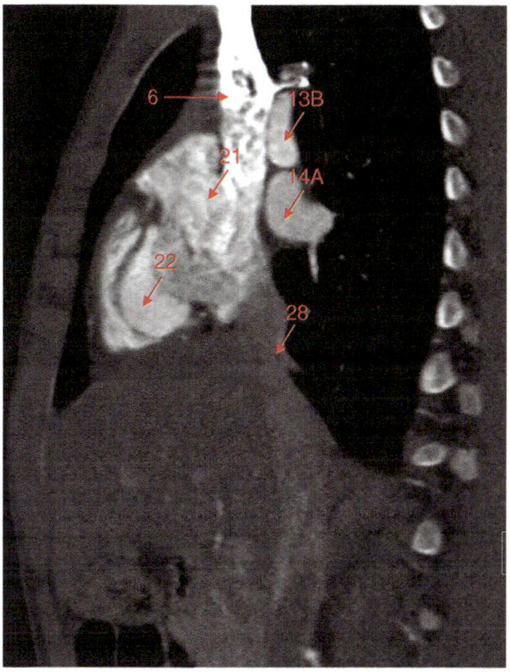

Fig. 3.41 6—SVC, 13B—Right pulmonary artery; 14A—Right superior pulmonary vein; 21. Right atrium; 22. Right ventricle, 28—IVC

Part 2: MRI Anatomy (Figs. 3.43–3.50)

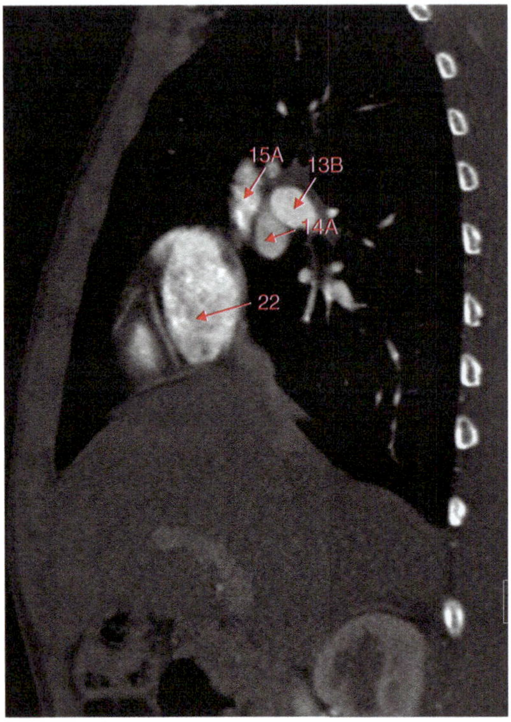

Fig. 3.42 13B—Right pulmonary artery; 14A—Right superior pulmonary vein; 15A. Right atrial appendage; 22. Right ventricle

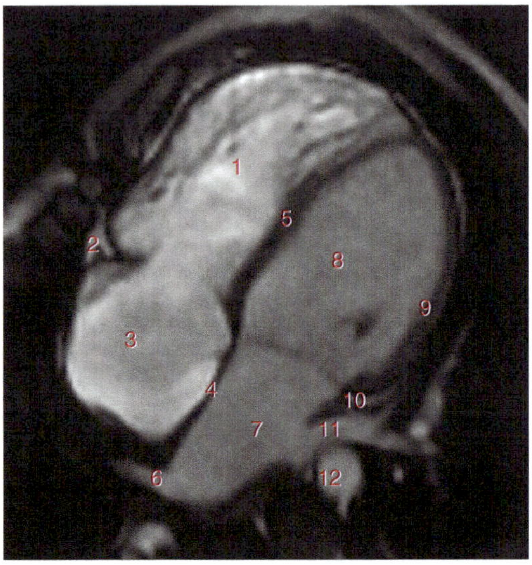

Fig. 3.44 Four-chamber plane. 1—Right ventricle; 2—Right AV groove with RCA; 3—Right atrium; 4—Intertribal septum; 5—Inferior interventricular septum; 6—Right pulmonary vein; 7 Left atrium; 8 Left ventricle; 9—Anterolateral LV wall; 10—Left AV groove with LCX; 11—Left pulmonary vein; 12—Descending aorta

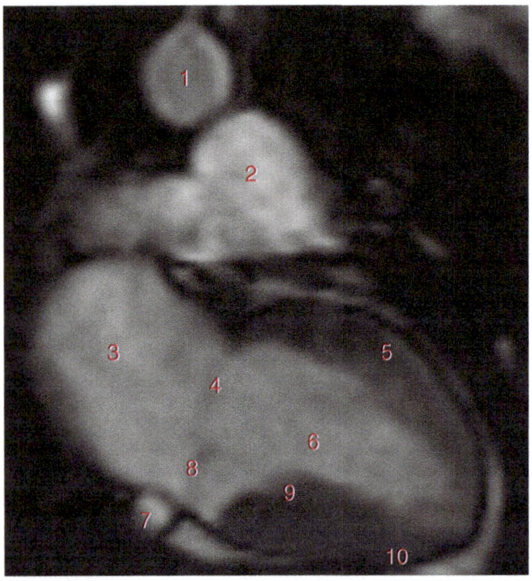

Fig. 3.43 Two-chamber view. 1—Aorta; 2—Pulmonary artery; 3—Left atrium; 4—Anterior mitral leaflet; 5—Anterior LV wall; 6—Left ventricle; 7—Coronary sinus; 8—Posterior mitral leaflet; 9 Posterior papillary muscle; 10—Inferior LV wall

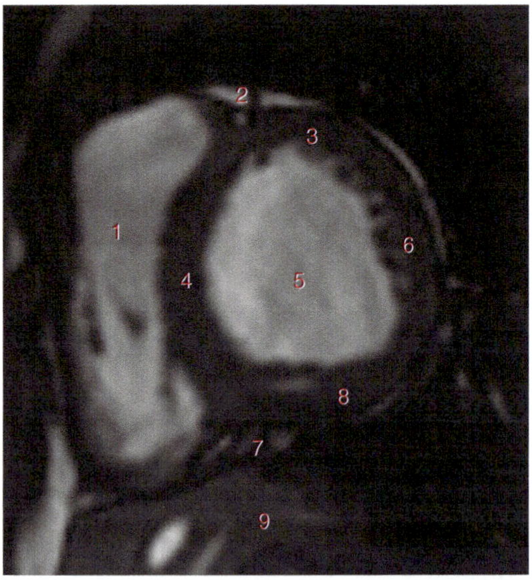

Fig. 3.45 Mid short-axis plane. 1—RV; 2—Anterior interventricular groove with LAD, 3—Anterior LV wall; 4—Interventricular septum; 5—LV; 6—Lateral LV wall; 7—Posterior interventricular groove with the posterior descending artery (PDA); 8—Inferior LV wall; 9—Liver

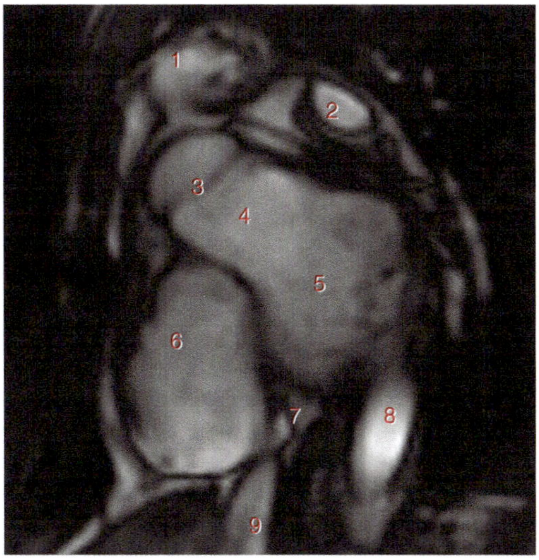

Fig. 3.46 Basal short-axis view. 1—Pulmonary artery; 2—Pulmonary vein; 3—Aortic valve; 4—LVOT; 5—LV; 6—RV; 7—Posterior interventricular groove; 8—Descending aorta; 9—IVC

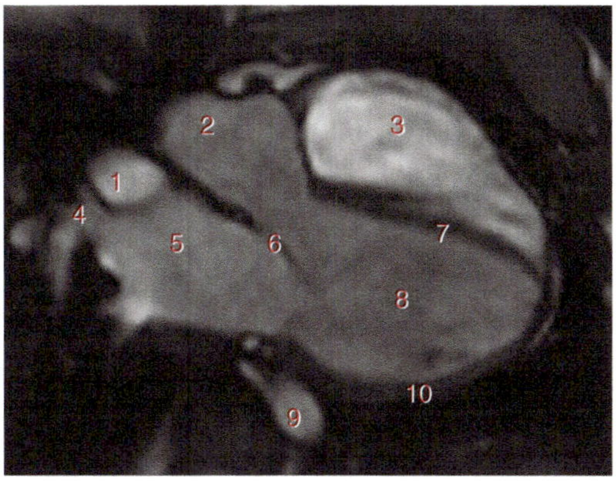

Fig. 3.47 LV outflow (three-chamber) view. 1—SVC; 2—Aorta; 3—Right ventricle; 4—Right upper pulmonary vein; 5—Left atrium; 6—Anterior mitral leaflet; 7—Anterior interventricular septum; 8—Left ventricle; 9—Descending aorta; 10—Inferolateral LV wall

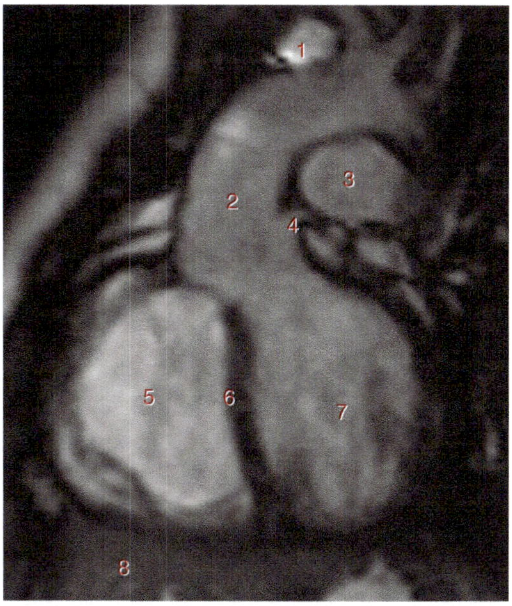

Fig. 3.48 Second LVOT view (planned perpendicular to interventricular septum with the long axis through aorta from three-chamber view). 1__SVC; 2__Ascending aorta; 3__Branch pulmonary artery; 4__Aortic sinus; 5__Right ventricle; 6__Inter-ventricular septum; 7__Left ventricle; 8__Liver

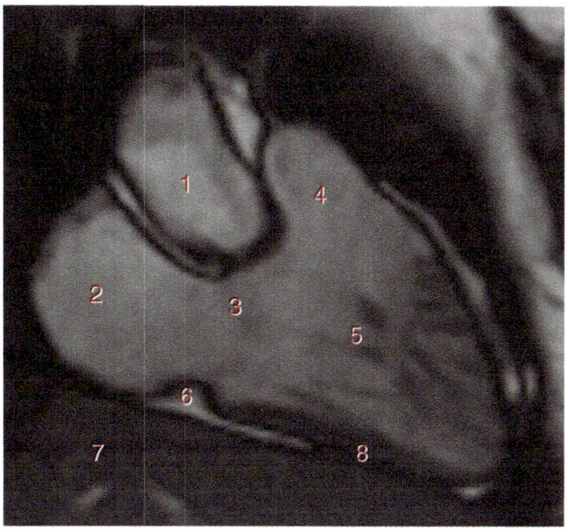

Fig. 3.49 Right side two-chamber view. 1—Ascending aorta; 2—Right atrium; 3—Tricuspid valve; 4—Right ventricle outflow (RVOT); 5—Right ventricle; 6—Right atrioventricular groove; 7—Liver; 8—Inferior right ventricle wall

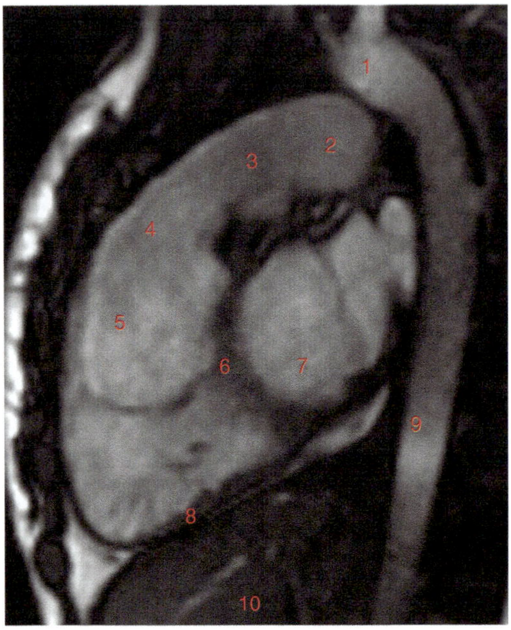

Fig. 3.50 RVOT view. 1—Arch of aorta; 2—Main pulmonary artery; 3—Pulmonary valve; 4—Right ventricle outflow; 5—Right ventricle; 6—Interventricular septum; 7—Left ventricle; 8—Inferior right ventricle wall; 9—Descending aorta; 10—Liver

Technical Aspects of Pediatric Cardiac CT

4

Hemant B. Telkar, Amol Dikshit, and Ramiah Rajeshkannan

4.1 Introduction

CT angiography (CTA) became an important tool for assessing pediatric congenital heart disease (CHD) post 2D echo in an era when 4 slice CT was launched in 2000 in India. Demonstrating anomalies became much easier with the advancement of technology from 16 slices to 64 slices and greater. Newer scanners image faster with better temporal and spatial resolution, greater anatomic coverage per rotation, more consistent enhancement while using a lesser volume of intravascular contrast material, and higher-quality 2D reformation and 3D reconstruction owing to the acquisition of an isotropic data set.

Cardiac CT (CCT) mainly helps in the analysis of complex cardiovascular anatomic features before surgery and to demonstrate post-treatment complications. It also helps in assessing extracardiac systemic and pulmonary arterial and venous structures.

H. B. Telkar (✉)
Infinity Medical Centre, Next to Gandhi (MGM) hospital, Parel, Mumbai, India

A. Dikshit
Infinity Medical Centre, Parel, Mumbai, India

R. Rajeshkannan
Department of Radiology, Amrita School of Medicine, Amrita Institute of Medical Sciences and Research Centre, Amrita Vishwa Vidyapeetham, Kochi, Kerala, India

The purpose of the chapter is to understand the technical requirements involved in the good acquisition of data at minimal radiation dose.

4.2 Common Indications for Pediatric CCT

Cardiac CT (CCT) is used when echocardiography fails to evaluate extracardiac structures, such as the pulmonary arteries, pulmonary veins, and the aortic arch and great vessels due to acoustic window limitations [1] (Fig. 4.1).

Catheter-directed cardiac angiography is limited by its 2D nature and difficulties in simultaneous evaluation of the systemic and pulmonary vascular systems.

Compared with CCT, cardiac catheterization has a higher complication rate owing to its invasive nature (Fig. 4.2), typically requires a larger volume of intravascular contrast material, has a more frequent need for general anesthesia, and often imparts greater radiation dose to the patient [2].

The role of CT in the evaluation of pediatric CHD has now been widely accepted clinical indications for which the benefits of imaging outweigh the risks in the following conditions:

- CHD known or suspected on the basis of echocardiographic findings, when further imaging is needed to characterize extracardiac anoma-

R. Rajeshkannan et al. (eds.), *CT and MRI in Congenital Heart Diseases*,
https://doi.org/10.1007/978-981-15-6755-1_4

lies before the intervention. The distal pulmonary arteries, pulmonary veins, aortic arch, and great vessels generally are inadequately characterized on 2D echocardiography.
- Postoperative evaluation of CHD patients who have a variety of suspected treatment-related complications. CT quickly displays evidence of a variety of CHD surgery-related complications and numerous other medical conditions, such as pulmonary embolism, pneumonia, pleural and pericardial effusion, and pneumothorax.
- 3D printing using CT data can be very useful for preoperative planning of complex CHD like double outlet right ventricle (DORV) and transposition of great arteries (TGA), especially in older children.
- Can be useful before a reoperation to assess altered anatomic features related to previous surgery and to know the relationship between sternal wires and cardiac structures.

CT as the first line of investigation has now been established in:

(a) Evaluation of suspected vascular ring or sling [3]
(b) Suspected aortopulmonary collateral arteries in patients with severe right ventricular outflow tract obstruction [4]
(c) Suspected coronary artery anomalies (Fig. 4.3)

The role of CT in the evaluation of intracardiac anomalies has been limited since imaging of the pediatric patient is performed without heart rate control, often without breath-hold, poor spatial and temporal resolution of old non-ECG gated CT scans. Although that situation is chang-

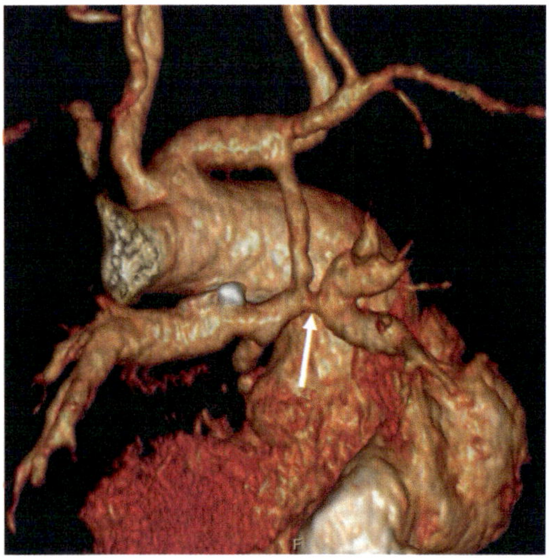

Fig. 4.1 Posterior oblique VRT image of a patient with pulmonary atresia shows widely patent Blalock Taussig shunt with focal right pulmonary artery stenosis (arrow). Pulmonary artery branches and aortopulmonary collaterals are better assessed by CT than echo

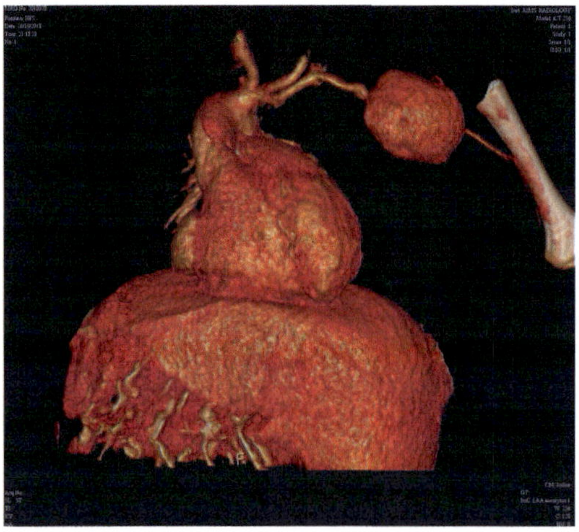

Fig. 4.2 CCT demonstrates a puncture site pseudoaneurysm after cardiac catheterization in a case of heterotaxy syndrome

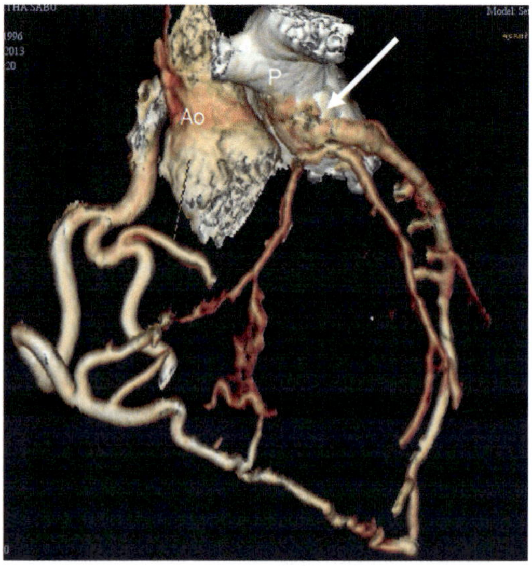

Fig. 4.3 ECG-gated CCT shows aberrant left coronary artery origin (arrow) from the pulmonary artery (ALCAPA). *Ao* ascending aorta; *P* Pulmonary artery

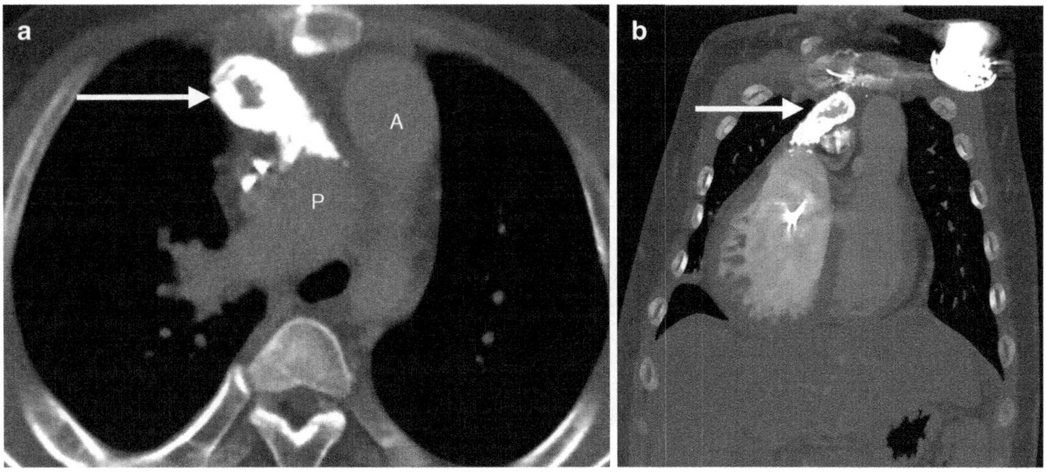

Fig. 4.4 Axial and coronal MIP CT in a patient with transposition having pacemaker shows tight stenosis with calcification of RV to pulmonary artery conduit (arrow)

ing owing to advances in MDCT scanners and ECG-gating techniques.

Because CT involves ionizing irradiation, preference should be given to Magnetic Resonance Imaging (MRI) whenever possible. However, the major advantages of CT over MRI lie within the rapid evaluation of the airways and lung parenchyma in conditions such as vascular rings, pulmonary arterial sling, or absent pulmonary valve syndrome. CT is preferred over MRI in patients with a pacemaker (Fig. 4.4).

4.3 Technical Requirements for Pediatric Cardiac CT

The following are the preferred technical requirements for doing high-quality pediatric cardiac CT:

- 64-slice MDCT scanner and above
- Gantry rotation time of below 400 ms
- Adaptive multisegment reconstruction or dual-source CT
- ECG gating capabilities
- Dual-head contrast injector for saline flush
- Workstation with automatic curved multiplanar reformation and 3D data segmentation and analysis capabilities
- Well-trained and experienced CT technicians knowledgeable in radiation exposure

4.4 Technical Parameters for a Successful Cardiac CT

Before scan, while the patient is in the waiting area:

- Clear instructions should be given to the child about the gantry environment such as the table movement while doing the scan and warm sensation while injecting contrast media.
- Importance of strict immobilization during the scan.
- Instruction about breath-hold for older children.
- Inquiry about previous surgical procedures will help in optimizing the scan and contrast timing.
- Removing all metallic objects.
- Securing good IV line.

4.4.1 Intravenous (IV) Access

After establishing that there is no contraindication for iodinated contrast, an IV line is established in a leg vein, since upper limb contrast injection may produce streak artifacts from the contrast in the SVC obscuring the mediastinal vasculature especially right pulmonary artery and vein (Fig. 4.5). The IV line needs to be flushed properly and tested because of the greater risk of

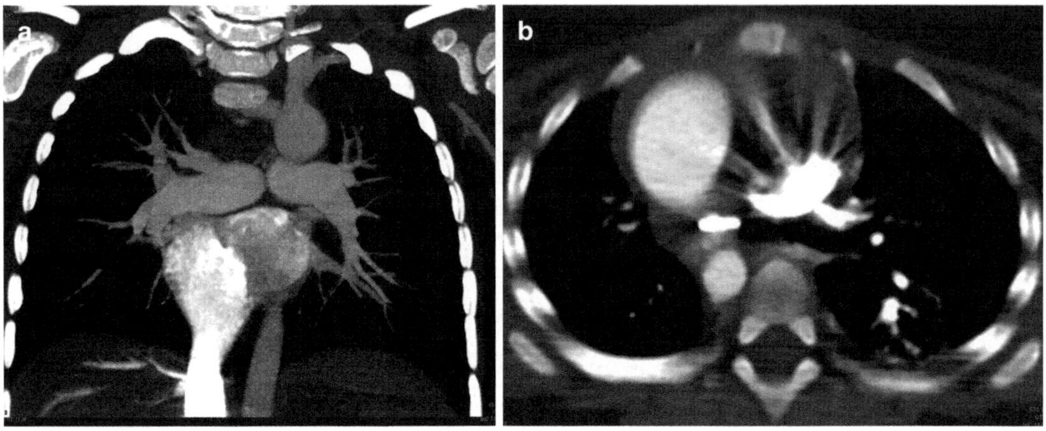

Fig. 4.5 (**a**) Shows good opacification of pulmonary arteries with lower limb contrast injection. (**b**) Shows streak artifacts from dense contrast in the left SVC due to upper limb injection

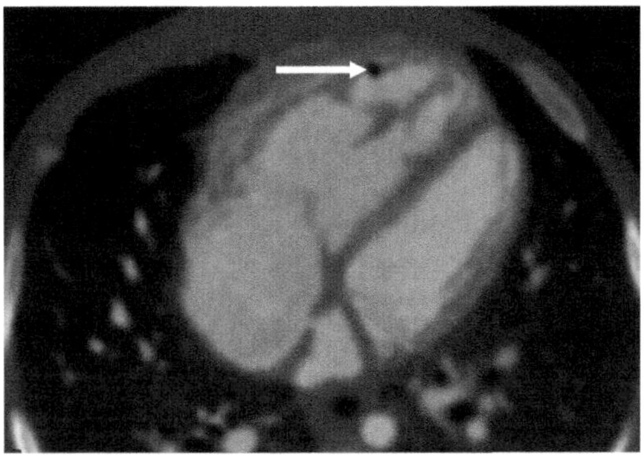

Fig. 4.6 Axial CT shows a small air pocket (arrow) in the right ventricle

contrast extravasation. A 24 G IV cannula is used for children less than 2 years of age and a 22 G IV cannula is used in older children.

It is essential to avoid any injection of air during the scan procedure (Fig. 4.6). All air bubbles should be removed when connecting the catheter to the power injector. Because many children with CHD have right to left shunt, air injection through venous access could cause air systemic embolism, possibly with fatal consequences. It is also important to note that since IVC blood will be directed to the systemic circulation in post-Glenn shunts, any air bubble from lower limb injection has a chance for systemic embolism in these patients.

4.4.2 Sedation

Some of neonates can undergo CT imaging using a "feed and wrap" approach [5]. However, the majority of pediatric thoracic CTA typically requires sedation. A good-quality CT scan can be performed under sedation, as quiet breathing rarely causes appreciable respiratory artifacts [6, 7] (Fig. 4.7).

The CT scan can be done under oral sedation with pedicloryl (Trichlorofos) (relative contraindication is SPO2 less than 70) for children 6 months to 5 years of age (or till 15 kg of weight). Oral sedation syrup pedicloryl has to be given after IV accesses with a maximum dose of not more than 1 ml/Kg body weight. Oral swab dipped in dextrose can be given for sucking and it usually takes about1 hr. for the child to sleep.

Children older than 5 years of age may allow the imager to instruct them orally. The term "vocal anesthesia" refers to the process of gaining the child's confidence by repeated reassurance and guidance before the start of the scan and leading to the child subsequently following the instruction during the scan. However, short IV sedation can be used if the child is not cooperative.

A variety of forms of sedation have been described for pediatric thoracic CTA, and include oral and rectal chloral hydrate [8], IV and intranasal midazolam [9, 10], and IV pentobarbital [11].

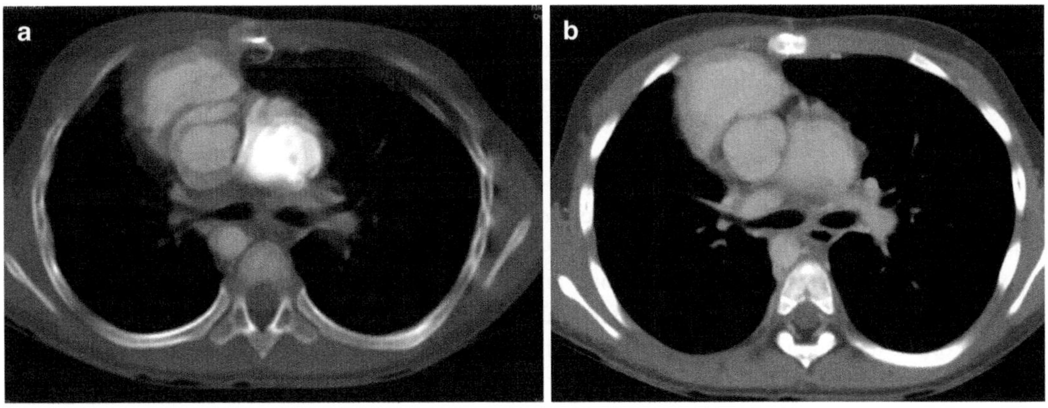

Fig. 4.7 (**a**) Shows severe respiratory movement artifact as the baby cried during contrast injection. (**b**) Repeat second run CT shows good image quality

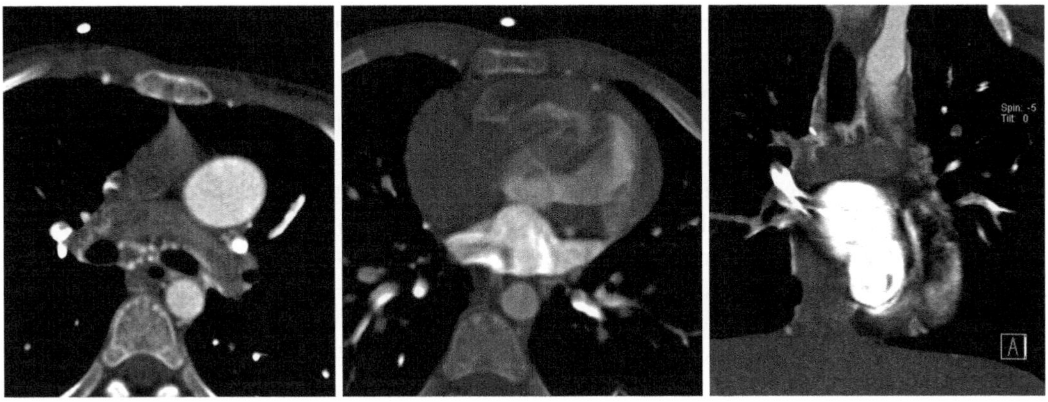

Fig. 4.8 Poor BDGS opacification due to large saline bolus

4.4.3 Fasting

The child is kept fasting for about 2 h before the scan for the non-anesthetic procedure and 4 h for an anesthetic procedure.

4.4.4 Contrast Media

IV line to be flushed slowly at the time of the scan. Low-osmolar or iso-osmolar intravascular iodinated contrast agents (300 mg Iodine/mL or greater) are recommended. Contrast dose is 2 ml per kg body weight followed by 5–10 ml of saline chaser is recommended to clear contrast from peripheral veins. It is preferable to use only a smaller volume of saline chase to maintain adequate contrast opacification of both ventricles in complex CHD cases (Fig. 4.8). Larger saline volume may be needed to washout the right heart chamber for coronary artery study.

Dual-head power injector is preferable to hand injection to achieve homogeneous and consistent intravascular enhancement [12].

Contrast Injection rates:

	Flow rate
Children less than 2 years of age, 24 G IV cannula	0.8–1.5 ml/s
Children more than 2 years of age, 22 G IV cannula	1.5–2 ml/s

Some authors have advocated dilution of contrast material, such as a 1:1 ratio of contrast material and normal saline solution, to minimize streak artifact [13].

Sufficient opacification of the right heart can be obtained by split-bolus injection in which an initial bolus of contrast medium is followed by a 70%:30% saline-to-contrast medium mixture and a final saline chaser [14].

It is important to be familiar with the congenital cardiac anatomy and surgical history before contrast administration. For example, it is preferable to use a dual-injection technique using an upper extremity vein and a dorsal foot/femoral vein in order to simultaneously opacify both upper and lower extremity circulation in a post-Fontan patient or for assessment of post-atrial switch baffle integrity [15, 16].

4.4.5 CT Angiography Procedure

After the preparation, the child is positioned supine and feet first on the scanner. Babies are covered adequately to avoid the risk of hypothermia. To optimize image quality, both hands should be raised above the head. If ECG gating is required, leads are placed in an appropriate position and the tracing to be assessed for good R wave.

CT angiogram starts with taking a low dose frontal scout topogram for further planning.

Non-contrast-enhanced CT has to be done if indicated, for example, when active bleeding or a tumor is suspected. Otherwise, a plain scan should be avoided to reduce the radiation dose.

4.4.6 Timing of CTA Scan

The optimal timing of CTA image acquisition varies depending on anatomy, age, hemodynamic status, previous surgical procedures, and clinical indication for imaging [6].

Three methods of timing CT image acquisition with the IV contrast injection are commonly used to assure satisfactory vascular enhancement:

1. Test dose injection: Exact arrival time of contrast can be calculated by small test dose injection of about 5 ml contrast followed by repeated acquisition at the level of interest (e.g., pulmonary artery or ascending aorta). The time delay between the test dose injection to good opacification of intrathoracic vasculature can be used to plan high-resolution full-volume CTA [17]. The disadvantages of this method include increased volume of contrast material administered (e.g., in neonates 5 ml may be the total dose of contrast) and increased examination time.
2. Fixed delay: Empirical delay after initiation of the contrast injection. Siegel described a delay of 12–15 s for patients weighing less than 10 kg and a delay of 20–25 s for heavier patients [13]. This method is not commonly used as the peak contrast opacification depending on many factors including the rate of injection, cardiac status, and presence of shunts.
3. Automated bolus detection methods. The commonly used method is real-time contrast bolus tracking. It has three steps:
   (a) Pre-monitoring: Single axial section typically at the level of MPA bifurcation is taken to plan the monitoring phase. A very low dose can be used for this scan. A region of interest is placed within a vascular structure of interest. A region of interest may be placed on the right side of the heart for evaluation of the pulmonary arteries and on the left side of the heart for evaluation of the thoracic aorta.
   (b) Monitoring: Following the monitoring delay, repetitive low-dose images are obtained every 1–1.5 s at the same level after the contrast injection. Diagnostic image acquisition is triggered at a specified attenuation threshold, typically between 100 HU and 200 HU. Monitoring delay is the time duration between the start of contrast injection and the start of the monitoring scan. During this phase, no scan is acquired to reduce the total radiation dose. This delay is given for the contrast to reach from peripheral vein to thoracic vessel of interest. For younger babies, this delay is about 4–5 s and for older babies for evaluation of aortic

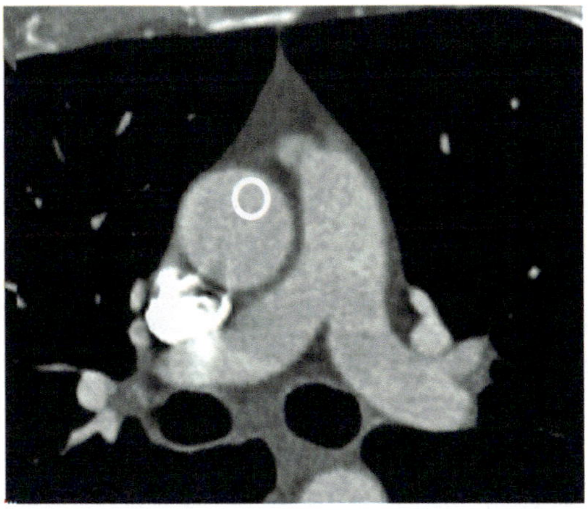

Fig. 4.9 Monitoring phase. The region of interest (ROI) for contrast arrival monitoring should be kept away from SVC streak artifact to prevent premature triggering

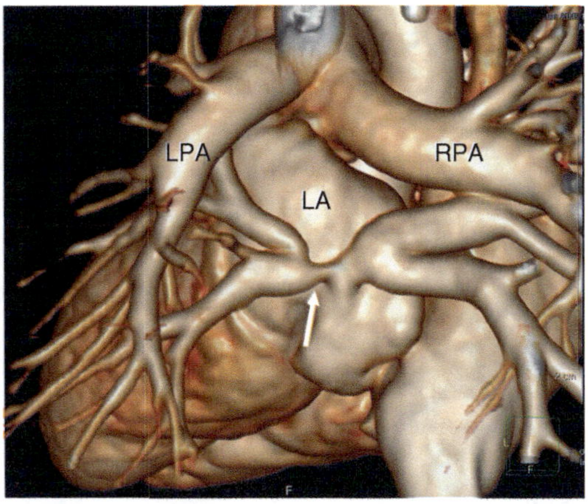

Fig. 4.10 Posterior oblique CT VRT shows tight pulmonary venous stenoses (arrow) following TAPVC repair. Limited scan range is sufficient to demonstrate the clinical question

anomalies, it can be as long as 10 s. The ROI can be placed away from SVC to prevent premature triggering due to streak artifact from dense contrast in SVC (Fig. 4.9).

(c) Angio scan: Scan delay is the duration between the peak contrast opacification reaching the set threshold (100–200 HU) to the actual start of the spiral scan. During this phase, table will move from monitoring plane to whole chest scan, and breathing instruction will be given. Scan delay should be kept as minimum as possible and is typically set at about 4–6 s.

CT angio scan parameters used are as follows:

- Dose: 80–100 kVp; 50–100 mAS
- Gantry rotation time: fastest time possible from the scanner, ideally less than 300 ms
- Detector collimation: Since reconstructed slice thickness cannot be thinner than collimation thickness, it should be kept as minimum as possible (e.g., 64 × 0.6 mm for 64 slice scanner). Higher image noise due to thin collimation can be overcome by increasing the reconstructed slice thickness by using multiplanar reformats.
- Pitch: Depending on the scanner, 1–1.5 is used

4.4.7 Scan Range

The scan range is decided according to the indication. Generally, a whole thoracic coverage from apex to just below the diaphragm is sufficient (Fig. 4.10). However, extended scans can be considered in conditions like Abernathy syndrome, anomalous pulmonary vein, and IVC anomalies (Fig. 4.11).

4.4.8 Single-Phase Versus Multiphase CT Angio

To demonstrate simple aortic anomalies like coarctation, single-phase CT angio may be sufficient. Due to various reasons, the desired vessel may not opacify in the first run (Fig. 4.12). In order to get good homogenous opacification of both pulmonary and systemic circulation, CTA may need to be repeated two or rarely three times (Fig. 4.13). From a practical point of view, a second run can be planned for all cases. After seeing good inline images of the first run, the second phase can be terminated immediately.

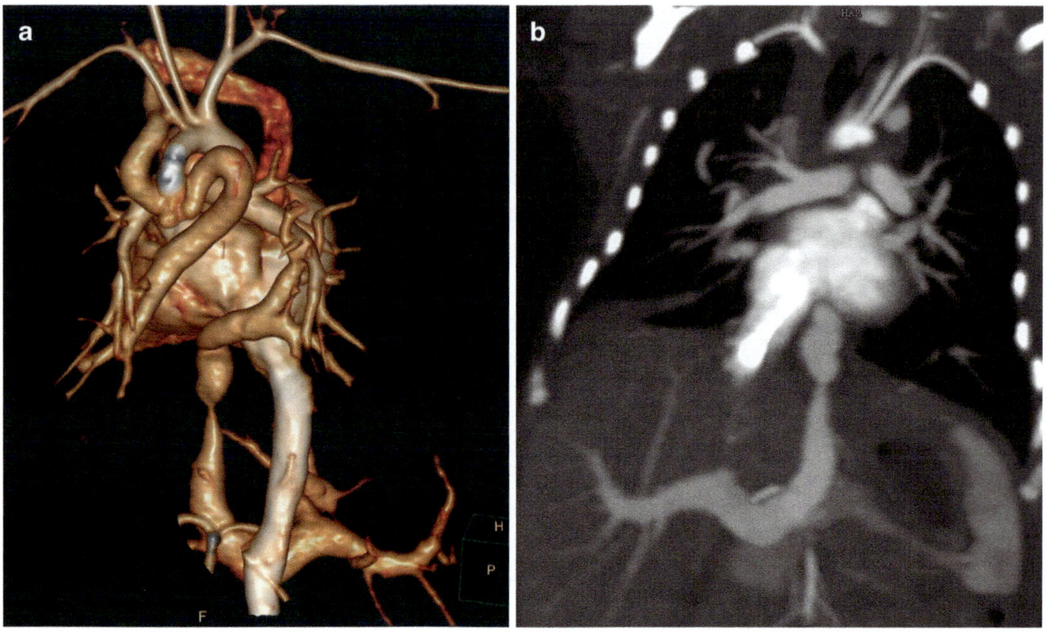

Fig. 4.11 Posterior view VRT (**a**) and coronal MIP (**b**) show mixed TAPVC with left-sided pulmonary veins draining into the left innominate vein and right-sided veins draining into the portal vein. CT scan needs to be extended till the lower border of the liver in a suspected case of infra cardiac anomalous pulmonary venous drainage

4.4.9 ECG-Gated Versus Non-ECG Gated Study

This is an important and common point of discussion.

4.4.9.1 Non-ECG Gated Scan

The non-ECG gated study is generally sufficient for the majority of cases (Fig. 4.14). An ECG-gated study is recommended if the coronary arteries are to be assessed; however, it is found in practice that the non-gated study is sufficient to answer certain specific questions such as variants and anomalies of the coronary artery, e.g., crossing RVOT [18]. Some reports suggest that coronary anatomy is in fact better seen on the non-ECG gated exam rather than ECG-gated study since heart rate and breath-hold are not optimized for coronary imaging.

ECG-gated CTA: Facilitates potentially motion-free evaluation of the heart (including intracardiac structures), coronary arteries, and great vessels. Heart rate limitations are noted if the gated study is planned (Oral ground tablet of propranolol 10 mg one tablet in a dose of 1–2 mg/ per kg can be given if the heart rate is more than 100 bpm). Younger children with severe heart disease are often critically ill. The use of beta-blockers to lower the heart rate should thus be avoided because of reduced coronary blood flow and blood pressure.

ECG synchronization can be performed with three different acquisition modes: retrospectively ECG-gated spiral CT, prospectively ECG-triggered sequential CT, and prospectively ECG-triggered high-pitch helical CT (only in dual-source CT).

4.4.9.2 Retrospective ECG-Gated Spiral Scan

In retrospective ECG-gated CT, data acquisition continues throughout the cardiac cycle along with ECG tracing. To ensure good temporal resolution in single-source CT, a low pitch (0.2) with multi-segment reconstruction is required. A point of critical difference between adult scans and pediat-

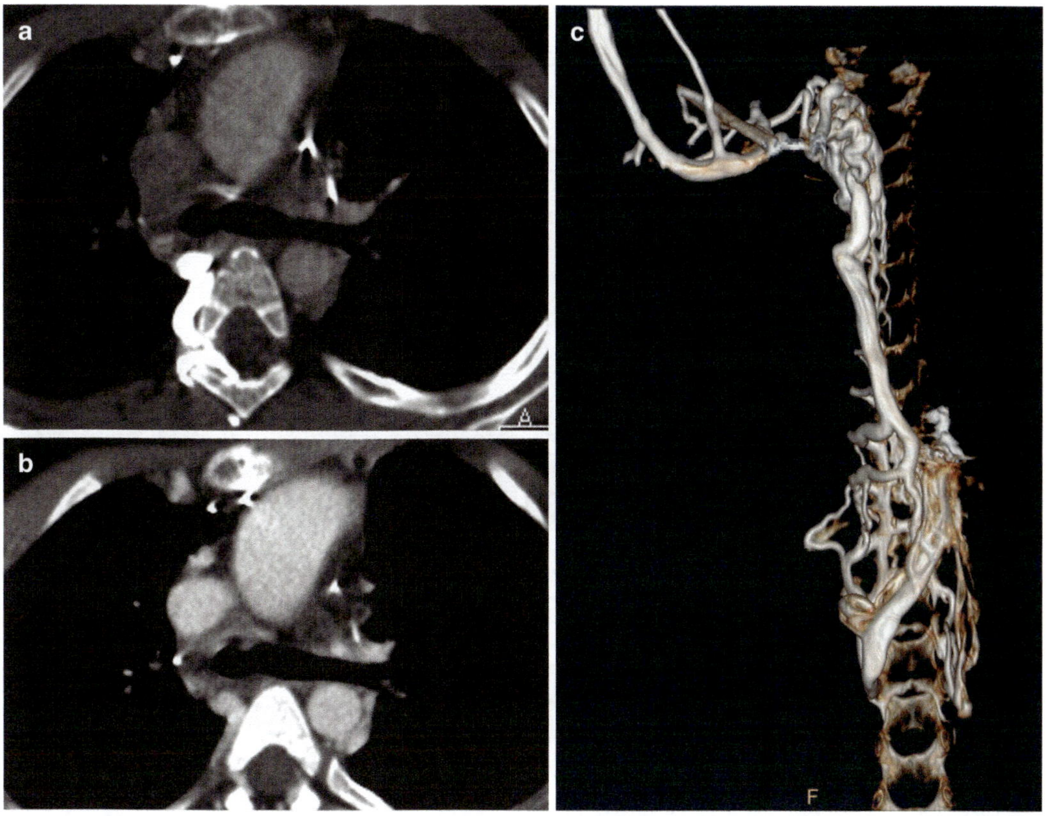

Fig. 4.12 Due to extensive venovenous collaterals following BDGS, most of the contrast injected from right upper limb shunted to lower body lead to poor opacification of thoracic vessels in the first run (**a**). All structures are better seen in the second run (**b**. VRT image of the first run shows extensive collaterals (**c**)

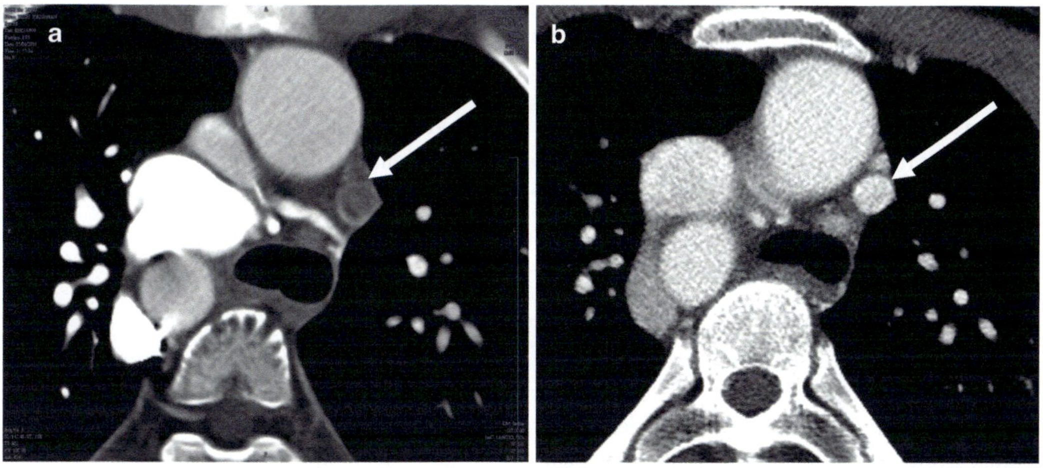

Fig. 4.13 Right upper limb contrast injection leads to poor opacification of left SVC (arrow) in the first run (**a**) and is better opacified in the second run (**b**)

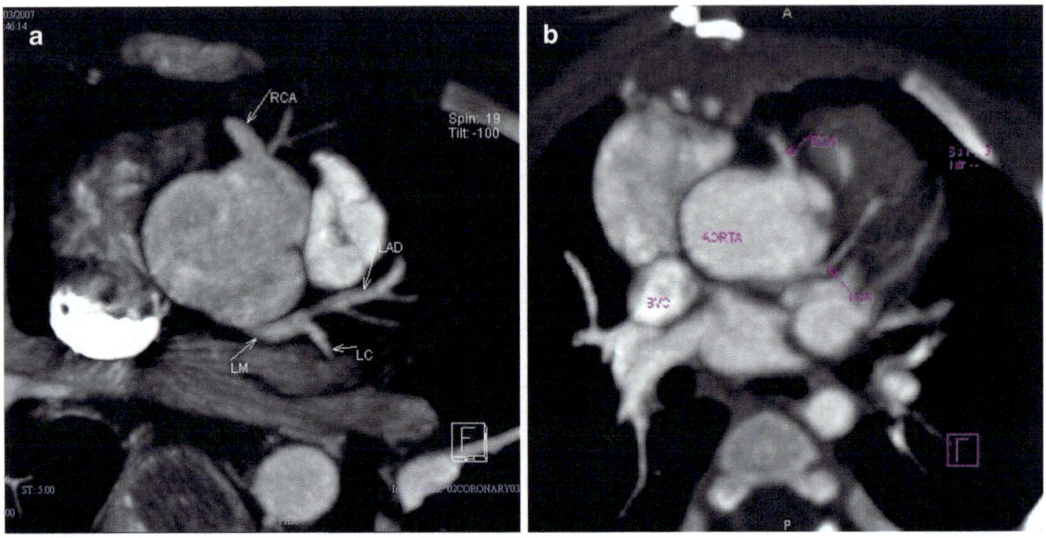

Fig. 4.14 ECG-gated CT (**a**) shows better resolution with good visualization of coronary arteries. Non-gated CT (**b**) can show proximal coronary artery

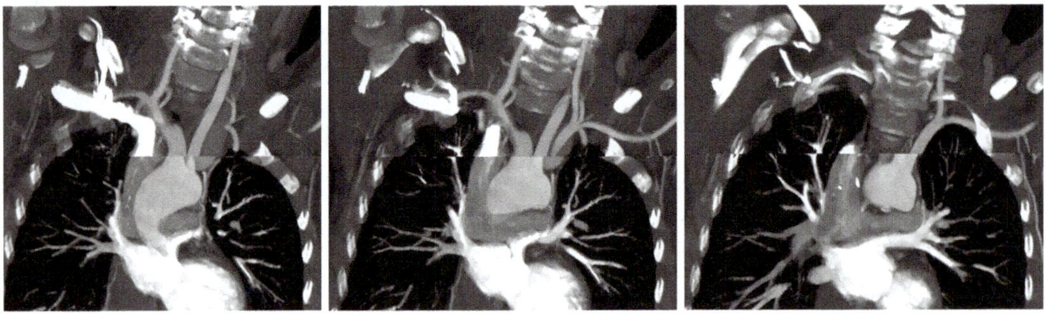

Fig. 4.15 Two station step and shoot axial CT with coronal reformation shows an abrupt change in contrast density in a case of BDGS. Movement of the child just prior to the start of the scan leads to improper coverage of thoracic structures

ric scans is that the end-systolic phase is preferred with a heart rate above 80 bpm since this phase is less susceptible to motion artifacts [19].

4.4.9.3 Prospective ECG-Gated Sequential Scan

This "step and shoot" method is characterized by applying maximum tube current at a pre-defined phase in the R-R cycle, with complete cessation of radiation output during the remainder of the cardiac cycle as the table moves to the next position in the *z*-direction. Data is acquired at end-systole using an absolute (ms) trigger delay as opposed to a relative (percentage) trigger delay [20] to ensure maximum image quality. The protocol traditionally used for calcium scoring can be used for this acquisition. In this step and shoot scan, a significant time delay between the table position leads to inhomogeneous contrast opacification (Fig. 4.15).

Disadvantages of ECG gating in pediatric patients include:

(a) Increased radiation dose (three times the non-gated dosage, due to the use of lower pitch, higher tube current, and retrospective gating techniques).
(b) Increased scan time.
(c) Good control of the heart rate needed. In babies with cyanotic CHD, cardiac rhythm is much higher than normal, generally between 100 and 140 bpm.

(d) ECG-gated acquisition is much slower than non-gated acquisitions, causing more respiratory artifacts.

4.4.9.4 Prospectively ECG-Triggered High-Pitch Helical CT

The use of dual-source CT addresses some of the abovementioned limitations. With this method, two X-ray tubes and the corresponding detectors are placed 90° to each other on the rotating gantry. The advantages of dual-source technology are marked improvement in temporal resolution, faster scan, and a reduction in radiation dose. The improved temporal resolution of dual-source CT facilitates accurate diagnosis, usually without β-blockade to reduce heart rate [21–23].

For assessing coronary arteries in patients with complex CHD, Ben Saad et al. and Goo have devised a "Combo" CT protocol. This includes a non-gated spiral examination of the entire thorax followed by a limited ECG-triggered CTA focusing on the conotruncal region [24, 25].

> **Practical points**
> Methods to improve temporal resolution in ECG-gated CT:
>
> - Selecting fastest gantry rotation
> - Using multisegment reconstruction—using the scan data from more than one heart cycle
> - Using dual-source CT if available

4.5 Processing the Raw Data

From the CT raw data, images are processed at the axial plane with sub-millimeter slice thickness with an increment of about 50% overlap to achieve isotropic voxels. Smooth kernel reconstruction algorithm is used for general purpose and sharper kernel to assess stents and calcified segments. For better resolution, a small field of view limited to mediastinal vasculature is recommended.

4.6 Image Reconstruction

Various image reformatting techniques including curved planar reconstruction, maximum intensity projection (MIP), minimum intensity projection (MinIP), and volume-rendering technique (VRT) are used to get all the clinically relevant information (Fig. 4.16).

4.7 Keep Radiation to Minimum (ALARA)

Pediatric thoracic CTA doses quoted in the literature vary greatly from 1 to 2 mSv to more than 10 mSv.

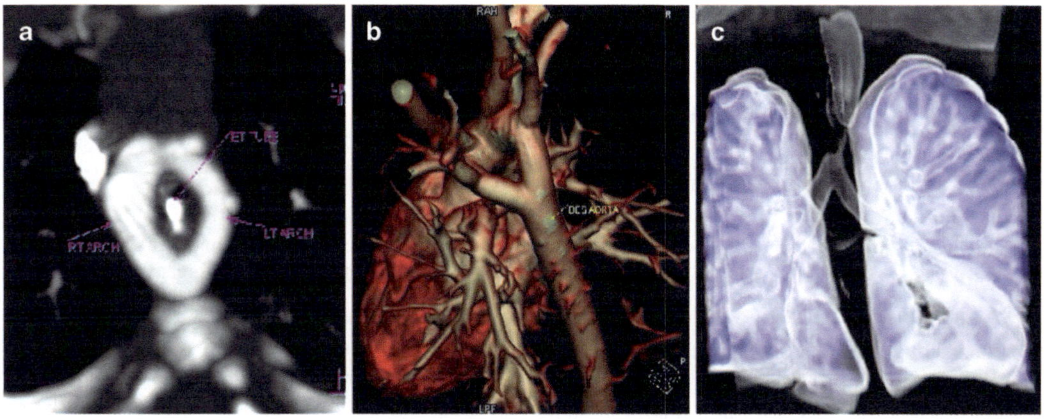

Fig. 4.16 Oblique axial MIP (**a**), VRT (**b**) and MinIp (**c**) images demonstrate a double aortic arch causing airway compression

A variety of techniques have proved effective in lowering radiation exposure, including decreasing tube current and potential, increasing pitch and table speed, avoiding multiphasic imaging, and minimizing scan coverage. Rotational tube current modulation, a form of automatic exposure control, can be used to further lower radiation exposure. With this technique, a noise index is set by the operator, and the tube current is continuously adjusted to minimize radiation exposure while an acceptable signal-to-noise ratio is maintained [26, 27].

Reducing the kilovoltage from 120 to 80 kVp decreases the radiation dose by 65% at a constant current setting, as radiation dose varies with the square of kV.

The other advantage of 80 kV settings is the possibility for reduction of the amount of contrast medium injection because low kilovoltage is more sensitive to contrast (iodine has a high atomic number) than standard 120 or 140 kV settings.

As a rule of thumb, use 80 kVp for patients with weight less than 15 kg and 100 kVp for weight more than 15 kg.

When imaging large vessels, like aorta and pulmonary arteries, a lower current can be used. If the target vessel is small, such as diminutive aortopulmonary collateral arteries, a higher current is required for proper delineation of these small structures from the background noise.

Automatic dose modulation mode to be used to give the right amount of mAs.

4.8 Documentation and Storage of Data

Although in the era of PACS, there is little need for prints, many imaging centers still print CT images for conveying data sets to referring cardiologists and cardiac surgeons.

Newer CT scanners generate isotropic data sets with voxels measuring less than 1 mm in the *x*-, *y*-, and *z*-planes. Archiving the entire raw data occupies a huge amount of storage space. A combination of 2D multiplanar and 3D maximum-intensity-projection and volume-rendered images are most commonly used for storage and communication.

With advances in CT scanners and software, a variety of high-quality 2D reformatted and 3D reconstructed images can be generated that aid in the understanding of complex cardiovascular anatomy. Two-dimensional multiplanar reformations can in any plane be generated with resolution comparable with that of axial images. Coronal and sagittal images are also used to document information about cardiovascular structures, particularly structures that traverse the *z*-axis, which may not be apparent on axial images.

4.9 3D Printing

It can be very useful for preoperative planning and evaluation of postoperative changes [28]. But due to cost factors, its use is still restricted to certain complex cases and institutes.

Key Points

- The endpoint of Cardiac CT imaging should be diagnostically readable data set and not smooth beautiful looking images.
- Pediatric thoracic CTA typically requires sedation as quiet breathing rarely causes appreciable respiratory artifacts.
- Cardiac CT is used when echocardiography fails to evaluate extracardiac structures.
- The non-ECG gated study generally suffice for the majority of cases of pediatric CCT.
- With the advent of new-generation scanner like dual-source technology with marked improvement in temporal resolution, faster scan, and a reduction in radiation dose, CT can be used for a comprehensive assessment of both intra- and extra-cardiac anatomy.

References

1. Hopkins KL, Patrick LE, Simoneaux SF, Bank ER, Parks WJ, Smith SS. Pediatric great vessel anomalies: initial clinical experience with spiral CT angiography. Radiology. 1996;200:811–5.
2. Lee T, Tsai IC, Fu YC, et al. Using multidetector-row CT in neonates with complex congenital heart disease to replace diagnostic cardiac catheterization for anatomical investigation: initial experiences in technical and clinical feasibility. Pediatr Radiol. 2006;36:1273–82.

3. Taylor AM. Cardiac imaging: MR or CT? Which to use when. Pediatr Radiol. 2008;38(suppl 3):S433–8.
4. Rajeshkannan R, Moorthy S, Sreekumar KP, Ramachandran PV, Kumar RK, Remadevi KS. Role of 64-MDCT in evaluation of pulmonary atresia with ventricular septal defect. AJR Am J Roentgenol. 2010 Jan;194(1):110–8.
5. Windram J, Grosse-Wortmann L, Shariat M, Greer ML, Crawford MW, Yoo SJ. Cardiovascular MRI without sedation or general anesthesia using a feed-and -sleep technique in neonates and infants. Pediatr Radiol. 2011;42:183–7.
6. Leschka S, Oechslin E, Husmann L, et al. Pre- and postoperative evaluation of congenital heart disease in children and adults with 64-section CT. Radiographics. 2007;27:829–46.
7. Lee KH, Yoon CS, Choe KO, et al. Use of imaging for assessing anatomical relationships of tracheobronchial anomalies associated with left pulmonary artery sling. Pediatr Radiol. 2001;31:269–78.
8. Goo HW, Park IS, Ko JK, et al. CT of congenital heart disease: normal anatomy and typical pathologic conditions. Radiographics. 2003;23:S147–65.
9. Tsai IC, Chen MC, Jan SL, et al. Neonatal cardiac multidetector row CT: why and how we do it. Pediatr Radiol. 2008;38:438–51.
10. Choo KS, Lee HD, Ban JE, et al. Evaluation of obstructive airway lesions in complex congenital heart disease using composite volume-rendered images from multislice CT. Pediatr Radiol. 2006;36:219–23.
11. Siegel MJ. Multiplanar and three-dimensional multi-detector row CT of thoracic vessels and airways in the pediatric population. Radiology. 2003;229:641–50.
12. Frush DP, Herlong JR. Pediatric thoracic CT angiography. Pediatr Radiol. 2005;35:11–25.
13. Kim TH, Kim YM, Suh CH, et al. Helical CT angiography and three-dimensional reconstruction of total anomalous pulmonary venous connections in neonates and infants. AJR. 2000;175:1381–6.
14. Kerl JM, Ravenel JG, Nguyen SA, et al. Right heart: split-bolus injection of diluted contrast medium for visualization at coronary CT angiography. Radiology. 2008;247(2):356–64. 57
15. Greenberg SB, Bhutta ST. A dual contrast injection technique for multidetector computed tomography angiography of Fontan procedures. Int J Cardiovasc Imaging. 2008;24:345–8.
16. Saremi F, Kang J, Rahmanuddin S, Shavelle D. Assessment of post-atrial switch baffle integrity using a modified dual extremity injection cardiac computed tomography angiography technique. Int J Cardiol. 2013;162(2):e25–7.
17. Spevak PJ, Johnson PT, Fishman EK. Surgically corrected congenital heart disease: utility of 64-MDCT. AJR. 2008;191:854–61.
18. Goo HW, Park IS, Ko JK, Kim YH, Seo DM, Yun TJ, et al. Visibility of the origin and proximal course of coronary arteries on non-ECG-gated heart CT in patients with congenital heart disease. Pediatr Radiol. 2005;35:792–8.
19. Goo HW. State of the art CT imaging techniques for congenital heart disease. Korean J Radiol. 2010;11:4–18.
20. Arnoldi E, Hohnson TR, Rist C, Wintersperger BJ, Sommer WH, Becker A, Becker CR, Reiser MF, Nikolaou K. Adequate image quality with reduced radiation dose in prospectively triggered coronary CTA compared with retrospective techniques. Eur Radiol. 2009;19:2147–55.
21. Leschka S, Stolzmann P, Schmid FT, et al. Low kilovoltage cardiac dual-source CT: attenuation, noise, and radiation dose. Eur Radiol. 2008;18:1809–17.
22. Ropers U, Ropers D, Pflederer T, et al. Influence of heart rate on the diagnostic accuracy of dual source computed tomography coronary angiography. J Am Coll Cardiol. 2007;50:2393–8.
23. Jin KN, Park EA, Shin CI, Lee W, Chung JW, Park JH. Retrospective versus prospective ECG-gated dual-source CT in pediatric patients with congenital heart disease: comparison of image quality and radiation dose. Int J Cardiovasc Imaging. 2010;26:63–73.
24. Ben Saad M, Rohnean A, Sigal-Cinqualbre A, et al. Evaluation of image quality and radiation dose of thoracic and coronary dual-source CT in 110 infants with congenital heart disease. Pediatr Radiol. 2009;39:668–76.
25. Goo HW, Yang DH. Coronary artery visibility in free breathing young children with congenital heart disease on cardiac 64-slice CT: dual-source ECG-triggered sequential scan vs. single source non-ECG-synchronised spiral scan. Pediatr Radiol. 2010;40(10):1670–80.
26. Lerner CB, Frush DP, Boll DT. Evaluation of a coronary-cameral fistula: benefits of coronary dual-source MDCT angiography in children. Pediatr Radiol. 2008;38:874–8.
27. Dillman JR, Hernandez RJ. Role of CT in the evaluation of congenital cardiovascular disease in children. AJR. 2009;192:1219–31.
28. Kappanayil M, Koneti NR, Kannan RR, Kottayil BP, Kumar K. Three-dimensional-printed cardiac prototypes aid surgical decision-making and preoperative planning in selected cases of complex congenital heart diseases: early experience and proof of concept in a resource-limited environment. Ann Pediatr Card. 2017;10:117–25.

Scan Techniques for Pediatric Cardiac MRI

5

Ramiah Rajeshkannan

5.1 Introduction

To plan effective management of congenital heart disease, one needs the clearest understanding of the anatomy and pathophysiology. Echocardiography and angiography are the traditional imaging modalities used to diagnose congenital heart disease. Although echocardiography and catheter angiography are the dominant imaging modalities in patients with congenital heart disease, Cardiac Magnetic Resonance Imaging (CMR) and computed tomography (CT) are valuable noninvasive adjuncts.

The direct multiplanar image capability of MR imaging allows the precise depiction of the complex and often unexpected cardiac and extracardiac arterial and venous morphologies present.

To obtain good-quality CMR images in children, it is essential to adjust the technical parameters of the pulse sequences to the small size and fast heart rates of the patients.

Electronic Supplementary Material The online version of this chapter (https://doi.org/10.1007/978-981-15-6755-1_5) contains supplementary material, which is available to authorized users.

R. Rajeshkannan (✉)
Department of Radiology, Amrita School of Medicine, Amrita Institute of Medical Sciences and Research Centre, Amrita Vishwa Vidyapeetham, Kochi, Kerala, India
e-mail: rajeshkr@aims.amrita.edu

It is important to understand that "the child not a small adult", when it comes to paediatric cardiovascular MRI. The smaller anatomy requires greater spatial resolution, higher heart rates need a greater temporal resolution. Paediatric patients may be sedated or uncooperative rendering breath-hold imaging strategies useless.

This chapter is a summary of the primary techniques used in CMR for both paediatric and adult congenital heart diseases.

5.2 Paediatric CMR Set-Up

The preparation of the child is critical prior to taking the patient into the MRI room.

These include:

- Clear instructions about the gantry environment such as the amount of noise while doing the scan.
- Importance of strict immobilization [1, 2].
- The parents should be briefly interviewed with regard to MR contraindications and also informed about the study and may themselves be anxious.
- Similar to all MRI exams, standard questionnaires for the pacemaker, implanted device, or other foreign materials inside the body which can cause severe local artefacts lead to discontinuation of study is a must (Fig. 5.1). All cos-

R. Rajeshkannan et al. (eds.), *CT and MRI in Congenital Heart Diseases*,
https://doi.org/10.1007/978-981-15-6755-1_5

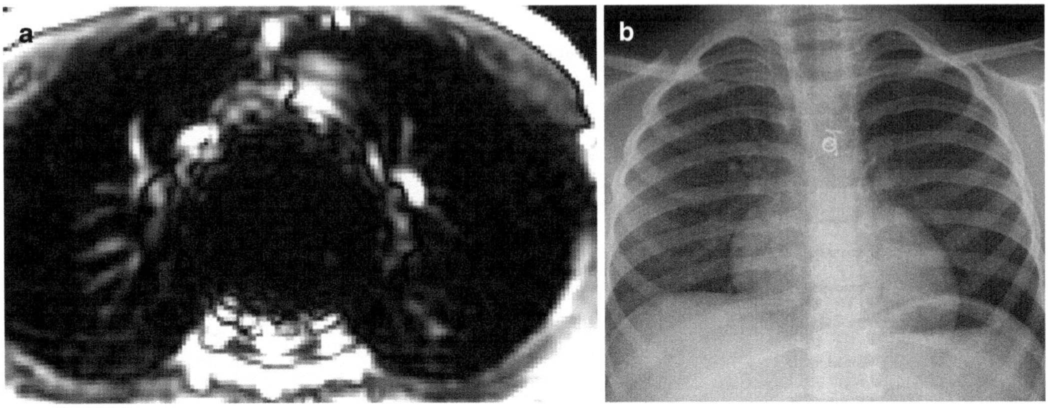

Fig. 5.1 (**a**) Axial SSFP MR image showing severe susceptibility artefact obscuring most of the mediastinal vasculature. (**b**) Chest radiograph showing small embolization coil

metics, make-up, and jewellery need to be removed. Cosmetics often have a metallic base and can cause artefacts in the image or can cause local burns [3].
- Secure IV line if contrast study is needed.

Patients must be kept warm within the colder MRI room environment. Since the temperature inside the scanner is very low for the children, especially for neonates and smaller infants, it is important to understand that any prolongation of study in a small child carries a significant risk of hypothermia.

- A cheerful and well-lit MRI room and surroundings is helpful to reassure and prepare paediatric patients.
- Colourful paintings and cartoons in the preparation area and inside the scanner room will comfort the older child who may be apprehensive at the prospect of a study while awake.
- Good lighting within the room ensures continuous assessment of the child. A dimmer switch enables the light to be dimmed to facilitate sleep in small children when needed.

5.3 Sedation/Anaesthesia

The challenge of Cardiac MRI examination to the patient is a long scan time, need for strict immobilization, repeated breath-holds at the same point of the respiratory cycle, over a period of perhaps 45–60 min. The patient has to do this in a very strange environment within a long tunnel, in a very noisy surrounding, while being covered with coils, ECG leads, and respiratory bellows. Most children above 7–10 years old can cooperate for the procedure if they are trained well before the exam. However, sedation or general anaesthesia may be required in those children too young to cooperate adequately.

Neonates and small infants can be scanned during natural sleep. This can be achieved by:

- Keeping the child in a fasting state for 2–3 h.
- Feeding just before the exam, "feed and sleep" technique [4].
- Swaddling of the child in a warm sheet.
- Commercially available vacuum-shaped support bags may help to immobilize the child.

The choice between sedation and general anaesthesia with endotracheal intubation depends on individual institutional and patient preference. It depends on many factors, including the age of the child, the type of information needed and the scan time, availability of MR scanner time, expertise availability of the anaesthesiology team, and anaesthesia equipment. Endotracheal intubation with pharmacologically induced paralysis is needed if breath-holding is desirable [5]. The anaesthetist can be asked to temporarily cease ventilation to do "breath-hold" scans. Prolonged, multiple breath-holds are required, thus adequate pauses for ventilation control between breath-holds are required, to ensure that hypoxia and hypercapnoea are avoided.

Intravenous sedation is a preferred alternative to intubation amongst parents and anaesthesiologists and has two important requirements:

- Anaesthesiologists experienced in administering intravenous sedation in patients with congenital heart disease
- Ability to modify the MR sequences for free-breathing acquisition

The main drawbacks of scanning with deep sedation are an unprotected airway and reliance on spontaneous respiratory effort with the associated risks of aspiration, airway obstruction, and hypoventilation [6]. Sedation with free-breathing is more physiological than with general anaesthesia which may use positive pressure ventilation and breath-holding. This is particularly important in evaluating near-physiological circulation and calculation of pulmonary blood flow in patients with Fontan circulation.

Among children undergoing sedation for CT and MRI, Malviya et al. found a 2.9% incidence of hypoxemia and failure rate of 7% in children who received sedation [7] compared to the 100% successful scan in children receiving general anaesthesia, with a 0.7% incidence of laryngospasm. Even though general anaesthesia is a more expensive procedure than sedation, it is an important tool in the successful completion of MRI scanning with minimal adverse events [8] (Table 5.1).

Table 5.1 Imaging under sedation versus general anaesthesia (GA)

Parameter	Sedation	GA
Scanning method	Free-breathing sequences	Breath-hold
Scan time	Long	Short
Data interpretation	Near physiological	Altered physiology
Image quality	Blurred images	Better image quality

Generally, most of the anaesthesia doctors and technical staffs are not used to the high magnetic field environment. Proper training of all the staff members are needed regarding the safety procedures required to handle the metal objects inside the scan room. Assembling a fixed team that will be routinely responsible rather than having many anaesthesiologists rotate through MRI will improve care.

MRI compatibility is required for all equipment used for anaesthesia, monitoring, and kept in the scan room. Monitoring routinely includes limb lead ECG, pulse oximetry, and blood pressure. Additional requirements include inspiratory and expiratory gas analysis used in anaesthetized child. Temperature monitoring should be available especially while scanning neonates and infants.

If the special anaesthetic machines designed to operate within the MRI room are not available, the anaesthetic equipment can be kept directly outside the scan room, with all gas lines passing through waveguides installed for this purpose.

5.4 Patient Positioning and Coil Placement

Most MRI systems have specific cardiac or torso coils to do cardiac scan. Multi-element phased array coils with parallel imaging capability are preferred. These coils have both anterior and posterior elements, which require accurate positioning, critical for adequate signal reception. If available, dedicated paediatric flex coils with maximum elements can be used.

Small babies can be scanned with adult head or knee coil to get the maximum signal-to-noise ratio.

Coil selection also depends on the appropriate clinical indication and the desired field of view (FOV). For a suspected anomalous coronary artery in an infant, a smaller size coil is preferred. In a larger patient with suspected systemic vasculitis, one should use a larger body phased array coil to screen the entire thoracic and abdominal aorta [9].

5.5 ECG Placement

The R wave of the ECG is typically used to generate a trigger signal indicating the beginning of the cardiac cycle with the initiation of ventricular systole. CMR pulse sequence events are timed relative to that trigger to acquire data at specific time points within the cardiac cycle.

With the advent of vectorcardiogram (VCG) triggering system, the technical difficulties associated with obtaining accurate cardiac triggering and gating for cardiac MR examinations have been essentially eliminated. These systems use the spatial information in a vector cardiogram to improve R wave detection in the MR environment and improve and isolate the R wave signal from the magneto-hydrodynamic effects of blood flowing in the aorta. Coupled with fibre-optic hardware, the VCG system provides clinically reliable and robust ECG-triggering for all patients.

Before attaching the electrodes, the skin should be shaved if excess hair and cleaned with alcoholic pads or an abrasive gel to improve surface contact. Only MR compatible ECG leads to be used.

The optimal lead position also varies depending on the location, orientation, and size of each individual's heart. The goal is to obtain a well-defined and relatively high-amplitude QRS complex in which the R upstroke of ventricular depolarization is significantly larger than the T wave of the cardiac cycle, so that image triggering will occur consistently at the same point within the cycle.

ECG leads can be placed on the right side in patients with dextrocardia if left side tracing is not satisfactory [9]. If the intra-cardiac anatomy is significantly distorted as in the criss-cross heart or univentricular heart, ECG leads may have to be positioned in an unusual location. In cases of difficulties due to pericardial effusion and a weak ECG signal, peripheral pulse gating can be used.

Before placing the coil, the quality of the ECG trace should be checked for high amplitude R wave distinct from the tall T wave. It is well worth the time taken to get a good signal. If the tracing is unsatisfactory, restart and reposition the electrodes to get good signals rather than hurrying into the study acquisition.

Furthermore, care should be taken to recheck the ECG signal once the patient has entered the bore of the magnet as interference from voltages produced by the flow of the blood in the magnetic field (the magnetohydrodynamic effect) can distort the signal obtained, so that the R wave may no longer be clearly defined [10].

Peripheral pulse triggering, which can be obtained from MRI-compatible optical fingertip pulse monitors, provides a less-preferred but often adequate alternative if a satisfactory ECG signal cannot be obtained. It is also useful in patients with cardiac arrhythmias, because the premature beats do not produce a peripheral pulse, and therefore ignored during the scan.

For safety reasons, the ECG leads should not be allowed to form loops, because of the risk of burns from the induction of a current by the strong RF power used in MRI.

5.6 Breath-Holding Versus Free-Breathing Scan

Paediatric cardiac MRI can use three different methods of respiration:

1. Breath-holding in an awake and cooperative child
2. General anaesthesia with endotracheal intubation and controlled ventilation
3. Free-breathing

In the first two instances, MRI can be done with suspended respiration to reduce respiratory motion.

In cases of difficulties due to profound respiratory motion, an abdominal band can be used to reduce artefacts. While doing MRI with endotracheal intubation, additional scans with 100% oxygen can be performed to assess pulmonary vasoreactivity in cases like pre-Fontan assessment.

If the child is not cooperative for breath-hold and in sedated patients free-breathing MRI sequences can be used (Fig. 5.2) [11]. Good-

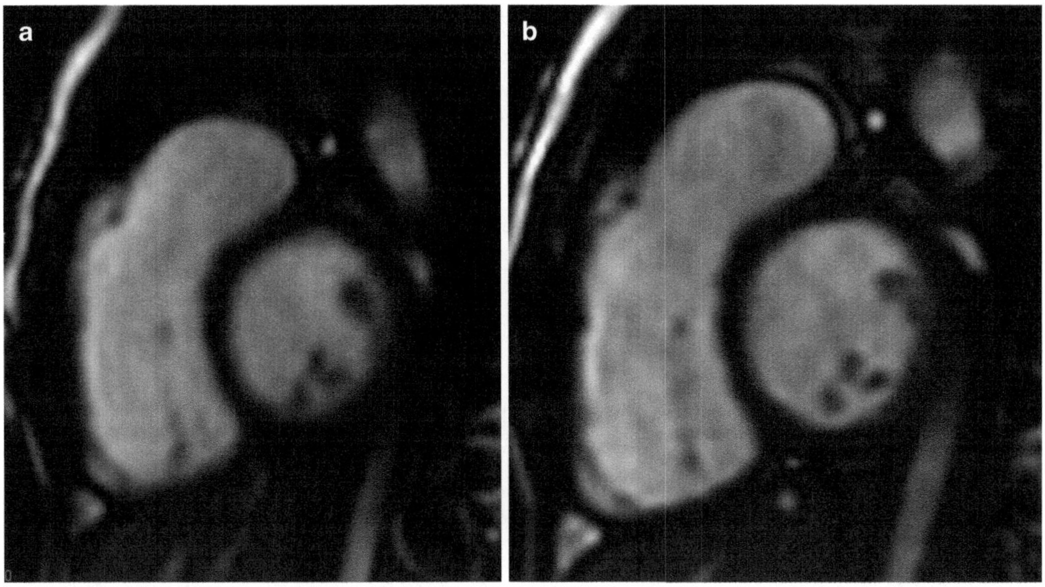

Fig. 5.2 Free-breathing cine MRI image (**a**) showing minimal blurring compared to breath-hold sequence, (**b**) but gives diagnostic quality

quality free-breathing scans can be done by increasing the number of averages or number of excitations (NEX) to 3–4. Reducing the slice thickness and FOV is also helpful. If the parallel imaging is not available with multiple NEX, then it can be removed and the scan time can be significantly reduced by reducing the phase FOV %. While doing free-breathing cine sequences, one should keep an eye on the SAR value which will rapidly rise during the prolonged acquisition.

Practical Tips

Following changes recommended for free-breathing MRI:

- Three to four NEX—to compensate respiratory misregistration
- Reduced slice thickness and FOV—for better resolution
- Reduce flip angle—to reduce SAR
- Reduce phase FOV and use parallel imaging—to reduce scan time

Free-breathing MRI can be done with navigator gating, in which the diaphragmatic position is tracked continuously while imaging is acquired when the diaphragm is at a particular predetermined position (Fig. 5.3). Navigator gating is mainly used for 3D imaging of the heart and coronary arteries using bright blood SSFP sequence and for delayed myocardial enhancement sequence. The navigator planning of column placement can be improved by:

- Positioning over a diaphragmatic edge where the edge will move along the column during the respiratory cycle.
- Columns intersect the right dome of the diaphragm.
- Care must be taken to ensure that the columns (and the slice-selective excitations used to produce them) do not extend into a region of interest as signal loss from the navigator pulse excitation will interfere with visualization of the affected tissue.

The advantages are that the free-breathing imaging combines information from multiple heartbeats, averages the information, and reflects the physiology of contractility and flow across inspiration and expiration [12]. Disadvantages include a long scan time and lower resolution images. The calculation of ventricular function may be limited.

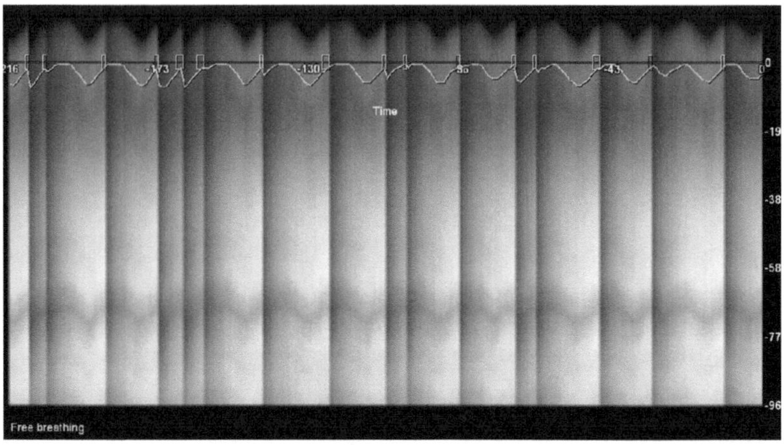

Fig. 5.3 During navigator gating, the diaphragmatic position is tracked continuously (blue line) while imaging is acquired (yellow boxes) when the diaphragm is at a particular predetermined position

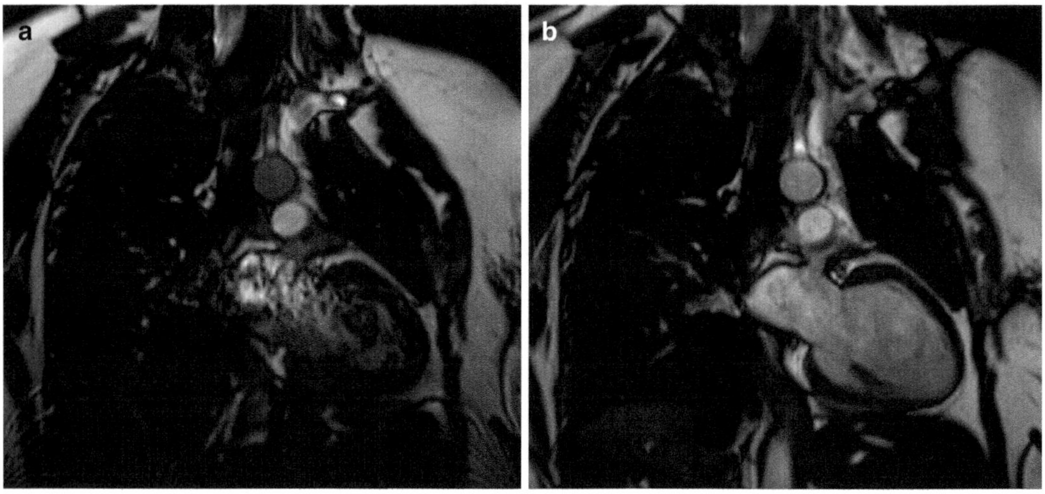

Fig. 5.4 (**a**) Shows severe artefacts over the heart. They are removed by proper shimming in (**b**)

5.7 MRI Scanner

Most paediatric cardiac MRIs are performed on 3 T or 1.5 T field strength. In general, 3 T scanner yields a higher signal-to-noise ratio and therefore allows for better spatial resolution, improved clinical performance of coronary angiography, contrast-enhanced angiography, myocardial tagging, and myocardial perfusion imaging sequences. SAR is increased at 3 T. The T1 time is also increased at 3 T and protocols from 1.5 T need to be changed before being incorporated into a 3 T scanner. MR imaging at 3 T may produce off-resonance artefacts and dielectric shading artefacts. CMR at 3 T, thus, requires protocol optimization, careful shimming, and adjustment of the RF pulses to prevent artefacts (Fig. 5.4).

5.8 Contrast Media for MRI

Contrast media or agents denote extrinsic substances that are intended to improve the image contrast of the target tissues from the background [13]. Generally, Gadolinium (Gd)-based contrast media is injected with a maximum dose of 0.2 mmol/kg for MRA and to assess myocardial scar using late Gd enhancement (LGE) sequence.

The use of gadolinium-based contrast agents needs to be carefully managed, especially considering the risk of nephrogenic systemic fibrosis (NSF) and the potential for Gd deposits that are observed in brain tissue after repeated administrations [14, 15]. Since infants have reduced GFR, extra care should be taken while selecting the total contrast dose.

5.9 MRI Acquisition Protocol

A standard paediatric cardiac MRI examination will start with the initial screening of the patient and setting up of cardiac gating (and possible intravenous access for contrast administration). This will be followed by MRI with initial quick "scout" localizing images and a stack of relatively rapid "survey" images through the chest in all three orthogonal planes to obtain an initial overview of the heart and the associated intrathoracic anatomy. After identifying the location of the axes of the ventricles in three dimensions, basic static and cine images are acquired of the heart in standard short- and long-axis orientations, as well as various optional images, as indicated by the specific clinical questions.

A relatively small (20–26-cm) field of view, a sufficiently large matrix, and thin sections are recommended in children to get good spatial resolution.

5.10 CMR Pulse Sequences

These are specialized software programmes that define the type, magnitude, and timing of the RF pulses. Depending on these factors, sequences can be of several types. Basic pulse sequences currently used for cardiac imaging can be generally divided into dark blood (black blood) and bright blood techniques. Black *blood imaging* used in CMR is based on spin-echo imaging and the b*right blood imaging* is based on GRE imaging. Other commonly used techniques include MR angiography, phase contrast MRI and viability imaging.

5.10.1 Black Blood Sequences

These techniques make fast-flowing blood to appear dark for anatomic delineation of the blood vessel lumen and cardiac chambers [16]. Examples of this technique include conventional spin-echo (SE), breath-hold turbo or fast spin-echo (TSE, FSE), and half-Fourier turbo spin-echo sequences with double inversion recovery (IR) pulses to suppress blood signal (HASTE, double-IR TSE/FSE). For dark blood sequences, the effective repetition time (TR) should be approximately 85%–90% of the patient's R-R interval.

Black blood MR imaging techniques have the advantage of being less susceptible to artefacts from the metallic implanted devices such as stents, embolization coils, occluder devices, and sternal wires.

5.10.2 Bright Blood Cine Imaging

ECG-gated cine images are most frequently acquired using standard spoiled gradient echo (SPGR) or balanced steady-state free precession (b-SSFP) pulse sequences. Compared with SPGR, b-SSFP sequences are less sensitive to slow-flow artefacts and allow for a faster acquisition and better discrimination between the blood pool and the myocardium. However, bSSFP sequences are more influenced by the inconsistencies of the magnetic field [17].

As an important difference to echocardiography, these cine images, with few exceptions, are not acquired in real time, but are assembled over many cardiac cycles so that a temporal correlation of cardiac events with the coinciding beat-to-beat electrocardiogram is not possible.

The fast heart rates in children require a high temporal resolution (20–60 ms) for accurate ventricular volume measurements. If a segmented k-space technique is used, the number of lines or views per segment must be reduced to a higher heart rate to achieve sufficient temporal resolution.

Real-time cine sequence (MR echo) is a reasonable alternative for evaluation of ventricular function in children who cannot sustain breath-hold or with arrhythmias [18].

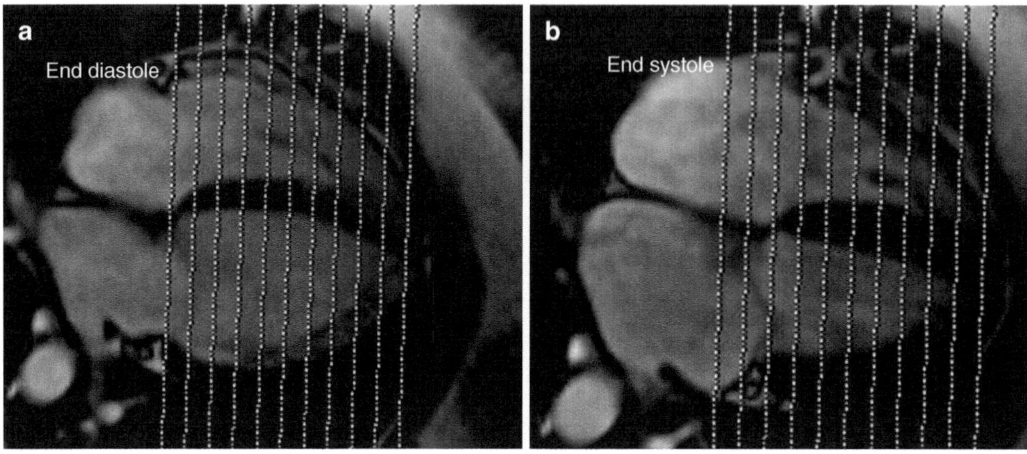

Fig. 5.5 Importance of planning short-axis cine from end-diastolic reference frame. Four-chamber cross-reference for short-axis cine showing basal slices through the ventricle on end-diastolic image (**a**). Due to AV valve excursion, most basal slices moved to atria on end-systolic image (**b**)

Cine imaging can be performed in any plane to assess the dynamic function of any structure, including the outflow tracts, valves, and great arteries. Furthermore, short-axis cine images, acquired in equal-width slices, perpendicular to the long axis of the heart from base to apex, or similar long-axis imaging in an axial plane, can be used to accurately assess cardiac function and measure the ventricular volumes.

For accurate quantification, short-axis cine are planned from end-diastolic four-chamber and two-chamber planes covering from AV valve level to apex using a minimum of 10–12 slices (Fig. 5.5). Minimum 20–24 phases covering the entire cardiac cycle is useful to correctly identify end-diastolic and systolic frames. Increasing the flip angle (up to 60°) can increase the blood-myocardial contrast. TE is kept short to improve the blood signal (Table 5.2).

Table 5.2 Key points for planning short-axis cine for volume calculation

Planning from end-diastolic four-chamber and two-chamber cine
Minimum 10–12 slices
6–8 mm thick slices without gap
Increase flip angle to 60°
Keep TE short (<1.5 ms)
20–24 phases

5.10.3 MR Angiography

MR angiography is a bright blood technique that produces a luminogram of entire thoracic vasculature. It can be done either with or without contrast injection.

5.10.3.1 Contrast MRA

Gadolinium-based contrast media are generally used in MRA. Dual head injector capable of injecting as low as 0.1 ml/s incremental rate is recommended to image small children where the total dose may be only 1–2 ml.

Technique

The Gd-enhanced 3D MR angiography is performed with a section thickness of 1.2–2.4 mm, a field of view of 220 mm, and a matrix of 256 × 160. CE-MRA should be acquired during breath-hold in order to minimize motion artefacts in a relatively short acquisition time [19]. Parallel imaging acquisition techniques allow to reduce the scan time.

MRA images are usually obtained in a coronal orientation to cover the entire chest with a minimum number of slices, but also can be obtained in a sagittal oblique orientation to assess the aortic arch.

Contrast Timing

For MR angiography, we use a double dose of gadolinium-based contrast material (0.2 mmol/kg body weight).

The exact timing of the MR angiographic image acquisition is crucial for obtaining images with a high signal-to-noise ratio. This can be achieved with three different methods:

- Fixed delay: scan can be started about 5–10 s after contrast injection depending on the vessels of interest.
- Test dose injection: Exact arrival time of contrast can be calculated by small test dose injection followed by repeated acquisition using "time-resolved" MR angiography (TRICKS), which consists of a series of consecutive short 3D volume acquisitions. This technique also gives important information about the sequential filling of different chambers and conduits. The time delay between the test dose injection to good opacification of intrathoracic vasculature can be used to plan high-resolution MRA.
- Automated bolus detection methods. Newer softwares allow real-time MR fluoroscopic monitoring of contrast arrival into the vessel of interest. Centric "k-space" encoding acquisition method capture the precise timing of first-pass peak contrast enhancement to correspond with the high contrast portion of MRA acquisition. To ensure that all vessels including the systemic veins are enhanced, imaging is repeated three to four times.

TRICKS MRA can be done using one-fourth of the total Gd dose followed by high-resolution MRA with the rest of the contrast (Video 5.1).

When the TRICKS MRA sequence is not available, multislice MR perfusion can be used to assess sequential chamber opacification in complex CHD (Video 5.2).

Despite the fast acquisition using CE-MRA approaches, it is important to note that these techniques are not ECG-gated, resulting in motion blurring of the aortic root, coronary arteries, and cardiac chambers.

5.10.3.2 Non-contrast MRA

Respiratory navigator gated ECG triggered 3D SSFP sequences can be used to acquire high-resolution MRA images. The isotropic 3D SSFP data allow arbitrary reconstruction of images in any plane desired, without any loss of spatial resolution [20]. Even though 3D SSFP can be acquired without contrast, scanning after contrast media injection gives better blood pool signals. A spectrally selective fat saturation pulse and a T2 preparatory pulse are used to increase the contrast among blood, fat, and myocardium.

5.10.4 Phase-Contrast Velocity Mapping Imaging

Complete technical aspects of phase-contrast imaging are described in Chapter 20. However, salient aspects are discussed in this section.

Phase-contrast acquisitions are sensitive to the speed of flow, and the velocity encoding parameters should be carefully selected to avoid aliasing artefacts. To prevent partial volume artefacts, slice thickness and slab orientation should be appropriately chosen. Images have to be positioned perpendicular to the vessel flow with the isocenter of acquisition positioned in the centre of the vessel. Acquisitions can be performed during a single breath-hold or in free-breathing using multiple averages.

5.10.5 Myocardial Viability Imaging

The evolution of delayed enhancement PSIR sequence has placed CMR as the major contender for assessing myocardial viability. The pulse sequence consists of an inversion recovery prepared T1 weighted gradient echo image in which the normal viable myocardium is nulled following an appropriately selected inversion pulse. Non-viable and scarred tissue appears bright. Selecting the correct inversion time is critical to differentiate non-viable from viable myocardium (Fig. 5.6).

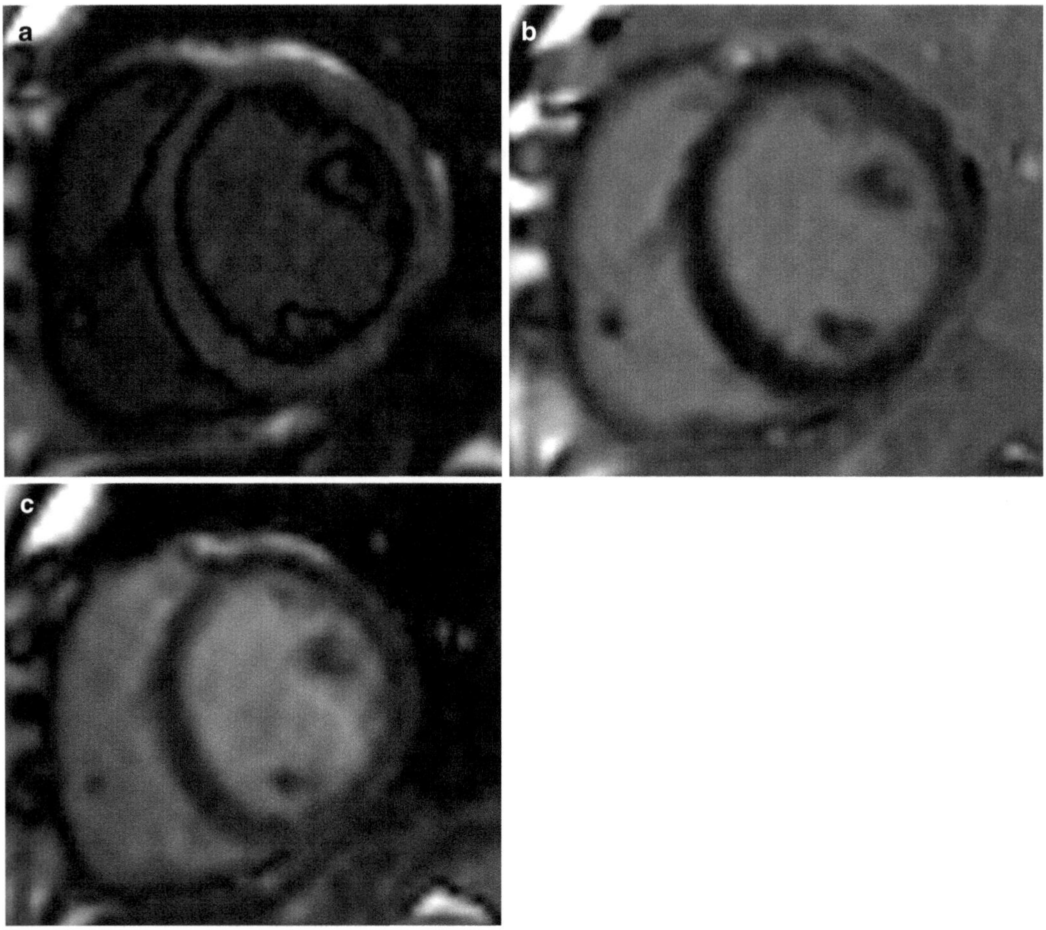

Fig. 5.6 (**a**) LGE image acquired with lower TI value shows bright myocardium, which may be misinterpreted as scar tissue. MRI using PSIR sequence (**b**) and higher TI image (**c**) showed normal myocardial suppression

5.11 MRI Imaging Planes

The main cardiac imaging planes are oblique to one another. Commonly used cardiac imaging planes are short axis (horizontal two-chamber), horizontal long axis (four-chamber), and vertical long axis (vertical two-chamber).

From the localizer images, true axial sections are taken initially. The vertical long-axis view is prescribed from the axial image. The long axis is the line from the centre of the mitral valve orifice to the left ventricular apex. From the vertical long-axis view, four-chamber view is taken. Using these last two images, short-axis view is taken. Note that the initial horizontal long axis view that is prescribed from a vertical long-axis image is only approximate; a true four-chamber view should be prescribed from the short-axis view (Fig. 5.7). Right-side two-chamber view planned similar to the left side (Fig. 5.8).

Double-oblique (oblique-sagittal) planes through the pulmonary trunk and aorta (Figs. 5.9 and 5.10.) are useful for demonstrating the pulmonic and aortic valves and outflow tracts The three-chamber view can be prescribed from the left ventricular outflow tract slice of a short-axis view. This view displays the aortic and mitral valves immediately adjacent to one another. The second LVOT view is planned perpendicular to interventricular septum with the long axis through aorta from the three-chamber view (Fig. 5.11).

This view is very useful to assess residual VSD after intracardiac repair for TOF as well to assess

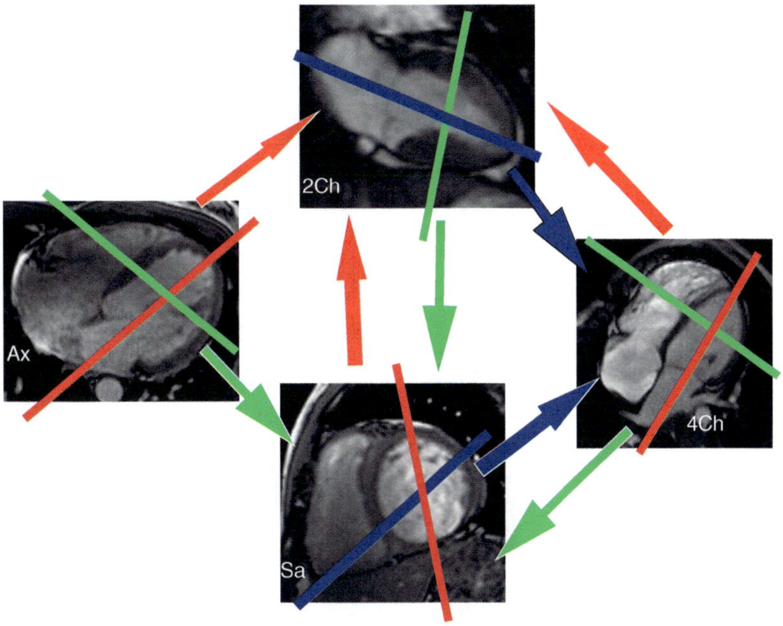

Fig. 5.7 Workflow for CMR imaging planes. Each scan plane is planned from two differently angled reference images using a double oblique technique. Red lines and arrows indicate the methods to acquire the two-chamber view. Similarly, for short axis and four-chamber planes are marked in green and blue colour, respectively

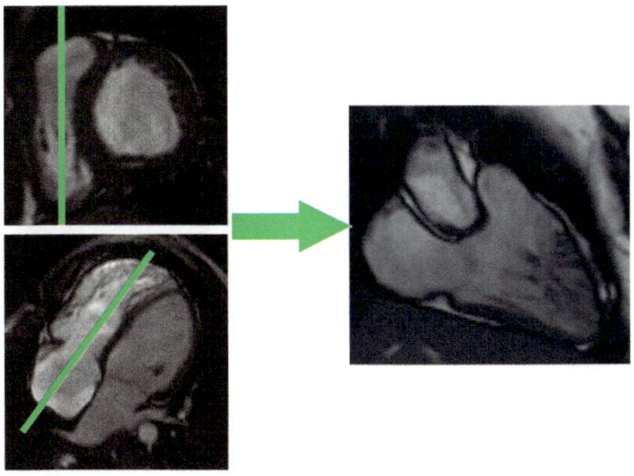

Fig. 5.8 RV two-chamber view is prescribed from four-chamber and SA views

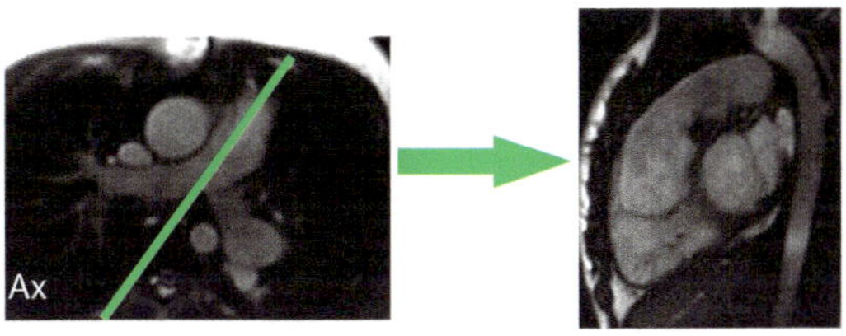

Fig. 5.9 RV outflow view is planned from the axial image through the main pulmonary artery

LV-to-aorta route in complex CHD like DORV (Fig. 5.12). Figure 5.13 demonstrates the planning for two-, three-, and four-chamber views from short-axis view. Many of the complex cardiac anatomy can be assessed by contiguous axial, coronal and sagittal cine stack images without any gap (Fig. 5.14, Video 5.3, 5.4, and 5.5).

5.12 Standard CMR Pulse Sequences for CHD

Following CMR pulse sequences are used for CHD imaging. The selection of sequences is on case-by-case basis:

- 2D SSFP cine: Axial, coronal, sagittal stack (No gap): 2Ch, 4Ch, short axis, RVOT, LVOT
- Black blood: Axial, coronal, sagittal stack (No gap)
- Gd MRA—coronal
- ECG-gated 3D SSFP—coronal or axial (Video 5.6)
- 2D PSIR—short axis
- PC flow study: Asc. Aorta, Dec aorta, MPA, RPA, LPA, SVC, Pulmonary veins

Common MRI pulse sequences used in the author's centre are available in a supplementary movie file (Video 5.7, 5.8, 5.9, 5.10, 5.11, 5.12, 5.13, 5.14, 5.15, 5.16, 5.17, 5.18, 5.19, 5.20, and 5.21).

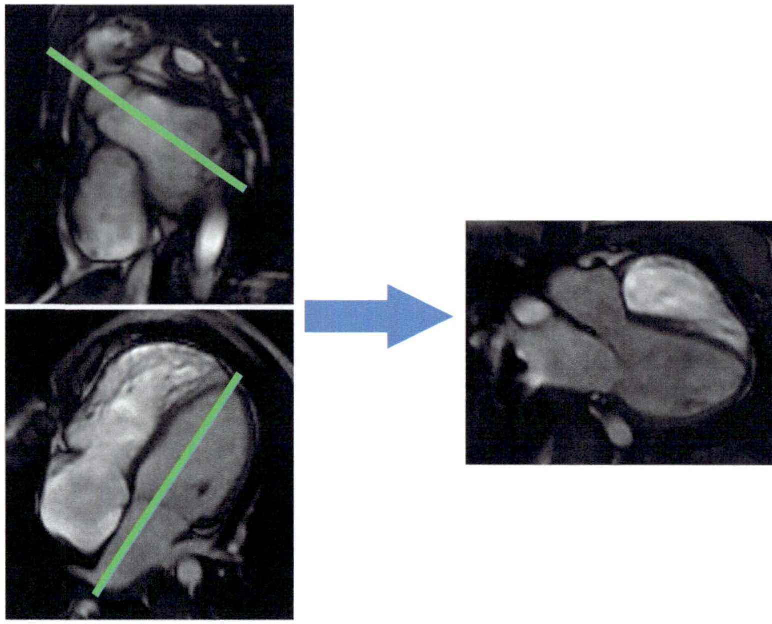

Fig. 5.10 LVOT (three-chamber) view is planned from four-chamber and basal short-axis views

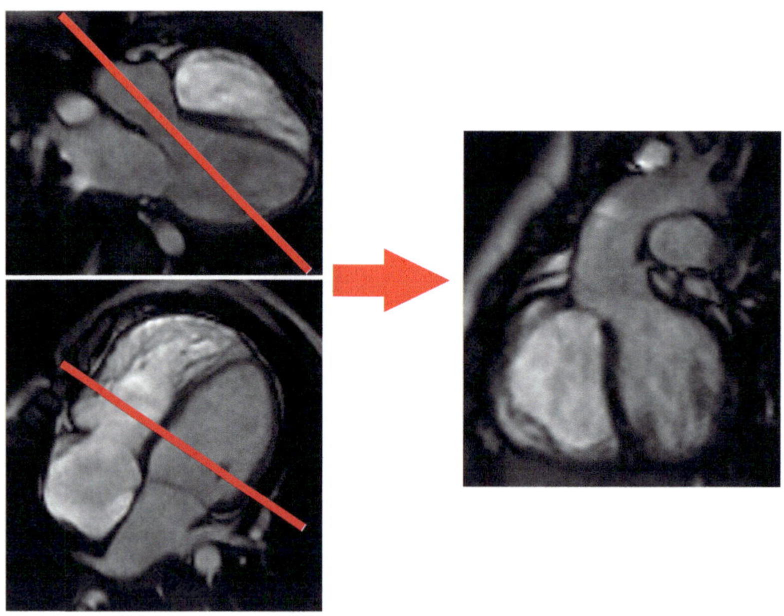

Fig. 5.11 Second LVOT view is planned perpendicular to interventricular septum with the long axis through aorta from three-chamber view

5.13 Postprocessing

Using many commercially available software, the segmentation of the blood pool and myocardial border can be performed manually, or by using automated signal thresh-holding techniques. End-diastolic and end-systolic frames are selected by looking at maximal and minimal ventricular dilatation, respectively.

Using a manual segmentation process, simple endocardial contour is drawn and the trabeculae ignored and papillary muscles are included in the blood pool for more efficient and reproducible contouring (Fig. 5.15) [21].

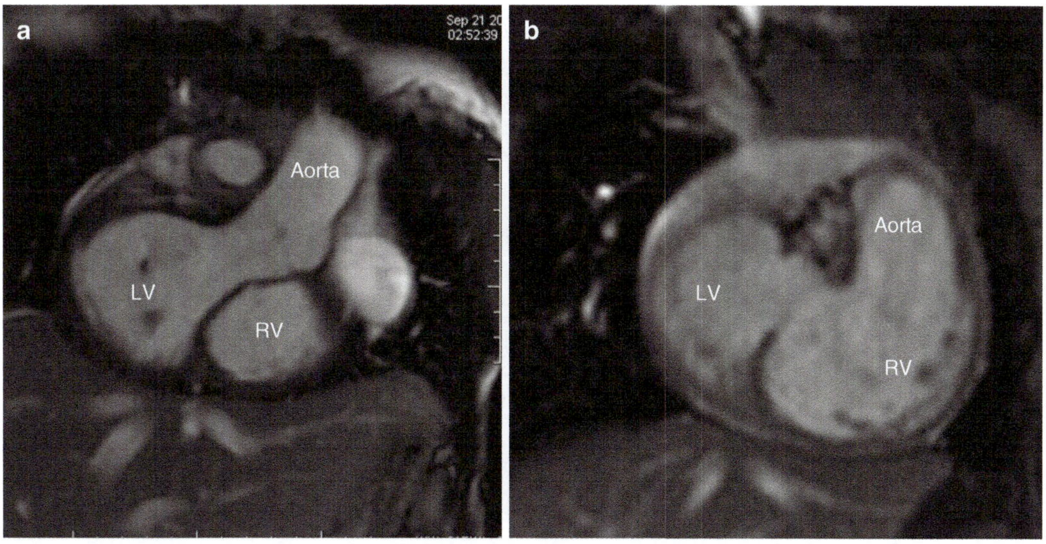

Fig. 5.12 Usefulness of second LV outflow view perpendicular to interventricular septum for assessing LV to aorta route. (**a**) Shows a clear path between the LV and aorta. (**b**) Demonstrates the conal tissue between the LV to aorta

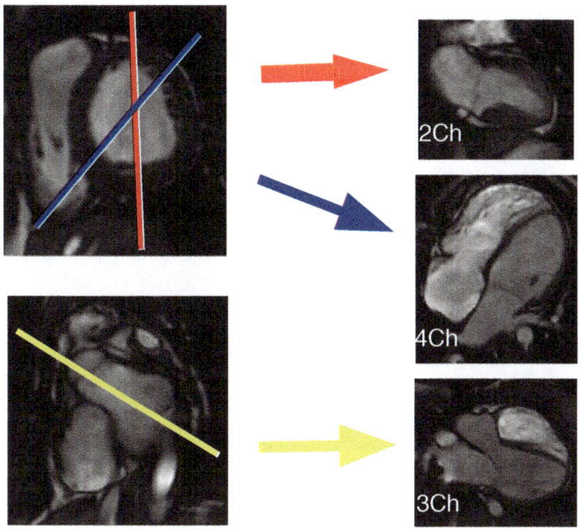

Fig. 5.13 Short-axis reference image showing planning for two-, three-, and four-chamber views

Tracing these structures will yield smaller ventricular volumes, with little change in stroke volume but a higher ejection fraction. Though theoretically more accurate, this approach is time-consuming in the absence of a reliable automated system and may reduce measurement reproducibility.

Sievers et al. showed that faster determination of right and left ventricular volumes and ejection fractions without loss of the accuracy can be achieved by tracing just outside these small papillary muscles and trabeculae [22].

Studies had shown that contouring in axial stack images were more reproducible than short-axis images for right ventricular volumes [23, 24] (Table 5.3).

In conditions like post-TOF follow-up cases, RV can dilate beyond the atrioventricular groove, when it appears as a "shoulder" surrounding the right atrium in the basal short axis. In these cases, end-diastolic RV volume will be underestimated unless the short-axis tracing starts outside the atria. (Fig. 5.16).

Cross-referencing the ventricular short-axis images with long-axis images and observing wall motion in a cine fashion facilitates accurate determination of the atrioventricular and semilunar valves planes (Figs. 5.17 and 5.18). To help discriminate ventricle from atria, atrioventricular excursion should be estimated by cross-referencing short-axis slices against each long axis acquisition. Ventricles have thicker myocardium than atria. Identifying the coronary artery in the AV groove and AV valve in the cavity can be used to differentiate the atrial section from the ventricular section. It is also important to note that atria are bigger during ventricular systole than diastole (Table 5.4).

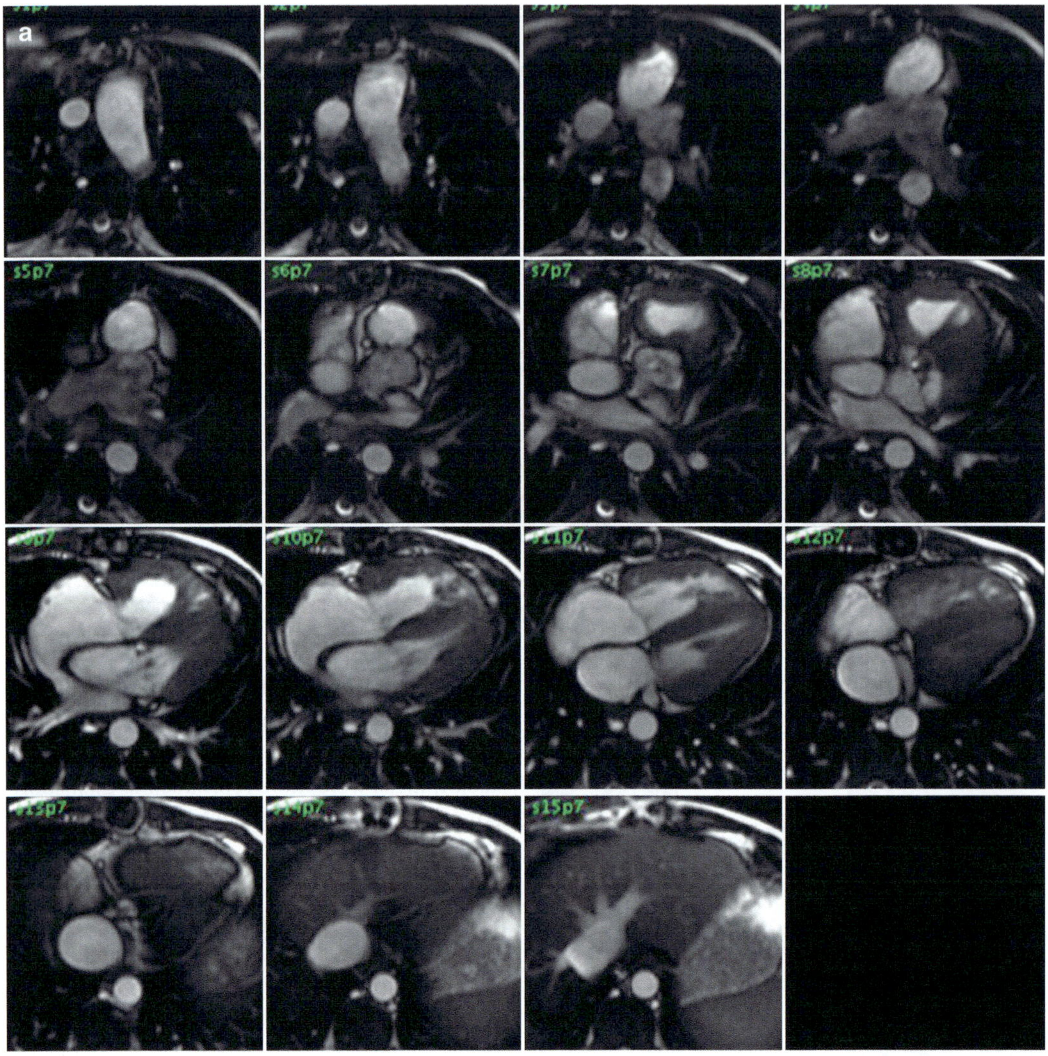

Fig. 5.14 Axial (**a**), coronal (**b**) and sagittal (**c**) cine stack images showing complete cardiac morphology in a post-Senning's case

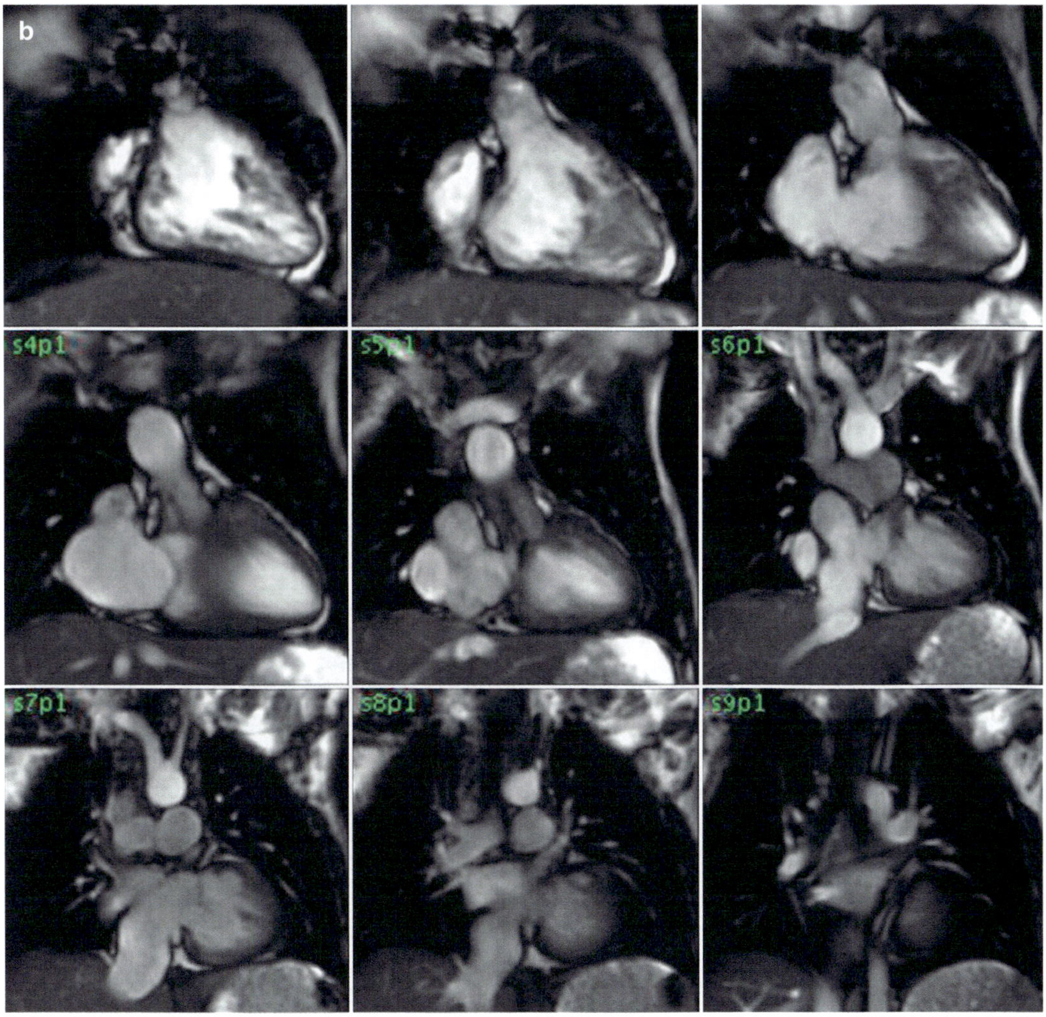

Fig. 5.14 (continued)

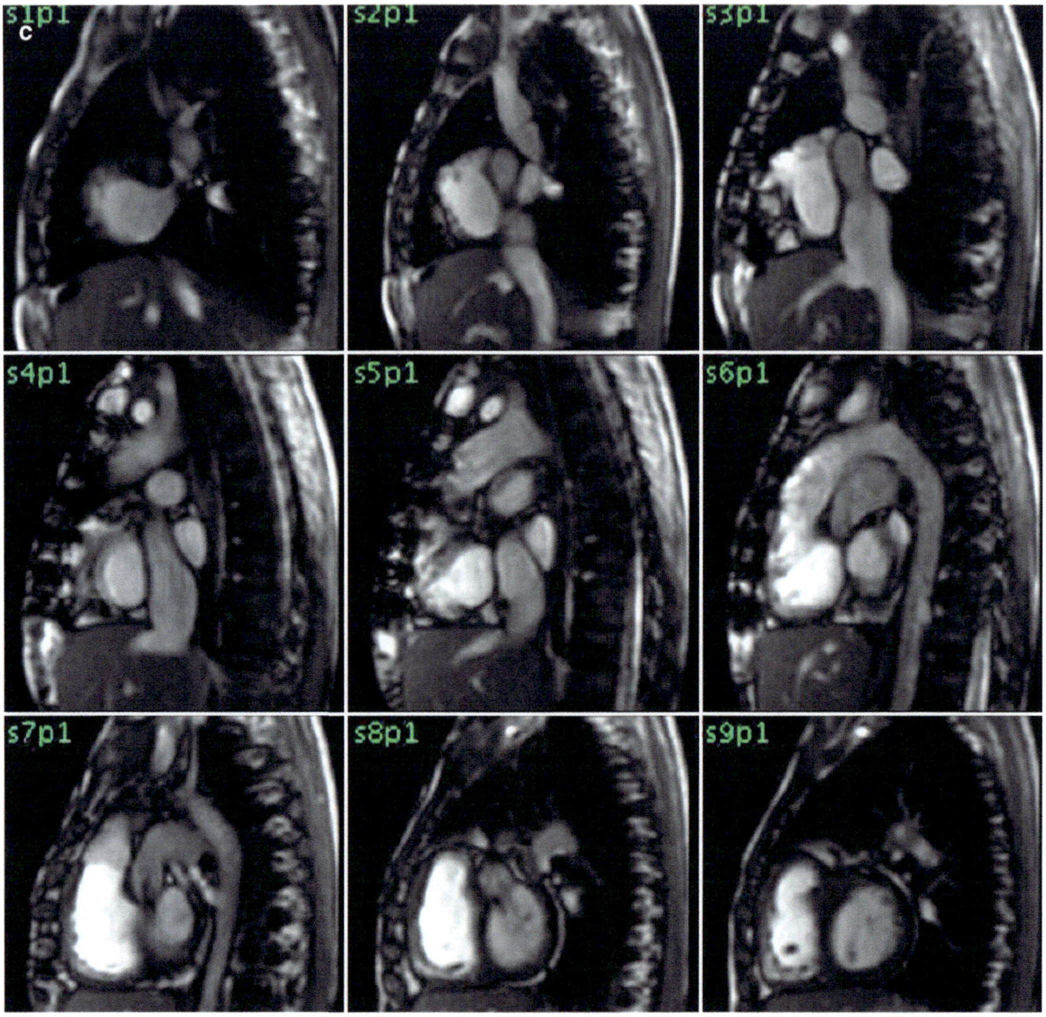

Fig. 5.14 (continued)

Short-axis evaluation of ventricular volume requires extra care in basal slice contouring, and it is helpful to use the cross-reference of two- and four-chamber planes together. In end-systolic (ES) phase, since atrioventricular valvular plane moves towards the apex, endocardial contour that can be drawn in end-diastolic (ED) phase may not be drawn in ES phase at a most basal slice (Fig. 5.17). In addition, there may be different endocardial contours along the valvular plane between the ED and ES phases. The final reconstructed volumetric 3D image from postprocessing needs to be assessed for respiratory misregistration artefacts (Fig. 5.19).

To achieve high quality and reliability, each centre should maintain a rigorous and consistent approach to imaging and analysis.

Normative data on ventricular parameters by CMR are available for children [25, 26].

5.14 MR Imaging Safety

The strong magnetic environment has the potential to pose serious risks to patients and MRI staff in several ways. Injuries can result from the static magnetic field (projectile impact injuries), very rapid gradient-field switching (induction of

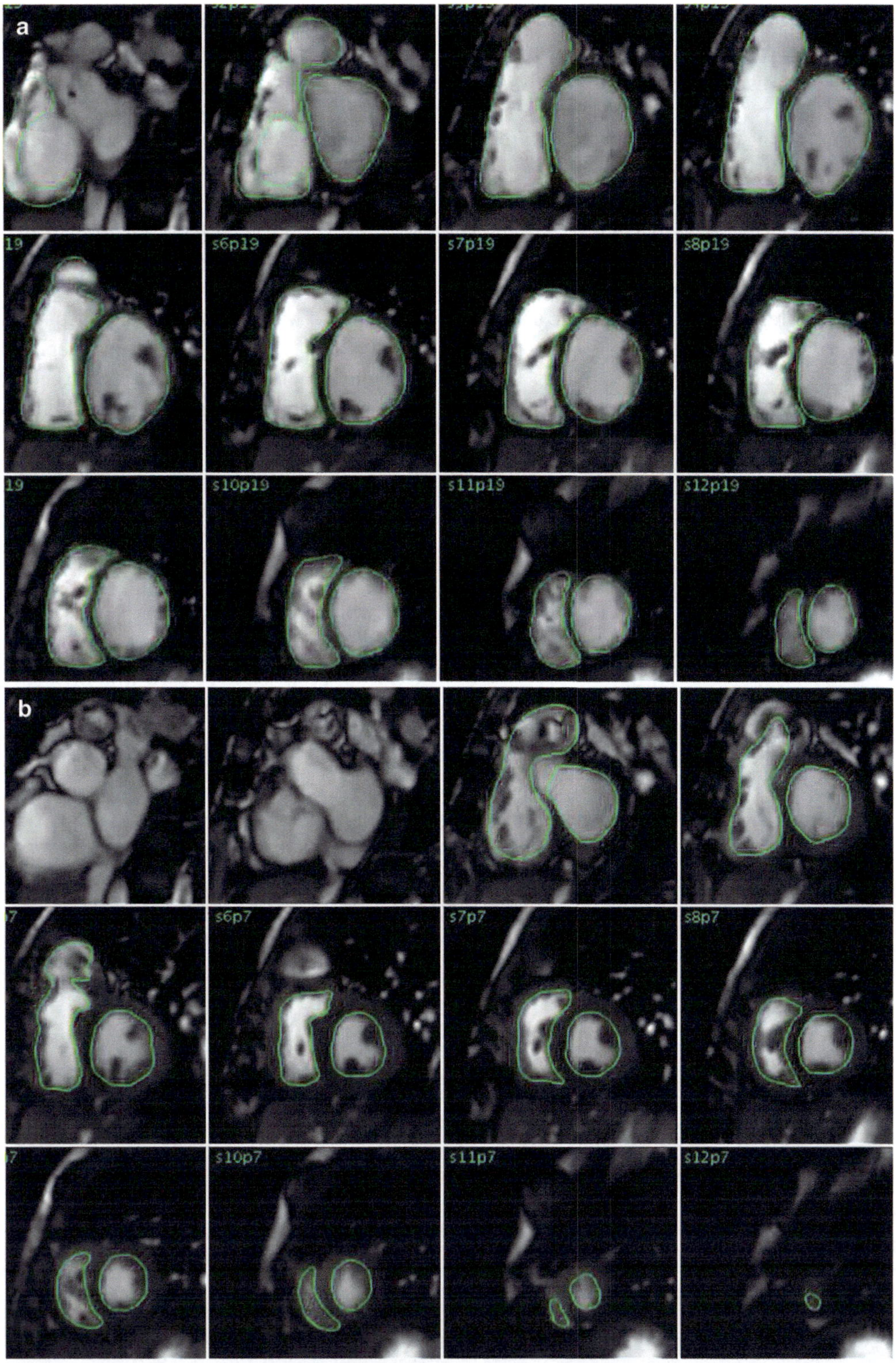

Fig. 5.15 End-diastolic (**a**) and end-systolic (**b**) frames of short-axis cine showing the contouring for volumetry calculations

electric currents leading to peripheral nerve stimulation), RF-energy deposition (heating of the imaged portion of the body), and acoustic noise [27].

Prior to shifting the patient into the MRI room, the physician and technologists should review the patient' s history and safety screening form to identify implanted devices that may be hazardous in the CMR environment or produce image artefact. If in doubt a screening radiograph of the chest or other region of concern may be useful to identify any metal implants.

Furthermore, many metallic objects in the normal uncontrolled medical environment, such as gas canisters, intravenous poles, or scissors, maybe quite magnetizable and can cause injury to the patient (or damage to the MRI system) if they are inadvertently brought close to the system.

Table 5.3 Differences between short-axis versus axial segmentation process

	Short axis	Axial
Pulmonary valve plane	Better	Poor
AV valve plane	Poor	Better
Respiratory depth variation	Less	More
Interobserver variation	High	Less
Acquisition planning	Difficult	Easy
Assessment of RWMA*	Better	Difficult

*RWMA - Regional wall motion abnormalities

To avoid these problems, all metal objects to be used in (or around) the MRI suite must first be carefully screened for magnetic risk, and all metal objects must be removed from both the patient and the medical personnel before they are allowed near the MRI system.

The use of MR-safe or compatible equipment (stethoscopes, wheelchairs, O2 cylinders, infusion pumps, monitors, etc.) with clear labeling of such in the scanner area reduces this risk further.

The RF magnetic fields used in MRI can be on the order of tens of kilowatts, strong enough to induce currents that can cause heating sufficient to damage tissue if loops of wire, such as the ECG monitoring leads used for cardiac gating are in contact with the skin. To minimize the risk of such injury, any monitoring leads should be as short as possible, without any loops, and only ECG leads designed to be used with MRI should be employed.

Many implanted cardiac pacemakers are sensitive to magnetic fields and may have their func-

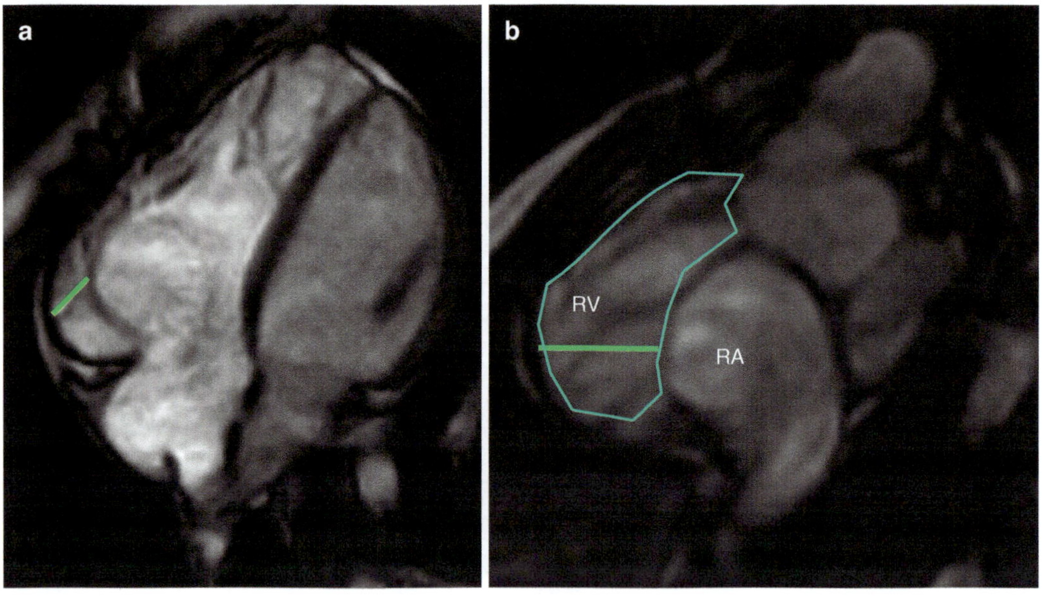

Fig. 5.16 Four-chamber reference image (**a**) showing the part of basal RV extending beyond AV valve plane requiring to contour the RV outside the atrium as shown in (**b**)

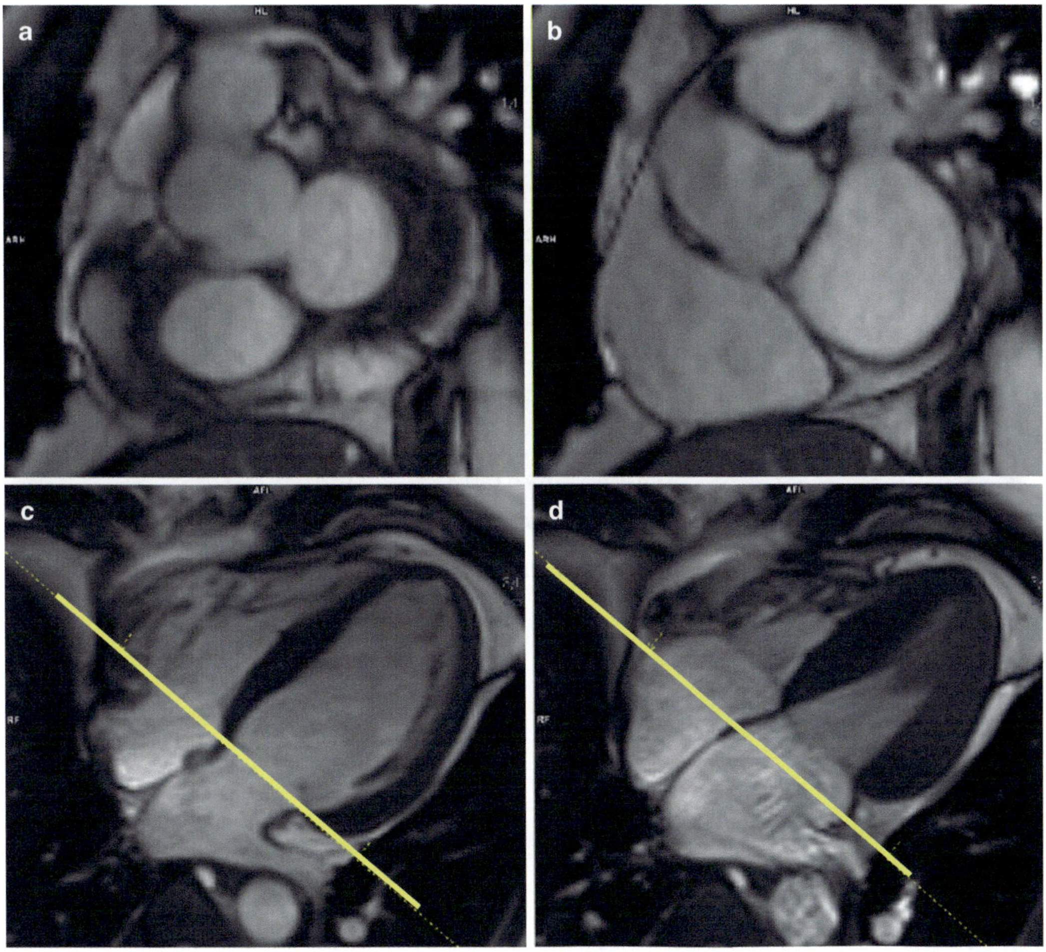

Fig. 5.17 Short-axis end-diastolic (**a**) and end-systolic (**b**) cine phase with corresponding four-chamber reference slice on end-diastolic phase (**c**) shows that the slice passes through ventricles. But the slice moved to atria level on end-systole (**d**)

tion altered by exposure to even a weak magnetic field, such as that in the vicinity of an MRI system. In the past, a cardiac implantable electronic device (CIED) was considered an absolute MRI contraindication. Due to recent technical developments, clinical reports have indicated that MRI can be performed safely under certain specific and controlled conditions, even in patients with CIED [28, 29].

Table 5.4 Differentiation between atrium and ventricle on basal short-axis cine

Characteristics	Atrium	Ventricle
Myocardial thickness	Thin	Thick
Size on ventricular systole compared to diastole	Bigger	Smaller
Relationship to coronary artery in the AV groove	More basal	More apical
Relationship to AV valve in the cavity	More basal	More apical

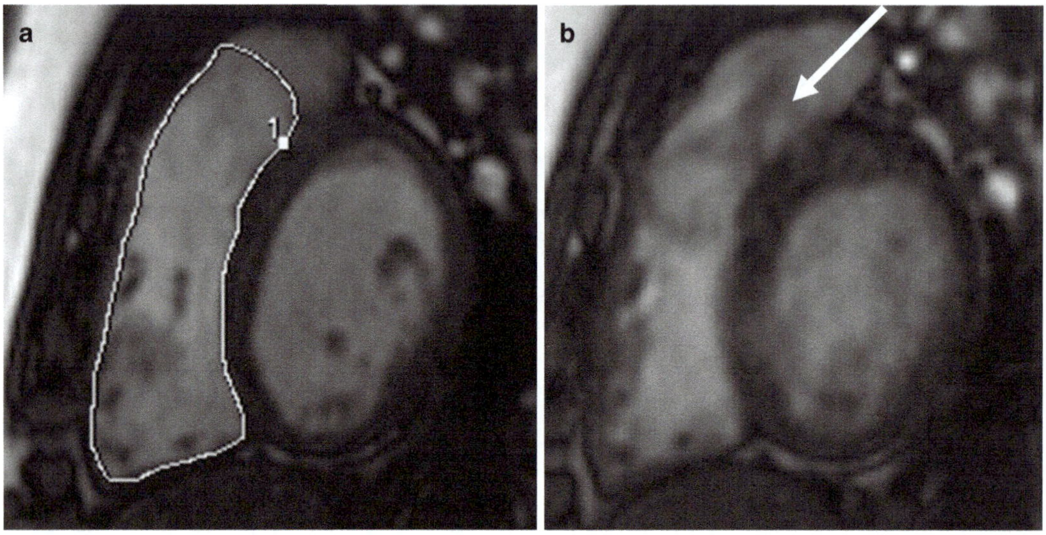

Fig. 5.18 (a) Contouring at basal short-axis frame is facilitated by viewing the full cine images. Arrow in (b) shows the level of the pulmonary valve

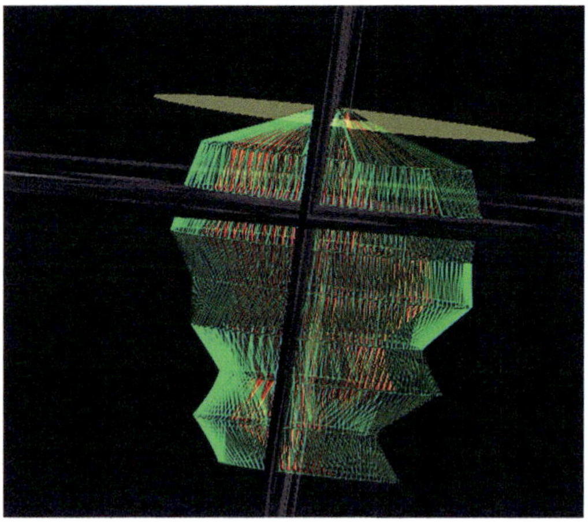

Fig. 5.19 Reconstructed 3D image from the final contouring shows significant respiratory misregistration artefacts limiting the accuracy of the values

References

1. Fratz S, Hess J, Schuhbaeck A, Buchner C, Hendrich E, Martinoff S, Stern H. Routine clinical cardiovascular magnetic resonance in paediatric and adult congenital heart disease: patients, protocols, questions asked and contributions made. J Cardiovasc Magn Reson. 2008;10:46.
2. Bailliard F, Hughes ML, Taylor AM. Introduction to cardiac imaging in infants and children: techniques, potential, and role in the imaging work-up of various cardiac malformations and other pediatric heart conditions. Eur J Radiol. 2008;68:191–8.
3. Shellock FG, Spinazzi A. MRI safety update 2008: part 2, screening patients for MRI. Am J Roentgenol. 2008;191:1140–9.
4. Windram J, Grosse-Wortmann L, Shariat M, Greer ML, Crawford MW, Yoo SJ. Cardiovascular MRI without sedation or general anesthesia using a feed-and -sleep technique in neonates and infants. Pediatr Radiol. 2011;42:183–7.
5. Odegard KC, DiNardo JA, Tsai-Goodman B, Powell AJ, Geva T, Laussen PC. Anaesthesia considerations for cardiac MRI in infants and small children. Pediatr Anesth. 2004;14:471–6. https://doi.org/10.1111/j.1460-9592.2004.01221.x.
6. Fogel MA, Weinberg P, Parave E, Harris C, Montenegro L, Concepcion M. Safety and efficacy of deep sedation in infants, children and adolescents undergoing cardiac magnetic resonance. J Pediatr. 2008;152:534–9.
7. Malviya S, Voepel-Lewis T, Eldevik OP, Rockwell DT, Wong JH, Tait AR. Sedation and general anaesthesia in children undergoing MRI and CT: adverse events and outcomes. Br J Anaesth. 2000;84:743–8.
8. Adam L, Dorfman MD, Odegard KC, Powell AJ, et al. Risk factors for adverse events during cardiovascular magnetic resonance in congenital heart disease. J Cardiovasc Magn Reson. 2007;9:793–8.
9. Fratz S, Chung T, Greil GF, et al. Guidelines and protocols for cardiovascular magnetic resonance in children and adults with congenital heart disease: SCMR expert consensus group on congenital heart disease. J Cardiovasc Magn Reson. 2013;15:51.

10. Boxt LM. Cardiac MR imaging: a guide for the beginner. Radiographics. 1999;19(4):1009–25. discussion 1026–8
11. Simonetti OP, Cook S. Technical aspects of pediatric CMR. J Cardiovasc Magn Reson. 2006;8(4):581–93.
12. Johansson B, Babu-Narayan SV, Kilner PJ. The effects of breath-holding on pulmonary regurgitation measured by cardiovascular magnetic resonance velocity mapping. J Cardiovasc Magn Reson. 2009;11:1.
13. Bhargava R, Hahn G, Hirsch W, et al. Contrast enhanced magnetic resonance imaging in pediatric patients: review and recommendations for current practice. Magn Reson Insights. 2013;6:95–111.
14. Runge VM. Safety of approved MR contrast media for intravenous injection. J Magn Reson Imaging. 2000;12:205–13.
15. Tibussek D, Rademacher C, Caspers J, et al. Gadolinium brain deposition after macrocyclic gadolinium administration: a pediatric case-control study. Radiology. 2017;285(1):223–30.
16. Simonetti OP, Finn JP, White RD, Laub G, Henry DA. Black-blood T2-weighted inversion recovery MR imaging of the heart. Radiology. 1996;199:49–57.
17. Carr J, Simonetti O, Bundy J, Li D, Pereles S, Finn J. Cine MR angiography of the heart with segmented true fast imaging with steady-state precession. Radiology. 2001;219:828–34.
18. Kellman P, Chefd'hotel C, Lorenz CH, et al. High spatial and temporal resolution cardiac cine MRI from retrospective reconstruction of data acquired in real time using motion correction and resorting. Magn Reson Med. 2009;62(6):1557–64.
19. Masui T, Katayama M, Kobayashi S, et al. Gadolinium- enhanced MR angiography in the evaluation of congenital cardiovascular disease pre- and postoperative states in infants and children. J Magn Reson Imaging. 2000;12(6):1034–42.
20. Sorensen TS, Korperich H, Greil GF, Eichhorn J, Barth P, Meyer H, Pedersen EM, Beerbaum P. Operator-independent isotropic three-dimensional magnetic resonance imaging for morphology in congenital heart disease: a validation study. Circulation. 2004;110:163–9.
21. Winter M, Bernink F, Groenink M, Bouma B, van Dijk A, Helbing W, Tijssen J, Mulder B. Evaluating the systemic right ventricle by CMR: the importance of consistent and reproducible delineation of the cavity. J Cardiovasc Magn Reson. 2008;10:40.
22. Sievers B, Kirchberg S, Bakan A, Franken U, Trappe HJ. Impact of papillary muscles in ventricular volume and ejection fraction assessment by cardiovascular magnetic resonance. J Cardiovasc Magn Reson. 2004;6(1):9–16.
23. Fratz S, Schuhbaeck A, Buchner C, Busch R, Meierhofer C, Martinoff S, Hess J, Stern H. Comparison of accuracy of axial slices versus short-axis slices for measuring ventricular volumes by cardiac magnetic resonance in patients with corrected tetralogy of fallot. Am J Cardiol. 2009;103:1764–9.
24. Alfakih K, Plein S, Bloomer T, Jones T, Ridgway J, Sivananthan M. Comparison of right ventricular volume measurements between axial and short axis orientation using steady-state free precession magnetic resonance imaging. J Magn Reson Imaging. 2003;18:25–32.
25. Sarikouch S, Peters B, Gutberlet M, Leismann B, Kelter-Kloepping A, Koerperich H, Kuehne T, Beerbaum P. Sex-specific pediatric percentiles for ventricular size and mass as reference values for cardiac MRI: assessment by steady-state free-precession and phase-contrast MRI flow. Circ Cardiovasc Imaging. 2010;3:65–76.
26. Buechel EV, Kaiser T, Jackson C, Schmitz A, Kellenberger CJ. Normal right and left ventricular volumes and myocardial mass in children measured by steady state free precession cardiovascular magnetic resonance. J Cardiovasc Magn Reson. 2009;11:19.
27. Nazarian S, Hansford R, Rahsepar AA, et al. Safety of magnetic resonance imaging in patients with cardiac devices. N Engl J Med. 2017;377:2555–64.
28. Roguin A. Magnetic resonance imaging in patients with implantable cardioverter-defibrillators and pacemakers. J Am Coll Cardiol. 2009;54:556–7.
29. Ainslie M, Miller C, Brown B, Schmitt M. Cardiac MRI of patients with implanted electrical cardiac devices. Heart. 2014;100:363–9.

Sequential Segmental Approach to CHD

6

Ramiah Rajeshkannan

6.1 Introduction

Recent advances in the technique of multidetector CT angiography (CTA) and cardiac magnetic resonance imaging (CMR) have stimulated the interest of radiologists in the diagnosis of congenital heart disease and encouraged the reappraisal of classifications and definitions used by cardiologists and cardiac surgeons. Different systems of classification and nomenclature have been described.

A standardised approach to congenital heart disease (CHD) is preferable as the number of individual lesions that can coexist within malformed hearts are considerable. If these alleged complex lesions are approached in a simple and straightforward fashion, none need to be difficult to understand and describe.

Earlier description and categorisation of CHD in the 1960s by Richard Van Praagh from USA and Maria Victoria de la Cruz from Mexico City were based on the topographic arrangements of the atrium, ventricles, and great arteries, thus developing the concept of concordance and discordance [1–3].

An alternative classification system known as sequential segmental analysis, which was developed in Europe by Anderson and colleagues, incorporates fundamental characteristics of the Van Praagh segmental classification system but emphasises the junctional variations across the atrioventricular (AV) and ventriculo-arterial (VA) connections also [4, 5].

There are still major differences of opinion as how best to cope with certain conditions, such as patients with splenic syndromes.

It is important that the system we use for describing a CHD should have more clarity, and the concept of sequential and segmental approach appears more appropriate at this point in time. This method is commonly used to facilitate communication between physicians from various specialties who are involved in diagnosing and managing these patients. By and large, there is no right or wrong way of describing the hearts, simply different ways.

The remainder of this chapter offers a step-by-step guide for using the sequential segmental analysis system to report key imaging findings that allow accurate diagnosis and appropriate management of CHD.

Four different CMR cases of visceral heterotaxy with full reports are available at online-only video files.

Electronic Supplementary Material The online version of this chapter (https://doi.org/10.1007/978-981-15-6755-1_6) contains supplementary material, which is available to authorized users.

R. Rajeshkannan (✉)
Department of Radiology, Amrita School of Medicine, Amrita Institute of Medical Sciences and Research Centre, Amrita Vishwa Vidyapeetham, Kochi, Kerala, India
e-mail: rajeshkr@aims.amrita.edu

R. Rajeshkannan et al. (eds.), *CT and MRI in Congenital Heart Diseases*,
https://doi.org/10.1007/978-981-15-6755-1_6

6.2 Basic Concepts of Sequential and Segmental Approach

This system is based on three different facets of the cardia, namely (1) morphology of the cardiac components, (2) the way they are connected together, and (3) the relations between them.

Basically, the heart is considered as a segmented structure and has three building blocks or regions, namely the atriums, the ventricular mass, and the great arterial trunks with two junctions between them namely atrioventricular and ventriculo-arterial [6]. Each region is partitioned into the left- and right-sided component.

First visceroatrial situs is established by determining the thoraco-abdominal visceral positions and arrangements of morphological right and left atrium. Then each segment of the cardiac structure is assessed in a sequential manner in the direction of blood flow, i.e. starting from systemic and pulmonary venous blood flow, both atria, atrioventricular valves, ventricles, semilunar valves and finally the great arteries.

A catalogue is then made of all associated cardiac and, where pertinent, non-cardiac malformations including the orientation of cardiac apex and the position of the heart in relation to the sternum.

It is important to note that the right- and left-sided cardiac chambers are defined by their intrinsic morphology rather than by location within the chest. For example, if a patient's right atrium is on the left side, it should still be called the (morphological) right atrium because it has the characteristic structure of a right atrium. So the term morphologic left or morphologic right is used to indicate that the characteristic structure is meant without any implication about the actual location of the structure.

6.3 Morphologic Features of Different Cardiac Chambers

6.3.1 Atria

Anatomically each atrium has three segments: appendage, venous component, and the interatrial septum. Since the venous connection to the atria are highly variable in the setting of CHD, morphologic right and left atria are identified mainly by the morphology of the appendages.

The morphologically right atrial appendage has the shape of a blunt triangle (tongue shape), and its cavity has a broad base with the remainder of the atrium (Fig. 6.1). The junction is marked externally by the terminal groove and internally by the terminal crest. Its most significant feature

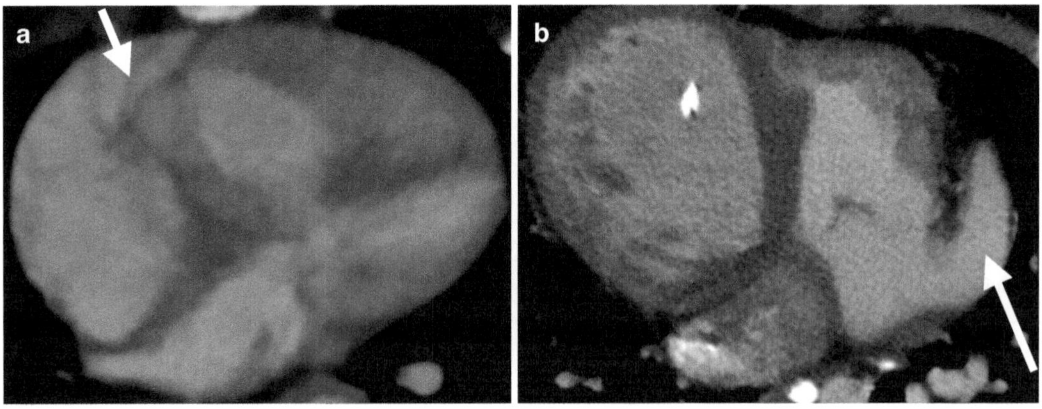

Fig. 6.1 (**a**) The morphologically right atrial appendage (arrow) has the shape of a blunt triangle (tongue shape), and its cavity has a broad base with the remainder of the atrium. (**b**) The left atrial appendage (arrow) is typically narrower than the right and has a tubular, fingerlike configuration and its connection to the atrium is also narrower

is that the pectinate muscles lining the appendage extend all round the parietal atrioventricular junction. The septal surface on the RA side consists of superior and inferior limbic bands. The supradiaphragmatic IVC and coronary sinus usually drain into morphological RA. Eustachian and Thebesian valves commonly guard the entrances of IVC and coronary sinus.

The left atrial appendage is typically narrower than the right and has a tubular, finger-like configuration with several lobes. Its connection to the atrium is also narrower, and the pectinate muscles are confined within the appendage. The posterior aspect of the morphologically left vestibule, also containing the coronary sinus, being smooth-walled as it merges with the pulmonary venous component. Important differences between the morphological right and left atrium are summarised in Table 6.1.

Why should we need to differentiate morphologic LA from RA?

Since the major conduction system of the heart namely sinoatrial (SA) node and atrioventricular (AV) node are located on the morphological RA, changes in atrial morphology will alter these pathways and may affect the surgical management. For example, in patients having right isomerism with normal systemic and pulmonary venous drainage to either side of heart, the presence of two SA nodes can lead to additional conduction pathways [7].

Table 6.1 Differences between morphological right and left atrium

Character	Morphological RA	Morphological LA
Appendage	Blunt triangle (tongue like)	Tubular (finger like)
Appendageal orifice with atrium	Wide	Narrow
Pectinate muscles	Extend up to AV junction	Confined to appendage
Crista terminalis	Present	Absent
Fossa ovalis and limbus	Present	Absent
IVC and coronary sinus	Usually drain into RA	No

6.3.2 Ventricles

Description of ventricles, no matter how malformed they may be, is facilitated by analysing their three components. These are:

(a) Inlet—extending from the atrioventricular junction to the distal attachment of the atrioventricular valvar tension apparatus.
(b) Apical trabecular component—extending from the papillary muscle to the apex.
(c) Outlet component—supporting the leaflets of the arterial valve.

Out of these three components, it is the apical trabecular component that is almost universally present in normal as well as in malformed and incomplete ventricles [4]. The RV has coarse trabeculations and LV has fine trabeculations with smooth wall. The tricuspid valve always goes with RV and has three leaflets. Mitral valve is attached to LV and has only two leaflets without septal attachment. The tricuspid valve is positioned closer to the apex in comparison to the mitral valve (Fig. 6.2). The moderator band, extending from the base of the papillary muscle to the septum, is present only in the RV. On the LV side mitral—aortic valve fibrous continuity is present, whereas conus muscle bundle separates the tricuspid valve and pulmonary valve on the RV (Fig. 6.3) (Table 6.2).

In the morphological right ventricle of a normal heart, irrespective of its position in space, only the palmar surface of the right hand can be placed on the septal surface such that the thumb occupies the inlet and the fingers fit into the outlet. The palmar surface of the left hand then fits in comparable fashion within the morphological left ventricle. Using CTA or MR angiography (MRA), the hand rule is best applied by using either a three-dimensional hollow view rotated so that the right ventricular side of the septum is visible or, alternatively, a vertical long-axis image is obtained with oblique multiplanar reconstruction at an angle that allows visualisation of the outflow tract [8] (Fig. 6.4).

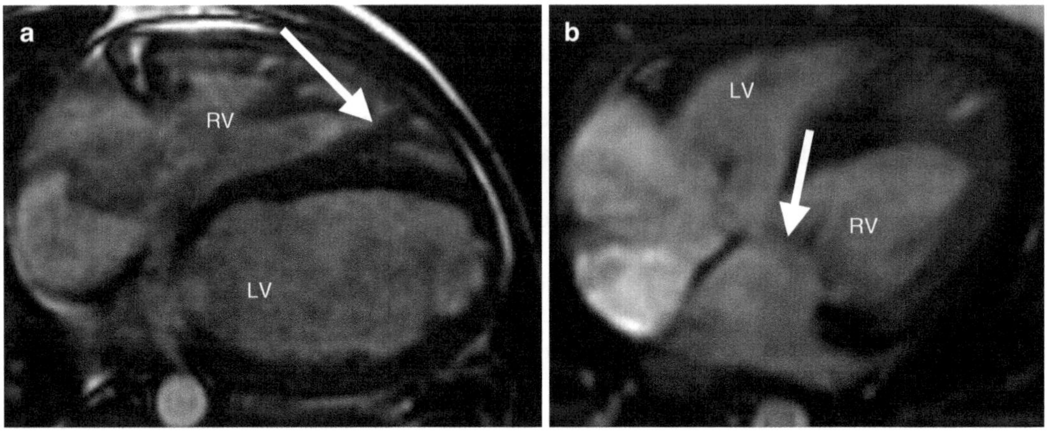

Fig. 6.2 Irrespective of their location (right-sided RV in **a**, left-sided RV in **b**) morphological right and left ventricle have characteristic anatomic features. Moderator band (arrow in **a**) and more apically placed tricuspid valve compared to mitral valve (arrow in **b**) are features of RV. Smooth septal surface is seen at LV side

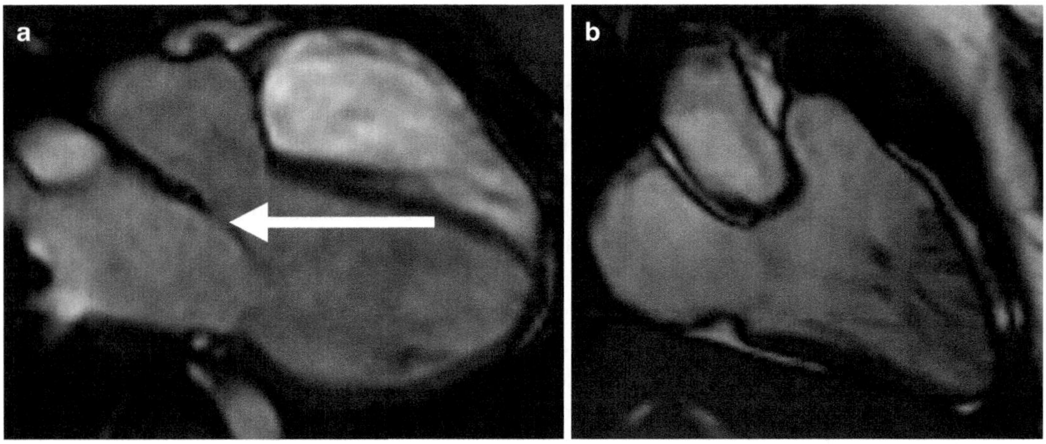

Fig. 6.3 (**a**) LV three-chamber view shows aorto-mitral fibrous continuity (arrow). (**b**) RV inlet–outlet view shows absent tricuspid–pulmonary valve fibrous continuity

Why should we need to differentiate morphologic LV from RV?

In conditions like LTGA (L-Transposition of Great Arteries), the physiology of pulmonary and systemic circulation may be normal. But since the morphologic RV is connected to aorta, it cannot withstand the systemic pressure and eventually fails in the adult life.

6.3.3 Great Arteries

Aorta and pulmonary artery can be easily identified by their branching pattern. Ascending aorta gives off three major branches and continues as descending aorta, whereas the main pulmonary artery divides early into two branches. Aortic sinuses can be identified by recognising the origin of coronary arteries from them. In almost all cases, the aortic arch crosses superior to the bifurcation of the pulmonary arteries.

The position of the greater mass of the heart, with respect to the sternum, is described by using the prefix levo (leftward), dextro (rightward), or meso (centre) in combination with the noun position. The abnormalities in cardiac position can be either primary or secondary to changes in the lungs, bones, or other extracardiac structures. For example, right lung collapse leads to dextroposed heart with normal leftward orientation of apex without any intrinsic cardiac abnormalities. However, when describing cardiac abnormality in relation to the base-apex long axis then the prefix is combined with the root word cardia. So dextrocardia is defined as a right-sided heart with long axis directed rightward resulting from a developmental anomaly. The term dextroversion in situs solitus is used when the cardiac apex fails to pivot to the left and the heart appears to have twisted to the right [9]. It is important to note that on CT and MRI, the cardiac base-apex is better defined in coronal images than axial.

Table 6.2 Differences between morphological right and left ventricle

Character	Morphological RV	Morphological LV
Moderator band	Present	Absent
Trabeculations	Coarse and irregular	Thin and fine
Septal surface	Coarse due to attachment of the septal papillary muscle	Smooth
AV valve	Tricuspid	Bicuspid
Septal attachment of AV valve	More apical	More basal
Continuity between AV valve and semilunar valve	Discontinuous by infundibulum	Fibrous continuity
Septal and parietal band	Present	Smooth superior septal surface

6.4 Anatomical Analysis of Each Segment

The sequential segmental approach to CHD consists of the following six steps:

I. Determining the visceroatrial situs
II. Ascertain atrioventricular junction and arrangement of AV valves
III. Determining the orientation of the ventricular loop
IV. Analysing ventriculo-arterial connections
V. Determining the origin and position of the great vessels
VI. Related intra- and intersegmental abnormalities

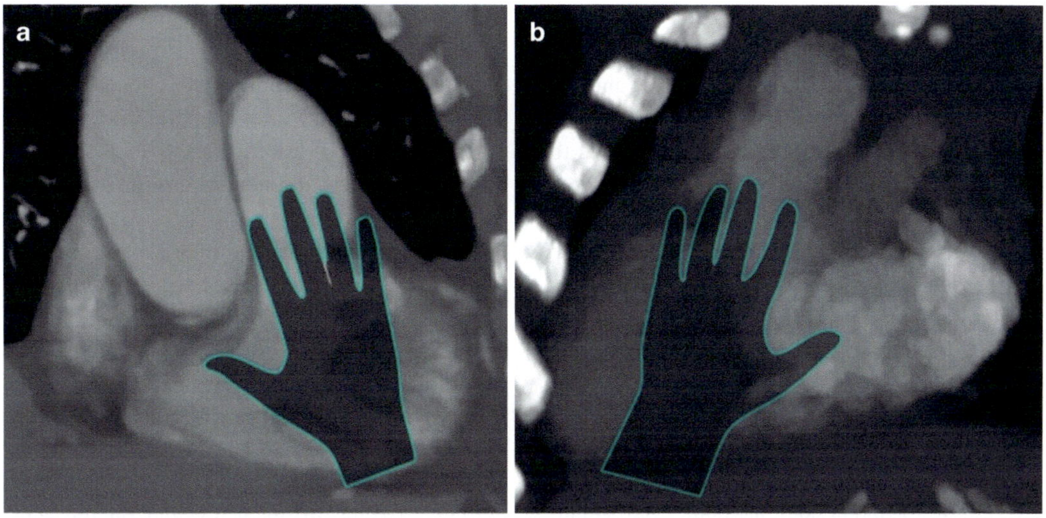

Fig. 6.4 Coronal oblique cardiac CT image with a superimposed hand shows how the hand rule is used to determine the orientation of the ventricular loop. While viewing the heart from the anterior to the posterior direction, the viewer imagines placing a hand into the morphologic right ventricle with the palm against the interventricular septum, the thumb in the right ventricular inflow tract, and the fingers in the outflow tract. If this exercise can be performed with the right hand (**a**), a D-loop is present; if it can be performed only with the left hand (**b**), an L-loop is present

Along with this analysis, Van Praagh's three-part notation consisting of letters separated by commas and encompassed by a set of braces is used to succinctly describe the three cardiac segments. This is detailed as:

I. Visceroatrial Situs (X, _, _)

Description of visceroatrial situs consists of three parts: visceral situs, thoracic (bronchopulmonary), and atrial situs. Three different anatomic configurations may be observed: situs solitus (normal) depicted as (S, _, _), situs inversus (inverted) depicted as (I, _, _) or situs ambiguous (ambiguous) depicted as (A, _, _).

The term situs refers to the position of the heart and viscera relative to midline. The Latin term situs solitus means the site or situation that is usual, ordinary, or customary.

The first step in the assessment of the cardiac anatomy is to locate and identify the morphological left and right atria based on the appearance of their appendages. However, sometimes the appendages are not reliably identifiable on cross-sectional imaging, and the localisation of noncardiac organs is more helpful for determining the correct situs.

(a) Visceral Situs

In the normal anatomic configuration (visceral situs solitus), the largest lobe of the liver and IVC are on the right side, and the spleen, stomach, and aorta are on the left. Situs inversus indicates the mirror-image location of the viscera relative to situs solitus. Situs ambiguous, or heterotaxia, is defined as an abnormal arrangement of organs and vessels as opposed to the orderly arrangement typical of situs solitus and situs inversus. In contrast to individuals with situs solitus or situs inversus with dextrocardia, those with situs ambiguous have congenital heart disease in 50%–100% of cases [10].

The two major subcategories of situs ambiguous are polysplenia and asplenia. Polysplenia (left isomerism) is characterised in general by midline or ambiguous location of the majority of the abdominal organs and multiple spleens (Fig. 6.5).

Situs ambiguous with asplenia (right isomerism) is characterised by the ambiguous location of the abdominal organs and absence of the spleen (Fig. 6.6). Patients with aplenia have a 99%–100% prevalence of CHD that is much more severe than that seen with polysplenia and the other situs anomalies [11].

As per venoatrial concordant rule, IVC is located on the side of the morphologically right appendage and the abdominal aorta lies to opposite sides of the spine [12]. When there is isomerism, then the great vessels usually lie to the same side of the spine, with the IVC in anterior position in those with right isomerism, and posterior, or with the azygos vein posterior, in those having left isomerism (Fig. 6.7). However, as shown in Fig. 6.7d, exceptions can occur. Interrupted IVC with azygos continuation is a feature of left isomerism.

(b) Thoracic Situs

Description of thoracic situs includes the morphology of right and left main bronchus, the relationship between the corresponding pulmonary arteries, and the number of lobes in the lung. The right main bronchus is shorter, wider, and more vertical compared to the left main bronchus. Right bronchus divides early to give rise to upper lobe bronchus.

Right upper lobe bronchus is located above the right pulmonary artery (eparterial bronchus) whereas the left side bronchus is located below the corresponding pulmonary artery (hyparterial bronchus) (Fig. 6.8).

The right side lung has three lobes compared to two lobes on the left side.

(c) Atrial Situs

Morphological right and left atria are identified primarily based on the intrinsic features of the appendages as describes earlier.

As per viscero-atrial concordant rule, the morphological right atrium is located on the same side as liver, eparterial bronchus, and morphological right lung [2]. Morphological left atrium is located on the side of spleen, hyparterial bronchus, and bilobed lung.

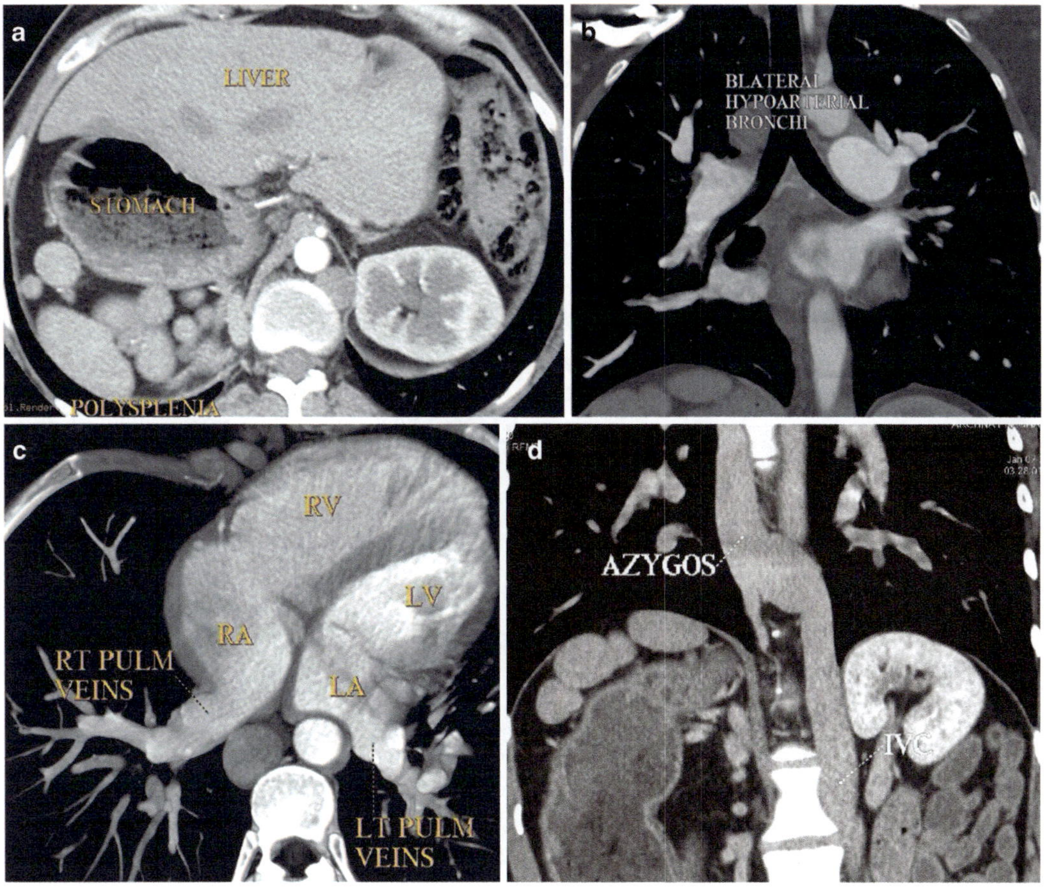

Fig. 6.5 Case of left isomerism showing multiple spleens on the right side (**a**), bilateral hyparterial bronchus (**b**), anomalous pulmonary venous connection to the right-sided atrium (**c**) and azygos continuation of IVC (**d**)

Left isomerism is usually indicated by bilateral LA appendages, bilateral bilobed lungs, interruption of the IVC, multiple spleens and pulmonary veins that drain into both the right- and the left-sided atria.

When there is right isomerism, bilateral RA appendages, bilateral trilobed lungs, a large symmetric liver, absent spleen, and total anomalous pulmonary venous return are frequently observed.

Practical Pearls

Viscero-atrial concordant rule: the visceral situs is highly predictive of the atrial situs.

Venoatrial concordance rule: The atrium which is directly connected to IVC is morphological RA.

Right isomerism: At the level of the diaphragm, IVC is anterior to the aorta.

Left isomerism: IVC/azygos vein lies posterior to the aorta.

II. Atrioventricular Junction

In order to analyse accurately the morphology of the atrioventricular junction, it is necessary to know the atrial arrangement and the morphology of the ventricular mass so as to establish which atrium is connected to which ventricle. With this information in hand, it is possible to define the specific patterns of connection across the AV junctions and to determine the morphology of the valves guarding the atrioventricular junctions.

Atrioventricular (AV) connection can be either biventricular or univentricular. When the two atria are connected to two good size ventricles then it is called biventricular connection. In uni-

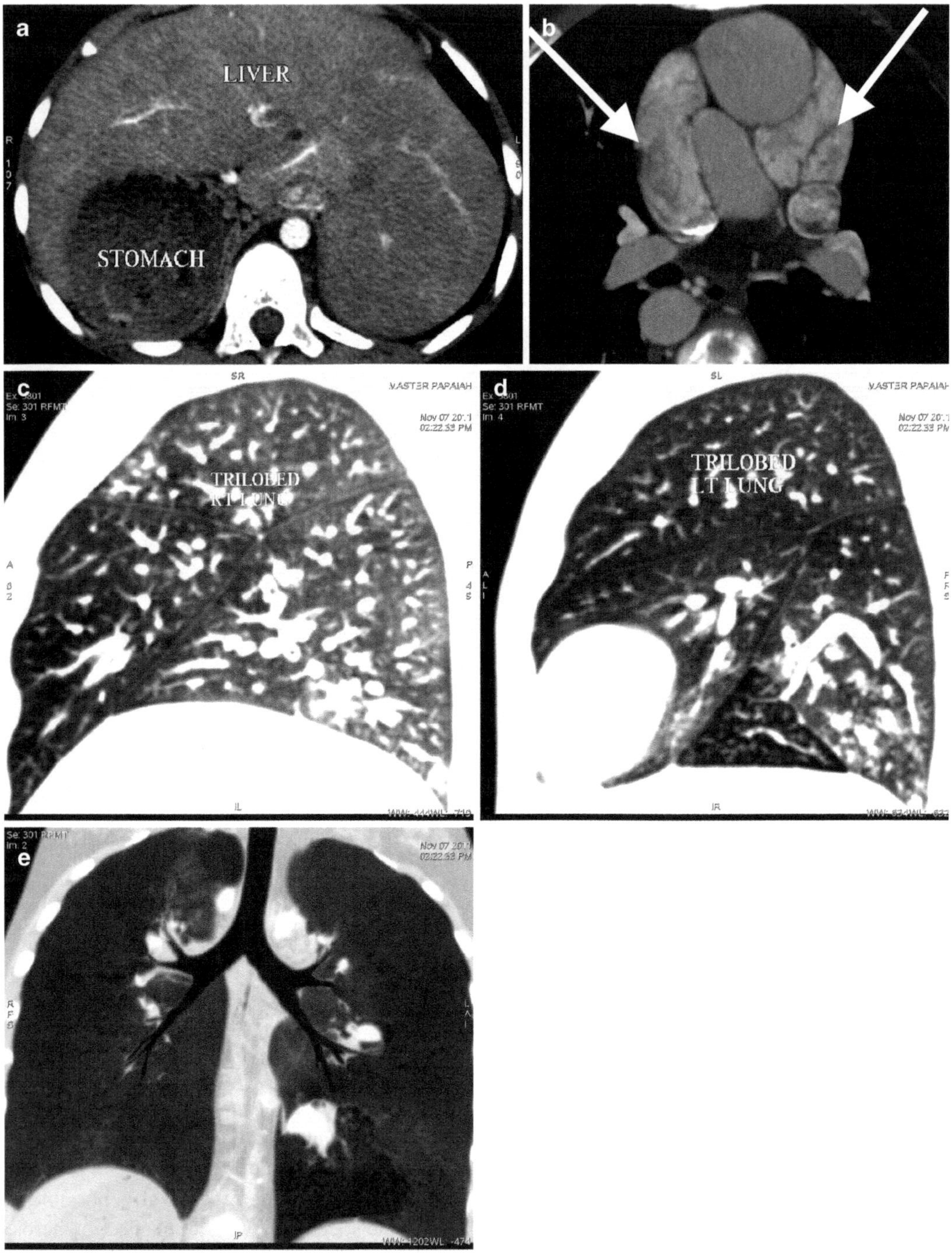

Fig. 6.6 Visceroatrial concordance in right isomerism. (**a**) Shows situs ambiguous with right side stomach and absent spleen. Both atrial appendages show right-sided morphology (arrows in **b**). Both side lungs are trilobed (**c**, **d**) with both bronchi showing right-sided morphology (**e**)

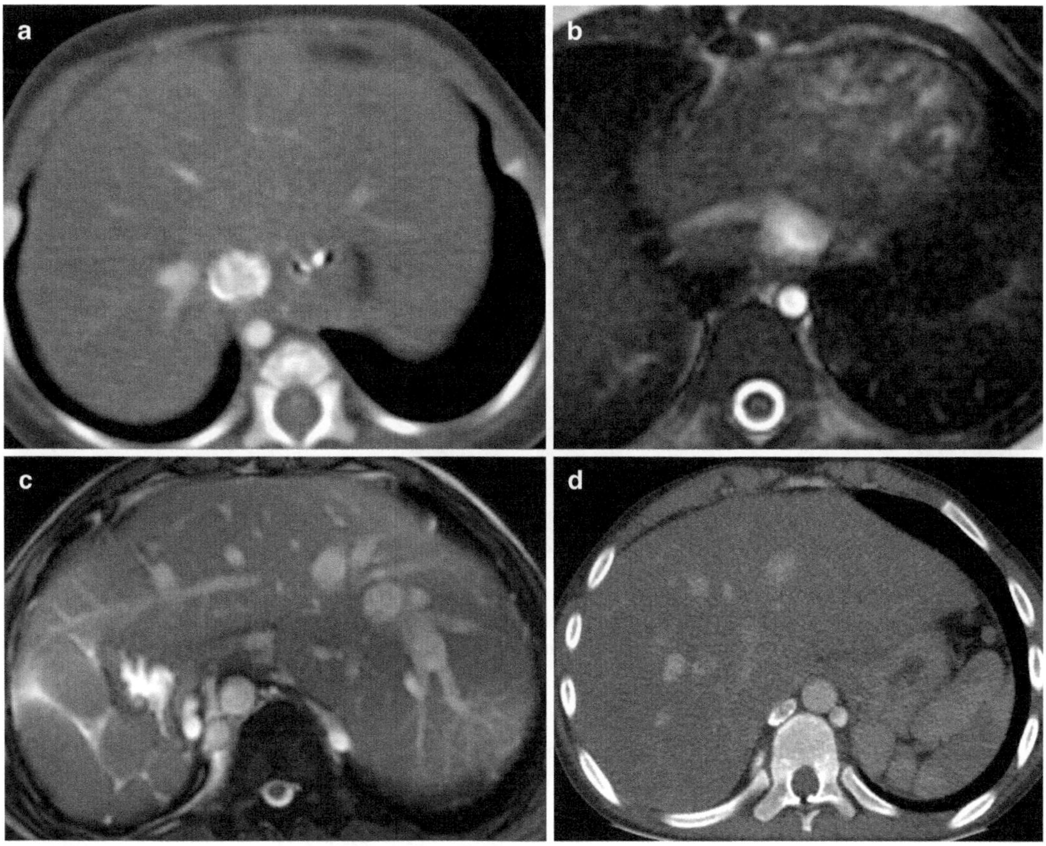

Fig. 6.7 Relationship between abdominal aorta and IVC at the level of diaphragm in situs anomalies. (**a**, **b**) Cases with right isomerism shows the IVC and aorta on the same side of the spine with IVC located anteriorly. (**c**). Patient with left isomerism shows azygos continuation of IVC posterior to the aorta on the same side. (**d**) Patient with left isomerism shows side-by-side location of aorta and azygos vein

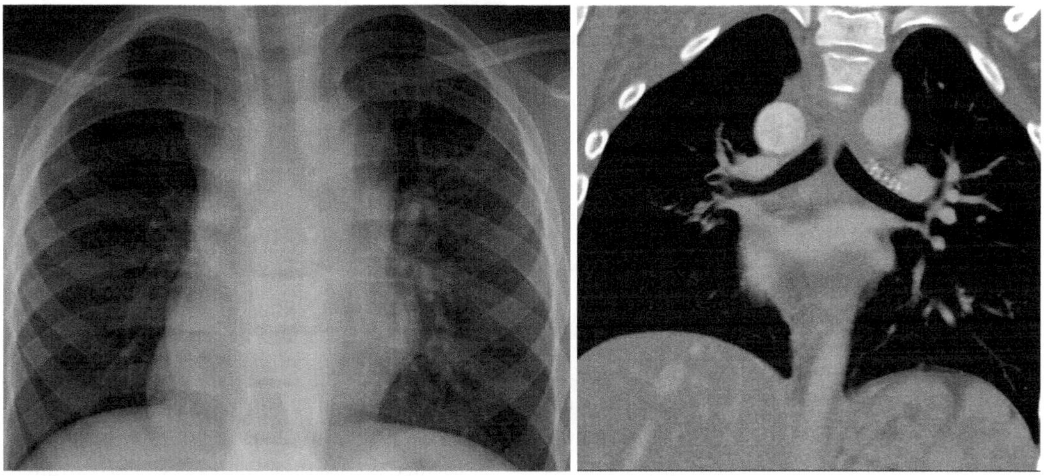

Fig. 6.8 Chest X-ray shows bilateral long bronchi without early branch suggesting left-sided morphology. Coronal reformatted CT confirms bilateral hyparterial bronchi

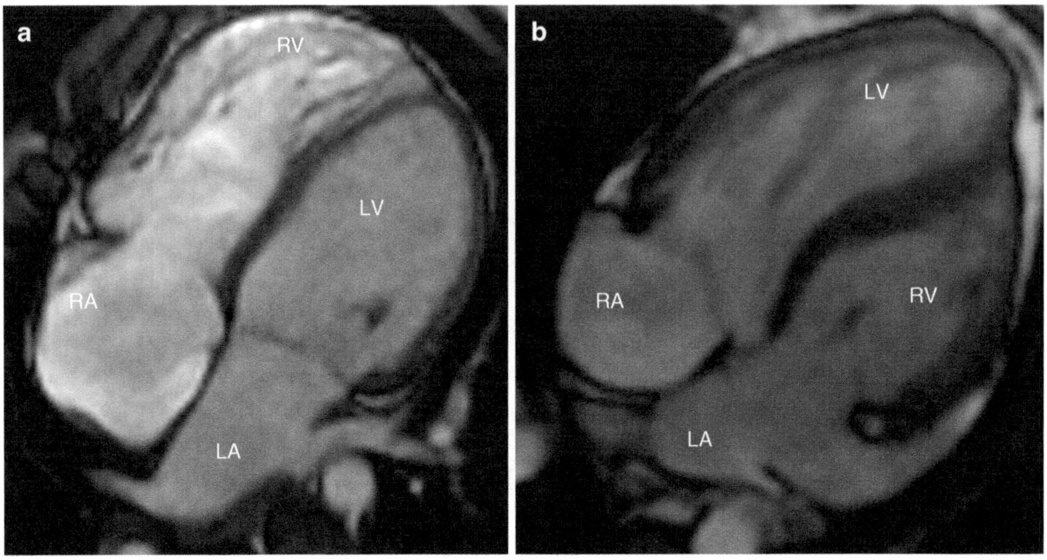

Fig. 6.9 Biventricular AV connection. (**a**) Concordant AV connection. (**b**) Discordant AV connection, in which RA is connected to LV and LA is connected to RV. LV can be identified by the smooth septal surface and more basal attachment of its AV valve

ventricular AV connection, only one of the ventricles, if indeed two are present, is in communication with the atrial cavities.

(A) Biventricular Connection

In the concordant connection, the right atrium is connected to the right ventricle and the left atrium to the left ventricle. In a discordant connection, the right atrium is connected to the left ventricle and the left atrium to the right ventricle (Fig. 6.9). In atrial isomerism, the term ambiguous connection is used. So it can be right isomeric atria with biventricular connection or left isomeric atria with biventricular connection. Rarely both AV valves may be fused to form a common valve with five leaflets.

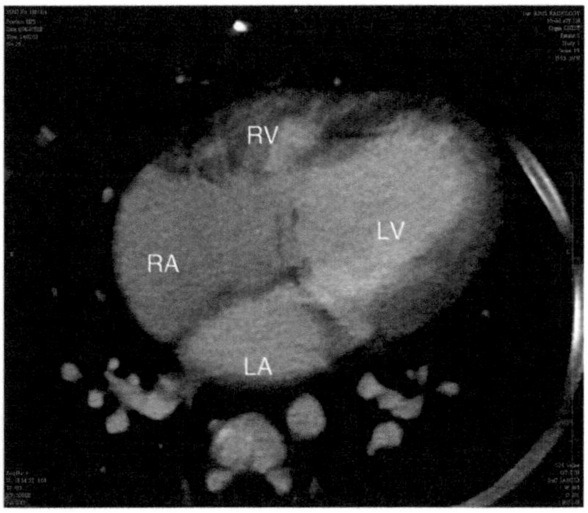

Fig. 6.10 Double inlet LV (DILV). Both atria are draining into LV with hypoplastic RV located anteriorly

(B) Univentricular Connection

Three types of univentricular AV connections can be seen:

(a) Double inlet ventricle (LV or RV), i.e. the two AV valves open into a single ventricle. Here the cavities of right- and left-sided atrial chambers are connected directly to the same ventricle (Fig. 6.10).
(b) Atresia of one of the AV valves (tricuspid or mitral atresia) (Figs. 6.11 and 6.12). In the univentricular heart, the dominant ventricle is usually left ventricle.
(c) Very rarely, one of the atrioventricular connections is absent and the solitary atrioventricular junction, via a straddling valve, is connected to two ventricles. This arrangement is uniatrial but biventricular.

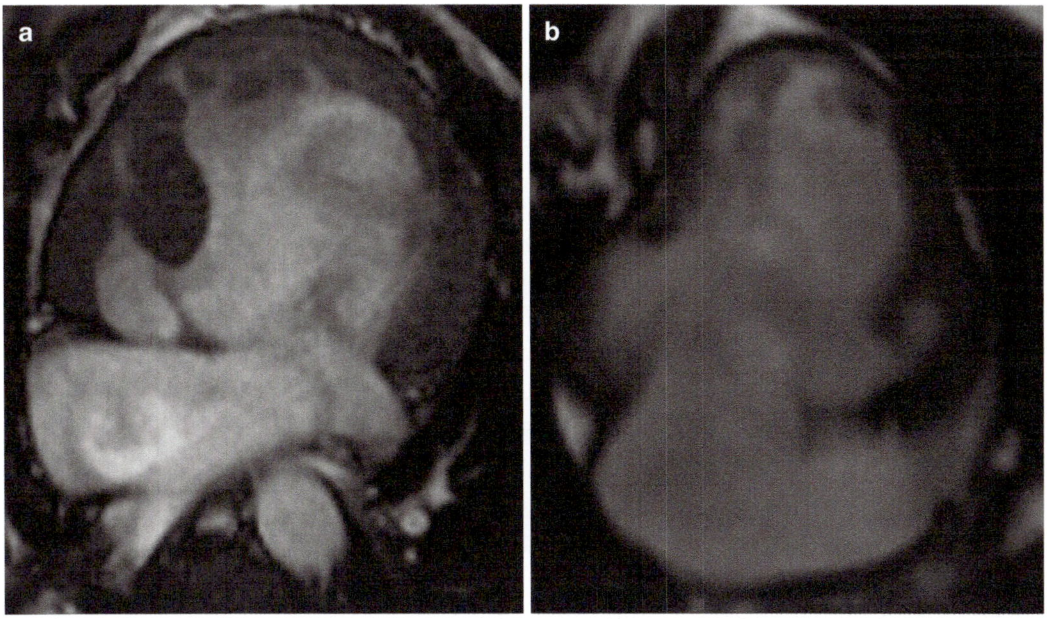

Fig. 6.11 Absent AV connection. (**a**) Shows Tricuspid atresia and (**b**) shows mitral atresia

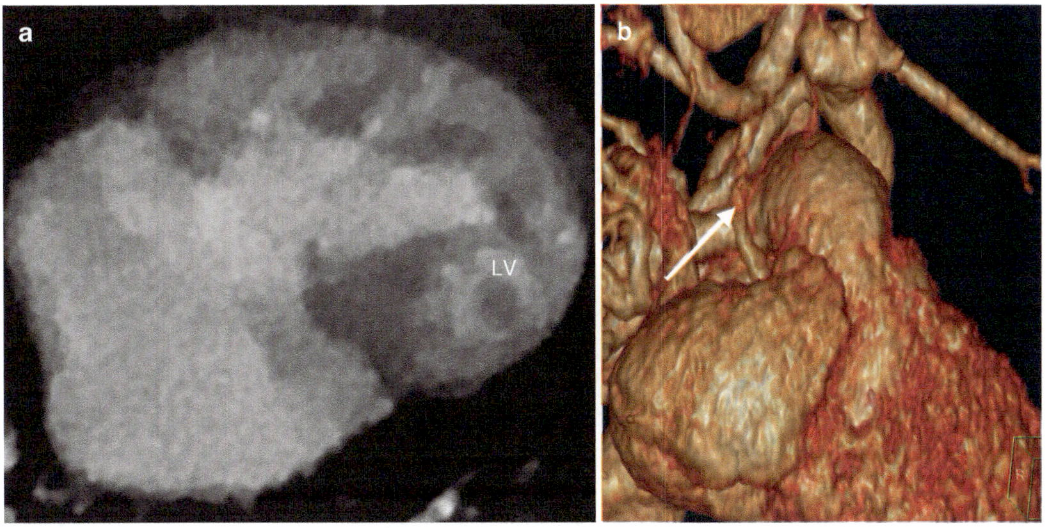

Fig. 6.12 Oblique axial CT image (**a**) shows hypoplastic left heart (LV) with mitral atresia. VRT image (**b**) of the same child shows hypoplastic ascending aorta (arrow)

Practical Pearls
Types of AV connection:

(A) Biventricular: concordant, discordant, right isomeric, or left isomeric
(B) Univentricular: DILV, DIRV, mitral atresia, or tricuspid atresia
(C) Uniatrial biventricular

Arrangement of AV Valves
The morphology of the AV valves guarding the overall atrioventricular junctional area is independent of the patterns that depend on the way that the myocardium of both atriums is joined to the ventricular myocardium around the entirety of the atrioventricular junctions.

The right- and left-sided atrioventricular junctions may be guarded by two patent valves, by one patent valve and one imperforate valve, by a common valve (Fig. 6.13), or by straddling and overriding valves.

Straddling indicates anomalous insertion of tensor apparatus (chordae tendineae and papillary muscles) of AV valve into the contralateral ventricle, either along its septum or its free wall. Overriding indicates abnormal alignment or connection of AV valve in which one valve annulus opens into another ventricle through a VSD. In the overriding AV valve, the atrioventricular junction is connected to ventricles on both sides of an interventricular septum.

III. Determining the Orientation of the Ventricular Loop (_, X, _)
During embryologic development, the primitive heart is like a tube, consisting of several segments that eventually give rise to the main cardiac components. During development, the tube folds over itself normally to the right (D-loop) with the right ventricle on the right side of the left ventricle. If the tube curves towards the left, the right ventricle is positioned leftward of the left ventricle, forming an L-loop [13].

On imaging, if the morphological RV (MRV) is located on the right side of morphological LV (MLV), then the letter D can be assigned to denote the presence of a D-loop (_, D, _). If the MRV is leftward of the left ventricle, it indicates an L-loop, and the letter L can be assigned (_, L, _) (Fig. 6.14).

To apply "Hand rule", we can use 3D reconstructed CT or MR angio image and view the heart from anterior to posterior direction. If we imagine placing our hand in the MRV with the palm against interventricular septum with the thumb pointing towards the inlet and fingers in

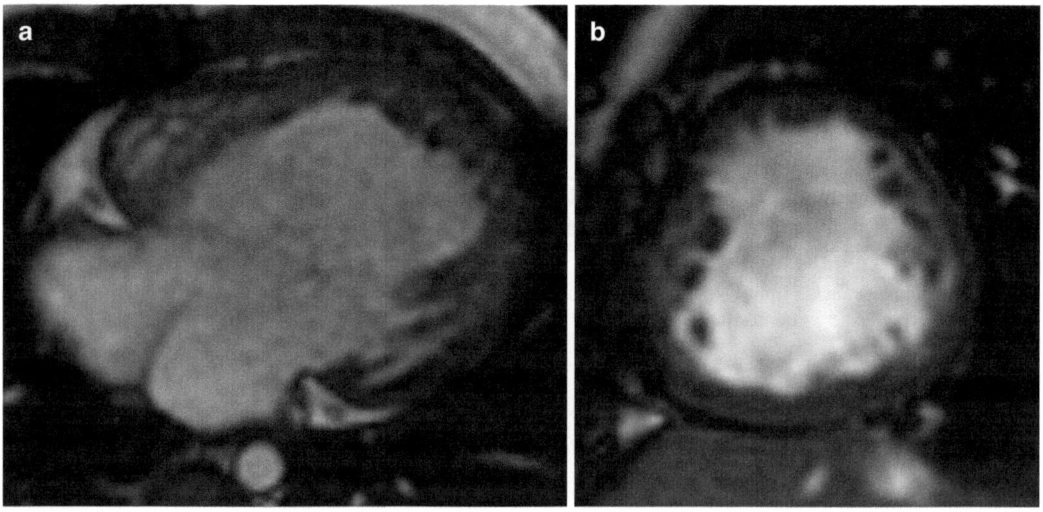

Fig. 6.13 Common AV canal defect. Four chamber (**a**) and short axis (**b**) MRI shows large primum ASD and inlet VSD, single large ventricle of indeterminate morphology with common AV valve

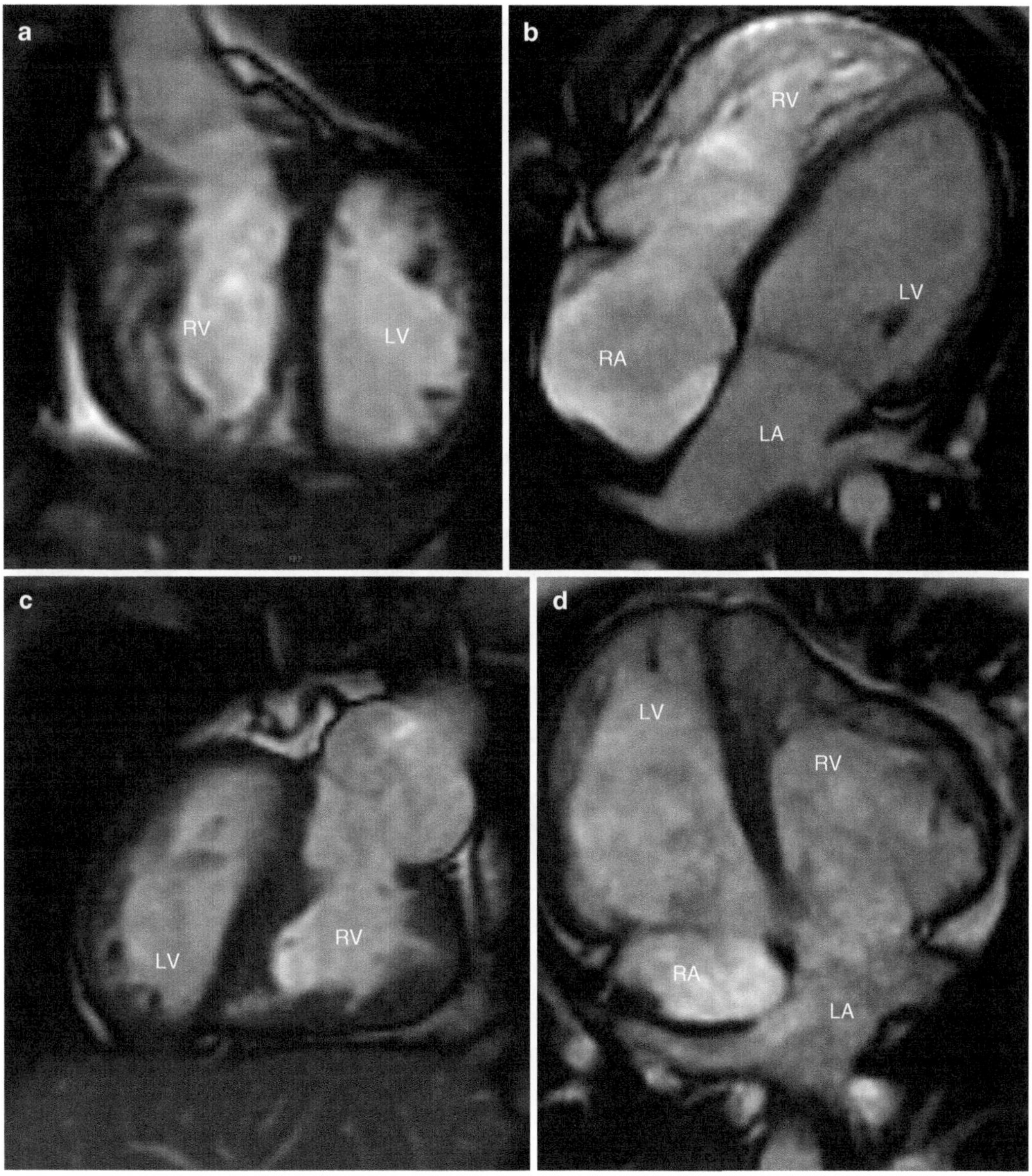

Fig. 6.14 In D-loop, RV is located on the right side of LV (**a**, **b**). In L-loop, RV is located on the left side of LV (**c**, **d**)

the outflow tract. If this can be performed with the right hand, it indicates a D-loop; if it can be performed only with the left hand, an L-loop is present [8] (Fig. 6.4).

Using the "Loop rule", the ventricular loop orientation can be predicted based on the location and relationship of semilunar valves. If the aortic valve is located on the right side of the pulmonary valve, it indicates D-loop; whereas left-sided aortic valve indicates L-loop [14].

Rarely, the cardiac chambers and great arteries show unexpected spatial relationships for the given segmental connections, and the atrioventricular blood flow axes spiral each other due to clockwise or counterclockwise rotation of ventricles along their long axis. This leads to supero-inferiorly related ventricles with the morphological right ventricle located superiorly (Fig. 6.15). With further twisting, the atrioventricular connection may appear crisscrossed [15,

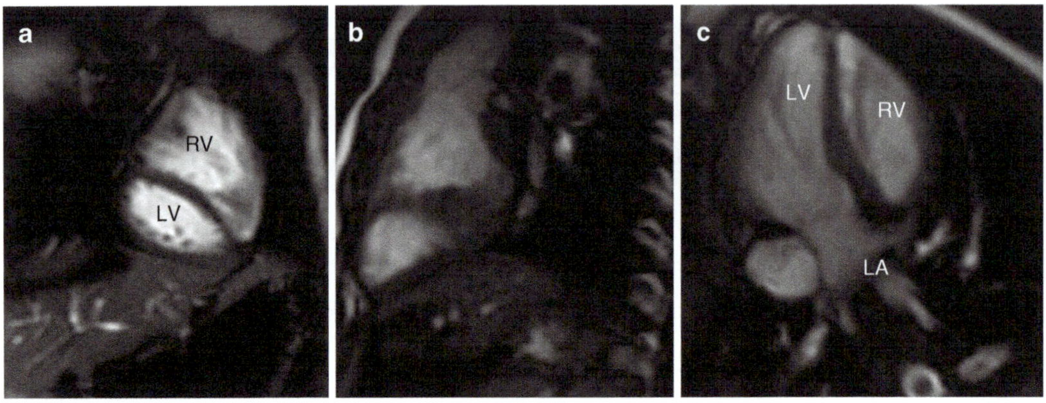

Fig. 6.15 Superoinferiorly related ventricles. Coronal (**a**), sagittal (**b**), and axial (**c**) MRI images show superiorly located RV, posteriorly placed LA, and anteroinferiorly located LV

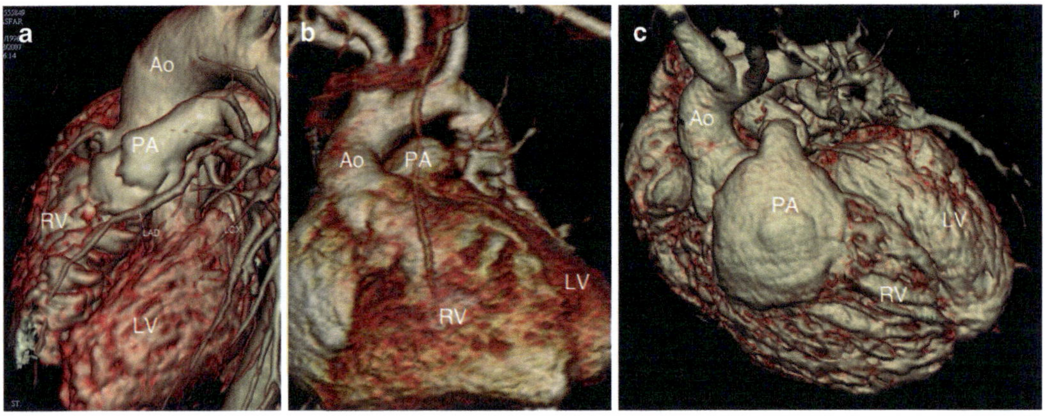

Fig. 6.16 Ventriculo-arterial connection. (**a**) Concordant connection where aorta (AO) comes from LV and PA from RV. (**b**) Discordant connection (TGA)—Aorta from RV and PA from LV. (**c**) Double outlet RV (DORV)—both great vessels from RV

16]. It may be seen with all kinds of atrioventricular and ventriculo-arterial connections.

Practical Pearls

D-loop: Morphological RV on right side of LV

L-loop: Morphological RV on the left side of LV

Loop rule

D-loop is associated with right-sided aortic valve in relation to the pulmonary valve.

L-loop is associated with left-sided aortic valve.

IV. Analysing Ventriculo-Arterial Connections

Similar to the analysis of the AV junctions, it is necessary to describe the way the arteries take origin from the ventricles and the nature of the semilunar valves guarding the ventricular arterial junctions. There are four possible types of ventriculo-arterial connections namely concordant, discordant, double outlet ventricle, and single outlet (Figs. 6.16 and 6.17).

In concordant ventriculo-arterial connection, the aorta arises from MLV and the pulmonary artery (PA) from MRV, be the ventricles complete

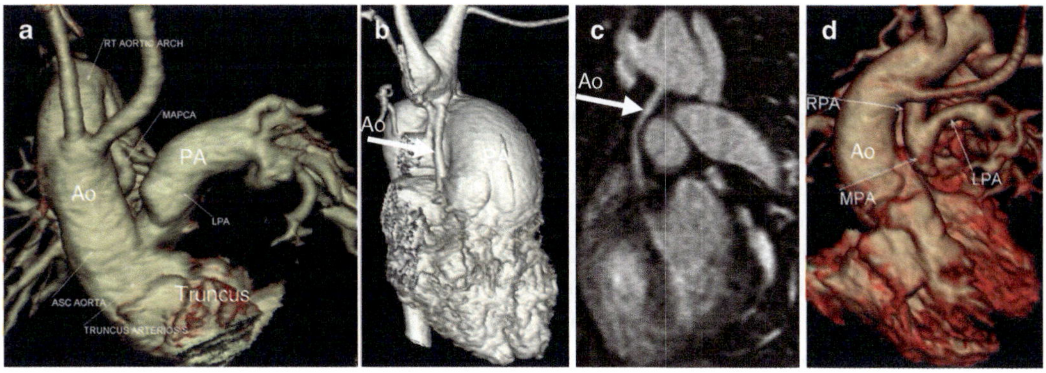

Fig. 6.17 Single outlet ventriculo-arterial connection. (**a**) In truncus arteriosus, solitary arterial trunk from the ventricles supply both aorta and pulmonary arteries. (**b**, **c**) In aortic atresia, aortic branches are supplied through PDA. (**d**) In pulmonary atresia, aorta supplies the pulmonary artery branches

or incomplete. The term discordance is used when the aorta is connected to RV and the PA to the LV as in the transposition of great arteries [17].

In double outlet connection, one valve is entirely connected with a ventricle and over 50% of the ring of the other valve is connected to the same ventricle as in double-outlet RV (DORV) [18] or double-outlet LV (DOLV) [19].

If only one great artery arises from both ventricles, it is called as single outlet connection (Fig. 6.17). The single outlet can be either a common trunk (truncus arteriosus) or a solitary trunk (aortic or pulmonary atresia). The term common trunk is used when both ventricles are connected via a common arterial valve to one trunk that gives rise directly to the coronary arteries, at least one pulmonary artery, and the majority of the systemic circulation.

Similar to overriding AV valves, the degree of override of an arterial valve determines the precise origin of the arterial trunk from the ventricular mass, the overriding valve, being assigned to the ventricle supporting the greater part of its circumference. For example, if more than half of an overriding pulmonary valve was connected to an RV, when the aorta is connected to LV, it is called as concordant connections. If more than half the overriding aortic valve was connected to the right ventricle in this situation, then the term double outlet connection is used. Basal short-axis planes that are perpendicular to interventricular septum are useful to demonstrate the ventriculo-arterial relationship especially when there is VSD with overriding of an artery (Fig. 6.18).

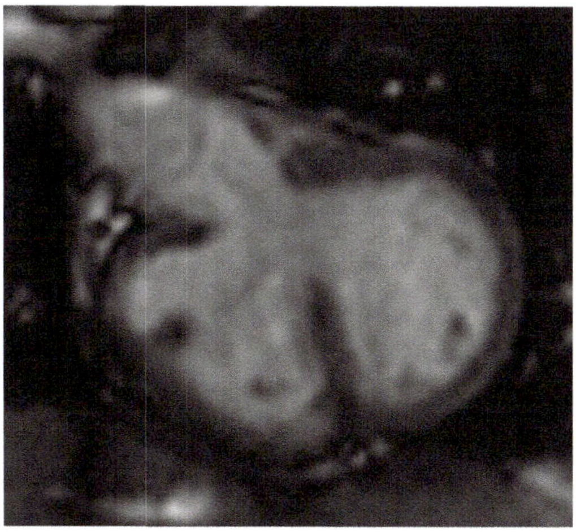

Fig. 6.18 Outflow view taken perpendicular to interventricular septum demonstrates the relationship between the VSD and aorta

Practical Pearls
Types of ventriculo-arterial connections:

1. Concordant
2. Discordant (TGA)
3. Double-outlet ventricle (DORV/DOLV)
4. Truncus arteriosus
5. Solitary trunk (aortic atresia/pulmonary atresia)

V. Determining the Position and Relation of the Great Vessels (_, _, X)

As per Van Praagh et al., the embryonic aortic valve is located anterior to the pulmonary valve. When the normal ventricular loop is formed, the valves become side by side with the aortic valve to the right. A muscle (conus) is present beneath the arterial valves causing discontinuity with the AV valves. Normally, the muscle under the aortic valve resorbs whereas the subpulmonary conus continues to grow. This leads to a rightward and posterior position of the aortic valve with mitro-aortic fibrous continuity. The pulmonary valve is then located anteriorly and on the left of the aortic valve, with a muscular discontinuity with the tricuspid valve. During development, the semilunar valves undergo about 150-degree dextrorotation [20].

Maldevelopment of these positioning of great vessels leads to conotruncal anomalies. There are four possible types of conal anatomy: subpulmonary conus (normal), subaortic conus (TGA) (Fig. 6.19), bilateral conus (DORV) (Fig. 6.20a), and bilaterally absent conus (DOLV) (Fig. 6.20b).

Great arterial relationships are usually described at valvar level, and many systems for nomenclature have been constructed on this basis (Fig. 6.21). In situs solitus (_, _, S), the aortic valve is rightward and posterior to the pulmonary valve. When the aorta maintains its normal posterior relation to the MPA but has an inverted position leftward of the MPA, the letter I is assigned to denote situs inversus, designated as (_, _, I).

If the aorta is anterior and right of the MPA, the anomaly is described as dextro (D) transposition of the great vessels (Complete TGA) (_, _, D-TGV). In levo (L) transposition (congenitally corrected TGA) the aorta is anterior to and leftward of the MPA, which is denoted as (_, _, L-TGV).

If the ventricular origin of a great vessel cannot be established, or if the great vessels arise from a single ventricle as in DORV, the term malposition of the great arteries (MGA) is used. Compared to transposition, in malposition, the aorta is neither anterior or posterior to MPA rather it is right or leftward. Generally, the term transposition is used when there is discordant ventriculo-arterial connection and malposition indicates other abnormal ventriculo-arterial connections [21]. The term “Anatomically corrected malposition” is used to describe concordant VA connections with parallel great arteries [22].

From the stance of positions of the arterial trunks, the possibilities are either for the pulmonary trunk to spiral round the aorta as it ascends from the base of the ventricles or for the two trunks to ascend in a parallel fashion. Spiralling trunks are associated most frequently with concordant ventriculo-arterial connections and parallel trunks with discordant or double outlet connections,

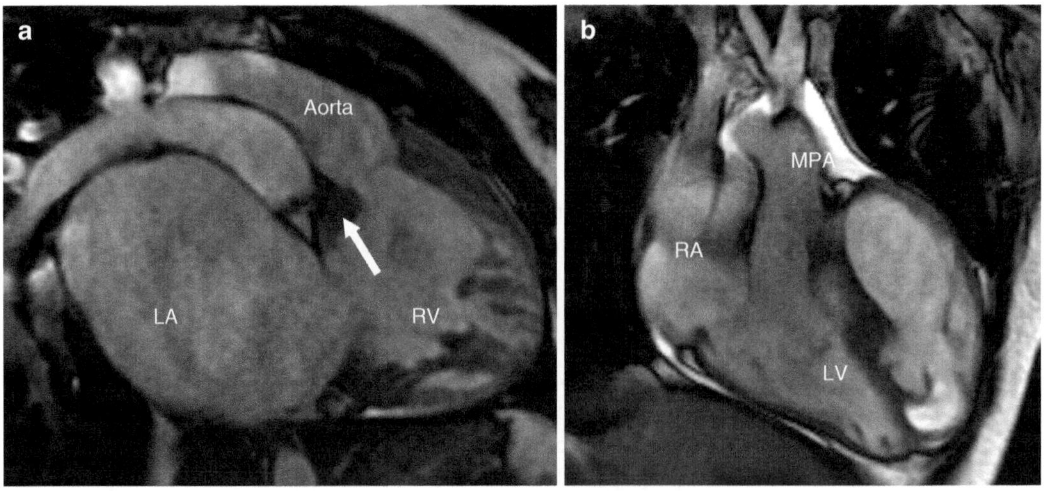

Fig. 6.19 Case of LTGA showing subaortic conus (**a**) and no subpulmonary conus (**b**)

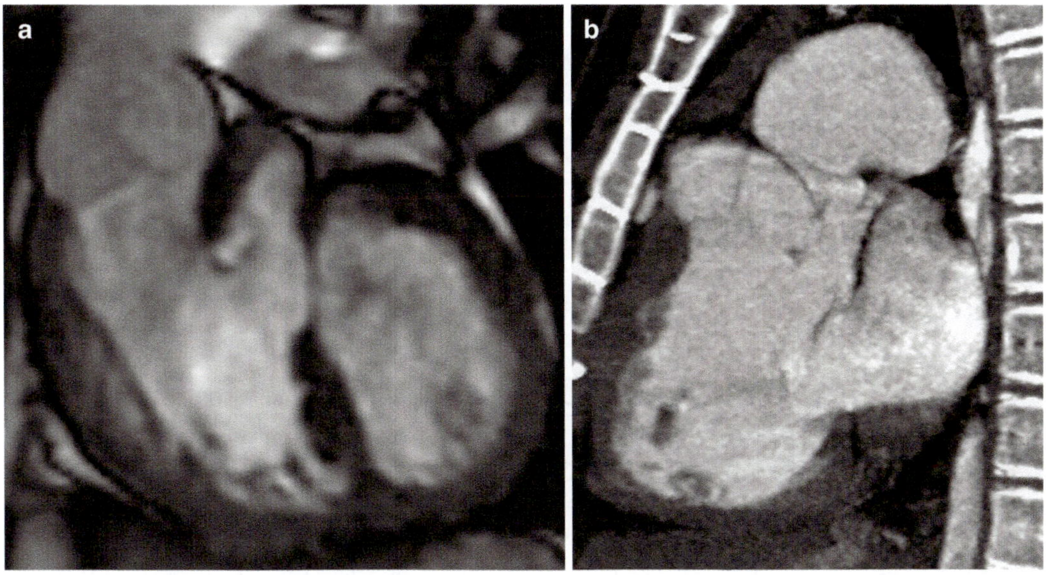

Fig. 6.20 Conal tissue is seen below both aorta and pulmonary trunk in a case of DORV (**a**), no conal tissue is seen below both great arteries in a case of DOLV (**b**)

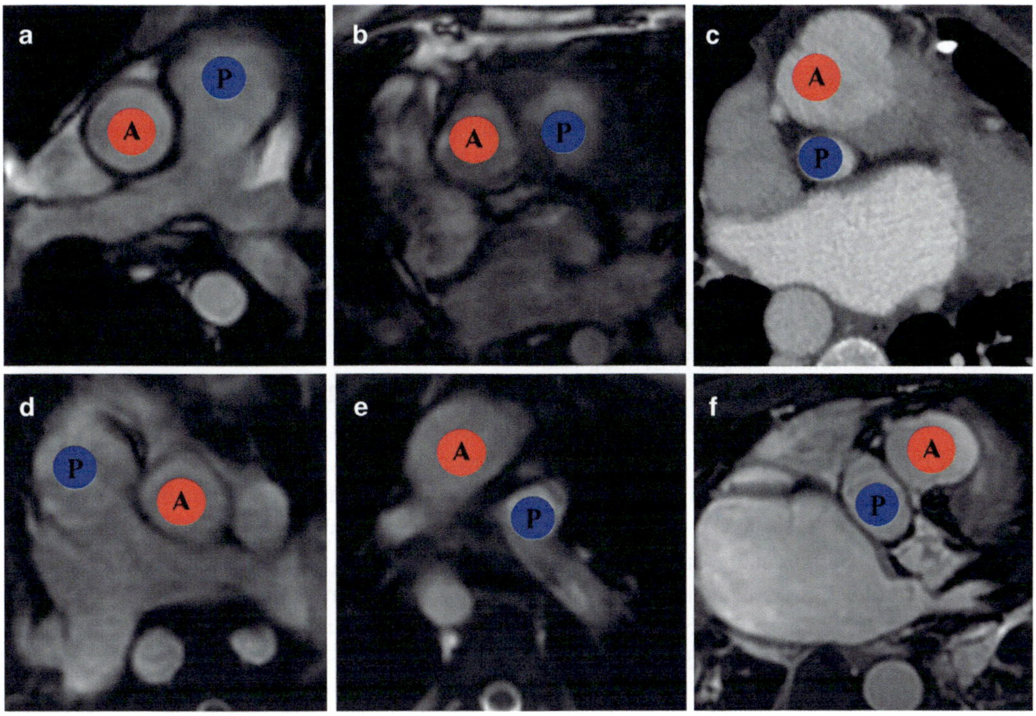

Fig. 6.21 Great arterial relationship at the level of the semilunar valve annulus. (**a**) Situs solitus (normal)—aorta is right and posterior to PA. (**b, c**) Side by side and anteroposterior-related great arteries are common in DORV. (**d**) Situs Inversus—Aorta is left and posterior. (**e**) DTGA—aorta is right and anterior. (**f**) LTGA—aorta is left and anterior

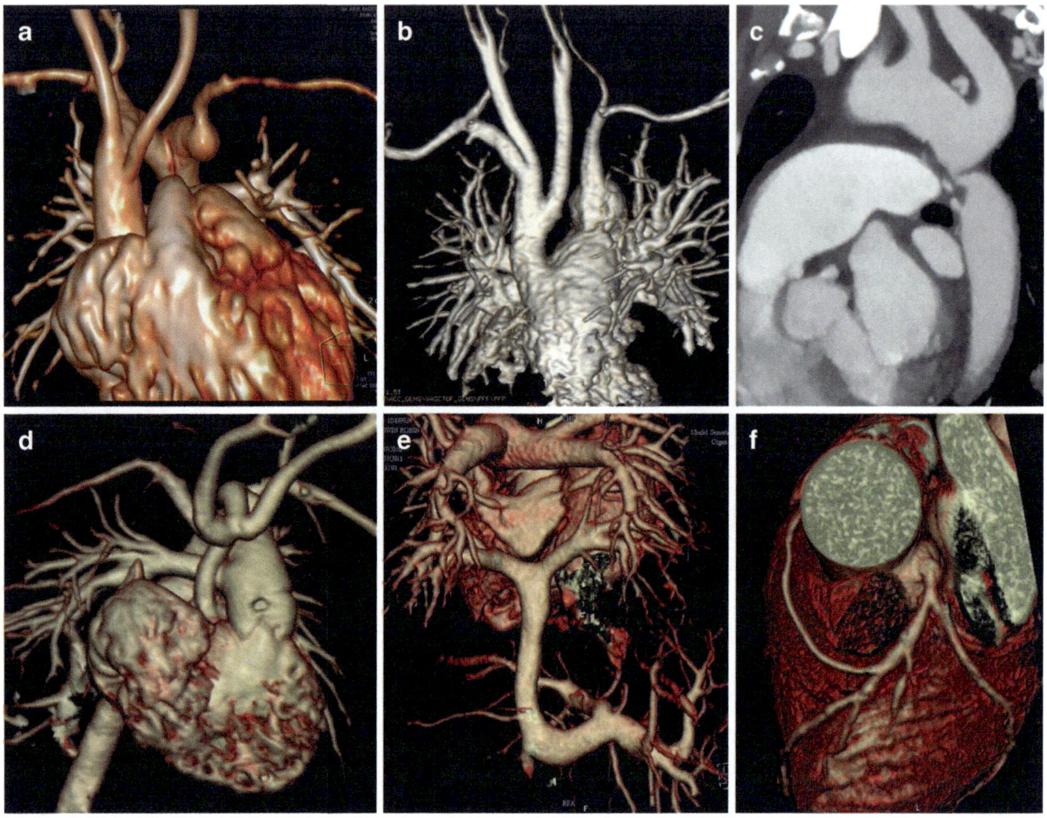

Fig. 6.22 Some of the extracardiac anomalies associated with congenital heart disease includes right aortic arch with aberrant left subclavian artery (**a**), interrupted aortic arch (**b**), coarctation of the aorta (**c**), hypoplastic ascending aorta (**d**), anomalous pulmonary venous connection to the portal vein (**e**), and coronary artery anomalies (**f**)

The side of the aortic arch depends on whether it passes to the right or the left of the trachea. The position of the descending aorta is defined relative to the vertebral column.

Practical Pearls

Relationship between aorta and MPA at valve level:

Normal: Aorta is right and posterior to MPA
DTGA: Aorta is right and anterior
LTGA: Aorta is left and anterior
Situs inversus: Aorta is left and posterior
DORV: Side by side or anteroposterior great arteries

VI. Associated Intra- and Intersegmental Abnormalities

There are many anomalies within each segment of the heart that can accompany any possible combination of above described normal or abnormal connections (Fig. 6.22). Such anomalies are frequently major lesions that influence the surgical approach and have profound physiologic significance.

Table 6.3 Common associated intra- and intersegmental anomalies

Cardiac segmental region	Examples of anomalies
I. Visceroatrial situs	(a) Systemic veins
	Double SVC and left SVC
	Interrupted IVC
	Retro-aortic left innominate vein
	Coronary sinus anomalies
	(b) Pulmonary veins
	Total or partial anomalous pulmonary venous drainage
	Stenosis
	Levoatrial cardinal vein
	(c) Atria
	Atrial septal defect (ASD)
	Cor triatriatum
	Juxtaposed atrial appendage
	(d) Airways
	Tracheal bronchus
	Airway narrowing caused by abnormal vessel
	(e) Abdominal viscera
	Multiple or absent spleen
	Malrotation of gut, biliary atresia
II. Atrioventricular junction	AV canal defects
	Mitral or tricuspid regurgitation/stenosis
	Ebstein anomaly
III. Ventricles	Ventricular septal defect (VSD)
	Hypoplastic right or left ventricle
	Double chamber right ventricle
IV. Ventriculao-arterial connection	Aortic or pulmonary stenosis/regurgitation
	Sub-pulmonary or subaortic membrane
V. Great vessel	Supravalvar aortic stenosis (William syndrome)
	Coronary artery anomalies
	Coarctation/interrupted aorta
	Aortopulmonary window
	Patent ductus arteriosus (PDA)
	Vascular rings and slings
	Major aortopulmonary collateral artery (MAPCA)

Some of the common associated anomalies are listed in Table 6.3.

6.5 Conclusion

The sequential segmental approach emphasises the proximal-to-distal positions and relationships of cardiac chambers and great vessels. This approach facilitates the detection and characterisation of even complex congenital heart diseases (Figs. 6.23 and 6.24).

It is important for imagers to become familiar with these terminologies and anomalies, the spectrum of their manifestations, and their significance. The use of common language is important to communicate with cardiac physicians and surgeons. There are exceptions to every rule in medicine, so the general rules described in the chapter should be used with an appropriate clinical setting.

Acknowledgement Figures 6.5 and 6.6 are provided by Dr. Vijaya Bhaskar Nori, Vista imaging centre, Hyderabad, India.

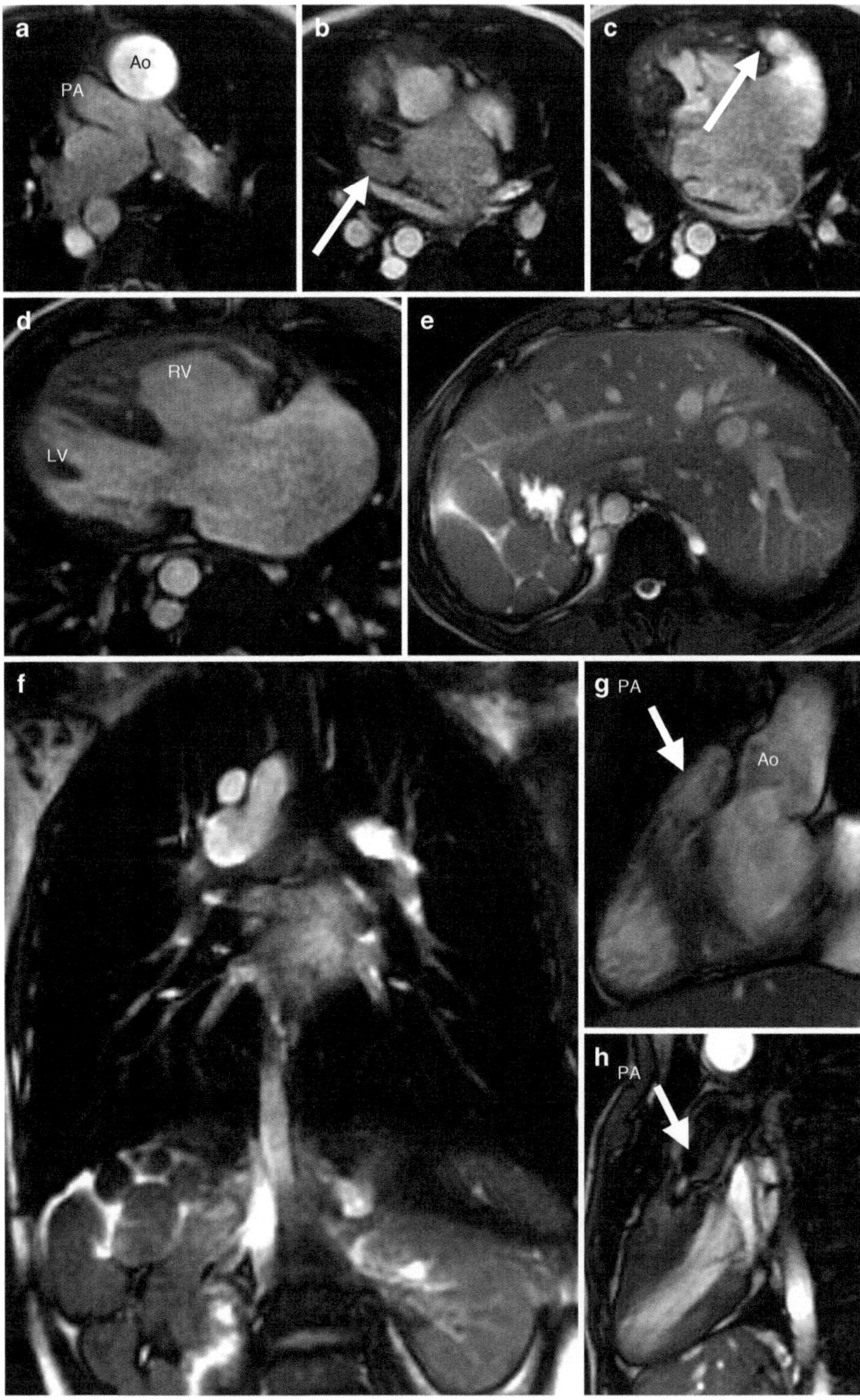

Fig. 6.23 Comprehensive CMR assessment in a case of left isomerism. Axial SSFP images (**a**–**e**) show L posed aorta, dextrocardia, L-loop ventricles (RV on left of LV), both atrial appendages having left-sided morphology (arrows in **b**, **c**), common AV valve, common atrium, azygos continuation of IVC, situs ambiguous and polysplenia. (**f**) Shows polysplenia and bilateral hyparterial bronchus. (**g**) Shows double outlet right ventricle. (**h**) Shows subpulmonary obstruction. *Ao* aorta; *LV* left ventricle; *PA* pulmonary artery trunk; *RV* right ventricle

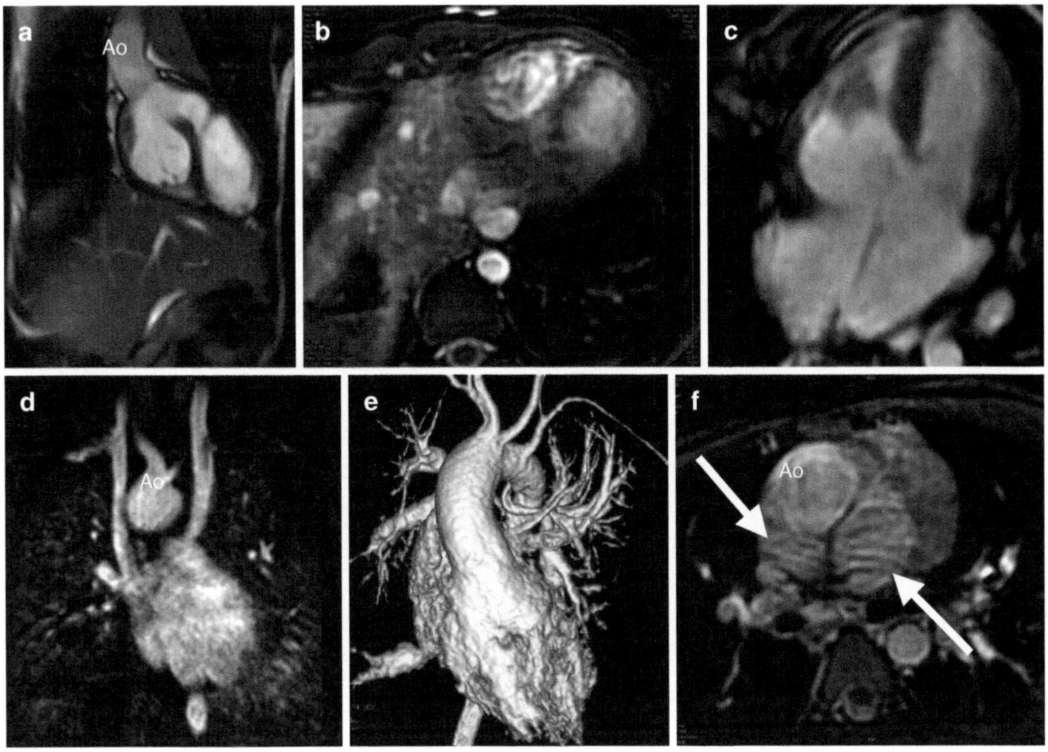

Fig. 6.24 A case of situs ambiguous, asplenia with IVC located anterior to the aorta and the same side (**a**, **b**). (**c**) Shows common AV septal defect with large primum ASD and inlet VSD. MRA shows double SVC and pulmonary atresia (**d**, **e**). Axial 3D SSFP image shows juxtaposed atrial appendages both having right-sided morphology (arrows in **f**). *Ao* aorta

References

1. Van Praagh R. The segmental approach to diagnosis in congenital heart disease. In: Bergsma D, editor. Birth defects original article series, National Foundation—March of Dimes, vol. 8. Baltimore: Williams & Wilkins; 1972. p. 4–23.
2. De la Cruz MV, Nadal-Ginard B. Rules for the diagnosis of visceral situs, truncoconal morphologies and ventricular inversions. Am Heart J. 1972;84:19–32.
3. Van Praagh R. Terminology of congenital heart disease: glossary and commentary. Circulation. 1977;56(2):139–43.
4. Anderson RH, Becker AE, Freedom RM, et al. Sequential segmental analysis of congenital heart disease. Pediatr Cardiol. 1984;5:281–8.
5. Anderson RH, Shirali G. Sequential segmental analysis. Ann Pediatr Cardiol. 2009;2(1):24–35.
6. Lapierre C, Déry J, Guérin R, Viremouneix L, Dubois J, Garel L. Segmental approach to imaging of congenital heart disease. Radiographics. 2010;30(2):397–411.
7. Uemura H, Ho SY, Devine WA, Kilpatrick LL, Anderson RH. Atrial appendages and venoatrial connections in hearts with patients with visceral heterotaxy. Ann Thorac Surg. 1995;60:561–9.
8. Erica KS, Gary HD, Richard K, et al. Describing congenital heart disease by using three-part segmental notation. Radiographics. 2013;33:E33–46.
9. Tonkin IL. The definition of cardiac malpositions with echocardiography and computed tomography. In: Friedman WF, Higgins CB, editors. Pediatric cardiac imaging. Philadelphia: Saunders; 1984. p. 157–87.
10. Ghosh S, Yarmish G, Godelman A, et al. Anomalies of visceroatrial situs. AJR. 2009;193:1107–17.
11. Fulcher AS, Turner MA. Abdominal manifestations of Situs anomalies in adults. Radiographics. 2002;22:1439–56.
12. Brandt PW, Calder AL. Cardiac connections: the segmental approach to radiologic diagnosis in congenital heart disease. Curr Probl Diagn Radiol. 1977;7:1–35.
13. Manner J. The anatomy of cardiac looping: a step towards the understanding of the morphogenesis of several forms of congenital cardiac malformations. Clin Anat. 2009;22(1):21–35.

14. Van Praagh R. The importance of segmental situs in the diagnosis of congenital heart disease. Semin Roentgenol. 1985;20(3):254–71.
15. Anderson RH. Criss-cross hearts revisited. Pediatr Cardiol. 1982;3(4):305–13.
16. Anderson RH, Shinebourne EA, Gerlis LM. Crisscross atrioventricular relationships producing paradoxical atrioventricular concordance or discordance: their significance to nomenclature of congenital heart disease. Circulation. 1974;50(1):176–80.
17. Warnes CA. Transposition of the great arteries. Circulation. 2006;114(24):2699–709.
18. Ebadi A, Spicer DE, Backer CL, Fricker FJ, Anderson RH. Double-outlet right ventricle revisited. J Thorac Cardiovasc Surg. 2017;154:598–604. https://doi.org/10.1016/j.jtcvs.2017.03.049.
19. Brandt PW, Calder AL, Barratt-Boyes BG, Neutze JM. Double outlet left ventricle: morphology, cineangiocardiographic diagnosis and surgical treatment. Am J Cardiol. 1976;38(7):897–909.
20. Van Praagh R, Layton WM, Van Praagh S. The morphogenesis of normal and abnormal relationships between the great arteries and the ventricles: pathologic and experimental data. In: Van Praagh R, Takao A, editors. Etiology and morphogenesis of congenital heart disease. Mount Kisco, NY: Futurama; 1980. p. 271–316.
21. Van Praagh R, Van Praagh S. Isolated ventricular inversion: a consideration of the morphogenesis, definition and diagnosis of nontransposed and transposed great arteries. Am J Cardiol. 1966;17(3):395–406.
22. Cavalle-Garrido T, Bernasconi A, Perrin D, Anderson RH. Hearts with concordant ventriculoarterial connections but parallel arterial trunks. Heart. 2007;93:100–6.

Part II

Imaging in Congenital Heart Disease

Congenital Aortic Anomalies

7

Alpa Bharati and Ramiah Rajeshkannan

7.1 Introduction

Aortic diseases are one of the most common indications for cross-sectional imaging studies in congenital heart diseases. They account for 15–20% of all congenital cardiovascular malformations [1]. As with other congenital heart diseases (CHDs), aortic diseases can occur in isolation or as a spectrum of other complex CHDs. Many of the arch anomalies may be incidentally seen on imaging done for other reasons. These include aberrant right or left subclavian artery origin with a retro-esophageal course or a cervical aortic arch. This chapter will concentrate on significant aortic anomalies that would need definitive medical or surgical intervention. The commonest aortic diseases covered in this chapter are subdivided into root anomalies, arch anomalies and genetic anomalies.

Aortic root anomalies:

- Truncus arteriosus
- Transposition of great arteries
- Sinus of Valsalva aneurysm (with or without rupture)
- Aorto-pulmonary window
- Supravalvar membrane (Williams syndrome)
- Aorta to LV fistula
- Aortic valve anomalies
- Ascending aortic atresia

Arch anomalies:

- Anomalous location of arch
- Hypoplastic arch
- Coarctation of aorta
- Interrupted arch
- Double aortic arch
- Persistent fifth arch
- Double lumen aorta

Genetic anomalies:

- Marfan syndrome
- Aortic tortuosity syndrome

Electronic Supplementary Material The online version of this chapter (https://doi.org/10.1007/978-981-15-6755-1_7) contains supplementary material, which is available to authorized users.

A. Bharati (✉)
BJ Wadia Hospital for Children, Holy Family Hospital, Mumbai, India

R. Rajeshkannan
Department of Radiology, Amrita School of Medicine, Amrita Institute of Medical Sciences and Research Centre, Amrita Vishwa Vidyapeetham, Kochi, Kerala, India

7.2 Normal Embryology

The human aorta and its arch vessels develop from the aortic sac and the primitive paired aortic arches. Chronologically, the first arch appears first and sixth arch appears last. There is no fifth arch in humans and hence the arches that contribute to developing the aorta, arch vessels and the pulmonary arteries are from the aortic sac and paired arches 1, 2, 3, 4 and 6.

R. Rajeshkannan et al. (eds.), *CT and MRI in Congenital Heart Diseases*,
https://doi.org/10.1007/978-981-15-6755-1_7

The first arch gives rise to the right and left dorsal aorta which fuse caudally to form a single dorsal aorta (Fig. 7.1a) The second arch arises between the first arch and the primitive heart. Both the first and second arches and the intervening dorsal aorta degenerate and third and fourth arches begin to appear and become the major source of blood supply from the heart (Fig. 7.1b).

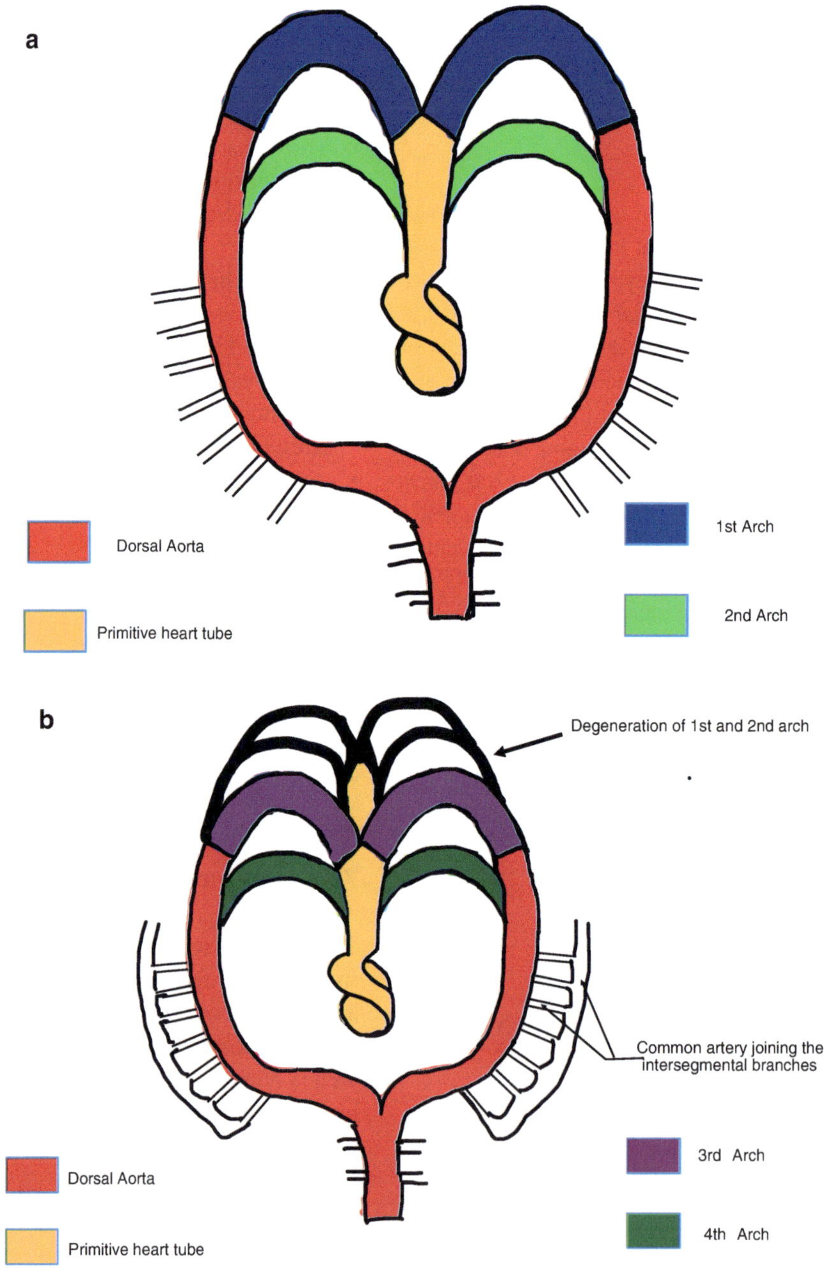

Fig. 7.1 Cartoons show different stages of aortic embryology

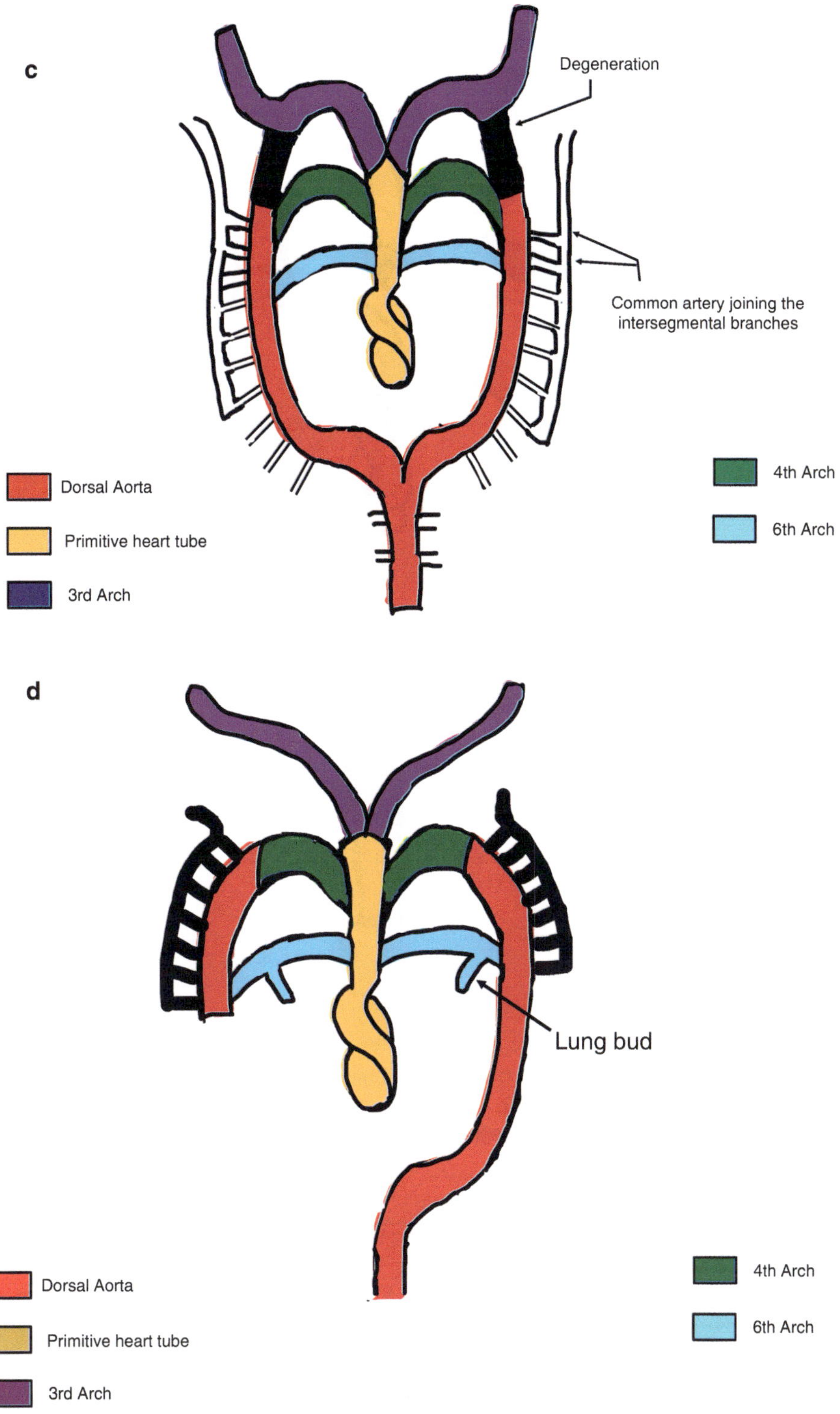

Fig. 7.1 (continued)

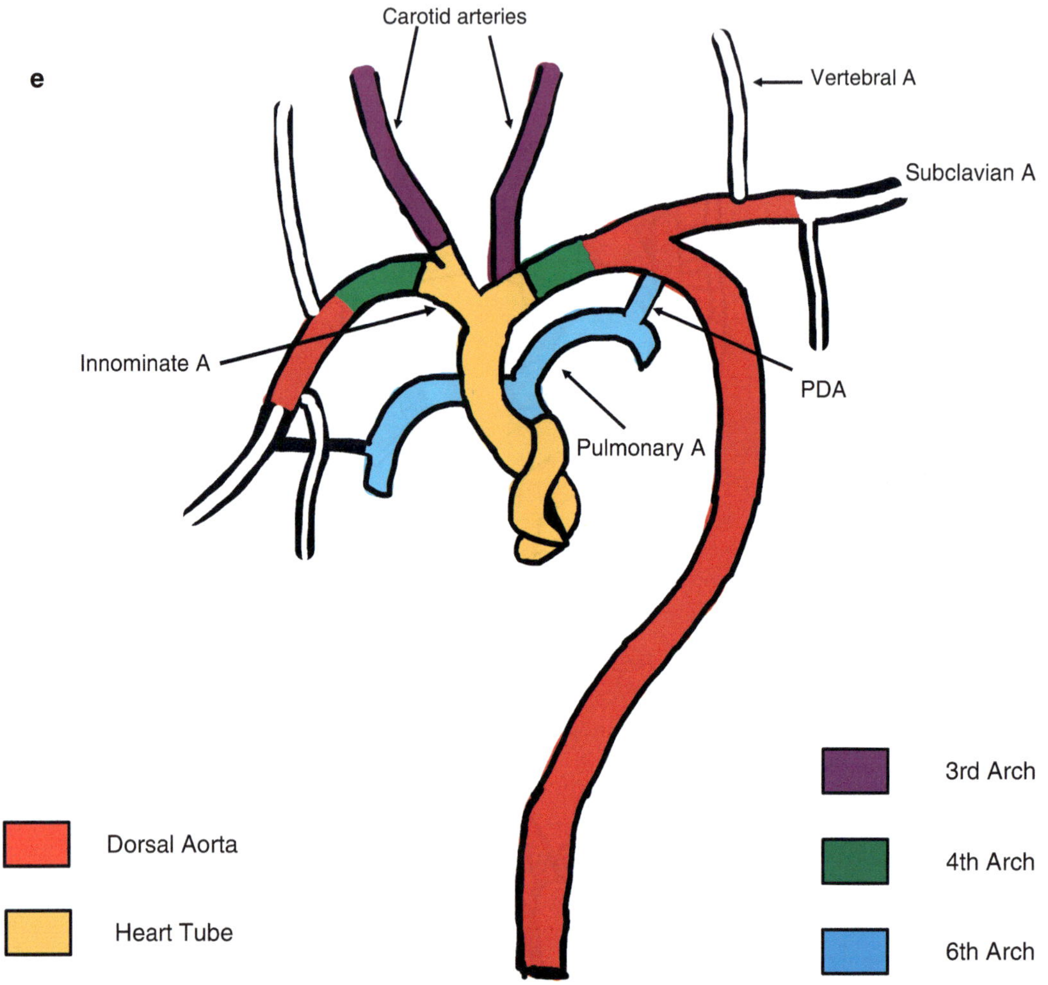

Fig. 7.1 (continued)

Eventually, the dorsal arch between the third and fourth arches on either side also degenerates. The aortic sac now gives rise to the third arch vessels, which grow cranially to form the bilateral common carotid arteries (Fig. 7.1c).

Meantime, the fourth and sixth arches continue to communicate with the dorsal aorta on either side along with elongation of the dorsal aorta between the fourth and sixth arches. The sixth arch comes to lie at the level of pulmonary buds and gives rise to pulmonary arterial branches. These supply the growing lung buds and form the definitive pulmonary arteries (Fig. 7.1d).

The dorsal aorta also gives rise to seven intersegmental arteries, of which all but the seventh degenerate. A common communicating artery, connecting the seven intersegmental arteries develops and continues to grow cranially eventually fusing with the contralateral common communicating artery forming the vertebrobasilar system (Fig. 7.1a–e).

The seventh intersegmental artery grows into the upper limb buds forming the bilateral subclavian arteries (Fig. 7.1e).

Later the right dorsal aortic segment between the right subclavian artery and the left-sided dorsal aorta degenerates resulting in the definitive left aortic arch with right subclavian artery as its first arch vessel (Fig. 7.1e).

Internal separation of the common aortic sac takes place separating the aorta and the pulmonary trunk. The communication between the sixth arch on the left side and the dorsal aorta persists as the ductus arteriosus which eventually fuses postnatally (Fig. 7.1e).

Key points on embryology:

- Aortic sac forms the aortic root, ascending aorta, proximal brachiocephalic trunk and the aortic arch up to the origin of the left common carotid artery.
- Third arch forms the carotids.
- Fourth arch forms the part of the aortic arch between the left common carotid and left subclavian arteries on the left side and proximal right subclavian artery on the right side.
- Sixth arch forms the pulmonary arteries.
- Patent communication between the sixth left arch and left-sided dorsal aorta forms the ductus arteriosus. The communication between the right sixth arch and dorsal aorta degenerates resulting in no communication between the right subclavian artery and the right pulmonary artery.
- The seventh intersegmental artery on either side contributes to forming the bilateral subclavian arteries.

7.3 Imaging Protocols

7.3.1 CT Aortogram

A CT angiogram gives an excellent depiction of the thoracic aorta and pulmonary arteries. Using the newer fast scanners, CT imaging can be done without ECG gating but scanners with lower rotation speeds need ECG gating with contrast preferably being injected via the lower limb venous access. The lower limb venous access avoids streaking artefacts from dense contrast in the region of the aortic root and proximal thoracic aorta. In our institute, we usually use non-ionic contrast with 350 mg% iodine concentration. Contrast is injected via the lower limb at a flow rate of approximately 2–3 ml/s using a 24G or lesser gauge venous access. Patients are scanned after short sedation using ketamine or propofol in the presence of an anaesthetist. Contrast dose is approximately 1.3 ml/kg followed by an equal amount of saline chase. Contrast is injected using injector to maintain uniform flow rate except in neonates especially of low birth weight in whom hand-injection of contrast is used due to small doses required. CT is preferred over MRI in view of short scan times and a small dose of sedation needed compared to MRI.

7.3.2 MR Angiogram

MRI is recommended if flows are to be assessed or ventricular size, function and volumes need to be assessed. Since many patients would be infants or even neonates, hypothermia within the MR room must be considered. Other parameters to consider before a MRI, include the child's status of hydration and taking precautions to avoid hypotension and hypoglycaemia, especially in neonates. The imaging should preferably be done with day-care admission with appropriate hydration and maintaining glucose levels in the neonate. A good anaesthesia support should also be insisted. The MRI protocol should be tailored to answer specific medical or surgical questions which will help reduce imaging time and maintain SAR within acceptable limits in neonates. MR imaging protocol should include black-blood imaging for anatomy and cine and flow imaging for functional evaluation. Dynamic MR angiography is done using gadolinium-based contrast in a dose of 0.2 ml/kg. Oblique sagittal imaging sections, through a plane bisecting the aortic arch in the axial plane, provides a good profile view of the aorta. A non-contrast 3D whole-heart imaging can be included where details of origin and course of proximal coronary arteries are required.

All follow-up post-operative imaging is done on MRI to prevent repeated exposure to radiation and for serial assessment of ventricular morphology and function and flows across valves and vessels as required.

7.4 Aortic Root Anomalies

7.4.1 Truncus Arteriosus

Truncus arteriosus (TA) is a conotruncal anomaly. It occurs due to a lack of adequate separation of the aorta and pulmonary trunk. This results in a condition where there is a common vascular channel arising from normal sized ventricles with a common valve overriding a VSD. It is a rare congenital heart disease accounting for approximately 7 per 100,000 live births [2]. It is associated with genetic mutations of 22q11 and DiGeorge syndrome. It is also one of the three most common conditions associated with gestational and pregestational diabetes [3, 4].

Pathophysiology: Truncus arteriosus is characterised by common truncal valve overriding a VSD and a common vascular outflow trunk draining the well-formed right and left ventricles. There is mixing of blood at the level of VSD. This blood circulates through both the pulmonary and systemic circulation as well as the coronaries. In antenatal life, the pulmonary vascular resistance (PVR) is high and most of the blood gets shunted to the systemic circulation. Postnatally the PVR decreases leading to excessive shunting of blood to the lung parenchyma. An increase in the pulmonary blood flow (PBF) leads to increasing cyanosis and congestive heart failure. The pathology is further worsened if there is associated truncal valve stenosis or regurgitation or a coexistent aortic interruption, coarctation or aortic hypoplasia. In the absence of treatment, there is continuous increased pulmonary blood flow which results in permanent damage to the pulmonary vascular bed followed by a further increase in PVR causing increasing cyanosis and eventually leading to death.

TA is thus a form of critical congenital heart disease predominantly presenting in the neonatal period, mostly within the first few weeks of life. It's pathology is influenced largely by the extent of PBF, PVR, coexistent truncal valve stenosis or regurgitation and aortic interruption, hypoplasia or coarctation. Almost 50% of the cases of TA can show truncal valve stenosis or regurgitation and almost 10% are reported to have critical coarctation [5–7]. Almost always patients with TA will not survive in the absence of corrective surgery. Surgical correction of TA involves separating the pulmonary artery (PA) from the common trunk and connecting it to the right ventricle (RV) through an RV–PA conduit. Delineation of the pulmonary arterial anatomy is therefore of utmost importance. If there are associated anomalies of the arch or truncal valve, it is usually corrected in the same sitting. In cases where immediate surgical correction is not possible, banding of the pulmonary arteries is done to reduce the blood flow to the lung and surgical correction is done after the required growth of the infant is achieved. In the absence of any cardiac intervention, most patients die before the age of 1 year whereas with early surgical intervention, almost 80% show survival up to the age of 20 years. Repeat surgery is however needed in almost 75% of cases. Most patients subsequently would out-grow the RV–PA conduit causing RV outflow tract (RVOT) obstruction. Other causes for surgical re-intervention include repair or replacement of the valve or to relieve the aortic restenosis. These invariably require long-term follow-up [8, 9].

Imaging Truncus arteriosus is well diagnosed on a 2D echocardiogram. Stenosis and regurgitation across the truncal valve are also better assessed on 2D echo. Further imaging is usually warranted for cases where there is ambiguity regarding the type of truncus arteriosus and for better delineation of the aorta and branch pulmonary arteries and the coronaries.

Imaging in truncus arteriosus can be accomplished by CT or MRI if echocardiography is insufficient. The choice of imaging depends on the specific medical or surgical questions that need to be assessed. An isolated anatomical delineation is sufficiently and quickly done on contrast CT angiography, whereas assessment of flows through pulmonary arteries, assessment of truncal valve anatomy, flow and regurgitation and ventricular size and function will need an MRI. Since most of these patients would present in the neonatal period, it is important to keep in mind the high risk of longer duration of sedation and complications of hypothermia and hypotension-hypoglycaemia, before an MRI procedure is undertaken. Keeping the same in mind, a quick CT angiogram may be preferred over MRI especially in neonates with weight less than 3 kg.

Imaging will show a single common outflow valve also called the truncal valve which invariably overrides a malaligned VSD (Fig. 7.2a, b).

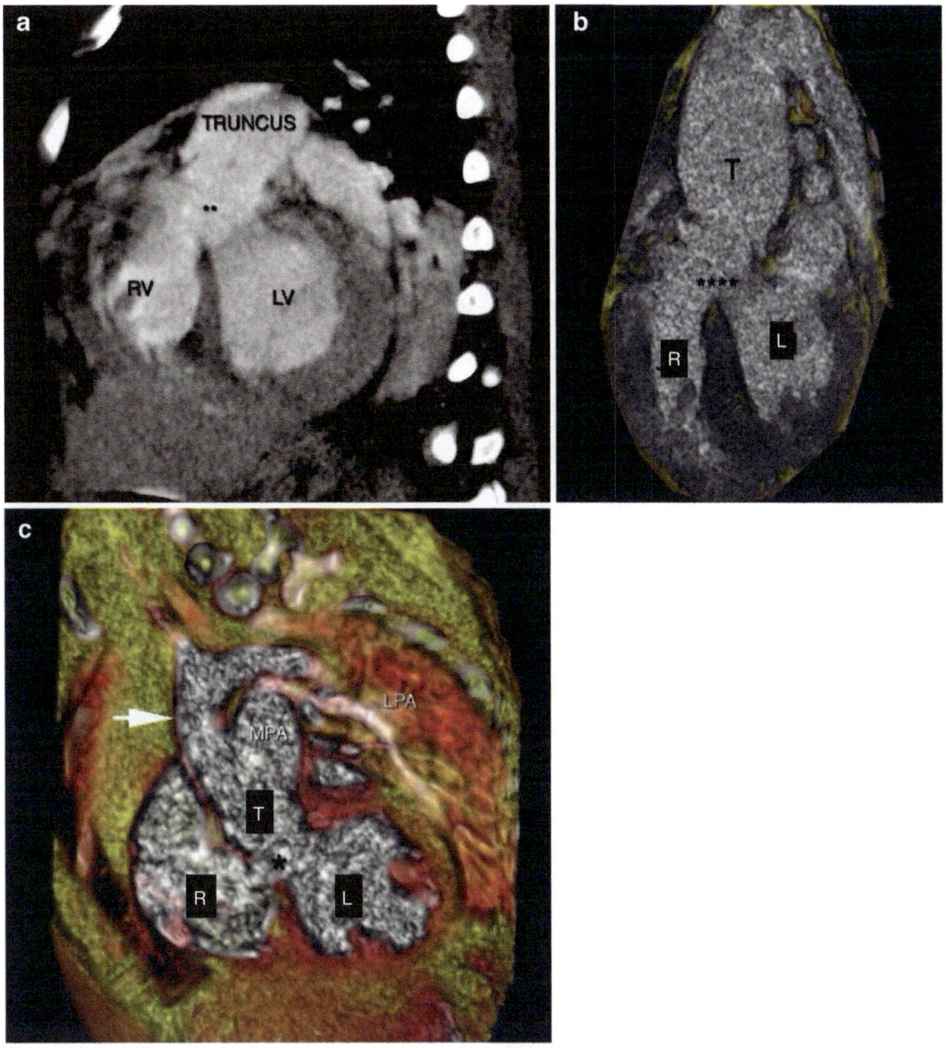

Fig. 7.2 (**a**) Image in basal short axis view shows a common truncus overriding a VSD (**). (**b**) Volume-rendered image in the oblique coronal plane shows the dilated truncus (T) overriding the VSD (****). *R* right ventricle; *L* left ventricle. (**c**) VR image in the basal short axis view shows type I truncus arteriosus with common truncus (T) giving rise to MPA and aorta (white arrow). The LPA is seen arising from the MPA. VSD is marked with (*), *R* right; *L* left ventricle. (**d**) Type I truncus arteriousus. Stack of short-axis view. Tracing the truncus from left to right shows the truncus overriding the VSD, giving rise to the MPA which bifurcates to the LPA and RPA. The aortic arch is complete and normal in calibre. (**e**) Truncus arteriosus type II. Basal short axis view shows the origin of truncus overriding the VSD in the first image. As we trace the truncus in the same short-axis view, the separate origins of the pulmonary artery (R and L) are seen from the truncus (T). Tracing the truncus in the short-axis view provides the most accurate assessment of the type of truncal anatomy especially helping to differentiate type I and type II truncus arteriosus. (**f**) A case of truncus arteriosus type III shows focal stenosis at the site of origin of LPA (black arrow). Asterisks (**) represent the VSD. (**g**) Volume-rendered image in type IV truncus arteriosus shows aortic interruption with a short gap (arrowhead in i) between the ascending aorta (AA) and descending thoracic aorta (DTA). Image ii on the right shows the right and left pulmonary arteries (R and L) arising from the truncus and a short PDA (arrowhead in ii) supplying the descending thoracic aorta (DTA). (**h**) MPR view of the truncus giving rise to the MPA (P). The measurement of the distance from the truncal valve to the origin of the first pulmonary arterial branch is important for surgical planning. It can be done on MPR or curved reformatted images. (**i**) Axial image shows severe stenosis of the origin and proximal left bronchus (black arrowhead) in a case of truncus arteriosus due to the dilated right pulmonary artery. *TA* truncus arteriosus

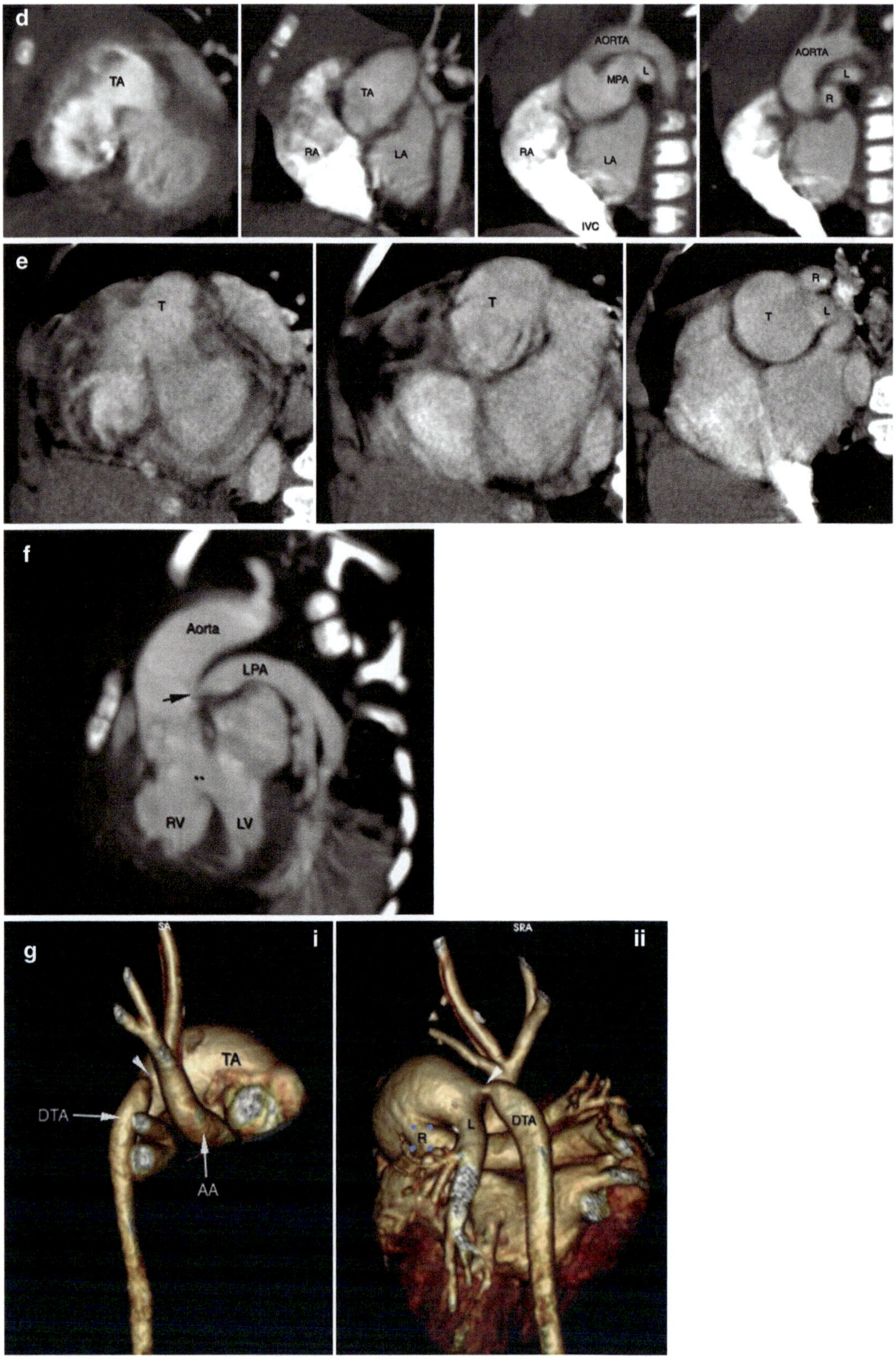

Fig. 7.2 (continued)

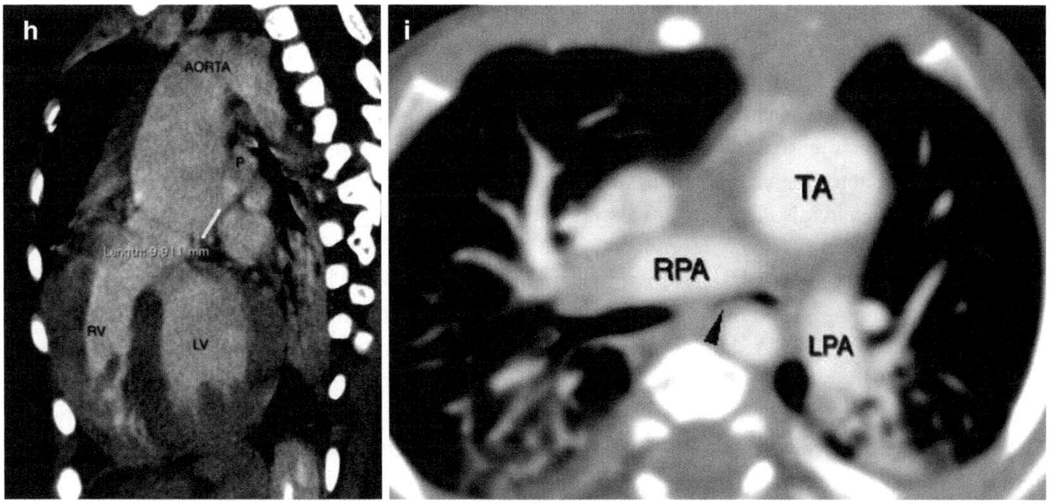

Fig. 7.2 (continued)

The valve may be committed more to either the right or left ventricle or be equally committed to both ventricles. After a variable length, the common vascular trunk divides into the aorta and pulmonary arteries. The pattern of origin of pulmonary arteries decides the type of truncus arteriosus. It was first classified as Collett and Edwards and later modified by Van Praagh who included arch anomalies in the classifications system.

The modified classification by Van Praagh is as under:

- Type I—MPA arises from the truncus and gives rise to the right and left branch pulmonary arteries (Fig. 7.2c, d).
- Type II—MPA is absent, the right and left pulmonary arteries arise from the truncus, in close proximity to one another (Fig. 7.2e).
- Type III—MPA is absent, the right and left pulmonary arteries arise from the truncus and their origins are widely separated from one another (Fig. 7.2f).
- Type IV—truncus arteriosus is associated with interrupted arch (Fig. 7.2g).

The truncus is dilated with truncal valve being stenosed or more often leaking. The valve leaflets are commonly thickened and dysplastic. Truncal valve may be monocuspid, bicuspid, tricuspid or quadricuspid of which the tricuspid valve is the most common. After variable length, the truncus gives rise to either the main pulmonary artery (MPA) or directly the branch pulmonary arteries and thereafter continues as the aorta. It may be difficult to differentiate type I and type II truncus on axial imaging alone and it is best to evaluate the same on multiplanar reconstructed images especially on the short axis view (Fig. 7.2d). The distance of the origin of the first/main pulmonary artery from the truncal valve is crucial in surgical planning (Fig. 7.2h). Similarly, the course of the coronaries is also vital as they arise from the common trunk and need to be committed to the aorta post-repair. The branch pulmonary arteries are usually dilated in truncus arteriosus with overflow in the pulmonary bed. There can be bronchial narrowing due to the dilated branch pulmonary arteries. The same must be looked for on CT in all cases of truncus arteriosus (Fig 7.2i).

Truncus can be associated with an interrupted arch with a distal arch being supplied by the PDA (Fig. 7.2g). In such cases, the truncus may appear to be bifurcating or trifurcating with large PDA between the PA and descending aorta. This is best evaluated on sagittal images which will show the extent of interruption in profile. Valve anatomy is best assessed on cine MRI.

Pre-operative imaging of truncus arteriosus should delineate the type of truncus arteriosus, the anatomy of the pulmonary arteries including the presence or absence of MPA, distance of origins of branch pulmonary arteries as they arise from the truncus in type 2–type 4, distance of the first pulmonary artery from the truncal valve and description of the interrupted arch if present. Any other associated anomalies like venous drainage anomalies must be looked for. It is vital to also look for any compression of the underlying tracheo-bronchial tree (Fig. 7.2i). Coronary anomalies are important in pre-operative planning. Besides these, the size and location of the VSD and PDA should be defined.

Surgery is invariably required to treat the condition preferably in the neonatal age group. Surgical correction involves committing the truncal valve to the LV and communicating the pulmonary artery to the RV through a valved homograft. With time, the homograft may show stenosis with or without valvar stenosis or regurgitation.

Post-operative imaging is thus often required to look for restenosis of the repaired pulmonary valve, assessment of stenosis of the pulmonary conduit and RV function and morphology. The extent of pulmonary valve regurgitation and stenosis is best assessed by flow analysis on MRI. Additionally, bi-ventricular function and size, especially RV volumes and ejection fraction are also best assessed by MRI using cine imaging. MRI can assess the total PBF as well as differential flow in each lung, percentage of truncal valve regurgitation and quantitatively assess bi-ventricular size and ejection fraction.

7.4.2 Aorto-Pulmonary Window (AP Window: APW)

APW constitutes approximately 0.2–0.6% of all cardiac malformation [10–12]. It is a condition where there is abnormal communication between the MPA and the proximal aorta in the presence of two separate outflow valves, each one committed to the aorta and pulmonary artery. The presence of two separate valves distinguishes it from the truncus arteriosus. APW is commonly associated with arch anomalies, ASD, tetralogy of Fallot, aortic origin of the right pulmonary artery and occasionally with VSD, TGA or atresia of the aortic, pulmonary or tricuspid valves [13–16]. APW is classified into proximal, distal and total defects [17]. Proximal defects (type A) are the commonest (Fig. 7.3a). They are small and located close to the semilunar valves. Distal APW (type B) is closer to the level where aorta gives off its arch vessels and pulmonary bifurcation. The total defect (type C) is a large defect encompassing the proximal and distal segments due to the absence of the entire aorto-pulmonary septum [17]. Although small defects can be asymptomatic, most patients present early in life due to large left to right shunt causing increased pulmonary blood flow (PBF) and features of pulmonary overload such as respiratory difficulty, failure to thrive and tachypnea. If it is untreated, the increased PBF invariably leads to pulmonary hypertension and onset of pulmonary vascular disease and death (Fig. 7.3b) (Videos 7.1, 7.2, 7.3, 7.4, 7.5, and 7.6). Almost all patients would need surgical correction or catheter-based device closure of the defect. Associated aortic arch anomalies and other CHDs if any decide the medical or surgical course and management.

Imaging: Most of the time, a 2D echocardiogram is sufficient for the diagnosis of APW, and additionally a catheter angiogram is done to assess the pulmonary vascular resistance. Cross-sectional imaging may be required only when echo imaging is sub-optimal. In such times, CT can demonstrate accurately the type and size of defect, arch anatomy and the orientation and bifurcation anatomy of the pulmonary arteries and the anatomy of the coronaries. CT can additionally also reveal bronchial compression due to dilated branch pulmonary arteries. The role of MRI in the evaluation of APW in routine practice is not defined though it may be of value when there are associated CHDs.

7.4.3 Transposition of Great Arteries (TGA)

Transposition of great arteries is a ventriculo-arterial discordance where the morphological RV gives rise to the aorta and morphological LV gives rise to the pulmonary artery. TGA can be corrected or uncorrected. For uncorrected TGA, an additional shunt is mandatory for survival. TGA is covered in detail in Chap. 16.

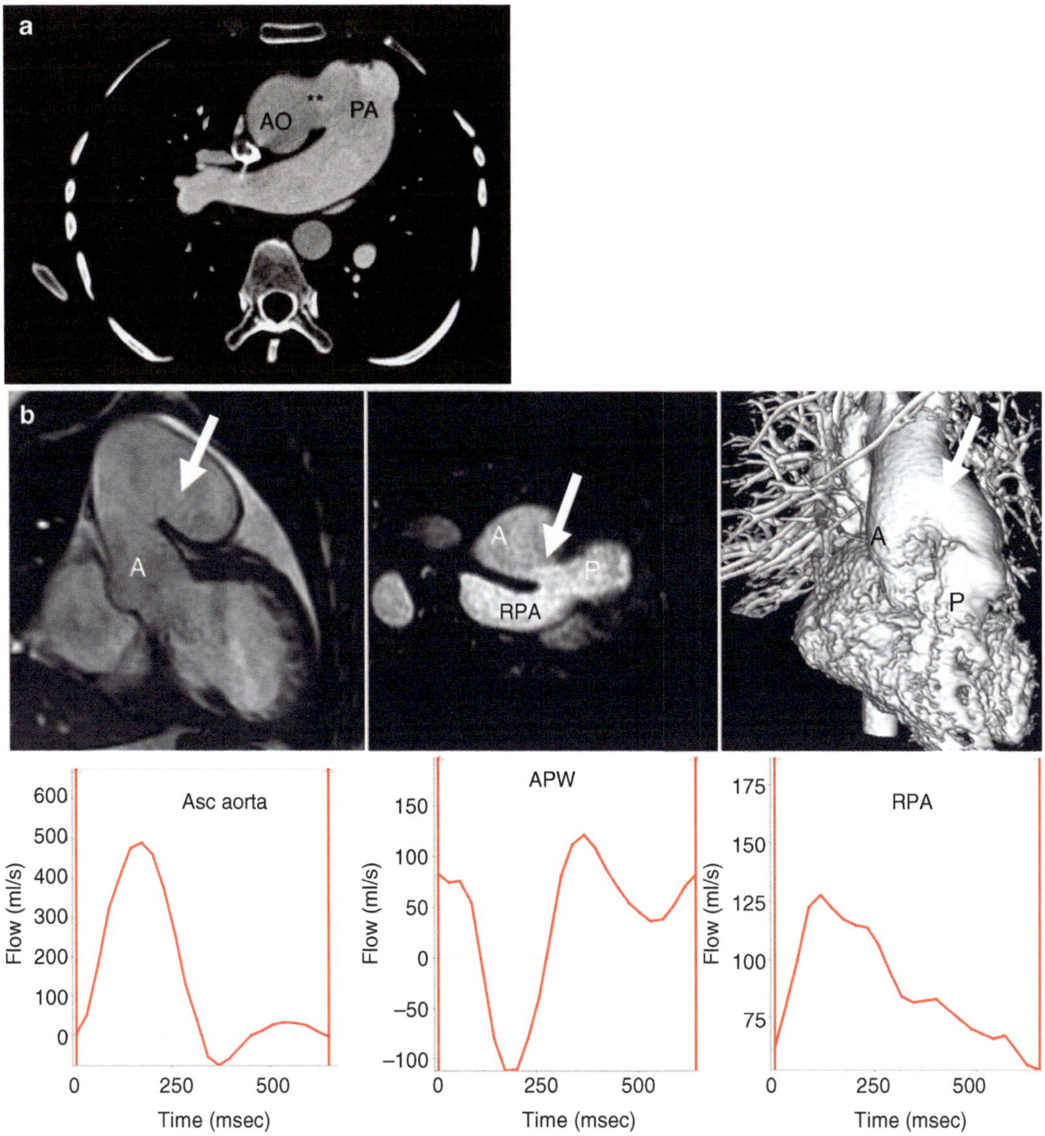

Fig. 7.3 (**a**) Large proximal type of APW. A wide communicating channel (**) is seen connecting the proximal aorta (AO) with the pulmonary artery (PA). (**b**) A 41-year-old patient with dyspnoea and cyanosis. MRI shows large aorto-pulmonary window (arrow) with a bidirectional (predominantly right–left) shunt. Absent left pulmonary artery; dilated main pulmonary artery continuing as right pulmonary artery (RPA). RPA PC flow pattern suggests severe pulmonary hypertension. *A* aorta; *APW* aortopulmonary window; *P* pulmonary artery (Ref to Videos 7.1 to 7.6)

7.4.4 Sinus of Valsalva Aneurysm

Sinus of Valsalva (SOV) aneurysms accounts for 0.1–3.5% of congenital heart defects [18, 19]. It is commonly associated with membranous VSD. It is believed to occur due to inadequacy in the elastic lamina at the junction of the aortic media and annulus fibrosus or due to lack of elastic tissue as seen in Marfan disease or Ehlers–Danlos syndrome. Rarely it can become sufficiently aneurysmal and rupture. SOV aneurysm most commonly involves the right coronary sinus (70–90%) (Fig. 7.4), followed by non-coronary sinus (10–20%) and it least commonly affects the left coronary sinus (<5%) [18]. SOV aneurysm may be incidentally discovered or may present as rupture with sudden severe aortic insufficiency and heart failure [20]. Such cases present usually as young

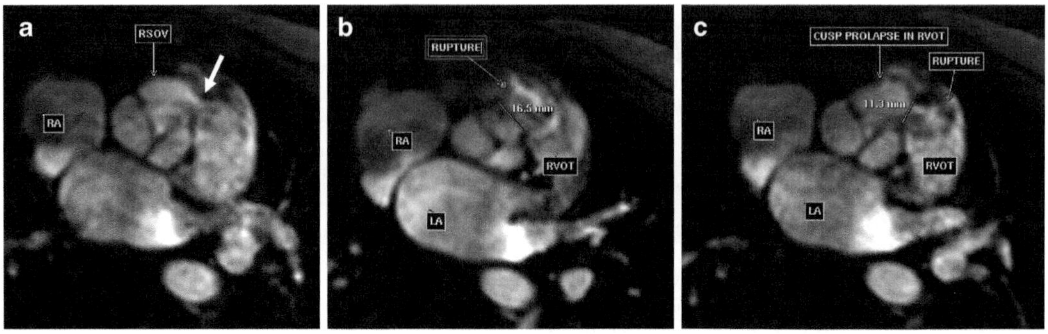

Fig. 7.4 (**a**, **b**) Serial cross-sectional MR images at the aortic valve level shows ruptured right sinus of Valsalva (RSOV) aneurysm with associated septal defect (white arrow) causing left to right shunt from the ruptured sinus to the right ventricular outflow tract (RVOT). (**c**) Shows turbulent blood flow at the site of rupture into the RVOT. It also shows the dilatation of the right coronary sinus with the prolapse of the right coronary cusp into the RVOT

adults with sudden onset dyspnea, chest pain or collapse due to abrupt onset of left-to-right shunt. Almost 50% of cases of SOV aneurysms can develop varying degrees of aortic regurgitation [21]. Other complications include thrombus formation within the aneurysm with the risk of stroke, compromise of coronary ostia with myocardial ischemia or infarction [22–24], mass effect on the adjoining structures namely the right ventricular outflow tract (RVOT) and impairment of mitral or tricuspid valve function [25]. Other notable associated malformation with SOV aneurysm includes a bicuspid aortic valve [26].

MRI is excellent to depict the flow pattern and quantification of shunt. The difference between the total forward flow in the MPA distal to the shunt and the total flow in the aorta distal to the rupture will give the excess flow in the MPA.

Imaging usually is warranted in complex cases to demonstrate the extent of defect in the aortic sinus and its location. An MRI using flow estimation sequences can give additional information about the degree of shunting. MRI is often a preferred modality due to lack of radiation and its ability to assess aortic and other valvar functions as well as the size and function of the right and left ventricles. Many patients are young adults; hence, MR imaging can be performed without any sedation for a comprehensive evaluation of the ventricular size and function, valvar function and accurate assessment of the shunt. MRI however lacks the spatial resolution possible on CT imaging. Both imaging techniques give excellent information about the mass effect of the aneurysm on the adjoining structures, especially the RVOT and depiction of thrombus if any. Ruptured SOV aneurysm has been classified depending on the site of origin and leak by Sakakibara and Konno in 1962 [27]. It has been further modified by HW Guo et al. in 2013 into a simple modified version for surgical planning [28]. On imaging, an SOV aneurysm is diagnosed if it shows origin above the aortic annulus, a saccular shape and normal size of adjoining aorta and aortic root [29]. Specific information that must be provided in SOV aneurysm rupture include—size of the aneurysm in comparison to the other normal cusp, size of the ruptured site, location of the site of rupture, the site of the leak, its distance from the coronary artery and mass effect or obstruction to the surrounding structures. Further information about associated anomalies like a concurrent VSD or complications such as thrombus, myocardial perfusion defect or scar can be assessed. The site and size of rupture and coronary anatomy help in deciding if a percutaneous closure of the leak is possible. Surgical planning is also heavily based on anatomical features of the SOV aneurysm. In unruptured cases, the size of aneurysm more than 50% than the other normal sinuses or distortion of the surrounding structures have been recommended for surgical repair [30].

7.4.5 Supravalvar Aortic Stenosis

Supravalvar aortic stenosis (SVAS) is the rarest lesion of the left ventricular outflow tract obstructions (LVOTOs). It is a focal or diffuse narrowing of the aorta starting at the sino-tubular junction and often involving the entire ascending aorta (15% of cases). The other entities in LVOTO group are bicuspid aortic valve, aortic coarctation and subaortic stenosis. SVAS is commonly associated with Williams–Beuren syndrome, an autosomal dominant multisystemic disorder that may manifest with SVAS (71% of cases), mitral valve prolapse and pulmonary artery stenosis (Fig. 7.5a) [31].

2D echo remains the modality of choice for the depiction of the supravalvar aortic stenosis though CT/MRI can help in adult cases where the window for echo imaging is difficult to obtain especially to demonstrate associated pulmonary artery lesions (Fig. 7.5b). The membrane-like lesion is seen as a focal area of severe narrowing

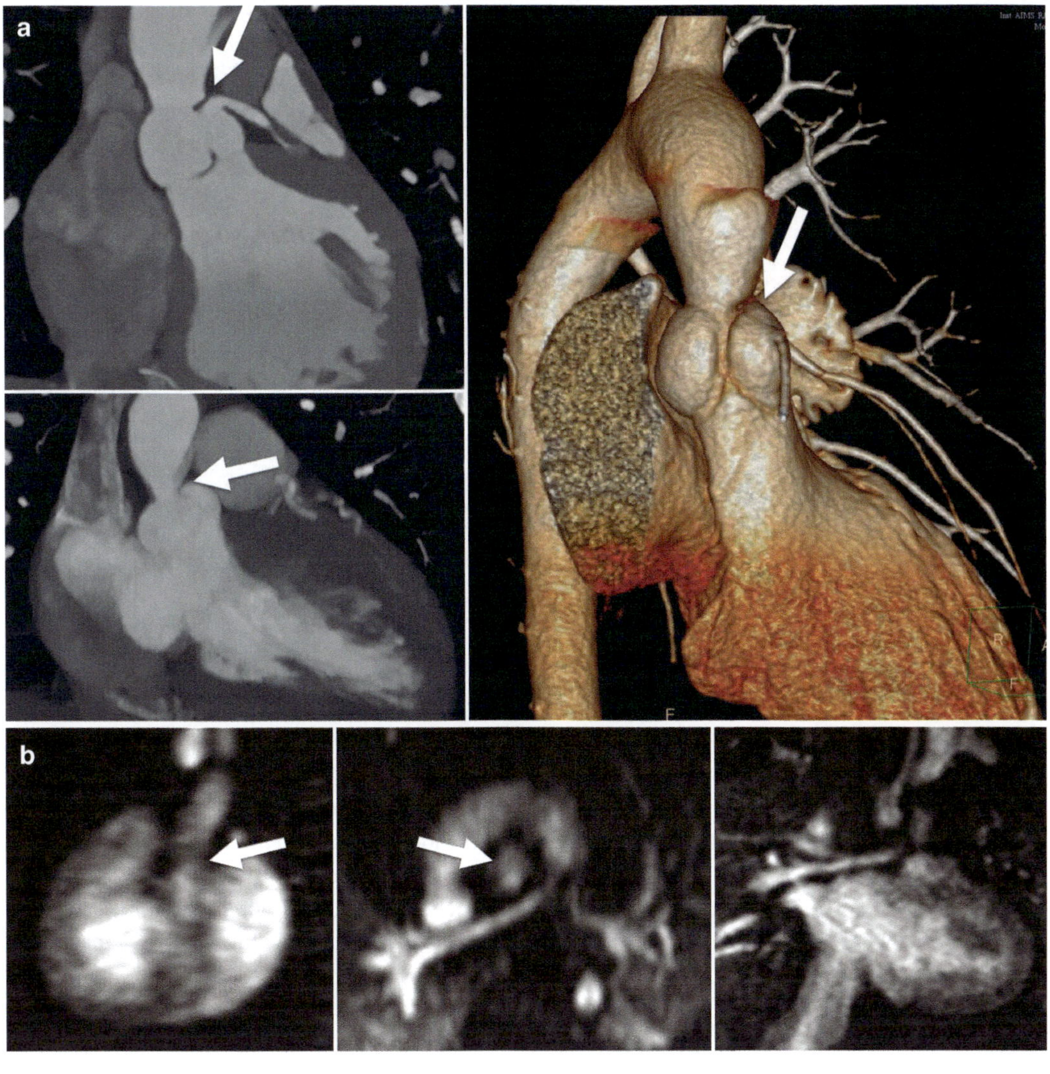

Fig. 7.5 (**a**) An 18-year-old male with Williams syndrome. ECG-gated CT angio shows discrete ridge-like supravalvar aortic stenosis with LV hypertrophy. (**b**) MR angiogram in a non-Williams phenotype shows moderate supravalvar discrete fibro muscular type aortic stenosis (arrow) with bilateral peripheral pulmonary stenosis. (**c**) True axial imaging multiplanar reconstruction shows severe stenosis of the aortic lumen at the ST junction. The diameter is measured in the left lower image in the true axial plane of the aorta. The purple line in the left upper and right-sided image represents the cut-plane. (**d**) Severe stenosis at the ST junction (White arrow) is seen with severe LVH (white asterisk). Also noted is a PDA (black arrowhead). (**e**) A 19-year-old male with supravalvar aortic stenosis shows ectatic dilatation of the left main coronary artery (LM) demonstrated on axial MIP image

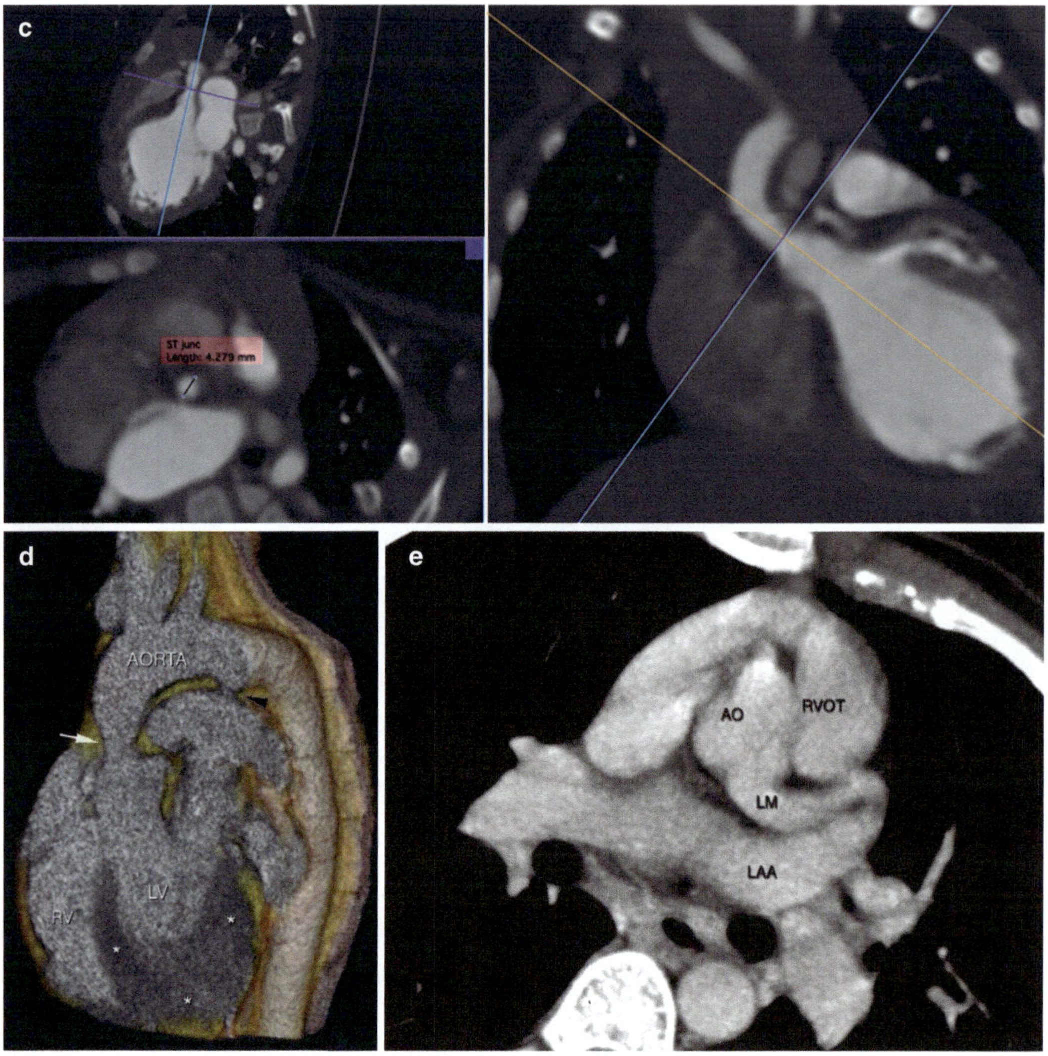

Fig. 7.5 (continued)

of the aorta usually at or just above the level of the ST junction (Fig. 7.5b). The luminal diameter of the aorta must be measured in the true axial plane of the aorta. The membrane may result in eccentric narrowing of the ascending aorta or ST junction. A prominent jet beyond the site of stenosis can be demonstrated on MRI. In adult patients, there would be LVH depending on the extent of stenosis (Fig. 7.5c). Ectatic dilatation of the coronaries may be seen as the flow is diverted to the coronaries instead of the ascending aorta (Fig. 7.5d). A dedicated CT coronary angiogram with wider coverage to include the entire thoracic aorta is therefore useful in these cases. Dilated and ectatic coronaries along with LVH can result in chest pain in these individuals. Management involves surgical resection of the membrane; however, once LVH has set in, it is difficult to reverse the same. This condition is associated with poor forward flow to the developing aorta and may lead to a hypoplastic arch and ascending aorta.

7.4.6 Aorta to LV Fistula

It is a rare anomaly that shows a vascular channel communicating between the proximal aorta and the LV mimicking the physiology of aortic regurgitation (AR). A small fistula may be left as it is but a larger fistula needs surgical closure (Fig. 7.6a, b).

7.4.7 Aortic Valve Anomalies

Aortic valve anomalies include congenital aortic stenosis and valve leaflet anomalies such as monocuspid, bicuspid and quadricuspid aortic valves. Congenital aortic stenosis can be seen as an isolated condition or associated with a hypoplastic left heart. There is a reduced forward flow of blood into the aorta which may be associated with a hypoplastic aortic arch. Often the stenosis causes significant pressure gradient across the stenotic valve which can cause the ascending aorta to dilate to variable extent. Follow-up of these cases associated with aortic dilatation is needed to assess the risk of potential rupture. MR angiography with flow studies can be used to non-invasively image these patients for both aortic valve pathology and extent of aortic dilatation. Besides left ventricular function can be accurately assessed which can aid in follow-up and decision-making.

7.4.8 Ascending Aortic Atresia

Ascending aortic atresia is usually associated with hypoplasia of left ventricle and or mitral/aortic valve in the majority of the cases as a part of hypoplastic left heart syndrome (HLHS). But rarely it may be associated with ventricular septal defect (VSD) and a reasonably developed LV, as the VSD provides an outflow for the left ventricle. The hypoplastic ascending aorta and the coronary arteries receive usually low-pressure diastolic retrograde flow via the ductus arteriosus and aortic arch (Fig. 7.7) (Videos 7.7, 7.8, 7.9, 7.10, 7.11, 7.12, 7.13, and 7.14). Compared to HLHS, this small subset of patients with VSD and adequate LV shows excellent long-term survival by primary bi-ventricular repair [32, 33].

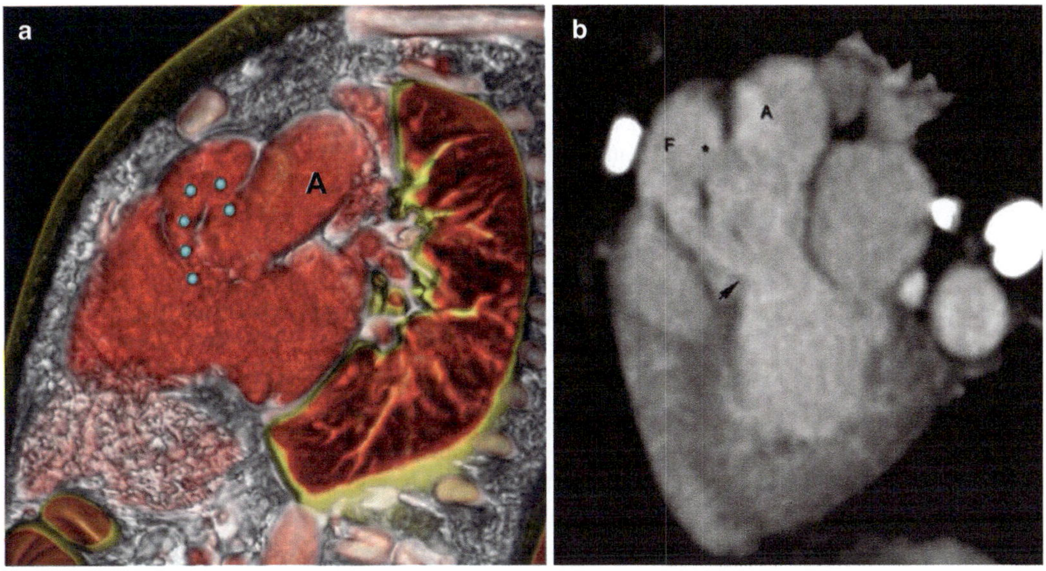

Fig. 7.6 (**a**) Volume-rendered image showing aorta to LV fistulous communication. The tract is marked by blue dots. *A* aorta. (**b**) MPR image of the same case shows the site of communication of fistula with aorta marked in asterisk and its site of communication with the LV marked by black arrowhead. *F* fistula; *A* aorta

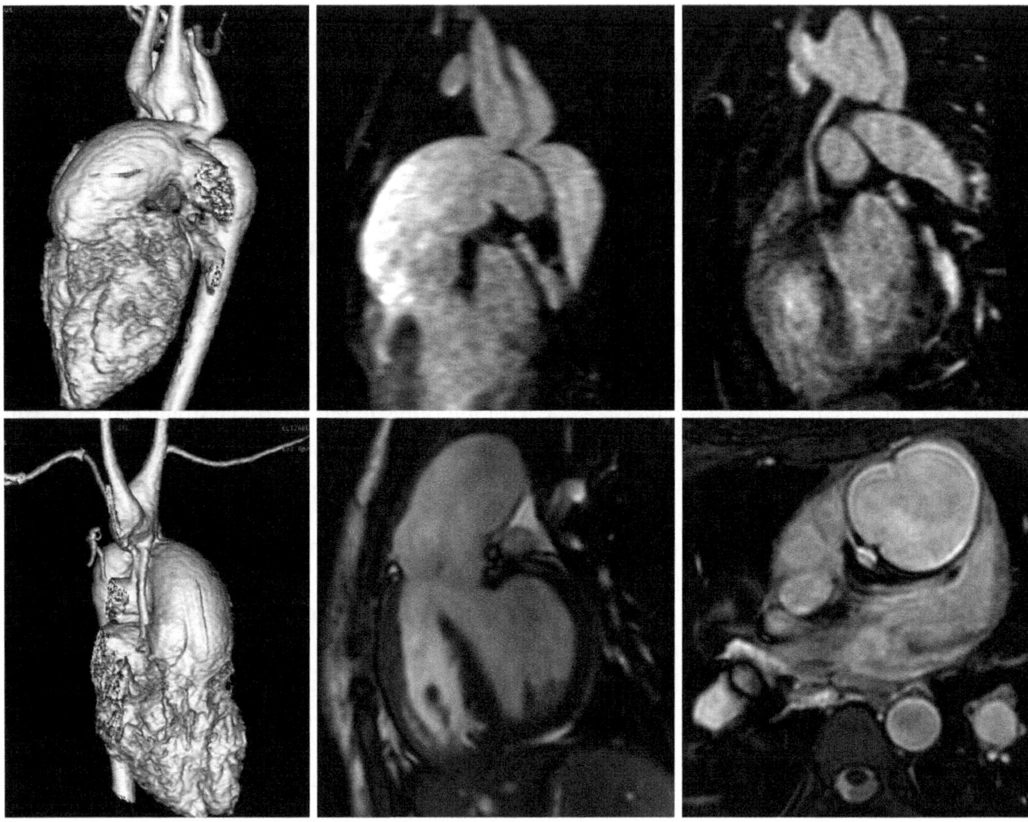

Fig. 7.7 Hypoplastic ascending aorta and aortic valve atresia in a 16-year-old girl (Full description is available in the videos 7.7 to 7.14)

7.5 Aortic Arch Anomalies

A significant number of arch anomalies and variants are known along with variation in sidedness. The arch is considered right-sided if it curves over the right bronchus and left-sided if it arches over the left bronchus. Variable arch anomalies resulting in vascular loops such as the aberrant origin of subclavian arteries, double arch, cervical arch, circumflex aorta, Kommerell's diverticulum form a spectrum of vascular rings which will be covered in Chapter 8.

This section will predominantly highlight arch anomalies involving hypoplasia, coarctation, interruption of the aorta and congenital ductus arteriosus aneurysm.

7.5.1 Hypoplastic Aortic Arch

Aortic arch is considered as hypoplastic if the proximal arch diameter is less than 60% of the diameter of the ascending aorta or of the distal arch is less than 50% of the ascending aorta [34, 35] and of the isthmus being less than 40% of the ascending aorta [36]. Since these measurements can only be applied in those cases who show normal ascending aortic size, comparing the arch diameters with established normal sizes for the given height and weight of the patient is recommended. The aortic diameters have to be obtained in a plane truly perpendicular to the aorta. CT and MRI with their multiplanar capabilities can provide appropriate perpendicular sections of the aortic lumen using two orthogonal planes. Aorta or any other cardiac structure is considered normal if it lies within two standard deviations (SD) above or below the mean. One standard deviation across the mean will encompass almost 68% of the normal population and 2SD comprises of almost 95% of the normal population. Outliers above the 2SD are considered dilated, and below the 2SD considered as hypoplastic or stenotic. Mean values are calculated as *z*-scores which are more established on 2D echocardiography than on cross-sectional imaging. CT and MRI data have been published for normal expected aortic sizes and can be used for evaluation [37, 38].

Hypoplastic arch can be seen in association with reduced LV outflow conditions resulting in poor forward flow in the aorta, such as hypoplastic left heart, aortic stenosis or mitral stenosis as well as with septal defects and PDA [39]. A hypoplastic arch is often associated with coarctation of the aorta.

On imaging, the hypoplastic arch is reduced in calibre and may often be elongated (Fig. 7.8a, b). It often shows a tenting in its mid part. Often there is an associated coarctation. There may be associated reduced calibre of the rest of the thoracic aorta. A differential for the hypoplastic arch in older children would be arteritis-induced narrowing. Clinical presentation is usually sufficient for suspecting vasculitis; however, rarely vasculitis presenting in early childhood, below 5 years of age, can present a clinical dilemma where imaging can play a role in distinguishing the two entities and providing necessary information for the extent of disease affection in cases of vasculitis. Vasculitis often shows multi-vessel involvement especially the subclavian arteries and to variable extent of other arch vessels. The presence of plaques, especially calcific plaques, and surrounding vessel wall thickening are characteristics of vasculitis and are absent in cases of congenital hypoplasia. The presence of plaques, wall thickening and involvement of origin of other vessels should prompt a diagnosis of vasculitis rather than arch hypoplasia. MR angiography can also be useful in cases of vasculitis as it can

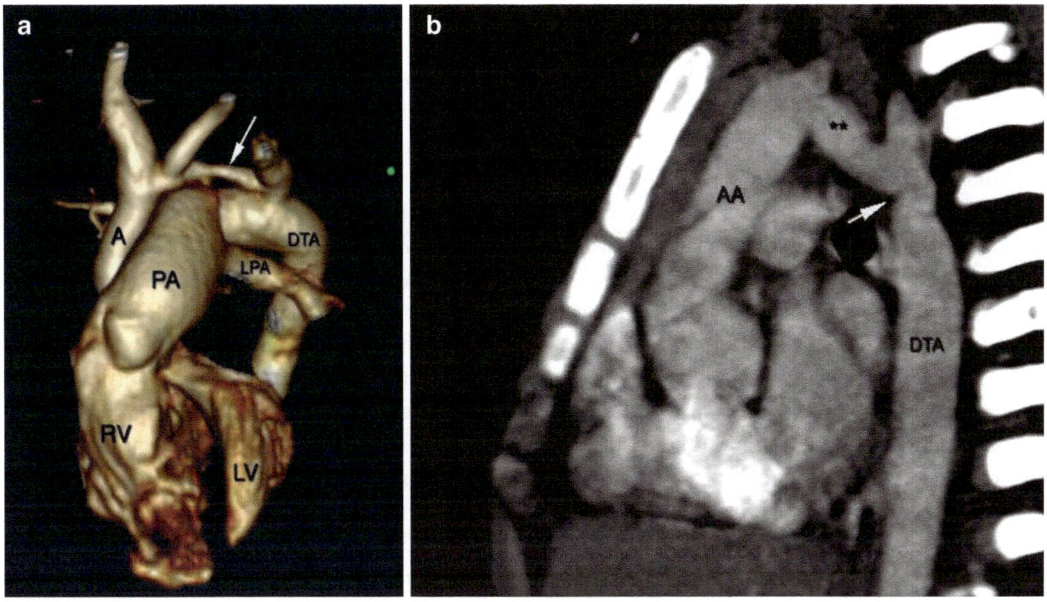

Fig. 7.8 (**a**) Volume-rendered blood pool image shows small-sized LV with reduced calibre of the ascending aorta and hypoplastic aortic arch (white arrow). There is associated dilatation of the pulmonary artery (PA) and preserved calibre of the descending thoracic aorta (DTA). (**b**) MPR oblique sagittal image shows elongated and hypoplastic arch (double asterisk) with terminal tortuosity and ductal coarctation. *AA* ascending aorta; *DTA* descending thoracic aorta

depict surrounding vessel wall edema and inflammation; otherwise, a regular ECG-gated CT imaging of the aorta would suffice.

7.5.2 Coarctation of Aorta

Coarctation accounts for 4%–8% of congenital heart defects and has a prevalence of approximately 4 per 10,000 live births [40, 41]. Coarctation of the aorta is a severe narrowing of the aorta close to the level of the ductus arteriosus. There is often a shelf-like membrane causing luminal stenosis. This can be located proximal, at the level or distal to the ductus arteriosus [42] thus resulting in pre-ductal, ductal or post-ductal coarctation, respectively. It is often associated with varying extent of narrowing of the surrounding isthmus or a hypoplastic arch. Bicuspid aortic valve is the most common association. Two theories have been postulated in the development of coarctation. One believes the proliferation of abnormal ductal tissue along the aortic isthmus as the cause for aortic narrowing; however, it fails to explain the concurrent cause of aortic and isthmic narrowing so often associated with coarctation. The second theory proposes abnormal hemodynamics resulting in poor antegrade flow in the aorta in utero as a cause of coarctation which also explains the co-existence of arch and isthmic hypoplasia [36, 43]. Coarctation is rarely seen in a right aortic arch, and if present, it is commonly associated with an aberrant left subclavian artery [44]. Although most cases of coarctation are sporadic, there is a strong genetic association [42].

Clinically pre-ductal coarctation presents during infancy and post-ductal often presents after the neonatal period or in adulthood. Mild cases present insidiously in adulthood as perfusion is maintained through collateral circulation from intercostal, internal mammary, thyrocervical, thoracoacromial and scapular arteries which supply the descending thoracic aorta [42].

Aortic coarctation is well diagnosed on echocardiography. CT- or MRI-based aortogram is usually required to look for the location, severity of the stenosis (Fig. 7.9a, b), extent of isthmic and arch hypoplasia if any and extent of post-stenotic dilatation (Fig. 7.9c, d). The extent or length of post-stenotic dilatation is an indication of the extent or severity of stenosis. Multiple thoracic collaterals, namely the intercostal arteries often are dilated and shunt blood to the aorta distal to the coarctation. CT also delineates the distance of the segment of coarctation from the last arch vessel, usually the ipsilateral subclavian artery (Fig. 7.9c, d). Both these measurements can be accurately given on CT imaging. For all aortic measurements, the internal luminal diameter is measured in the true axial plane (Fig. 7.9e). This is achieved by either reconstructing the true cross-section using two orthogonal planes or by using curved multiplanar reconstruction by drawing a central line through the vessel along its length. The internal luminal diameter of the stenotic segment needs to be measured in the true axial plane of the aorta (Fig. 7.9e).

Coarctation repair can be done by either catheter balloon angioplasty or by surgical reconstruction. Common surgical methods of correction include resection of the stenosed segment followed by end-to-end anastomosis, angioplasty using subclavian flap and extended end-to-end or end-to-side anastomosis [45]. If the coarctation is in close proximity to the subclavian artery, stenting may be difficult and surgical correction may be preferred. A vital measurement therefore on CT or MR angiography imaging would be the distance of the coarctation from the last arch vessel (Fig. 7.9f). In the case of an associated aberrant subclavian artery, the distance from the same may be mentioned. Severe stenosis also may not be amenable to cather balloon angioplasty due to a higher risk of aortic rupture. Such patients are best treated by surgical correction. Often the adjoining subclavian artery may be used for reconstruction and it would be worthwhile to mention the diameter of the subclavian arteries. Cross-sectional imaging can also delineate the presence or absence of any adjoining aortic tortuosity which may result in a difficult trans-catheter approach (Fig. 7.9a, b).

Aortic coarctation repair after surgery has led to improving the lifespan of patients to 35–50 years [46]. Complications that appear post-repair include restenosis of the repaired segment and aneurysm formation (Fig. 7.9g, h). The patients also are prone to hypertension and increased risk of coronary artery disease, stroke and heart failure [46, 47].

The severity of coarctation of the aorta can be assessed by evaluating the collateral flow circulation by phase-contrast (PC) MRI. Normally flow volume in the proximal descending aorta is approximately 7% higher than in the distal thoracic aorta, but in patients with coarctation, there may be greater blood flow distally due to retrograde collateral blood flow into the aorta from the intercostal arteries and other aortic branches. The amount of flow in descending aorta at the level of diaphragm minus flow volume just distal to the coarctation segment gives the exact volume of collateral flow. The presence of collateral flow indicates a hemodynamically significant coarctation. MRI and PC flow studies can be used in complex coarctation cases (Fig. 7.9i) (Videos 7.15, 7.16, 7.17, 7.18, 7.19, 7.20, and 7.21)

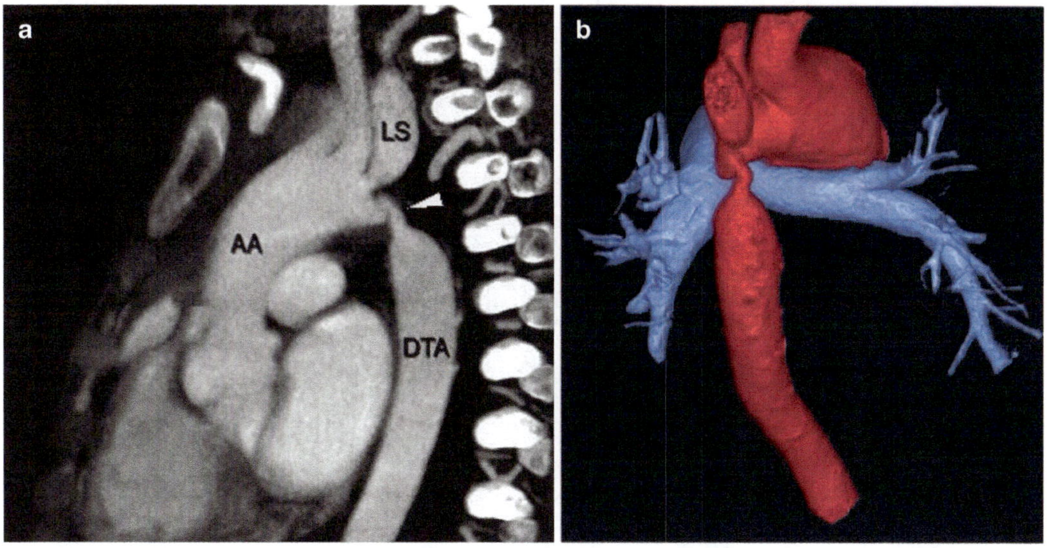

Fig. 7.9 (**a**) Severe short segment coarctation of the aorta (white arrowhead), just beyond the origin of the left subclavian artery (LS). Note the tortuosity of the segment of coarctation making it a difficulty subset for catheter balloon dilatation or stenting. (**b**) Volume-rendered image of (**a**) better delineates the tortuosity of the segment of coarctation as seen from the posterior aspect. Red—aorta, blue—pulmonary arteries. (**c**) Volume-rendered image shows severe focal coarctation of the aorta (White arrow) with post-stenotic dilatation (yellow arrowheads) for a length of almost 2 cm suggesting severe gradient across the stenotic segment. Its length from the left subclavian artery measures approximately 8 mm. The measurements are best obtained on MPR or curved multiplanar reformatted images. (**d**) MPR image of the same case as (**c**) shows severe focal coarctation of aorta (White arrowhead) due to shelf-like membrane causing severe luminal narrowing and long segment of post-stenotic dilatation. *AA* ascending aorta. (**e**) MPR images are used to obtain true perpendicular plane for aortic luminal measurement. The site of coarctation is measured in the axial plane demarcated as purple plane in the oblique sagittal image in upper left-hand side and coronal image on the right side. The axial image represented in the lower left side is the true axial plane of the site of coarctation. Luminal measurement is shown in black line. (**f**) Oblique sagittal reformatted image shows the aorta in profile with post-ductal focal coarctation. There is significant length of aorta beyond the origin of left subclavian artery and no tortuosity, a favourable case for trans-catheter balloon dilatation. (**g**) Smooth area of long segment narrowing in a case of balloon angioplasty of aortic coarctation (arrowhead). (**h**) volume-rendered reconstruction shows long segment irregular narrowing of the aortic arch (white arrowheads) following surgical repair of hypoplastic arch and ductal coarctation. (**i**) Thirty-year-old male patient with severe discrete coarctation of aorta with large PDA and pulmonary hypertension. Cine images and phase contrast flow study provided the detailed physiology of circulation in the pulmonary arteries and aorta, which was used to guide further treatment plans. Post-coarctation stenting CMR showed an increment of 34% in absolute pulmonary blood flow and a moderate improvement in bi-ventricular function (not shown here) (Ref to Videos 7.15 to 7.21)

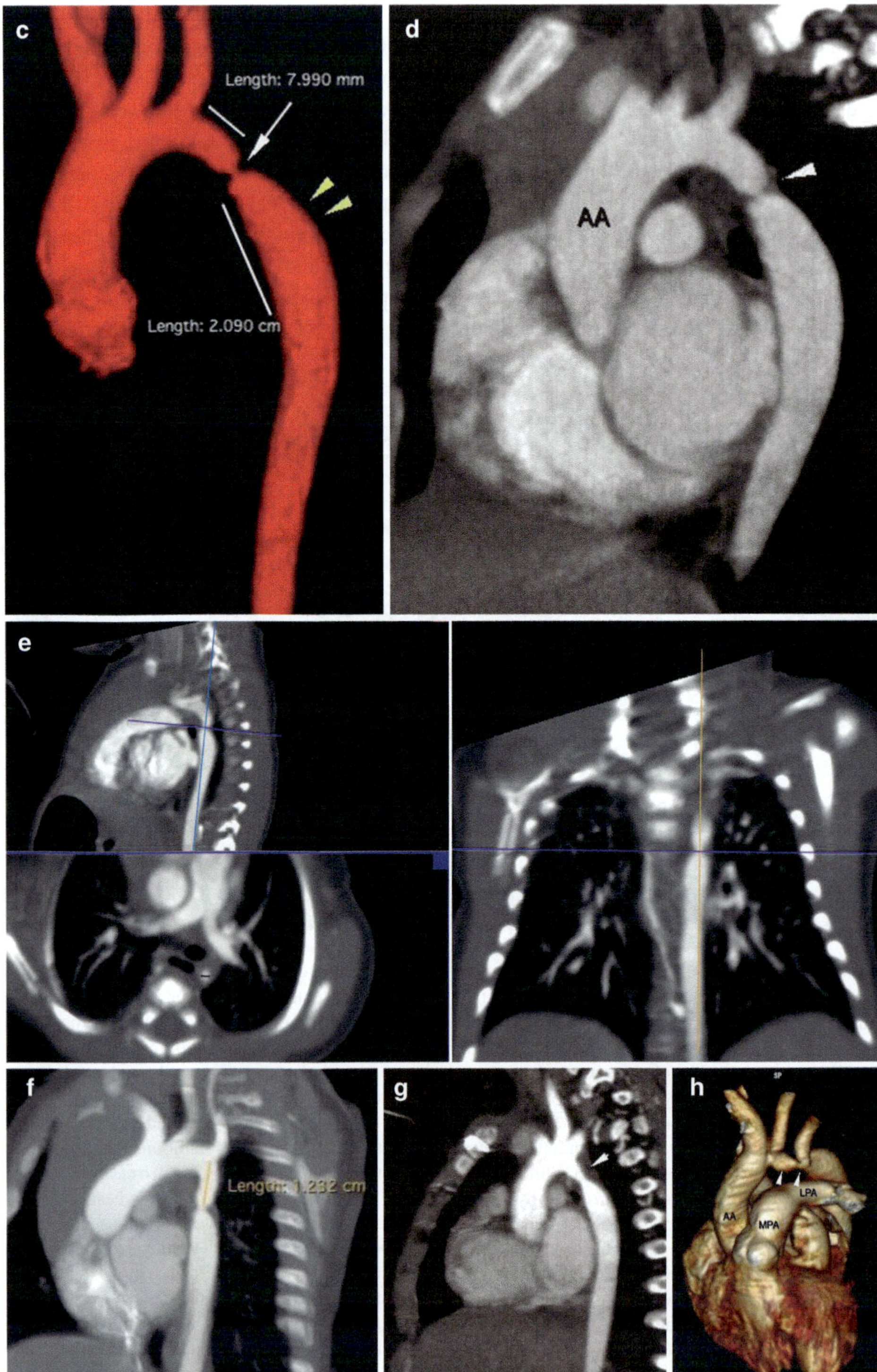

Fig. 7.9 (continued)

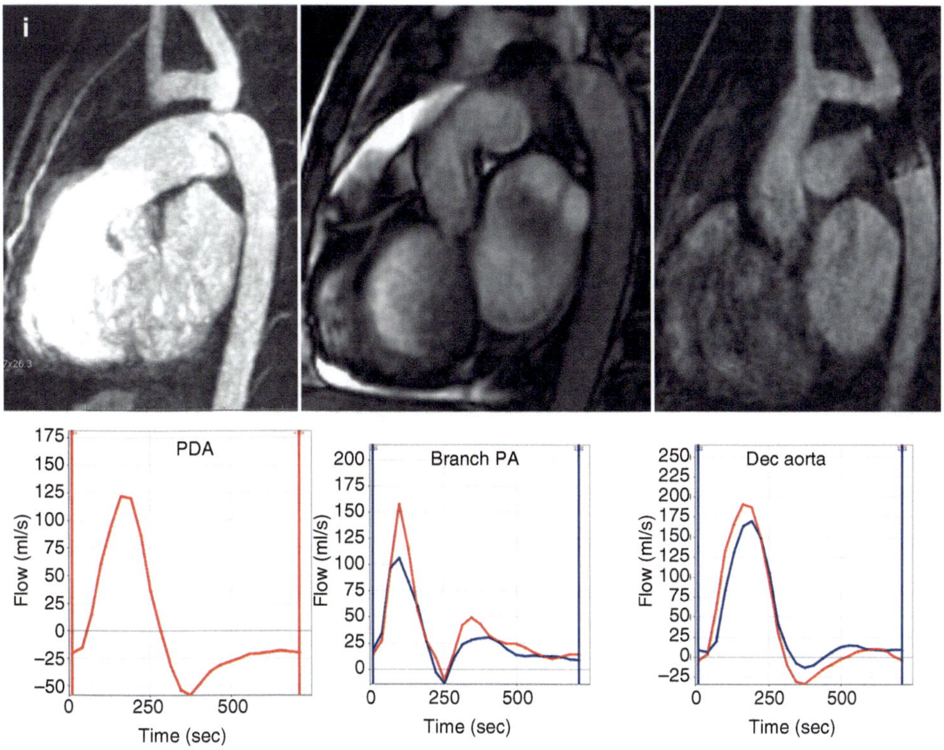

Fig. 7.9 (continued)

7.5.3 Interrupted Aortic Arch

Interrupted aortic arch is a condition where there is complete luminal discontinuity between the proximal and distal aorta with or without an atretic fibrotic band [48]. It represents approximately 1.5% of congenital heart disease cases [49]. It is almost always associated with a PDA and is often seen with a large VSD and may be associated with APW and truncus arteriosus [50]. The clinical presentation is usually within the first 2 weeks of life, often with cardiac failure.

Interrupted aortic arch is classified into three types depending on the site of discontinuity:

- Type A—interruption occurs distal to the origin of the left subclavian artery (Fig. 7.10a, b).
- Type B—interruption occurs between the left common carotid and left subclavian artery origin (Fig. 7.10c).
- Type C—interruption occurs between the innominate artery and the left common carotid arteries.

Of these, type B is the commonest, and type C the least common [36, 51]. Type B and C are postulated to result from poor forward flow in the aorta during foetal life [50]. Type B is often associated with bicuspid aortic valve, posteriorly deviated conal septum causing subaortic stenosis and VSD. Other associations include microdeletion of chromosome 22q11.2 and DiGeorge syndrome [36].

Surgical repair is the only corrective measure for these patients. Pre-surgical evaluation by cross-sectional imaging must provide detailed information regarding the type of interruption, diameters of the proximal and distal aorta, length of interruption (Fig. 7.10d) as well as the size of PDA and anatomic details of the arch vessels [52]. Additionally, there may be associated smaller calibre of proximal aorta and v-shaped orientation of the arch vessels (Fig. 7.10c). This can be visual-

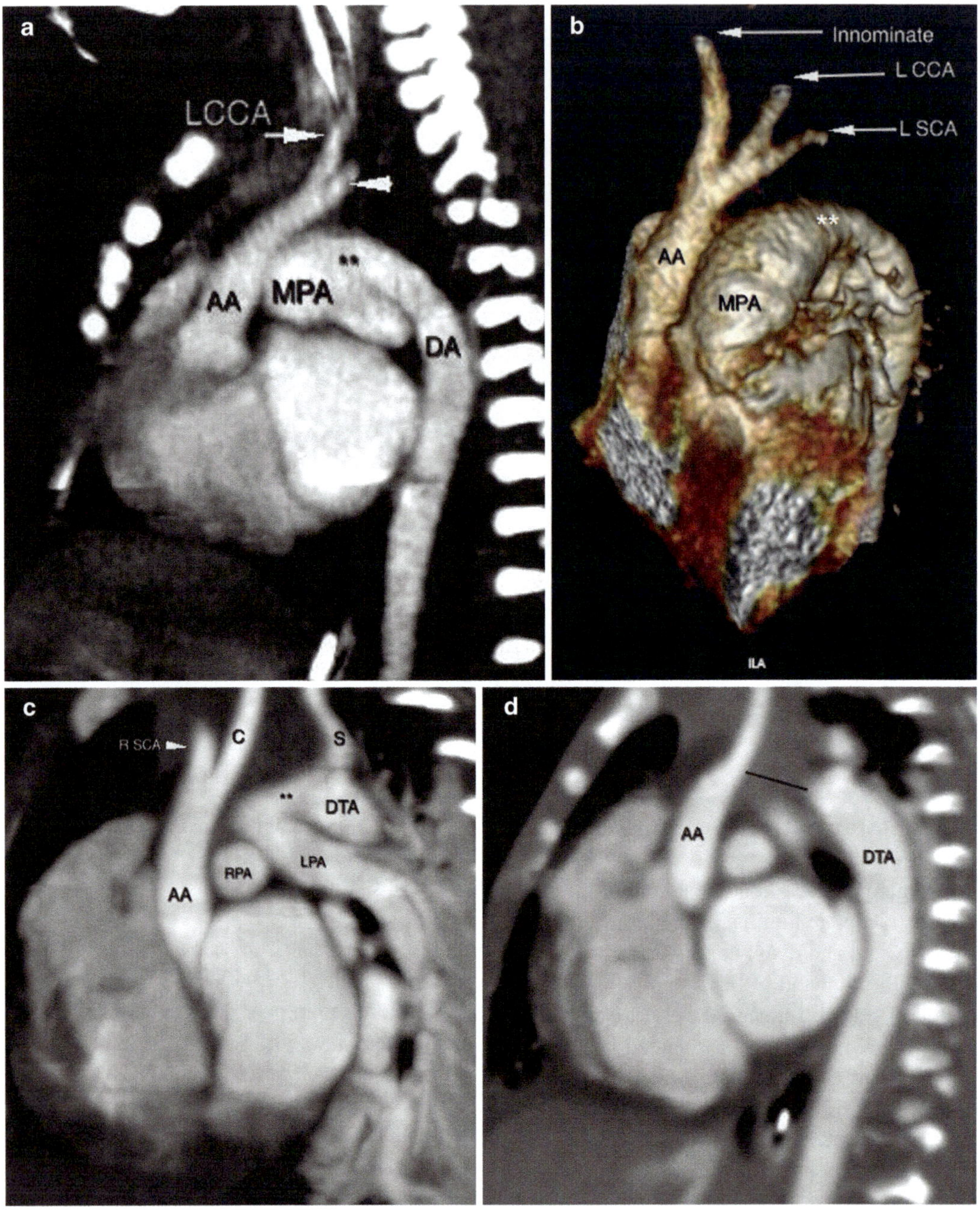

Fig. 7.10 (**a**) MPR oblique sagittal reconstructed image shows type A interruption. Interruption is distal to the left subclavian artery (arrowhead). The descending aorta (DA) is supplied by PDA (double black asterisk). (**b**) Volume-rendered image of the same case as (**a**), shows type A interruption with MPA supplying the descending aorta through the PDA (double white asterisk). (**c**) Oblique sagittal reconstruction shows type B interruption. The ascending aorta (AA) ends on bifurcating to the right subclavian artery (R SCA). PDA (**) is seen supplying the descending aorta (DTA). LPA is seen in profile and RPA in the cross section. Note the V-shaped orientation of the arch vessels. (**d**) Same case as (**c**); Oblique sagittal reconstruction shows the measurement of the distance between the ascending and descending aorta (black line)

ised on both CT angiography as well as on MR Imaging. MR imaging can further contribute by providing a detailed evaluation of both ventricular outflow tracts and cardiac function. Black-blood imaging technique in the oblique sagittal plane can show the proximal arch and the origins of the arch vessels and non-oblique sagittal images shows the PDA in profile as it courses antero-posteriorly. On non-oblique, true sagittal plane, the antero-posteriorly placed large PDA may be mistaken for a complete arch, multiplanar imaging is thus warranted to prevent this fallacy [52]. MR imaging is also useful in post-operative follow-up imaging due to a lack of ionising radiation and simultaneous assessment of the cardiac function. In older children, long-term post-repair follow-up MRI is safely possible without ionising radiation. MRI in older children may also score over 2D echocardiography which may be limited due to poor echo windows. Common post-operative complications include graft stenosis or aneurysm [52].

7.5.4 Congenital Ductus Arteriosus Aneurysm

Congenital ductus arteriosus aneurysm (DAA) is a rare condition characterised by saccular or tubular dilation of ductus arteriosus and is an important cause of extrinsic compression on the airways, producing stertorous breathing in the newborn [53, 54].

Ductus arteriosus aneurysm likely develops in the third trimester and may be the result of abnormal intimal cushion formation or defective elastin in the ductus arteriosus.

Congenital DAA is generally asymptomatic and often goes unnoticed in the majority of the neonates.

Symptoms are due to complications like spontaneous rupture, thromboembolism, infection, erosion into airways or compression of adjacent thoracic structures [54].

In our series, the symptoms of DAA subsided within 3–5 days in the three neonates managed conservatively (Fig. 7.11). Serial echocardiograms showed thrombus formation and obliteration of the cavity in these cases over a period of 6 weeks to 3 months.

The authors of this retrospective review have recommended surgical excision of DAA in case of persistence of PDA beyond the neonatal period, or propagation of thrombus into adjacent vessels, or thromboembolism, or significant compression of adjacent structures, or when associated with connective tissue disorder [55].

7.6 Genetic Anomalies Affecting the Aorta

7.6.1 Marfan Syndrome

Marfan syndrome is a connective tissue disorder affecting multiple organ systems. It occurs due to the mutation of fibrillin-1 gene. It shows autosomal dominant inheritance with 25–30% sporadic mutations [56]. It is estimated to affect 2–3 per 10,000 persons [57]. Although it is a multisystem disease, the most common cause of death in these patients is related to cardiovascular affection resulting in aortic aneurysm, dissection and congestive cardiac failure [56].

As part of the connective tissue disorder, there is cystic medial necrosis of the aortic wall with disruption of the elastic lamina. It initially causes dilatation of the aortic root and may progress to aneurysm, dissection or rupture.

The aortic root consists of three parts—the aortic annulus, aortic sinuses and the sino-tubular junction (Fig. 7.12a). The aortic annulus is the site of attachment of the aortic valve leaflets and the junction of the aorta with the ventricles. The sinuses are the dilated portions of the root and the sino-tubular junction is the distal portion of the root from where the aorta assumes its true tubular form. Annulo-aortic ectasia is one of the most crucial manifestations of Marfan syndrome. It results in dilatation of the aortic root, first affecting the sinuses, then progressing to involve the sino-tubular junction (STJ) and finally the annulus [56] (Fig. 7.12b). The progressive annulo-aortic ectasia causes a lack of valvar coaptation and varying degrees of aortic regurgitation (AR) which further leads to aortic dilatation and often dissection. Ascending aortic

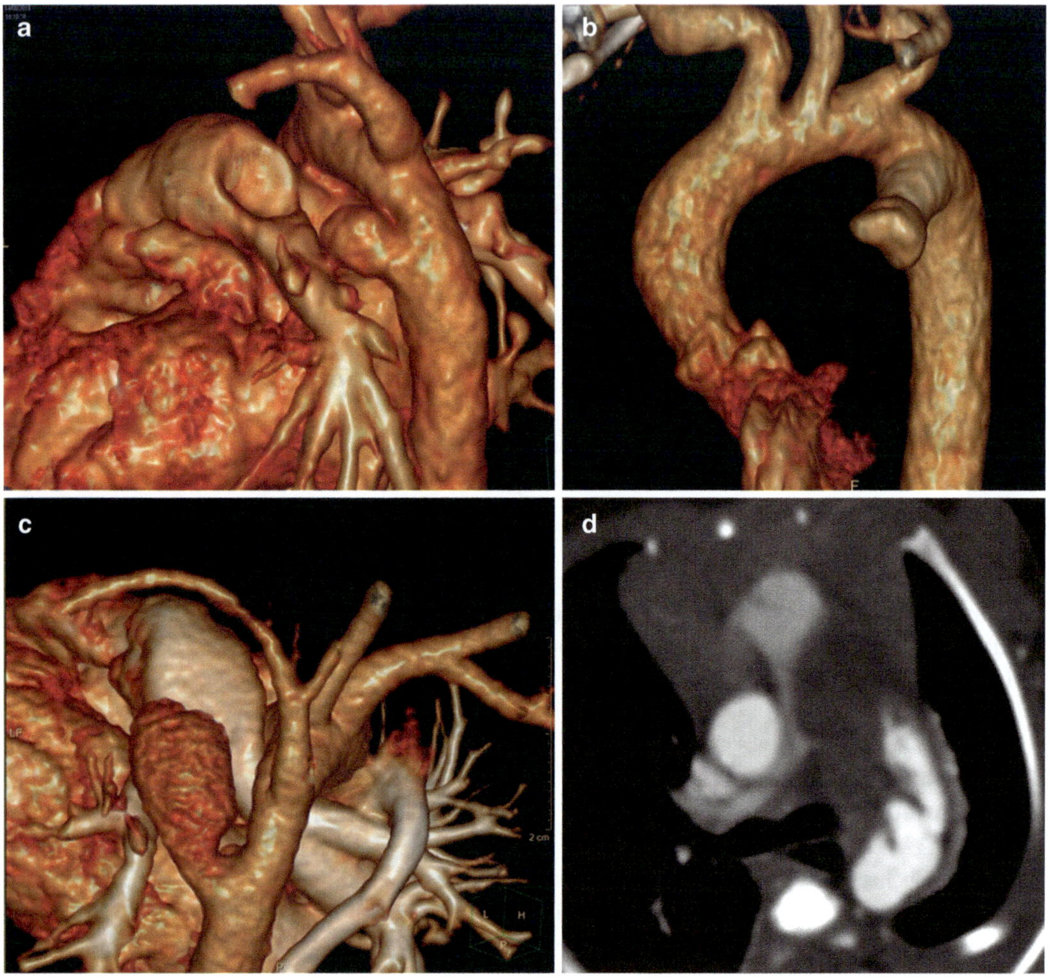

Fig. 7.11 Three different neonates with ductal diverticulum (**c**, **d** are the same baby). Note the large peripheral thrombus indenting the pulmonary artery (**d**). On follow-up echo (not shown), all babies showed complete thrombosis of the aneurysm

aneurysm can also occur in the absence of annulo-aortic ectasia. The aneurysms in Marfan syndrome also tend to enlarge more rapidly than atherosclerotic disease [58].

CT or MR imaging using ECG gating can demonstrate the dilated aortic root with loss of normal angulation at the sino-tubular junction (Fig. 7.12d). There is often a fusiform dilatation of the aortic root and ascending aorta. The patients are younger and imaging rarely shows changes of atherosclerosis such as intimal thickening, plaques or calcification. Other connective tissue disorders such as Ehlers–Danlos disease may show similar appearance and cannot be differentiated on imaging the aorta alone. It is recommended to check the aortic diameter in Marfan syndrome and offer prophylactic surgery when indicated. Aortic root diameter more than 5.5 cm in adults and 5 cm in children has been considered an indication for prophylactic surgery. Annual follow-up in patients diagnosed with Marfan disease is recommended to enable early detection of aneurysm formation and dissection. Prophylactic surgery is recommended if aortic diameter exceeds 1 cm per year and there is a family history of dissection.

ECG-gated CT imaging with retrospective gating or ECG-gated MR imaging is recommended. Cross-sectional imaging will show the exact extent of aortic dilatation, tethering of aortic leaflets and lack of coaptation in cases of aortic valve insufficiency [56]. MR imaging will additionally quantify the extent of aortic regurgitation, ventricular function and flow data (Fig. 7.12d) (Videos 7.22, 7.23, 7.24, and 7.25). Valve-sparing annuloplasty repair is often done to preserve the native aortic valve by placing an annular ring at the aortic root to curtail further dilatation and aortic insufficiency. CT can accurately evaluate the ring for its placement and valves for their coaptation.

Another complication in Marfan syndrome is aortic dissection where blood seeps into the aortic intima–media creating a false lumen. The lumen is discerned by the presence of an intimal flap that can be demonstrated on post-contrast CT imaging. Often the false lumen may be completely thrombosed and difficult to see on post-contrast imaging. In such cases, indirect signs such as hyper-dense tissue in the aortic wall, presence of

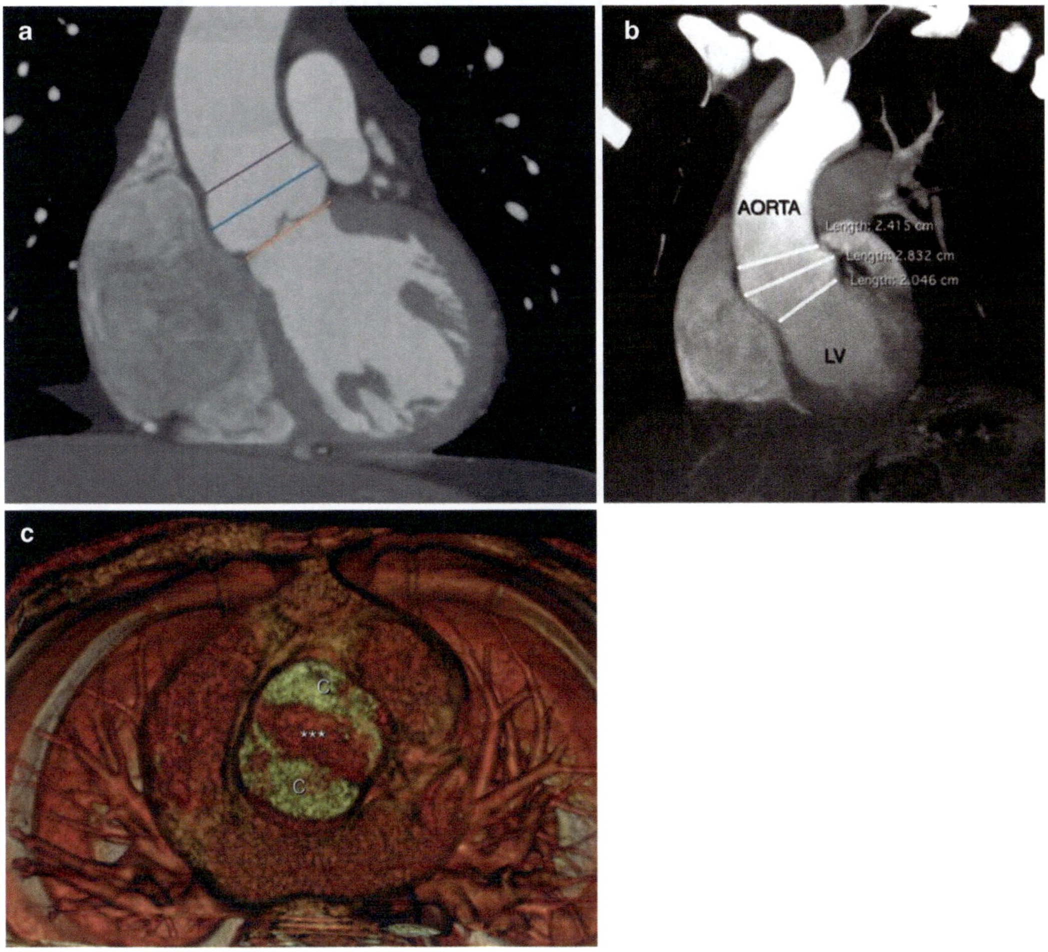

Fig. 7.12 (**a**) Normal aorta. The lines represent sites at which true perpendicular plane of the aortic root is to be measured. The orange line corresponds to the level of the aortic annulus, the blue line represents the sinuses, the purple line is the sino-tubular junction (STJ). (**b**) Marfan syndrome; A 4-year-old male child shows dilatation of the aortic annulus, sinuses and the sino-tubular junction. (**c**) Same case as (**b**). The volume-rendered CT image shows a bicuspid aortic valve. C—valve cusp, asterisk in white represents the valve opening. (**d**) A 13-year-old male with Marfan syndrome. MRI shows severe pectus excavatum, aortic root dilatation with aortic regurgitation, mitral valve prolapse with mitral regurgitation and dilated left atrium and left ventricle (Ref to Videos 22 to 25)

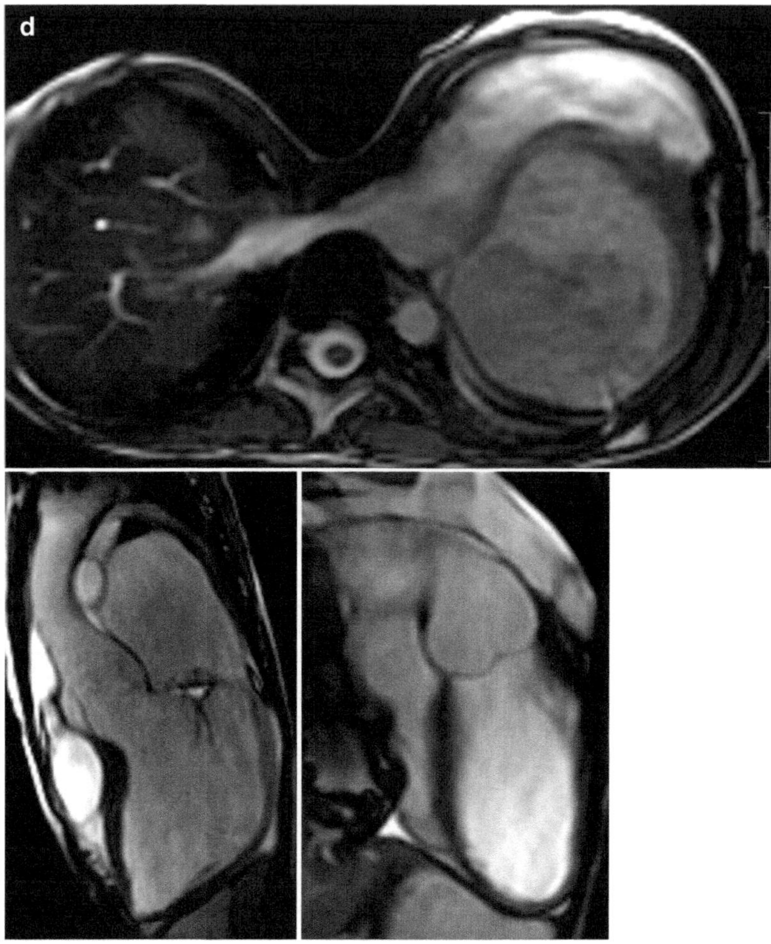

Fig. 7.12 (continued)

mediastinal hematoma, infarction in regions supplied by the aortic arch branch vessels and pericardial haemorrhage can help in suspecting dissection [59]. Using Stanford's classification, all dissections involving the ascending aorta need surgical correction, and those with an arch or distal aortic dissection can be medically managed. The false lumina may be one, two or three in number resulting in complex aortic dissection. Bentall's procedure is used for surgical correction. It involves aortic root replacement with graft repair of ascending aorta and coronary reimplantation. Exact aortic diameters and the origin and proximal coronary arteries are well delineated on ECG-gated CT and dedicated MR aortogram. Images evaluated using multiplanar reconstruction in both CT and MRI are most useful in obtaining true cross-sectional diameters as well as to assess existing complications and the origin and course of the coronaries. MR imaging thus scores over CT imaging as it does not involve ionising radiation.

7.6.2 Arterial Tortuosity Syndrome (ATS)

It is an autosomal recessive genetic disorder affecting the connective tissue [60]. It affects the large and mid-sized arteries which include the aorta, arch vessels as well as the main and branch pulmonary arteries. The vessels affected are exceptionally elongated and tortuous in course. Pulmonary arteries may be dilated and may also show areas of narrowing. These findings can easily be detected on CT or MR imaging (Fig. 7.13a, b) [61].

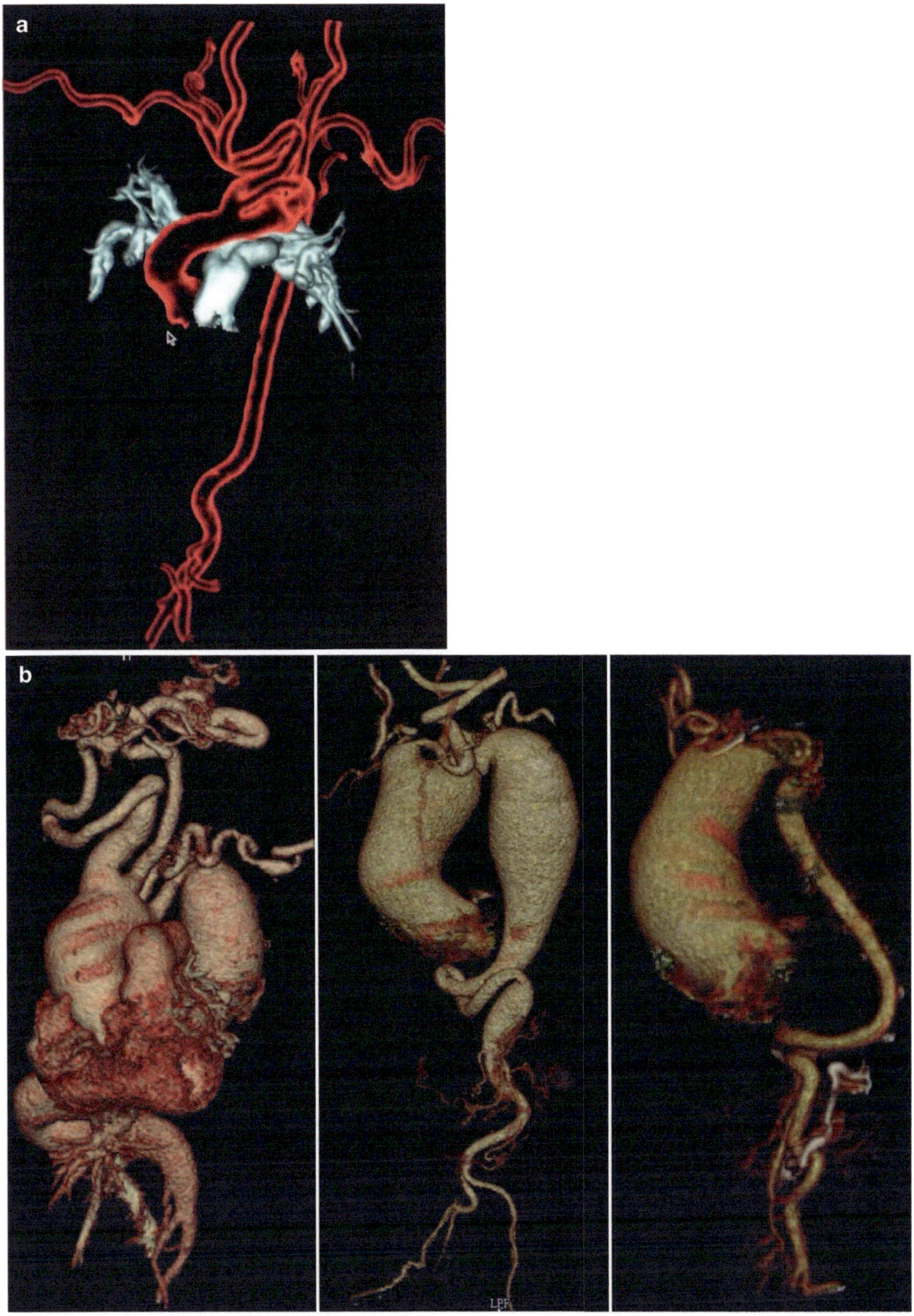

Fig. 7.13 (**a**) Volume-rendered image in Arterial Tortuosity Syndrome shows extensive tortuosity of the aortic arch vessels along with elongation and ectatic course of the aortic arch. (**b**) Arterial tortuosity caused by Fibulin 4 mutation in three different children show grossly dilated and tortuous aorta and its branches

References

1. Goldmuntz E. The epidemiology and genetics of congenital heart disease. Clin Perinatol. 2001;28:1–10.
2. Moorman A, Webb S, Brown NA, Lamers W, Anderson RH. Development of the heart: (1) formation of the cardiac chambers and arterial trunks. Heart. 2003 Jul;89(7):806–14.
3. McElhinney DB, Driscoll DA, Emanuel BS, Goldmuntz E. Chromosome 22q11 deletion in patients with truncus arteriosus. Pediatr Cardiol. 2003 Nov-Dec;24(6):569–73.
4. Yang T, Chen L, Wang L, et al. Risk of congenital heart defects in offspring exposed to maternal diabetes mellitus: an updated systematic review and meta-analysis. Arch Gynecol Obstet. 2019; https://doi.org/10.1007/s00404-019-05376-6.
5. Marcelletti C, McGoon DC, Mair DD. The natural history of truncus arteriosus. Circulation. 1976 Jul;54(1):108–11.
6. Niwa K, Perloff JK, Kaplan S, Child JS, Miner PD. Eisenmenger syndrome in adults: ventricular septal defect, truncus arteriosus, univentricular heart. J Am Coll Cardiol. 1999 Jul;34(1):223–32.
7. Tlaskal T, Hucin B, Kucera V, Vojtovic P, Gebauer R, Chaloupecky V, Skovranek J. Repair of persistent truncus arteriosus with interrupted aortic arch. Eur J Cardiothorac Surg. 2005 Nov;28(5):736–41.
8. Reller MD, Strickland MJ, Riehle-Colarusso T, Mahle WT, Correa A. Prevalence of congenital heart defects in metropolitan Atlanta, 1998-2005. J Pediatr. 2008 Dec;153(6):807–13.
9. Kalavrouziotis G, Purohit M, Ciotti G, Corno AF, Pozzi M. Truncus arteriosus communis: early and midterm results of early primary repair. Ann Thorac Surg. 2006 Dec;82(6):2200–6.
10. Tiraboschi R, Salomone G, Crupi G, Manasse E, Salim A, Carminati M, et al. Aortopulmonary window in the first year of life: report on 11 surgical cases. Ann Thorac Surg. 1988;46:438–41.
11. Blieden LC, Moller JH. Aorticopulmonary septal defect: an experience with 17 patients. Br Heart J. 1974;36:630–5.
12. Richardson JV, Doty DB, Rossi NP, Ehrenhaft JL. The spectrum of anomalies of aortopulmonary septation. J Thorac Cardiovasc Surg. 1979;78:21–7.
13. Redington AN, Rigby ML, Ho SY, Gunthard J, Anderson RH. Aortic atresia with aortopulmonary window and interruption of the aortic arch. Pediatr Cardiol. 1991;12:49–51.
14. Shore DF, Ho SY, Anderson RH, de Leval M, Lincoln C. Aortopulmonary septal defect coexisting with ventricular septal defect and pulmonary atresia. Ann Thorac Surg. 1983;35:132–7.
15. Duca V, Sulliotti G, Maggio C. Corsello transposition of the great arteries and aortopulmonary window in the same patient: clinical report and follow-up. Pediatr Cardiol. 2002;23:474–5.
16. Kutsche LM, Van Mierop LH. Anatomy and pathogenesis of aorticopulmonary septal defect. Am J Cardiol. 1987 Feb 15;59(5):443–7.
17. Mori K, Ando M, Takao A, Ishikawa S, Imai Y. Distal type of aortopulmonary window. Report of 4 cases. Br Heart J. 1978 Jun;40(6):681–9.
18. Chang CW, Chiu SN, Wu ET, Tsai SK, Wu MH, Wang JK. Transcatheter closure of a ruptured sinus of valsalva aneurysm. Circ J. 2006;70:1043–7. https://doi.org/10.1253/circj.70.1043.
19. Conde CA, Meller J, Donoso E, Dack S. Bacterial endocarditis with ruptured sinus of Valsalva and aorticocardiac fistula. Am J Cardiol. 1975;35:912–7. https://doi.org/10.1016/0002-9149(75)90128-9.
20. McKay R, Anderson RH, Cook AC. The aorto-ventricular tunnels. Cardiol Young. 2002;12:563–80. https://doi.org/10.1017/S1047951102001038.
21. Feldman DN, Roman MJ. Aneurysms of the sinuses of valsalva. Cardiology. 2006;106:73–81.
22. Fujiwara R, Noguchi T, Morii I, et al. Acute myocardial infarction and cardiogenic shock caused by a huge right valsalva sinus aneurysm. Circ J. 2014;78:1264–5. https://doi.org/10.1253/circj.CJ-13-1476.
23. Lijoi A, Parodi E, Passerone GC, Scarano F, Caruso D, Iannetti MV. Unruptured aneurysm of the left sinus of valsalva causing coronary insufficiency: case report and review of the literature. Tex Heart Inst J. 2002;29:40–4.
24. Weinreich M, Yu PJ, Trost B. Sinus of valsalva aneurysms: review of the literature and an update on management. Clin Cardiol. 2015;38:185–9. https://doi.org/10.1002/clc.22359.
25. Hanna MF, Malguria N, Saboo SS, et al. Cross-sectional imaging of sinus of valsalva aneurysms: lessons learned. Diagn Interv Radiol. 2017;23(5):339–46. https://doi.org/10.5152/dir.2017.16522.
26. Xenikakis T, Malliotakis P, Barbetakis N, Manousakis E, Hassoulas J. Congenital malformations of the aortic root: bicuspid aortic valve in combination with unruptured aneurysm of the left sinus of valsalva and aberrant left coronary artery. Hellenic J Cardiol. 2008;49:288–91.
27. Sakakibara S, Konno S. Congenital aneurysm of the sinus of valsalva anatomy and classification. Am Heart J. 1962;63(3):405–24.
28. Guo H-W, Xiong H, Xu J-P, Wang X-Q, Hu S-S. A new and simple classification for sinus of valsalva aneurysms and the corresponding surgical procedure. Eur J Cardiothorac Surg. June 2013;43(6):1188–93.
29. Ring WS. Congenital heart surgery nomenclature and database project: aortic aneurysm, sinus of valsalva aneurysm, and aortic dissection. Ann Thorac Surg. 2000;69:S147–63.
30. Vural KM, Sener E, Tasdemir O, Bayazit K. Approach to sinus of valsalva aneurysms: a review of 53 cases. Eur J Cardiothorac Surg. 2001;20:71–6. https://doi.org/10.1016/S1010-7940(01)00758-8.
31. Aboulhosn J, Child JS. Left ventricular outflow obstruction: subaortic stenosis, bicuspid aortic valve,

supravalvular aortic stenosis, and coarctation of the aorta. Circulation. 2006;114:2412–22.
32. Jagia P, Sharma A, Gupta SK, Guleria M. Aortic atresia with normal sized left ventricle. Indian J Radiol Imaging. 2016 Oct-Dec;26(4):521–3.
33. Esmaeilzadeh M, Naderi N, Tabaei AS. Aortic atresia with normally developed left ventricle in a young adult. Cardiol J. 2011;18:304–6.
34. Backer CL, Mavroudis C. Congenital heart surgery nomenclature and database project: patent ductus arteriosus, coarctation of the aorta, interrupted aortic arch. Ann Thorac Surg. 2000;69(suppl 4):S298–307.
35. Moulaert AJ, Bruins CC, Oppenheimer-Dekker A. Anomalies of the aortic arch and ventricular septal defects. Circulation. 1976;53(6):1011–5.
36. Hanneman K, Newman B, Chan F. Congenital variants and anomalies of the aortic arch. RadioGraphics. 2017;37(1):32–51.
37. Hegde SV, Lensing SY, Greenberg SB. Determining the normal aorta size in children. Radiology. 2015;274(3):859–65.
38. Kaiser T, Kellenberger CJ, Albisetti M, Bergsträsser E, Valsangiacomo Buechel ER. Normal values for aortic diameters in children and adolescents: assessment in vivo by contrast-enhanced CMR-angiography. J Cardiovasc Magn Reson. 2008;10(1):56.
39. Ho SY, Anderson RH. Coarctation, tubular hypoplasia, and the ductus arteriosus: histological study of 35 specimens. Br Heart J. 1979;41(3):268–74.
40. Hoffman JI, Kaplan S. The incidence of congenital heart disease. J Am Coll Cardiol. 2002;39(12):1890–900.
41. Bjornard K, Riehle-Colarusso T, Gilboa SM, Correa A. Patterns in the prevalence of congenital heart defects, metropolitan Atlanta, 1978 to 2005. Birth Defects Res A Clin Mol Teratol. 2013;97(2):87–94.
42. Karaosmanoglu AD, Khwaja RDA, Onur MR, Kalra MK. CT and MRI of aortic coarctation: pre- and postsurgical findings. Am J Roentgenol. 2015;204(3):W224–33.
43. Rudolph AM, Heymann MA, Spitznas U. Hemodynamic considerations in the development of narrowing of the aorta. Am J Cardiol. 1972;30(5):514–25.
44. Ming Z, Aimin S. Right aortic arch with coarctation in Chinese children. Pediatr Radiol. 2008;38(5):511–7.
45. Kpodonu J, Ramaiah VG, Rodriguez-Lopez JA, Diethrich EB. Endovascular management of recurrent adult coarctation of the aorta. Ann Thorac Surg. 2010;90:1716–20.
46. Verheugt CL, Uiterwall CS, Grobbee DE, Mulder BJ. Long term prognosis of congenital heart defects: a systematic review. Int J Cardiol. 2008;131:25–32.
47. Kische S, Schneider H, Akin I, et al. Technique of interventional repair in adult thoracic aortic coarctation. J Vasc Surg. 2010;51:1550–9.
48. Reardon MJ, Hallman GL, Cooley DA. Interrupted aortic arch: brief review and summary of an eighteen-year experience. Tex Heart Inst J. 1984;11:250–9.
49. Collins-Nakai RL, Dick M, Parisi-Buckley L, Fyler DC, Castaneda AR. Interrupted aortic arch in infancy. J Pediatr. 1976;88:959–62.
50. Gruber PJ, Epstein JA. Development gone awry: congenital heart disease. Circ Res. 2004;94(3):273–83.
51. Kimura-Hayama ET, Meléndez G, Mendizábal AL, et al. Uncommon congenital and acquired aortic diseases: role of multidetector CT angiography. Radiographics. 2010;30:79–98.
52. Dillman JR, Yarram SG, D'amico AR, Hernandes RJ. Interrupted aortic arch: spectrum of MRI findings. Am J Roentgenol. 2008;190(6):1467–74.
53. Koneti NR, Kanchi V, Kandraju H, Jaishankar S. Symptomatic aneurysm of ductus arteriosus in neonates. Ann Pediatr Cardiol. 2011;4(2):159–63. https://doi.org/10.4103/0974-2069.84659.
54. Das BB, Solowiejczyk DE, Kamath V, Sharma J. Congenital ductus arteriosus aneurysm presenting with stridor in a newborn. J Perinatol. 2002;22:179–80.
55. Dyamenahalli U, Smallhorn JF, Geva T, Fouron JC, Cairns P, Jutras L, et al. Isolated ductus arteriosus aneurysm in the fetus and infant: a multi-institutional experience. J Am Coll Cardiol. 2000;36:262–9.
56. Ha HI, Seo JB, Lee SH, Kang J-W, Goo HW, Lim T-H, Shin MJ. Imaging of Marfan syndrome: multisystemic manifestations. RadioGraphics. 2007;27(4):989–1004.
57. Pyeritz RE, McKusick VA. The Marfan syndrome: diagnosis and management. N Engl J Med. 1979;300:772–7.
58. Posniak HV, Olson MC, Demos TC, Benjoya RA, Marsan RE. CT of thoracic aortic aneurysms. RadioGraphics. 1990;10:839–55.
59. Fisher ER, Stern EJ, Godwin JD 2nd, Otto CM, Johnson JA. Acute aortic dissection: typical and atypical imaging features. RadioGraphics. 1994;14:1263–71.
60. Coucke PJ, Willaert A, Wessels MW, Callewaert B, Zoppi N, et al. Mutations in the facilitative glucose transporter GLUT10 alter angiogenesis and cause arterial tortuosity syndrome. Nat Genet. 2006;38:452–7.
61. Rajeshkannan R, Kulkarni C, Kappanayil M, et al. Imaging findings in a distinct lethal inherited arteriopathy syndrome associated with a novel mutation in the FBLN4 gene. Eur Radiol. 2014;24:1742–8.

Vascular Rings and Slings

8

Elizabeth Joseph, Linu Kuruvilla, Binita Chacko, and Aparna Irodi

8.1 Introduction

This chapter describes anomalous vascular anatomy that forms a ring or sling around the trachea and esophagus which could result in its compression. The embryology, clinical presentation, imaging findings, and management options of vascular rings and slings are explained. Easy to understand embryological line diagrams and practical tips are provided for radiologists.

Robert E Gross introduced the term "vascular ring" in 1945. He described two complete vascular rings in the superior mediastinum, which caused compression of the trachea from the anterior aspect and esophagus from the posterior aspect [1]. Vascular rings could be an isolated finding or it could be associated with other congenital cardiac abnormalities or chromosomal abnormalities. Vascular rings form 1% of all congenital cardiac abnormalities [2]. Multidetector CT with its three-dimensional (3D) capabilities and 3D MRI angiogram helps in the identification, characterization, and management of vascular rings and slings better than two-dimensional conventional imaging techniques such as chest radiograph, barium swallow, and conventional angiography.

The most widely used classification for the vascular ring is by Carl Backer and Constantine Mavroudis [3]. Anatomically, vascular rings can be complete or incomplete. Complete vascular ring fully encircles the trachea and esophagus. Incomplete or partial vascular ring partially encircles the trachea and esophagus. The different types of vascular rings and slings are listed below:

A. Double aortic arch. Both arches could be patent or one of the arches could be atretic with fibrous remnant.
B. Left aortic arch with aberrant right subclavian artery and retroesophageal diverticulum of Kommerell.
C. Right aortic arch with aberrant left subclavian artery and retroesophageal diverticulum.
D. Right or left circumflex aorta.
E. Left aortic arch with aberrant right subclavian artery without diverticulum of Kommerell.
F. Right aortic arch with aberrant left subclavian artery without diverticulum of Kommerell.
G. Right arch with mirror-image branching and left ductus arteriosus or left ligamentum arteriosum.
H. Innominate artery compression syndrome.
I. Pulmonary sling.

The first four types listed above are complete vascular rings and the last five types listed above are incomplete vascular rings. The Kommerrell's

E. Joseph (✉) · L. Kuruvilla · B. Chacko · A. Irodi
Department of Radiology, Christian Medical College and Hospital, Vellore, Tamil Nadu, India

R. Rajeshkannan et al. (eds.), *CT and MRI in Congenital Heart Diseases*,
https://doi.org/10.1007/978-981-15-6755-1_8

diverticulum itself could be large enough to cause independent compression of the esophagus and trachea. The left aortic arch with left ductus or left ligamentum arteriosum and, the right aortic arch with mirror-image branching and right ductus or right ligamentum arteriosum do not form vascular rings.

8.2 Embryology

Classical Rathke's diagram (Fig. 8.1) explains the development of the aortic arch and its branches. During the third to eighth week of gestation, six pairs of arches appear and disappear between the dorsal and ventral aorta in a craniocaudal fashion. The two ventral aortae fuse to form the aortic sac. The two dorsal aortae fuse to form the descending thoracic aorta. The first, second, and fifth arches disappear. A remnant of the first arch forms the maxillary artery, while a remnant of the second arch forms the hyoid and stapedial arteries. The third arch forms the common carotid and proximal part of the internal carotid arteries. The right fourth arch forms part of the right subclavian artery and the left fourth arch forms the aortic arch. The fifth arch regresses spontaneously. The right sixth arch gives rise to the right pulmonary artery and the left sixth arch forms the distal main pulmonary artery, left pulmonary artery, and ductus arteriosus.

The aortic sac forms part of the ascending aorta and right innominate artery. The dorsal aorta forms part of the right subclavian artery on the right side and, part of the left aortic arch and descending aorta on the left side. The right subclavian artery is formed by part of the right fourth arch, right dorsal aorta, and right seventh intersegmental artery. The left subclavian artery is formed by the left seventh intersegmental artery. The normal left aortic arch is formed by aortic

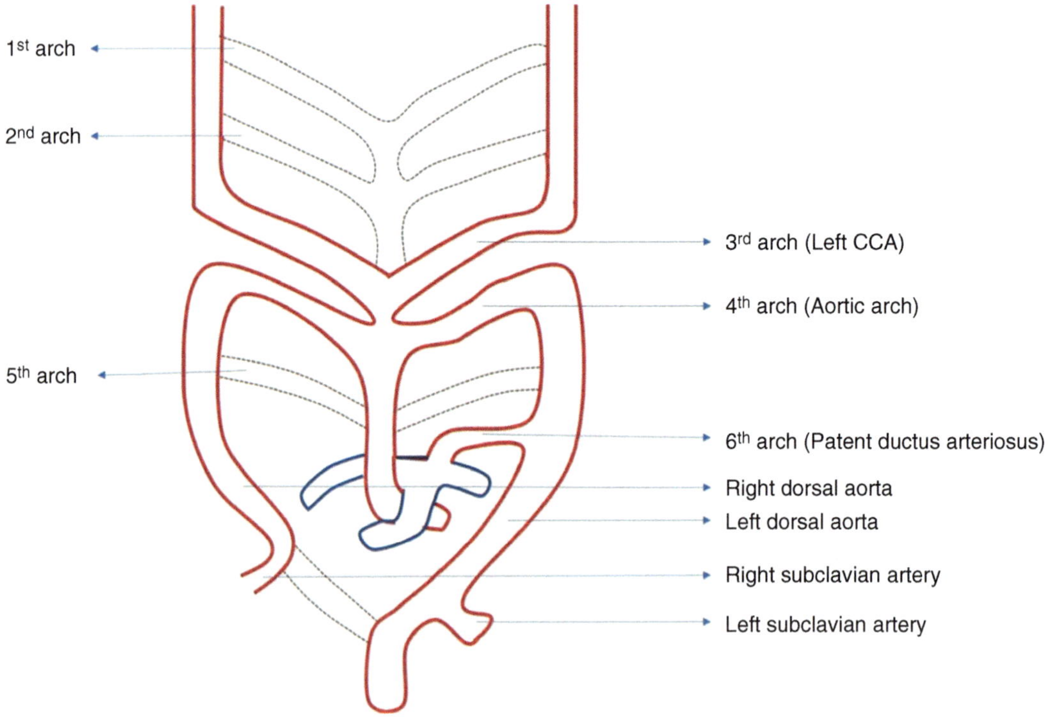

Fig. 8.1 Classical Rathke's diagram showing the development of the aortic arch and its branches. Interrupted brown lines represent arches/part of arches that normally disappear. Red and blue continuous lines represent arches/part of arches which normally persists

sac, left fourth arch, and part of the left dorsal aorta (Fig. 8.3) [4]. The truncus arteriosus forms proximal ascending aorta and proximal main pulmonary artery.

Vascular rings and slings are well explained by Edwards hypothesis of double aortic arch development with carotid and subclavian artery branches in both arches and ductus arteriosus in both sides (Fig. 8.2). The aortic system, pulmonary system, and ductus arteriosus are represented by red, blue, and brown lines, respectively in Figs. 8.2, 8.3, 8.4, 8.7, 8.9, 8.11, 8.14, 8.17, and 8.19. The solid line represents segments that persist and the interrupted line represents segments that involute/become atretic. The development of normal left aortic arch with left-sided ductus/ligamentum arteriosus is shown in Fig. 8.3.

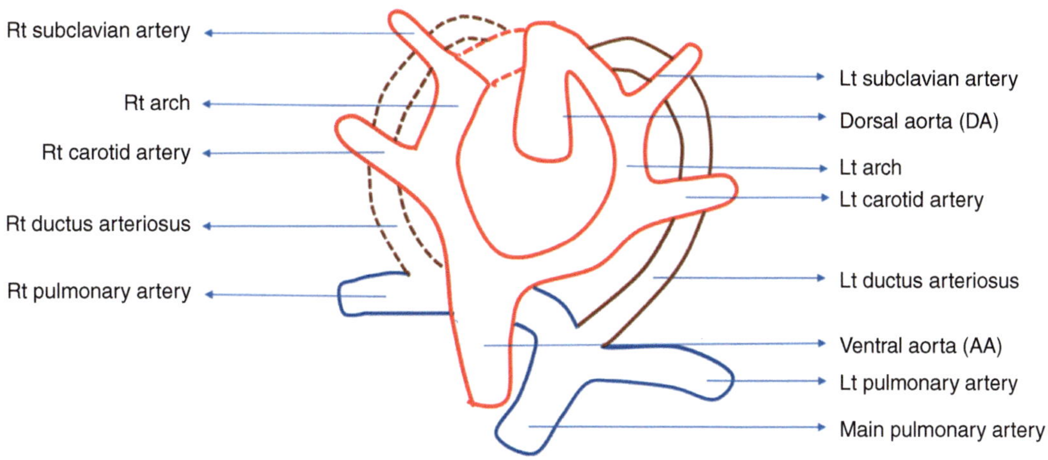

Fig. 8.2 Edward's hypothesis of double aortic arch development

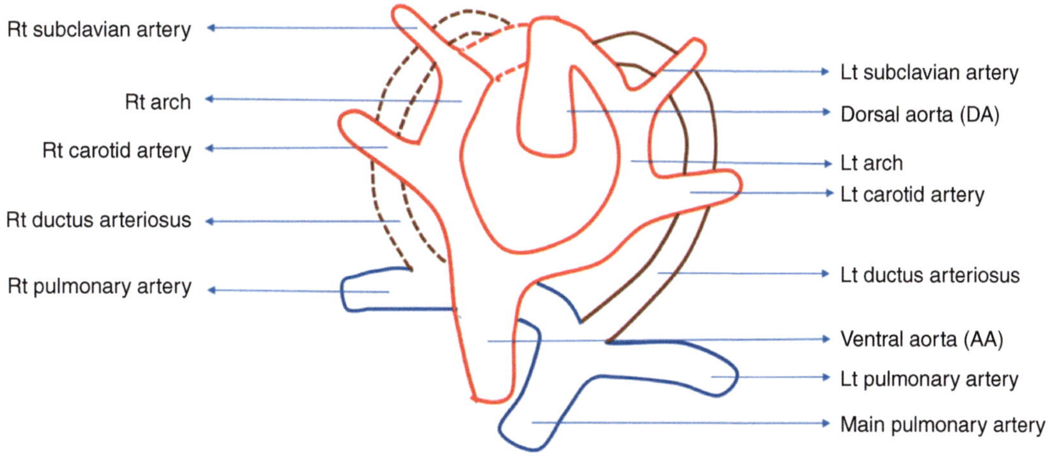

Fig. 8.3 Embryological development of normal left arch. The interrupted brown line represents involuted right-sided ductus arteriosus. The continuous brown line represents persisting left-sided ductus arteriosus/ligamentum arteriosum. The interrupted red line between the right subclavian artery and descending aorta represents the involuted portion of the right arch

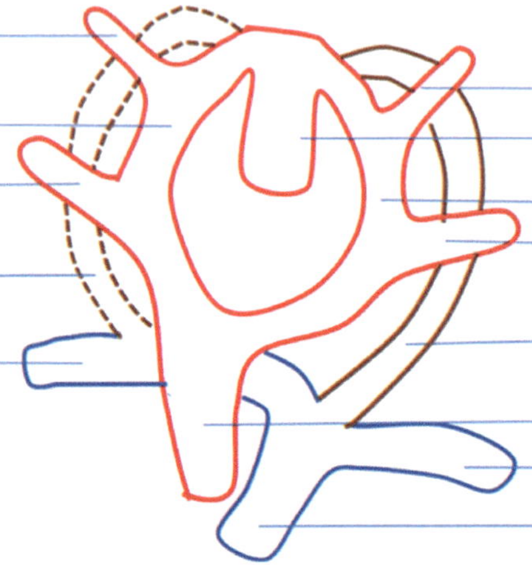

Fig. 8.4 Embryological development of double aortic arch with both arches patent. The continuous lines represent the part that persists to form the double aortic arch. The interrupted brown line represents the right ductus arteriosus which usually involutes

8.3 Types of Vascular Rings and Slings

8.3.1 Double Aortic Arch

Two main subtypes:

1. Double aortic arch with both arches patent
2. Double aortic arch with atresia or hypoplasia of one arch with fibrous remnant

8.3.1.1 Double Aortic Arch with Both Arches Patent

Introduction

They are complete vascular rings that occur due to the persistence of both right and left fourth aortic arches. They compress the trachea and esophagus partially or completely, by encasing them. They are usually symptomatic by the early months of life [5]. It is the most common type of complete vascular ring with an incidence of 46–76% among all causes of vascular rings [6].

Embryology (Fig. 8.4)

A double aortic arch results when both fourth arches persist to connect the trunco-aortic sac to the dorsal aorta. The arches can persist entirely (Shuford and Syber classification Type 1), or a part of it (usually the left arch) can become atretic or hypoplastic (Shuford and Syber classification Type 2) [6, 7]. Usually, only one of the six arches persists (solid brown line in Fig. 8.4) as ductus arteriosus [4].

Morphology

The ascending aorta divides into two branches, a left and a right aortic arch that join posteriorly to form the descending aorta. The left arch passes anteriorly and to the left of the trachea. The right aortic arch passes to the right and then posterior to the esophagus to join the descending aorta, forming a vascular ring. The ligamentum arteriosum and descending aorta usually remain on the left. The ligamentum arteriosum or the ductus arteriosus is located at the junction of the aortic arch and the descending aorta. From each arch arise a carotid artery and a subclavian artery. The arches are usually unequal in size, the right arch is generally dominant [6]. The right arch is usually larger and higher than the left arch. The descending aorta is usually contralateral to the dominant arch, with the most common configuration being a larger, higher right arch, left-sided descending thoracic aorta, and left-sided ligamentum arteriosum [4]. The descending aorta may be on the left, right, or midline.

Double aortic arch is not commonly associated with other congenital heart diseases [8]. It can be rarely seen in patients with the tetralogy of Fallot, transposition of the great arteries, cervical arch, common arterial trunk, and coarctation of the aorta.

Pathophysiology

The trachea and esophagus may be compressed as they are completely encircled by the two arches. The clinical presentation is usually in infants and children, dating from birth. Wheezing, stridor exacerbated by crying, tachypnea, cyanosis, and dysphagia are common manifestations [4].

Imaging Findings

Chest radiograph (CXR) findings:

Indentation on both sides of the trachea and widened right paratracheal stripe may be seen. Lateral chest radiograph may show anterior bowing of the lower trachea.

CT and MRI findings (Figs. 8.5 and 8.6):

Cross-sectional imaging (CT and MRI) is the best modality to assess both aortic arches and their branching patterns. An axial image through the level of the branch arteries will show symmetry of the common carotid and subclavian arteries—the "figure of four sign." Narrowing of the trachea can be visualized both on the axial and volume-rendered images of the airway. Dilatation of the proximal thoracic esophagus cephalad to the vascular ring may be noted. Phase-contrast sequences on MRI can quantitate which arch has more flow when the arches are codominant [8].

Practical Tips

The "figure of four" sign (symmetric aortic arch branching pattern at the level of branch arteries) distinguishes this entity from other vascular rings and slings.

Treatment

The surgical approach is via a thoracotomy on the side of the descending aorta and to divide the nondominant arch and ligamentum arteriosum. If the arches are equal, the approach is to divide the posterior arch. A median sternotomy is preferred for those patients who require additional cardiac procedures.

Despite good surgical outcomes, persistent respiratory symptoms are frequent postoperatively, perhaps due to earlier compression-related maldevelopment of the trachea and major airways [9].

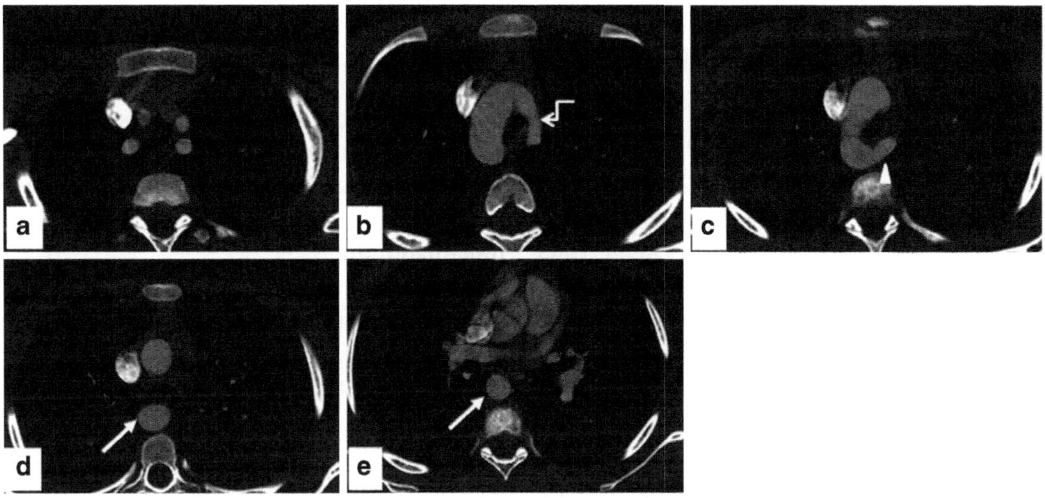

Fig. 8.5 Axial images of CT angiogram showing a double aortic arch with a hypoplastic left arch completely encircling the trachea and esophagus. "Figure of four" sign is demonstrated in the image (**a**) at the level of the origin of the aortic branches. The curved white arrow in image (**b**) represents the smaller left aortic arch. The white arrowhead in image (**c**) represents the posterior anastomosis of both arches. The white arrow in images (**d**, **e**) shows the descending thoracic aorta lying in the midline

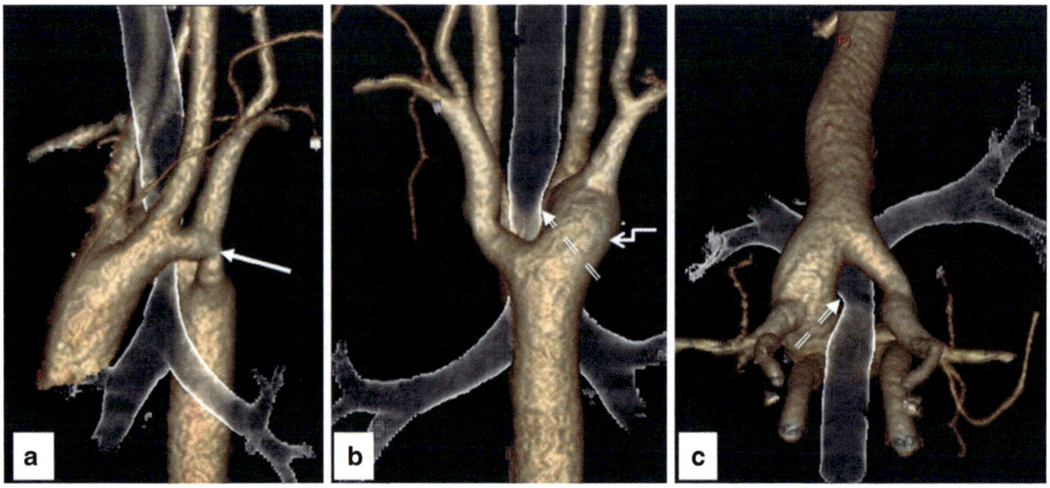

Fig. 8.6 Volume reconstruction of the CT angiogram shown in Fig. 8.5 above. The white arrow in image (**a**) shows the hypoplastic left aortic arch with the left common carotid and left subclavian arteries arising from it. The curved white arrow in image (**b**) shows the larger right aortic arch with the right common carotid and right subclavian arteries arising from it. The double-line white arrow in images (**b**, **c**) shows the tracheal compression at the level of the double aortic arch. Indentation is more on the right side as shown in image (**c**)

8.3.1.2 Double Aortic Arch with Atresia or Hypoplasia of One Arch with Fibrous Remnant

Introduction

Double aortic arch with atresia of a segment of the arch, replaced with fibrous cord is a form of incomplete double aortic arch. It is a less common cause of a symptomatic vascular ring. Atresia of the distal left aortic arch segment is far more common than of the distal right aortic arch [10].

Embryology and Morphology (Fig. 8.7)

Atresia of the left arch can involve different segments. There are two classifications, Shuford and Sybers classification into subtypes 1 to 4 [7] and Garti et al. classification into types A to D [11]. These classifications are essentially the same.

In subtype 1/type A, atresia is in the distal left arch, between ductus and descending aorta, and the atretic fibrous cord inserts in a diverticulum of the descending aorta. The left ductus/ligamentum arteriosum extends from the left pulmonary artery to the anterior left arch and not the descending aortic diverticulum.

In subtype 2/type B, atresia occurs between the ductus and the left subclavian artery, the atretic fibrous cord, and the ductus/ligamentum arteriosum inserts in the descending aortic diverticulum [12].

In subtype 3/type C, atresia occurs between the left common carotid artery and left subclavian artery.

In subtype 4/type D, atresia occurs in the anterior portion of the left arch, proximal to the left common carotid artery.

Pathophysiology

As in the case of other complete vascular rings, this anomaly has the potential of producing stridor, wheezing, or dysphagia [9].

Imaging Findings

CXR findings:

Can vary according to the type. Indentation on the right side of the trachea by the right arch and widening of the right paratracheal stripe can be seen.

CT and MRI findings (Fig. 8.8a, b):

A double aortic arch has symmetric common carotid and subclavian arteries originating from each arch on an axial section just above the level of the arches (the *four-vessel* or *four-artery sign*) with more posterior location of the proximal left

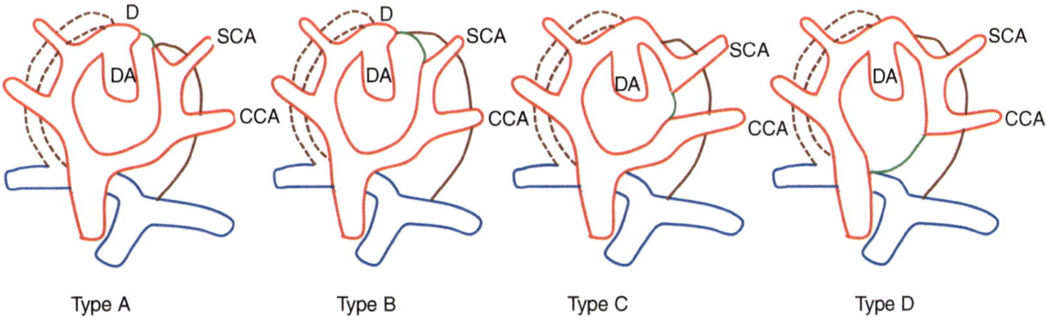

Fig. 8.7 Embryology and morphology of subtypes of double aortic arch with atresia of different segments of the left arch, replaced with fibrous ligament. The green line represents the atretic segment in the left arch. *DA* descending aorta; *D* aortic diverticulum; *SCA* subclavian artery; *CCA* common carotid artery

arch and the presence of a diverticulum of the descending aorta commonly.

The type A variant needs to be distinguished from a right aortic arch with mirror-image branching (please refer to type A in Figs. 8.7 and 8.19). In the right aortic arch with mirror-image branching, there is an involution of the segment between the left ductus and descending aorta (not atresia). In the right arch with mirror-image branching, the presence of a left brachiocephalic artery arising from the arch results in asymmetry at the level of the arches with a more anterior position of the left brachiocephalic artery and absence of a descending aortic diverticulum. The incomplete double aortic arch with distal left arch atresia forms a complete vascular ring, unlike a right aortic arch with mirror-image branching [4].

The type C double aortic arch needs to be differentiated from the right aortic arch with aberrant left subclavian artery (the distinguishing features have been illustrated in Fig. 8.8. Please also refer to type C in Figs. 8.7 and 8.17) [9].

Practical Tips

This condition is commonly mistaken for the right aortic arch with mirror-image branching. The asymmetric branching pattern at the level of the arch of aorta, presence of a left brachiocephalic artery, the relative anterior position of the arch, and absence of a descending aortic diverticulum helps distinguish a right aortic arch with mirror-image branching from an incomplete double aortic arch.

Treatment

In atresia between the left common carotid and the left subclavian artery (type C), the surgeon has to ligate the atretic portion of the left arch in addition to the ligamentum arteriosum. Division of ligamentum arteriosus alone will not provide adequate relief of bronchial compression [9].

8.3.2 Left Aortic Arch with Aberrant Right Subclavian Artery and Kommerrell's Diverticulum

Introduction

Aberrant right subclavian artery is the most common anomaly associated with a left aortic arch with a prevalence of 0.7–2% and female predominance [13]. Kommerrell's diverticulum (KD) is a funnel-shaped dilatation at the origin and proximal aberrant right subclavian artery. Becker et al. defined KD as dilatation more than 1.5 times the size of the distal right subclavian artery. The incidence of KD in the aberrant right subclavian artery varies 7–52% in adults in different studies [14, 15]. The location could be behind the esophagus in 80%, between the esophagus and trachea in 15%, and behind the trachea in 5% [16].

Embryology (Fig. 8.9)

Aberrant right subclavian artery results from the regression of the right arch, between the right subclavian and right common carotid arteries

a

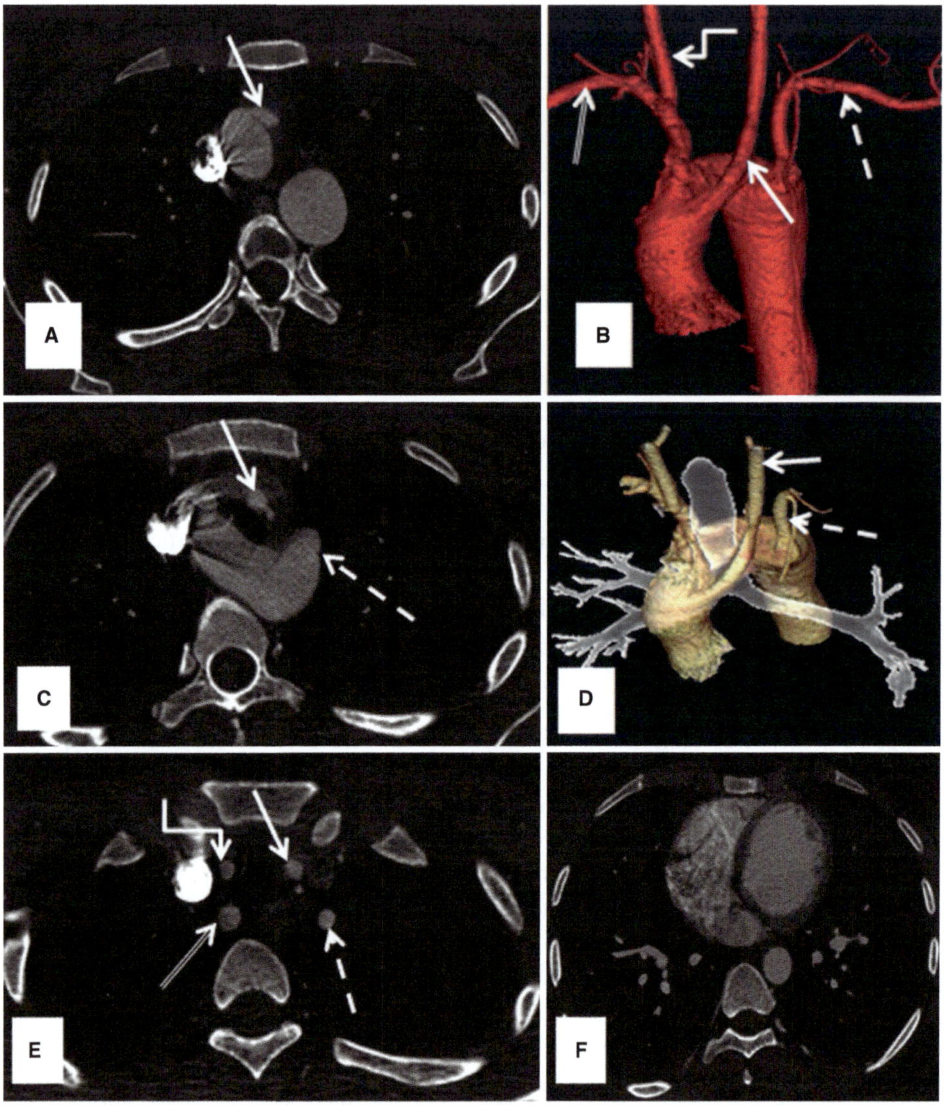

Fig. 8.8 (**a**) Axial and 3D reconstructed images showing a double aortic arch with an atretic left arch (Type C). The white arrows show the left common carotid artery as the first branch from the ascending aorta followed by the right common carotid (white curved arrows) and right subclavian artery (white double-line arrows). There is an aberrant course of the left subclavian artery arising from the ectatic retroesophageal portion of the aorta (broken-white arrows). Unlike a double aortic arch, there is asymmetry of the origin of the aortic arch branches with an absent "figure of four" sign (image "E"). The descending aorta is seen to the left of the spine in image "F." Mild compression of the distal trachea is demonstrated in image "D." (**b**) This figure illustrates differentiating features between "Type C" double aortic arch with atretic left arch (A–E) and right aortic arch with aberrant left subclavian artery (F–J). The black arrow represents the right common carotid artery, the white arrow represents the right subclavian artery, broken black arrow represents the left common carotid artery, and the broken white arrow represents the left subclavian artery. (Images A–E) "Type C" double aortic arch with atretic left arch showing Symmetric arrangement of vessels around the trachea at the thoracic inlet (Image A), posterior deflection of the proximal left common carotid artery (Image B), tethering of the left common carotid artery to the trachea (Image C), circumflex arch or retroesophageal arch (Image C and D) and bilateral tracheal indentation (Image E). (Images F–J) Right aortic arch with aberrant left subclavian artery showing asymmetric arrangement of vessels around the trachea at the thoracic inlet (Image F), with more distance between the common carotid and subclavian arteries on the left side as compared to the right side. There is no posterior deflection or tethering of the proximal part of the left common carotid artery to the trachea in images G and H. The aortic arch does not have a retroesophageal course in images H and I. Instead, the descending aorta traverses on the right side adjacent to the esophagus. There is indentation on only the right lateral wall of the trachea in image J

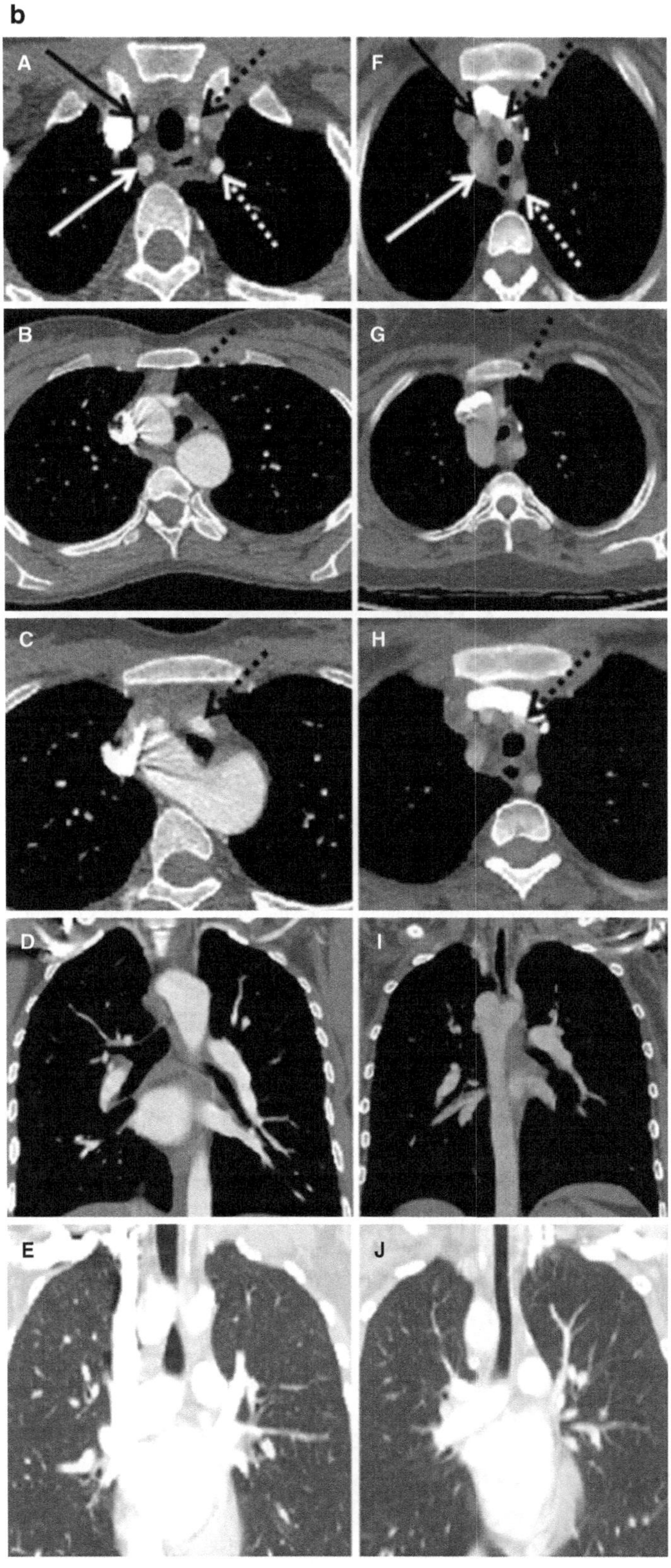

Fig. 8.8 (continued)

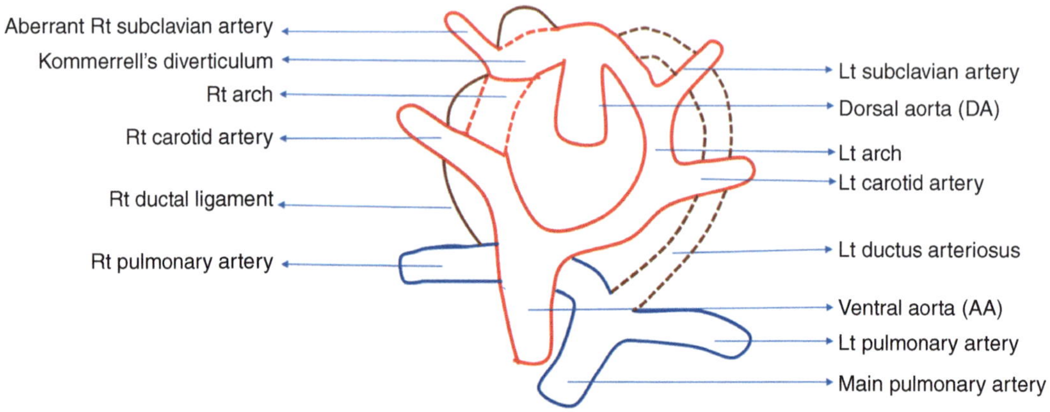

Fig. 8.9 Embryological development of left aortic arch with aberrant right subclavian artery and Kommerrell's diverticulum. The right-sided ligamentum arteriosum persists and the left-sided ductus arteriosus involutes

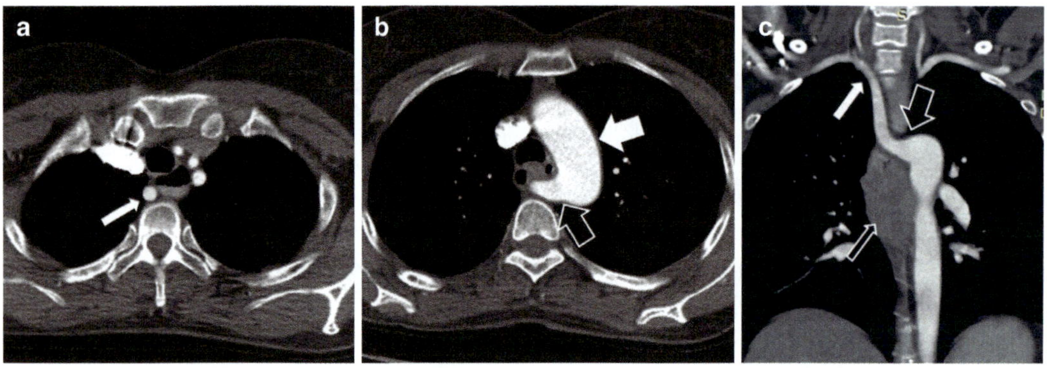

Fig. 8.10 Left Aortic Arch with Aberrant Right Subclavian Artery and Kommerrell's Diverticulum. Contrast-enhanced CT images in the axial (**a**, **b**) and coronal planes (**c**) showing a normal left aortic arch (short thick arrow in **b**) with aberrant right subclavian artery (long thin arrow in **a**, **c**) arising from Kommerrell's diverticulum (short thick open arrow in **b**, **c**). The esophagus is compressed from the posterior aspect by the left aortic arch and diverticulum. This was an incidental finding in a patient with upper to mid-thoracic esophageal carcinoma (long thin open arrow)

(CCA), with the distal dorsal right aorta forming the retroesophageal proximal portion of the right subclavian artery. KD is thought to be due to the persistence of the component of the right sixth arch that forms the ductus arteriosus. Ligamentum arteriosum or ductus arteriosus on the right side connects the KD to the right pulmonary artery forming a vascular ring.

Clinical Features

The vascular ring in the left aortic arch with aberrant right subclavian artery and Kommerrell's diverticulum is usually a loose ring. The patients are usually asymptomatic.

Imaging Findings

CXR findings:

Oblique shadow above the aortic arch on the frontal chest radiograph.

CT and MRI findings (Fig. 8.10):

The aberrant right subclavian artery originates from the Kommerrell's diverticulum arising from the proximal descending thoracic aorta and located posterior to the esophagus.

Practical Tips

The presence of Kommerrell's diverticulum in an aberrant right subclavian artery indicates a vascular ring completed by ligamentum arteriosum or ductus arteriosus on the right side [13]. The absence of Kommerrell's diverticulum in an aberrant right subclavian artery indicates the absence of vascular ring as the ligamentum arteriosum or ductus arteriosum is on the left side.

8.3.3 Right Aortic Arch with Aberrant Left Subclavian Artery and Kommerrell's Diverticulum

Introduction

The right aortic arch with aberrant left subclavian artery has a prevalence of 0.04–0.4% with male predominance [13, 17]. Kommerrell's diverticulum (KD), although originally described in the context of the left aortic arch with aberrant right subclavian artery, is also used in the context of the right aortic arch with aberrant left subclavian artery. KD is very commonly seen in these patients with incidence up to 100% in CT studies [15]. This finding forms a complete vascular ring as it is completed by ductus arteriosum or ligamentum arteriosum on the left side.

Embryology (Fig. 8.11)

Right aortic arch with aberrant left subclavian artery develops due to the regression of the embryonic left fourth arch (between the left common carotid artery and subclavian artery) and left sixth arch, and the persistence of the right fourth aortic arch. KD results from the failure of the regression of the dorsal segment of the left fourth primitive arch.

Clinical Features

The vascular ring in the right aortic arch with aberrant left subclavian artery and Kommerrell's diverticulum is usually loose rings and patients are usually asymptomatic. Dilatation of KD may result in dysphagia, dyspnea, wheezing, cough, or chest pain. Increased risk of rupture and dissection has been reported in 19–53% [18].

Imaging Findings (Fig. 8.12)

CXR findings:

Right aortic knuckle with a slight deviation of the trachea to the left side.

BA swallow:

Posterior compression of the esophagus.

CT and MRI findings:

Aberrant left subclavian artery originates as the last branch of the right aortic arch from a diverticulum with retroesophageal course across the midline to the left side. The Kommerrell's diverticulum is usually rounded in shape and larger in the right aortic arch unlike conical shape in the left aortic arch.

Management

Management options for KD are based on the anatomy, symptoms, comorbidities of the patient, and available surgical expertise [16, 19].

Surgical intervention is considered when the diameter of the diverticulum orifice is more than 30 mm, and/or the diameter of the descending aorta adjacent to the diverticulum is more than 50 mm.

Practical Tips

Symptoms in this condition are secondary to the diverticulum rather than the primary pathology.

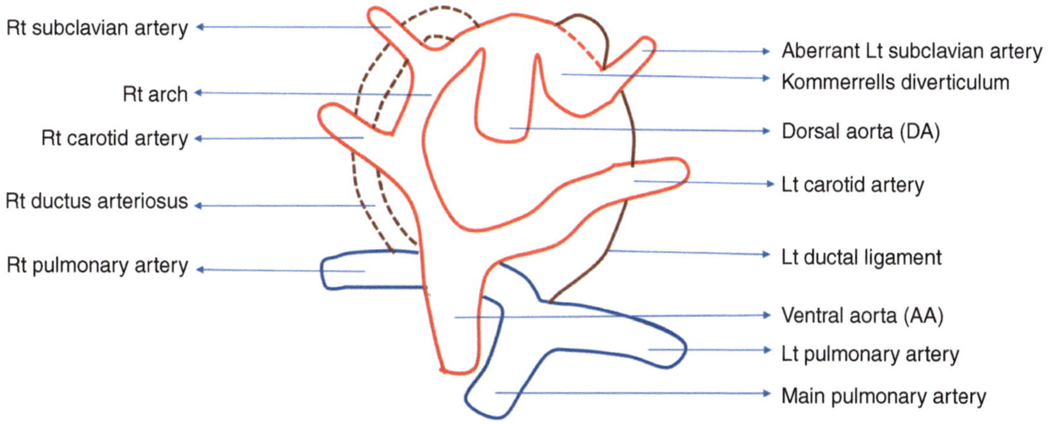

Fig. 8.11 Right-sided aortic arch with Kommerrell's diverticulum and aberrant left subclavian artery. The left-sided ligamentum arteriosum persists and the right-sided ductus arteriosus involutes

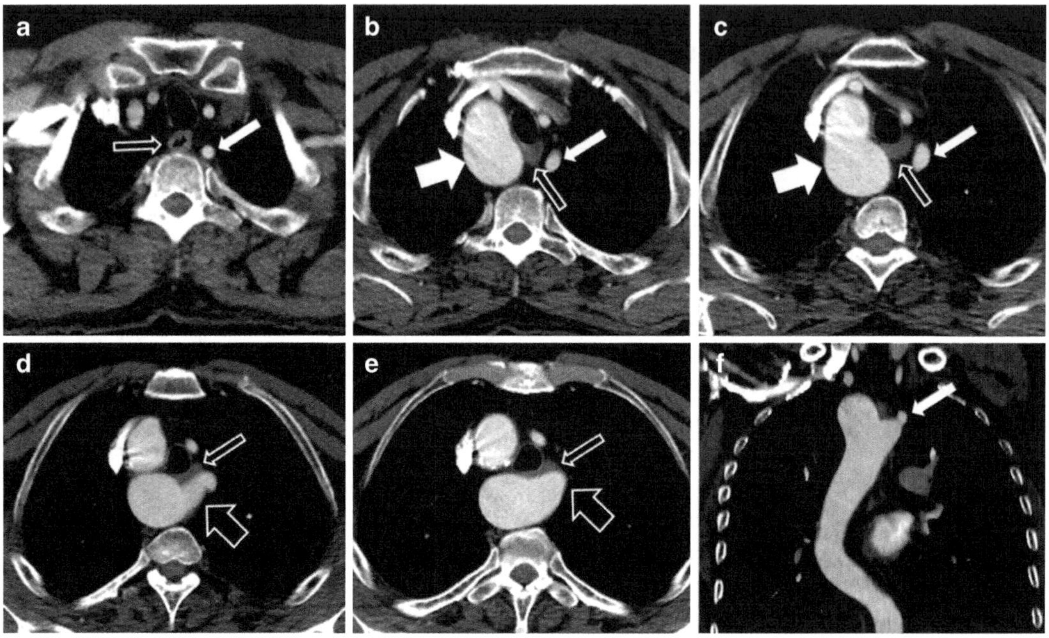

Fig. 8.12 Right aortic arch with aberrant left subclavian artery arising from Kommerrell's diverticulum. Cranial to caudal axial (**a**–**e**) and coronal (**f**) CT sections show. Right aortic arch (short thick arrow) with aberrant left subclavian artery (long thin arrow) arising from Kommerrell's diverticulum (short open arrow). Esophagus (long open arrow) is compressed from posterior aspect by the right aortic arch and diverticulum

8.3.4 Right Circumflex Aorta and Left Circumflex Aorta

Introduction

Circumflex aorta is a rare anomaly in which the aortic arch itself crosses the midline posterior to the esophagus and above the level of the carina. After crossing the midline, the aorta gives off a diverticulum with ligamentum arteriosus or ductus arteriosus which connects to the pulmonary artery forming a vascular ring. If there is a left aortic arch with the right descending aorta and right ductus arteriosus or ligamentum arteriosum, it is left circumflex aorta. If there is a right aortic arch and left descending aorta with left ductus arteriosus or ligamentum arteriosum, it is right circumflex aorta. The right circumflex aorta is more common than left circumflex aorta [13, 20, 21].

Embryology

Right circumflex aorta results from regression of left fourth arch between the subclavian artery and carotid artery, persistence of left sixth arch forming ductus arteriosus, and persistence of the left dorsal aorta. Left circumflex aorta results from the regression of right fourth arch, persistence of the right sixth arch forming ductus arteriosus, and persistence of right dorsal aorta.

Clinical Features

Patients presents early with stridor, dyspnea, respiratory infection, and feeding difficulties due to tracheobronchial and esophageal compression.

Imaging Findings (Fig. 8.13)

CXR findings:

Widening of the superior mediastinum to both sides.

BA swallow:

Indentation in the upper esophagus on the side of the arch and another oblique indentation running from the side of the arch to contralateral side at the expected level of aortic arch on AP view and posterior indentation in the upper esophagus on lateral view seen.

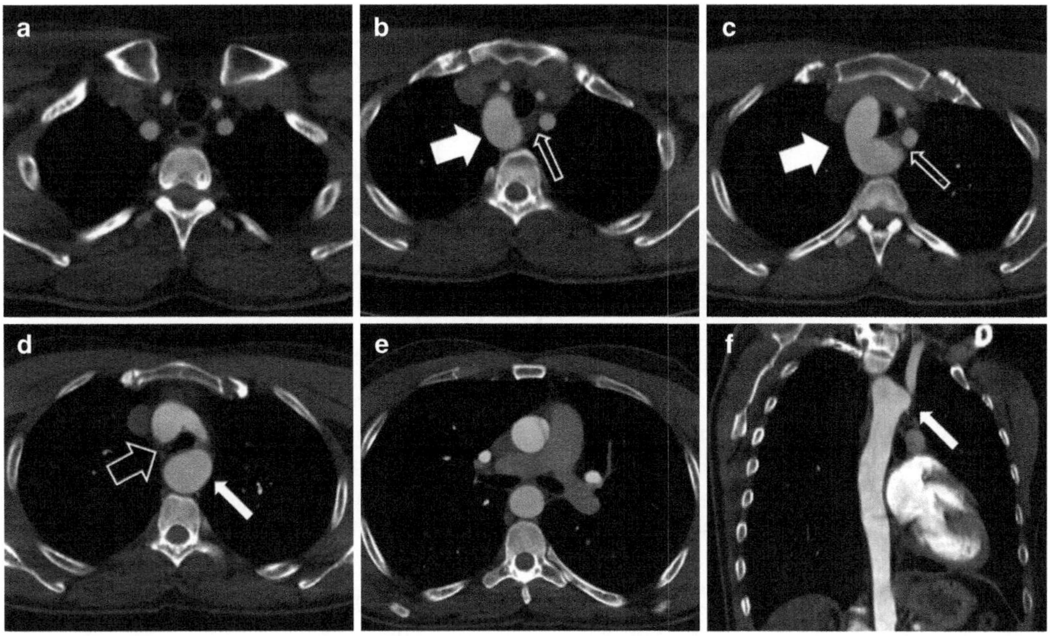

Fig. 8.13 Circumflex aortic arch. Cranial to caudal axial (**a**–**e**) and coronal (**f**) CT sections show. Circumflex right aortic arch (short thick arrow) crossing the midline to the left side with aortic diverticulum (long thin arrow). Trachea is compressed from the right anterior aspect (short open arrow) and the esophagus is compressed from the right lateral and posterior aspect (long open arrow) by the right circumflex aorta. Left-sided ligamentum arteriosum was present on surgery

CT and MRI findings:

Aortic arch crosses the midline posterior to the esophagus and descending thoracic aorta is on the side opposite to the arch. Aortic diverticulum is seen at the proximal descending aorta (Fig. 8.13).

Practical Tips

Look for aortic arch itself crossing the midline posterior to the esophagus (not aberrant subclavian artery) with descending aorta to the opposite of the arch. It resembles a right aortic arch with aberrant left subclavian artery arising from a diverticulum and, double arch with atresia of the left arch.

Treatment

Aortic uncrossing procedure may be needed in addition to the division of ligamentum arteriosum to relieve the patient's symptoms. In the aortic uncrossing procedure, the distal aortic arch is divided and retroesophageal segment is brought anterior to the trachea and anastomosed to the ascending aorta.

8.3.5 Left Aortic Arch with Aberrant Course of Right Subclavian Artery

Introduction

Left aortic arch with aberrant right subclavian artery has a reported prevalence of 0.5–2% and is the most common anomaly of the aortic arch [22].

It is usually isolated, but can rarely be associated with other congenital anomalies like coarctation of the aorta, VSD, or PDA. Patients with trisomy 21, DiGeorge, and Edwards syndromes are also reported to have a high prevalence of this anomaly [23].

Embryology (Fig. 8.14)

It results from the regression of the right arch, between the right subclavian and right common carotid arteries (CCA), with the distal dorsal right aorta forming the retroesophageal proximal portion of the right subclavian artery.

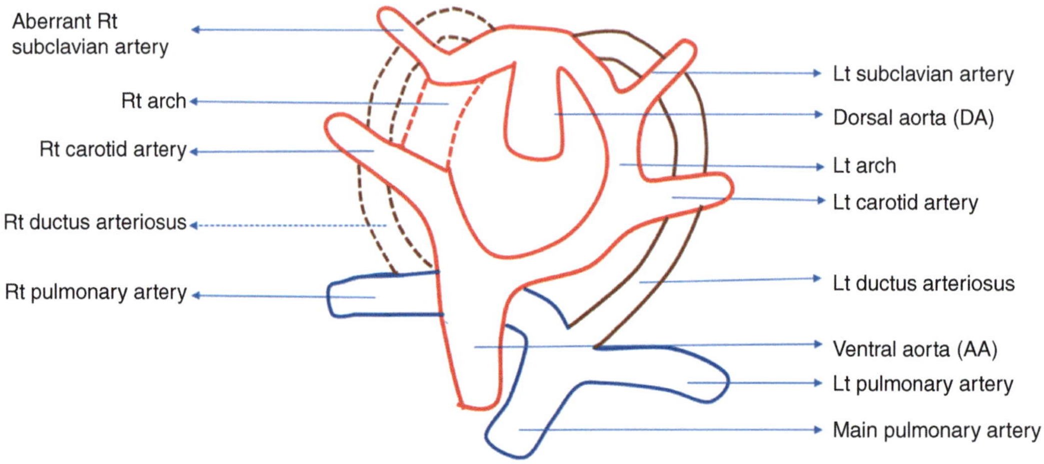

Fig. 8.14 Embryology of left aortic arch with an aberrant course of the right subclavian artery. The left-sided ductus arteriosus/ligamentum arteriosus persists and the right-sided ductus arteriosus involutes

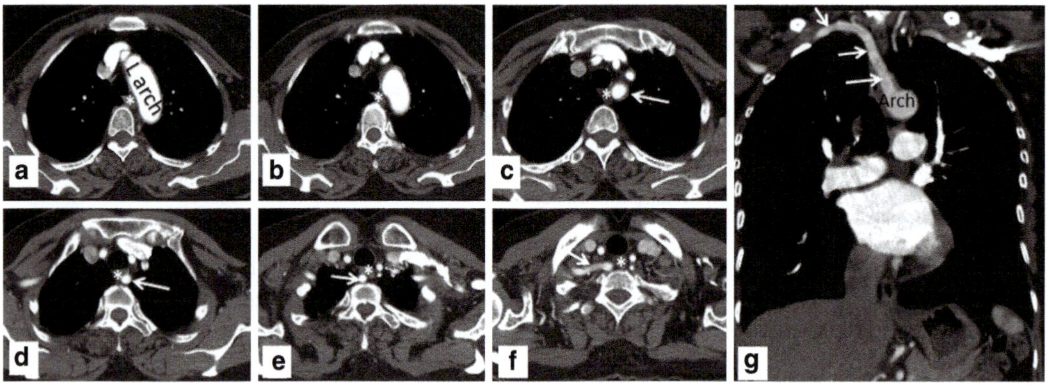

Fig. 8.15 Left aortic arch with aberrant right subclavian artery. Caudo-cranial axial (**a**–**f**) and coronal (**g**) CT sections show. Left aortic arch with aberrant right subclavian artery. Normal left-sided arch (L arch) is seen with the aberrant origin of the right subclavian artery (arrows) as the last branch of the aortic arch which traverses posterior to the esophagus (*) to supply the right upper limb

Clinical Features

It is usually asymptomatic and incidentally found. If symptomatic, may present in childhood with stridor and in the fifth or sixth decade with dysphagia [24]. Around 10% of people with this anomaly may have dysphagia lusoria due to extrinsic compression of the posterior aspect of the esophagus by the anomalous course of the aberrant right subclavian artery [25]. Dysphagia has been reported to be more common in people with Kommerell's diverticulum or when associated with truncus bicaroticus (common origin of the carotid arteries) or very close origin of carotid arteries. Dysphagia is also hypothesized to be related to atherosclerotic changes in older individuals [26].

Imaging Features (Figs. 8.15 and 8.16)

CXR findings:

CXR is insensitive to depict abnormalities of the aortic arch. CXR abnormalities were found in only 20% of patients presenting with dysphagia related to vascular rings [27].

Barium swallow:

Extrinsic indentation on the left lateral and posterior aspect of the barium column in the esophagus.

CT and MRI findings:

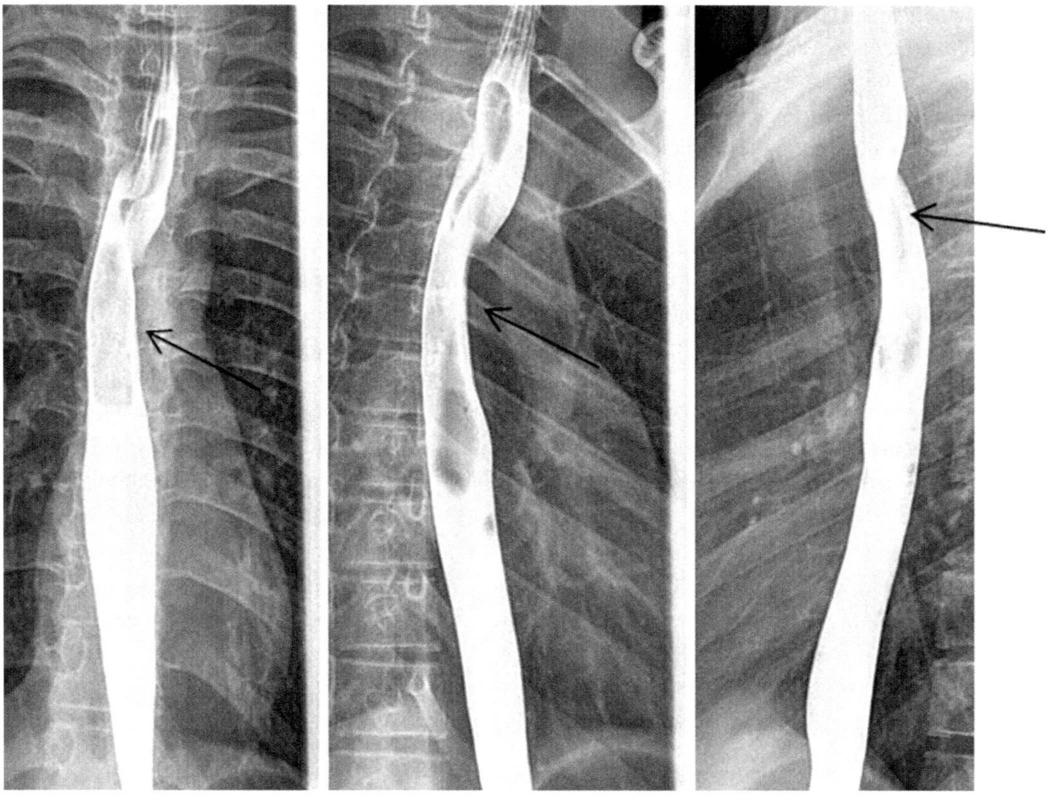

Fig. 8.16 AP and lateral views of Barium swallow images showing extrinsic indentation (arrows) on the left lateral and posterior aspect of the barium column in the esophagus due to the aberrant right subclavian artery

The aberrant right subclavian artery is the last branch of the aortic arch, arising after the left common carotid artery and courses obliquely from left (and inferior) to the right (and superior), posterior to the esophagus, to supply the right arm.

Practical Tip
In the presence of a retroesophageal diverticulum, the ligamentum arteriosum is usually on the side opposite to the arch and forms a vascular ring. In the absence of the diverticulum, ligamentum arteriosum is usually on the same side as the arch and typically does not form a vascular ring [4].

This anomaly may pose problems when surgeries like esophagectomy or other procedures like tracheostomy or transradial catheter angiogram are being performed.

Treatment
In symptomatic patients, many surgical techniques have been described for the division of the aberrant right subclavian artery with reconstruction of blood flow to the right arm.

8.3.6 Right Aortic Arch with Aberrant Course of Left Subclavian Artery Without Retroesophageal Diverticulum

Introduction
This anomaly of aberrant left subclavian artery arising from right aortic arch is described as type 2 right aortic arch and is more common than type 1 right aortic arch (mirror-image branching) and type 3 right aortic arch (isolated left subclavian

artery which arises from the pulmonary artery through the ductus arteriosus).

Embryology (Fig. 8.17)

Right arch with aberrant left subclavian artery develops due to regression of embryonic left fourth arch (between the left common carotid artery and subclavian artery), and left sixth arch and persistence of the right fourth aortic arch. Therefore, left dorsal aorta does not form part of descending aorta and there is no retroesophageal diverticulum.

Clinical Features

This anomaly is rarely symptomatic and mostly an incidental finding on imaging.

Imaging Features

CXR findings:

Indentation on the right side of the lower trachea, with no indentation on the left side.

Barium swallow:

Extrinsic indentation on the right lateral and posterior aspect of the barium column in the esophagus, by the right arch and the retroesophageal aberrant left subclavian artery.

CT and MRI findings:

In this anomaly, first artery arising from the right-sided arch is the left CCA, followed by right CCA, right subclavian artery and the last branch is the left subclavian artery, which courses from right to left and caudal to cranially, posterior to the esophagus [28] (Fig. 8.18).

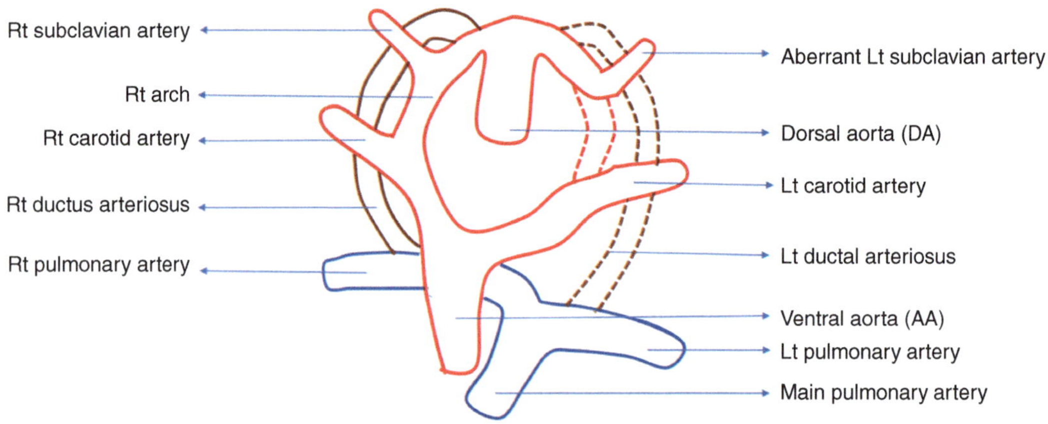

Fig. 8.17 Embryology of right aortic arch with an aberrant course of the left subclavian artery. The right-sided ductus arteriosus/ligamentum arteriosus persists and the left-sided ductus arteriosus involutes

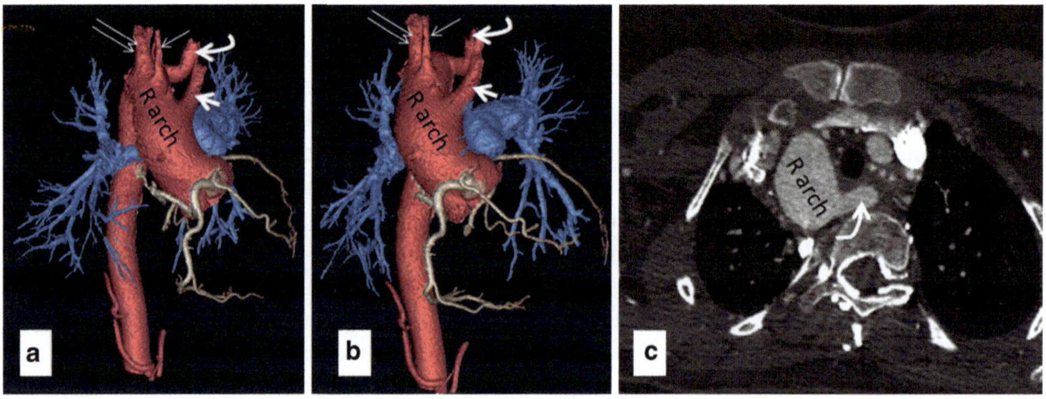

Fig. 8.18 Right aortic arch with aberrant left subclavian artery without retroesophageal diverticulum. Volume-rendered (**a**, **b**) and axial (**c**) contrast-enhanced CT images showing right-sided aortic arch (R arch), left CCA (short thick arrow) as the first branch, followed by right CCA (thin single arrow), right subclavian artery (thin double arrows) and the aberrant left subclavian artery (curved arrow) as the last branch which has a retroesophageal course as depicted on the axial image

Practical Tip
Although other associated cardiac anomaly is rare in the right aortic arch with aberrant left subclavian artery, some studies have reported stenosis in carotid or subclavian arteries and this has to be actively looked for [29].

Unlike in patients with a retroesophageal diverticulum, here the ligamentum arteriosum is either absent or right-sided and so, does not form a vascular ring.

8.3.7 Right Aortic Arch with Mirror-Image Branching

Introduction
The right aortic arch with mirror-image branching is less common as compared to the right aortic arch with an aberrant left subclavian artery. In these cases, the aortic arch is right-sided with the left innominate artery arising as its first branch. The left innominate artery later bifurcates into the left common carotid and left subclavian arteries. The second and third branches of the aortic arch are the right common carotid and right subclavian arteries, respectively [30].

Embryology
This anomaly results from the regression of the left fourth branchial arch between the left ductus and dorsal aorta. The ductus arteriosus is usually on the left side, originating from the left innominate artery and coursing anteriorly without forming a vascular ring. Occasionally, the ductus may be on the right side or bilateral. Although in most cases, the right arch with mirror-image branching does not form a vascular ring, rarely it may, when the left ductus arises from the descending thoracic aorta (Fig. 8.19) and courses posterior to the esophagus toward the left pulmonary artery [31].

Clinical Features
Since there is no vascular ring in these cases, the right aortic arch with mirror-image branching on its own is asymptomatic. However, 98% of these cases are associated with congenital heart diseases and hence, become symptomatic due to the same. The congenital heart diseases associated with this condition are usually cyanotic and include tetralogy of Fallot, truncus arteriosus, tricuspid atresia, double-outlet right ventricle, and transposition of the great arteries.

Imaging Features (Fig. 8.20)

CXR findings:

Indentation on the right side of the trachea.

CT and MRI findings:

The right aortic arch courses between the superior vena cava (SVC) and the trachea and esophagus, but does not form a vascular ring. The first branch of the aortic arch is the left innominate artery, followed by the right common carotid

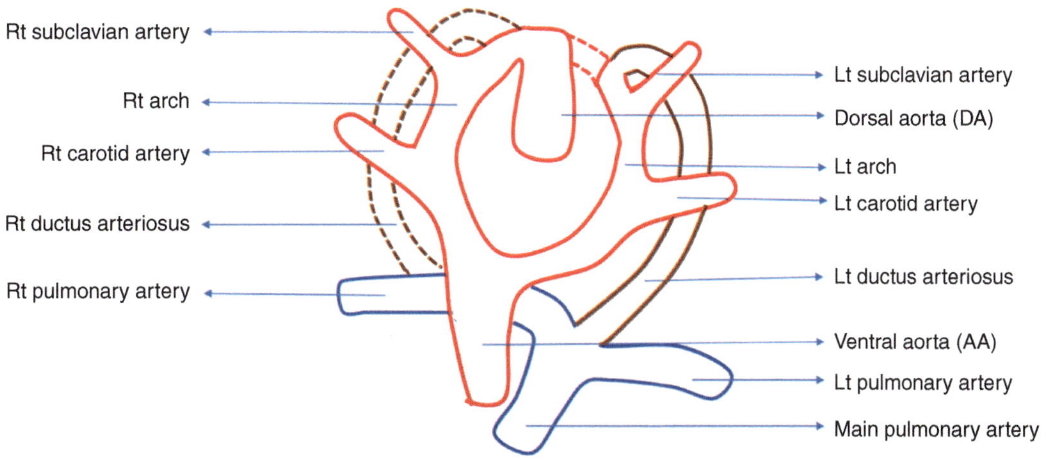

Fig. 8.19 Right-sided aortic arch with mirror-image branching and PDA on the left

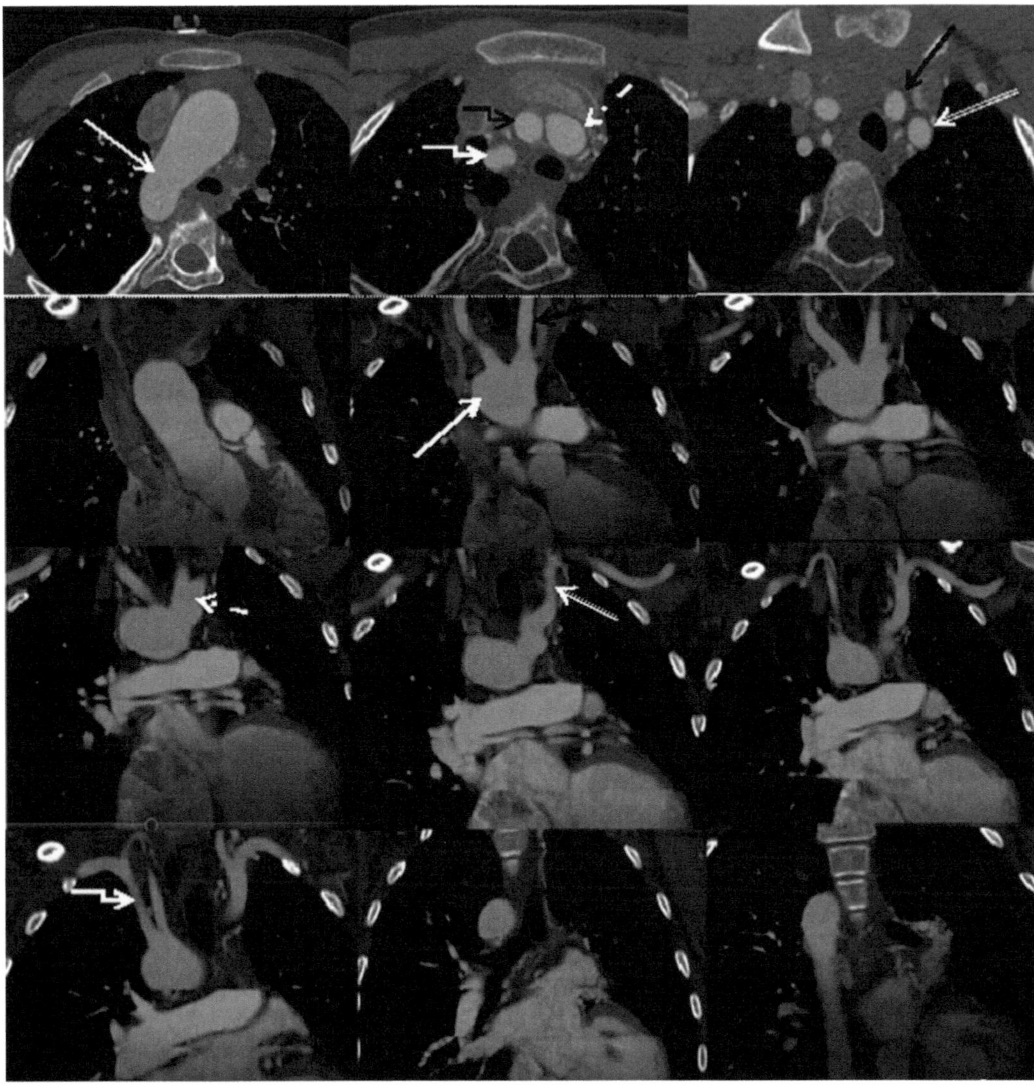

Fig. 8.20 Right arch with mirror-image branching—Axial and coronal images of a patient with Tetralogy of Fallot. The aortic arch (white arrow) and the descending aorta are on the right side. The first branch from the aortic arch is the left innominate artery (broken-white arrow), which later divides into the left common carotid (black arrow) and left subclavian arteries (double-line white arrow). The next branch is the right common carotid artery (curved black arrow) and the last branch is the right subclavian artery (curved white arrow)

and right subclavian arteries. The arch and descending thoracic aorta are on the right side. Both CT and MRI can demonstrate right aortic arch and its mirror branching pattern in an excellent way. MRI can be used in patients in whom CT is contra-indicated due to radiation risk or due to contra-indications to injection of contrast.

CT and MRI can also help in assessing other associated congenital heart diseases, which are seen in 98% of these cases.

Practical Tip
Always look for associated congenital heart disease, which can be seen in 98% of such cases.

Treatment
Isolated right aortic arch with mirror-image branching does not require any treatment. Treatment is directed toward any associated congenital heart disease.

8.3.8 Innominate Artery Compression Syndrome

Introduction
Innominate artery compression syndrome is also known as brachiocephalic artery compression syndrome and is a condition seen in infants where the innominate artery causes compression of the trachea as it courses anterior to it.

Clinical Features
Presentation is usually in the first year of life in the form of respiratory distress, cough, recurrent pulmonary infections, and stridor [32]. With growth, the origin of the innominate artery moves toward the right side and hence, most children outgrow any tracheal compression.

Imaging Findings (Fig. 8.21)
CXR findings: Compression on the anterior aspect of the trachea, seen on lateral CXR.

CT and MRI findings:

The brachiocephalic or innominate artery normally takes its origin toward the left side of the trachea in children and usually does not cause any tracheal compression. However, in some cases, this innominate artery may cause narrowing or compression of the trachea as it crosses anterior to it at the level of the thoracic inlet. CT and MRI show the tracheal narrowing and its relation to the innominate artery in a better way. CT and MRI can provide 3D images that are helpful, especially if surgery is being planned.

Practical Tips
This condition causes tracheal compression in infancy due to its location on the left side. As children grow older, the origin shifts toward the right side of the trachea relieving the compression.

Treatment
Since most children outgrow any tracheal compression, treatment is usually conservative. Surgery is done in cases with severe respiratory distress or with multiple recurrent pulmonary infections [32]. Surgical repair usually includes aortopexy and fixation of the aortic arch along with the fixation of the innominate artery to the sternum [33]. Innominate artery reimplantation is another surgical option [34].

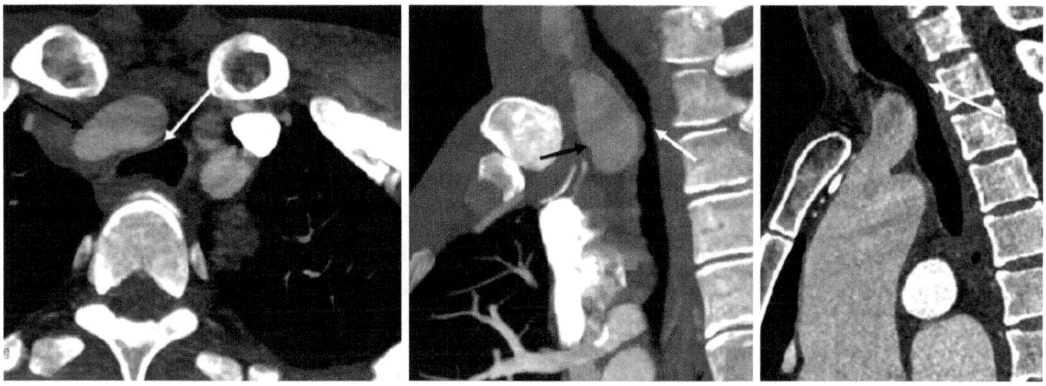

Fig. 8.21 Innominate artery compression syndrome. Axial and sagittal oblique CT images showing the right innominate artery (black arrow) coursing anterior to the trachea and compressing the tracheal lumen (white arrow). Image courtesy: Dr. Jagia, AIIMS, Delhi

8.3.9 Pulmonary Sling

Introduction

Pulmonary sling or aberrant left pulmonary artery is a rare anomaly where the left pulmonary artery arises from the posterior aspect of the right pulmonary artery rather than from the main pulmonary artery, courses above the right main bronchus and between the trachea and esophagus to reach the left pulmonary hilum, thereby causing compression of these structures.

Classification

Type 1: In these cases, the carina is at its normal level (T4–T5 vertebral level) and the bronchial branching pattern is normal [35]. This type is further divided into type 1A and type 1B, depending on the presence (type 1A) or absence (type 1B) of a tracheal bronchus on the right side. In type 1 pulmonary sling, there is usually narrowing of the distal trachea or right main bronchus, thereby leading to hyperinflation of the right lung. These patients may also have tracheobronchomalacia.

Type 2: In these cases, the pulmonary sling is associated with an abnormal bridging bronchus and carina at a lower level than normal (at T6 vertebral level). This type is also further divided into types IIA and IIB.

In type IIA, the right upper lobe bronchus is normal, while a bridging bronchus from the left main bronchus supplies the right middle and lower lobes. In type IIB, the normal right bronchial tree is absent and a bridging bronchus arises from the left main bronchus to supply the right lung.

Type II is more common than type I and is usually associated with long-segment tracheal stenosis due to complete cartilaginous rings with resultant bilateral lung hyperinflation.

Morbidity and mortality are higher in type 2 than in type 1 [36].

Clinical Features

Clinical features are usually apparent in the neonatal or infantile period. The most common presenting features are usually due to tracheal compression and include respiratory distress, stridor, or wheeze. Cough and recurrent pulmonary infections may also be seen. Symptoms of esophageal compression like vomiting and feeding difficulties are less common but may be seen. Occasionally, type 1 cases may be asymptomatic and detected incidentally in adults.

Imaging Findings (Fig. 8.22a, b)

CXR findings:

CXR may show tracheal compression along with hyperinflation of the right lung in type 1 pulmonary sling. There may be bilateral lung hyperinflation along with long-segment tracheal compression and a low-placed tracheal carina in type 2 pulmonary sling.

Barium swallow:

Can show impression on the anterior wall of the mid-thoracic esophagus (at the level of the carina).

CT and MRI findings:

Show the aberrant left pulmonary artery arising from the posterior aspect of the right pulmonary artery and also help to assess any right main bronchial, tracheal, or esophageal compression. CT and MRI can also be used to look for any other associated pulmonary or cardio-vascular anomalies which are common in type 2 pulmonary sling.

Practical Tips

Pulmonary sling also needs consideration when chest radiograph shows unilateral or bilateral hyperinflation of the lungs.

Treatment

Treatment of type 1 pulmonary sling includes reimplantation of aberrant left pulmonary artery [37]. In type 2 pulmonary sling, treatment for long-segment tracheal stenosis is also required along with reimplantation of the left pulmonary artery. Tracheal stenosis can be treated by tracheoplasty or grafts.

8.4 Conclusion

Salient CT/MRI features of vascular rings and slings are given in Table 8.1. Identification of vascular ring can be difficult even on

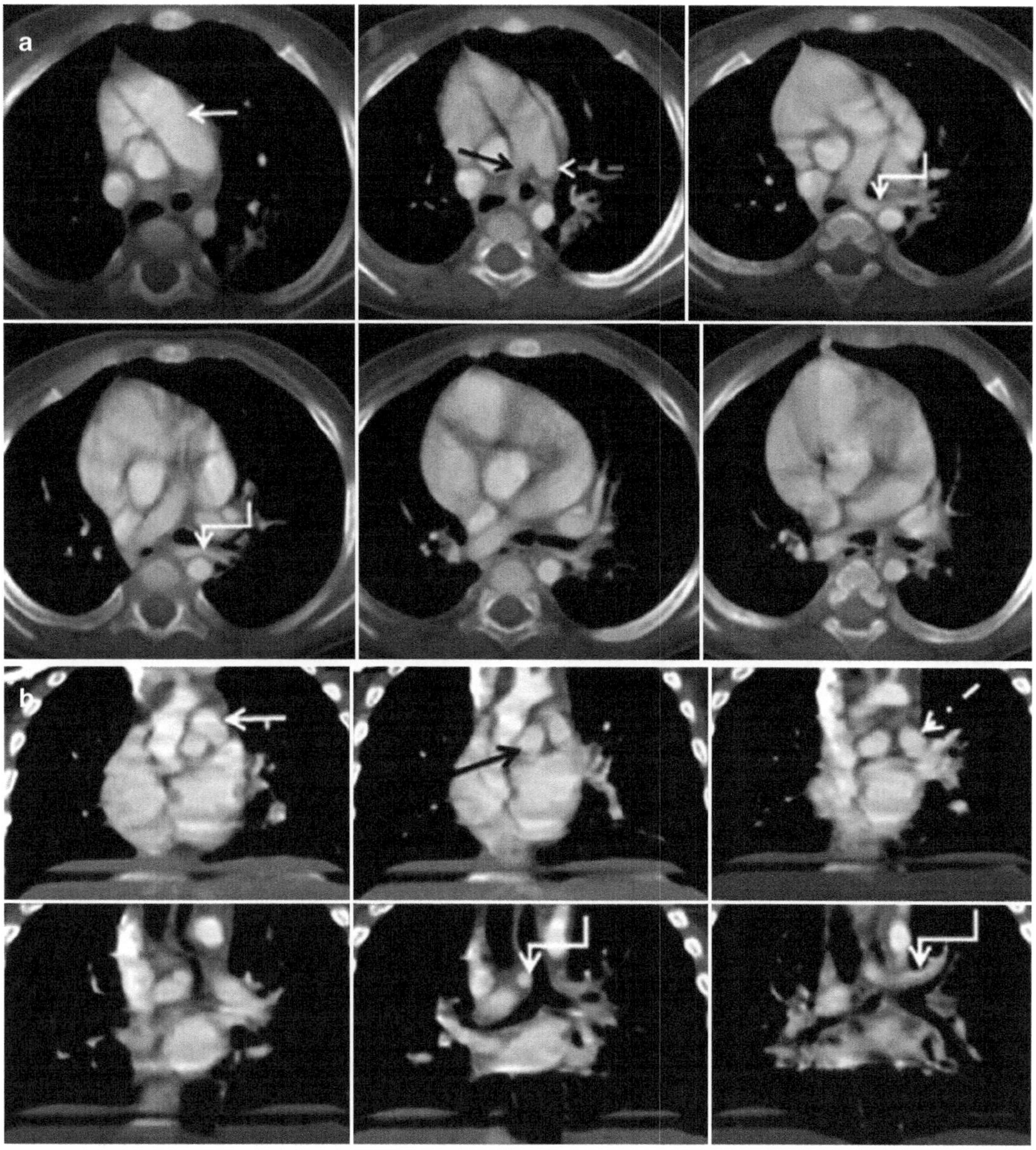

Fig. 8.22 (**a**) Pulmonary sling—Images show the main pulmonary artery (white arrow) dividing into the right (black arrow) and left (broken-white arrow) pulmonary arteries. Inferiorly, an accessory pulmonary artery is seen (curved white arrow) arising from the right pulmonary artery and coursing between the trachea and esophagus to reach the left pulmonary hilum. (**b**) Coronal images of the same patient

cross-sectional imaging if the ring has atretic segments which are fibrous structures that are not readily visible, unlike opacified vessels. The secondary signs which are pointers toward a vascular ring are four vessel sign, distorted subclavian artery sign, diverticulum of Kommerell, ductal diverticulum on the opposite side of the aortic arch and descending aorta on the opposite of aortic arch [38]. We hope that we have simplified the challenging topic of vascular rings and slings with practical tips and easy to understand line diagrams depicting the embryological basis of different types of vascular rings and slings.

Table 8.1 Salient CT/MRI imaging features of vascular rings and slings

Name of condition	CT/MRI findings
Double aortic arch with both arches patent	An axial image through the level of the branch arteries will show symmetry of the common carotid and subclavian arteries—the "figure of four sign." Phase-contrast sequences on MRI can quantitate which arch has more flow when the arches are codominant.
Double aortic arch with atresia or hypoplasia of one arch with fibrous remnant	"Figure of four" sign with more posterior location of the proximal left arch and the presence of a diverticulum of the descending aorta is commonly seen.
Left aortic arch with aberrant right subclavian artery and Kommerrell's diverticulum	The aberrant right subclavian artery arises from the proximal descending thoracic aorta and originates from the Kommerrell's diverticulum which is located posterior to the esophagus.
Right aortic arch with aberrant left subclavian artery and Kommerrell's diverticulum	Aberrant left subclavian artery originates as the last branch of the right aortic arch from a diverticulum with retroesophageal course. The diverticulum is usually rounded in shape and larger in the right aortic arch unlike the conical shape in the left aortic arch.
Left aortic arch with an aberrant course of the right subclavian artery without Kommerrell's diverticulum	The aberrant right subclavian artery is the last branch of the aortic arch, arising after the left common carotid artery and courses obliquely from left (and inferior) to the right (and superior), posterior to the esophagus, to supply the right arm.
Right aortic arch with an aberrant course of the left subclavian artery without retroesophageal diverticulum	The first artery arising from the right-sided arch is the left CCA, followed by right CCA, right subclavian artery and the last branch is the left subclavian artery, which courses from right to left and caudal to cranially, posterior to the esophagus.
Right aortic arch with mirror-image branching	Right-sided aortic arch which courses between the superior vena cava (SVC) and the trachea and esophagus, but does not form a vascular ring. The first branch of the aortic arch is the left innominate artery, followed by the right common carotid and right subclavian arteries. The arch and descending thoracic aorta are on the right side. Look for associated congenital heart diseases, which are seen in 98% of these cases.
Innominate artery compression syndrome	Origin of the brachiocephalic or innominate artery toward the left side of the trachea causing narrowing or compression of the trachea as it crosses anterior to it at the level of the thoracic inlet. Chest radiograph (especially in lateral projection) may show compression of the trachea anteriorly. CT and MRI show the tracheal narrowing and its relation to the innominate artery in a better way.
Pulmonary sling or aberrant left pulmonary artery	The left pulmonary artery arises from the posterior aspect of the right pulmonary artery rather than from the main pulmonary artery, courses above the right main bronchus, and between the trachea and esophagus to reach the left pulmonary hilum. There may be compression of the lower part of the trachea, right main bronchus, or the esophagus. It is classified into types 1 and 2, depending upon the tracheobronchial division pattern. Associated pulmonary or cardio-vascular anomalies are common in type 2 pulmonary sling.

References

1. Gross RE. Surgical relief for tracheal obstruction from a vascular ring. N Engl J Med. 1945;233:586–90.
2. Ganie IS, Amod K, Reddy D. Vascular rings: a radiological review of anatomical variations. Cardiovasc J Afr. 2016;27(1):30–6.
3. Backer CL, Mavroudis C. Congenital heart surgery nomenclature and database project: patent ductus arteriosus, coarctation of the aorta, interrupted aortic arch. Ann Thorac Surg. 2000;69(4 suppl):S298–307.
4. Hanneman K, Newman B, Chan F. Congenital variants and anomalies of the aortic arch. Radiographics. 2017;37:32–51.

5. Fenández-Tena A, Martínez-González C. Double aortic arch diagnosed in a 44-year-old woman with recurring respiratory infections. Respir Med Case Rep. 2017 Feb 28;20:176–8.
6. Quail MA, Piers SYH, Daubeney EF. Vascular rings, pulmonary slings, and other vascular abnormalities. Diagnosis and management of adult congenital heart disease. 3rd ed. London: Elsevier; 2018. p. 429–39.
7. Shuford WH, Sybers RG, Weens HS. The Angiographic features of double aortic arch. Am J Roentgenol. 1972;116(1):125–40.
8. Poletto E, Mallon MG, Stevens RM, Avitabile CM. Imaging review of aortic vascular rings and pulmonary sling. J Am Osteopath Coll Radiol. 2017;6(2):83–5.
9. Khalfan A, Rebecca G, Karamlou T, William WG, Mc Crindle BW. Management and outcomes of double aortic arch in 81 patients. Pediatrics. 2006;118(5):e1336–41.
10. Adachi I, Krishnamurthy R, DLS M. A double aortic arch mimicking a right aortic arch with an aberrant subclavian artery. J Vasc Surg. October 2011;54(4):1151–3.
11. Garti J, Aygen MM, Vidne B. Type C double aortic arch—double aortic arch with aberrant left subclavian artery. Cardiovasc Radiol. 1978;1:143–5.
12. Schlesinger AE, Krishnamurthy R, Sena LM, Guillerman RP, Chung T, DiBardino DJ, Fraser CD Jr. Incomplete double aortic arch with atresia of the distal left arch: distinctive imaging appearance. Am J Roentgenol. May 2005;184(5):1634–9.
13. Priya S, Thomas R, Nagpal P, Sharma A, Steigner M. Congenital anomalies of the aortic arch. Cardiovasc Diagn Ther. 2018;8(Suppl 1):S26–44.
14. Backer CL, Russell HM, Wurlitzer KC, Rastatter JC, Rigsby CK. Primary resection of Kommerell diverticulum and left subclavian artery transfer. Ann Thorac Surg. 2012;94(5):1612–7.
15. Ichikawa T, Koizumi J, Tanno K, Okochi T, Nomura T, Shimura S, Imai Y. Kommerell diverticulum in adults: evaluation of routine CT examinations. Tokai J Exp Clin Med. 2016 Jun 20;41(2):65–9.
16. Barranhas AD, Indiani JM, Marchiori E, Santos AA, Rochitte CE, Nacif MS. Atypical presentation of Kommerell's diverticulum. Arq Bras Cardiol. 2009 Dec;93(6):e88–90.
17. Criado T. A new look at Kommerell: recent insights on aortic diverticula. Vasc Dis Manag. 2016;13(7):E156–65.
18. Guido HW, van Bogerijen GHW, Patel HJ, Eliason JL, Criado E, Williams DM, Knepper J, Yang B, Deeb GM. Evolution in the management of aberrant subclavian arteries and related Kommerell diverticulum. Ann Thorac Surg. 2015;100:47–53.
19. Tanaka A, Milner R, Ota T. Kommerell's diverticulum in the current era: a comprehensive review. Gen Thorac Cardiovasc Surg. 2015 May;63(5):245–59.
20. Pandey NN, Shaw M, Sachdeva S, Gulati GS, Kothari SS. Circumflex retroesophageal left aortic arch with right ductus arteriosus: a rare complete vascular ring diagnosed on computed tomography angiography. Ann Pediatr Cardiol. 2020;13(1):98–9.
21. Russell HM, Rastatter JC, Backer CL. The aortic uncrossing procedure for circumflex aorta. Oper Tech Thorac Cardiovasc Surg. 2013 Jul 11;18(1):15–31.
22. Türkvatan A, Büyükbayraktar FG, Olçer T, Cumhur T. Congenital anomalies of the aortic arch: evaluation with the use of multidetector computed tomography. Korean J Radiol. 2009;10(2):176–84.
23. Fehmi Yazıcıoğlu H, Sevket O, Akın H, Aygün M, Özyurt ON, Karahasanoğlu A. Aberrant right subclavian artery in down syndrome fetuses. Prenat Diagn. 2013;33(3):209–13.
24. Puri SK, Ghuman S, Narang P, Sharma A, Singh S. CT and MR angiography in dysphagia lusoria in adults. Indian J Radiol Imaging. 2005;15(4):497–501.
25. Janssen M, Baggen MG, Veen HF, et al. Dysphagia lusoria: clinical aspects, manometric findings, diagnosis, and therapy. Am J Gastroenterol. 2000;95(6):1411–6.
26. Polguj M, Chrzanowski Ł, Kasprzak JD, Stefańczyk L, Topol M, Majos A. The aberrant right subclavian artery (arteria lusoria): the morphological and clinical aspects of one of the most important variations: a systematic study of 141 reports. Sci World J. 2014;2014:1–6.
27. Branscom JJ, Austin JHM. Aberrant right subclavian artery. Findings seen on plain chest roentgenograms. Am J Roentgenol. 1973;119(3):539–42.
28. Hernanz-Schulman M. Vascular rings: a practical approach to imaging diagnosis. Pediatr Radiol. 2005 Oct;35(10):961–79.
29. Arazińska A, Polguj M, Szymczyk K, Kaczmarska M, et al. Right aortic arch analysis - anatomical variant or serious vascular defect? BMC Cardiovasc Disord. 2017;17(1):102.
30. McElhinney DB, Hoydu AK, Gaynor JW, et al. Patterns of right aortic arch and mirror-image branching of the brachiocephalic vessels without associated anomalies. Pediatr Cardiol. 2001;22:285–91.
31. Knight L, Edwards JE. Right aortic arch. Types and associated cardiac anomalies. Circulation. 1974;50:1047–51.
32. Friedman E, Kennedy A, Neitzschman HR. Innominate artery compression of the trachea: an unusual cause of apnea in a 12-year-old boy. South Med J. 2003 Nov;96:1161–4.
33. Gross RE, Neuhauser EB. Compression of the trachea by an anomalous innominate artery: an operation for its relief. Am J Dis Child. 1948 Apr;75(4):570–4.
34. Hawkins JA, Bailey WW, Clark SM. Innominate artery compression of the trachea: treatment by reimplantation of the innominate artery. J Thorac Cardiovasc Surg. 1992;103(4):678–82.
35. Wells TR, Gwinn JL, Landing BH, Stanley P. Reconsideration of the anatomy of sling left pulmonary artery: The association of one form with bridging bronchus and imperforate anus. Anatomic and diagnostic aspects. J Pediatr Surg. 1988;23(10):892–98.

36. Siripornpitak S, Reddy GP, Schwitter J, Higgins CB. Pulmonary artery sling: anatomical and functional evaluation by MRI. J Comput Assist Tomo. 1997;21(5):766–8.
37. Newman B, Cho Y. Left pulmonary artery sling–anatomy and imaging. Seminars in Ultrasound, CT and MRI. 2010;31(2):158–70.
38. Gould SW, Rigsby CK, Donnelly LF, McCulloch M, Pizarro C, Epelman M. Useful signs for the assessment of vascular rings on cross-sectional imaging. Pediatr Radiol. 2015;45(13):2004–6.

Radiological Review of Coronary Artery Anomalies

9

Archita Goel, Bhavana Nagabhushana Reddy, and Sanjaya Viswamitra

9.1 Introduction

Coronary artery anomalies are an important cause of sudden cardiac death in a young individual. These anomalies are difficult to diagnose without radiological tests. CT coronary angiography alerts radiologists and cardiologists to variations of the anatomy of the coronary arteries. Electrocardiographically (ECG)-gated multidetector row computed tomography (CT) allows the accurate and noninvasive depiction of the origin, course, and termination of coronary artery anomalies and is superior to conventional angiography in delineating the ostial origin and proximal path of an anomalous coronary artery [1]. In this chapter, we review the normal anatomy as well as various variants and anomalies of the coronary arteries.

9.2 Normal Anatomy of the Coronary Arteries

Normally, only two main coronary arteries or coronary systems are present, the left and the right, which originate from the right and left coronary sinuses of Valsalva of the aortic root, respectively (Fig. 9.1) [2]. The posterior sinus also commonly referred to as the "noncoronary sinus" rarely gives rise to the coronary arteries. The right sinus is anterior and the left is posterior in location, hence the location of the sinuses are anatomic misnomers [3].

Coronary arteries can be divided into segments. A standardized approach to coronary segmentation, a reporting scheme proposed by the American Heart Association and adapted for cross-sectional imaging in a Society of Cardiovascular Computed Tomography report, improves description and communication of findings (Fig. 9.2) [4, 5].

The four main coronary arteries evaluated at CT are the right coronary artery (RCA), the left main coronary artery (LMCA), the left anterior descending (LAD) artery, and the left circumflex (LCx) artery [3].

9.2.1 Coronary Artery Dominance

The right ventricle is almost always supplied by the RCA. The anterior portion of the ventricular system and anterior wall of the left ventricle (LV) is supplied by the left coronary artery. The supply of the remainder of the LV varies depending upon coronary dominance [3]. The dominance is determined by which artery supplies the posterior descending artery (PDA) and the posterolateral ventricular branch (PLVB). Right dominance is

A. Goel (✉) · B. N. Reddy · S. Viswamitra
Department of Radiology, Sri Sathya Sai Institute of Higher Medical Sciences, Whitefield, Bengaluru, Karnataka, India
e-mail: Archita.g@sssihms.org.in

R. Rajeshkannan et al. (eds.), *CT and MRI in Congenital Heart Diseases*,
https://doi.org/10.1007/978-981-15-6755-1_9

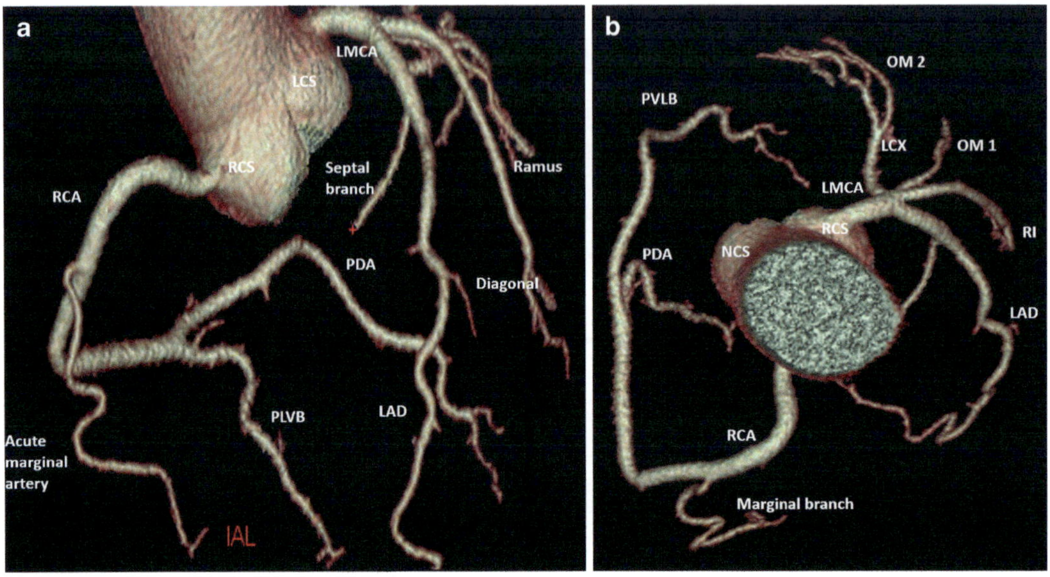

Fig. 9.1 (**a**, **b**) Normal origin of coronary arteries. Volume-rendered image shows the right coronary artery (RCA) arising from the right coronary sinus (RCS) of Valsalva while the left main coronary artery (LMCA) arising from the left coronary sinus (LCS) of Valsalva. The noncoronary sinus (NCS) gives no coronary artery. *PDA* posterior descending artery; *PLVB* posterior left ventricular branch; *LAD* left anterior descending artery; *LCX* left circumflex artery; *OM* obtuse marginal branches

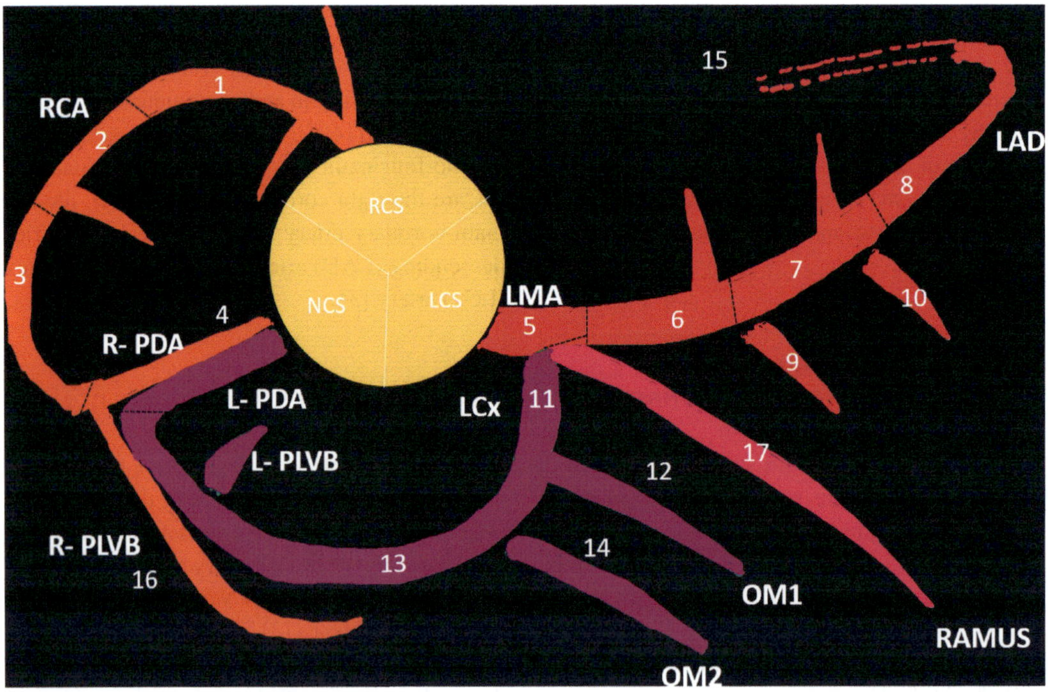

Fig. 9.2 SCCT coronary segmentation diagram. 1-proximal RCA, 2-mid RCA, 3-distal RCA, 4-PDA, 5-LMCA, 6-proximal LAD, 7-mid LAD, 8-distal LAD, 9-first diagonal, 10-second diagonal, 11-proximal LCx, 12-first obtuse marginal, 13-distal LCx, 14-second obtuse marginal, 15-posterior lateral ventricular branch from LCx (L-PLVB), 16-posterior lateral ventricular branch from RCA (R-PLVB),17-ramus intermedius

seen in approximately 85% of individuals where PDA and PLVB are supplied by RCA. Left dominance is seen in 7–8% of individuals where PDA and PLVB are supplied by LCx. Codominance is seen in the remaining 7–8%, where the inferior interventricular septum is supplied by branches from both distal RCA and distal LCx arteries [1].

9.2.2 Right Coronary Artery (RCA)

It originates from the right sinus of Valsalva and courses along the right atrioventricular septum and at least reaches the "acute margin" of the heart [3].

The RCA is divided into three segments—proximal, middle, and distal segments (Fig. 9.3).

Proximal RCA extends from the ostium of the RCA to one-half the distance to the acute margin of the heart. The conus branch arises from the proximal RCA in around 50–60% of cases and supplies the right ventricular outflow tract. The sinoatrial (SA) nodal branch arises from proximal RCA in approximately 50–60% of individuals (Fig. 9.4). In the rest of the individuals, it

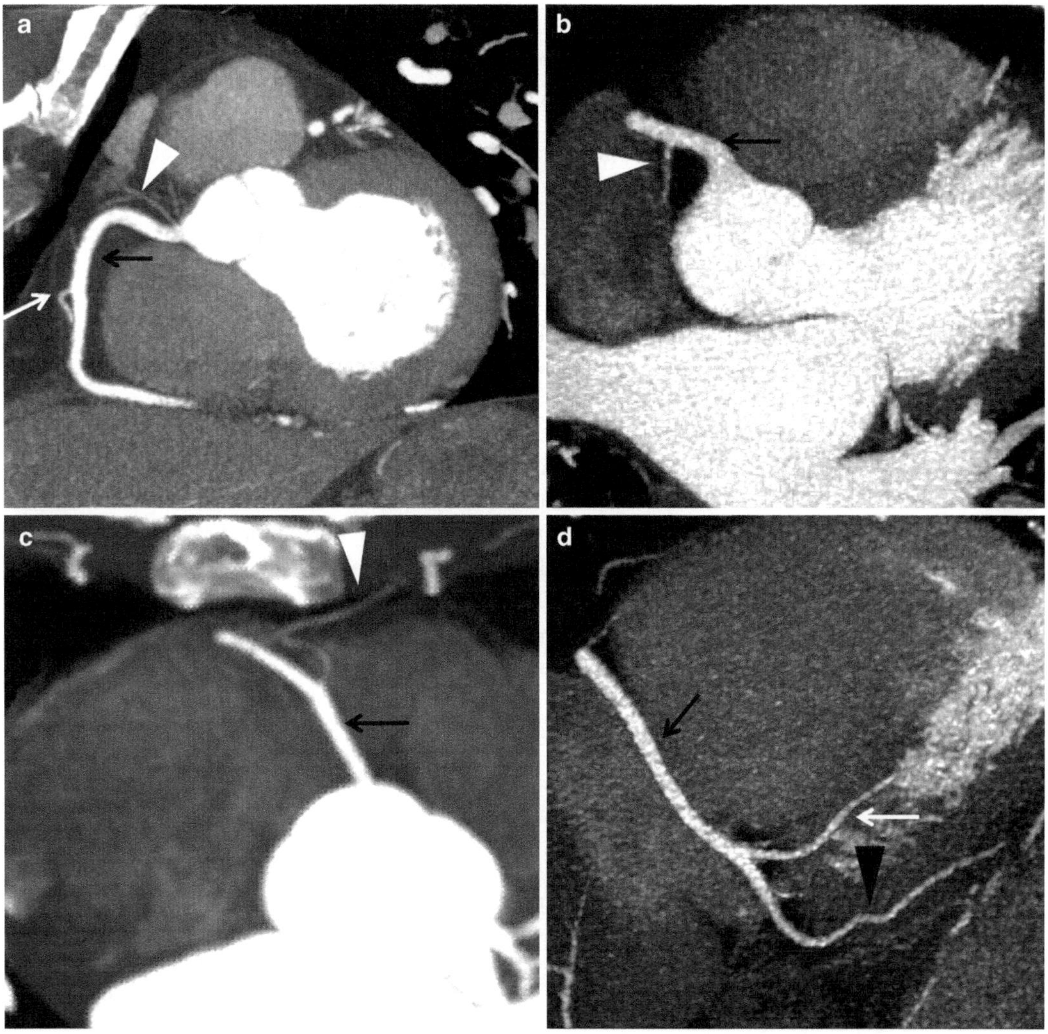

Fig. 9.3 MIP Oblique short axis (**a**), oblique axial (**b, c**) images show the RCA (black arrow in **a, b, c**) and its branches. White arrow (**a**) indicates the acute marginal branch, white arrowhead (**a, b**) indicates the sinoatrial nodal branch, white arrowhead (**c**) indicates the conus branch, white arrow (**d**) indicates PDA, black arrowhead (**d**) indicates posterior lateral ventricular branch

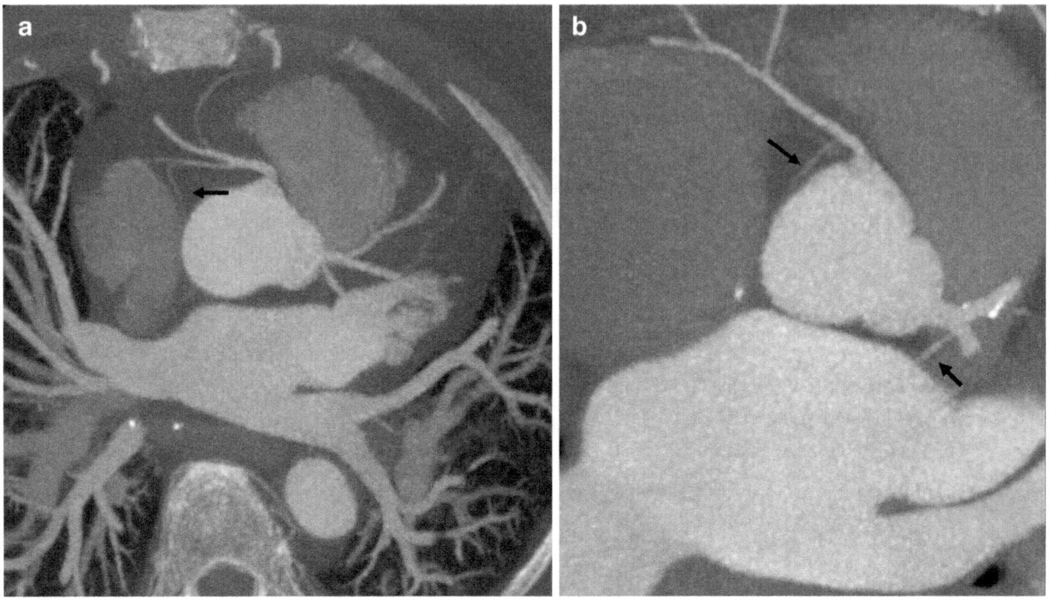

Fig. 9.4 CTA axial MIP images show the origin of SA nodal branch from RCA (**a**) and duplication of SA nodal branch arising from RCA and LCx

arises either from proximal LCx or distal RCA [3, 4].

Mid-RCA extends from the end of proximal RCA to the acute margin of the heart. Acute marginal artery arises from mid-RCA and supplies the right ventricular free wall [3, 4].

Distal RCA extends from the end of mid-RCA to the origin of the PDA. In the right dominant system, the PDA (R-PDA) and PLVB (R-PLVB) arise from the RCA and supply the inferior and infero-septal segments of the LV [2, 3]. Atrioventricular (AV) nodal branches arise from distal RCA from crux cordis at the base of the heart in 90% of cases [3, 4].

9.2.3 Left Main Coronary Artery (LMCA)

It is a segment of the left coronary system which originates from the left coronary cusp giving two primary subdivisions: the left anterior descending and the left circumflex artery (Fig. 9.5) [2].

9.2.4 Left Anterior Descending Artery (LAD)

The LAD is a segment of the left coronary system which is characterized by its course along the anterior interventricular groove (Fig. 9.5) [2]. Its branches are the septal perforator and diagonal branches [3].

The septal perforator branches supply the anterior two-thirds of basal interventricular septum and rest of the entire septum. The diagonal branches supply the anterior left ventricular wall [3].

Usually, the LAD reaches the cardiac apex; however, this is not always so. In such instances, the distal territory may be supplied by unusually long diagonal or right coronary branches [2].

The LAD can be divided into proximal, mid, and distal segments. Proximal LAD extends from the end of the left main coronary artery to the first large septal or D1 (first diagonal), whichever is most proximal. Mid-LAD extends from the end of proximal LAD to one-half the distance to the

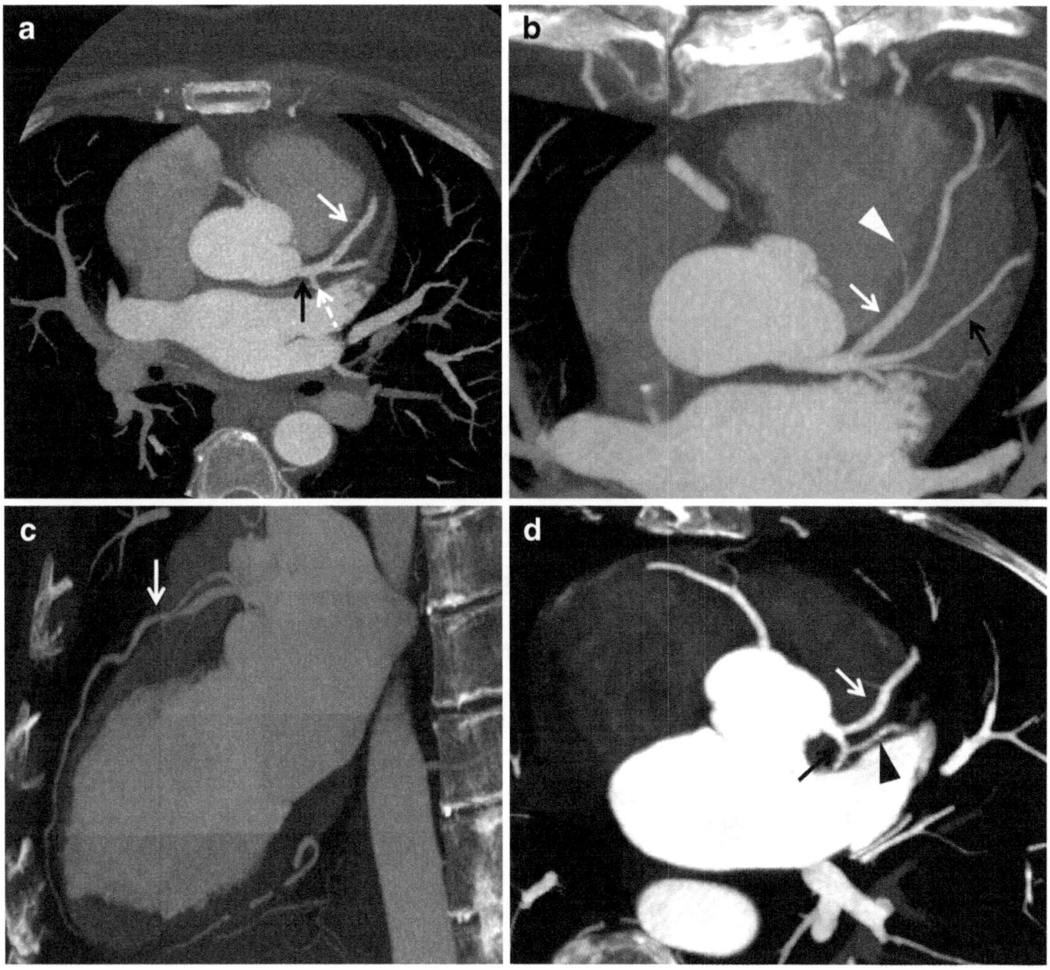

Fig. 9.5 Oblique axial (**a**, **b**) and vertical long-axis (**c**) MPR images. LMCA (black arrow in **a**) bifurcating into the left anterior descending (LAD) artery (white arrow) and the left circumflex (LCx) artery (dotted white arrow). The normal LAD artery (white arrow in **c**) coursing in the epicardial fat of the interventricular groove toward the LV apex. White arrowhead (**b**) shows the septal branch. Black arrow (**b**) shows the ramus intermedius. Oblique axial (**d**) image shows LMCA bifurcating into the left anterior descending (LAD) artery (white arrow) and the left circumflex (LCx) artery (black arrow). The left circumflex (LCx) artery (black arrow) is giving rise to the obtuse marginal branch (black arrowhead)

apex. Distal LAD extends from the end of mid-LAD to the end of LAD [4].

9.2.5 Left Circumflex Artery (LCx)

LCX is a segment of the left coronary system characterized by its course in the left-sided atrioventricular groove (Fig. 9.5). It usually supplies the lateral wall of the left ventricle and variable portions of the inferior wall through the obtuse marginal and posterolateral branches, respectively [3].

The LCX can be divided into two segments—proximal and distal. The proximal segment extends from the end of LMCA to the origin of the first obtuse marginal branch (OM1). The distal segment extends from distal to the OM1 branch to the end of the vessel or origin of the PDA (L-PDA). The LCx continues in the posterior AV groove and gives rise to PDA (L-PDA) and PLVB (L-PLVB) in left dominant or codominant circulation [3]. In some individuals, the distal LCX continues as an obtuse marginal branch.

9.2.6 Ramus Intermedius (RI)/(Medianus)

Sometimes, instead of bifurcating into the LAD and LCx, LMCA trifurcates into LAD, LCx, and ramus intermedius (Figs. 9.1 and 9.5). Ramus intermedius supplies the lateral and inferior walls, which are otherwise supplied by diagonal or obtuse marginal branches [3].

9.3 Normal Variants

9.3.1 Right Superior Septal Perforator

It refers to septal perforator that arises from the proximal RCA or the right sinus of Valsalva and supplies the anterior septum. Similar to the conus artery, it can act as a source of collateral in proximal LAD disease [3].

9.3.2 Supernumerary Coronary Ostia

In some patients, small branches may arise directly from the ascending aorta instead of arising from the RCA or LMCA (Fig. 9.6). Examples include separate origins of LCx and LAD from left coronary conus with no LMCA and direct origin of the conal artery from the aorta. Accurate knowledge of coronary ostia is extremely important for coronary catheterization [3].

9.3.3 Myocardial Bridging

Normally a coronary artery has an epicardial course [3]. Myocardial bridging is a congenital anomaly in which a segment of a coronary artery takes a "tunneled" intramuscular course under a "bridge" of overlying myocardium (Fig. 9.7) [6]. The middle segment of LAD is

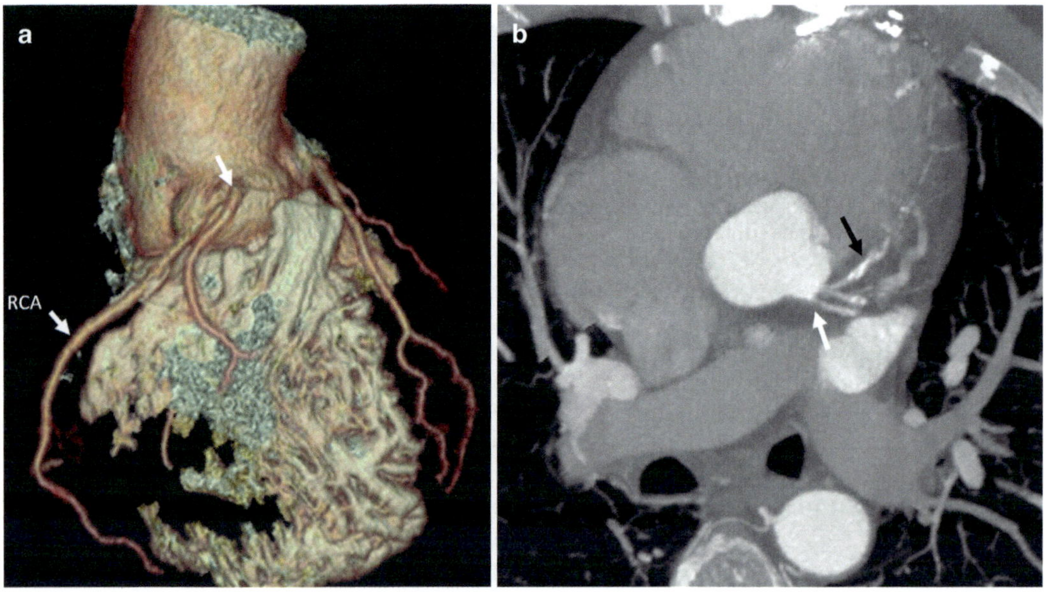

Fig. 9.6 (**a**) A 22-year-old male patient with tetralogy of Fallot. CT VR image shows the origin of the conal artery (white arrow) separate from RCA and directly from the right coronary sinus. (**b**) Another 54-year-old male patient with coronary artery disease status post CABG, axial MIP image shows short LMCA bifurcating into LAD (black arrow) and RI; and separate origin (white arrow) of LCX from the left coronary cusp

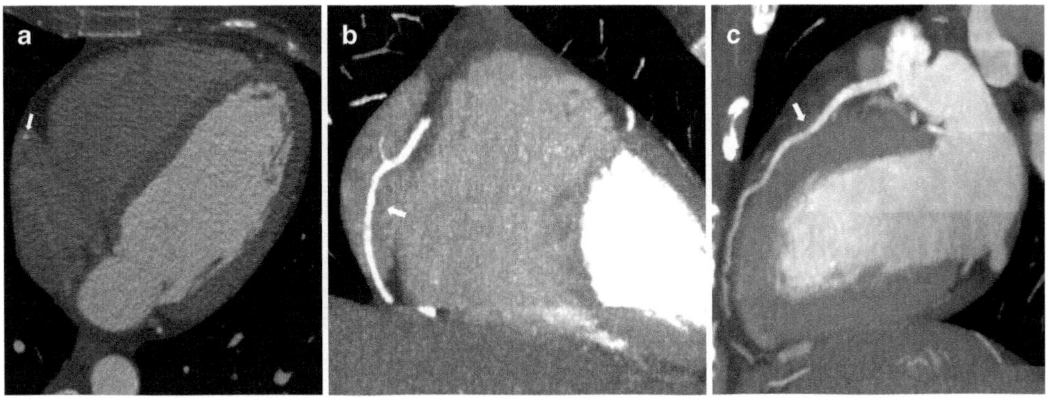

Fig. 9.7 A 25-year-old male patient with atypical chest pain. (**a**, **b**) CTA images show RCA coursing through the atrial myocardium (white arrow). (**c**) A 40-year-old male patient with coronary artery disease. CTA image showed incidental finding of myocardial bridging in mid LAD (white arrow)

most commonly involved, followed by RCA and LCX [7].

A typical myocardial bridge has been reported to have depth of 1–10 mm and length of 10–30 mm [6, 8]. LAD myocardial bridges have been divided into two types—superficial and deep. In superficial bridges, LAD runs in the interventricular groove where a muscle bundle crosses it at an angle or perpendicularly. This type accounts for 75% of cases. In the deep bridges, LAD dives into the interventricular septum on the side of the right ventricle. A longitudinal muscle bundle from the right ventricular apex crosses the LAD segment transversely or obliquely. Deep bridges may cause twisting of the tunneled arterial segment during the cardiac cycle resulting in hemodynamic compromise [6, 9].

A myocardial loop is a subset of myocardial bridging where an epicardial artery or vein (less common) courses through a segment of atrial myocardium (Fig. 9.7). Myocardial loop usually involves distal LCX and distal RCA and has a length of 10–15 mm and a thickness of 0.1–0.3 mm [6, 7].

On coronary angiography, the systolic compression of the tunneled segment of the coronary artery is termed as "milking" effect with "step down" and "step up" demarcation of the involved area [10].

Clinical Presentation Though most patients are asymptomatic, angina, myocardial ischemia, acute coronary syndromes, left ventricular dysfunction and stunning, arrhythmias, and sudden cardiac death have been reported in a few cases [6].

As the coronary arteries are filled mainly during diastole, systolic compression of the artery does not usually affect myocardial perfusion significantly. However, during tachycardia the diastolic filling shortens and compromises in systolic filling having a greater effect [11]. Some studies show that compression of the tunneled arteries continues in diastole as well, affecting the myocardial perfusion which may cause these symptoms [6, 12, 13].

The bridged segment of the artery shows sparing from atherosclerotic changes due to changes in the endothelium. However, these endothelial changes along with systolic compression may predispose the bridged segment to coronary vasospasm and thrombus formation [6, 14–17]. The segment of the artery proximal to the bridged segment shows accelerated atherosclerosis [6, 14]. Variations in symptoms depending upon the length and depth of the tunneled artery have been shown in Fig. 9.8 [10].

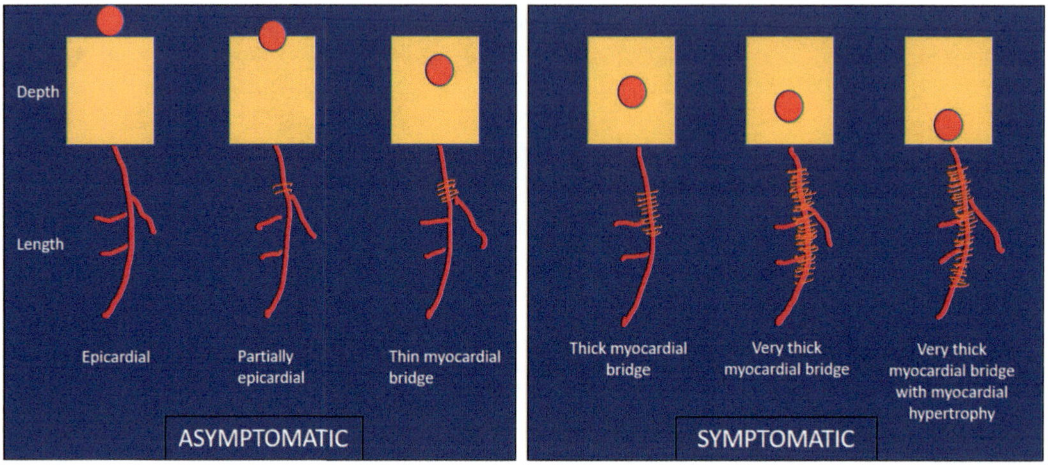

Fig. 9.8 Diagram shows variations in symptoms based on the depth of the myocardial bridge and length of the tunneled arterial segment

Treatment Patients thought to be developing symptoms due to myocardial bridging can be treated:

- Medically with beta-blockers and non-dihydropyridine calcium-channel blockers [6, 18]. Nitrates are contraindicated as they accentuate systolic compression of the vessel [6, 19].
- Surgical myotomy and coronary artery bypass graft surgery are reserved for patients with refractory symptoms [6].

9.4 Coronary Anomalies

The clinical manifestations of coronary artery anomalies vary in severity, with some anomalies presenting as sudden cardiac death and others being benign. Cardiovascular computed tomography (CT) has emerged as the standard of reference for the identification and characterization of coronary artery anomalies. Classification of coronary artery anomalies based on hemodynamic significance is illustrated in Table 9.1 [20].

Anomalies of coronary arteries can also be classified based on their origin, course, and termination (Table 9.2) [1].

Table 9.1 Classification of coronary artery anomalies based on hemodynamic significance

Hemodynamically significant anomalies	Hemodynamically less significant anomalies
Coronary ostial stenosis or atresia	Duplication of artery duplication
Origin from the pulmonary artery	High origin from the aorta
Origin of coronary artery from ventricle	Origin from the aorta in an anomalous position, including arteries that arise from the contralateral cusp or contralateral artery
Coronary artery fistula	Origin from other systemic vascular structures
Inter-arterial course	Anomalies of course: pre-pulmonic, trans-septal, or retro-aortic course; Shepherd's crook right coronary artery
	Systemic termination

9.5 Hemodynamically Significant Anomalies

9.5.1 Coronary Ostial Stenosis or Atresia (COSA)

COSA represents a spectrum of rare congenital developmental diseases. Important defining features of COSA are illustrated in Table 9.3.

Table 9.2 Classification of coronary anomalies based on origin, course, and termination

Anomalies of origin	Anomalies of course	Anomalies of termination
High takeoff	Myocardial bridging	Coronary artery fistula
Multiple ostia	Duplication of artery	Coronary arcade
Single coronary artery	Pre-pulmonic	Extracardiac termination
Anomalous origin of coronary artery from the pulmonary artery	Trans-septal	
Coronary artery origin from opposite or noncoronary cusp with anomalous course	Retro-aortic	
Coronary ostial stenosis or atresia	Inter-arterial/malignant	
Anomalous origin of the coronary artery from the ventricle	Shepherd's crook RCA	

Table 9.3 Features of COSA

Ostial location	Proximal course	Atretic segment
Absent	Normal location (epicardial)	Ostial
Normal location	Intramural course of ectopic artery (proximal stenotic trunk courses within the aortic wall and crosses over to the correct side of the heart after taking a tangential direction off the ostium).	Proximal
Ectopic (aortic or otherwise)		

Congenital atresia of the left coronary artery is more common than RCA. Ostial dimple/coronary ostial remnant may be present which is usually followed distally by the atretic proximal coronary stem and a blind distal trunk [21].

In all patients with congenital coronary artery atresia or right/left-sided coronary artery occlusion, three major inter-coronary collateral pathways (Fig. 9.9) (pre-conal, retro-conal, and retro-aortic collaterals) provide circulation between the right and left coronary systems. These are summarized in Table 9.4 [22, 23].

Only one or two full diameter connecting collateral vessels are present without stenosis at the transition of supplying and receiving vessels. This is in contrast to the postnatally acquired collaterals which are numerous, may arise from septal, atrial, or infundibular branches and have a smaller diameter than the distal receiving vessel (step-up phenomenon). Atherosclerotic changes/stenosis are usually present in the recipient vessels of postnatally acquired collaterals [21].

Clinical Presentation Patients may be asymptomatic if the vascular collaterals are adequate [21]. If collaterals are inadequate, they may present with sudden cardiac death, syncope, failure to thrive, and myocardial infarctions in pediatric age group and dyspnoea on exertion and angina in older patients [24].

Cardiac anomalies such as supra-valvular aortic stenosis, pulmonary stenosis, ventricular septal defect may be associated with COSA [24].

Treatment Treatment depends on patient symptoms.

- Asymptomatic patients can be treated conservatively.
- Coronary artery reconstruction is the treatment of choice in symptomatic patients.
- In the pediatric age group, coronary artery bypass grafting has been tried with saphenous venous graft and internal mammary artery with variable results.
- LMCA reconstruction using the baffle of the ascending aorta has also been successful [24, 25].

COSA should be differentiated from the single coronary artery where only single ostium is present and no discontinuity of branch vessels is seen [21]. Vieussens' arterial ring (VAR) can also be present with a single coronary artery (VAR type 3) [22].

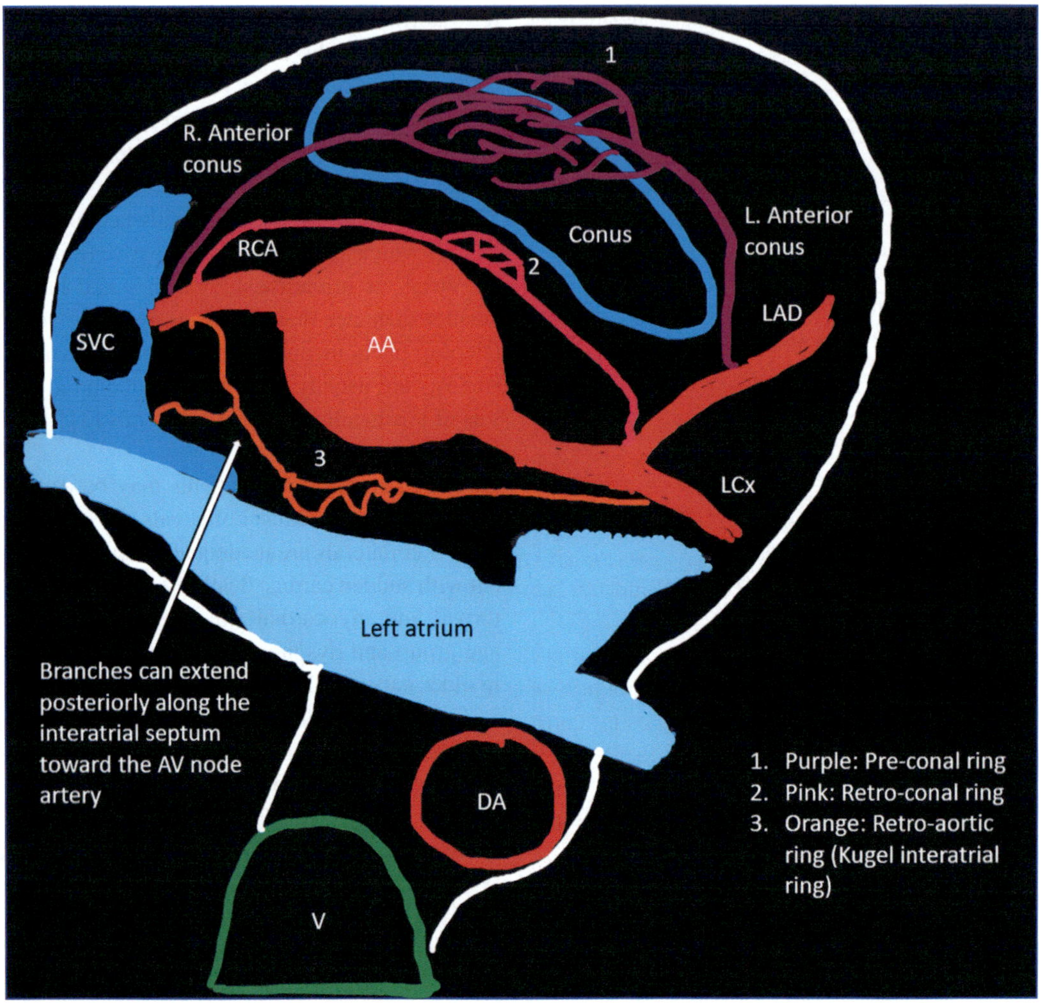

Fig. 9.9 Diagram shows major inter-coronary collateral pathways. AA-ascending aorta, DA-descending aorta, SVC-superior vena cava, V-vertebra

9.5.2 Anomalous Origin of the Coronary Artery from a Ventricle

Anomalous origin of the coronary artery from the right or left ventricle is a rare anomaly. Due to the retrograde flow of blood from the coronary artery into the same ventricle, the patients develop symptoms due to coronary steal phenomenon. Collaterals develop from the contralateral coronary artery. Blood flows during systole and diastole in right ventricular origin and during diastole in left ventricular origin. Coronary ostial stenosis may be present in the artery with left ventricular origin due to dysplastic aortic leaflet [21, 26, 27].

9.5.3 Anomalous Origin of the Coronary Artery from the Pulmonary Artery

Anomalous origin of the coronary artery from the pulmonary artery (ALCAPA) is one of the most serious congenital coronary artery anomalies. In the most common form of this disease, the LCA arises from the pulmonary artery and the RCA arises normally from the aorta (Bland–White–

Table 9.4 Major inter-coronary collateral pathways

Major collateral pathway	Named collaterals	Course	Connections
Pre-conal/ Vieussens' arterial ring	Right anterior conus artery from RCA or aorta (most constant) and Left anterior conus artery (from LMCA and LAD)	Pre-conal	Between RCA and proximal LAD/LMCA or aorta and LMCA/proximal LAD.
Retro-conal ring	-	Collateral course in inter-arterial space between the main pulmonary artery and the ascending aorta.	Between RCA and left coronary arteries
Retro-aortic collateral	Kugel anastomotic artery (arises from distal branches of atrio-ventricular nodal artery)	Interatrial septum	Between proximal LCX and/or RCA, and the distal coronaries.

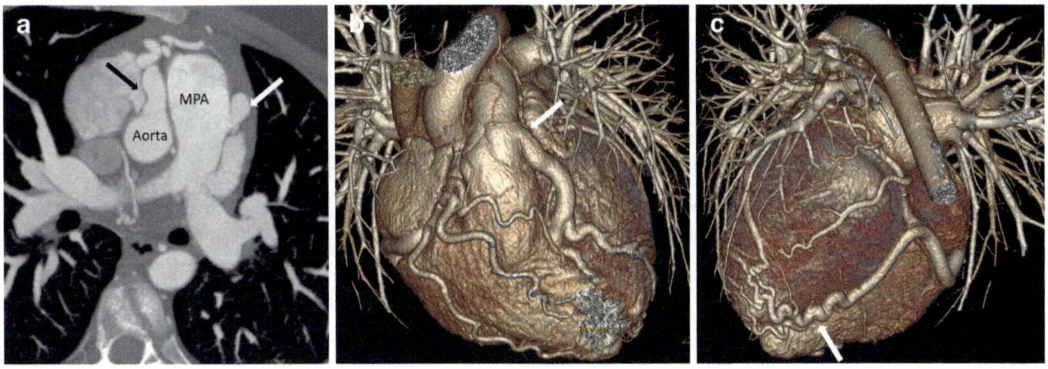

Fig. 9.10 A 10-year-old male child with dyspnea on exertion for 5 years. (**a**) Axial CT image shows the origin of LMCA from MPA (white arrow). RCA is dilated and tortuous and arises from the aorta (black arrow). (**b**) VRT image shows dilated LMCA arising from MPA (white arrow). (**c**) VRT image shows multiple dilated collaterals from PDA draining into diagonal branches of LAD (white arrow)

Garland syndrome) (Fig. 9.10) [1]. ALCAPA is of two types—Infant and Adult type. Differentiating features of the two types are illustrated in Table 9.5 [28].

Clinical Presentation During the neonatal period, as the pulmonary artery pressure is equivalent to the pressure in ascending aorta, no significant symptoms are present. As pulmonary vascular resistance falls, blood flows from the aorta to the RCA, RCA to LMCA (through inter-coronary collaterals), and in a retrograde fashion into the pulmonary artery. This results in "steal" of blood flow from the myocardium. Patients usually present with symptoms of myocardial ischemia or with left ventricular volume overload due to left-to-right shunting in the first few weeks of life with worsening of symptoms with a fall in pulmonary vascular resistance. Massive cardiomegaly is usually present [20]. Pathophysiologic changes in infant and adult type of ALCAPA are summarized in Table 9.6 [28].

Imaging features of ALCAPA on CT angiography (CTA) and magnetic resonance imaging (MRI) are summarized in Table 9.7 [28–34].

Treatment Treatment of ALCAPA consists of the reconstruction of dual coronary anatomy. Once the diagnosis of ALCAPA is made, surgery must be done as soon as possible. Following surgical techniques are devised:

Table 9.5 Differentiating features of Infant and adult type ALCAPA

Features	Infant type	Adult type
Onset of symptoms	8 weeks after birth	Asymptomatic/later in life
Clinical symptom	Failure to thrive, sweating, dyspnoea, pallor	Asymptomatic
Outcome	Congestive heart failure, mitral insufficiency secondary to myocardial infarction, 90% death in first year	Chronic myocardial infarctions, ventricular dysrhythmias, mitral insufficiency, sudden cardiac death
ECG	Ischemic changes	Left ventricular hypertrophy/ ischemic changes
RCA	Mildly dilated	Markedly dilated
Collaterals	Insufficient	Multiple collaterals present

- Coronary artery reimplantation into the aorta.
- Takeuchi repair: Flap of anterior wall of the main pulmonary artery is created followed by the creation of an intrapulmonary conduit from the left coronary ostia to the aorta.
- Ligation of the left coronary artery from the pulmonary artery, along with coronary artery bypass grafting using internal mammary artery or the saphenous vein. This procedure is preferred in adult type ALCAPA [1, 35, 36].
- In patients with severe post-capillary pulmonary hypertension, transcatheter percutaneous embolization of the LMCA at its origin from the main pulmonary artery can be done followed by anti-congestive medications. Coronary artery bypass is done after the resolution of post-capillary pulmonary hypertension [37].

Table 9.6 Flowchart shows document. pathophysiology of ALCAPA

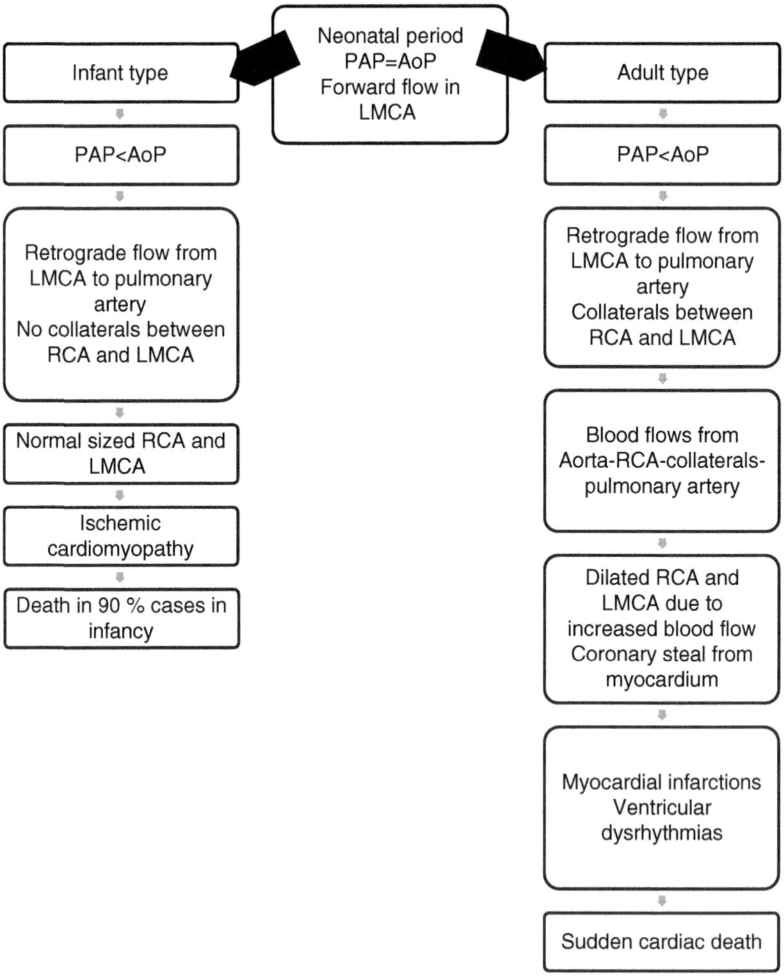

AoP= Ascending aorta pressure, PAP= Main Pulmonary artery pressure

Table 9.7 Table Imaging features of ALCAPA on CTA and MRI

CTA	• Visualisation of origin of LMCA from main pulmonary artery • Dilated and tortuous RCA • Collaterals from RCA to left coronary artery • Left ventricular hypertrophy and dilatation • Dilated bronchial arteries supplying left coronary artery.
MRI	• All anatomical findings that are appreciated on CTA • Lack of early enhancement of ALCAPA followed by late enhancement due to retrograde flow in ALCAPA from RCA (Myocardial steal) • Wall motion abnormalies • Myocardial scar detection and quantification • Mitral valve insufficiency and prolapse secondary to myxomatous degeneration. • Post operative perfusion defects on adenosine stress perfusion imaging seen in left coronary artery compromise. • Post op reversible perfusion defects in the presence of normal coronary artery may represent microvascular disease/consequence of collateral circulation prior to surgery.

9.5.4 Inter-arterial/Malignant course

Anomalous course of a coronary artery may be present when a coronary artery arises from the contralateral coronary artery or coronary cusp (either a left artery arising from a right artery or cusp or a right artery arising from a left artery or cusp) (Figs. 9.11 and 9.12). These courses are stated in Table 9.8 and described later in the text [20]. Anomalous RCA arising from the left sinus of Valsalva most commonly follows an inter-arterial course [38].

Clinical Presentation Patients with an inter-arterial course of the coronary artery may be asymptomatic, may present with atypical chest pain, dyspnoea on exertion, ventricular arrhythmias, or sudden cardiac death (SCD). SCD risk is higher when the left coronary arteries are involved. Few morphological features increase the risk of SCD (Fig. 9.13). These are (a) slit-like coronary ostium, (b) an acute angle between the anomalous coronary artery and the aorta (sharp angle of takeoff), and (c) an intramural aortic segment (proximal arterial segment courses within the tunica media of aortic wall). Here, the proximal artery is narrow in caliber with an elliptical shape [20, 39].

During physical exercise, there is kinking of the acute takeoff angled anomalous vessel, lateral compression of the intramural segment by the aorta, intermittent closure of the slit-like orifice, and compression of the inter-arterial segment by the aorta and pulmonary artery. The most significant life-threatening feature is the intramural course and its length [39–42].

Treatment Surgical repair may be required in patients with an inter-arterial course with otherwise unexplained ischemia. Following surgical techniques can be employed [20, 39, 43]:

- Unroofing of the coronary artery with the creation of neo ostium can be done in the intramural variant.
- Reimplantation of an aberrant coronary artery with the negligible intramural course.
- Pulmonary artery translocation-done in the artery with an inter-arterial course with no intramural segment and the single coronary artery.
- Percutaneous coronary intervention.

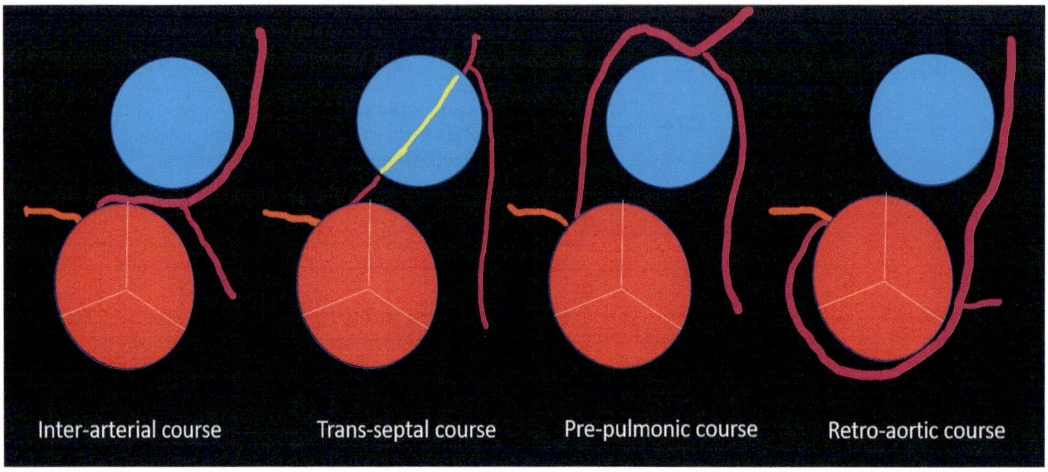

Fig. 9.11 Diagram shows the anomalous course of LMCA

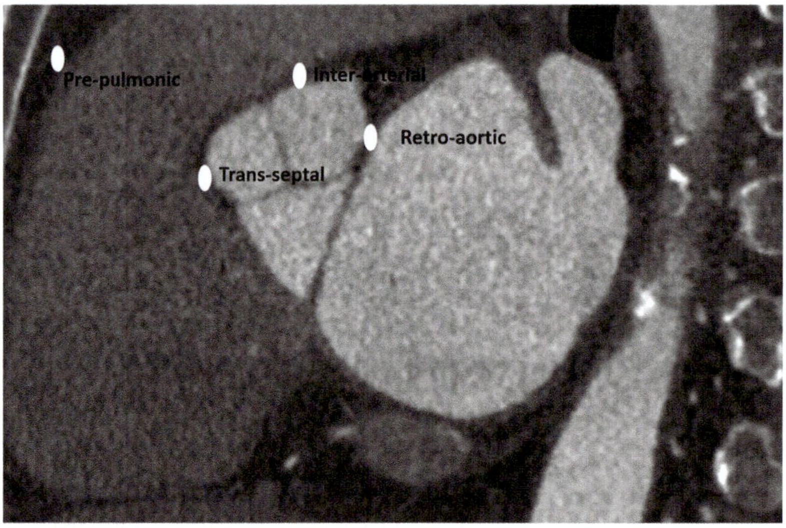

Fig. 9.12 CTA MIP thin image shows various anomalous courses of coronary artery

Table 9.8 Anomalous course of coronary arteries

Anomalous course	Description
Pre-pulmonic	Anterior to the right ventricular outflow tract
Inter-arterial	Between the aorta and pulmonary artery
Trans-septal	More caudal in position to inter-arterial course
Retro-aortic	Posterior to aorta

9.5.5 Coronary Arterial Fistula

A coronary artery fistula (CAF) is a rare coronary anomaly accounting for 0.3% of congenital heart diseases. Normally a coronary artery terminates in the capillary bed of myometrium. In CAF, an abnormal vascular communication exists between the coronary arteries with cardiac chambers or any of the systemic or pulmonary vessels, without an intervening capillary net-

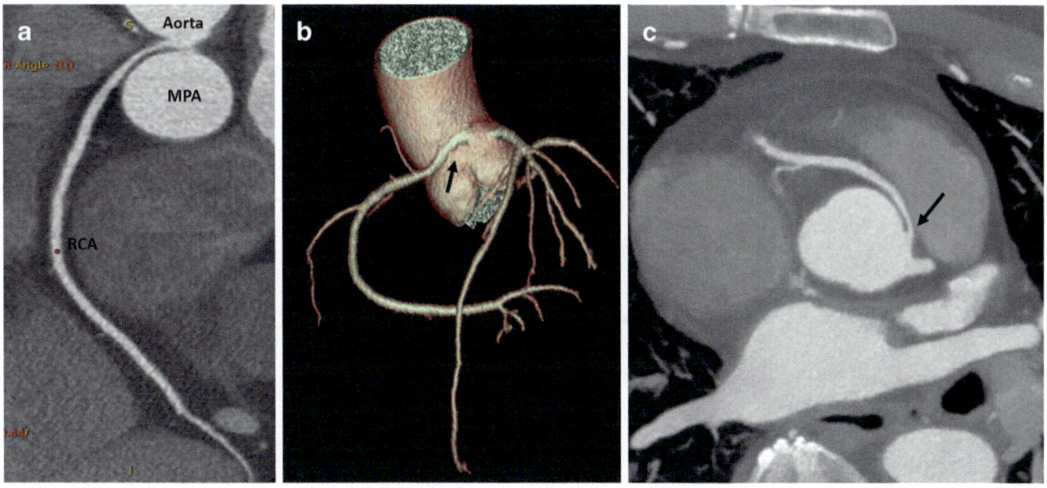

Fig. 9.13 A 67-year-old male patient with dyspnoea on exertion for 5 months. CTA shows inter-arterial course of RCA (**a**). RCA is arising from the left coronary cusp (black arrow) (**b, c**) and has slit-like ostia with acute angulation (**c**) (black arrow)

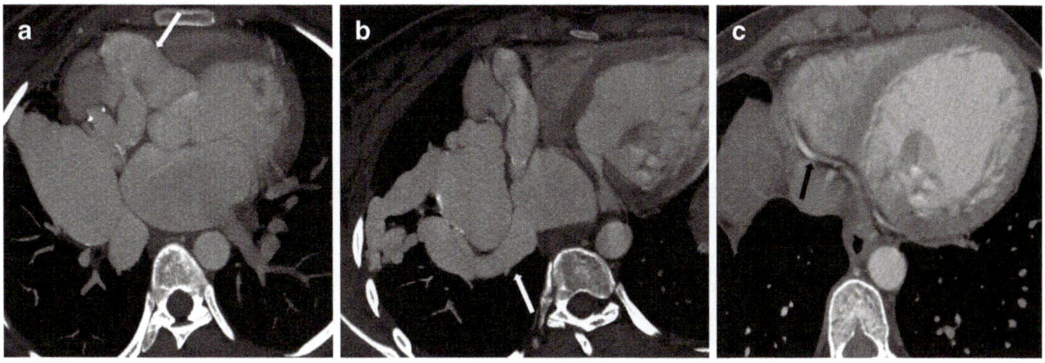

Fig. 9.14 A 22-year-old female patient with dyspnea on exertion. CTA shows a fistulous tract arising from the RCA (white arrow, **a**) and draining in the right superior pulmonary vein (white arrow, **b**). Distal RCA (black arrow, **c**) is normal in caliber

work (Figs. 9.14 and 9.15) [38, 44]. Classification of CAF is described in Table 9.9 [44–46].

Coronary cameral fistula is the most common type of CAF where coronary artery terminates in one of the cardiac chambers, followed by coronary artery to pulmonary artery fistulas (15%–30% of all CAFs) and coronary artery to coronary sinus fistulas (7% of all CAFs) [44, 47–49]. The right coronary artery (RCA) is the most common origin site of CAFs, accounting for 50%–55% of cases followed by LAD [44, 50]. The most common drainage site is the right ventricle (45% of cases), followed by the right atrium (25%) and the pulmonary artery (15%) [44].

A coronary cameral fistula must be differentiated from an aorto-atrial tunnel (described later in the text).

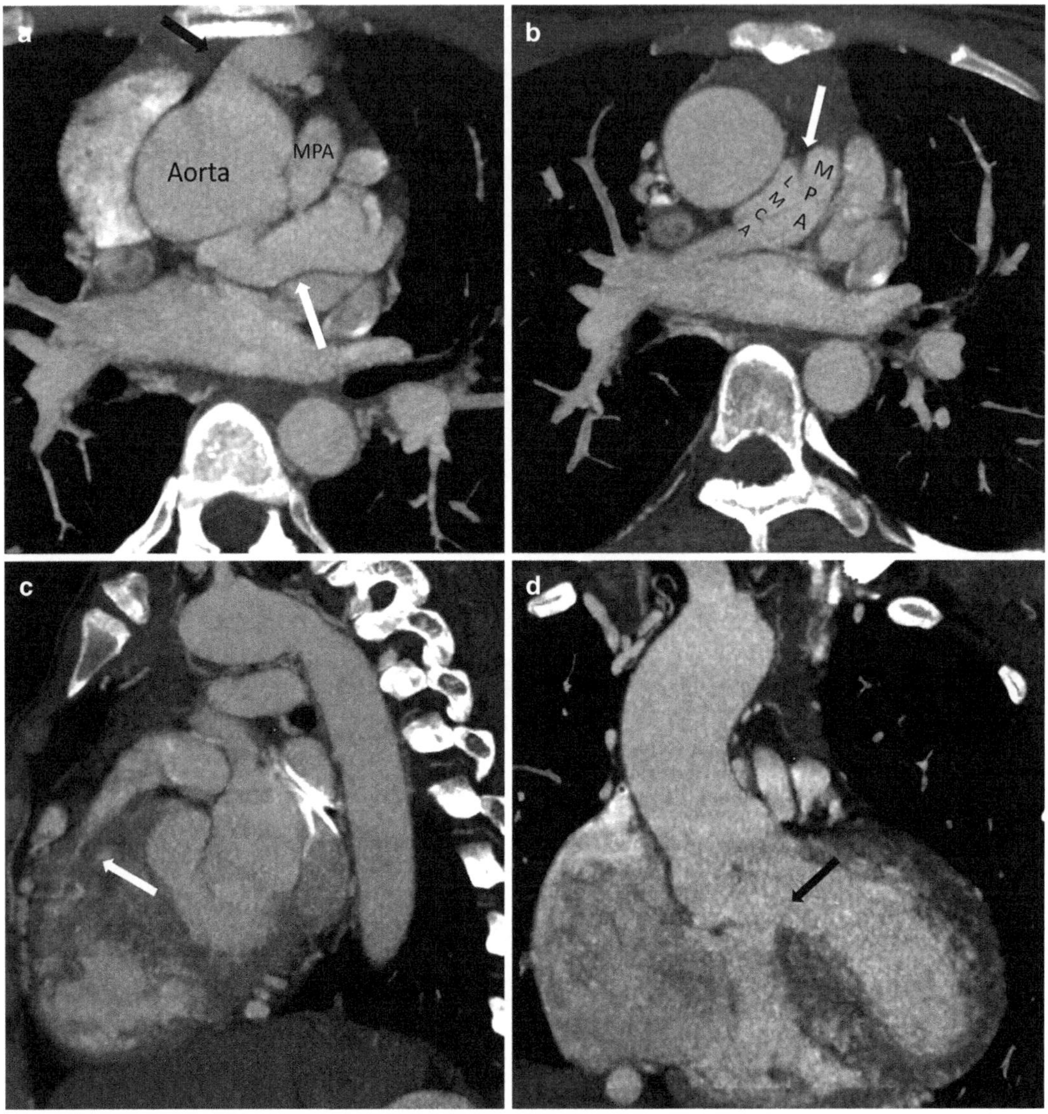

Fig. 9.15 A 26-year-old female patient with tetralogy of Fallot. (**a**) Axial MIP thin image shows dilated and tortuous LMCA (white arrow). RCA is also dilated (black arrow). (**b**) Communication of LMCA with MPA is seen (white arrow). (**c**) MIP sagittal image shows Infundibular pulmonary stenosis and (**d**) subaortic ventricular septal defect (VSD) with overriding aorta

Clinical Presentation CAFs can affect hemodynamic parameters and may lead to various complications, including myocardial ischemia (due to steal phenomenon), heart failure, arrhythmia, and infective endocarditis in adults [44].

As the pathophysiology of a CAF depends on the resistance of the fistulous connection and the site of fistula termination, accurate imaging assessment of the origin and drainage site of CAFs is crucial. A shunt to low-pressure structures may dilate the coronary arteries leading to the formation of an aneurysm [44].

A shunt leading into a right cardiac chamber result in an increased volume of the right heart with pulmonary arterial hypertension. Shunt leading to the left cardiac chamber results in volume overload of the left heart and with left ventricular hypertrophy. In left-to-left shunt,

Table 9.9 Classification of coronary arterial fistulas

Classification	Description
Etiology	• Congenital • Acquired: (i) Iatrogenic: secondary to by PCI, CABG, cardiac surgeries, permanent pacemaker insertion, myocardial biopsy (ii) Disease-related: secondary to Kawasaki disease, acute myocardial infarction, cardiomyopathy, tumor (iii) Trauma-related (iv) Radiation injury
Origin	RCA/LCA/both/anomalous coronary artery
Segment of CAF origin	• Sakakibara type A: Proximal coronary segment is dilated till the origin of fistula; distal artery is normal. • Sakakibara type B: CAF arises from distal native vessel; entire coronary artery is dilated.
Drainage site	• Coronary cameral fistula: CAF drains in cardiac chamber • Coronary arteriovenous fistula: CAF drains in pulmonary artery, coronary sinus, vena cavas, bronchial vessels, or other extracardiac veins.
Mode of termination	• Macro-fistula: Fistulous vessel is seen on angiography • Micro-fistula: Contrast blush visible instead of discrete fistulous vessel.
Number of fistulous tracts	Single or multiple
Complexity	Simple CAF: single origin and single drainage fistula present. Complex CAF: involves entangled blood vessels with multiple fistulous structures.
Presence of associated anomaly	Isolated CAF: no accompanying anomaly CAF associated with other cardiac anomalies such as ventricular septal defect, patent ductus arteriosus, tetralogy of Fallot, valvular disease, etc.

runoff from the aorta mimics aortic regurgitation [46].

Compared with other imaging modalities, CT angiography is useful for the evaluation of CAFs because of its shorter acquisition time and higher temporal and spatial resolutions. Post-procedure complications can be identified by comparing pre- and postprocedural images. Table 9.10 summarizes the utility of CTA [44].

Treatment Treatment depends on patient symptoms:

- Asymptomatic patients may not require any intervention.
- Treatment is however required for large hemodynamically significant fistulas. Treatment options include surgical ligation and percutaneous transcatheter closure. Table 9.11 summarizes treatment preferences [44].

Table 9.10 Utility of CTA in coronary arterial fistulas

Pre-operative assessment	Post-procedure evaluation
Number and location of fistula origins	Post-operative residual leakage or recanalization
Number and location of fistula drainage sites	Persistent dilatation of coronary artery or ostium/aneurysm formation
Course and size of fistulous tract	Formation of thrombus
Fistula complexity: angulations, tortuosity, associated connection with other structures	Migration of coil or device
Other associated anomalies	Myocardial ischemia, infarction
	Complication due to transcatheter procedures
	Coronary artery spasm, dissection, or perforation

Table 9.11 Treatment options in coronary arterial fistulas

Indications of surgical treatment	Indications of percutaneous transcatheter closure
• Large symptomatic fistula • Presence of multiple communications and drainage sites • Tortuous and aneurysmal fistulous arteries • Requirement for simultaneous distal bypass • Large vascular branches that can be accidentally embolized	• Proximal origin of fistula • Single drainage site • Non-tortuous vessel • Distal portion of fistula easily accessible with the closure device • Termination of fistula away from normal coronary arteries • In patients with high risk of perioperative complications • Absence of associated cardiac disorders

9.5.6 Aorto-Atrial Tunnel

Aorto-atrial tunnel is a rare entity. Aorto-right atrial (ARAT) and aorto-left atrial tunnels (ALAT) have been described wherein an extra-cardiac vascular tubular connection exists between one of the aortic sinuses and the right atrium or left atrium, respectively [51–53].

Various theories have been proposed to explain the embryological basis of the anomaly. The most accepted theory is the congenital weakness in the media layer of the aortic wall with tunnel formation, which gradually enlarges over time due to intra-aortic high pressure; and ultimately ruptures into the low-pressure atrial chamber. ARAT arising from the right sinus courses anterior and that arising from the left sinus courses posterior to the aorta based on anatomical proximity to the right atrium (Fig. 9.16). Aneurysmal dilatation of the sinonodal artery is another possible explanation for the development of the tunnel [51]. ARAT results in left-to-right shunt at the level of the right atrium [52].

An aorto-atrial tunnel does not follow the course of a normal coronary artery and does not give myocardial branches. Both coronary arteries are seen arising separately away from the tunnel or from the tunnel itself which differentiates it from coronary cameral fistulas. Complete visual-

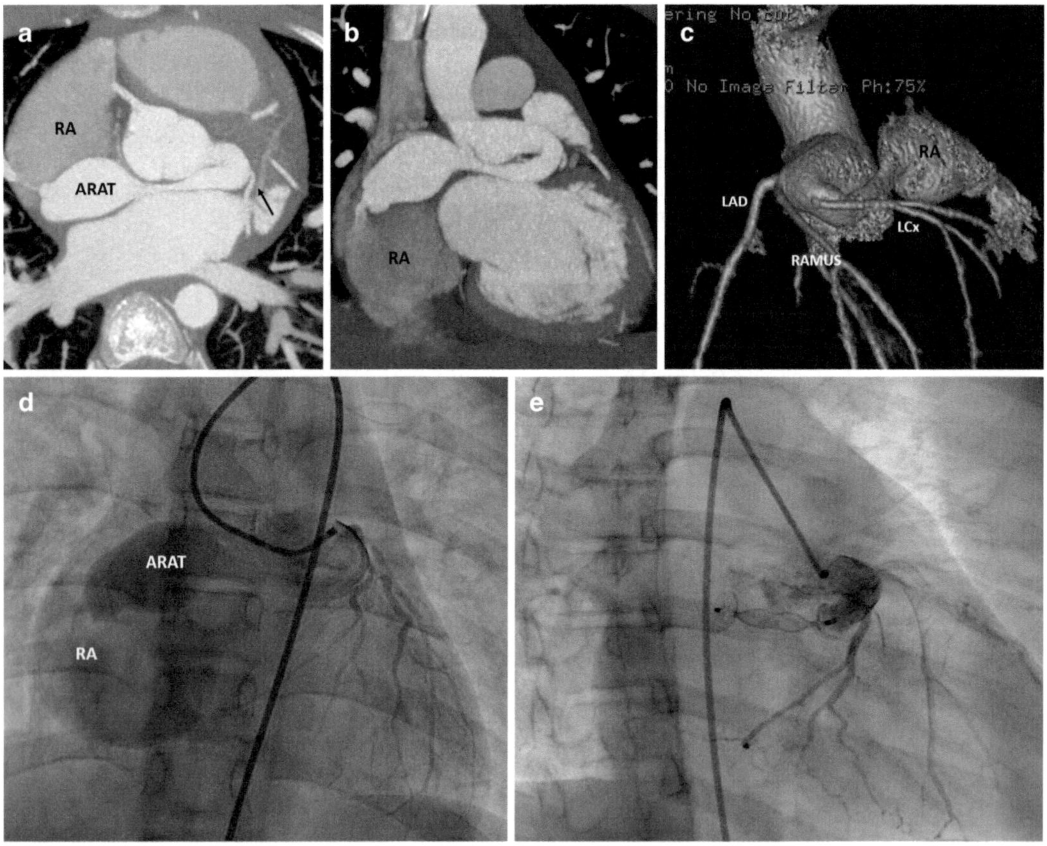

Fig. 9.16 A 13-year-old female child with recurrent respiratory tract infection, exertional palpitation, and dyspnoea on exertion for 4 years. CTA MIP thin images show vascular tunnel (ARAT) arising from left sinus coursing posterior to the aorta and draining in the right atrium (RA) (**a**, **b**). VRT image shows LAD and LCx arising separately from the tunnel (**c**). Catheter angiography shows the filling of RA through ARAT (**d**). Transcatheter vascular plug closure of the ARAT done (**e**)

ization of the extracardiac tunnel draining into the right atrium differentiates it from the ruptured sinus of Valsalva aneurysms [51, 54].

Clinical Presentation Patients with ARAT may be asymptomatic or can have dyspnoea on exertion, palpitations, or recurrent respiratory tract infections [51]. Patients with ALAT have variable presentation ranging from being asymptomatic to having a congestive cardiac failure [53]. If left untreated, complications are likely to occur. These include wall calcifications, aneurysmal dilatation, spontaneous rupture, ventricular overload, aortic valve insufficiency, infective endocarditis, congestive cardiac failure, and increase surgical mortality [52].

Treatment Treatment options include:

- Percutaneous transcatheter closure, coil embolization.
- Ligation under controlled hypotension or repair under cardiopulmonary bypass.
- Reimplantation of the coronary artery with a part of the tunnel into the respective sinus of Valsalva if the coronary artery is arising from the tunnel [51, 52].

9.6 Hemodynamically Less Significant Anomalies

9.6.1 Duplication

Duplication of the LAD and RCA arteries have been reported with LAD duplication being more common than RCA. Duplication of the LAD artery consists of a short LAD artery, which courses and terminates in the anterior interventricular sulcus without reaching the apex, and a long LAD artery, which originates from either the LAD artery proper or the RCA, then enters the distal anterior interventricular sulcus and courses to the apex [1, 55]. Based on these, the duplication of LAD can be divided into four angiographic subtypes. (Table 9.12) [38, 56].

Table 9.12 LAD duplication subtypes

Types	Description
Type I	Short LAD runs in the anterior interventricular septum (AIVS) and gives off all major proximal septal perforators. Long LAD runs in the AIVS, descends on the left ventricular side of the AIVS, and re-enters the distal AIVS to reach the apex.
Type II	Short LAD runs in AIVS and gives off all major proximal septal perforators. Long LAD descends over the right ventricular side before re-entering the AIVS.
Type III	Short LAD runs in AIVS and gives off all major proximal septal perforators. Long LAD has an intramyocardial course in the ventricular septum.
Type IV	Short LAD originates from LMCA and gives off major septal perforators and diagonal branches. Long LAD arises from the RCA.

Duplicate LAD may have a pre-pulmonic, trans-septal, or inter-arterial course [20]. Whenever duplication of LAD is present in a patient planned for coronary artery bypass graft surgery, the cardiac surgeon should be forewarned regarding its presence, to avoid incorrect placement of arteriotomy and achieve appropriate myocardial perfusion [1, 55].

A diagonal branch running parallel to the LAD artery may mimic duplicate LAD. Such a diagonal branch takes over the course of the distal LAD artery similar to the long LAD but without re-entering into the anterior interventricular sulcus [1].

Clinical Presentation It is a benign anomaly. Patients are usually asymptomatic unless inter-arterial course with high-risk factors is present.

Treatment As the anomaly is hemodynamically insignificant, no treatment is required.

9.6.2 High Origin/High "Takeoff"

A high coronary artery origin is defined as the origin of a coronary artery more than 1 cm above the sino-tubular junction (Fig. 9.17) [20, 57].

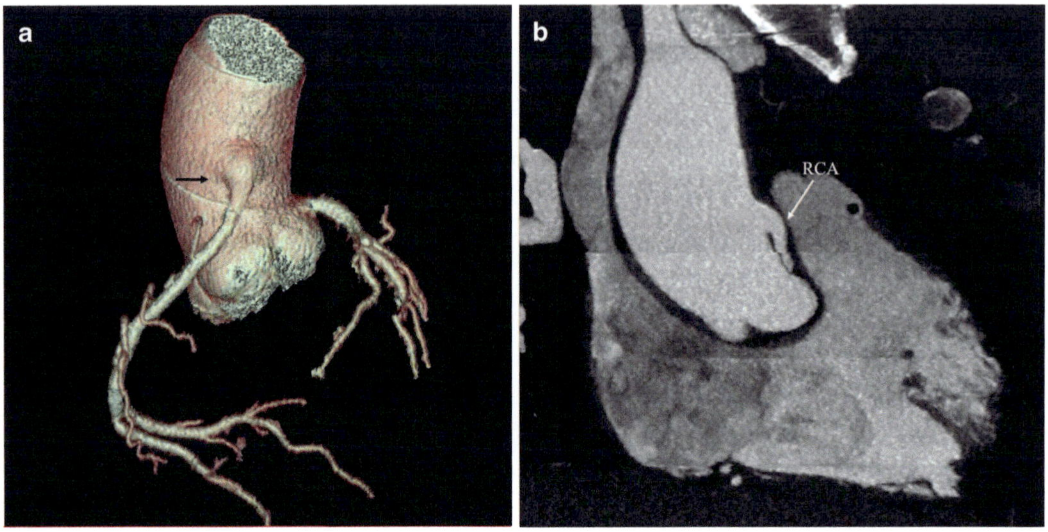

Fig. 9.17 A 54-year-old male patient with coronary artery disease. Prospective ECG-gated-CTA showed incidental finding of high takeoff (arrow) of RCA from ascending aorta (**a**, **b**)

Clinical presentation: Though this anomaly has no hemodynamic significance, it is clinically important due to the following reasons [20, 57, 58]:

- Selective catheterization of a coronary artery with a high origin may be difficult.
- The presence of High takeoff of coronary artery, if unrecognised, may be injured during aortotomy for aortic valve surgery or ascending aortic replacement.
- Cross-clamping of the aorta below a high-origin coronary artery may result in unsuccessful induction of cardioplegia.

High origin of RCA has been more commonly reported than LMCA and is frequently associated with the presence of aortic bicuspid valve [20, 58]. Higher position of a coronary ostium may be associated with a higher risk of coronary hypoperfusion as maximum coronary diastolic perfusion is facilitated by the sinuses of Valsalva [59].

Treatment This most often does not require treatment unless clinically associated with hypoperfusion.

9.6.3 Single Coronary Artery (SCA)

It is a rare anomaly seen in 0.0024%– 0.044% of the population [60]. In this anomaly, a single coronary artery arises with a single ostium from the aortic trunk without discontinuity of branch vessels (Fig. 9.18) [1, 21]. It may either divide into two branches and have a distribution similar to RCA and LCA or have a distribution other than that of the normal coronary arterial tree [1, 61].

Lipton et al. classified isolated single coronary artery based on site of origin and anatomical distribution on angiography (Table 9.13) [60, 62, 63]. This classification was modified by Yamanaka and Hobbs (Table 9.14) [38].

Based on the course of SCA from one side of the heart to the other, Lipton groups II and III have been further designated with A, B, P, S, or C suffixes (Table 9.14) [38, 60].

Clinical Presentation Patients with this anomaly are at an increased risk of sudden cardiac death if a major coronary branch has an interarterial course. Type R-II-B SCA has been reported to cause sudden death during exercise. The main pathophysiological cause behind this

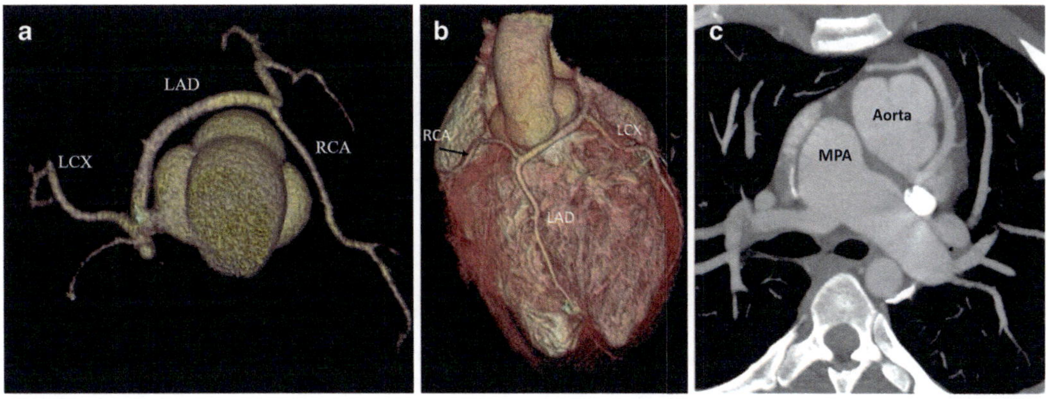

Fig. 9.18 A 25-year-old male patient with double outlet right ventricle and L-Transposition of great arteries. (**a**, **b**) CTA VR images show a single coronary artery arising from a single ostium on the left side, RCA is arising from LAD. (**c**) Axial CT MIP image shows that aorta is to the left and anterior to the main pulmonary artery (MPA)

Table 9.13 Lipton classification of single coronary artery

Lipton classification	R—Solitary vessel originates from the right sinus	L—Solitary vessel originates from the left sinus
I	A solitary vessel follows the course of either a normal right or left coronary artery. R-I: Large RCA gives rise to LAD artery. L-I: Dominant LCx gives off PDA, right atrial and ventricular branches.	
II	Solitary coronary artery arises from right or left coronary sinus and gives off a large trunk that crosses at the base of the heart to reach the site of normal contralateral artery	
III	SCA arises from the right sinus of Valsalva. LCx and LAD arise separately from the common trunk	

is probable kinking and compression of the LMCA (arising from RCA) due to increase angulation caused by aortic dilatation during exercise [60].

Proximal stenosis of a single coronary artery may result in extensive myocardial infarctions in the absence of an ability to develop collateral channels [1].

Treatment Treatment depends on patient symptoms:

Table 9.14 Suffixes of Lipton group II and III based on the course of SCA

Suffixes	Description of SCA course
A	Anterior to the great vessels
P	Posterior to the great vessels
B	Between the aorta and the pulmonary artery
S	Part of courses through the interventricular septum
C	Combination of different routes

- No treatment is required in asymptomatic patients.
- Pulmonary artery translocation may be performed in patients with an inter-arterial course of the isolated single coronary artery without intramural segment. In this procedure, the pulmonary artery confluence is repositioned away from the coronary artery either laterally or anteriorly to decompress it [39, 43].

9.6.4 Pre-pulmonic Course

A pre-pulmonic course refers to the anomalous course of a major coronary artery anterior to the pulmonary outflow tract or pulmonary artery. The most common artery with a pre-pulmonic course is LMCA. RCA with anomalous origin from LMCA or LAD may take a pre-pulmonic course [20].

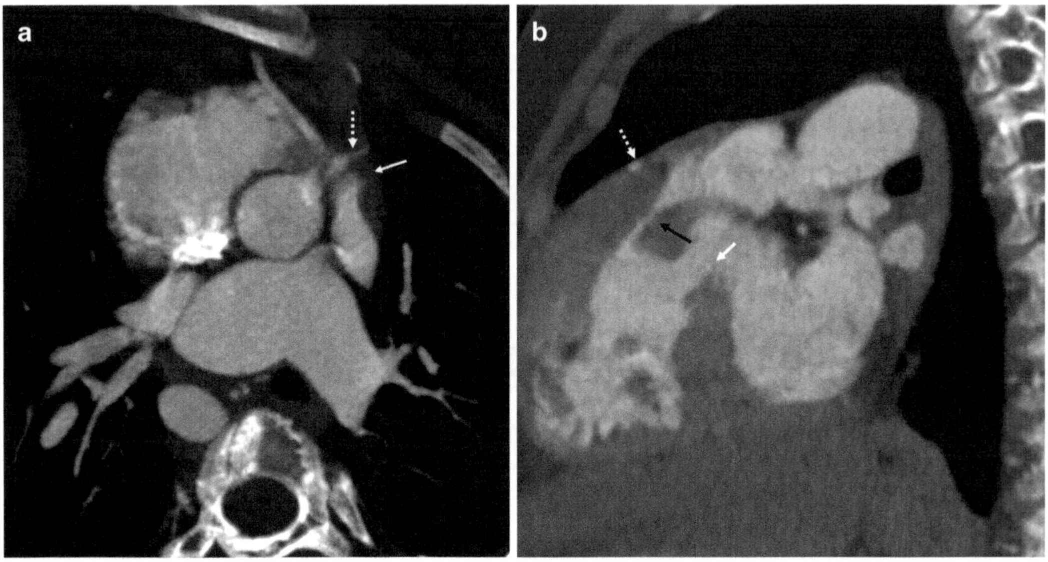

Fig. 9.19 A 10-year-old male patient with tetralogy of Fallot. (**a**) Axial CT MIP images show LAD (dotted arrow) arising from the right coronary sinus and crossing right ventricle outflow tract (RVOT—solid white arrow). (**b**) Sagittal CT MIP images show pre-pulmonic course of LAD (dotted arrow), infundibular pulmonary stenosis (black arrow) and subaortic VSD (solid white arrow)

Clinical Presentation Usually, patients are asymptomatic. However, angina has been reported in some patients [20, 64]. In patients with tetralogy of Fallot, the pre-pulmonic course of a coronary artery can complicate the surgical approach to correction of right ventricular outflow tract stenosis (Figs. 9.11, 9.12 and 9.19) [20, 65].

Treatment Usually, the anomaly is hemodynamically insignificant and no treatment is required. Medical management for vasospasm is done in patients with angina [64].

9.6.5 Trans-Septal Course

Sometimes a coronary artery with anomalous origin from the contralateral artery or cusp passes through the septal myocardium, below the level of the pulmonary valve (Figs. 9.11 and 9.12). Such an anomalous course has been described as a trans-septal course. The trans-septal artery courses downwards below the crista supraventricularis (hammock sign at conventional angiography), is surrounded by the septal myocardium and does not have a slit-like orifice differentiating it from the inter-arterial course [1, 20, 38, 66]. The most common arteries with trans-septal courses are LAD or LMCA [20].

Clinical Presentation It is essentially a benign anomaly. However, cases with chest pain, syncope, arrhythmias, and myocardial ischemia have been reported [63, 67].

Treatment Treatment depends on the clinical presentation of the patient:

- No treatment is required in asymptomatic patients.
- Coronary artery bypass grafting has been successfully tried in symptomatic patients with SCA with the trans-septal course [67].

9.6.6 Retro-Aortic Course

A retro-aortic artery usually arises from the RCA or right coronary cusp and supplies the distribution of the LMCA or LCX artery. It courses in the space between the posterior aorta (the noncoronary cusp) and the interatrial septum (Fig. 9.20) [20, 68].

Clinical Presentation Patients are asymptomatic. As a retro-aortic coronary artery partially encircles the aortic valve, it may get injured during aortic valve surgeries [20, 69].

Treatment As the anomaly is hemodynamically insignificant, no treatment is required.

9.6.7 Acute Takeoff of LCx

An angle of ≤45° between LMCA and LCx as observed on left anterior oblique/caudal and/or right anterior oblique/caudal conventional angiography projections is termed as an acute takeoff of LCx. It occurs due to the distal origin of LCx from LMCA followed by a backward proximal course. The origin and length of LMCA should be described in the report. This anatomical variant may pose difficulties in selective coronary catheterization of LCx [59, 70].

9.6.8 Shepherd's Crook RCA

In this variant, the RCA takes a tortuous and high course, usually immediately after it originates from the aorta. As it is difficult to pass a catheter beyond the kink of the shepherd's crook, percutaneous transcatheter coronary angioplasty (PTCA) is difficult in shepherd's crook RCA with lower primary success rates. Hence, in a patient with

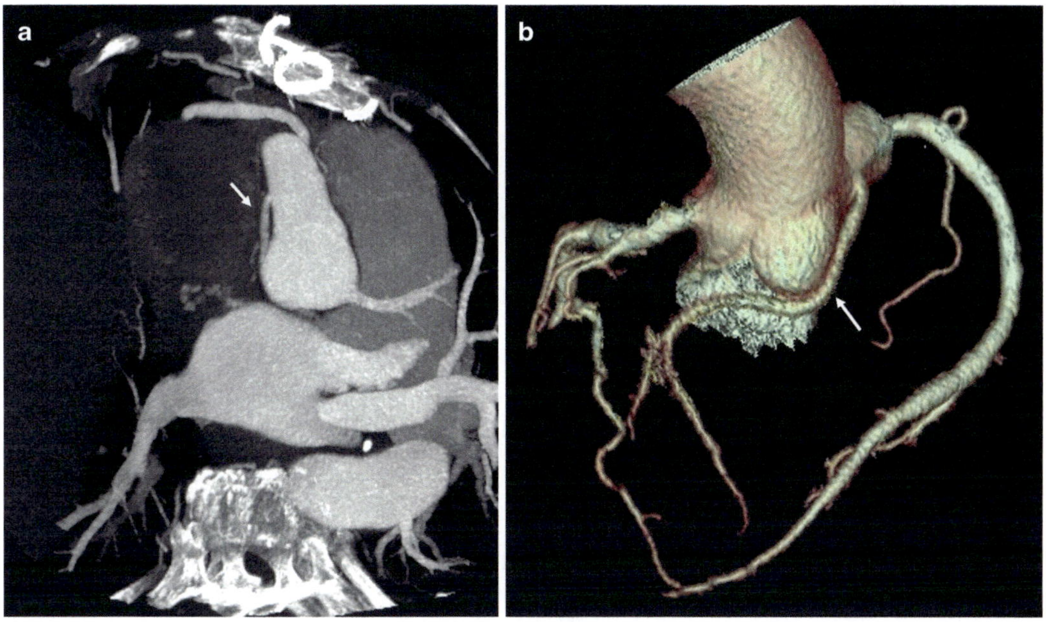

Fig. 9.20 A 62-year-old female patient with right sinus of Valsalva aneurysm presenting with atypical chest pain. (**a**) Axial CT image shows an incidental finding of LCx arising from the right sinus of Valsalva (arrow). (**b**) CT VR image shows retro-aortic course of LCx (arrow)

multiple vessel disease, alternative surgical options can be tried. The acuteness of the angle at the kink and the distance from the RCA origin should be described in the report [20, 71, 72].

9.6.9 Coronary Arcade

Coronary arcade refers to communication between the RCA and the LCA identified angiographically in the absence of coronary artery stenosis. A prominent straight vascular connection is seen between two unobstructed major arteries, at or near the level of the crux, in contrast to the tortuous collateral vessels that are seen between the patent vessel and the obstructed vessel in case of coronary artery stenosis [1, 73, 74].

9.6.10 Extracardiac Termination

Vascular connections between the coronary and extracardiac vessels such as the bronchial, internal mammary, superior and inferior diaphragmatic, intercostal, pericardial, anterior mediastinal, and esophageal arteries may exist, which become hemodynamically significant only when the two arterial systems have pressure gradient. In coronary artery disease, these vascular connections allow blood to flow from bronchial arteries to the coronary arteries [1].

9.7 Conclusion

While reporting a coronary CT, a specific constellation of potential implications should be kept in mind for each specific variant. Thorough familiarity with the anatomic pattern, variants, anomalies and clinical significance of each anomalous condition are necessary to categorize each anomaly, understand its importance, and forewarn the cardiologist and cardiac surgeons regarding the same.

References

1. Kim SY, Seo JB, Do KH, et al. Coronary artery anomalies: classification and ECG-gated multidetector row CT findings with angiographic correlation. Radiographics. 2006;26(2):317–34. https://doi.org/10.1148/rg.262055068.
2. Angelini P. Normal and anomalous coronary arteries: definitions and classification. Am Heart J. 1989;117(2):418–34. https://doi.org/10.1016/0002-8703(89)90789-8.
3. Young PM, Gerber TC, Williamson EE, Julsrud PR, Herfkens RJ. Cardiac imaging: part 2, normal, variant, and anomalous configurations of the coronary vasculature. AJR Am J Roentgenol. 2011;197(4):816–26. https://doi.org/10.2214/AJR.10.7249.
4. Raff GL, Abidov A, Achenbach S, et al. SCCT guidelines for the interpretation and reporting of coronary computed tomographic angiography. J Cardiovasc Comput Tomogr. 2009;3(2):122–36. https://doi.org/10.1016/j.jcct.2009.01.001.
5. Austen WG, Edwards JE, Frye RL, et al. A reporting system on patients evaluated for coronary artery disease. Report of the ad hoc committee for grading of coronary artery disease, council on cardiovascular surgery, American Heart Association. Circulation. 1975;51(4 Suppl):5–40. https://doi.org/10.1161/01.cir.51.4.5.
6. Lee MS, Chen CH. Myocardial bridging: an up-to-date review. J Invasive Cardiol. 2015;27(11):521–8.
7. Polacek P, Kralove H. Relation of myocardial bridges and loops on the coronary arteries to coronary occulsions. Am Heart J. 1961;61:44–52. https://doi.org/10.1016/0002-8703(61)90515-4.
8. Angelini P, Trivellato M, Donis J, Leachman RD. Myocardial bridges: a review. Prog Cardiovasc Dis. 1983;26(1):75–88. https://doi.org/10.1016/0033-0620(83)90019-1.
9. Ferreira AG Jr, Trotter SE, König B Jr, Décourt LV, Fox K, Olsen EG. Myocardial bridges: morphological and functional aspects. Br Heart J. 1991;66(5):364–7. https://doi.org/10.1136/hrt.66.5.364.
10. Tarantini G, Migliore F, Cademartiri F, Fraccaro C, Iliceto S. Left anterior descending artery myocardial bridging: a clinical approach. J Am Coll Cardiol. 2016;68(25):2887–99. https://doi.org/10.1016/j.jacc.2016.09.973.
11. Bourassa MG, Butnaru A, Lespérance J, Tardif JC. Symptomatic myocardial bridges: overview of ischemic mechanisms and current diagnostic and treatment strategies. J Am Coll Cardiol. 2003;41(3):351–9. https://doi.org/10.1016/s0735-1097(02)02768-7.
12. Erbel R, Rupprecht H-J, Junbo GE, Gerber T, Görge G, Meyer J. Coronary artery shape and

flow changes induced by myocardial bridging. Echocardiography. 1993;10:71–7. https://doi.org/10.1111/j.1540-8175.1993.tb00013.x.

13. Ge J, Erbel R, Rupprecht HJ, et al. Comparison of intravascular ultrasound and angiography in the assessment of myocardial bridging. Circulation. 1994;89(4):1725–32. https://doi.org/10.1161/01.cir.89.4.1725.
14. Ge J, Jeremias A, Rupp A, et al. New signs characteristic of myocardial bridging demonstrated by intracoronary ultrasound and Doppler. Eur Heart J. 1999;20(23):1707–16. https://doi.org/10.1053/euhj.1999.1661.
15. Masuda T, Ishikawa Y, Akasaka Y, Itoh K, Kiguchi H, Ishii T. The effect of myocardial bridging of the coronary artery on vasoactive agents and atherosclerosis localization. J Pathol. 2001;193(3):408–14. https://doi.org/10.1002/1096-9896(2000)9999:9999<::AID-PATH792>3.0.CO;2-R.
16. Ishii T, Asuwa N, Masuda S, Ishikawa Y. The effects of a myocardial bridge on coronary atherosclerosis and ischaemia. J Pathol. 1998;185(1):4–9. https://doi.org/10.1002/(SICI)1096-9896(199805)185:1<4::AID-PATH50>3.0.CO;2-3.
17. Ciampricotti R, el Gamal M. Vasospastic coronary occlusion associated with a myocardial bridge. Cathet Cardiovasc Diagn. 1988;14(2):118–20. https://doi.org/10.1002/ccd.1810140213.
18. Schwarz ER, Klues HG, Vom Dahl J, Klein I, Krebs W, Hanrath P. Functional, angiographic and intracoronary Doppler flow characteristics in symptomatic patients with myocardial bridging: effect of short-term intravenous beta-blocker medication. J Am Coll Cardiol. 1996;27(7):1637–45. https://doi.org/10.1016/0735-1097(96)00062-9.
19. Ishimori T, Raizner AE, Chahine RA, Awdeh M, Luchi RJ. Myocardial bridges in man: clinical correlations and angiographic accentuation with nitroglycerin. Cathet Cardiovasc Diagn. 1977;3(1):59–65. https://doi.org/10.1002/ccd.1810030107.
20. Shriki JE, Shinbane JS, Rashid MA, et al. Identifying, characterizing, and classifying congenital anomalies of the coronary arteries. Radiographics. 2012;32(2):453–68. https://doi.org/10.1148/rg.322115097.
21. Angelini P. Congenital coronary artery ostial disease: a spectrum of anatomic variants with different pathophysiologies and prognoses. Tex Heart Inst J. 2012;39(1):55–9.
22. Doğan N, Dursun A, Özkan H. Vieussens' arterial ring: a rare coronary variant anatomy. Diagn Interv Radiol. 2019;25(2):109–13. https://doi.org/10.5152/dir.2019.17449.
23. Saremi F, Goodman G, Wilcox A, Salibian R, Vorobiof G. Coronary artery ostial atresia: diagnosis of conotruncal anastomotic collateral rings using CT angiography. JACC Cardiovasc Imaging. 2011;4(12):1320–3. https://doi.org/10.1016/j.jcmg.2011.09.018.
24. Musiani A, Cernigliaro C, Sansa M, Maselli D, De Gasperis C. Left main coronary artery atresia: literature review and therapeutical considerations. Eur J Cardiothorac Surg. 1997;11(3):505–14. https://doi.org/10.1016/s1010-7940(96)01121-9.
25. Mullins CE, el-Said G, DG MN, Cooley DA, Treistman B, Garcia E. Atresia of the left coronary artery ostium. Repair by saphenous vein graft. Circulation. 1972;46(5):989–94. https://doi.org/10.1161/01.cir.46.5.989.
26. Pirelli L, Yu PJ, Srichai MB, Khvilivitzky K, Angelini P, Grau JB. Ectopic origin of left coronary ostium from left ventricle, with occlusive membrane: a previously unreported anomaly, with an embryologic interpretation. Tex Heart Inst J. 2008;35(2):162–5.
27. Shen TC, Chou HH, Tsai KT. Ectopic and atretic ostium of left main coronary artery: from interleaflet triangle between left and noncoronary cusps. Tex Heart Inst J. 2012;39(1):60–2.
28. Peña E, Nguyen ET, Merchant N, Dennie C. ALCAPA syndrome: not just a pediatric disease. Radiographics. 2009;29(2):553–65. https://doi.org/10.1148/rg.292085059.
29. Khanna A, Torigian DA, Ferrari VA, Bross RJ, Rosen MA. Anomalous origin of the left coronary artery from the pulmonary artery in adulthood on CT and MRI. AJR Am J Roentgenol. 2005;185(2):326–9. https://doi.org/10.2214/ajr.185.2.01850326.
30. Horisaki T, Yamashita T, Yokoyama H, Urasawa K, Kitabatake A. Three-dimensional reconstruction of computed tomographic images of anomalous origin of the left main coronary artery from the pulmonary trunk in an adult. Am J Cardiol. 2003;92(7):898–9. https://doi.org/10.1016/s0002-9149(03)00913-5.
31. Takenaga M, Matsuda J, Miyamoto N, Ikushima I, Koiwaya Y. Magnetic resonance imaging of bland-white-Garland syndrome—a case of anomalous origin of the left coronary artery from the pulmonary trunk in a 22-year-old woman. Jpn Circ J. 1998;62(3):219–21. https://doi.org/10.1253/jcj.62.219.
32. Secinaro A, Ntsinjana H, Tann O, et al. Cardiovascular magnetic resonance findings in repaired anomalous left coronary artery to pulmonary artery connection (ALCAPA). J Cardiovasc Magn Reson. 2011;13(1):27. https://doi.org/10.1186/1532-429X-13-27.
33. Gutgesell HP, Pinsky WW, DePuey EG. Thallium-201 myocardial perfusion imaging in infants and children. Value in distinguishing anomalous left coronary artery from congestive cardiomyopathy. Circulation. 1980;61(3):596–9. https://doi.org/10.1161/01.cir.61.3.596.
34. Hurwitz RA, Caldwell RL, Girod DA, Brown J, King H. Clinical and hemodynamic course of infants and children with anomalous left coronary artery. Am Heart J. 1989;118(6):1176–81. https://doi.org/10.1016/0002-8703(89)90006-9.
35. Li D, Zhu Z, Zheng X, et al. Surgical treatment of anomalous left coronary artery from pulmonary artery in an adult. Coron Artery Dis. 2015;26(8):723–5. https://doi.org/10.1097/MCA.0000000000000286.
36. Naimo PS, Fricke TA, d'Udekem Y, et al. Surgical intervention for anomalous origin of left coronary

artery from the pulmonary artery in children: a long-term follow-up. Ann Thorac Surg. 2016;101(5):1842–8. https://doi.org/10.1016/j.athoracsur.2015.11.020.
37. Trivedi KR, Assaidi A, Macé L, Cuisset T, Fraisse A. Management of anomalous origin of the left coronary artery from the pulmonary artery in an adult with ischemic cardiomyopathy and pulmonary hypertension. Ann Thorac Surg. 2014;98(2):e41–3. https://doi.org/10.1016/j.athoracsur.2014.04.055.
38. Yamanaka O, Hobbs RE. Coronary artery anomalies in 126,595 patients undergoing coronary arteriography. Catheter Cardiovasc Diagn. 1990;21(1):28–40. https://doi.org/10.1002/ccd.1810210110.
39. Gräni C, Kaufmann PA, Windecker S, Buechel RR. Diagnosis and management of anomalous coronary arteries with a malignant course. Interv Cardiol. 2019;14(2):83–8. https://doi.org/10.15420/icr.2019.1.1.
40. Maron BJ, Haas TS, Ahluwalia A, Murphy CJ, Garberich RF. Demographics and epidemiology of sudden deaths in Young competitive athletes: from the United States National Registry. Am J Med. 2016;129(11):1170–7. https://doi.org/10.1016/j.amjmed.2016.02.031.
41. Basso C, Maron BJ, Corrado D, Thiene G. Clinical profile of congenital coronary artery anomalies with origin from the wrong aortic sinus leading to sudden death in young competitive athletes. J Am Coll Cardiol. 2000;35(6):1493–501. https://doi.org/10.1016/s0735-1097(00)00566-0.
42. Eckart RE, Scoville SL, Campbell CL, et al. Sudden death in young adults: a 25-year review of autopsies in military recruits. Ann Intern Med. 2004;141(11):829–34. https://doi.org/10.7326/0003-4819-141-11-200412070-00005.
43. Brothers JA, Frommelt MA, Jaquiss RDB, Myerburg RJ, Fraser CD Jr, Tweddell JS. Expert consensus guidelines: anomalous aortic origin of a coronary artery. J Thorac Cardiovasc Surg. 2017;153(6):1440–57. https://doi.org/10.1016/j.jtcvs.2016.06.066.
44. Yun G, Nam TH, Chun EJ. Coronary artery fistulas: pathophysiology, imaging findings, and management. Radiographics. 2018;38(3):688–703. https://doi.org/10.1148/rg.2018170158.
45. Reddy G, Davies JE, Holmes DR, Schaff HV, Singh SP, Alli OO. Coronary artery fistulae. Circ Cardiovasc Interv. 2015;8(11):e003062. https://doi.org/10.1161/Circinterventions.115.003062.
46. Mangukia CV. Coronary artery fistula. Ann Thorac Surg. 2012;93(6):2084–92. https://doi.org/10.1016/j.athoracsur.2012.01.114.
47. Dodge-Khatami A, Mavroudis C, Backer CL. Congenital heart surgery nomenclature and database project: anomalies of the coronary arteries. Ann Thorac Surg. 2000;69(4 Suppl):S270–97. https://doi.org/10.1016/s0003-4975(99)01248-5.
48. Kugelmass AD, Manning WJ, Piana RN, Weintraub RM, Baim DS, Grossman W. Coronary arteriovenous fistula presenting as congestive heart failure. Cathet Cardiovasc Diagn. 1992;26(1):19–25. https://doi.org/10.1002/ccd.1810260106.
49. Okwuosa TM, Gundeck EL, Ward RP. Coronary to pulmonary artery fistula-diagnosis by transesophageal echocardiography. Echocardiography. 2006;23(1):62–4. https://doi.org/10.1111/j.1540-8175.2006.00116.x.
50. Pathak R, Giri S, Hwang I, Alsafwah S. Multiple coronary-cameral fistulas to the left ventricle arising from both coronary arteries. J Community Hosp Intern Med Perspect. 2016;6(3):31190. https://doi.org/10.3402/jchimp.v6.31190.
51. Gajjar T, Voleti C, Matta R, Iyer R, Dash PK, Desai N. Aorta-right atrial tunnel: clinical presentation, diagnostic criteria, and surgical options. J Thorac Cardiovasc Surg. 2005;130(5):1287–92. https://doi.org/10.1016/j.jtcvs.2005.07.021.
52. Sai Krishna C, Baruah DK, Reddy GV, Panigrahi NK, Suman K, Kumar PV. Aorta-right atrial tunnel. Tex Heart Inst J. 2010;37(4):480–2.
53. Paul SK, Gajjar TP, Desai NB. Aorto-left atrial tunnel: a rare entity. Ann Thorac Surg. 2013;95(5):e121–2. https://doi.org/10.1016/j.athoracsur.2012.11.009.
54. Sreedharan M, Baruah B, Dash PK. Aorta-right atrial tunnel—a novel therapeutic option. Int J Cardiol. 2006;107(3):410–2. https://doi.org/10.1016/j.ijcard.2005.01.056.
55. Yoshikai M, Kamohara K, Fumoto H, Kawasaki H. Dual left anterior descending coronary artery: report of a case. Surg Today. 2004;34(5):453–5. https://doi.org/10.1007/s00595-003-2733-x.
56. Nasrin S, Cader FA, Haq MM, Shafi MJ. Type IV dual left anterior descending coronary artery: a case report. BMC Res Notes. 2017;10(1):659. https://doi.org/10.1186/s13104-017-2984-z.
57. Thakur R, Dwivedi SK, Puri VK. Unusual "high take off" of the right coronary artery from the ascending aorta. Int J Cardiol. 1990;26(3):369–71. https://doi.org/10.1016/0167-5273(90)90096-n.
58. Palomo AR, Schrager BR, Chahine RA. Anomalous origin of the right coronary artery from the ascending aorta high above the left posterior sinus of valsalva of a bicuspid aortic valve. Am Heart J. 1985;109(4):902–4. https://doi.org/10.1016/0002-8703(85)90657-x.
59. Villa AD, Sammut E, Nair A, Rajani R, Bonamini R, Chiribiri A. Coronary artery anomalies overview: the normal and the abnormal. World J Radiol. 2016;8(6):537–55. https://doi.org/10.4329/wjr.v8.i6.537.
60. Desmet W, Vanhaecke J, Vrolix M, et al. Isolated single coronary artery: a review of 50,000 consecutive coronary angiographies. Eur Heart J. 1992;13(12):1637–40. https://doi.org/10.1093/oxfordjournals.eurheartj.a060117.
61. Smith JC. Review of single coronary artery with report of 2 cases. Circulation. 1950;1(5):1168–75. https://doi.org/10.1161/01.cir.1.5.1168.
62. Lipton MJ, Barry WH, Obrez I, Silverman JF, Wexler L. Isolated single coronary artery: diagnosis, angiographic classification, and clinical signifi-

cance. Radiology. 1979;130(1):39–47. https://doi.org/10.1148/130.1.39.
63. Glushko T, Seifert R, Brown F, Vigilance D, Iriarte B, Teytelboym OM. Transseptal course of anomalous left main coronary artery originating from single right coronary orifice presenting as unstable angina. Radiol Case Rep. 2018;13(3):549–54. https://doi.org/10.1016/j.radcr.2018.02.009.
64. Sanford GB, Molavi B, Sinha AK, Garza L, Angelini P. Single coronary artery with prepulmonic coursing left main coronary artery manifesting as prinzmetal's angina. Tex Heart Inst J. 2007;34(4):449–52.
65. Davis JT, Teske DW, Allen HD, Cohen DM, Schauer GM. Anomalous course of the left main coronary artery in tetralogy of Fallot. Ann Thorac Surg. 1996;61(1):229–31. https://doi.org/10.1016/0003-4975(95)00742-3.
66. Angelini P. Coronary artery anomalies—current clinical issues: definitions, classification, incidence, clinical relevance, and treatment guidelines. Tex Heart Inst J. 2002;29(4):271–8.
67. Johnson JN, Bonnichsen CR, Julsrud PR, Burkhart HM, Hagler DJ. Single coronary artery giving rise to an intraseptal left coronary artery in a patient presenting with neurocardiogenic syncope. Cardiol Young. 2011;21(5):572–6. https://doi.org/10.1017/S1047951111000606.
68. Garg N, Tewari S, Kapoor A, Gupta DK, Sinha N. Primary congenital anomalies of the coronary arteries: a coronary: arteriographic study. Int J Cardiol. 2000;74(1):39–46. https://doi.org/10.1016/s0167-5273(00)00243-6.
69. Castillo JG, Sanz J, Fischer GW, Bowman K, Filsoufi F. Management of anomalous left circumflex artery encircling the aortic annulus in a patient undergoing multivalvular surgery. J Card Surg. 2009;24(6):667–9. https://doi.org/10.1111/j.1540-8191.2009.00930.x.
70. Angelini P, Trujillo A, Sawaya F, Lee VV. "Acute takeoff" of the circumflex artery: a newly recognized coronary anatomic variant with potential clinical consequences. Tex Heart Inst J. 2008;35(1):28–31.
71. Gossman DE, Tuzcu EM, Simpfendorfer C, Beck GJ. Percutaneous transluminal angioplasty for shepherd's crook right coronary artery stenosis. Cathet Cardiovasc Diagn. 1988;15(3):189–91. https://doi.org/10.1002/ccd.1810150313.
72. Nesto RW, Sassower MA. PTCA of "shepherd's crook" right coronary arteries with a new shape of guiding catheter. Cathet Cardiovasc Diagn. 1993;29(1):70–3. https://doi.org/10.1002/ccd.1810290115.
73. Voci G, Patel RB, Trivedi AD, Patel PV, Burris AC, Ruby SR. Angiographic demonstration of congenital intercoronary communication in normal adults. Am J Cardiol. 1987;59(12):1205–6. https://doi.org/10.1016/0002-9149(87)90880-0.
74. Kruskal JB, Hartnell GG. Nonatherosclerotic coronary artery disease: more than just stenosis. Radiographics. 1995;15(2):383–96. https://doi.org/10.1148/radiographics.15.2.7761642.

10 Imaging in Pulmonary Atresia with Ventricular Septal Defect

Yashpal Rana and Ramiah Rajeshkannan

10.1 Introduction

Pulmonary atresia with ventricular septal defect (PA-VSD), as a unique term, has been proposed by the international nomenclature committee of Congenital Heart Surgery Nomenclature and Database Project and is defined as a group of congenital cardiac malformations in which there is lack of luminal continuity between either ventricle and the pulmonary arteries along with a defect in the interventricular septum [1, 2]. This defect may be best considered as an extreme form of classic Tetralogy of Fallot (TOF) which consists of the tetrad of right ventricular outflow tract (RVOT) stenosis, malaligned conotruncal ventricular septal defect (VSD), overriding of the aorta and right ventricular hypertrophy (RVH). In contrast, PA-VSD consists of atresia of RVOT and part or all of the central pulmonary arteries along with the remaining three findings of classic TOF. The complexity of pulmonary blood flow and challenging management sets PA-VSD apart from classic TOF. The pulmonary blood supply originates most commonly from a patent ductus arteriosus (PDA) or from major aortopulmonary collateral arteries (MAPCAs), which connect the systemic circulation with the pulmonary arteries.

Other synonyms for this defect are "Type IV truncus arteriosus" and "Pseudotruncus arteriosus" [1, 3]. The intracardiac defect in PA-VSD may be TOF, double-outlet right ventricle (DORV), or transposition of the great arteries (TGA). Precise characterization of native pulmonary arteries and MAPCAs is of vital importance in managing patients with PA-VSD. MDCT and MRI along with 3D software have revolutionized noninvasive imaging of complex pulmonary blood supply in PA-VSD [4, 5] and have helped to achieve better surgical outcomes in recent years [6].

Three different MRI cases of PA-VSD with the full report are available at online-only video files.

Electronic supplementary material The online version of this chapter (https://doi.org/10.1007/978-981-15-6755-1_10) contains supplementary material, which is available to authorized users.

Y. Rana (✉)
U.N. Mehta Institute of Cardiology and Research Centre, Ahmedabad, Gujarat, India

Radiscan Diagnostics, Ahmedabad, Gujarat, India

R. Rajeshkannan
Department of Radiology, Amrita School of Medicine, Amrita Institute of Medical Sciences and Research Centre, Amrita Vishwa Vidyapeetham, Kochi, Kerala, India

10.2 Etiology

Etiology is unclear and remains multifactorial. Genetic, environmental, and familial factors may play a causative role. PA-VSD has been observed more often with DiGeorge syndrome and

R. Rajeshkannan et al. (eds.), *CT and MRI in Congenital Heart Diseases*,
https://doi.org/10.1007/978-981-15-6755-1_10

Chromosome 22q11 microdeletion. Other associations include VACTER, CHARGE, Alagille syndromes, and chromosomal anomalies such as Trisomy 13, Trisomy 21, and Deletion 5p. There is an increased incidence of PA-VSD in infants of diabetic mothers compared to non-diabetic mothers.

10.3 Embryology

The development of the arterial branches starts about day 27 of gestation. Pulmonary arteries develop from the sixth pharyngeal arch. Lungs have dual blood supply between the 27th and 50th days. Segmental arteries involute into pulmonary arteries and branches from the descending aorta become comparatively smaller and develop bronchial arteries. When the normal connection between heart and pulmonary arteries is disrupted blood supply to the lungs is maintained via PDA or systemic to pulmonary collaterals.

Van Praagh and coworkers suggested that the embryologic basis for PA-VSD was severe underdevelopment of the subpulmonary infundibulum (conus) [7]. The result is that the infundibulum is shifted; later it hypertrophies secondary to the marked obstruction that is created by the shift. The mechanism of underdevelopment may be partly related to increased absorption of the distal part of the infundibulum.

10.4 Morphology

Pulmonary atresia varies from plate-like atresia of the pulmonary valve to the absence of the valve which can include a variable-length of the main pulmonary artery (MPA). Further extension of MPA atresia to its bifurcation results in non-confluent central pulmonary arteries (PA). One can, thus, understand that the anatomic spectrum varies significantly. One form is that of atresia of the pulmonary valve, presence of MPA, and confluent normal-sized PA that are supplied by a PDA. Another is that there is atresia of MPA with diminutive and/or non-confluent PA and absent PDA, in which the pulmonary blood flow is solely provided by MAPCAs and bronchial arteries.

Pulmonary arterial supply is said to be unifocal when all the bronchopulmonary segments are supplied by the native pulmonary artery. Multifocal supply is when different bronchopulmonary segments of one lung are supplied from more than one source. The goal of surgery is to consolidate the blood supply to the lungs in a unifocal manner particularly for the multifocal supply.

VSD is usually large, malaligned, perimembranous type and can occasionally be of the infundibular type. Variable degree of aortic override and RVH develops as a consequence of hemodynamic effects. The specific intracardiac defect in PA-VSD may be TOF, DORV, or TGA.

The ascending aorta is dilated since it receives the entire biventricular cardiac output and the intrinsic aortopathy due to inherent medical abnormality. A right aortic arch can be seen in up to 50% cases of PA-VSD.

PA-VSD should be separately identified from pulmonary atresia-intact ventricular septum (PA-IVS) which has an absence of VSD along with hypoplasia of tricuspid valve and right ventricle (RV) or dilated RV with regurgitant tricuspid valve. The presence of coronary sinusoids is a characteristic feature of PA-IVS and it usually has no pulmonary arterial abnormalities.

10.5 Classification

The most widely accepted classification system has been proposed by Congenital Heart Surgeons Society based on the complexity of pulmonary blood supply which in turn indicates the complexity of surgical repair (Fig. 10.1) [1].

Type A: Native PAs present, pulmonary vascular supply through PDA, and no MAPCAs (Fig. 10.2).

Type B: Native PAs and MAPCAs present (Figs. 10.3 and 10.4).

Type C: No native PAs, pulmonary blood supply through MAPCAs only (Figs. 10.5 and 10.6).

Surgical approach for type B and C is similar except that more extensive unifocalization of MAPCAs will be needed in Type C before the total repair is achieved.

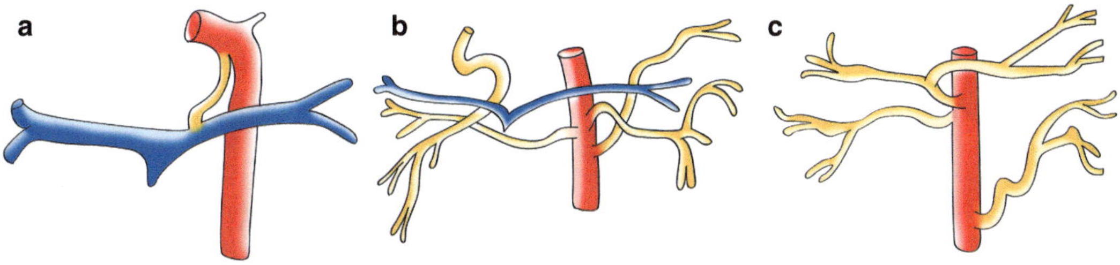

Fig. 10.1 Schematic representation of types of PA-VSD. (**a**) Type A. (**b**) Type B. (**c**) Type C

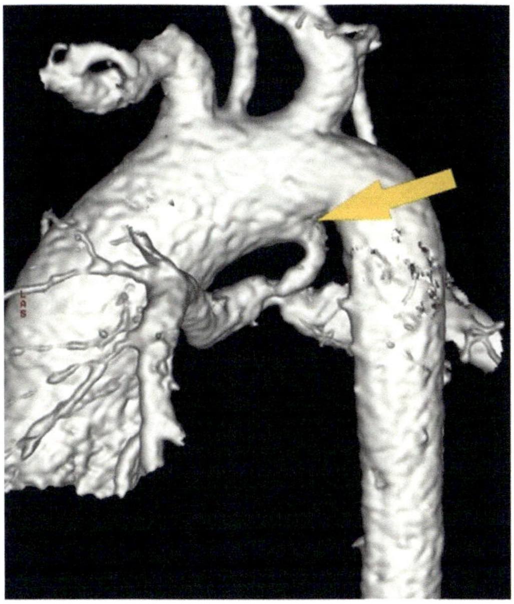

Fig. 10.2 Type A PA-VSD. Left oblique volume-rendered MR angiography image showing PDA (arrow) supplying confluent pulmonary arteries with stenosis at its pulmonary end

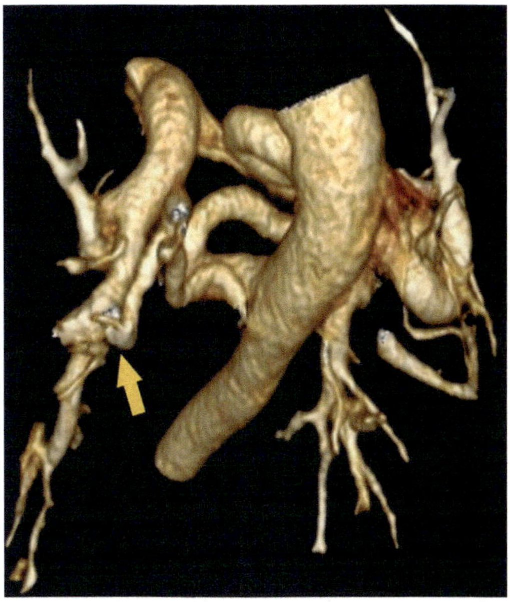

Fig. 10.3 Type B PA-VSD. Posterior oblique view volume-rendered CT image of another subject shows major aortopulmonary collateral artery (MAPCA) reinforcing right pulmonary artery (RPA) (arrow)

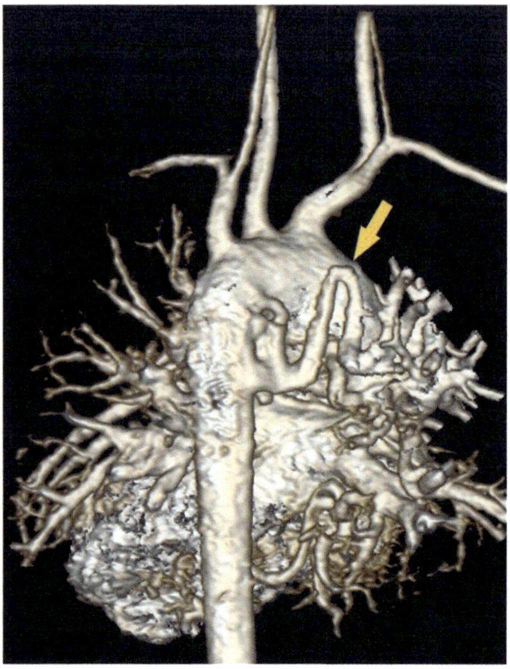

Fig. 10.4 Type B PA-VSD. Posterior oblique volume-rendered MR angiography image showing a MAPCA (arrow) to right lung

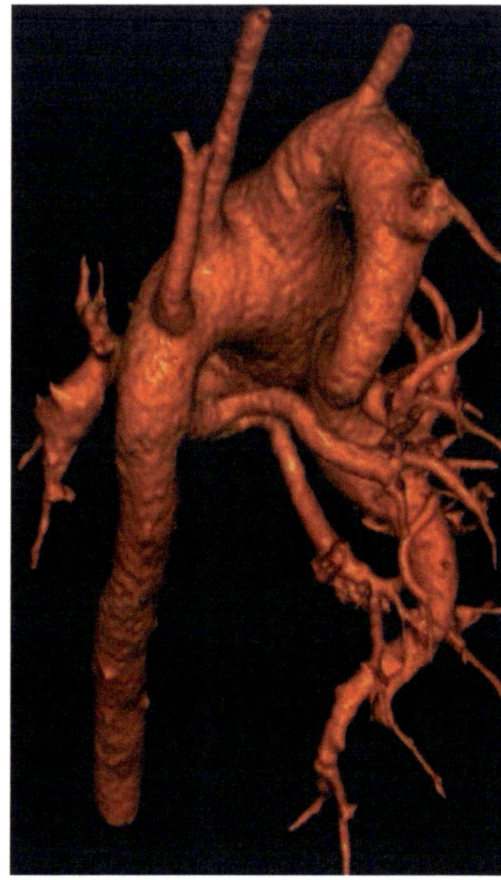

Fig. 10.5 Type C PA-VSD. Oblique volume-rendered CT image depicts multiple major aortopulmonary collateral arteries (MAPCAs) supplying both lungs with absent native pulmonary arteries

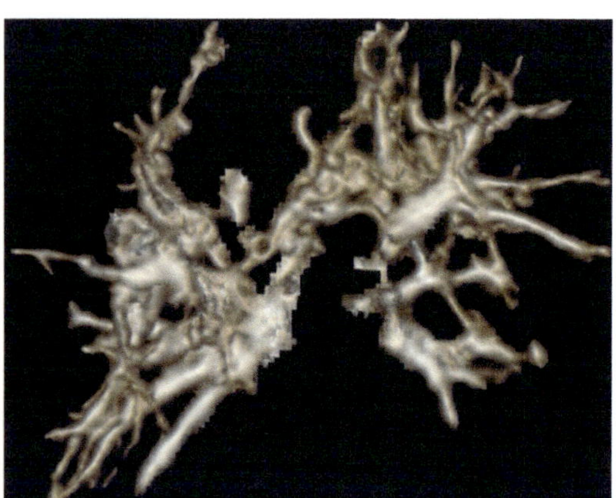

Fig. 10.6 Type C PA-VSD. Volume-rendered MR angiography image demonstrating multiple MAPCAs to both lungs

10.6 Pathophysiology

There is a complete mixing of pulmonary and systemic venous blood in the aorta through the large nonrestrictive VSD. Hence, the distribution of blood to the body, as opposed to the lungs, depends on the relative resistances offered by the two circulations. The pulmonary vascular resistance is a complex interplay of the number of collaterals, the extent of intrapulmonary anastomosis, and the presence of focal narrowing in the collaterals. Focal narrowing in the MAPCAs apparently protects the peripheral intra-acinar arteries from high flow and systemic pressure and prevents changes of excessive muscularity and intimal hyperplasia [8].

The discussion of pulmonary blood flow in PA-VSD includes the extent of atresia, PDA, native pulmonary artery(s) (NPA), aortopulmonary collaterals, and distal pulmonary vascular arborization.

PDA: PDA typically originates from either the undersurface of the arch or from the undersurface of the innominate artery. The PA is most commonly confluent and of an adequate size when the PDA is present. However, variations include bilateral PDA with non-confluent PA. PDA can also be absent in one-third of subjects and is associated with absent central PAs [9].

Major aortopulmonary collaterals (MAPCAs): They represent fetal primitive intersegmental arteries that originate from the descending aorta and have not involuted. They gain access to the lung through the hilum and connect with native pulmonary arteries in the mediastinum or at the lobar or subsegmental level. MAPCAs are seen in 30–65% of patients with PA-VSD [10] and are usually 2–6 in number, usually arise from the anterior wall of the aorta opposite the origin of the intercostal arteries. Aneurysmal dilatation and thrombus can occur in MAPCAs in long-standing cases.

Types of MAPCAs

1. They can be broadly classified as direct or indirect (on the basis of origin). Direct MAPCA arises directly from the thoracic or abdominal aorta and indirect MAPCA arises from a branch of aorta like internal mammary artery. Common sites of origin are from the descending thoracic aorta at the level of the carina, subclavian arteries, abdominal aorta, or coronary arteries.
2. Protected or unprotected (based on the presence or absence of stenosis). Many MAPCAs have stenosis either at diagnosis or may develop over some time during follow-up. The presence of stenosis can protect pulmonary vasculature from future pulmonary hypertension.
3. Single or dual supply (depending upon the pulmonary segments they supply). It is important to differentiate the MAPCA from bronchial artery, PDA and native PA (Tables 10.1, 10.2, and 10.3).

Pleural Pulmonary Collaterals: Rarely, intercostal arteries and other systemic branches supplying the thoracic wall can perfuse the intrapulmonary arteries across the pleural connections.

Bronchial Arteries: The bronchial arteries are usually normal in patients with PA-VSD, but occasionally they become an important source of supply to the pulmonary arterial system [12, 13].

Other sources of pulmonary blood supply include the mediastinal collaterals originating from the subclavian arteries and coronary–pulmonary collaterals from branches of coronary arteries through atrial, pericardial, and mediastinal branches [14].

Table 10.1 Difference between bronchial artery and MAPCAs [11]

Bronchial artery	MAPCAs
Gives off mediastinal branches and sometimes gives branches to the spinal cord.	Do not give branch to any other structure in the mediastinum.
Do not anastomose with native Pas.	They may anastomose with the native Pas.
Accompany bronchi and form a nutritive plexus around bronchi.	They may accompany bronchi but do not form a nutritive plexus around bronchi.
Connected to intercostal arteries.	Never connected to intercostal arteries.
Different elastic wall structure.	Most MAPCAs have an elastic wall structure resembling the pulmonary artery or aorta rather than bronchial arteries.

Table 10.2 Difference between PDA and MAPCAs

PDA	MAPCAs
Tendency to close during early infancy, hence a less reliable blood supply source beyond the first few days of life.	Stenosis occurs over a period of weeks to months, hence remain patent and is more reliable than PDA.
Usually straight and vertical.	Usually tortuous.
Does not branch.	May branch.
Anastomose with central PA.	Anastomose with peripheral PA.

Table 10.3 Difference between native PA and MAPCAs

Native PA	MAPCAs
Confluent except for when there is an interruption.	Non-confluent, multiple sites of origin—Arise from descending thoracic or abdominal aorta or other systemic arteries like subclavian arteries, coronary arteries.
Stenosis may be present, for example, at site of PDA insertion or sometimes in parenchymal branches.	Stenosis frequently observed.
Branches frequently supplies all lobes.	Supply limited to a few bronchopulmonary segments or lobes.
Focal aneurysm is rare.	Focal aneurysmal dilatation may occur in long-standing cases.
Usually straight.	Usually tortuous.
Runs anterior to bronchus in mediastinum.	Courses behind the bronchus.

10.7 Clinical Presentation

The age of presentation varies from newborn to late infancy depending upon the adequacy of the pulmonary blood supply. The modes of presentation consist of cyanosis, heart failure, or failure to thrive [15].

A duct-dependent circulation presents when the duct starts to constrict typically in the newborn. Severe hypoxia, acidosis, and shock ensue after the closure of PDA. Immediate resuscitation with prostaglandin E1 (PGE1) infusion will help to stabilize the patient. Since these patients also usually have good-sized NPAs neonatal repair is accomplished by a right ventricle to pulmonary artery (RV–PA) conduit.

Patients with more complex pulmonary blood flow via MAPCAs are less dependent on ductal flow, and usually present after 4–6 weeks of age with increasing cyanosis or signs of heart failure when progressive stenosis develops in MAPCAs. These babies will only have mild cyanosis as a newborn and will escape detection.

Patients with adequate and "balanced" pulmonary blood flow throughout the early infancy and may present during late infancy. Such patients may present with a heart murmur that was heard during routine physical examination. Cyanosis and heart failure are not clinically obvious.

10.8 Imaging Modalities

10.8.1 Chest X-Ray

The combination of concavity at the upper mid part of the left heart border due to hypoplastic or absent main pulmonary artery segment with the upward pointing of the cardiac apex due to right ventricular hypertrophy creates a boot shape appearance of the cardiac silhouette on chest X-ray. Right aortic arch, if present, can be diagnosed on chest X-ray. When MAPCAs supply the lungs, pulmonary vascular markings have a typical reticular pattern.

10.8.2 Echocardiography

Echocardiography is the initial modality of choice to delineate intracardiac defects but has limitations for the extracardiac vascular structures. Echocardiography has the advantage of evaluating the direction of blood flow in central PAs by color Doppler analysis. This helps to differentiate collateral flow from PDA from MAPCAs supply. The PDA joins the PA in the mediastinum and hence flow in the PA is antegrade. MAPCAs join PAs at the lung hilum, and hence, the flow in the central PAs will be retrograde [9, 16, 17]. Echocardiography is often of limited value in older children because of poor acoustic windows. Though echocardiography remains the first modality to be used in the evaluation of such patients, the use of other noninvasive modalities such as CT and MRI is increasingly used to define pulmonary blood flow and for a precise anatomic road map to surgeons. With regard to intracardiac anatomy, Beekman RP et al. found that MR imaging was superior to echocardiography for the evaluation of right ventricular hypertrophy and overriding aorta [18]. MRI also has an edge for postoperative evaluation of pulmonary arteries compared to echocardiography [19, 20].

10.8.3 Cardiac Catheterization

Catheter angiography is a useful technique to assess the blood supply to each bronchopulmonary segment before unifocalization surgery. Its disadvantages include that it is invasive, has a long procedure time, need for sedation, arterial puncture, and consequent vascular complications [21, 22]. The focus of catheterization has shifted from making the diagnosis to filling in missing information in the diagnosis such as the hemodynamic data regarding pulmonary blood supply.

10.8.4 MR Angiography (MRA)

Breath-hold ECG-gated cardiac MRI and contrast-enhanced MR angiography are emerging as ideal techniques for the evaluation of complex congenital heart disease and PAs. Cardiac MRI gives anatomic and functional information without exposing the patient to ionizing radiation or the risk of an adverse reaction to iodinated contrast material. Cine MR images can provide additional information about cardiac function, valve patency, and the hemodynamic significance of vascular stenosis [23, 24].

10.8.4.1 Assessment of Morphology

Contrast-enhanced 3D MR angiography (MRA) can delineate all sources of pulmonary blood supply as well as provide an accurate assessment of native pulmonary artery size for planning corrective surgery. Continuous stack of cine SSFP and black blood images with short breath-hold times provide a detailed anatomic and topologic assessment of the heart and great vessels. RPA is best measured at coronal oblique cine MRI or reformatted MRA sequences. LPA can be seen better at sagittal oblique cine MRI or reformatted MRA images. There is a good correlation between the reformatted MRA and catheter angiography in measuring the diameter and the cross-sectional area of branch pulmonary arteries and their stenoses. Axial cine bSSFP CMR is the best surgically measured correlate of PA branch size due to this being a measure of stretched diameter [25]. Holmqvist et al. reported 93% agreement between MRI and catheter angiography with regard to a finding of main pulmonary artery stenosis, 79% agreement with regard to that of right pulmonary artery stenosis, and 86% agreement with regard to that of left pulmonary artery stenosis [26].

10.8.4.2 Functional Assessment

ECG-gated cine MRI is useful to assess end-diastolic, end-systolic volumes, ejection fraction, and wall motion abnormalities. MRI becomes the gold standard especially to evaluate RV function. Phase-contrast MRI may also provide hemodynamic information about the pulmonary and systemic blood flow. The pulmonary to systemic blood flow ratio (QP/QS) in PA-VSD can be calculated in many ways. Total pulmonary blood flow to each lung (QP) can be estimated by measuring the pulmonary venous return through the individual pulmonary veins. QS can be calculated by summing up SVC and IVC flow or by subtracting the pulmonary venous flow from ascending aortic flow ($QP/QS = QPV/(QAO - QPV)$). Quantification of blood flow volume and assessment of the flow pattern of individual MAPCAs is possible using PC-MRI. The blood distribution between the right and left lungs can be accurately assessed by PC imaging of the branch pulmonary arteries or pulmonary veins (Fig. 10.7).

However, administering long sedation and anesthesia in critically ill children in the closed MR environment carries significant risks [22].

The decision to image with CT versus MRI should be based on institutional equipment, reporting experience, and the patient's ability to cooperate.

10.8.5 CT Angiography (CTA)

MDCT angiography can answer specific questions unanswered by echocardiography such as (1) confirmation of presence or absence of native PAs; (2) MAPCAs—number, size, distribution,

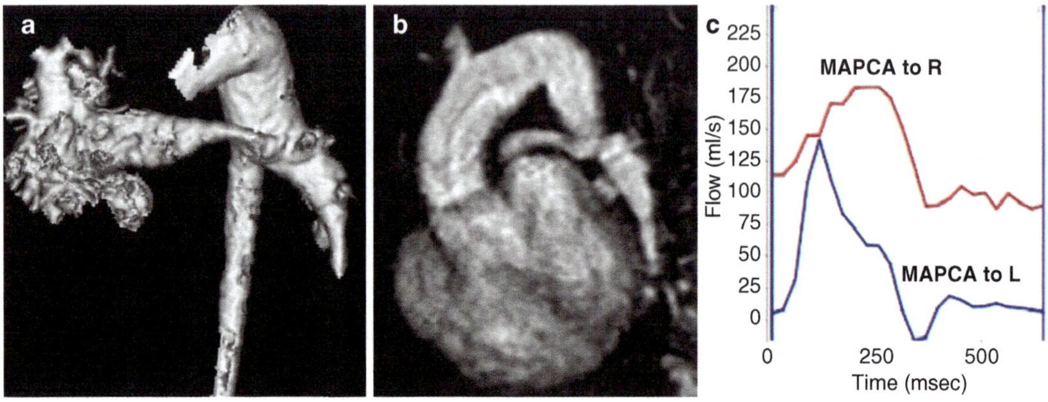

Fig. 10.7 Frontal volume-rendered image (**a**) and maximum-intensity-projection (MIP) (**b**). MR angiography images demonstrating a stenotic MAPCA to right lung and wide MAPCA to the left lung. Phase-contrast flow MRI demonstrating higher flow through the stenotic protected MAPCA compared to unprotected MAPCA to left lung suggesting Eisenmengerization of the left lung (**c**) (Ref to video file 1)

any stenosis in collateral vessel; (3) number of lung segments connected to native PAs; (4) lung segments with dual blood supply; and (5) coronary anatomy. Various studies have shown that MDCT is an accurate tool for evaluating PAs [22, 27–29].

10.8.5.1 Technical Factors

64 or higher versions of MDCT scanners are preferred. The radiation dose is kept to a minimum by reducing the kilovoltage and tube current appropriately and using automated dose regulation methods. ECG gating is not used routinely as not only does it increases radiation dose, it also significantly increases scan time, which produces more respiratory artifacts. Most of the extracardiac anatomy can be adequately depicted without ECG gating. Even though distal coronary arteries cannot be visualized without ECG gating, nongated MDCT images are sufficient to identify the origin and to evaluate the proximal course of the major coronaries, which is sufficient for management of these patients [30].

A short-term IV sedation is often required, particularly in children under 5 years of age. Whenever possible, a leg vein is preferable for contrast injection, to avoid streak artifacts from high-density contrast material in the upper limb veins. Contrast dose should be 1.5 mL/kg while contrast medium should be injected with a dual-head power injector at a rate of 1.5–2.0 mL/s for a 22-gauge cannula and 3.0 mL/s for a 20-gauge cannula. The use of a saline chaser serves to reduce the amount of contrast medium needed for CT angiography [31]. It is recommended to use 10–20 mL of saline at a rate equal to that of the contrast injection.

Using the bolus-tracking technique, the scanning can be started manually after seeing the contrast medium in the RV. A minimum delay of 4 s is used to start the scan after the contrast medium reaches the RV. Because of the presence of VSD in these infants, homogeneous contrast enhancement of both pulmonary and systemic arteries can be achieved consistently using this method.

10.8.5.2 Image Post-processing

Various image reformatting techniques including curved planar reconstruction, maximum intensity projection (MIP), minimum intensity projection (MinIP), and volume-rendering technique (VRT) are used to get all the clinically relevant information. Curved planar reformatting and MIP are primarily used to evaluate curved structures such as the PAs and MAPCAs. MinIP is used to evaluate the airway and lung parenchyma. For 3D reformatting of the complex anatomy, VRT is used. Thin-section multiplanar reformatting (MPR) is used for quantitative analysis of the structure in question.

10.9 MDCT and MRI Evaluation of PA-VSD

10.9.1 Pulmonary Arteries

Analysis of the pulmonary artery anatomy is the single most important aspect of diagnostic imaging of patients with PA-VSD. The confluent PAs, together with the abbreviated main pulmonary trunk, appears as a seagull in flight when seen in frontal view.

Following parameters must be carefully assessed:

(a) The length of the atretic segment
(b) Presence of pulmonary artery confluence
(c) The diameter of MPA, RPA, and LPA at the origin and the hilum
(d) Branch pulmonary artery stenosis (Fig. 10.8)
(e) Sources of pulmonary blood flow to each lung
(f) Number of bronchopulmonary segments supplied by native pulmonary arteries
(g) Distribution of each MAPCA

10.9.2 PDA

MDCT/MRI with 3D VRT can clearly delineate the PDA anatomy, its diameter, tortuosity, and stenosis if present. There is a high risk of stenosis of the pulmonary arteries at the PDA insertion site which can be clearly seen on cross-sectional imaging.

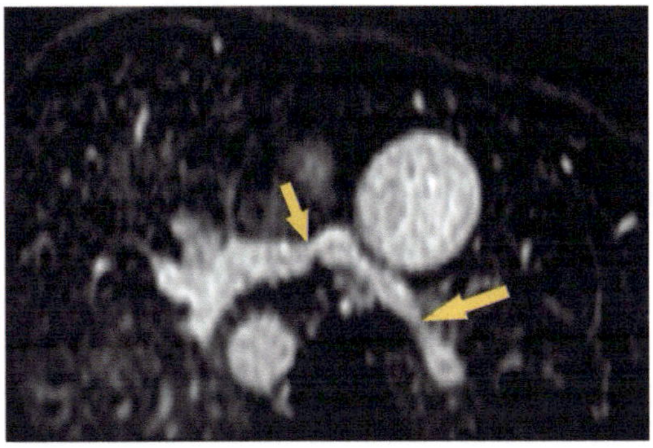

Fig. 10.8 Axial oblique maximum-intensity-projection (MIP) MR angiography image showing focal stenoses (arrows) at branch pulmonary arteries

10.9.3 MAPCAs

MDCT with 3D VRT has the potential to elucidate all the MAPCAs shown by invasive catheter angiography [32–34]. Using various MDCT post-processing techniques, the total number of MAPCAs and their origin, course, proximity to structures like veins and airways, and intrapulmonary connections can be easily assessed. The size of collaterals can also be described as—Large (>2 mm in diameter), Medium (1–2 mm in diameter), and small (<1 mm in diameter). In long-standing cases, aneurysmal dilatation of MAPCAs can occur (Fig. 10.9). Stenosis occurs in most MAPCAs, particularly at the aortic origin and pulmonary anastomotic sites (Fig. 10.10).

CTA/MRA can also delineate other sources of collateral flow like Pleural Pulmonary Collaterals, bronchial arteries, mediastinal collaterals originating from the subclavian arteries, and coronary–pulmonary collaterals from branches of coronary arteries through atrial, pericardial, and mediastinal branches [14] (Figs. 10.11 and 10.12).

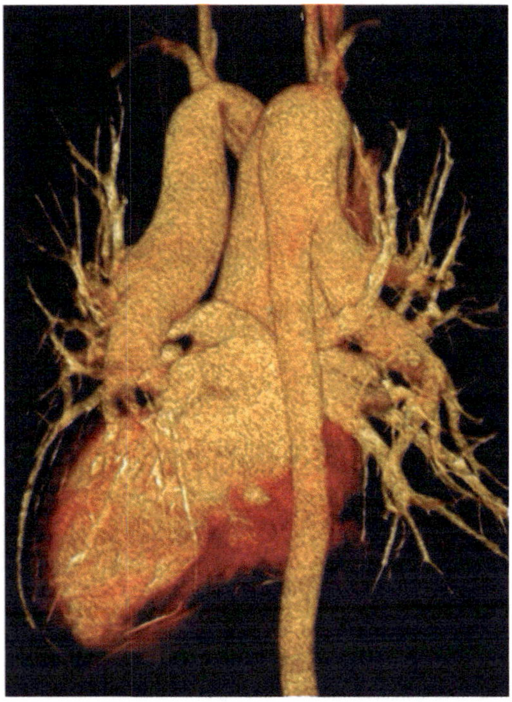

Fig. 10.9 Oblique lateral view of volume-rendered image shows aneurysmal dilatation of major aortopulmonary collateral artery (MAPCA) in Type C PA-VSD

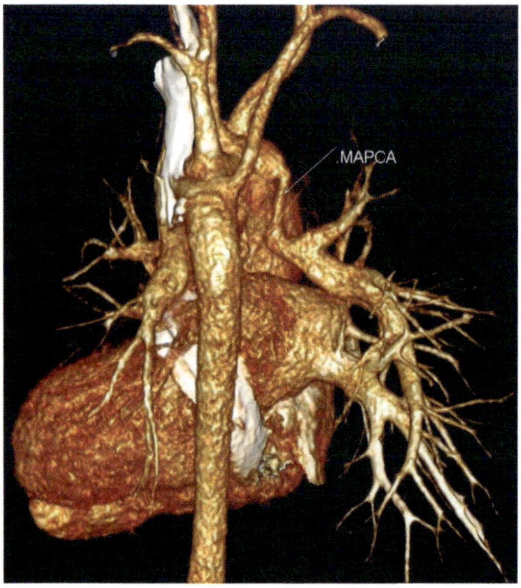

Fig. 10.10 Stenosis of major aortopulmonary collateral artery (MAPCA). Posterior oblique volume-rendered image shows tight stenosis of MAPCA

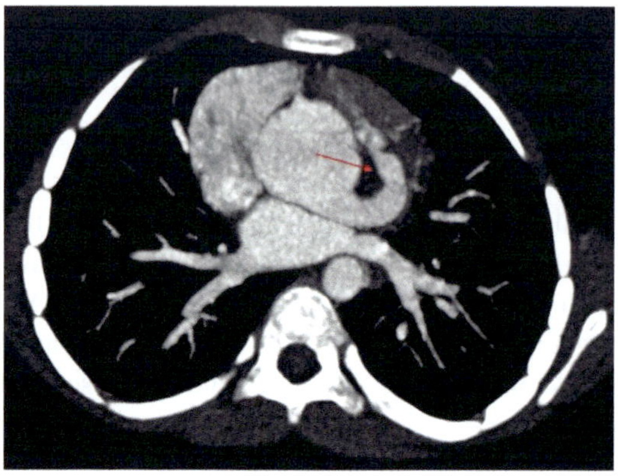

Fig. 10.12 Axial maximum-intensity-projection (MIP) CT image shows coronary to pulmonary collateral with severe stenosis at the pulmonary end (red arrow)

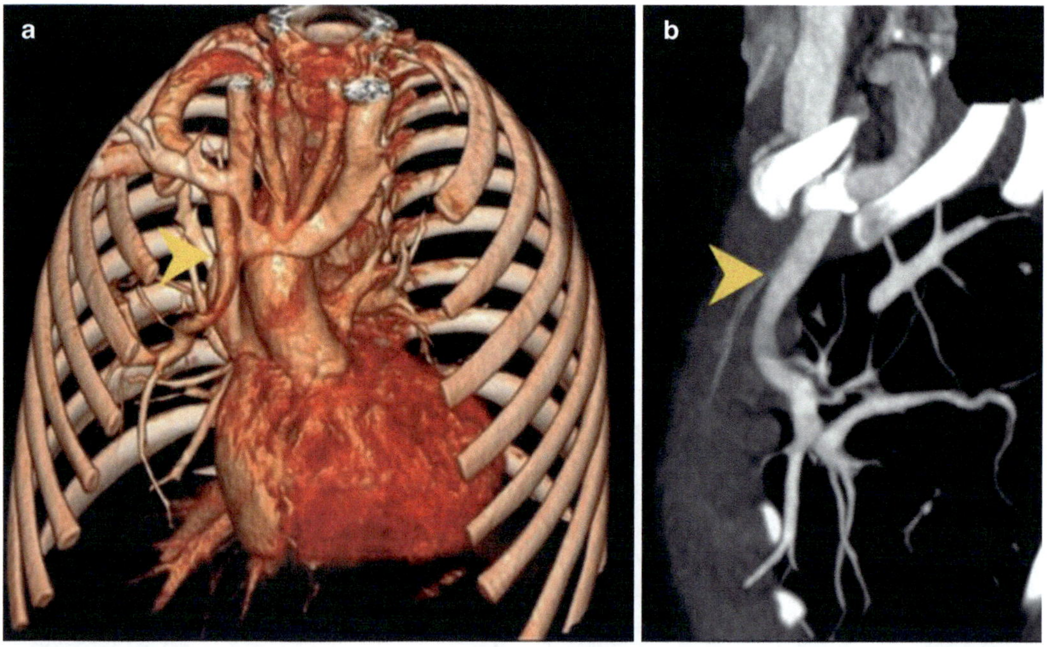

Fig. 10.11 Chest wall collaterals in PA-VSD. (**a**) Volume-rendered image. (**b**) Sagittal oblique maximum-intensity-projection (MIP) CT image shows hypertrophied right internal mammary artery (RIMA) supplying the right lung (arrowhead)

Several pulmonary artery indices that are described on catheter angiography can also be precisely measured on CTA/MRA.

10.9.4 Z-Score

The Z-score is defined as the number of SDs a measurement lies from the mean, allowing for a quantitative assessment of cardiovascular dimensions relative to the range of values normally observed. The Z-score represents a numerical value that clinicians can easily interpret with respect to the normal 95% range (approximately ± 2). Furthermore, the use of Z-scores can simplify comparisons of longitudinal cardiovascular change, because their values are adjusted to the mean and variation at any given age. The use of Z-scores can, therefore, allow for a more precise evaluation of vascular dimensions that severely alter cardiovascular dimensions. Lower than normal size of vessels is denoted by a negative Z-score.

Z = Observed dimension – Mean normal dimension / Standard deviation around mean normal dimension.

10.9.5 McGoon's Ratio

McGoon's ratio is calculated by dividing the sum of the diameters of the right pulmonary artery (RPA) and left pulmonary artery (LPA) (before their bifurcation as shown in Fig. 10.13), divided by the of aorta at the level above the diaphragm [DRPA / DDTAO) + (DLPA/DDTAO)]. An average value of 2.1 is noted in normal subjects. A ratio above 1.2 is associated with acceptable postoperative RV systolic pressure while a ratio below 0.8 is deemed inadequate for the complete repair of PA-VSD. VSD closure is deferred in such patients at the time of repair or they underwent aortopulmonary shunt procedure as a first stage [35, 36].

10.9.6 Nakata Index

Nakata PA index is calculated from the cross-sectional area (CSA) of PAs measured immediately proximal to the origin of upper lobe branches of the respective branch PAs [37]. The sum of the CSA of right and left PAs is divided by the body surface area (BSA) of the patient [Nakata index = CSA of RPA (mm^2) + CSA of LPA (mm^2)/BSA (m^2)]. A Nakata index of >150 mm^2/m^2 is acceptable for complete repair without a prior palliative shunt.

10.9.7 Total Neo-pulmonary Artery Index (TNPAI)

Nakata index has no provision for the additional vascular bed that will be added by unifocalization, hence it is of limited use for evaluation of the adequacy of PAs in single-stage repair strategy where unifocalization of several MAPCAs is followed by total repair in at the same operation.

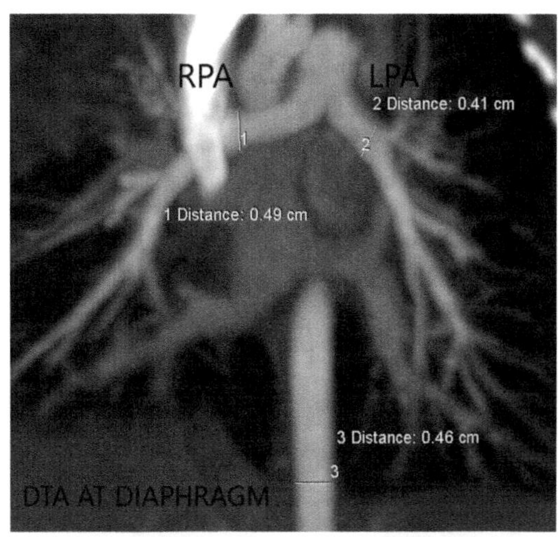

Fig. 10.13 McGoon ratio. Coronal maximum-intensity-projection (MIP) CT image shows a maximum diameter of right and left pulmonary arteries at pre-branching level and descending thoracic aorta at the diaphragm level

TNPAI is developed for such single-stage repair strategy as a composite index of native PAs and the MAPCAs that will be unifocalized, in order to determine whether the VSD could be closed at surgery [38]. The sum of the total MAPCAs index and Nakata index is called TNPAI. MAPCAs index is calculated by the addition of CSA of all significant MAPCAs divided by the BSA. A TNPAI index >200 mm^2/m^2 correlates well with low postoperative RV/LV pressure ratio and identifies patients who are clear candidates for VSD closure at the time of single-stage surgical repair.

The nature of the distal pulmonary vascular bed and pulmonary vascular resistance is not expressed in these calculations but these factors play an important role in postoperative RV pressure and in turn the hemodynamic outcome of surgical repair.

10.9.8 Lung Arborization (Distribution)

Before doing major corrective surgery in patients with PA-VSD, it is important to know the adequacy of the pulmonary blood flow in each bronchopulmonary segment. If both MAPCAs and NPAs supply a bronchopulmonary segment, ligations of MAPCAs do not affect lung arborization. If a bronchopulmonary segment is exclusively supplied by MAPCAs, then that segment needs to be unifocalized. It is important to know whether MAPCAs are communicating with NPAs or not. If they are communicating, the NPAs tend to be good-sized, and coiling or ligation of MAPCAs does not affect pulmonary blood flow once the antegrade flow is restored [39]. Communication between MAPCAs and NPAs can occur with central pulmonary arteries, at the hilum or major lobar branches, and segmental or subsegmental levels. Areas of poor arborization can be identified easily with MDCT.

10.9.9 Aortic Anomalies

MDCT/MRI has proven value in the accurate delineation of various associated aortic anomalies [40–42]. A right-sided aortic arch is seen in up to 25–50% of cases, more common than in classical TOF (Fig. 10.14). It may also be associated with an aberrant right or left subclavian artery, coarctation of the aorta, and double aortic arch [2, 43]. These variations are important to determine the surgical approach for a shunt.

10.9.10 Coronary and Intracardiac Abnormalities

The incidence of coronary artery anomalies in TOF is reported to be 2–10% [44]. Recognizing anomalous coronary artery preoperatively is important in surgical planning. Common coronary anomalies associated with PA-VSD are anomalous origin of the left anterior descending

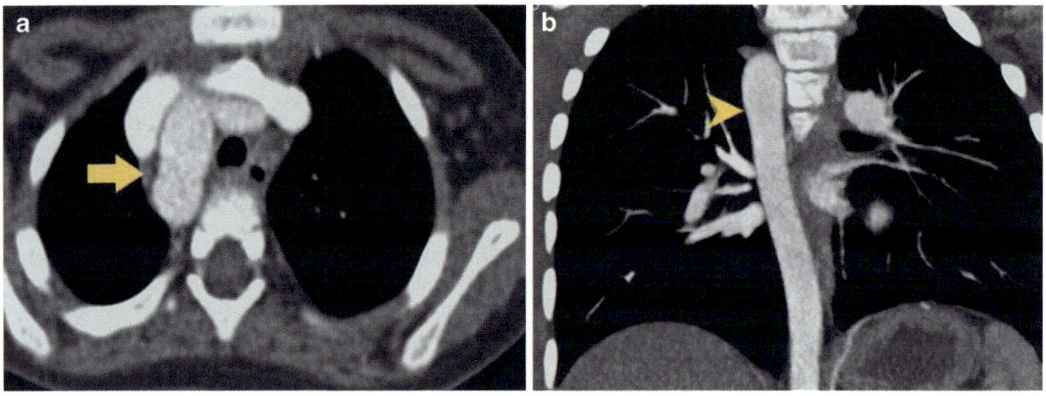

Fig. 10.14 Right aortic arch in PA-VSD. (**a**) Axial and (**b**) Coronal maximum-intensity-projection (MIP) CT images showing right aortic arch (arrow) and right descending thoracic aorta (arrowhead)

artery (LAD) from the right coronary artery (RCA) coursing anterior to the infundibulum of the RV, high origin of the coronary ostia, coronary artery to pulmonary-artery fistula, and anomalous RCA origin from the left aortic sinus [43]. One should be cautious in depicting the coronary anatomy pattern in PA-VSD because there is generally a clockwise rotation of the aortic root in such cases [30]. The sensitivity of ECG-gated MDCT in detecting coronary anomalies approaches 100% [45–47]. However, even non-ECG-gated MDCT in small children can provide confident identification of the osteo-proximal segments of the major coronary arteries [48].

Free-breathing respiratory navigator-gated, ECG-triggered, T2-prepared, 3D SSFP MR coronary angiography can be used to assess coronary anomalies even without injecting contrast medium. American heart association committee on cardiovascular imaging provides a level IIa recommendation for MR and CT angiography in the evaluation of coronary artery anomalies.

10.9.11 Septal Defects

All of these patients will have large sub-aortic VSD, which is usually of the membranous type. (Fig. 10.15). Small muscular VSD is difficult to see on MDCT but can be clearly seen on MRI. Ostium secundum–type atrial septal defect (ASD) or patent foramen ovale (PFO) is also common and can be visualized with MDCT/MRI.

10.9.12 Intracardiac Morphology

CT/MRI can delineate precise intracardiac morphology associated. The most common intracardiac morphology is mild overriding aorta into RV (TOF type). Less common types include aorta arising from right-sided RV as in D-TGA, left-sided RV as in L-TGA and large VSD amounting to single ventricle (Fig. 10.16).

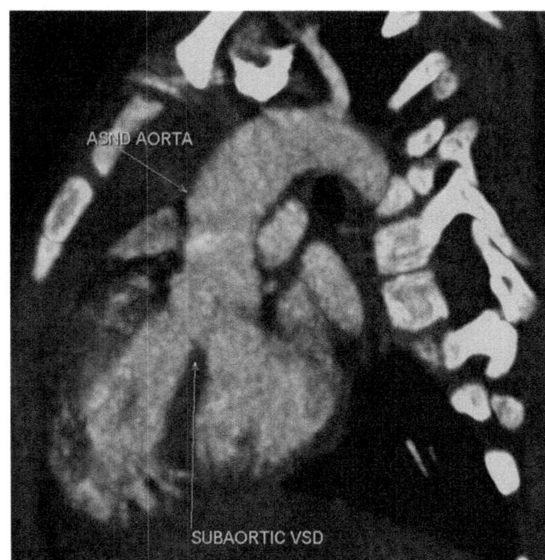

Fig. 10.15 Oblique sagittal maximum-intensity-projection (MIP) CT image shows subaortic ventricular septal defect (VSD) with aortic override

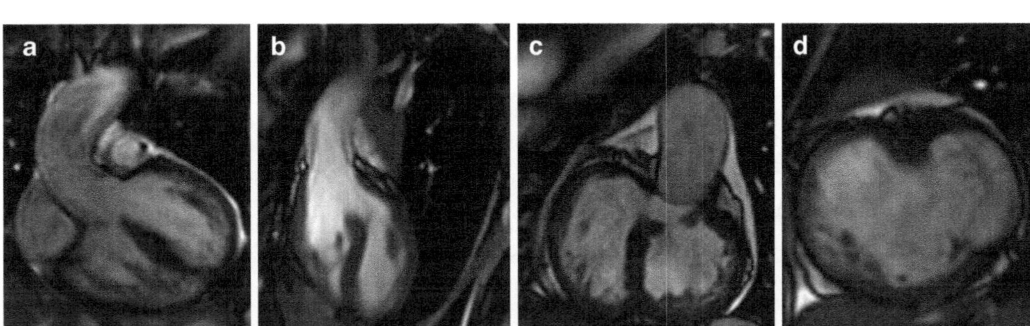

Fig. 10.16 SSFP images demonstrating different intracardiac morphologies associated with pulmonary atresia and VSD. The most common intracardiac morphology is mild overriding aorta into RV (TOF type) as in (**a**). Less common types include aorta arising from right-sided RV (**b**) as in D-TGA, left-sided RV (**c**) as in L-TGA and large VSD amounting to single ventricle (**d**)

10.9.13 Pulmonary and Systemic Venous System

Various studies have proven that MDCT is a highly accurate tool in showing thoracic venous anomalies [49–52]. Common venous anomalies associated with PA-VSD include partial and total anomalous pulmonary venous drainage (Fig. 10.17), left-sided superior vena cava (SVC), double SVC (Fig. 10.18), retro-aortic left innominate vein, and interrupted inferior vena cava (IVC). The presence or absence of communicating vein between the double SVC needs to be assessed.

10.9.14 Situs Anomalies

PA-VSD may be associated with asplenia, central liver, right-sided stomach, or left-sided IVC (Fig. 10.19).

10.10 Management

Components of Surgical Repair

(a) Placement of RV–PA conduit
(b) Unifocalization of MAPCAs
(c) VSD closure

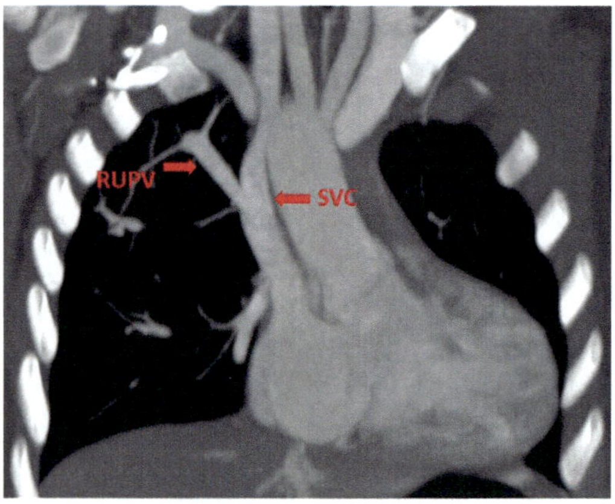

Fig. 10.17 PAPVC in PA-VSD. Coronal maximum-intensity-projection MIP CT image shows right upper lobe pulmonary vein (RUPV) drains into superior vena cava (SVC)

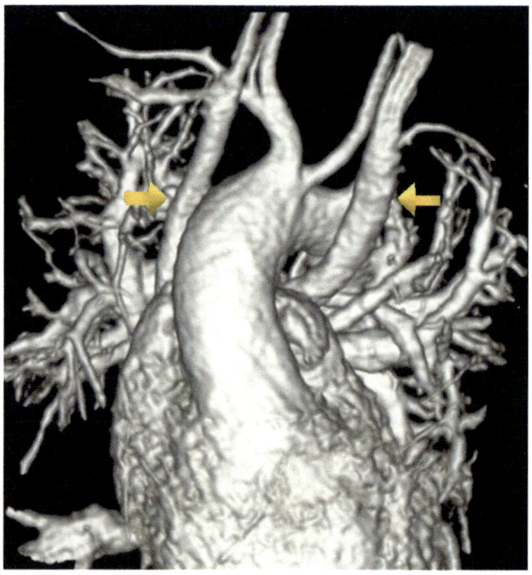

Fig. 10.18 Anterior oblique volume-rendered MR angiography image showing pulmonary atresia, aorta arising from anterior RV associated with double SVC (arrows)

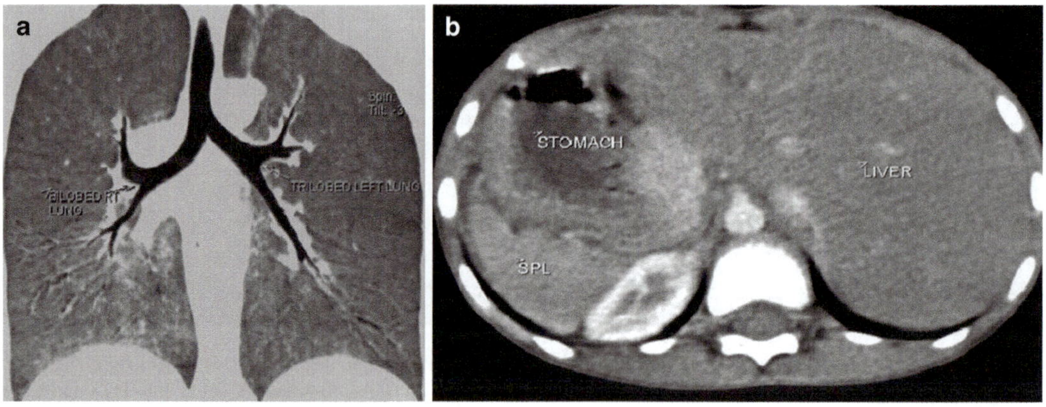

Fig. 10.19 Situs inversus in PA-VSD. (**a**) Minimum-intensity-projection (MinIP) image showing inverted bronchial branching pattern. (**b**) Axial image shows liver on left side, spleen and stomach on right side

These components are performed in single-stage or multi-stage depending on the anatomy and institutional policy.

General Principles of Surgical Repair

"Unifocalization" procedure aims to eliminate extracardiac sources of pulmonary arterial blood flow and a coalition of the largest possible number of pulmonary arterial segments so that they eventually can be incorporated into the RVOT [53] (Figs. 10.20 and 10.21). Connecting as many lung segments as possible to the blood flow from RV during early infancy is essential since the early attrition of these patients occurs during infancy and significant histologic changes occur in pulmonary vasculature during young age. At least 10–16 lung segments need to be connected to the RV–PA conduit in order to have satisfactory hemodynamic results after complete repair [54]. The development of the pulmonary vascular occlusive disease from unrestricted pulmonary blood flow from MAPCAs can develop as early as 4 weeks [55]. Adequacy of the pulmonary vascular bed and the pulmonary vascular resistance are the determinants of postoperative RV pressure which in turn has been closely correlated with surgical outcome.

Closure of VSD at the time of initial repair is desirable in order to avoid the need for further surgery. However, when there are concerns about the adequacy of the pulmonary vascular bed, it is advisable to defer VSD closure. Leaving the VSD unrepaired, helps to avoid supra-systemic RV pressure in the immediate postoperative period by allowing RV to decompress through the VSD. Over a period of months, pulmonary vascular development occurs and the VSD can be closed safely with sub systemic RV pressure. The strategy of delayed VSD closure has reduced operative mortality.

10.10.1 Single-Stage Versus Multi-Stage Approach

10.10.1.1 Single-Stage Approach

The current surgical approach attempts to perform MAPCAs unifocalization and cardiac repair at the same operation, through median sternotomy [56]. With the single-stage surgical repair strategy, it is important to ensure that pulmonary

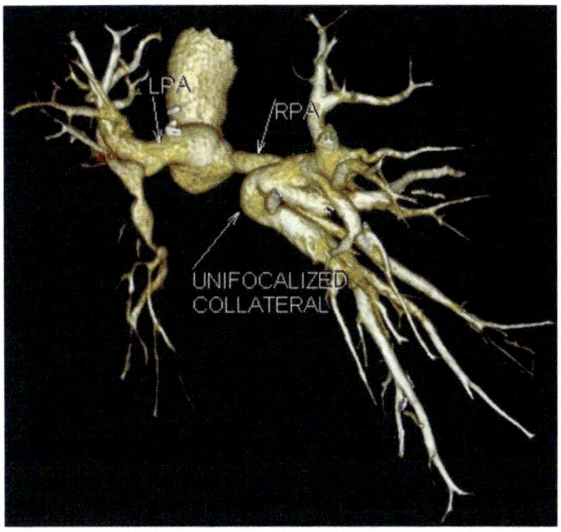

Fig. 10.21 Oblique volume-rendered CT image showing post-unifocalization of collateral to RPA

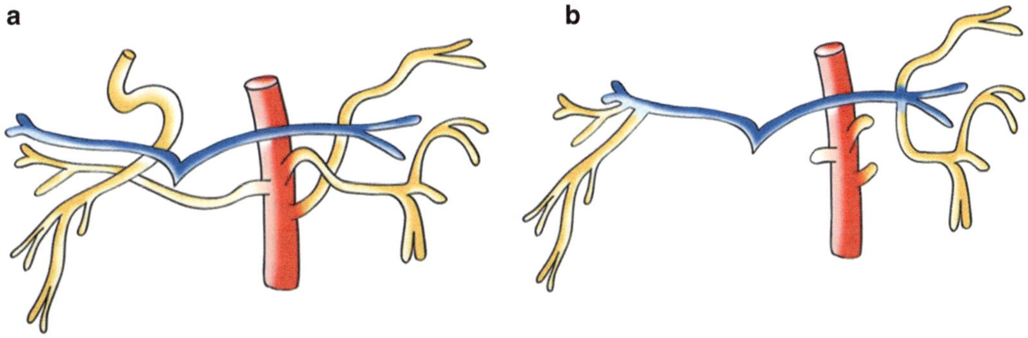

Fig. 10.20 Schematic representation of (**a**) pre- and (**b**) post-unifocalization

vasculature is adequate, both in diameter of proximal pulmonary vessels and development of distal pulmonary vascular bed, for the safe closure of VSD. Newborns with no PDA and adequate collateral dependent pulmonary blood supply with acceptable systemic oxygen saturations are the typical candidates for elective single-stage unifocalization and cardiac repair that is performed at about 3 months of age.

10.10.1.2 Multi-Stage Approach

A subgroup of patients who have relatively small NPAs is treated with systemic-to-pulmonary-artery shunt procedures [57, 58]. Commonly performed shunt procedures for PA-VSD include the aortopulmonary shunt or modified Blalock–Taussig shunt (subclavian artery to pulmonary artery), Glenn shunt (SVC to pulmonary artery), and RV–PA conduit. With absent mediastinal PAs, two modified Blalock–Taussig (BT) shunts are performed to each PA via bilateral thoracotomies. The VSD is typically left open at this first stage. Any possible unifocalization of MAPCAs will also be performed. A subsequent operation will be done to close the VSD, relieve any residual RVOT obstruction, and place a valved conduit.

10.10.1.3 Comparison Between Multi- and Single-Stage Repair

The choice between multi-stage and single-stage repair is dependent on the following various factors:

- Nature of PAs (small vs. adequate size)
- Pulmonary blood flow (duct-dependent or collateral-dependent PBF)
- Age of the patient at presentation
- Status of MAPCAs
- Surgical expertise and results of the institution

Single-stage repair allows for an early normalization of cardiovascular physiology by recruitment of all possible lung segments into RV-derived circulation as early in life as possible. As earlier discussed, early repair preserves pulmonary vascular bed, avoids the development of pulmonary vaso-occlusive disease in the lung segments exposed to systemic pressure via MAPCAs, and hypoplasia of the distal pulmonary vasculature in under-perfused lung segments. Evidence also suggests that long-term cardiac function is preserved by avoiding ventricular dysfunction from prolonged cyanosis and arrhythmias [59].

10.11 Postoperative Assessment Using MDCT and MRI

The value of MR imaging for postsurgical follow-up and planning of reintervention has been well demonstrated [60]. The use of MR imaging for close monitoring of a decrease in right ventricular function, pulmonary artery regurgitation, and other functional parameters is possible and provides objective information for the postoperative evaluation of surgical repair [61].

MDCT also has an expanding role in the comprehensive evaluation of postoperative congenital heart defects [62–65]. RVOT-PA conduit patency, anastomotic site stenosis, or conduit aneurysm can be assessed (Figs. 10.22, 10.23, and 10.24). However, MRI is the preferred method for regular follow-up imaging after an echo. It is especially very useful to assess residual VSD, biventricular function, and to look for myocardial scar. However, post-embolization coils may cause susceptibility artifacts limiting its assessment.

10.11.1 Aortopulmonary Shunts

Aortopulmonary shunts are used to increase the delivery of systemic blood to the lungs, thereby increasing blood oxygenation and decreasing cyanosis. They also help in enlarging the pulmonary arteries for a later stage repair. It is usually done within a few weeks after birth. Four types of aortopulmonary shunts include: (1) The classic Blalock–Taussig shunt: An end-to-side anastomosis between the subclavian artery and the pulmonary artery; (2) The Pott's shunt: Shunt between the LPA and the descending aorta; (3) The Waterston's shunt: Shunt between the RPA

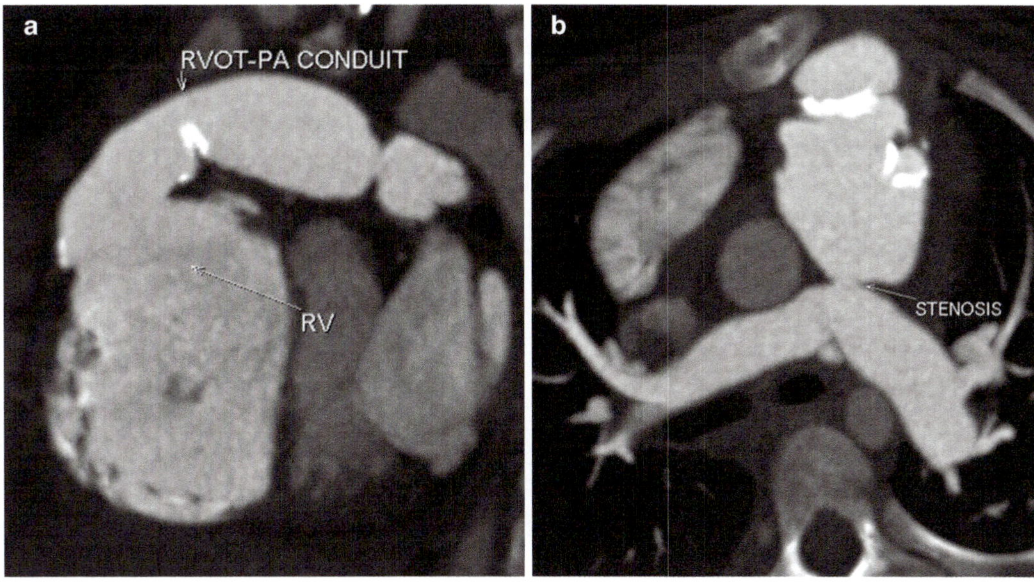

Fig. 10.22 RVOT-PA conduit stenosis. (**a**) Sagittal oblique and (**b**) Axial maximum-intensity-projection (MIP) CT images showing RVOT-PA conduit stenosis at the distal anastomotic site. Few calcifications also noted in conduit

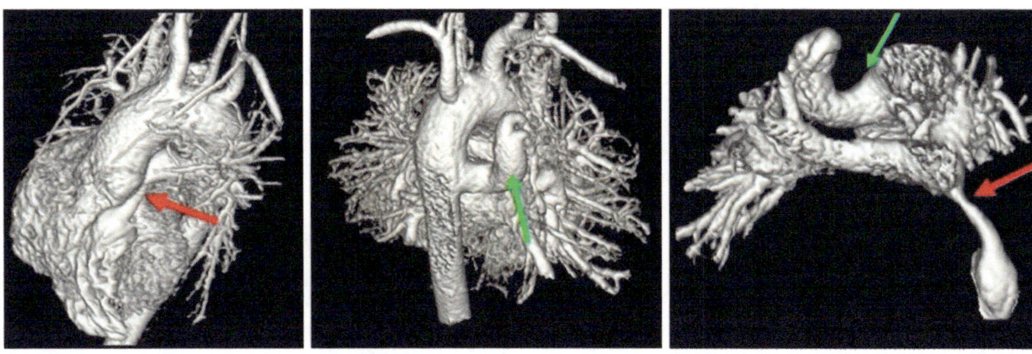

Fig. 10.23 A 27-year-old male with PA-VSD. Status post RV–PA conduit at 5 years of age. MRA showed tight stenosis in the conduit (red arrows) with large MAPCA (green arrows) communicating with native RPA

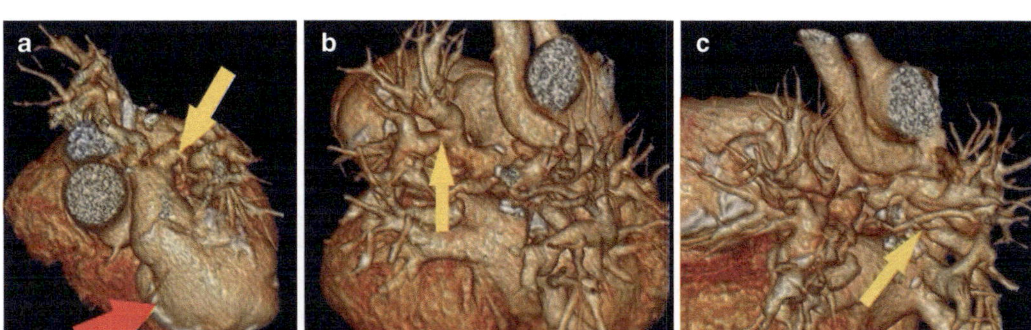

Fig. 10.24 Different views of VRT CTA images showing post-unifocalization changes with aneurysmal dilatation of RVOT and RV to PA conduit (red arrow in **a**) with multiple stenoses at branch PA and anastomotic sites (yellow arrows)

and the ascending aorta; and (4) The modified Blalock–Taussig (BT) shunt: Shunt between one of the branch pulmonary arteries and major branches of the aortic arch (subclavian or innominate artery) with a Gore-Tex tube graft. Among these aortopulmonary shunts, only the modified Blalock–Taussig shunt is performed currently.

Apart from shunt patency, complications of shunt procedures such as shunt stenosis, thrombosis, seroma, pulmonary artery distortion at the shunt insertion site, and shunt infection can be easily diagnosed with MDCT (Figs. 10.25, 10.26, 10.27, and 10.28). MDCT can also detect the rare complication of erosion of the shunt into adjacent viscera. Identification and localization of stenosis of pulmonary arteries distal to the shunt are critical for surgical decision-making regarding reintervention.

10.11.2 Classic Cavopulmonary Shunt (Glenn Operation)

The cavopulmonary shunt, or Glenn operation, is an end-to-side anastomosis between the divided RPA and superior vena cava (SVC), which is ligated between the anastomosis and the right atrium (RA). Not performed in the present scenario.

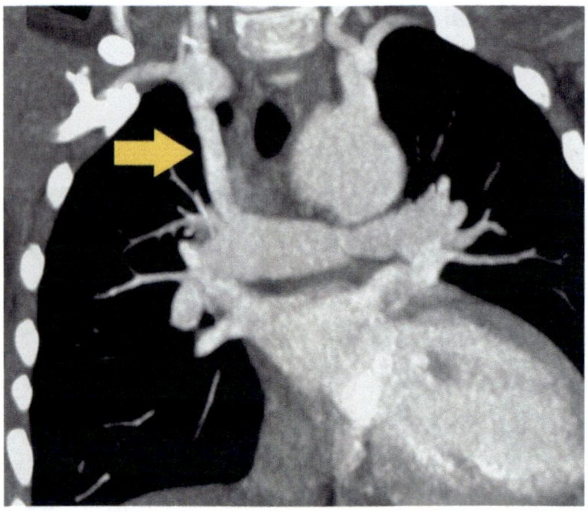

Fig. 10.25 Patent Blalock–Taussig (BT) shunt. Coronal oblique maximum-intensity projection (MIP) CT image shows patent right BT shunt (arrow) from right subclavian artery to right pulmonary artery (RPA)

10.11.3 The Bidirectional Glenn Shunt

The difference in the bidirectional Glenn shunt (BDGS) from the classic Glenn operation is that the RPA is not ligated so that SVC blood flows into both the branch pulmonary arteries (end-to-side anastomosis between the SVC and the undivided RPA). It is less likely to endanger pulmonary vascular obstructive disease compared with systemic–pulmonary shunts, and there is minimal distortion of pulmonary artery architecture. It is better tolerated, and preservation of the pulmonary artery confluence makes the Fontan procedure easier. BDGS is generally performed between 2 and 6 months of life. Complications of the procedure include excessive venous pressure in the SVC with subsequent cerebral edema; pulmonary artery stenosis and thrombosis; and, rarely, protein-losing enteropathy secondary to high pressure in the thoracic duct and intestinal lymphatics.

MDCT can depict the patency of the shunt and in addition, also show the veno-venous collaterals that develop.

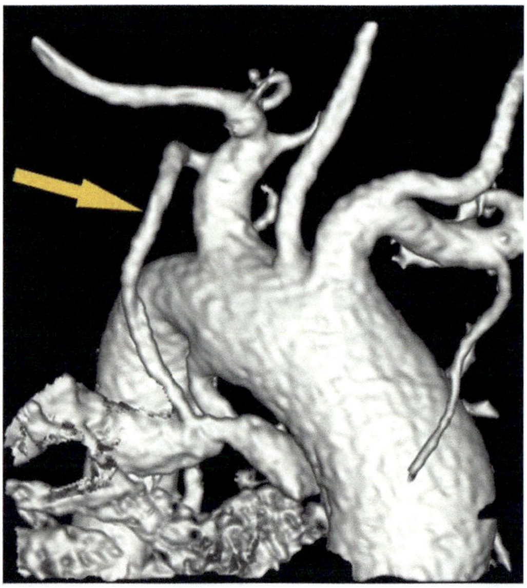

Fig. 10.26 Right oblique volume-rendered (**a**) MR angiography image demonstrating patent BT shunt (arrow) joining confluent pulmonary arteries

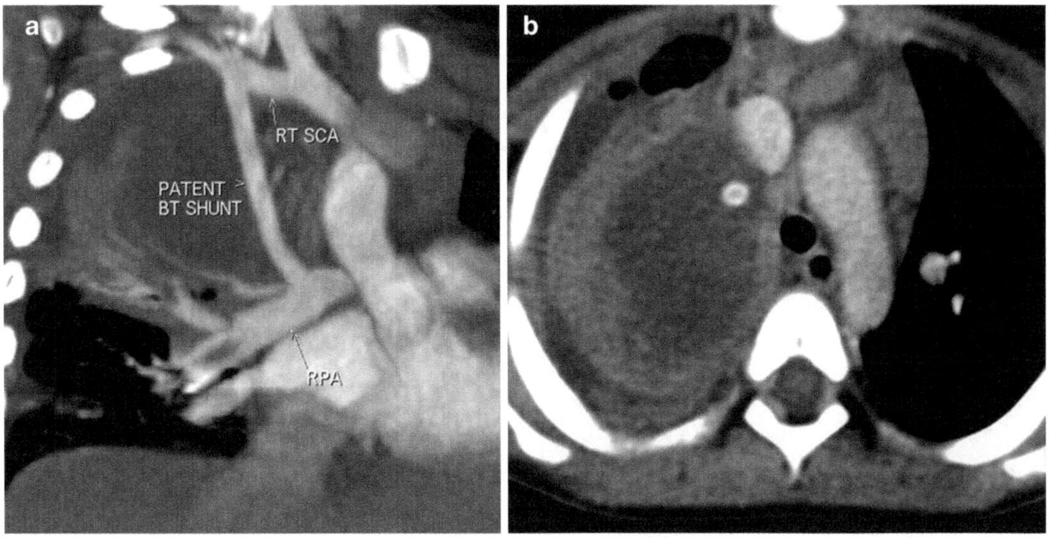

Fig. 10.27 Blocked Blalock–Taussig (BT) shunt. A) Coronal oblique and B) Axial maximum-intensity projection (MIP) CT images show occluded right BT shunt from right subclavian artery to right pulmonary artery (RPA)

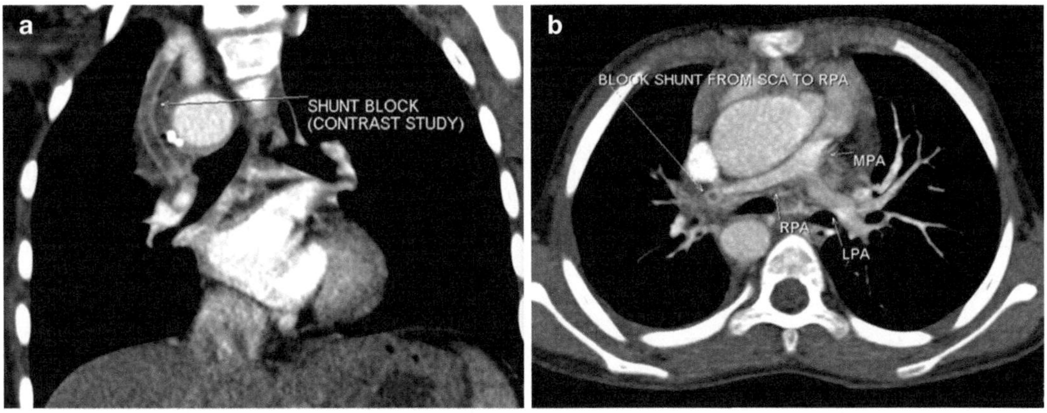

Fig. 10.28 Complication of Blalock–Taussig (BT) shunt. (**a**) Coronal and (**b**) Axial maximum-intensity-projection (MIP) CT images showing perigraft seroma surrounding right BT shunt

10.11.4 Fontan Procedure

The Fontan procedure is the complete right heart bypass, in which venous return from the SVC and inferior vena cava (IVC) are diverted to the PAs (Fig. 10.29). It can be performed either as staged palliation (bidirectional Glenn shunt followed by IVC-to-PA anastomosis at a later age) or as a single-stage procedure in selected cases. This is the final palliative procedure for PA-VSD that is not amenable to biventricular repair. Anatomic complications include narrowing of the Glenn anastomotic site or stenosis of the IVC-to-PA conduit.

Note should be made that to evaluate Fontan circuit patency on MDCT, a delayed run in routine CT protocol to show the patency of Fontan circuit. Another alternative way is to inject contrast simultaneously from upper and lower limb veins to achieve uniform opacification in both circuits at the same time.

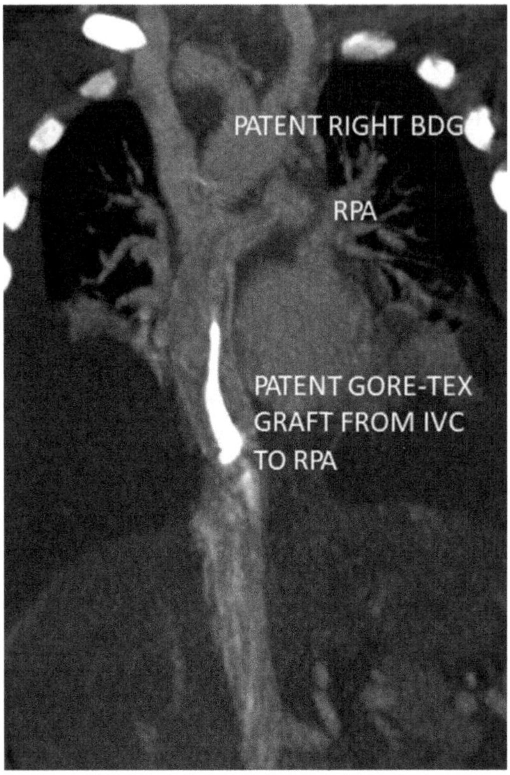

Fig. 10.29 Coronal maximum-intensity projection (MIP) CT image shows patent fontan circuit—right superior vena cava (SVC)-to-right pulmonary artery (RPA) bidirectional Glenn (BDG) shunt and inferior vena cava (IVC)-to-RPA

10.12 Limitations of MDCT

The main disadvantage of MDCT is radiation exposure, a factor to be considered particularly in regard to children [66–70]. All efforts should be taken to keep radiation exposure as low as possible during scanning [71]. We found that all clinically relevant diagnostic information can be obtained using low dose non-ECG-gated MDCT. A drawback of non-ECG-gated MDCT compared with catheter angiography is that it is a relatively static imaging method best suited for morphologic assessment.

Key Points

- Variations in pulmonary blood supply make each patient of PA-VSD unique and warrant individualized planning of surgical strategies.
- MDCT and MRI technologies have proved to be an invaluable diagnostic and decision-making tool for the management of patients with PA-VSD.
- MDCT angiography can answer specific questions like the status of native PAs, PDA, mapping of MAPCAs, and isolated versus dual supply of lung segments.

References

1. Tchervenkov CI, Roy N. Congenital heart disease nomenclature and database project: pulmonary atresia - ventricular septal defect. Ann Thorac Surg. 2000;69:S97–S105.
2. O'Leary PW, Edwards WD, Julsrud PR, Puga FJ. Pulmonary atresia and ventricular septal defect. In: Allen HD, Driscoll DJ, Shaddy RE, Feltes TF, editors. Moss and Adam's heart disease in infants, children, and adolescents. Baltimore, MD: Lippincott Williams & Wilkins; 2008. p. 878–88.
3. Liao PK, Edwards WD, Julsrud PR, Puga FJ, Danielson GK, Feldt RH. The pulmonary blood supply in patients with pulmonary atresia and ventricular septal defect. J Am Coll Cardiol. 1985;6:1343–50.
4. Lee T, Tsai I, Fu Y, et al. Using multidetector-row CT in neonates with complex congenital heart disease to replace diagnostic cardiac catheterization for anatomical investigation: initial experiences in technical and clinical feasibility. Pediatr Radiol. 2006;36:1273–82.
5. Bean MJ, Pannu H, Fishman EK. Three-dimensional computed tomographic imaging of complex congenital cardiovascular abnormalities. J Comput Assist Tomogr. 2005;29:721–4.
6. McElhinney DB, Reddy MV, Hanley FL. Tetralogy of Fallot with major aortopulmonary collaterals: early total repair. Pediatr Cardiol. 1998;19:289–96.
7. Van Praagh R, Van Praagh S. The anatomy of common aorticopulmonary trunk (truncus arteriosus communis) and its embryologic implications: a study of 57 necropsy cases. Am J Cardiol. 1965;16:406.
8. Haworth SG, Rees PG, Taylor JFN, et al. Pulmonary atresia with ventricular septal defect and major aorta pulmonary collateral arteries: effect of systemic pulmonary anastomosis. Br Heart J. 1981;45:133–41.
9. Acherman RJ, Smallhorn JF, Freedom RM. Echocardiographic assessment of pulmonary blood supply in patients with pulmonary atresia and ventricular septal defect. J Am Coll Cardiol. 1996;28:1308–13.
10. Hofbeck M, Sunnegardh J, Burrows PE, et al. Analysis of survival in patients with pulmonic valve atresia and ventricular septal defect. Am J Cardiol. 1991;67:737–43.

11. Ellis K. The bronchial arteries and anomalous systemic arteries to the lungs in congenital heart and lung disease. In: Butler J, editor. The bronchial circulation. New York, NY: Marcel Dekker; 1992. p. 599–748.
12. Botenga ASJ. The significance of bronchopulmonary anastomosis in pulmonary anomalies: a selective angiography study. Radiol Clin Biol. 1969;38:309–28.
13. Liebow AA, Hales MR, Bloomer WE. Relation of bronchial to pulmonary vascular tree. In: Adams WR, Veith I, editors. Pulmonary circulation: an international symposium. New York, NY: Grune & Stratton; 1959. p. 79–98.
14. Diethelm E, Soto B, Nath PH, Bargeron LM, Kirklin JK. The pulmonary vascularity in patients with pulmonary atresia and ventricular septal defect. Radiographics. 1985;5:243–54.
15. Bull C, Somerville J, Ty E, Spiegelhalter D. Presentation and attrition in complex pulmonary atresia. J Am Coll Cardiol. 1995;25:491–9.
16. Smyllie JH, Sutherland GR, Keeton BR. The value of Doppler color flow mapping in determining pulmonary blood supply in infants with pulmonary atresia with ventricular septal defect. J Am Coll Cardiol. 1989;14:1759–65.
17. Mackie AS, Gauvreau K, Perry SB, Nido PJ, Geva T. Echocardiographic predictors of aortopulmonary collaterals in infants with tetralogy of Fallot and pulmonary atresia. J Am Coll Cardiol. 2003;41:852–7.
18. Beekman RP, Beek FJ, Meijboom EJ. Usefulness of MRI for the pre-operative evaluation of the pulmonary arteries in the tetralogy of Fallot. Magn Reson Imaging. 1997;15(9):1005–15.
19. Greenberg SB, Crisci KL, Koenig P, Robinson B, Anisman P, Russo P. Magnetic resonance imaging compared with echocardiography in the evaluation of pulmonary artery abnormalities in children with tetralogy of Fallot following palliative and corrective surgery. Pediatr Radiol. 1997;27(12):932–5.
20. Duerinckx AJ, Wexler L, Banerjee A, Higgins SS, Hardy CE, Helton G, Rhee J, Mahboubi S, Higgins CB. Postoperative evaluation of pulmonary arteries in congenital heart surgery by magnetic resonance imaging: comparison with echocardiography. Am Heart J. 1994;128:1139–46.
21. Boechat MI, Ratib O, Williams PL, et al. Imaging and MR angiography for assessment of complex tetralogy of Fallot and pulmonary atresia. Radiographics. 2005;25:1535–46.
22. Oguz B, Haliloglu M, Karcaaltincaba M. Pictorial review: paediatric multidetector CT angiography: spectrum of congenital thoracic vascular anomalies. Br J Radiol. 2007;80:376–83.
23. Prasad SK, Soukias N, Hornung T, et al. Role of magnetic resonance angiography in the diagnosis of major aortopulmonary collateral arteries and partial anomalous pulmonary venous drainage. Circulation. 2004;109:207–14.
24. Geva T, Greil GF, Marshall AC, Landzberg M, Powell AJ. Gadolinium-enhanced 3-dimensional magnetic resonance angiography of pulmonary blood supply in patients with complex pulmonary stenosis or atresia; comparison with x-ray angiography. Circulation. 2002;106:473–8.
25. Vijarnsorn C, Rutledge JM, Tham EB. Which cardiovascular magnetic resonance planes and sequences provide accurate measurements of branch pulmonary artery size in children with right ventricular outflow tract obstruction? Int J Cardiovasc Imaging. 2014;30:329–38.
26. Holmqvist C, Hochbergs P, Bjorkhem G, Brockstedt S, Laurin S. Pre-operative evaluation with MR in tetralogy of Fallot and pulmonary atresia with ventricular septal defects. Acta Radiol. 2001;42(1):63–9.
27. Goo HW, Park IS, Ko JK, et al. CT of congenital heart disease: normal anatomy and typical pathologic conditions. Radiographics. 2003;23:S147–65.
28. Westra SJ, Hill JA, Alejos JC, Galindo A, Boechat MI, Laks H. Three-dimensional helical CT of pulmonary arteries in infants and children with congenital heart disease. AJR. 1999;173:109–15.
29. Greil GF, Kuettner A, Schoebinger M, et al. Visualization of peripheral pulmonary artery stenosis using high-resolution multidetector computed tomography. Vasc Med. 2005;10:235–6.
30. Rajeshkannan R, Moorthy S, Sreekumar KP, Ramachandran PV, Kumar RK, Remadevi KS. Role of 64-MDCT in evaluation of pulmonary atresia with ventricular septal defect. AJR Am J Roentgenol. 2010 Jan;194(1):110–8.
31. Duddalwar VA. Multislice CT angiography: a practical guide to CT angiography in vascular imaging and intervention. Br J Radiol. 2004;77:S27–38.
32. Greil GF, Schoebinger M, Kuettener A, et al. Imaging of aortopulmonary collateral arteries with high-resolution multidetector CT. Pediatr Radiol. 2006;36:502–9.
33. Murai S, Hamada S, Yamamoto S, et al. Evaluation of major aortopulmonary collateral arteries (MAPCAs) using three-dimensional CT angiography: two case reports. Radiat Med. 2004;22:186–9.
34. Maeda E, Akahane M, Kato N, et al. Assessment of major aortopulmonary collateral arteries with multidetector-row computed tomography. Radiat Med. 2006;24:378–83.
35. Piehler JM, Danielson GK, McGoon DC, Wallace RB, Fulton RE, Mair DD. Management of pulmonary atresia with ventricular septal defect and hypoplastic pulmonary arteries by right ventricular outflow construction. J Thorac Cardiovasc Surg. 1980;80:552–67.
36. Blackstone EH, Kirklin JK, Bertranou EG, Labrosse CJ, Soto B, Bargeron LM Jr. Preoperative prediction from cineangiograms of postrepair right ventricular pressure in tetralogy of Fallot. J Thorac Cardiovasc Surg. 1979;78:542–52.
37. Nakata S, Imai Y, Takanashi Y, Kurosawa H, Tezuka K, Nakazawa M, Ando M, Takao A. A new method for the quantitative standardization of cross-sectional area of the pulmonary arteries in congenital heart diseases with decreased pulmonary blood flow. J Thorac Cardiovasc Surg. 1984;88:610–9.

38. Reddy MV, Petrossian E, McElhinney DB, Moore P, Teitel DF, Hanley FL. One stage complete unifocalization in infants: when should the ventricular septal defect be closed? J Thorac Cardiovasc Surg. 1997;113:858–68.
39. Kirklin JW, Bargeron LM Jr, Pacifico AD, Soto B, Kirklin JK. Management of the tetralogy of Fallot with large aortopulmonary collateral arteries. In: Godman MJ, editor. Paediatric cardiology, vol. 4. New York, NY: Churchill Livingstone; 1981. p. 483–91.
40. Siegel MJ. Multiplanar and three-dimensional multidetector row CT of thoracic vessels and airways in the pediatric population. Radiology. 2003;229:641–50.
41. Lee EY, Siegel MJ, Hildebolt CF, Gutierrez FR, Bhalla S, Fallah JH. MDCT evaluation of thoracic aortic anomalies in pediatric patients and young adults: comparison of axial, multiplanar, and 3D images. AJR. 2004;182:777–84.
42. Ghanaati H, Motevalli M, Tabib A, Almasi A, Noohi F. Multidetector CT evaluation of congenital heart disease: a pictorial essay. Iran J Radiol. 2007;4:209–16.
43. Bharati S, Paul MH, Idriss FS, Potkin RT, Lev M. The surgical anatomy of pulmonary atresia with ventricular septal defect: pseudotruncus. J Thorac Cardiovasc Surg. 1975;69:713–21.
44. Dabizzi RP, Teodori G, Barletta GA, Caprioli G, Baldrighi G, Baldrighi V. Associated coronary and cardiac anomalies in the tetralogy of Fallot: an angiographic study. Eur Heart J. 1990;11:692–704.
45. Manghat NE, Morgan-Hughes GJ, Marshall AJ, Roobottom CA. Multidetector row computed tomography: imaging congenital coronary artery anomalies in adults. Heart. 2005;91:1515–22.
46. Hekmat M, Rafieyian S, Foroughi M, Tehrani MM, Monfared MB, Hassantash SA. Associated coronary anomalies in 135 Iranian patients with tetralogy of Fallot. Asian Cardiovasc Thorac Ann. 2005;13:307–10.
47. Li J, Soukias ND, Carvalho JS, Ho SY. Coronary arterial anatomy in tetralogy of Fallot: morphological and clinical correlations. Heart. 1998;80:174–83.
48. Goo HW, Park IS, Ko JK, Kim YH, Seo DM, Yun TJ, et al. Visibility of the origin and proximal course of coronary arteries on non-ECG-gated heart CT in patients with congenital heart disease. Pediatr Radiol. 2005;35:792–8.
49. Agarwal PP, Seely JM, Matzinger FR. MDCT of anomalous unilateral single pulmonary vein. AJR. 2004;183:1241–3.
50. Gilkeson RC, Haaga JR, Ciancibello LM. Anomalous unilateral single pulmonary vein: MDCT findings. AJR. 2000;175:1464–5.
51. Lawler LP, Corl FM, Fishman EK. Multi-detector row and volume-rendered CT of the normal and accessory flow pathways of the thoracic systemic and pulmonary veins. Radiographics. 2002;22:S45–60.
52. Demos TC, Posniak HV, Pierce KL, Olson MC, Muscato M. Venous anomalies of the thorax. AJR. 2004;182:1139–50.
53. Ishibashi N, Shin'oka T, Ishiyama M, Sakamoto T, Kurosawa H. Clinical results of staged repair with complete unifocalization for pulmonary atresia with ventricular septal defect and major aortopulmonary collateral arteries. Eur J Cardiothorac Surg. 2007;32:202–8.
54. Shimazaki Y, Tokusan Y, Lio M, Nakano S, et al. Pulmonary artery pressure and resistance late after repair of tetralogy of Fallot with pulmonary atresia. J Thorac Cardiovasc Surg. 1990;100:425–40.
55. Reddy MV, Wong J, Liddicoat JR, et al. Altered endothelium dependent responses in lambs with pulmonary hypertension and increased pulmonary blood flow. Am J Physiol. 1996;271:H562–70.
56. Balaguru D, Dilawar M. Pulmonary atresia with ventricular septal defect: systematic review. Heart Views. 2007;8:52–61.
57. Rodefeld MD, Reddy VM, Thompson LD, et al. Surgical creation of aortopulmonary window in selected patients with pulmonary atresia with poorly developed aortopulmonary collaterals and hypoplastic pulmonary arteries. J Thorac Cardiovasc Surg. 2002;123:1147–54.
58. Tchervenkov CI, Salasidis G, Cecere R, et al. Onestage midline unifocalization and complete repair in infancy versus multiple-stage unifocalization followed by repair for complex heart disease with major aortopulmonary collaterals. J Thorac Cardiovasc Surg. 1997;114:727–37.
59. Joffe H, Georgakopoulos D, Celermajer DS, et al. Late ventricular arrhythmia is rare after early repair of tetralogy of Fallot. J Am Coll Cardiol. 1994;23:1146.
60. Soulen RL, Donner RM, Capitanio M. Postoperative evaluation of complex congenital heart disease by magnetic resonance imaging. Radiographics. 1987;7(5):975–1000.
61. Rebergen SA, Niezen RA, Helbing WA, van der Wall EE, de Roos A. Cine gradient-echo MR imaging and MR velocity mapping in the evaluation of congenital heart disease. Radiographics. 1996;16(3):467–81.
62. Siegel MJ, Bhalla S, Gutierrez FR, Billadello JB. MDCT of postoperative anatomy and complications in adults with cyanotic heart disease. AJR. 2005;184:241–7.
63. Leschka S, Oechslin E, Husmann L, et al. Preand postoperative evaluation of congenital heart disease in children and adults with 64-section CT. Radiographics. 2007;27:829–46.
64. Spevak PJ, Johnson PT, Fishman EK. Surgically corrected congenital heart disease: utility of 64-MDCT. AJR. 2008;191:854–61.
65. Sato Y, Matsumoto N, Komatsu S, et al. MDCT evaluation of the right ventricle–pulmonary artery bypass

stenosis in corrected tetralogy of Fallot. Int J Cardiol. 2007;115:267–9.
66. Brenner DJ, Hall EJ. Computed tomography: an increasing source of radiation exposure. N Engl J Med. 2007;357:2277–84.
67. Hollingsworth CL, Yoshizumi TT, Frush DP, et al. Pediatric cardiac-gated CT angiography: assessment of radiation dose. AJR. 2007;189:12–8.
68. McCollough CH, Bruesewitz MR, Kofler JM. CT dose reduction and dose management tools: overview of available options. Radiographics. 2006;26:503–12.
69. Brenner D, Elliston C, Hall E, Berdon W. Estimated risks of radiation-induced fatal cancer from pediatric CT. AJR. 2001;176:289–96.
70. Boxt LM. CT angiography in children: it is accurate, but is it safe? JACC Cardiovasc Imaging. 2008;1:340–2.
71. Saxena AK, Prasad K, Kaza RK. Reducing radiation dose to pediatric patients. AJR. 2005;185:1658.

Congenital Pulmonary Venous Anomalies

11

Megha M. Sheth

11.1 Introduction

Anomalous pulmonary venous drainage (APVD) is the drainage of one or more pulmonary veins outside the left atrium. It is crucial to detect these anomalies due to the strong association with congenital heart disease as well as other respiratory anomalies, which have significant implications for patient management. Routine application of CT combined with the relatively non-specific clinical presentation of APVD has resulted in the increased incidental detection of these anomalies. Knowledge is hence important for the imaging specialist is many a time the first person to make a diagnosis, as many of the pulmonary venous anomalies go unnoticed until adulthood.

There is a broad spectrum of pulmonary venous connections that deviate from the usual anatomy and ranges from normal variant drainage to anomalous pulmonary–systemic communications.

Furthermore, pulmonary veins are important locations of arrhythmogenic foci, and radiofrequency (RF) ablation of such sites are used in the treatment of refractory atrial fibrillation. Hence, an imaging road map of these veins is critical before any management.

This chapter will illustrate embryology, normal and variant pulmonary vein anatomy, and imaging findings of varied patterns of APVD.

Finally, we discuss in brief the post-operative cases.

11.2 Embryology of the Pulmonary Veins

Understanding embryology is vital in appreciating the spectrum of APVD. Lung development commences at approximately 26 days of gestation with the respiratory diverticulum, arising from the primitive foregut [1]. The associated venous plexus (splanchnic plexus) communicates with the systemic cardinal and umbilicovitelline veins, thus forming the initial route of pulmonary venous drainage. At 27–29 days, an out-pouching (Common pulmonary vein (CPV)) develops from the posterosuperior wall of the primitive left atrium [2]. This out-pouching subsequently begins to communicate with the pulmonary venous component of the splanchnic plexus. Side by side the systemic veins involute, and thus two separate venous systems and four separate pulmonary veins draining into the left atrium develop. Any aberration in this process leads to the various types of anoma-

Electronic Supplementary Material The online version of this chapter (https://doi.org/10.1007/978-981-15-6755-1_11) contains supplementary material, which is available to authorized users.

M. M. Sheth (✉)
U.N. Mehta Institute of Cardiology and Research Centre, Ahmedabad, Gujarat, India

R. Rajeshkannan et al. (eds.), *CT and MRI in Congenital Heart Diseases*,
https://doi.org/10.1007/978-981-15-6755-1_11

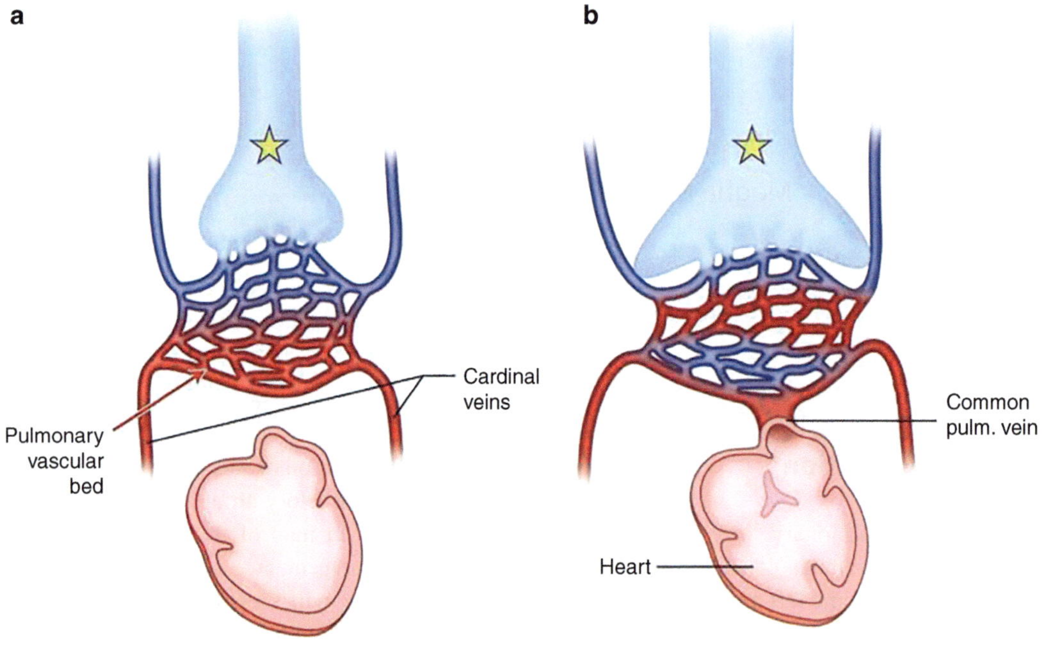

Fig. 11.1 (**a**) At post-conceptional Days 27–29, the primordial lung buds drain through a vascular bed to the cardinal veins, which will develop into systemic veins. (**b**) By Days 32–33, the common pulmonary vein forms from the left atrium and establishes a connection with the pulmonary venous circulation. Pulmonary venous connections to systemic veins begin to regress and pulmonary venous blood drains into the common pulmonary vein. At term systemic veins completely regress and four different pulmonary veins drain into the left atrium

lous venous drainage. Failure of incorporation of the normal pulmonary veins into the left atrium may also occur (cor triatriatum).

The schematic representation of pulmonary vein development has been done in Fig. 11.1a, b.

11.3 Normal Pulmonary Venous Anatomy

At the pulmonary hilum, the location of the superior pulmonary veins is anterior and inferior to the pulmonary arteries. The pulmonary veins traverse along the intersegmental septa while the segmental arteries traverse adjacent to the corresponding bronchus [3].

The pulmonary veins are not perfectly round but rather oval, the anteroposterior diameter being smaller than the superoinferior diameter, especially in the left veins [4, 5].

Practical Tips *The diameter of the pulmonary veins generally increases as they approach the left atrium, except for the left inferior pulmonary vein (LIPV), the diameter of which usually decreases as it enters the atrium, a finding that must be taken into consideration when evaluating possible stenosis at this location* [5] (Fig. 11.2).

Another feature of the pulmonary veins is that they have an intrapericardial portion in their central segment near the left atrium. The left superior pulmonary vein *(LSPV)* has the longest intrapericardial segment, which ranges from 11 to 13.7 mm; and the right inferior pulmonary vein *(RIPV)* has the shortest intrapericardial segment, which ranges from 4.5 to 11 mm [6].

The pulmonary veins are also covered with a myocardial layer known as "myocardial sleeves"

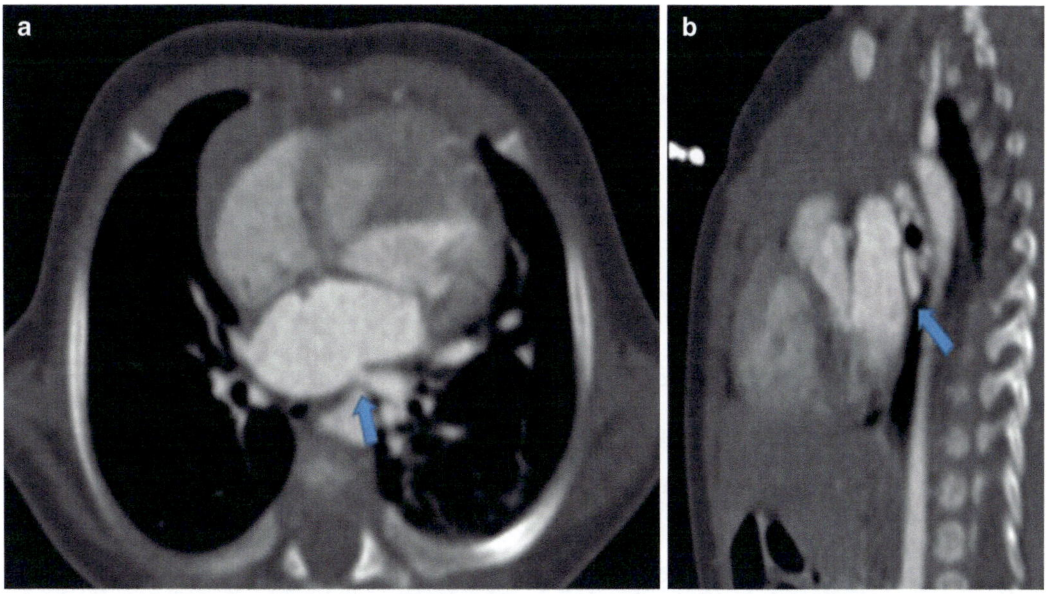

Fig. 11.2 Be careful while reporting stenosis of left inferior pulmonary vein. Axial (**a**) and sagittal (**b**) images showing mild normal anteroposterior narrowing of the left inferior pulmonary vein into the left atrium (arrow)

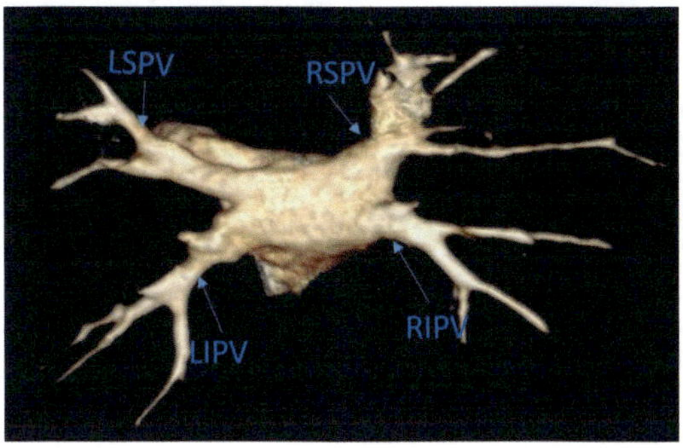

Fig. 11.3 CT VRT image (posterior view of the left atrium) showing the commonest arrangement of four pulmonary veins draining into LA

extending from the left atrium for an average length of 9.3 mm [7].

The usual commonest arrangement pattern of pulmonary veins consists of four separate pulmonary veins: right and left superior and inferior veins each, which drain individually into the left atrium (Fig. 11.3). Generally, the right superior pulmonary vein (RSPV) drains right upper and middle lobes of the lung, RIPV drains the right lower lobe; LSPV drains the left upper lobe including lingula and LIPV drains the left lower lobe. This anatomical arrangement is found in 60–70% of the population [8].

11.4 Normal Variant Pulmonary Venous Drainage

A wide variation of normal variant pulmonary venous drainage exists and is a common incidental finding. Normal variants typically consist of conjoined or accessory veins [9]. So the term normal variant is more suitable as it implies most common to least common patterns observed rather than an anomalous pulmonary venous drainage.

Figure 11.4 shows a schematic representation of normal and variant pulmonary venous drainage.

When the superior and inferior pulmonary veins on the same side unite to form a single confluence before entering the left atrium, it results in a conjoined vein and a single ostium (opening) into the left atrium. They are more common on the left. The common trunk can be long or short.

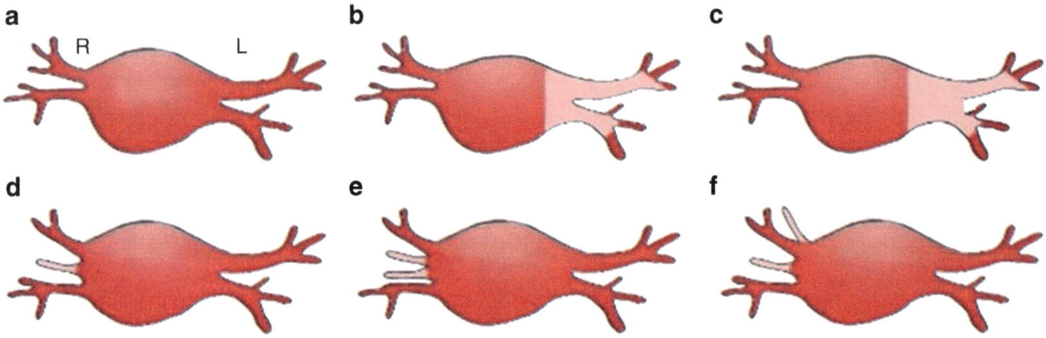

Fig. 11.4 Normal and variant pulmonary venous arrangements (**a**) is the commonest arrangement showing two right and two left pulmonary veins draining into LA; (**b**) shows a short left common trunk of LSPV and LIPV; (**c**) shows a long common trunk of LSPV and LIPV; (**d**) shows an accessory right middle lobe pulmonary vein; (**e**) shows two accessory right middle lobe pulmonary veins and (**f**) shows accessory right upper as well as right middle lobe pulmonary veins

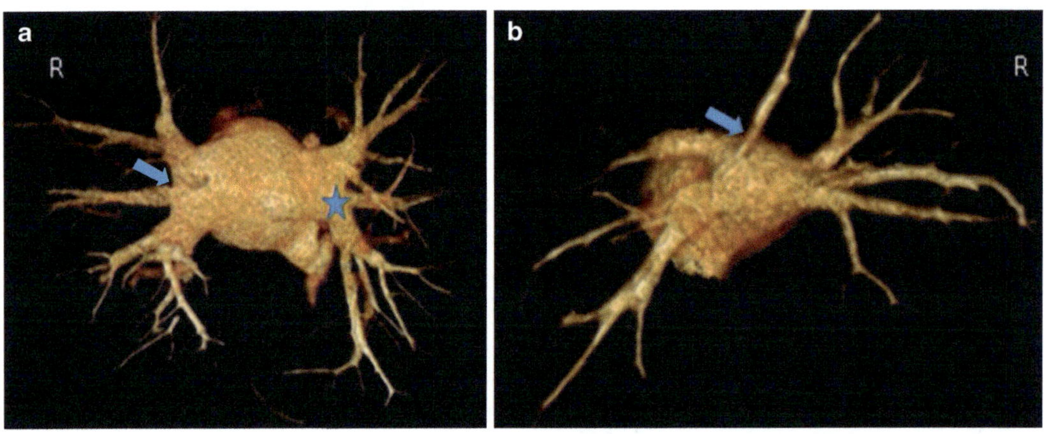

Fig. 11.5 (**a**) CT VRT image (posterior view of the left atrium) showing a variation wherein left-sided pulmonary veins form a common channel (indicated by blue star) and an accessory right middle lobe pulmonary vein (indicated by the blue arrow) draining separately into LA. (**b**) CT VRT image (posterior view of the left atrium) of another patient, showing accessory right upper lobe pulmonary vein (blue arrow) draining separately into LA

Accessory (or supernumerary) veins are separate from the superior or inferior pulmonary veins with an independent opening into the left atrium. These supernumerary variants usually have a narrower ostium than normal, contrary to a conjoined vein which has a large opening [10]. Accessory pulmonary veins may be seen in 30% of patients [11]. Again the supernumerary veins are more commonly observed on the right side, with a supernumerary vein draining right middle lobe more commonly observed in up to 26% patients than an accessory right upper lobe vein [11] (Fig. 11.5a, b).

Practical Tips *This road mapping of variants of pulmonary venous drainage patterns is very important prior to RF ablation in patients of refractory atrial fibrillation.*

11.5 Imaging Modalities

11.5.1 Chest Radiography

These are often done when a patient comes to any clinician for a primary examination. However, it may not lead to suspicion of anomalous drainage and is not useful for specific diagnoses.

11.5.2 Echocardiography

Echocardiography is the initial imaging technique of choice in the evaluation of congenital heart disease, including pulmonary venous anomalies [2].

However, evaluation of pulmonary veins may be suboptimal due to a limited field of view ("echo window") that may prevent the assessment of pulmonary venous structures peripheral to the expected location of the left atrial ostia. In addition, this imaging technique may not be able to completely characterize or even detect associated vascular anomalies.

Its advantage is that it gives real-time functional information like gradient at the site of the stenosis. It is also an operator-dependent modality and needs the expertise to suspect and diagnose anomalous venous drainage.

11.5.3 CT Scan

CT in our present scenario is a widely available modality that is best for imaging morphology in a breath-hold. It excellently depicts vascular structures other than the heart in the thorax [2, 12]. Additional benefits of this imaging technique when using newer MDCT scanners include very rapid imaging that may obviate patient sedation. 3D reconstructed images are excellent at depicting anomalous pulmonary venous structures and help a surgeon in planning surgery. The primary disadvantage of CT is that it requires the use of ionizing radiation. *With newer scanners, there are automated software and iterative reconstruction techniques available that help in reducing the ionizing radiation.* CT also requires the use of intravenous iodinated contrast material, which may adversely affect renal function or rarely result in acute allergic-like reactions.

CT Technique Regarding CT technique, as thin as possible detector collimation should be used to produce isotropically reformatted and 3D volume-rendered images.

Non-ionic low-osmolality (or iso-osmolality) iodinated contrast material (1.5–2.0 ml/kg) is typically administered IV using a power injector at injection rates ranging from 1 to 4 ml/s, depending on patient weight and quality of IV access.

CT image acquisition should be timed for maximum contrast opacification of the left atrium, with either bolus tracking or test bolus injection.

Practical Tips *It is important to acquire two phases of the dynamic CT exam to properly evaluate the pulmonary veins especially when there is suspicion of obstruction.*

The choice of the gated or non-gated scan depends on the individual protocol from institute to institute. *In general non-gated contrast CT is sufficient to delineate anomalous pulmonary venous drainage.*

When doing a CT scan for a suspected supracardiac APVD, it may be useful to inject contrast from the lower limb so that any contrast in a venous structure above the heart can clearly be identified as pulmonary venous origin in the first pass scan. This is particularly helpful when trying to differentiate LSVC from a vertical vein. The converse can be applied to infracardiac anomalies.

Despite the fact that most CT images are evaluated in the transverse plane (axial plane), evaluation of the pulmonary veins solely in this plane is a source of potential error. Pulmonary vein ostia can be quite close to one another, making adjacent ostia appear as one; or a common ostium may be mistaken for two separate ostia if only the branching divisions are appreciated. For this reason, the use of MPR is essential when the identification of the number and branching patterns of the pulmonary veins is necessary.

11.5.4 MRI

MR imaging can be used to evaluate congenital cardiopathies that cause pulmonary vein compromise without any ionizing radiation. Apart from obtaining morphological information, it has the added advantage of obtaining functional information [12].

Gadolinium-enhanced MR angiography (Gd-MRA) is the mainstay of anatomic evaluation. Ventricular volumetry with two-dimensional steady-state free-precession sequences and flow analysis with cine phase-contrast imaging provide physiologic information that may be used to calculate the degree of right heart enlargement and the shunt fraction, allowing to determine the functional importance of the lesion.

ECG gated 3D SSFP sequence is a good alternative to Gd-enhanced MRA. It can be done either with or without Gd contrast [13] (Fig. 11.6).

Drawbacks of MRI include the lengthy duration of the examination and it may be necessary to anesthetize the child. This requires specialized MR compatible anaesthesia trollies and other equipment for patient monitoring. It may be difficult to perform MR imaging in critically ill neonates, patients with claustrophobia, and those unable to cooperate because of their clinical condition.

11.6 Congenital Pulmonary Vein Anomalies

Commonly encountered abnormalities of the pulmonary veins are as follows:

1. Anomalies of pulmonary venous drainage
   (A) Total anomalous pulmonary venous drainage (TAPVD)
   (B) Partial anomalous pulmonary venous drainage (PAPVD)
   (C) Sinus venosus defect
   (D) Congenital pulmonary venolobar syndrome
   (E) Malposition of the septum primum
2. Pulmonary vein stenosis or atresia
   (A) Cor triatriatum
   (B) Congenital pulmonary vein atresia or stenosis
   (C) Recurrent pulmonary vein stenosis after repair of APVD
3. Miscellaneous abnormalities
   (A) Pulmonary varix
   (B) Meandering pulmonary vein

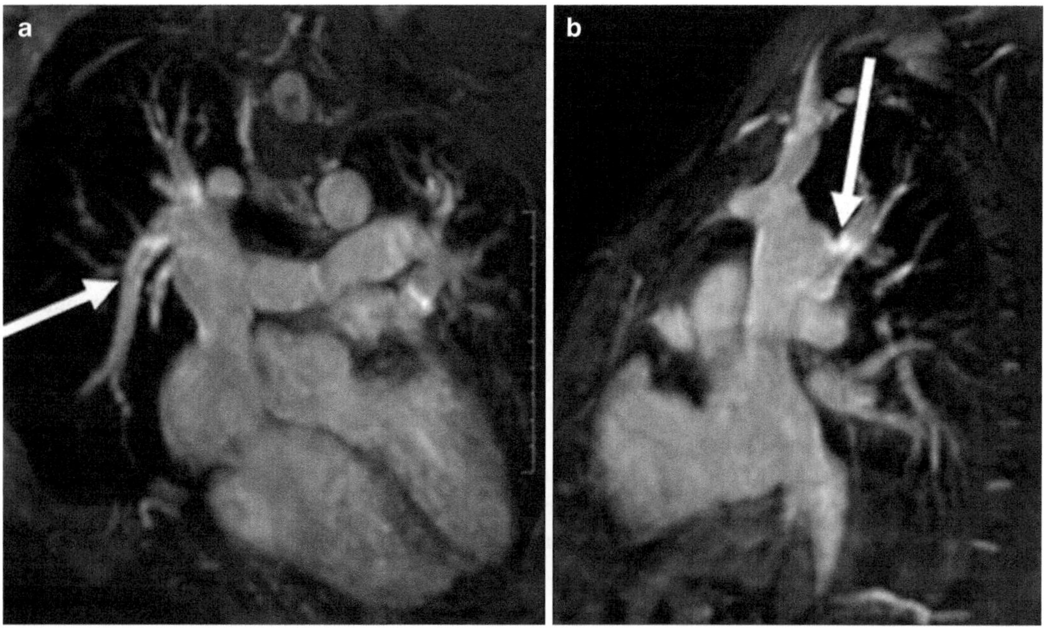

Fig. 11.6 Coronal oblique (**a**) and Sagittal oblique (**b**) MIP of 3D SSFP images showing partial anomalous pulmonary venous drainage into SVC (arrows). ECG gated non-contrast 3D SSFP is a good alternative to Gd-enhanced MRA (Ref to Video 11.1). Image courtesy: Dr. Ramiah Rajeshkannan, Amrita Institute of Medical Sciences, Kochi

(C) Levoatrial cardinal vein
(D) Pulmonary arteriovenous fistula

11.6.1 Total Anomalous Pulmonary Venous Drainage (TAPVD)

This refers to drainage of all four of the pulmonary veins to another cardiovascular structure other than the left atrium and accounts for about 2% of cardiac malformations [14].

Abnormal pulmonary venous return was first described as total anomalous pulmonary venous return (TAPVR) by Wilson [15].

Darling's classification (1957) is the most popular classification of TAPVD [16].

Four types exist, depending on the level of drainage:

- *Type 1—supracardiac:* This accounts for up to 55% of cases and is the most common. It typically involves the convergence of all four pulmonary veins behind the heart to form a common vein. This then drains into the left brachiocephalic vein and henceforth into the SVC.
- *Type 2—cardiac:* abnormal communication at the cardiac level: drainage occurs into the RA or coronary sinus.
- *Type 3—infracardiac:* drainage below the level of the heart or diaphragm, for example into the IVC, portal, or hepatic veins.
- *Type 4—mixed:* drainage at more than one level.

Herlong and colleagues [17] suggested a complete description of TAPVD including:

- Levels of connections—supracardiac, cardiac, infracardiac, or mixed.
- Presence or absence of obstruction.
- Cause of obstruction—extrinsic, intrinsic, or obstructive atrial septal communication.

Incidence—Sex ratio with supradiaphragmatic TAPVD is about equal. Male predominance (4:1) seen in infra diaphragmatic TAPVD.

The supracardiac type is the most common form of TAPVD (Figs. 11.7, 11.8, and 11.9). The pulmonary veins drain to a confluence (usually

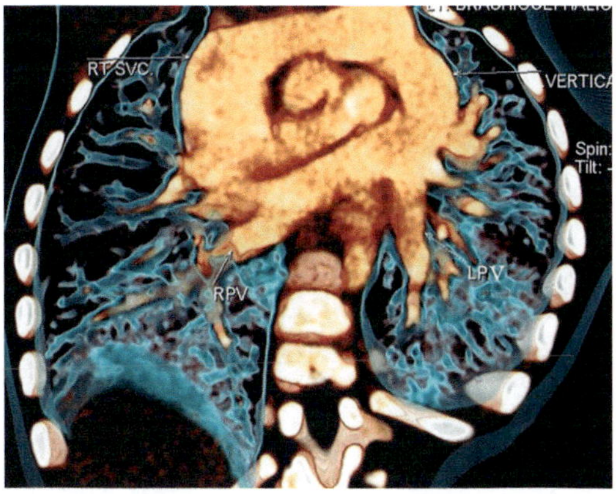

Fig. 11.7 VRT thin images showing non-obstructed supracardiac TAPVD

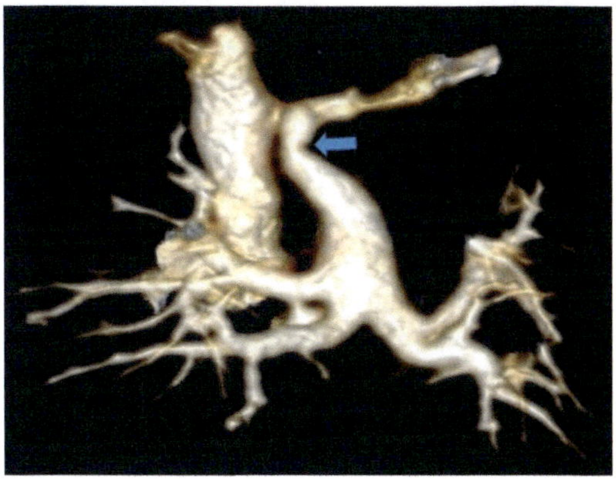

Fig. 11.8 VRT image showing obstructed supracardiac TAPVD, level of obstruction indicated by thick blue arrow

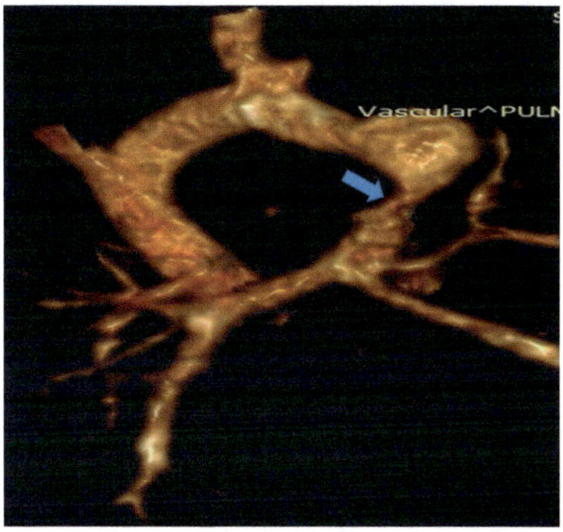

Fig. 11.9 VRT image showing obstructed supracardiac TAPVD, level of obstruction indicated by thick blue arrow

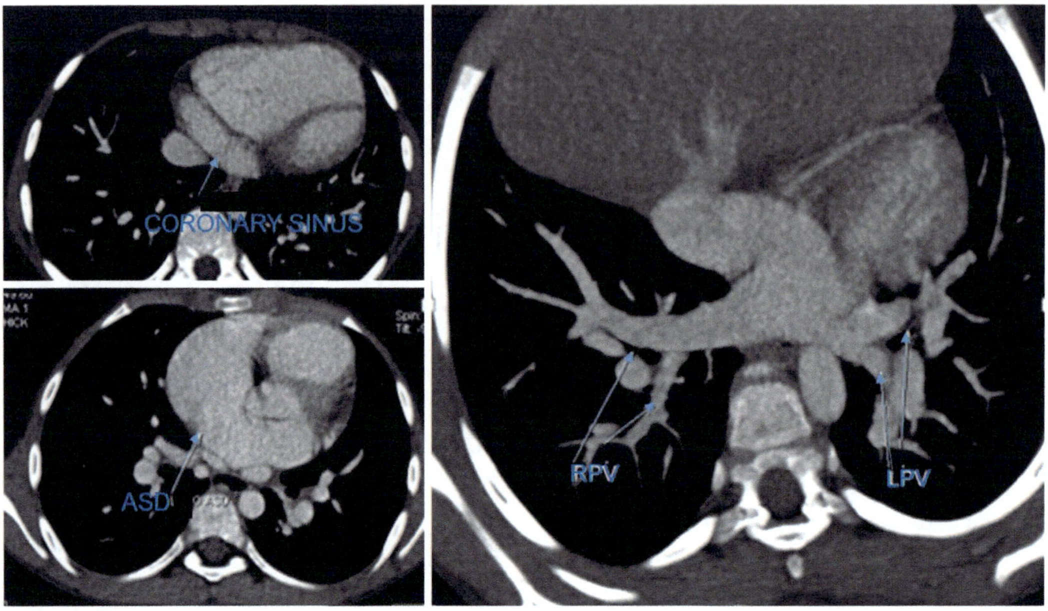

Fig. 11.10 Axial and MPR images showing cardiac TAPVD into coronary sinus

oriented horizontally) posterior to the left atrium (LA). An ascending vertical vein originates from this confluence and travels behind the left atrial appendage and, usually, anterior to the left pulmonary artery (LPA). However, occasionally this vein may travel posterior to LPA and may become trapped between the dilated artery and the left bronchus, leading to pulmonary venous obstruction. The vertical vein finally drains into the innominate vein. Occasionally, the site of the entrance to the innominate vein may also be narrowed, leading to obstruction. The innominate vein and SVC are dilated. The right heart is usually dilated due to volume overload. There is always an atrial septal defect or patent foramen ovale, which is the only source of flow to the left heart.

Practical Tips *In supracardiac TAPVD it is important to mention the presence or absence of obstruction along with the level and course of the anomalous channel.*

It is also important to mention the presence or absence of atrial septal defect and if present, the size of the atrial septal defect.

In the cardiac type of TAPVD (Fig. 11.10), the pulmonary venous confluence connects directly to the RA, usually through the coronary sinus (CS). The pulmonary veins and coronary sinus are significantly dilated, and echocardiography shows a characteristic "whale's tail" appearance. Obstruction is unusual in this form of TAPVD. Less common forms of intracardiac TAPVD include TAPVD directly to the right atrium.

In the infracardiac type of TAPVD (Figs. 11.11, and 11.12), the pulmonary venous confluence drains to systemic veins below the diaphragm. The confluence is usually posterior to LA and vertically oriented (sometimes described as an "inverted fir tree"). From here, a descending vein arises and passes through the esophageal hiatus. Most commonly, this vein connects to the portal vein (at the confluence of the splenic and superior mesenteric veins). Less often, the connection is to the ductus venosus, hepatic veins, or inferior vena cava (IVC). Patients with infracardiac TAPVD have a high prevalence (>90%) of obstruction. Such patients typically present as neonates with severe respiratory distress.

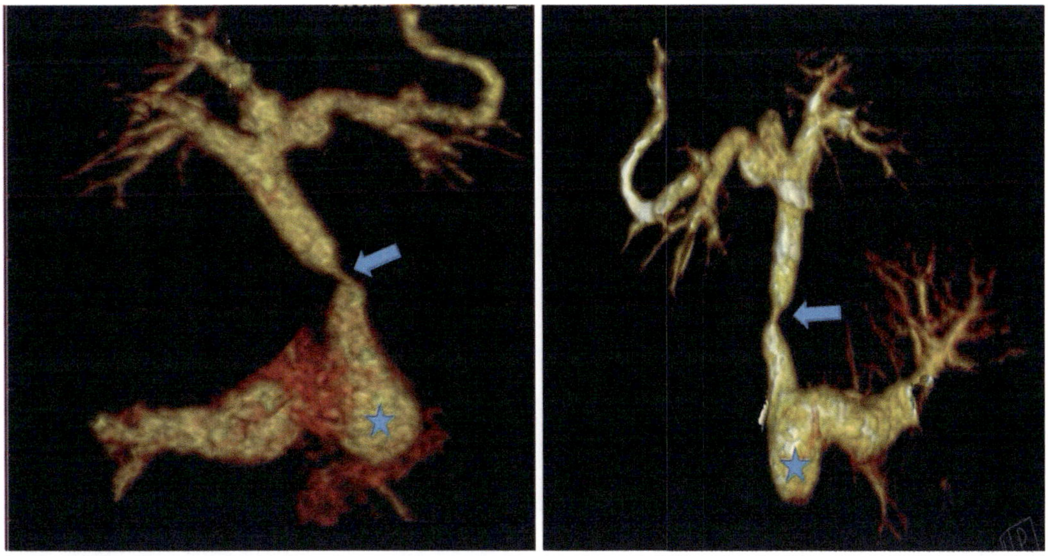

Fig. 11.11 VRT image showing obstructed infraracardiac TAPVD into the portal vein, thick blue arrow indicated severe narrowing at the level of diaphragmatic hiatus and blue star indicated drainage into the portal vein

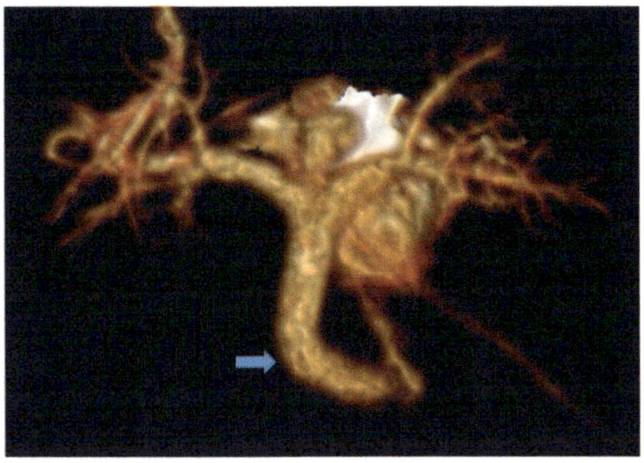

Fig. 11.12 VRT image showing obstructed infraracardiac TAPVD into ductus venosus, thick blue arrow indicates vertical channel

Practical Tips *Infracardiac TAPVD is considered obstructed TAPVD for all practical purposes.*

Patients with mixed TAPVD (Figs. 11.13, 11.14, and 11.15) have varying combinations of the three types described earlier. An example includes the connection of the right pulmonary veins to the coronary sinus and the connection of the left pulmonary veins to the innominate vein.

In patients with TAPVD, a right-to-left shunt is crucial for early survival and this manifests usually in the form of a patent foramen ovale or an atrial septal defect.

So the longevity in TAPVD is related to the size of the atrial septal defect—patients with larger atrial septal defects often surviving longer.

Intrinsic compression occurs due to abnormality in the wall of the anomalous venous channels whereas extrinsic compression may result in the narrowing of the venous structure. For example, when the anomalous venous channel to innominate vein passes between dilated LPA anteriorly and left bronchus posteriorly or anomalous venous connections to the SVC may be obstructed by RPA and trachea.

Another factor that may contribute to the impedance of pulmonary venous return is the length of the ascending or descending vertical venous pathway.

Patients of TAPVD without pulmonary venous obstruction are usually asymptomatic at birth. They may present with tachypnea, feeding difficulties, repeated respiratory tract infections, mild cyanosis. Gradually they develop right heart failure and pulmonary arterial hypertension (PAH).

Patients of TAPVD with obstruction present early in the neonatal period with symptoms of congestive cardiac failure, dyspnea, and severe

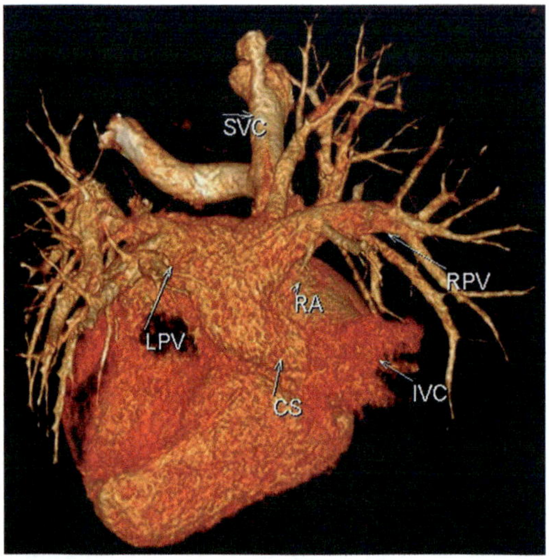

Fig. 11.13 VRT image showing mixed TAPVD with right upper lobe pulmonary veins draining into SVC and rest of pulmonary veins draining into the coronary sinus. *RPV* right pulmonary vein; *RA* right atrium; *LPV* left pulmonary vein; *CS* coronary sinus

cyanosis. Prompt surgical repair is essential, thus it is rarely encountered on CT or MRI. In the vast majority of cases, echocardiography is the mainstay of diagnosis and cross-sectional imaging is usually reserved for when the diagnosis is unclear or incomplete definition of the pulmonary veins at echocardiography [18].

TAPVD is commonly associated with other congenital cardiac lesions like TOF, TGA, Truncus Arteriosus, Tricuspid Atresia, Coarctation Of Aorta, HLHS, single ventricle. A large international multicentre study conducted by Seale et al. (n = 422) showed 14% of patients had associated cardiac lesions, and that if a definitive repair was not performed at the time of surgery this was an independent risk factor for death [19]. In addition, pre- and post-operative pulmonary vein obstruction or stenosis were also independent risk factors for death in multivariate analysis. This highlights the importance of accurate pre- and post-operative anatomical evaluation in this cohort of patients.

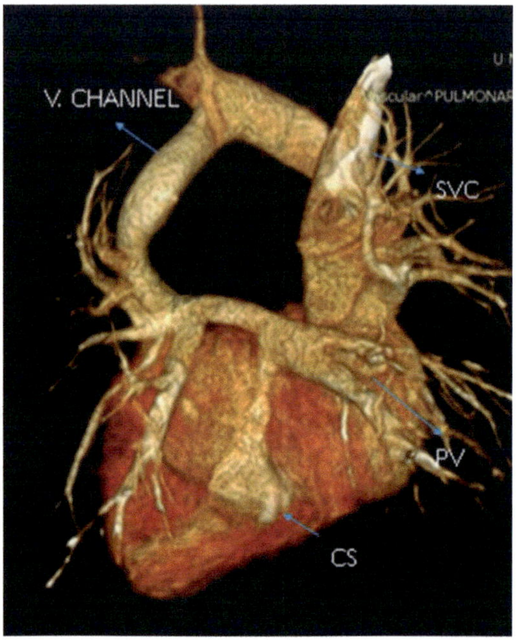

Fig. 11.14 VRT image showing mixed TAPVD with all pulmonary veins draining into SVC as well as into coronary sinus. *PV* pulmonary vein; *CS* coronary sinus; *V. CHANNEL* vertical channel

11.6.1.1 Imaging of TAPVD: Chest Radiography

The right heart is prominent in TAPVD because of the increased flow volume, but the *left atrium* remains normal in size. Types 1 and 2 result in cardiomegaly.

The supra cardiac variant (type 1) can classically depict a "*snowman appearance*" on a frontal chest radiograph, also known as "*figure of 8* heart" or "*cottage loaf heart*". The dilated vertical vein on the left, brachiocephalic vein on top, and the superior vena cava on the right form the head of the snowman; the body of the snowman is formed by the enlarged right atrium.

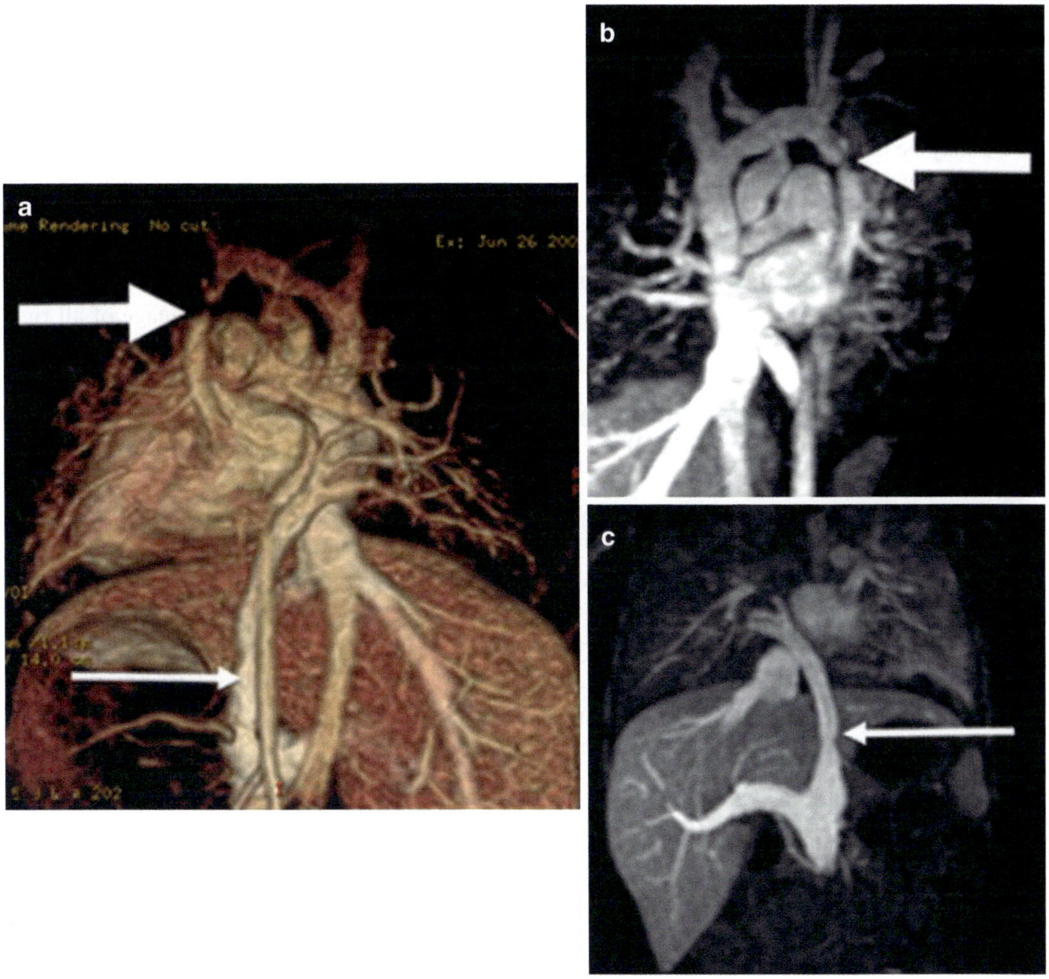

Fig. 11.15 Posterior oblique VRT (**a**), coronal MIP MRA images (**b**, **c**) demonstrating mixed TAPVC. Left pulmonary veins drain via a vertical vein into the left brachiocephalic vein with focal stenosis (thick arrow in **a**, **b**). Right pulmonary veins drain into the portal vein (thin arrow in **a**, **c**). (Ref to Video 11.2). Image courtesy: Dr. Ramiah Rajeshkannan, Amrita Institute of Medical Sciences, Kochi

Echocardiography May show blind-ended left atrium with no connecting veins.

CT/MRA

Direct visualization of anomalous venous return.

Cross-sectional imaging with CT scan accurately depicts the pathway of venous obstruction, the confluent chamber, the level or levels (if more than one) of abnormal drainage, presence or absence of stenosis/obstruction, presence and size of ASD, compression of the anomalous pulmonary channel. MDCT provides all this information over and above the underlying congenital heart disease.

An important point is that patients with TAPVD are usually neonates, who are potentially clinically unstable and require a short and efficient MR imaging study.

CT may be particularly advantageous in critically ill neonates with obstructive TAPVD. Non-gated CT allows accurate diagnosis with very short imaging times, avoiding the need for sedation, and maybe the modality of choice in such critically ill neonates.

11.6.2 Partial Anomalous Pulmonary Venous Drainage (PAPVD)

PAPVD represents the failure of one or more of the pulmonary veins to be incorporated into the left atrium. The anomalous veins empty instead into the systemic circulation. By definition, at least one pulmonary vein must drain normally into the left atrium, else this will be a total anomalous venous drainage.

The prevalence of PAPVD has been reported to be between 0.4% and 0.7% [12]. It is more common on the right side and results in a left-to-right shunt.

The right-sided pulmonary veins most often drain into the embryologic derivatives of the right cardinal vein, usually the superior vena cava (SVC) or inferior vena cava (IVC).

The most common form of PAPVD is the anomalous drainage of the RSPV into the SVC [20] (Figs. 11.16 and 11.17a). This frequently occurs at the junction of the SVC and RA [21]. Occasionally, drainage occurs at a higher level at the junction between the SVC and innominate vein above the level of the azygos vein, or into the azygos vein itself. Other right-sided pulmonary–systemic connections include drainage into the coronary sinus, IVC, or drainage of all right pulmonary veins into the RA.

Anomalous left-sided veins typically empty into derivatives of the left cardinal vein, most often the left innominate vein or the coronary sinus.

Up to 18.2% of PAPVD cases affect the left-sided pulmonary veins (Figs. 11.17a, 11.18, 11.19, and 11.20) [22]. The commonest pattern on the left is the LSPV connected to the left innominate vein [20]. In this condition, a vertically orientated vessel courses lateral to the aortic arch prior to draining into the left innominate vein. This anomalous vein can sometimes be misdiagnosed as a left-sided SVC on CT [20, 23]. Left SVC has no venous drainage from lungs and generally drains into the right atrium through the coronary sinus. The course of the lobar intraparenchymal veins may also be appreciated as they drain

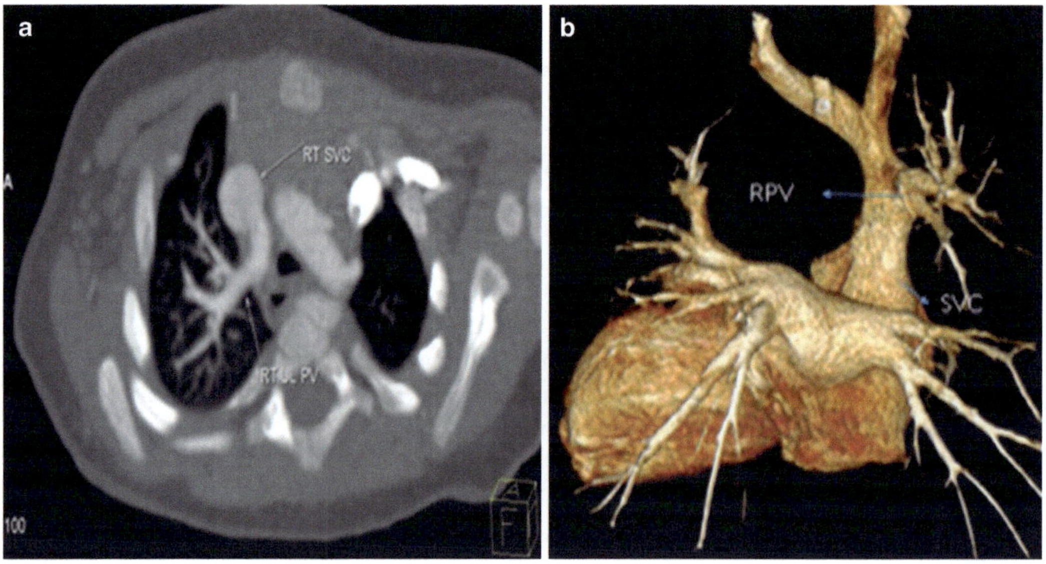

Fig. 11.16 Axial (**a**) and VRT (**b**) images showing PAPVD of right upper lobe pulmonary veins draining into SVC

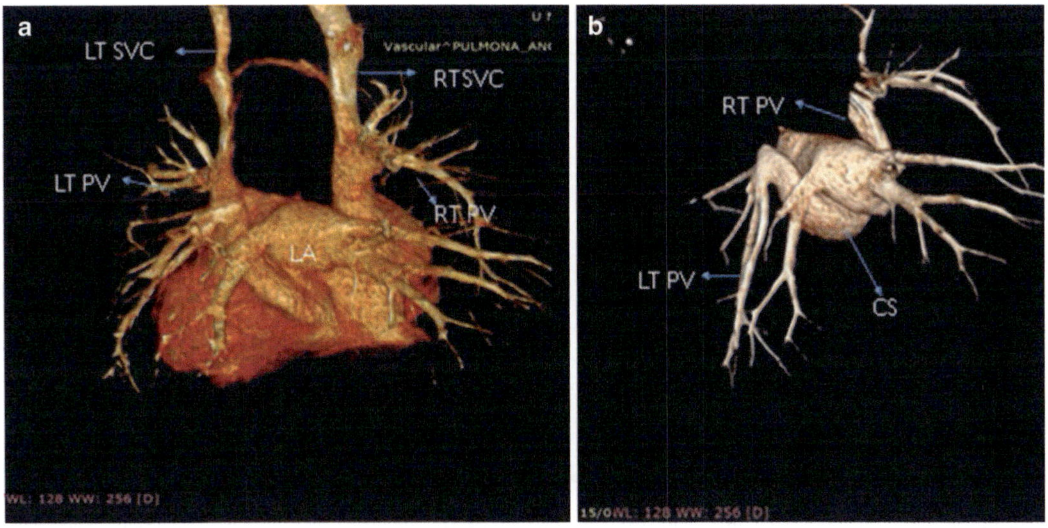

Fig. 11.17 VRT image showing (**a**) pre- as well as (**b**) post-operative case of PAPVD of right upper and left upper lobe pulmonary veins draining into right and left SVC. respectively. *PV* pulmonary vein; *RT* right; *LT* left; *CS* coronary sinus

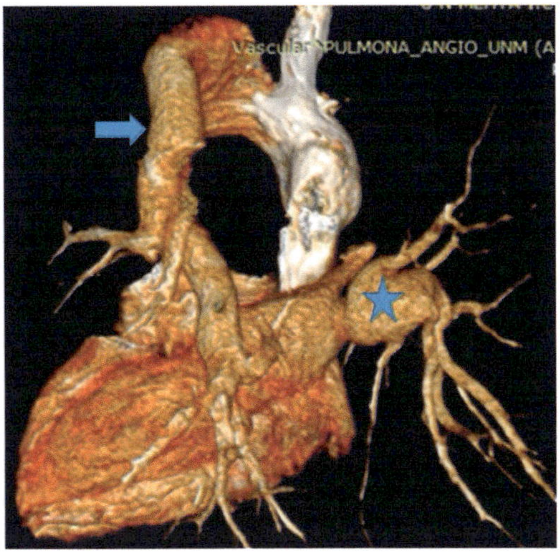

Fig. 11.18 VRT image showing PAPVD of left-sided pulmonary veins (blue arrow) draining into SVC. Venous varix (blue star) of right-sided pulmonary vein

into the anomalous vessel. A further feature of left upper lobe PAPVD is a normal or enlarged left innominate vein, whereas in a persistent left SVC the left innominate vein may be absent or small.

Other described left-sided connections include drainage into the hemiazygos vein or the coronary sinus [24].

Scrutiny of the pulmonary veins is important and the identification of less than four pulmonary veins connected to the left atrium should alert the reader to a diagnosis of PAPVD.

Practical Tips *Never rely only on the number of pulmonary veins draining into the left atrium; as even when there are four pulmonary veins draining into the left atrium there can be additional PAPVD that can be missed. Hence, it is imperative to follow the segmental sequential approach in the evaluation of each vessel carefully and tracing each pulmonary vein so as not to miss anything.*

In the presence of a left-to-right pulmonary shunt, enlargement of the right heart may occur due to increased volume loading, dependent on the presence of an intact atrial septum. In addition, the vessel receiving the anomalous vein may be enlarged and there may be asymmetry of the pulmonary veins. *The magnitude of the left-to-right shunt is dependent on the number of PAPVD.* In a series looking at single PAPVD, the shunt is modest (Q_p:Q_s ~ 1.3–1.6) associated with mild dilatation of the right ventricle [25]. This is the rea-

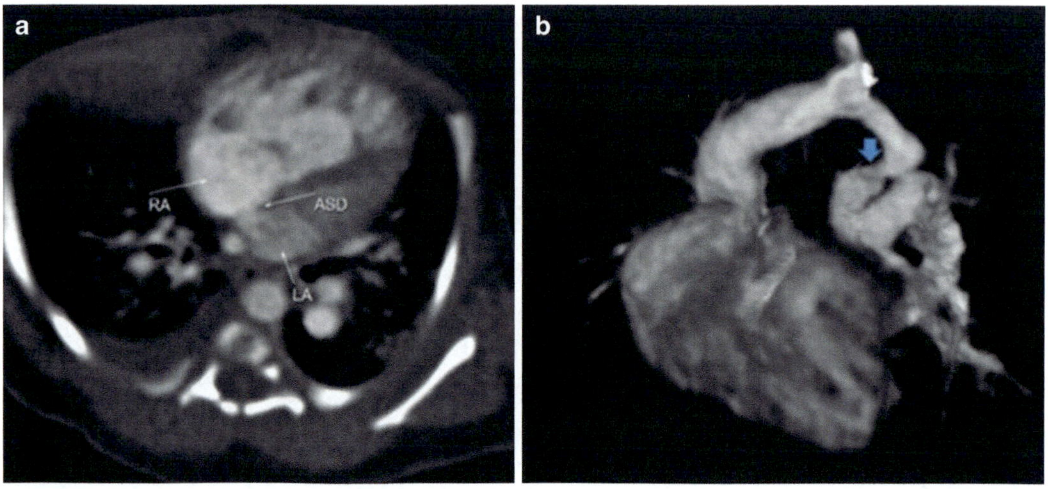

Fig. 11.19 Axial image (**a**) showing small ASD and VRT image (**b**) showing PAPVD of left-sided pulmonary veins draining via a tortuous channel into an innominate vein into SVC with mild compression along its course (arrow)

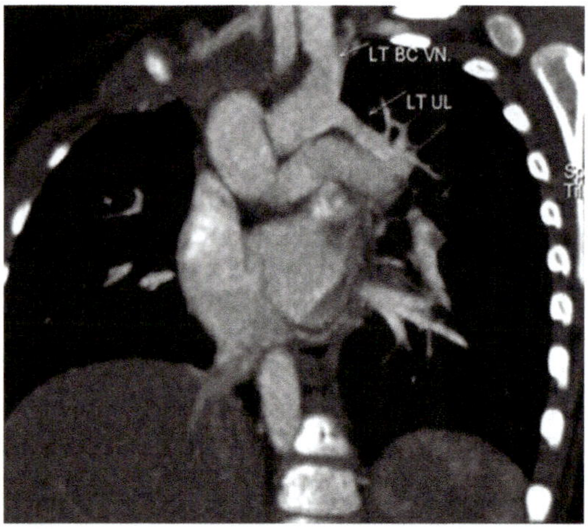

Fig. 11.20 MPR image showing PAPVD of left upper lobe pulmonary veins draining into the innominate vein

son why it goes unnoticed. If the shunt volume is large, then changes of pulmonary arterial hypertension develop. On top of volume loading to the right ventricle, APVD is one of the treatable causes of pulmonary hypertension in adults [26].

Effects of Longstanding Left-to-Right Shunts These include enlargement of the cardiac silhouette (in particular right ventricular dilatation), pulmonary plethora, right hilar vascular prominence, and dilatation of the central pulmonary arteries.

Congenital cardiac and thoracic anomalies, for example, thoracic hypoplasia and cardiac dextro/levoversion may also occur, the presence of which should prompt examination of the pulmonary venous anatomy.

One should make it a habit in sequential segmental approach to congenital heart diseases to have a thorough look at the pulmonary veins so as not to miss any anomaly.

11.6.2.1 Imaging of PAPVD: Chest Radiography

Patients with partial anomalous pulmonary venous drainage (PAPVD) often have non-specific cardiac or respiratory symptoms and are initially investigated with chest radiography, which can be completely normal. However, PAPVD should be suspected with the following findings: Unusual course of a central venous catheter or Focal mediastinal widening to the left of the aortic knob. This may be caused by an anomalous LSPV.

11.6.2.2 CT/MRA

Cross-sectional imaging with CT and MRI is widely used for the diagnosis of PAPVD in the adult population.

CT has superior spatial resolution and thus is useful in presurgical planning in complex lesions. However, MRI is often sufficient for diagnosis and has the advantage of providing functional assessment and shunt calculation. The amount of left-to-right shunting is quantified with cine phase-contrast flow analysis of the aorta and main pulmonary artery to estimate the Q_p/Q_s ratio.

11.6.3 Sinus Venosus Defect

Embryologically, sinus venosus defect is considered to represent the unroofing of the right pulmonary veins into the SVC or IVC. Thus, unroofing of the right upper pulmonary vein into the SVC is called sinus venosus defect of the SVC type (Figs. 11.21 and 11.22), while unroof-

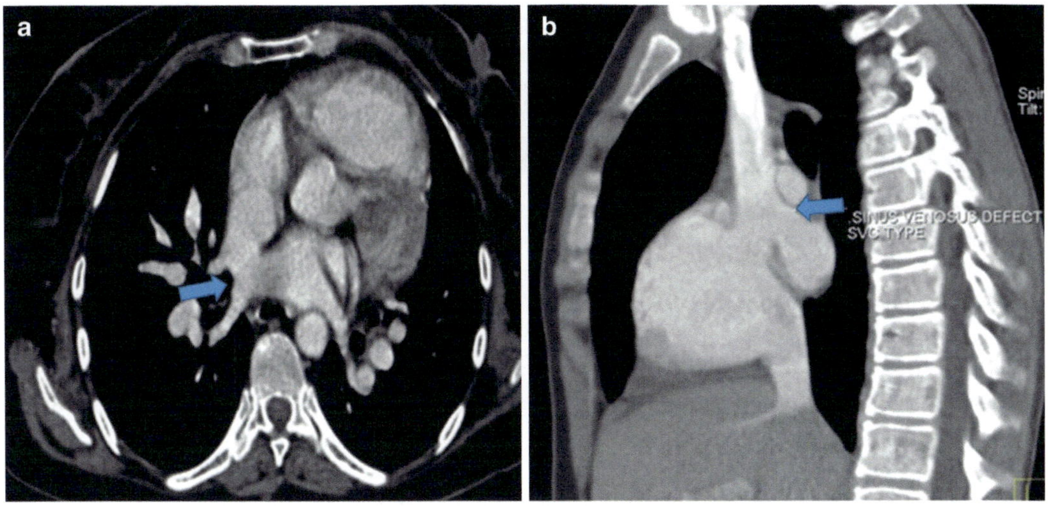

Fig. 11.21 A 21-year-old patient presented with unexplained pulmonary arterial hypertension. Axial (**a**) and sagittal (**b**) images showing SVC type of sinus venosus defect (indicated by thick blue arrow) with overriding of SVC

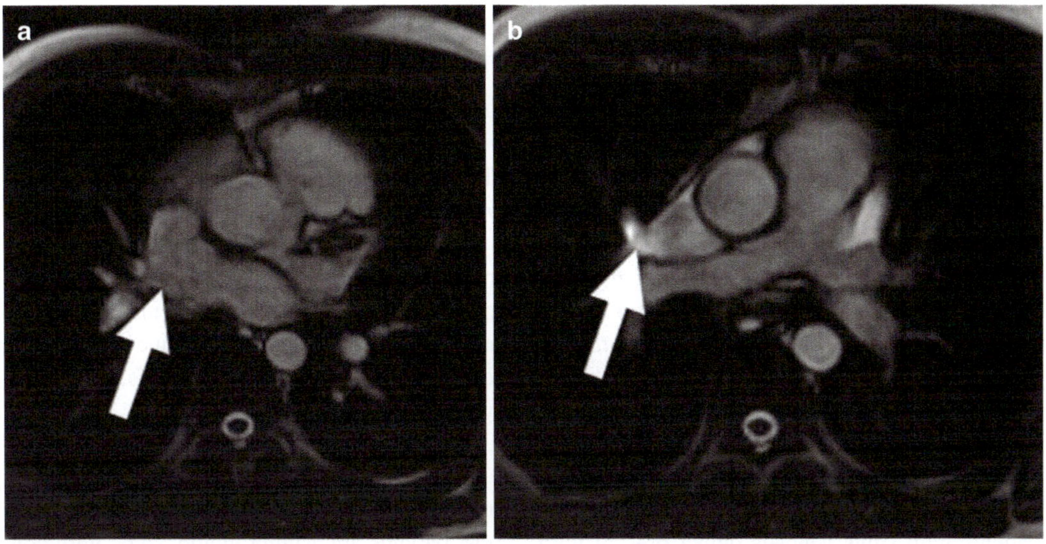

Fig. 11.22 Axial SSFP image showing sinus venous ASD (arrow in **a**), with anomalous drainage of the right upper pulmonary vein into SVC (arrow in **b**). Image courtesy: Dr. Ramiah Rajeshkannan, Amrita Institute of Medical Sciences, Kochi

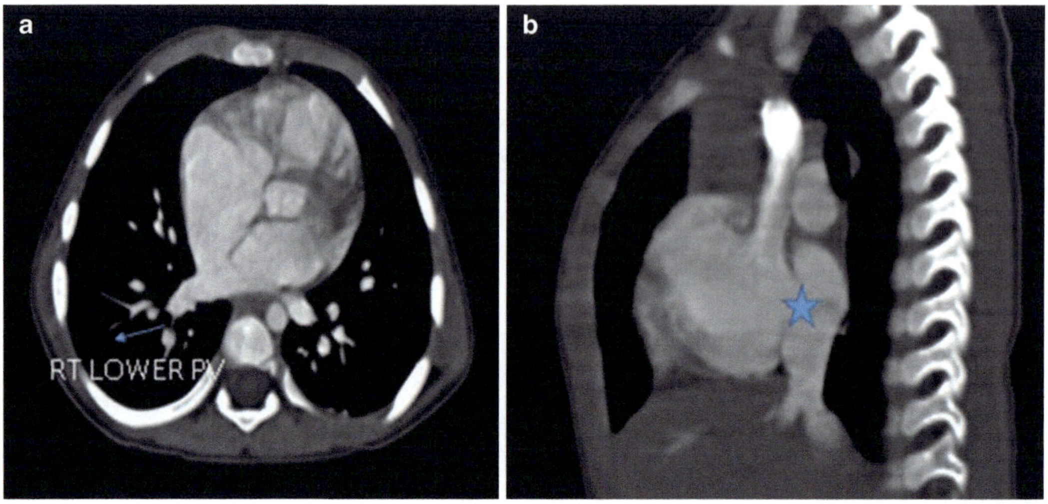

Fig. 11.23 Axial (**a**) and sagittal (**b**) images showing IVC type sinus venosus defect (blue star) with PAPVC of right lower lobe pulmonary vein and overriding of IVC

ing of the right lower pulmonary vein into the IVC is called sinus venosus defect of the IVC type (Fig. 11.23).

The term sinus venosus atrial septal defect is a misnomer since the true atrial septum is not involved in these defects. Sinus venosus defect is a defect in the wall that separates the SVC–right atrial junction from the posterior and superior aspect of the left atrium and is extra septal in location. In addition, owing to the unroofing of the RUPV into the SVC, the RUPV drains anomalously into the SVC, while the SVC overrides the sinus venosus defect and is committed to both atria.

The identification of these abnormalities has a significant bearing on surgical management [27].

Practical Tips *Occasionally, the patients with sinus venosus defect have an additional ostium secundum ASD and one should be careful to look for it.*

Functionally, the behaviour of sinus venosus defect is like that of a large atrial septal defect, producing a left-to-right shunt (RUPV to SVC). Patients with sinus venosus defect present with symptoms of right ventricular volume overload, including fatigue, dyspnea, and arrhythmias. Younger individuals are often asymptomatic and may present with a heart murmur.

Indications for CT/MR imaging include an unclear diagnosis or incomplete definition of involved pulmonary veins at echocardiography. In most cases, acquisition of functional information such as shunting and volumes typically is not clinically necessary, since the defect is almost always large and unrestrictive and the diagnosis alone is an indication for intervention.

11.6.4 Congenital Pulmonary Venolobar Syndrome

The term *congenital pulmonary venolobar syndrome* was first used by Felson [28] and refers to a wide spectrum of pulmonary developmental anomalies that may appear singly or in combination. The main components of congenital pulmonary venolobar syndrome are hypogenetic lung (including lobar agenesis, aplasia, or hypoplasia), partial anomalous pulmonary venous return, absence of pulmonary artery, pulmonary sequestration, systemic arterial supply to lung, absence of inferior vena cava. Although most patients are asymptomatic, some with concurrent cardiac anomalies or severe forms of pulmonary atresia or hypoplasia may have clinical symptoms at an early age. Surgical intervention may be required in selected cases involving recurrent infection, hemoptysis, and congestive heart failure or pulmonary hypertension due to excessive shunting [29, 30]. Identification of abnormal pulmonary and systemic vessels as well as tracheobronchial anomalies is essential for accurate diagnosis in the preoperative evaluation of affected patients.

11.6.4.1 Scimitar Syndrome

The scimitar is a curved traditional sword held by Persian and Turkish warriors, from which the syndrome receives its name.

Hypogenetic lung syndrome (scimitar syndrome) involves an anomalous pulmonary vein draining part or all of the right lung, emptying into the IVC either above or below the diaphragm (Fig. 11.24). The anomalous vein may on occasion drain into the hepatic veins, portal veins, azygous vein, coronary sinus, or right atrium. The anomalous vein is usually associated with various degrees of hypoplasia of the right lung and with a hypoplastic or aplastic pulmonary artery. The right lung may have abnormal lobation (frequently only two lobes), and the bronchial pattern may mimic that of the left lung [31]. About one-fourth of affected patients have associated congenital heart disease, most often a sinus venosus atrial septal defect. Reported associated anomalies include bronchogenic cyst, horseshoe lung, accessory diaphragm, and hernia.

11.6.4.2 Pulmonary Sequestrations and Variants

Pulmonary sequestration is defined as a segment of the lung parenchyma that is separated from the tracheobronchial tree and is supplied with blood from a systemic rather than a pulmonary artery [28, 32]. The blood supply usually comes from the descending thoracic aorta, but in about 20% of cases, it comes from the upper abdominal aorta, celiac artery, or splenic artery [32]. Sequestrations may be either intralobar or extralobar, the differences of which are summarized in Table 11.1.

There can be associated anomalies, the most common of which is a diaphragmatic hernia. Rare variants of sequestration such as bilateral sequestration and gastric or esophageal lung have been reported in both extra- and intralobar sequestrations.

11.6.4.3 Horseshoe Lung

Horseshoe lung is a rare congenital malformation in which, like a horseshoe kidney, an isthmus of pulmonary parenchyma extends from the right

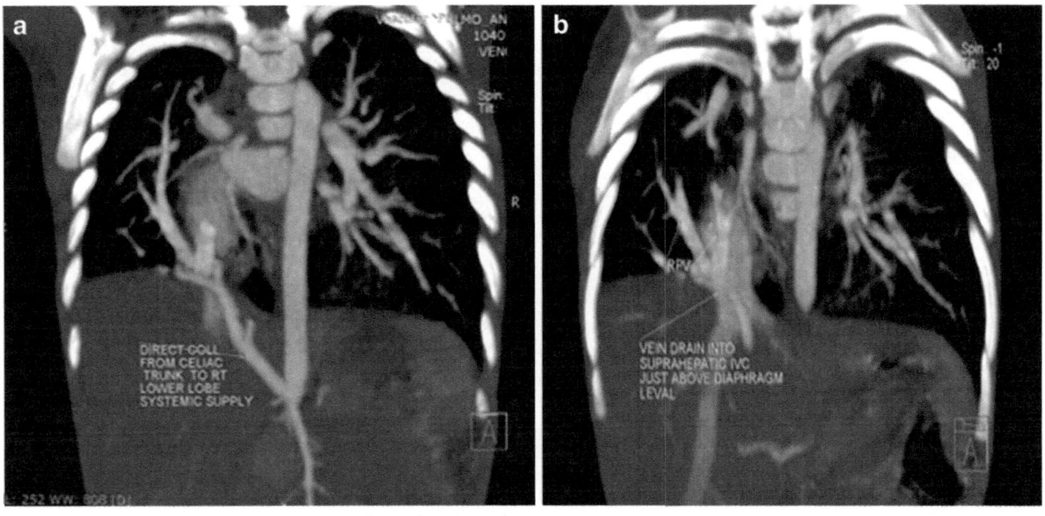

Fig. 11.24 Coronal MPR image showing a direct systemic supply from celiac trunk to right lower lobe (**a**) and right-sided pulmonary veins draining into suprahepatic IVC just above diaphragm level (**b**)—suggestive of scimitar syndrome

lung base across the midline behind the pericardium and joins the left lung parenchyma (Figs. 11.25a, b and 11.26) [29]. In most cases, horseshoe lung is associated with hypogenetic lung syndrome. Other associated findings include a hypoplastic right pulmonary artery, an abnormal systemic arterial supply from the aorta to the right lung, and bronchial sequestration. Right or left pulmonary artery branches can cross the midline to supply the isthmus:

- *Chest radiography* is non-specific and may show an enlarged right heart, small right hemithorax with mediastinal shift to the right, right-sided scimitar vein, recurrent lower lobe consolidation
- *CT* may show: right ventricular dilation and hypertrophy, anomalous pulmonary veins, e.g. scimitar vein, left vertical vein, sequestration with systemic arterial supply from the upper abdominal aorta, celiac trunk or SMA, small right lung with mediastinal shift to the right, horseshoe lung—right lung extends posteriorly to the heart, contiguous with the left lung
- *Cardiac MRI* In addition to CT, MRI allows the radiologist to measure the degree of left-to-right shunt via *phase-contrast* flow volumes, perform quantitation of right ventricular volumes and systolic function, identify systemic–pulmonary arterial supply with differential pulmonary perfusion

Table 11.1 Differences between intralobar and extralobar sequestration

Intralobar sequestration	Extralobar sequestration
Contained within the visceral pleura of the normal adjacent lung	Contained within a separate visceral pleural coat
More common (3:1)	Less common
More likely to be asymptomatic	More likely to be symptomatic
Venous drainage is commonly into pulmonary veins ➔ resulting in left-to-left shunt	Venous drainage is more commonly into the right side of the heart via the azygous vein, hemiazygous vein, or inferior vena cava (IVC) ➔ resulting in a left-to-right shunt

11.7 Malposition of the Septum Primum

The septum primum develops as a thin partition in the primitive atrium, dividing it into the right and left atria. This structure ultimately forms the thin flap valve of the fossa ovalis, while the septum secundum grows from the roof of the right atrium to the right of the septum primum. The septum secundum ultimately forms the thicker limbus of the fossa ovalis.

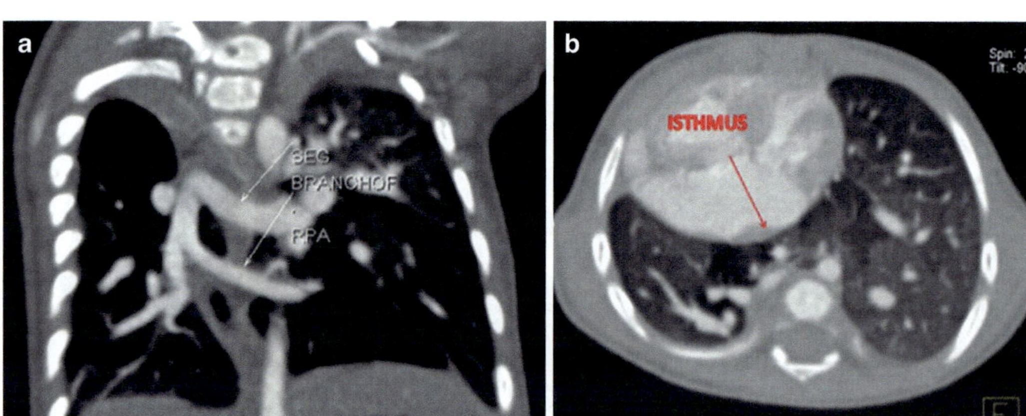

Fig. 11.25 Coronal MPR (**a**) and axial (**b**) images of a patient with congenital pulmonary venolobar syndrome showing horseshoe lung with isthmus posterior to heart and branches of right pulmonary artery crossing midline to supply the isthmus

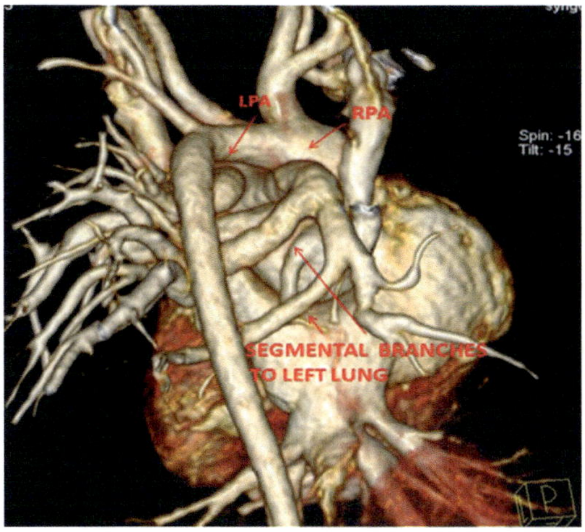

Fig. 11.26 VRT image of the same patient of congenital pulmonary venolobar syndrome showing branches of right pulmonary artery crossing midline to supply isthmus of horseshoe lung

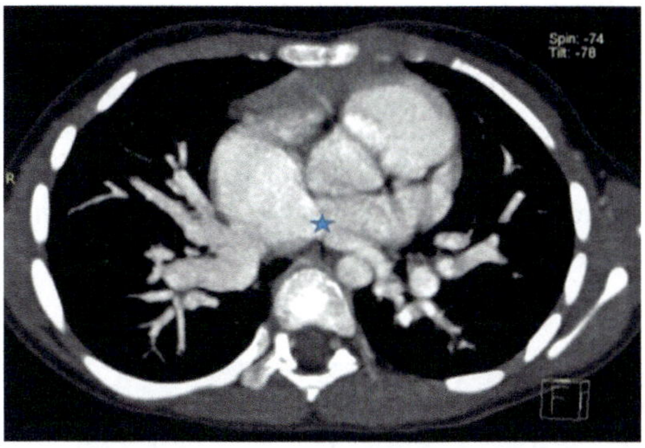

Fig. 11.27 Axial image of a 7-year-old male patient showing malaligned atrial septum (blue star) with resultant PAPVC of right-sided pulmonary veins into the right atrium

The right pulmonary veins drain just to the left of the cephalic attachment of the septum primum. Rarely, the septum primum may deviate leftward such that the normally connected right pulmonary veins drain anomalously to the right atrium (Fig. 11.27) [33]. With extreme degrees of malposition, even the left pulmonary veins may drain anomalously into the right atrium.

Malposition of the septum primum is typically associated with heterotaxy and polysplenia [33, 34]. The clinical picture is dominated by the presence of associated complex cardiac anomalies, which are frequent in patients with heterotaxy.

This defect is typically diagnosed with high-quality echocardiography; MR imaging and CT are usually not necessary to make the diagnosis. However, malposition of the septum primum may be encountered during imaging of complex cardiac defects and must be distinguished from other forms of PAPVD or TAPVD because the treatment is different, involving resection and repositioning of the atrial septum in a more normal position. Furthermore, when this anomaly occurs in the setting of heterotaxy syndromes, complex congenital heart defects are frequently associated and accurate definition of venous and arterial anomalies is necessary.

11.8 Meandering Pulmonary Vein

A meandering pulmonary vein can be generally defined as a vein that (a) has an anomalous variable or meandering course and (b) always drains into the left atrium. The latter criterion distinguishes it from PAPVD and scimitar veins; that is, the meandering pulmonary vein has no shunting, while PAPVD or a scimitar vein has a left-to-right shunt. Because the meandering pulmonary vein can be prominent in size, it can be easily mistaken for a scimitar *vein (pseudoscimitar syndrome)* on the chest radiograph when it occurs on the right [35]. The meandering pulmonary vein is often discovered incidentally and usually requires no treatment.

11.9 Levoatriocardinal Vein

Levoatriocardinal vein is defined as an abnormal pulmonary–systemic connection that is most commonly seen in association with obstructive left heart lesions. In this scenario, the vein serves as an alternative egress for pulmonary venous blood, providing a way of decompression of the left atrium. This anomaly was first reported in 1926 by McIntosh [36], although the term "levoatriocardinal vein" was first used by Edwards and DuShane in 1950 [37]. The term levoatriocardinal vein signifies left atrial communication with the cardinal system via a vein.

In the case of obstructive left heart lesions (e.g. hypoplastic left heart syndrome, cor triatriatum, congenital mitral stenosis), the pulmonary veins develop normal communication with the left atrium but can retain some form of primitive connection with the cardinal system. This persistent abnormal connection serves as a pop-off channel, allowing the pulmonary venous blood an alternative pathway to a systemic vein derivative of the cardinal system, such as an innominate vein, jugular vein, or superior vena cava (SVC), and forms the basis of a levoatriocardinal vein (Figs. 11.28a, b and 11.29).

Another entity that can be confused for a levoatriocardinal vein on imaging is a PLSVC [38]. This is, however, embryologically very different and is due to abnormal persistence of the left anterior cardinal vein. In the normal course of development, the left anterior cardinal vein regresses with the development of the left innominate vein. Persistence of the left anterior cardinal vein is the basis for PLSVC and is often associated with abnormal development of the innominate vein. This is the reason why some patients with PLSVC have a small or absent bridging vein [39]. The direction of blood flow in left SVC is towards the heart (vertically downwards), while that of LACV is away from the heart (vertically upwards). The direction of blood flow in the anomalous vessel can be assessed by colour Doppler or phase-contrast MR imaging. The left innominate vein is either absent or hypoplastic and works as a bridging vein in patients with left SVC. In the diagnosis of LACV, the presence of the left innominate vein is essential [39].

If an anomalous vein connects a pulmonary vein to a systemic vein but there is no connection between the pulmonary vein and left atrium, the diagnosis would more appropriately be termed "anomalous pulmonary venous drainage".

In the few sporadic cases in which a levoatriocardinal vein has been described in the absence of other cardiovascular abnormalities, the evaluation has been for an asymptomatic murmur or a clinically suspected atrial septal defect.

The shunting in a levoatriocardinal vein is usually left-to-right or bidirectional—especially in cases of increased pressure like Valsalva. Symptoms related to paradoxical embolism, such as transient ischemic attacks, can also occur in a bidirectional shunt [40].

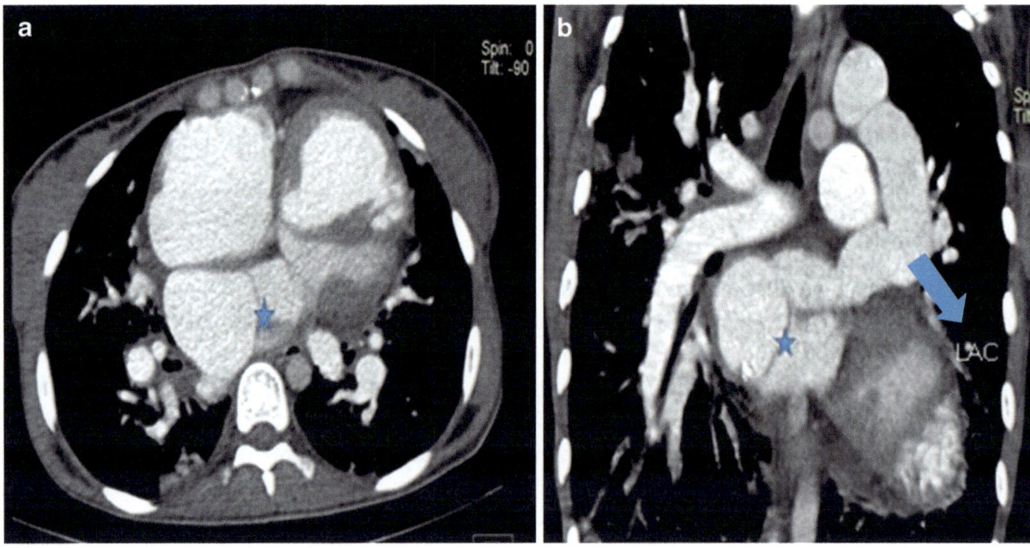

Fig. 11.28 Axial (**a**) and coronal (**b**) MPR images of an adult patient showing cor triatriatum (blue star, Loeffler's type 2) with persistent levoatrial cardinal vein (blue arrow)

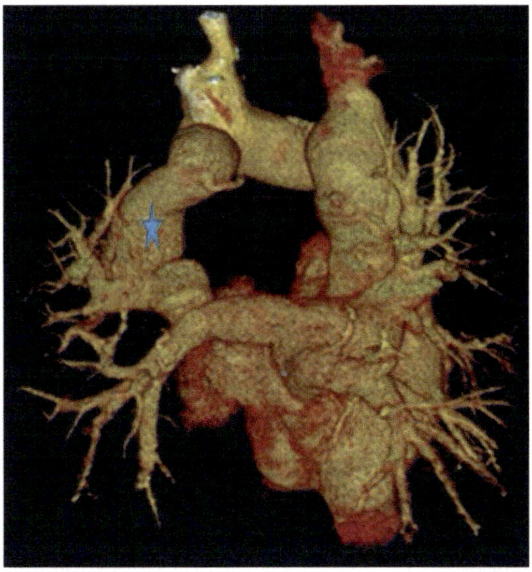

Fig. 11.29 VRT image of the same patient showing cor triatriatum with persistent levoatrial cardinal vein (blue star) between left upper lobe pulmonary vein and left innominate vein

11.10 Cor Triatriatum

Embryologically it develops when there is stenosis of connection between the common pulmonary vein and left atrium with resultant dilatation of the common pulmonary veins. This rare condition refers to the failure of incorporation of normal pulmonary veins into the left atrium [12] and accounts for up to 0.1% of congenital heart disease [41]. There is a separation of the left atrium into two chambers, separated by a thin, fenestrated membrane.

In classic cor triatriatum, there is an accessory chamber within the left atrium that represents the CPV (Fig. 11.28a, b).

This accessory chamber communicates with the left atrium through an opening that demonstrates varying degrees of stenosis. This is classified based on the size and the number of the openings in the accessory membrane into the left atrium. The most commonly used classification is the one developed by Loeffler [42]. According to that classification, cor triatriatum is divided into three distinct groups:

- Type 1 has no opening in the accessory membrane, with the proximal (posterior) left atrium draining into the right atrium
- Type 2 has one or more small restrictive openings (fenestrations), resulting in significant left ventricular inflow obstruction
- Type 3 has a large (nonrestrictive) opening in the membrane

No opening or 1 or more restrictive opening is commonly seen in the newborn, infants, and children. In the adult, cor triatriatum often contains a relatively wide opening.

The accessory chamber is always above the level of the left atrial appendage, a finding that allows differentiation of the membrane of cor triatriatum from a supravalvular mitral ring.

The posterior chamber drains the pulmonary veins and the anterior chamber (true left atrium) drains into the left ventricle via the mitral valve, overall resulting in an obstruction to the drainage of the pulmonary veins. Patients can present with failure to thrive and congestive heart failure.

Since shunts are not involved in the typical cor triatriatum, flow analysis and volumetry are generally not useful. The most important piece of information needed for management is the degree of pulmonary venous obstruction, which is determined by the flow gradient across the stenosis and by right ventricular pressures. The former may be estimated with MR imaging by using cine phase-contrast velocity flow mapping, while echocardiography provides an estimate of right ventricular pressure.

11.11 Pulmonary Vein Stenosis/Hypoplasia/Atresia

Congenital pulmonary vein stenosis and hypoplasia/atresia reflect a spectrum of the same abnormality and may affect an individual or multiple pulmonary veins. The abnormality may be focal or may involve a long segment of a pulmonary vein. They are rare causes of neonatal pulmonary edema that may be unilateral or bilateral. A recent study by Ou et al. determined that 64

SLICE-MDCT without gating more completely characterized pulmonary vein stenosis than did echocardiography in children [43].

Congenital pulmonary vein stenosis is associated with congenital heart disease in approximately 50% of affected patients.

The clinical presentation depends on the number of involved veins and the degree of pulmonary venous obstruction. Stenosis of a single pulmonary vein is generally well tolerated. With stenosis of all veins of one lung, there may be redirection of pulmonary arterial flow to the opposite lung. Pulmonary hypertension may occur. Bilateral pulmonary vein stenosis is poorly tolerated and is characterized by recurrent pulmonary infections, failure to thrive, hemoptysis, and pulmonary hypertension.

Atresia of the common pulmonary vein (CPV) is a rare anomaly thought to be due to failure of the CPV to establish a connection to the left atrium or regression of this connection after its establishment.

Chest radiographs of patients with congenital unilateral pulmonary vein stenosis or atresia may show a small lung and reticular opacities with Kerley B lines [44, 45].

It is difficult to definitively diagnose stenosis of individual pulmonary veins with echocardiography alone, particularly beyond the neonatal period. Thus, definitive imaging with MR imaging or CT is generally required. MR angiography and CT angiography both show pulmonary veins well, but CT does have a better spatial resolution. The characteristic CT findings are a small lung with ipsilateral mediastinal deviation, unilateral stenosis or absence of pulmonary venous drainage, and a small ipsilateral pulmonary artery (Fig. 11.30). The left atrial wall is completely smooth at the expected insertion site of the pulmonary vein. Abnormal confluent soft tissue can also be observed, which is due to the pulmonary-to-systemic venous collateral circulation [44]. The pulmonary parenchyma ipsilateral to pulmonary vein atresia shows radiologic features of pulmonary venous hypertension: interlobular

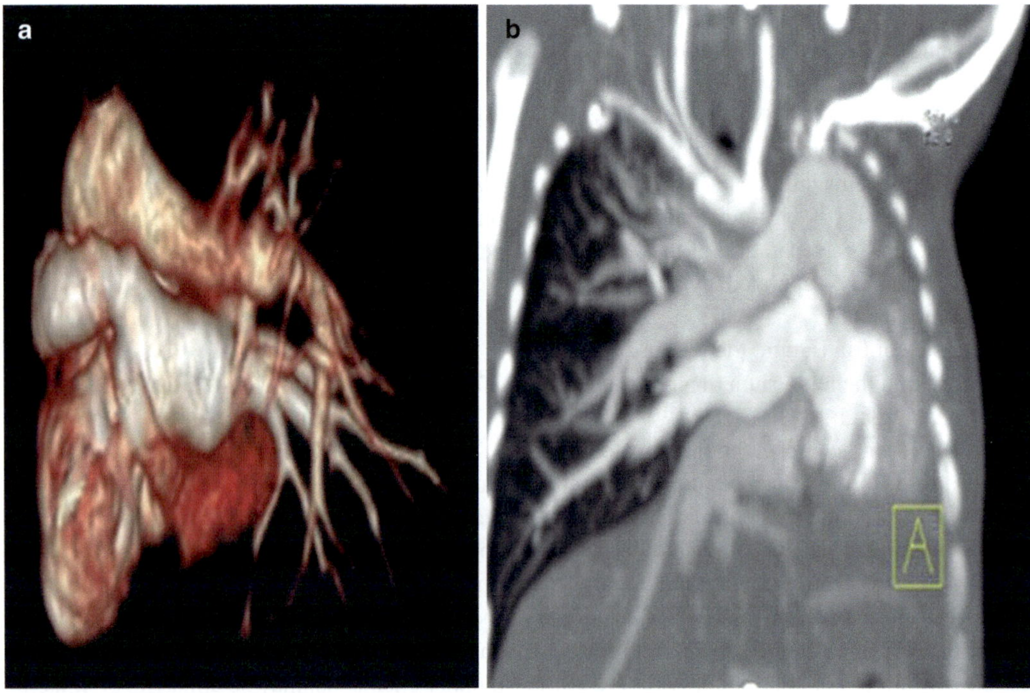

Fig. 11.30 VRT (**a**) and coronal (**b**) images of a patient showing complete agenesis of the left lung with absent left bronchus, LPA as well as LPV

septal thickening, peribronchovascular thickening, and ground-glass opacities [46] (Figs. 11.31, 11.32a, b, and 11.33).

Given the rarity of this anomaly and the degree of cardiorespiratory compromise, it is unusual that MR imaging may be needed or clinically feasible. Non-gated CT angiography may be the diagnostic modality of choice for confirming the diagnosis if needed. However, gadolinium-enhanced MR angiography is usually diagnostic and MR imaging provides additional functional information, such as pulmonary vein flow dynamics and differential pulmonary arterial flow.

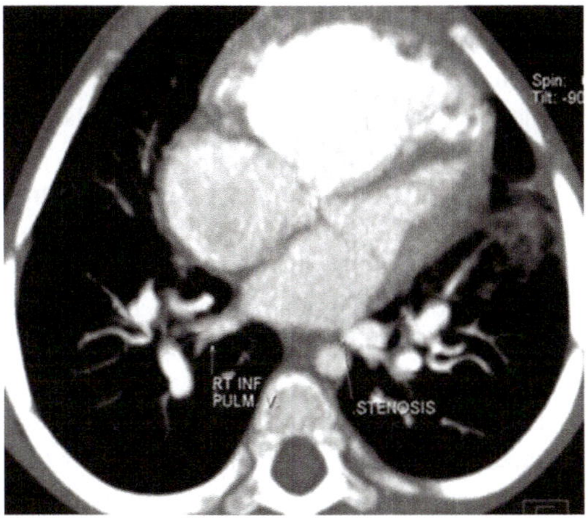

Fig. 11.31 Axial image of a patient showing stenosis at the drainage of left inferior pulmonary veins into left atrium with few Kerley's lines in visualized left lower lobe

11.12 Pulmonary Vein Varix

Pulmonary vein varix consists of a focal dilatation of a pulmonary vein segment that does not have an arterial connection, with the dilatation usually occurring close to the entrance of the vein into the left atrium [47, 48] (Fig. 11.18).

Generally, it is asymptomatic, though rarely may present with hemoptysis or thromboembolic disease.

Chest radiographic findings: mimics pulmonary nodule or mediastinal mass.

MDCT, especially when performed with 3D reconstruction or maximum intensity projection (MIP), facilitates the diagnosis [47, 48]. No treatment is needed for asymptomatic patients, but for symptomatic patients, surgical resection may be required [47].

11.13 Pulmonary Arteriovenous Malformation

By definition, it means an abnormal communication between a pulmonary artery and a pulmonary vein.

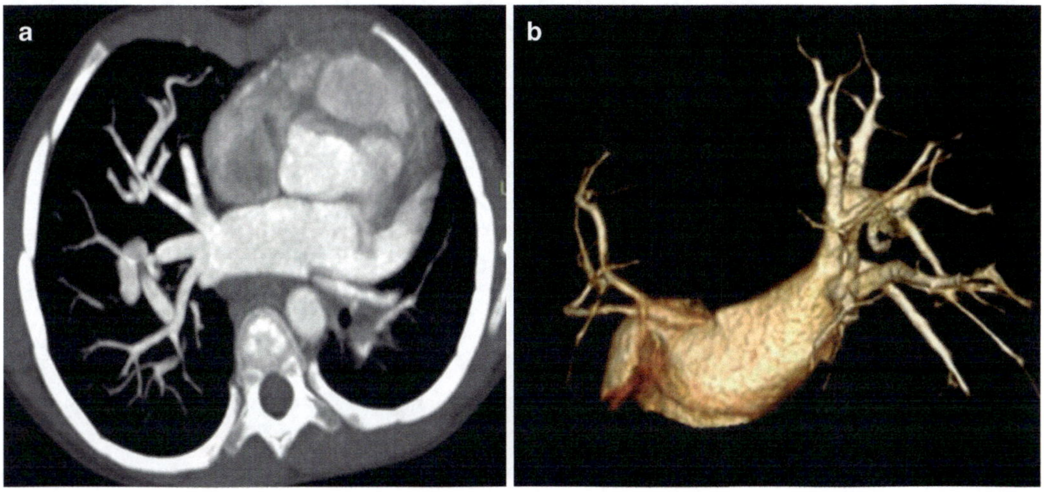

Fig. 11.32 Axial (**a**) and VRT (**b**) images of another patient showing severe stenosis at the drainage of left inferior pulmonary veins into the left atrium

The congenital form is the most common but acquired pulmonary arteriovenous malformation may develop in patients after surgery for cyanotic congenital cardiopathies (Glenn and Fontan procedures), in patients with chronic liver disease, and patients with a history of tuberculosis or actinomycosis. Pulmonary arteriovenous malformation can be single or multiple (Fig. 11.34). The anomaly is associated with Rendu–Osler–Weber syndrome (hereditary hemorrhagic telangiectasia) in as many as 60% of cases [49].

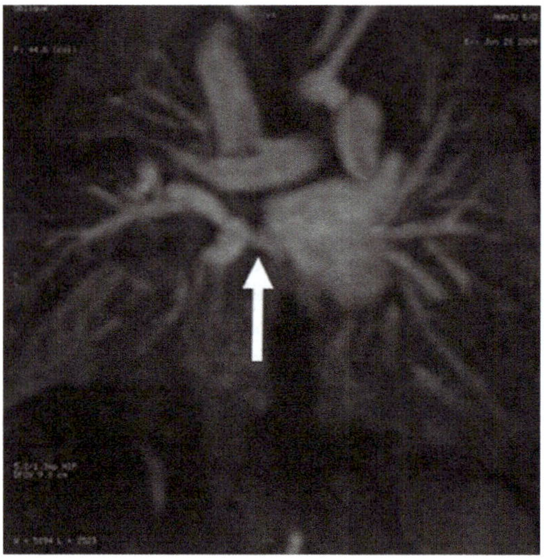

Fig. 11.33 Thin MIP MRA image showing focal stenosis (arrow) at the right pulmonary vein. Image courtesy: Dr. Ramiah Rajeshkannan, Amrita Institute of Medical Sciences, Kochi

The symptoms of this anomaly depend on the size of the lesion. Patients with pulmonary arteriovenous malformations smaller than 2 cm may be asymptomatic (1). If the malformation is larger or if there are multiple pulmonary arteriovenous malformations, the patient may present with hypoxemia, brain infarction or abscess, pulmonary haemorrhage, and paradoxical embolism [49]. More than 70% of all pulmonary arteriovenous malformations involve a single artery and a single vein, and as many as 50% of patients have more than one malformation [49].

Chest radiographic findings mimic a pulmonary nodule or mass.

Multidetector CT enables the detection and evaluation of the angioarchitecture and size of the lesion and is useful in post-treatment follow-up [47].

Pulmonary arteriovenous malformation requires treatment when the lesion is larger than 2–3 cm. Percutaneous transcatheter embolization is the treatment of choice.

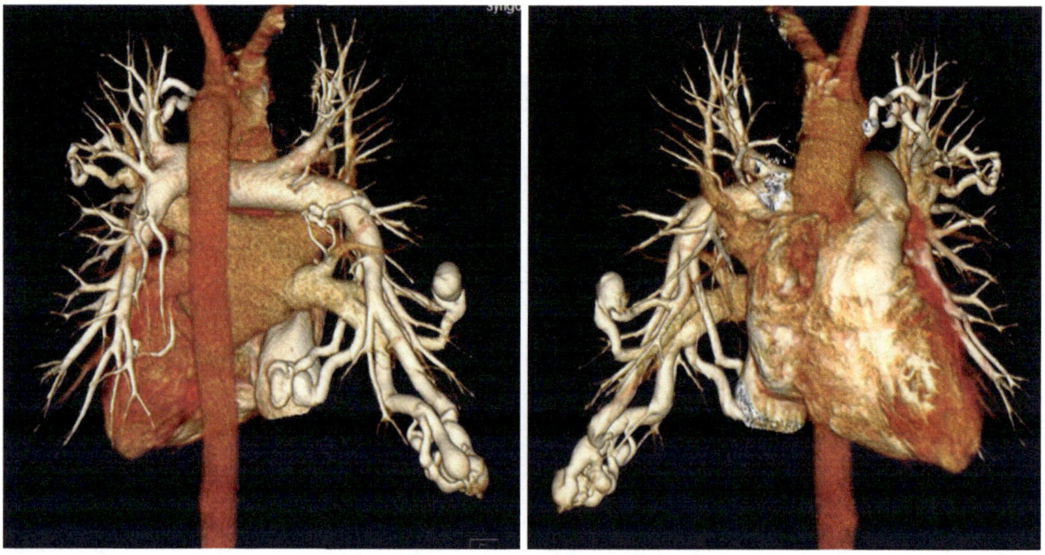

Fig. 11.34 VRT images showing multiple pulmonary AVMs on both sides

11.14 Post-operative TAPVD

Just a brief word on post-operative imaging of PAPVD and TAPVD. Corrective surgery is the definitive treatment for TAPVD. The goal of the surgery is to create an unobstructed egress of blood from pulmonary veins to the left atrium. The anomalous vertical vein is routinely ligated in supracardiac TAPVD but is controversial in infracardiac TAPVD. Pulmonary venous obstruction is the most significant cause of late morbidity and mortality after corrective surgery. It develops in 5–15% of patients within the first post-operative year where TAPVD is corrected using standard technique [50]. Echocardiography can depict the gradient in the case of pulmonary vein stenosis at the anastomotic site and MDCT/MRI is used as a supplementary tool to confirm the diagnosis (Figs. 11.17b, 11.35, 11.36, and 11.37).

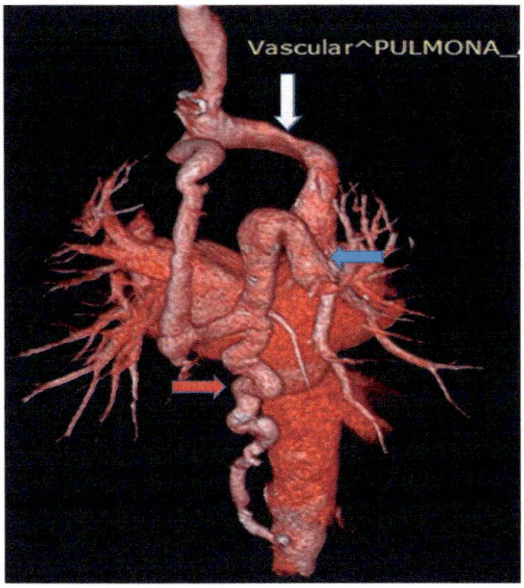

Fig. 11.35 VRT image showing post-operative case of PAPVD of right side pulmonary veins draining into the azygous system via collaterals. Occluded right innominate vein (blue arrow - right pulmonary vein, red arrow - azygous collaterals, white arrow - left innominate vein)

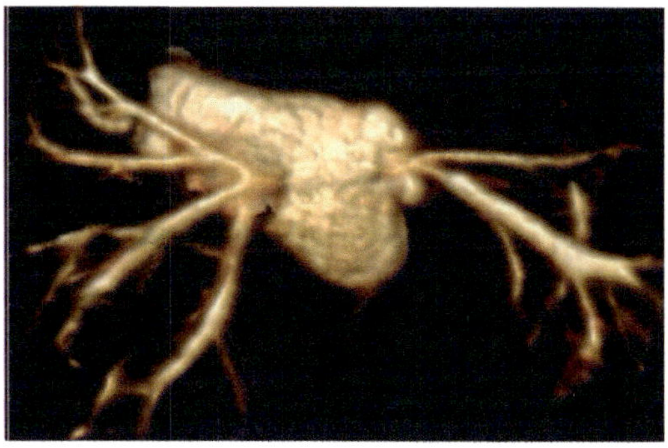

Fig. 11.36 VRT image of a 3-month-old patient with TAPVD repair showing severe stenosis at the drainage of both right and left pulmonary veins into the left atrium

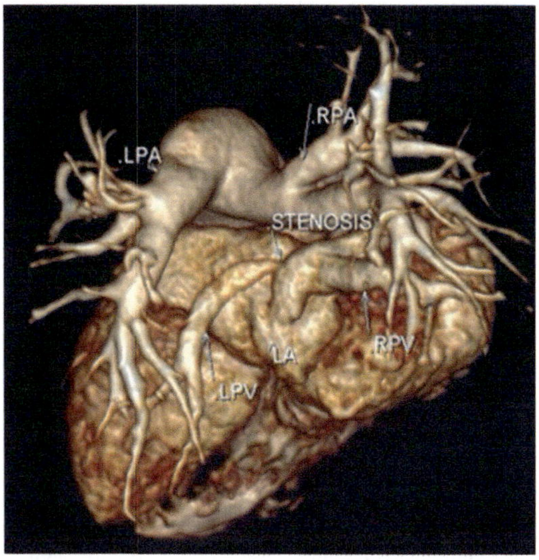

Fig. 11.37 VRT image of a patient who has undergone TAPVD repair showing stenosis at the drainage of left inferior pulmonary veins into a common chamber that opens into the left atrium

11.15 Summary

- We have reviewed the spectrum of common congenital pulmonary vein anomalies, their embryology, and clinical features and what information is desired from an advanced imaging study.

- Cross-sectional imaging—MR and CT are methods of choice for imaging of congenital pulmonary vein anomalies when echocardiography does not provide all the necessary information. We also get information about extracardiac structures from cross-sectional imaging.
- The golden rule is to follow the segmental sequential approach in evaluating any congenital heart disease and never stop when you find one or two major findings. Scrutiny of each structure is essential to miss none.
- In most patients, CT offers a better spatial resolution in a short period; the disadvantage of CT includes use ionizing radiation and lack of functional information.
- MR imaging provides precise anatomic as well as functional data without the use of ionizing radiation, but MR scanning takes more time which may not be suitable in critically ill neonates and infants with TAPVD.

Acknowledgement Figures 11.6, 11.15, 11.22, and 11.33 and Video files 11.1 and 11.2 are provided by Dr. Ramiah Rajeshkannan, Amrita Institute of Medical Sciences, Kochi, India.

References

1. Zylak CJ, Eyler WR, Spizarny DL, Stone CH. Developmental lung anomalies in the adult: radiologic-pathologic correlation. Radiographics. 2002;22:S25–43.
2. Latson LA, Prieto LR. Congenital and acquired pulmonary vein stenosis. Circulation. 2007;115(1):103–8.
3. Kirsch J, Kirby A, Williamson EE. Venous anatomy of the thorax. In: Ho VB, Reddy GP, editors. Cardiovascular imaging. St. Louis, MO: Elsevier; 2011. p. 1001.
4. Kato R, Lickfett L, Meininger G, et al. Pulmonary vein anatomy in patients undergoing catheter ablation of atrial fibrillation: lessons learned by use of magnetic resonance imaging. Circulation. 2003;107(15):2004–10.
5. Kim YH, Marom EM, Herndon JE II, McAdams HP. Pulmonary vein diameter, cross-sectional area, and shape: CT analysis. Radiology. 2005;235(1):43–9. discussion 49–50
6. D'Avila A, Scanavacca M, Sosa E, Ruskin JN, Reddy VY. Pericardial anatomy for the interventional electrophysiologist. J Cardiovasc Electrophysiol. 2003;14(4):422–30.
7. Hassink RJ, Aretz HT, Ruskin J, Keane D. Morphology of atrial myocardium in human pulmonary veins: a postmortem analysis in patients with and without atrial fibrillation. J Am Coll Cardiol. 2003;42(6):1108–14.
8. Ghaye B, Szapiro D, Dacher JN, Rodriguez LM, Timmermans C, Devillers D, et al. Percutaneous ablation for atrial fibrillation: the role of cross-sectional imaging. Radiographics. 2003;23:S19–33. discussion S48–50
9. Lacomis JM, Wigginton W, Fuhrman C, Schwartzman D, Armfield DR, Pealer KM. Multi-detector row CT of the left atrium and pulmonary veins before radiofrequency catheter ablation for atrial fibrillation. Radiographics. 2003;23:S35–48. discussion S48–50
10. Tsao H-M, Wu M-H, Yu W, Tai C-T, Lin Y-K, Hsieh M-H, et al. Role of right middle pulmonary vein in patients with paroxysmal atrial fibrillation. J Cardiovasc Electrophysiol. 2001;12(12):1353–7.
11. Schwartzman D, Lacomis J, Wigginton WG. Characterization of left atrium and distal pulmonary vein morphology using multidimensional computed tomography. J Am Coll Cardiol. 2003;41(8):1349–57.
12. Dillman JR, Yarram SG, Hernandez RJ. Imaging of pulmonary venous developmental anomalies. Am J Roentgenol. 2009;192(5):1272–85.
13. Sørensen TS, Körperich H, Greil GF, et al. Operator-independent isotropic three-dimensional magnetic resonance imaging for morphology in congenital heart disease. Circulation. 2004;110:163–9.
14. Ferguson EC, Krishnamurthy R, Oldham SAA. Classic imaging signs of congenital cardiovascular abnormalities. Radiographics. 2007;27(5):1323–34.
15. Wilson J, et al. A description of a very unusual formation of the human heart. Philos Trans R Soc Lond. 1798;88:346.
16. Darling RC, Rothney WB, Craig JM. Total pulmonary venous drainage into the right side of the heart: report of 17 autopsied cases not associated with other major cardiovascular anomalies. Lab Investig. 1957;6:44–64.
17. Herlong JR, Jaggers JJ, Ungerleider RM. Congenital heart surgery nomenclature and database project: pulmonary venous anomalies. Ann Thorac Surg. 2000;69:S56–69.
18. Vyas HV, Greenberg SB, Krishnamurthy R. MR imaging and CT evaluation of congenital pulmonary vein abnormalities in neonates and infants. Radiographics. 2012;32(1):87–98.
19. Seale AN, Uemura H, Webber SA, Partridge J, Roughton M, Ho SY, et al. Total anomalous pulmonary venous connection: morphology and outcome from an international population-based study. Circulation. 2010;122(25):2718–26.
20. Demos TC, Posniak HV, Pierce KL, Olson MC, Muscato M. Venous anomalies of the thorax. AJR Am J Roentgenol. 2004;182:1139–50.
21. Snellen HA, Van Ingen HC, Hoefsmit EC. Patterns of anomalous pulmonary venous drainage. Circulation. 1968;38(1):45–63.

22. Ammash NM, Seward JB, Warnes CA, Connolly HM, O'Leary PW, Danielson GK. Partial anomalous pulmonary venous connection: diagnosis by transesophageal echocardiography. J Am Coll Cardiol. 1997;29(6):1351–8.
23. Porres DV, Morenza OP, Pallisa E, Roque A, Andreu J, Martínez M. Learning from the pulmonary veins. Radiographics. 2013;33(4):999–1022.
24. Kivistö S, Hänninen H, Holmström M. Partial anomalous pulmonary venous return and atrial septal defect in adult patients detected with 128-slice multidetector computed tomography. J Cardiothorac Surg BioMed. 2011;6(1):126.
25. Dyme JL, Prakash A, Printz BF, Kaur A, Parness IA, Nielsen JC. Physiology of isolated anomalous pulmonary venous connection of a single pulmonary vein as determined by cardiac magnetic resonance imaging. Am J Cardiol. 2006;98(1):107–10.
26. Pauwaa S, Farzaneh-Far A. Isolated partial anomalous pulmonary venous return with intact atrial septum: a rare but treatable cause of pulmonary hypertension in adults. Eur Heart J Cardiovasc Imaging. 2014;15(7):830.
27. Van de Woestijne PC, Verberkmoes N, Bogers AJJC. Partial anomalous pulmonary venous connection (including scimitar syndrome). Multimed Man Cardiothorac Surg. 2013; https://doi.org/10.1093/mmcts/mmt001.
28. Felson B. Chest roentgenology. Philadelphia, PA: Saunders; 1973. p. 87–92.
29. Frank JL, Poole CA, Rosas G. Horseshoe lung: clinical, pathologic and radiologic features and a new plain film finding. AJR Am J Roentgenol. 1986;146:217–26.
30. Ellis K. Developmental abnormalities in the systemic blood supply to the lungs. AJR Am J Roentgenol. 1991;156:669–79.
31. Godwin JD, Tarver RD. Scimitar syndrome: four new cases examined with CT. Radiology. 1986;159:15–20.
32. Felker RE, Tonkin IL. Imaging of pulmonary sequestration. AJR Am J Roentgenol. 1990;154:241–9.
33. Van Praagh S, Carrera ME, Sanders S, Mayer JE, Van Praagh R. Partial or total direct pulmonary venous drainage to right atrium due to malposition of septum primum: anatomic and echocardiographic findings and surgical treatment—a study based on 36 cases. Chest. 1995;107(6):1488–98.
34. Tomar M, Radhakrishnan S, Shrivastava S. Partial or total anomalous pulmonary venous drainage caused by malposition of septum primum: echocardiographic description of a rare variant of anomalous pulmonary venous drainage. J Am Soc Echocardiogr. 2005;18(8):884.
35. Legras A, Guinet C, Alifano M, Lepilliez A, Regnard JF. A case of variant scimitar syndrome. Chest. 2012;142(4):1039–41.
36. McIntosh CA. Cor biatriatum triloculare. Am Heart J. 1926;1:735–44.
37. Edwards JE, DuShane JW. Thoracic venous anomalies. Arch Pathol (Chic). 1950;49:517–37.
38. Agarwal PP, Mahani MG, Lu JC, Dorfman AL. levoatriocardinal vein and mimics: spectrum of imaging findings. Am J Roentgenol. 2015;205:W162–71. https://doi.org/10.2214/AJR.15.14365.
39. Bernstein HS, Moore P, Stanger P, Silverman NH. The levoatriocardinal vein: morphology and echocardiographic identification of the pulmonary-systemic connection. J Am Coll Cardiol. 1995;26:995–1001.
40. Cullen EL, Breen JF, Rihal CS, Simari RD, Am-mash NM. Levoatriocardinal vein with partial anomalous pulmonary venous return and a bidirectional shunt. Circulation. 2012;126:e174–7.
41. Kokotsakis J, Anagnostakou V, Almpanis G, Paralikas I, Nenekidis I, Kratimenos T, et al. Cor triatriatum presenting as heart failure with reduced ejection fraction: a case report. J Cardiothorac Surg. 2011; 6:83.
42. Loeffler E. Unusual malformation of the left atrium: pulmonary sinus. Arch Pathol. 1949;48:371–6.
43. Ou P, Marini D, Celermajer DS, et al. Non-invasive assessment of congenital pulmonary vein stenosis in children using cardiac-non-gated CT with 64-slice technology. Eur J Radiol. 2008; https://doi.org/10.1016/j.ejrad.2008.02.006.
44. Pourmoghadam KK, Moore JW, Khan M, et al. Congenital unilateral pulmonary venous atresia: definitive diagnosis and treatment. Pediatr Cardiol. 2003;24(1):73–9.
45. Nasrallah AT, Mullins CE, Singer D, Harrison G, McNamara DG. Unilateral pulmonary vein atresia: diagnosis and treatment. Am J Cardiol. 1975;36(7):969–73.
46. Heyneman LE, Nolan RL, Harrison JK, McAdams HP. Congenital unilateral pulmonary vein atresia: radiologic findings in three adult patients. AJR Am J Roentgenol. 2001;177(3):681–5.
47. Lee EY, Boiselle PM, Cleveland RH. Multidetector CT evaluation of congenital lung anomalies. Radiology. 2008;247(3):632–48.
48. Vanherreweghe E, Rigauts H, Bogaerts Y, Meeus L. Pulmonary vein varix: diagnosis with multi-slice helical CT. Eur Radiol. 2000;10(8):1315–7.
49. Maldonado JA, Henry T, Gutiérrez FR. Congenital thoracic vascular anomalies. Radiol Clin North Am. 2010;48(1):85–115.
50. Caldarone CA, Najm HK, Kadletz M, Smallhorn JF, Freedom RM, Williams WG, Coles JG. Relentless pulmonary vein stenosis after repair of total anomalous pulmonary venous drainage. Ann Thorac Surg. 1998;66:1514–20.

CT and MRI of Simple Cardiovascular Shunts

12

Aparna Irodi, Binita Riya Chacko, Linu Kuruvilla, and Elizabeth Joseph

12.1 Introduction

Echocardiogram is the main modality for assessing simple cardiac shunts such as atrial septal defect (ASD), ventricular septal defect (VSD) and patent ductus arteriosus (PDA). Echocardiogram can assess most of the details required in the evaluation of these shunts (Table 12.1).

Contrast-enhanced CT is not primarily used to detect the shunts but is useful in evaluating associated anomalies like anomalous pulmonary venous drainage. Septal defects may be a part of more complex anomalies for which cross-sectional imaging may be performed. Shunts which are difficult to assess on echocardiogram like sinus venosus ASD or apical VSD are better assessed on CT.

MRI can again be used for similar indications like CT but has the additional advantage of accurate quantification of flows and ventricular function.

Table 12.1 Role of imaging in simple intracardiac shunts

Role of imaging in cardiac shunts
– Identify the presence of shunt
– Look for multiplicity, define the exact site and size of the shunt and its margins, relationships to the AV valves, veins and great arteries, thus defining the exact type
– Quantify flow across the shunts (i.e. assess hemodynamic significance)
– Status of AV and semilunar valves
– Accurate assessment of ventricular function
– Detailed account of associated anomalies
– Guide surgical or interventional management

12.2 Atrial Septal Defect (ASD)

12.2.1 Introduction

Figure 12.1 describes the embryology of interatrial septum. The incidence of atrial septal defects (ASD) is about 1.64 per 1000 live births, constituting 13% of all congenital heart diseases [1]. It is the next most common congenital heart defect after ventricular septal defect. Since ASDs may be relatively asymptomatic in the early stages, they are often detected incidentally in adults.

ASDs can be isolated or associated with other congenital heart anomalies. It can also be associated with syndromes like Lutembacher syndrome (ASD with mitral stenosis) and Holt–Oram syndrome (ASD with upper limb radial ray abnormalities).

A. Irodi (✉) · B. R. Chacko · L. Kuruvilla · E. Joseph
Department of Radiology, Christian Medical College and Hospital, Vellore, Tamil Nadu, India

R. Rajeshkannan et al. (eds.), *CT and MRI in Congenital Heart Diseases*,
https://doi.org/10.1007/978-981-15-6755-1_12

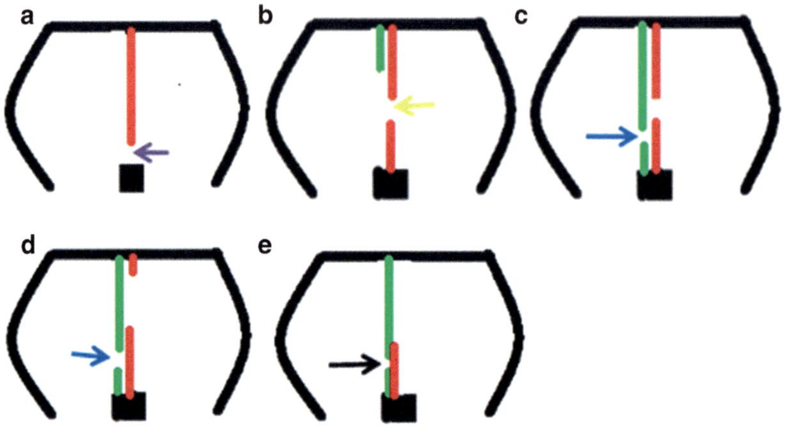

Fig. 12.1 Line diagrams showing the development of the inter-atrial septum. (**a**) The separation of the common primitive atrium into two atria in foetal life begins at about the fifth week of gestation when the septum primum (red) arises from the postero-superior part of the roof of the common primitive atrium and grows inferiorly towards the endocardial cushions (black) of the atrio-ventricular canal. There is a defect between the inferior end of the septum primum and the endocardial cushions, termed the ostium primum (purple arrow). (**b**) Following this, another membrane called the septum secundum (green) appears from the roof of the primitive atrium, towards the right side of the septum primum (red). By this time, another defect arises in the mid-part of the septum primum called the ostium secundum (yellow arrow), followed by closure of the ostium primum by fusion of the endocardial cushions (black). (**c**, **d**) The septum secundum (green) grows inferiorly and overlaps the ostium secundum. A defect is seen near the mid-part of the septum secundum, adjacent to the ostium secundum, called the foramen ovale (blue arrow). The foramen ovale is continuous with the ostium secundum. The superior part of the septum primum (red) partly regresses, while the inferior part of the septum primum forms the flap valve for foramen ovale which only allows blood from the right atrium to the left atrium. (**e**) After birth, pulmonary circulation is established, pulmonary and right heart pressures fall, left atrial pressure becomes higher than the right atrial pressure and the flap valve of the septum primum is compressed against the septum secundum with resultant functional closure of the foramen ovale. Anatomical closure of the foramen ovale occurs by about 6 months. An indentation forms towards the right atrial side of the closed foramen ovale called the fossa ovalis (black arrow).

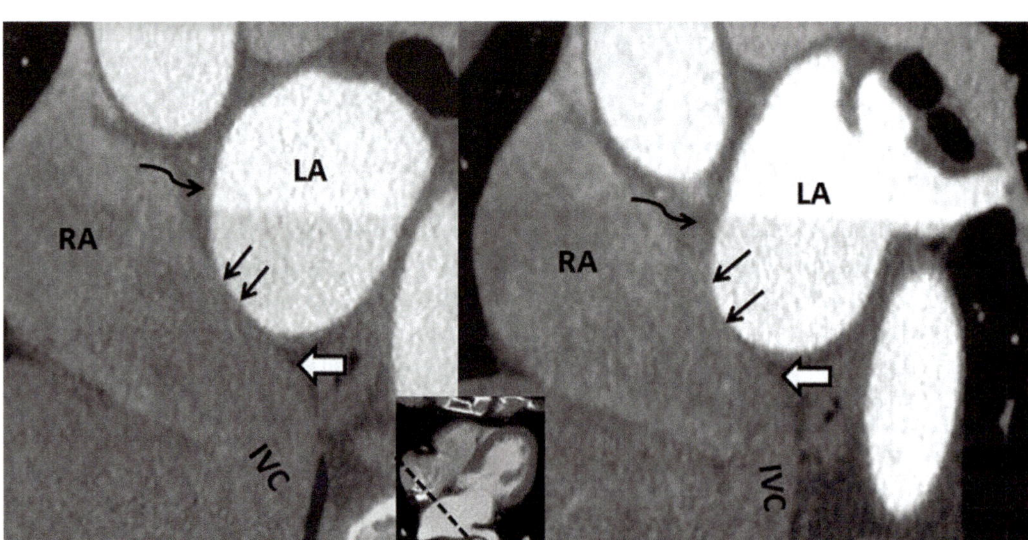

Fig. 12.2 CT reformatted images (short-axis images perpendicular to the inter-atrial septum (insert shows the plane of the image using dotted line), showing a normal inter-atrial septum and the superior (curved) and inferior (open white arrow) rims of the fossa ovalis formed by the septum secundum. Double black arrows point to the fossa ovalis. *RA* right atrium; *LA* left atrium; *IVC* inferior vena cava

12.2.2 Normal Anatomy of Inter-Atrial Septum (Fig. 12.2)

The normal inter-atrial septum is made up of the superior, posterior and inferior rims of the fossa ovalis which are formed by the septum secundum forming the inter-atrial groove. Fossa ovalis is the thin central portion of the inter-atrial septum and may not be well seen on thick section CT or MRI images and should not be mistaken to be an ASD. On MRI, an intact atrial septum thins gradually towards the site of signal intensity absence. However, in secundum ASD, the edge of the adjacent septum is thickened. The septum primum forms the floor of the fossa ovalis and antero-superiorly, overlaps the limbus which is mainly formed by the septum secundum. This septum primum flap of fossa ovalis is usually adherent to the limbus, thereby closing the foramen ovale. The size of fossa ovalis and the margins can differ in individuals.

12.2.3 Classification of ASD (Fig. 12.3)

1. Ostium secundum ASD
2. Ostium primum ASD
3. Sinus venosus ASD
4. Unroofed coronary sinus
5. Common atrial chamber
6. Patent foramen ovale (PFO)

12.2.4 Ostium Secundum ASD (Fig. 12.4)

This is the most common type of ASD and accounts for about 70% of all ASDs [2]. The defect is seen at the mid-part of the inter-atrial septum, in the region of the fossa ovalis. It occurs

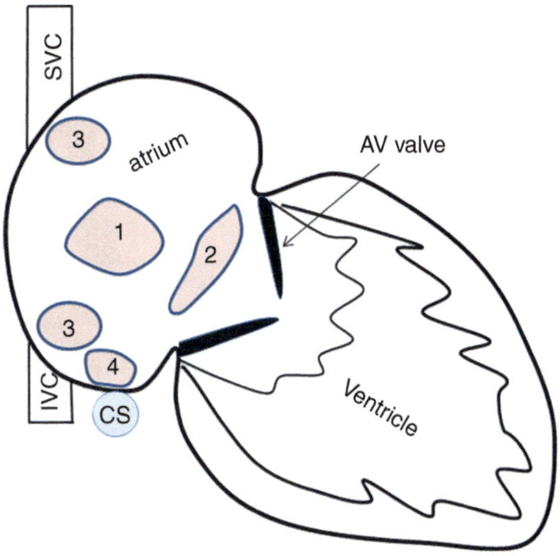

Fig. 12.3 Types of ASD. See the text for details. *CS* coronary sinus

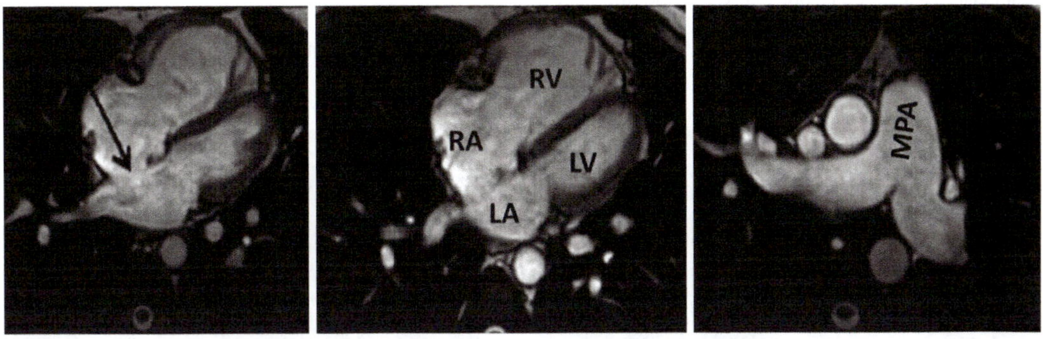

Fig. 12.4 Ostium secundum ASD—SSFP MRI images show an ostium secundum ASD (black arrow) with dilatation of the right atrium (RA) and right ventricle (RV) along with dilatation of the main pulmonary artery (MPA) as a result of pulmonary hypertension

due to increased resorption of the septum primum due to which the septum secundum fails to close the ostium secundum.

12.2.5 Ostium Primum ASD (Fig. 12.5)

This defect accounts for about 10–15% of all ASDs. An ostium primum ASD is seen at the antero-inferior end of the inter-atrial septum, near the atrio-ventricular valves. This defect develops due to failure of fusion between the lower end of the septum primum and the endocardial cushions. This defect can be associated with ventricular septal defects and defects in the atrio-ventricular valves, like a cleft in the anterior leaflet of the mitral valve.

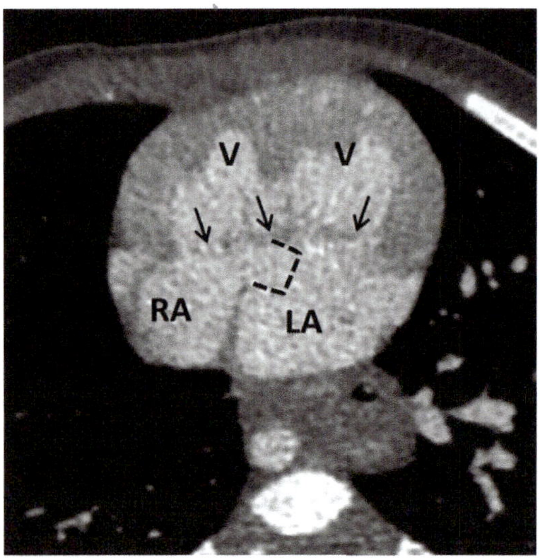

Fig. 12.5 Axial CT images showing an ostium primum type of ASD (dashed square bracket) in a patient with atrio-ventricular septal defect with a large VSD, single AV valve (small black arrows). This patient also had other anomalies like right-sided isomerism, total anomalous pulmonary venous connection and ventriculo-arterial discordance (not shown). *V* ventricles; *RA* right atrium; *LA* left atrium

12.2.6 Sinus Venosus ASD (Figs. 12.6 and 12.7)

They are the third most common type of ASDs. There is communication between cavo-atrial junction (superior vena cava (SVC) to right atrium) and the left atrium (superior sinus venosus ASD). Rarely, septal defect may be located at the junction of the inferior vena cava (IVC) and the right atrium (inferior sinus venosus ASD) [3].

It may be difficult to visualize sinus venosus ASD on transthoracic echocardiogram and transesophageal echocardiogram may be required. Sometimes, it may be identified on CT and MRI done to look for the cause of pulmonary hypertension or dilatation of right heart chambers.

This type of ASD is usually associated with partial anomalous pulmonary venous return (PAPVR), with usually the right upper lobe pulmonary vein draining into the SVC in superior sinus venosus type of ASD. Inferior sinus venosus ASD may be associated with PAPVR of right inferior pulmonary vein into the IVC.

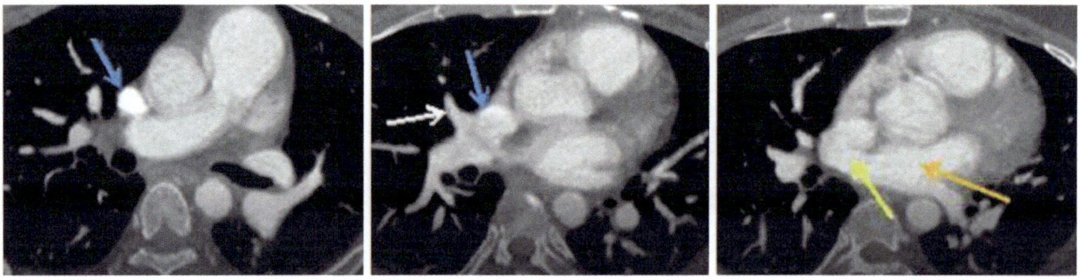

Fig. 12.6 Superior sinus venosus ASD with partial anomalous pulmonary venous return—axial CT images show the right upper lobe pulmonary vein (white arrow) draining into the superior vena cava (blue arrow) and an ASD (yellow arrow) at the level of entry of superior vena cava into the right atrium, due to which the superior vena cava is communicating with the left atrium (orange arrow) as well

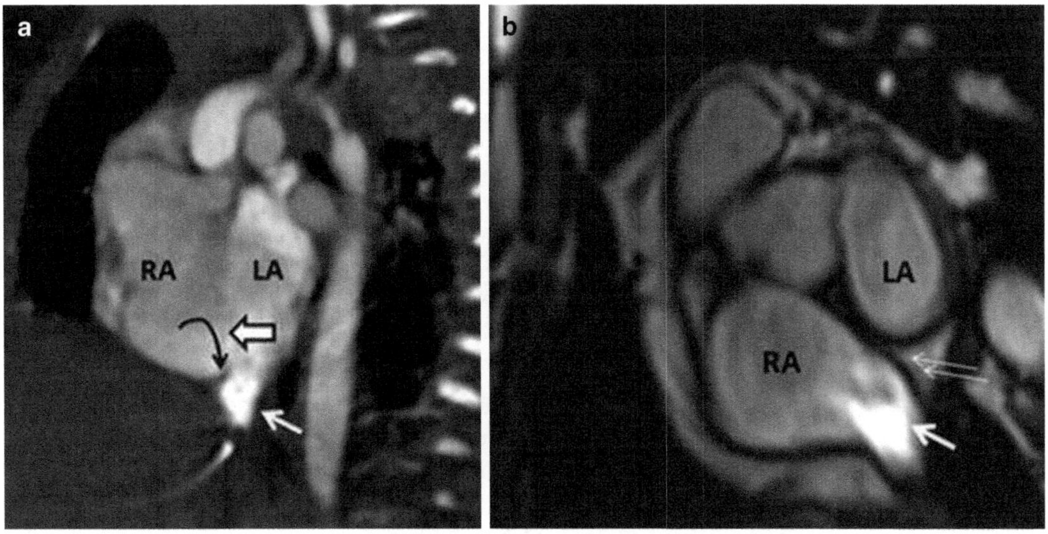

Fig. 12.7 Inferior sinus venosus ASD. Oblique sagittal reformatted CT image (**a**) shows the inferior vena cava (white arrow) draining into the right atrium (RA) and left atrium (LA). Prominent Eustachian valve (curved arrow) directs the contrast from the IVC through the ASD (open thick arrow) predominantly into the LA which is slightly more dense than the RA. Short-axis MRI image of another patient (**b**) for comparison showing the inferior vena cava (white arrow) draining normally into the right atrium (RA). There is no ASD in this case. Fat in the inter-atrial groove (double arrows) separates the RA and LA

12.2.7 Unroofed Coronary Sinus (Fig. 12.8)

This is a rare type of ASD where there is a communication between the coronary sinus and the left atrium. An unroofed coronary sinus is usually associated with a persistent left-sided SVC. There are four types of unroofed coronary sinus. Type 1 is a completely unroofed coronary sinus with persistent left-sided SVC. Type II is a completely unroofed coronary sinus without a persistent left-sided SVC. Type III is a partially unroofed coronary sinus defect in its mid-part, while type IV is a partially unroofed coronary sinus defect in its terminal part.

12.2.8 Common Atrium

The least common form of ASD is when there is a complete absence of the inter-atrial septum, with resultant formation of a common atrium. This type of defect is usually associated with other complex congenital heart anomalies.

12.2.9 Patent Foramen Ovale (PFO) (Figs. 12.9 and 12.10)

This occurs due to a lack of closure of the foramen ovale and is seen in up to 25% of the adult population [4]. A PFO is usually a very small communication between the right and left atria and as such, these patients very rarely develop volume overload of the right heart. However, these patients are at risk of developing paradoxical embolism and stroke. Occasionally, an anatomical defect may be seen in the region of the fossa ovalis even though there has been functional closure of the foramen ovale, a condition known as probe PFO. Some patients may have associated inter-atrial septal aneurysm.

12.2.10 Clinical Features

ASDs are left-to-right shunts which, even if large, are usually asymptomatic in early life and may become symptomatic even as late as the fifth or sixth decades of life. Patients may

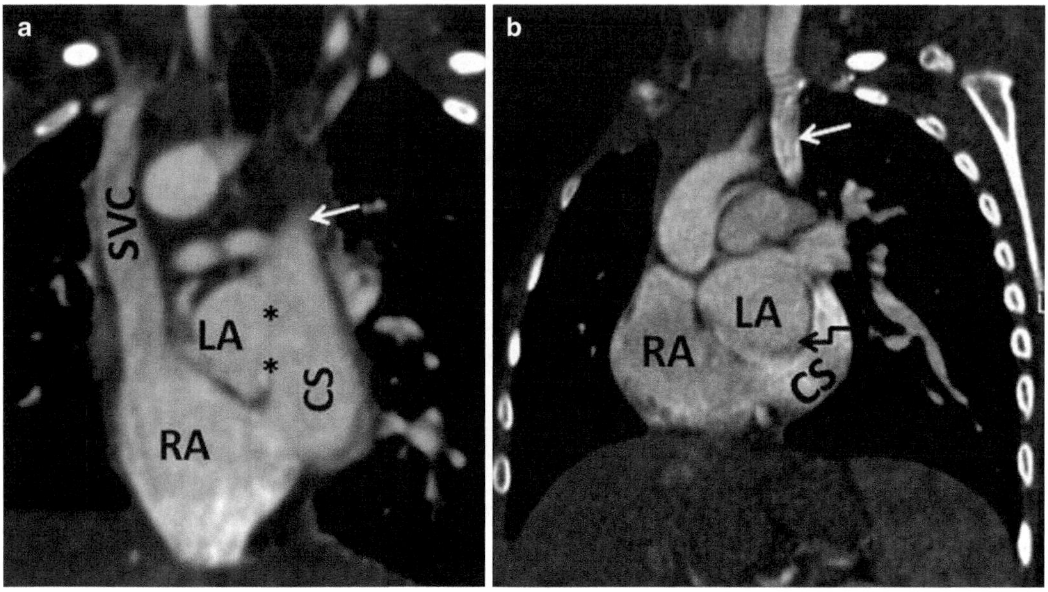

Fig. 12.8 (**a**) Left SVC with unroofing of the coronary sinus. Oblique coronal reformatted CT image showing left SVC (white arrow) (partly shown), draining into the coronary sinus (CS) with unroofing (**) of the coronary sinus, i.e. no wall between the roof of the coronary sinus and left atrium (LA). Coronary sinus drains into the right atrium (RA). Right SVC (SVC) also drains normally into the right atrium. (**b**) Intact roof of coronary sinus for comparison. Oblique coronal reformatted CT of another patient showing a persistent left-sided SVC (white arrow) which drains into the coronary sinus (CS) which in turn drains into the right atrium (RA). Note the intact roof of the coronary sinus (elbow black arrow), i.e. wall between the coronary sinus and left atrium (LA) in this case

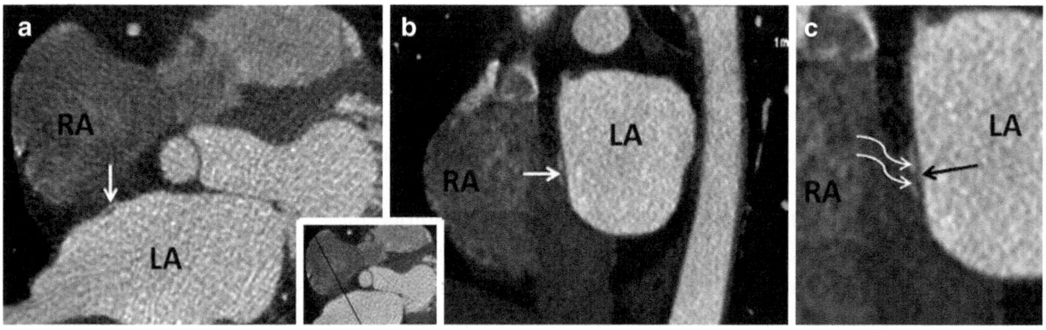

Fig. 12.9 Patent foramen ovale. Axial (**a**), short axis (**b**; insert shows the plane of **b**) and zoomed image (**c**) of the inter-atrial septum in short axis, show a patent foramen ovale (white arrows in **a**, **b**) as a slit-like extension of contrast into the inter-atrial septum (PFO tunnel) (curved arrows) at the level of fossa ovalis. Thin hypodense linear structure to the left atrial side of the PFO denoted by the black arrow in C is the flap valve (remnant of septum primum). In addition to pressure differences between right and left atrium, the length of the flap valve may determine the magnitude of shunting with more shunting occurring if the flap valve is shorter

develop exercise intolerance and atrial fibrillation. Later on, there may be a reversal of shunt due to the elevation of right heart pressures and pulmonary hypertension (Eisenmenger's syndrome).

12.2.11 Imaging Findings

Echocardiogram is the best imaging modality to diagnose an ASD. An echocardiogram can help to measure the size of an ASD, the direction of

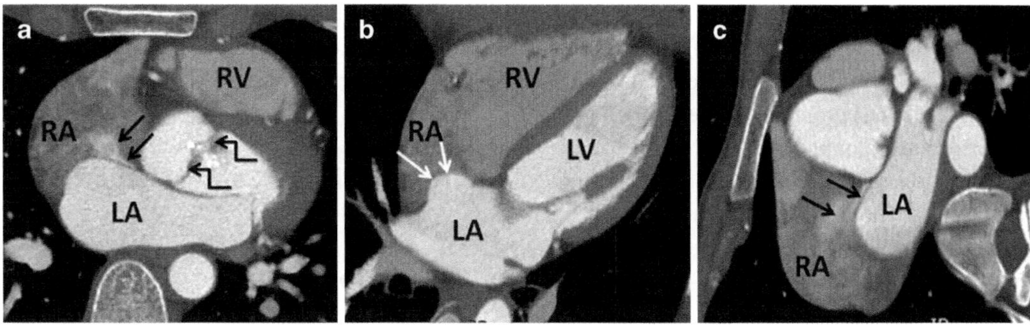

Fig. 12.10 Aneurysm of inter-atrial septum with PFO. Axial (**a**), 4 chamber (**b**), short axis (**c**) CT images showing aneurysm of inter-atrial septum (white arrows) which bulges towards the right atrium (RA). Oblique jet of contrast (black arrows) shows the shunting across the PFO. The oblique jet almost parallel to the inter-atrial septum helps to differentiate PFO from ASD where the jet is more perpendicular to the septum. This patient also had aortic stenosis with thickening and calcification of the aortic valve (elbow arrows). *LA* left atrium; *RV* right ventricle; *LV* left ventricle

shunt and whether there is any reversal and pulmonary hypertension. Echocardiogram is especially good at diagnosing PFOs and ostium secundum type of ASDs. Sinus venosus type of ASDs may not always be well seen on echocardiogram.

Chest radiographs may appear normal in small shunts. Larger shunts may show pulmonary plethora and eventually features of pulmonary hypertension. Right atrium and ventricle may be enlarged due to volume overload. The left atrium is usually not enlarged (unlike in VSD and PDA).

Inter-atrial septal defects can be well appreciated on CT as well. Thin fossa ovalis should not be mistaken for a septal defect. CT also helps in evaluating the rest of the heart and vascular structures for other associated anomalies. Passage of a jet of contrast-filled blood from the left to right atrium can help in visualizing the defect.

CT has a distinct advantage over echocardiogram in sinus venosus ASD where the defect may not be well appreciated on echocardiogram. Associated anomalies like partial anomalous pulmonary venous return are also well seen on CT.

Patients with ASD may develop pulmonary hypertension and reversal of shunt (Eisenmenger's syndrome) in later life, usually by about the fifth or sixth decades of life. Additional CT findings in such cases would include features of pulmonary hypertension like dilatation of the right atrium, right ventricle and the pulmonary arterial system. The main pulmonary artery is considered to be dilated when it measures more than 30 mm in maximum diameter or when its maximum diameter is equal to or more than the adjacent ascending aorta. The right ventricle is considered to be dilated when its maximum transverse diameter is equal to or more than that of the left ventricle. Echocardiogram is better than CT for the diagnosis of pulmonary hypertension since it assesses functional parameters as well as peak tricuspid regurgitation (TR) velocity and pulmonary artery acceleration time.

Ostium secundum ASD can usually be differentiated from a PFO by the appearance of the jet. PFOs are usually small communications and the contrast jet from the left to right atrium is at an angle or even parallel to the inter-atrial septum, rather than being perpendicular to the inter-atrial septum as in ostium secundum defects [5, 6]. Jet in PFO is at an angle to the inter-atrial septum due to the flap valve of the septum primum preventing the jet from being perpendicular to the inter-atrial septum.

The size of an ASD should ideally be measured in two dimensions, along the long-axis and short-axis of the defect. The size of ASD can be measured on transthoracic or trans-esophageal echocardiogram. Size can also be measured on MRI using through-plane phase-contrast imaging at the level of the jet of flow across the ASD. The thickness of the rim of tissue around an ASD needs to be measured as well. An ASD has an antero-superior rim (with the aortic valve), antero-inferior rim (with the tricuspid valve), postero-superior rim (with the SVC) and a postero-inferior rim (with the IVC). The absence of any rim or thickness of a rim less than 4 mm is a contra-indication for percutaneous closure of the ASD. Trans-esophageal echocardiography is usually used to assess the thickness of the rim of tissue around an ASD.

MRI can also be used to quantify the shunt volume non-invasively (see
the last section of this chapter).

12.2.12 Treatment

ASDs which are hemodynamically significant (Q_p:Q_s of more than 1.5) or have led to paradoxical embolism need to be closed. Surgical closure can be done. Ostium secundum ASDs measuring less than 40 mm in size and with more than 4 mm rim of tissue around the defect can be closed percutaneously with septal occluder devices. Isolated absence of the antero-superior (aortic) rim is not a contra-indication for per-cutaneous closure of an ostium secudum ASD.

Practical Tips

1. Sinus venosus ASDs may be associated with partial anomalous pulmonary venous return, usually involving the right superior pulmonary vein, and hence, has to be specifically looked for in all such cases.
2. Always look for an unroofed coronary sinus in patients with a persistent left-sided SVC and vice versa, since both of them can be associated with each other.
3. Ostium primum ASDs may be associated with ventricular septal defects and atrio-ventricular valve abnormalities like cleft in the anterior leaflet of the mitral valve.
4. In patients who undergo CT pulmonary angiogram for evaluation of pulmonary hypertension, partial anomalous pulmonary venous drainage with sinus venosus ASD should be actively looked for, as this can be missed on echocardiogram.

12.3 Ventricular Septal Defect (VSD)

12.3.1 Introduction

VSD is the presence of a defect in the interventricular septum (IVS) with a pathway between the left ventricle (LV) and right ventricle (RV).

VSD is the most common congenital heart disease in children, with a reported incidence of 2.62 per 1000 live births [1], occurring in up to 50% of children with congenital heart disease [1, 7] either in isolation or as a component of other lesions like tetralogy of Fallot, transposition of the great arteries, truncus arteriosus, AV canal defect or functionally single ventricular heart. In adults, VSD is the second most common congenital heart disease after bicuspid aortic valve [8].

2D and 3D echocardiogram is the main modality of imaging in evaluating the size and shape of VSD, thus helping in choosing ideal candidates for intervention or surgery and also in choosing the ideal devices.

12.3.2 Embryology (Figs. 12.11 and 12.12)

Conus and proximal third of the bulbus cordis merge with the primitive ventricle to form the ventricular cavity.

Outward growth of the apical components of the right and left ventricles and the hemodynamic forces result in the formation of the muscular part of the IVS, which extends upward towards the AV cushions (septum intermedium). The cephalic margin of the muscular IVS is concave, free and has a dorsal and ventral horn with the interventricular foramen at its upper margin.

Right and left bulbar ridges arise in the wall of the bulbar part of bulbo-ventricular cavity which fuse to form the bulbar septum. The bulbar septum grows inferiorly towards the muscular

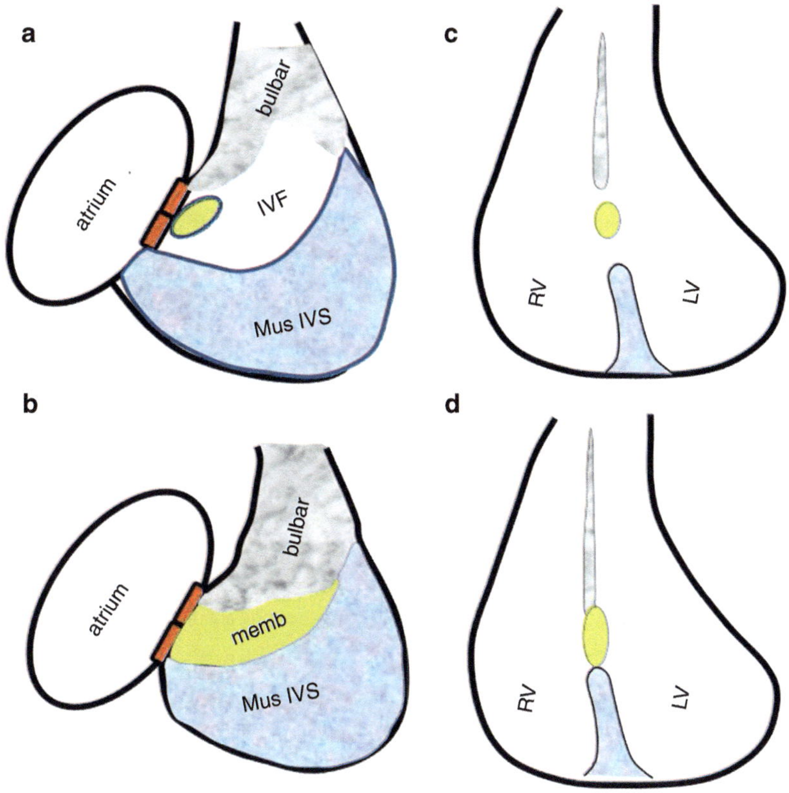

Fig. 12.11 Development of the interventricular septum. Muscular septum (Mus IVS) develops due to the outward growth of the primitive ventricles and hemodynamics forces of the blood flow in the ventricles. Bulbar septum (grey; bulbar) develops in the bulbar portion and grows towards the muscular septum, but does not meet it. Membranous septum (memb; yellow) develops as a proliferation from the endocardial cushion (brown)

septum but does not fuse with it, with a resultant persistent gap between the two.

This gap is filled by tissue proliferation from the right side of the AV cushion and from the bulbar ridges, which forms the membranous septum [9].

12.3.3 Normal Anatomy of Interventricular Septum (Figs. 12.13, 12.14, and 12.15)

- *Membranous septum* is composed of endocardium supported by fibrous tissue and is a small triangular or oval-shaped portion of the IVS located just inferior to the attachments of non-coronary and right coronary cusps of the aortic valve and between the inlet and outlet portions of the muscular IVS. The membranous portion is divided into the atrio-ventricular and interventricular portions by the attachment of the septal leaflet of the tricuspid valve. It is related to the central fibrous body, i.e. continuity of mitral, tricuspid and aortic valves.
- *Muscular septum* is a non-planar structure and can be divided into inlet, infundibular and trabecular parts:
  - The inlet portion is postero-inferior to the membranous septum and extends from the atrio-ventricular valves to the level of the apical chordal attachments.
  - The infundibular portion separates the RV and LV outflow tracts.
  - The trabecular portion is the largest part of the muscular septum and extends between the inlet and infundibular parts.

12.3.4 Pathophysiology of VSD

Depending on the location and size of the shunt and the pulmonary vascular resistance, different degrees of left to right shunt can occur and the hemodynamic significance depends on the amount of shunting and associated anomalies:

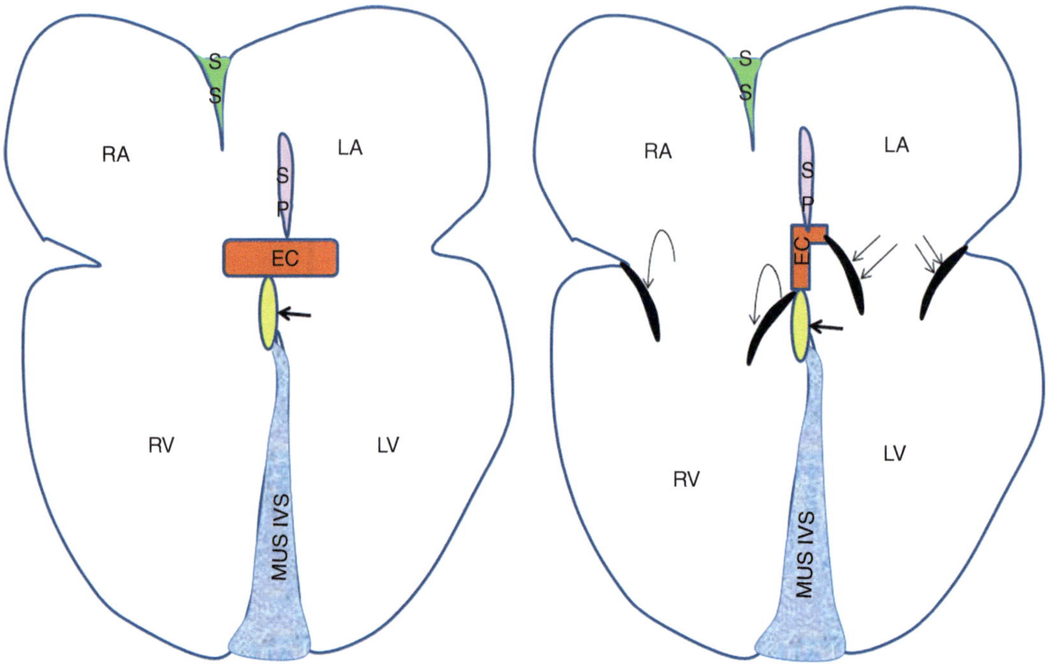

Fig. 12.12 The inter-atrial and interventricular septums do not meet the endocardial cushion in the same plane. Hence, part of the endocardial cushion (EC) also contributes to the membranous septum along with the proliferation from the endocardial cushion (yellow oval—short arrow). The septal leaflet of the tricuspid valve (curved arrows denote tricuspid valve) attaches more apically as compared to the mitral valve (double arrows) and is attached to the membranous septum at the junction of the parts derived from the endocardial cushion and the proliferation from the endocardial cushion (junction of orange and yellow portions in the figure). Due to these factors, the membranous IVS has two parts, the posterior part, which separates the left ventricle (LV) from the right atrium (RA) and the rest of it separates the right (RV) and left ventricles. Defect in the portion separating the LV and RA results in the Gerbode defect. *Mus IVS* muscular interventricular septum; *SP* septum primum; *SS* septum secundum

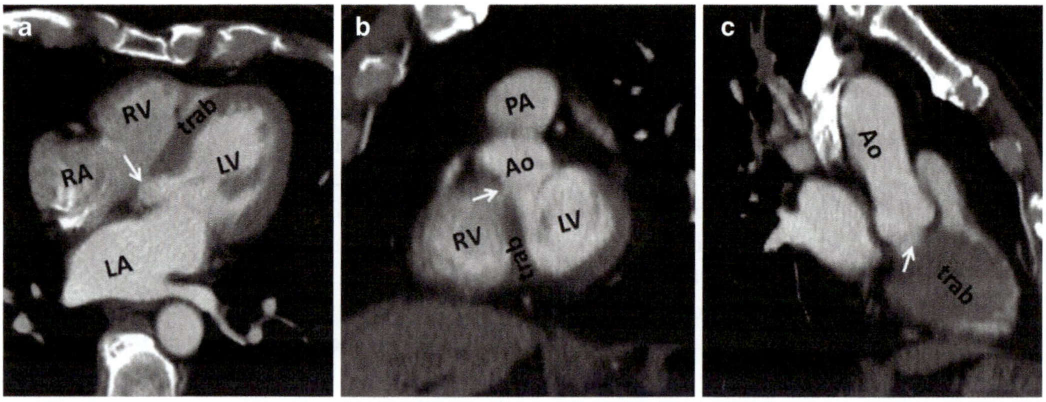

Fig. 12.13 Normal anatomy of the interventricular septum (IVS). Axial (**a**), oblique coronal (**b**) and oblique sagittal (**c**) images through the IVS, showing the membranous portion (white arrow) which is a small triangular or oval-shaped portion of the IVS located just inferior to the attachments of non-coronary and right coronary cusps of the aortic (Ao) valve. Trabecular portion (trab) is the largest portion of the IVS

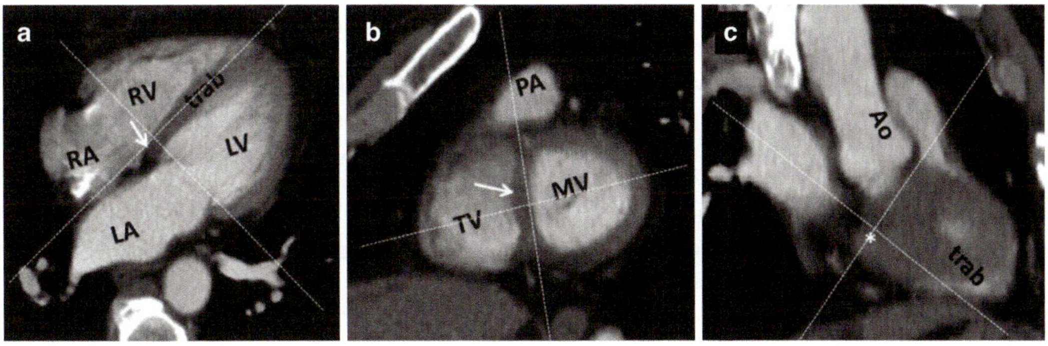

Fig. 12.14 Normal anatomy of the interventricular septum (IVS). Axial (**a**), oblique coronal (**b**) and oblique sagittal (**c**) images through the IVS with planes with respect to each other as shown with dotted lines, showing the inlet muscular portion (white arrow and white asterisk) which is a muscular portion of the IVS located postero-inferior to the membranous portion, postero-inferior to the tricuspid valve (TV) at the level where the tricuspid and mitral valve (MV) meet. Trabecular portion (trab) is the largest portion of the IVS

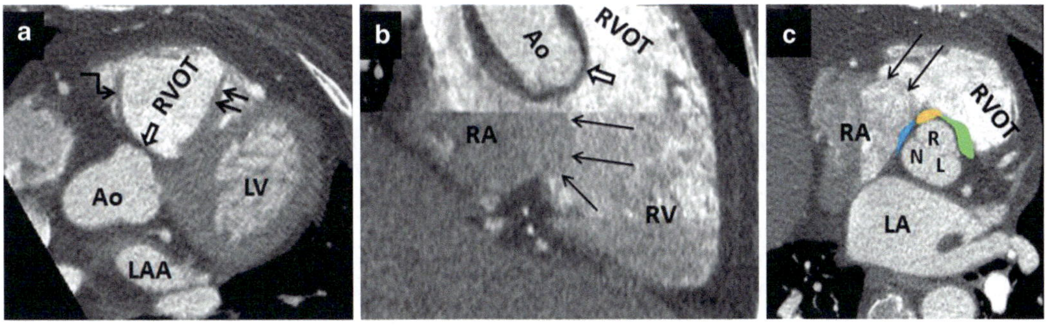

Fig. 12.15 Normal crista supraventricularis and outlet septum. Reformatted CT images in oblique axial (**a**), oblique sagittal (**b**) and double oblique (**c**) (**c** resembles the parasternal short-axis echocardiographic image), showing the parietal band (elbow arrow) and septal band (double black arrows) forming the posterolateral and posterior walls of the right ventricular outflow tract (RVOT). The junction of these two bands forms the crista supraventricularis (open arrow in **a**, **b**). Outlet defects are located superior to the crista supraventricularis and are also called as supracristal defects. Crista supraventricularis separates the tricuspid valve (thin long black arrows) from the pulmonary valve (not shown). The infundibular (green), membranous (orange) and atrio-ventricular septum (blue) are depicted. *R, L and N* right, left and non-coronary aortic cusps; *Ao* aorta; *RA* right atrium; *LA* left atrium; *LV* left ventricle; *LAA* left atrial appendage

- Approximately half of the VSDs are small (defect < 0.5 cm^2) which have less shunting with Q_p/Q_s usually being <1.5.
- Moderate-sized VSDs (defect of 0.5–1 cm^2) can allow more shunting with Q_p/Q_s of 1.5–2.
- Larger VSDs (defect >1 cm^2 or > 50–75% of the diameter of the aortic root) can be associated with larger shunts with Q_p/Q_s of more than 2 [10].

In restrictive VSD, shunt depends on the pressure gradient between ventricles which is maintained due to the small size of VSD. In large VSDs, pressure between ventricles may equalize, and shunt depends on the pulmonary and systemic vascular resistance.

The shunting results in volume overload in the pulmonary artery, left atrium and left ventricle which can be seen as dilatation of these chambers on imaging. Chronic pulmonary volume overload causes pulmonary vascular remodeling (smooth muscle proliferation, intravascular thrombosis) which in turn results in an increase in pulmonary vascular resistance. Eventually, when pulmonary pressure exceeds systemic pressure, there can be shunt reversal (i.e. right to left) and development of cyanosis which is termed as Eisenmenger syndrome.

Smaller sized and muscular VSDs have a high chance of spontaneous closure (varied reported incidence of 50–83% spontaneous closure). Larger and membranous and perimembranous VSDs have a lesser chance of closure [11].

Muscular VSDs close by ingrowth of muscle and fibrous tissue and membranous VSDs can close due to aneurysm formation in the septal leaflet of tricuspid valve which can get endothelialized. Prolapsed right aortic cusp can close outlet VSD. Aortic regurgitation can develop in outlet defects due to deficiency of the aortic valve support apparatus.

12.3.5 Complications of VSD

These include Eisenmenger's syndrome, infective endocarditis, aortic regurgitation, subaortic stenosis, congestive cardiac failure.

12.3.6 Classification

There are a lot of controversies regarding the classification of VSDs with two main different nomenclatures prevalent in different regions. The International Society for Nomenclature of Paediatric and Congenital Heart Disease has unified the major classification systems by using the location of VSD and its borders to classify VSDs (Table 12.2) which has been accepted by the 11th

Table 12.2 Types of VSD as proposed by the International Society for Nomenclature of Paediatric and Congenital Heart Disease and accepted by the 11th WHO Iteration of the International Classification of Diseases

Types of VSD
International Society for Nomenclature of Paediatric and Congenital Heart Disease classification of VSD based on the location of the defect in interventricular septum and margins of the defect as seen from morphological RV
1. Perimembranous central VSD
2. Inlet VSD without a common AV junction
– Inlet perimembranous VSD without AV septal malalignment and without a common AV junction
– Inlet perimembranous VSD with AV septal malalignment and without a common AV junction
– Inlet muscular VSD
3. Trabecular muscular VSD
– Midseptal
– Apical
– Postero-inferior
– Antero-superior
– Multiple ("Swiss cheese" appearance)
4. Outlet VSD
a. Outlet VSD without malalignment
• Outlet muscular VSD without malalignment.
• Doubly committed juxta-arterial VSD without malalignment.
– With a muscular postero-inferior rim
– With a fibrous postero-inferior rim (membranous extension)
b. Outlet VSD with anterior malalignment of outlet septum
• Outlet muscular VSD with anteriorly malaligned outlet septum.
• Outlet perimembranous VSD with anteriorly malaligned outlet septum.
• Doubly committed juxta-arterial VSD with anteriorly malaligned outlet septum.
– With a muscular postero-inferior rim
– With a fibrous postero-inferior rim (membranous extension)
c. Outlet VSD with posterior malalignment of the outlet septum
• Outlet muscular VSD with posteriorly malaligned outlet septum.
• Outlet perimembranous VSD with posteriorly malaligned outlet septum.
• Doubly committed juxta-arterial VSD with posteriorly malaligned outlet septum.
– With a muscular postero-inferior rim
– With a fibrous postero-inferior rim (membranous extension)

Iteration of International Classification of Diseases by WHO [12].

12.3.7 Imaging Findings

Plain chest radiograph can be normal in small shunts and show plethora in larger shunts. Later in life, features of pulmonary hypertension may develop. The left atrium and left ventricle are the chambers that can be dilated.

Again, echocardiogram is the mainstay for diagnosis and evaluation with CT and MRI used in certain situations where other anomalies are present or to detect lesions that are difficult to visualize on echocardiogram or to calculate the shunt fraction.

12.3.7.1 Central Perimembranous VSD (Figs. 12.16 and 12.17)

There is controversy in the literature regarding the term "perimembranous" as it refers more to the borders rather than the location. Synonyms include perimembranous, paramembranous, type 2 VSD, infracristal and subaortic VSD.

This is the most common type of VSD (75–80% of VSDs).

It occurs in the superior part of the IVS, just inferior to the aortic valve (commissure of right and non-coronary sinus) and just posterior to the septal leaflet of the tricuspid valve, at the junction of the inlet, trabecular and outlet portions of the septum. It is usually bordered by the fibrous continuity between an arterial semilunar valve (aortic valve in concordant connections) and the AV valve (usually the tricuspid valve). It can be surrounded only by fibrous tissue (i.e. true membranous VSD confined to the membranous septum) or extend to adjacent trabecular, inlet or outlet portions of the septum (peri or paramembranous) (Fig. 12.17).

The AV conduction band courses just below the postero-inferior rim and is vulnerable to injury during surgery.

12.3.7.2 Muscular: Trabecular VSD (Figs. 12.18 and 12.19)

Also called type 4 defect and accounts for approximately 20% of VSDs. This occurs along the muscular septum, distal to the attachment of the septal leaflet of the tricuspid valve, and is completely rimmed by muscle.

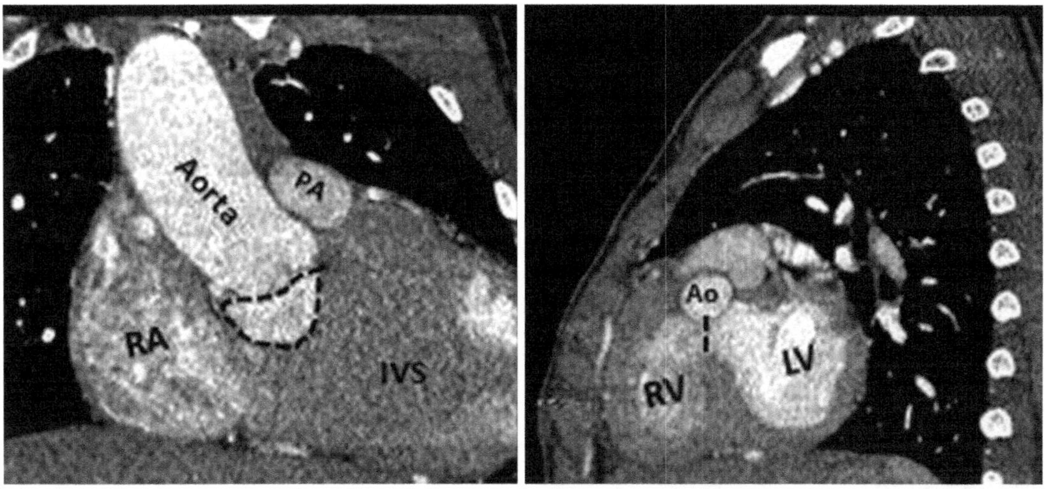

Fig. 12.16 Oblique coronal and oblique sagittal images (parallel and perpendicular to the IVS) showing a membranous VSD (dotted lines). Note that the VSD is just inferior to the aortic valve (*Ao* aorta)

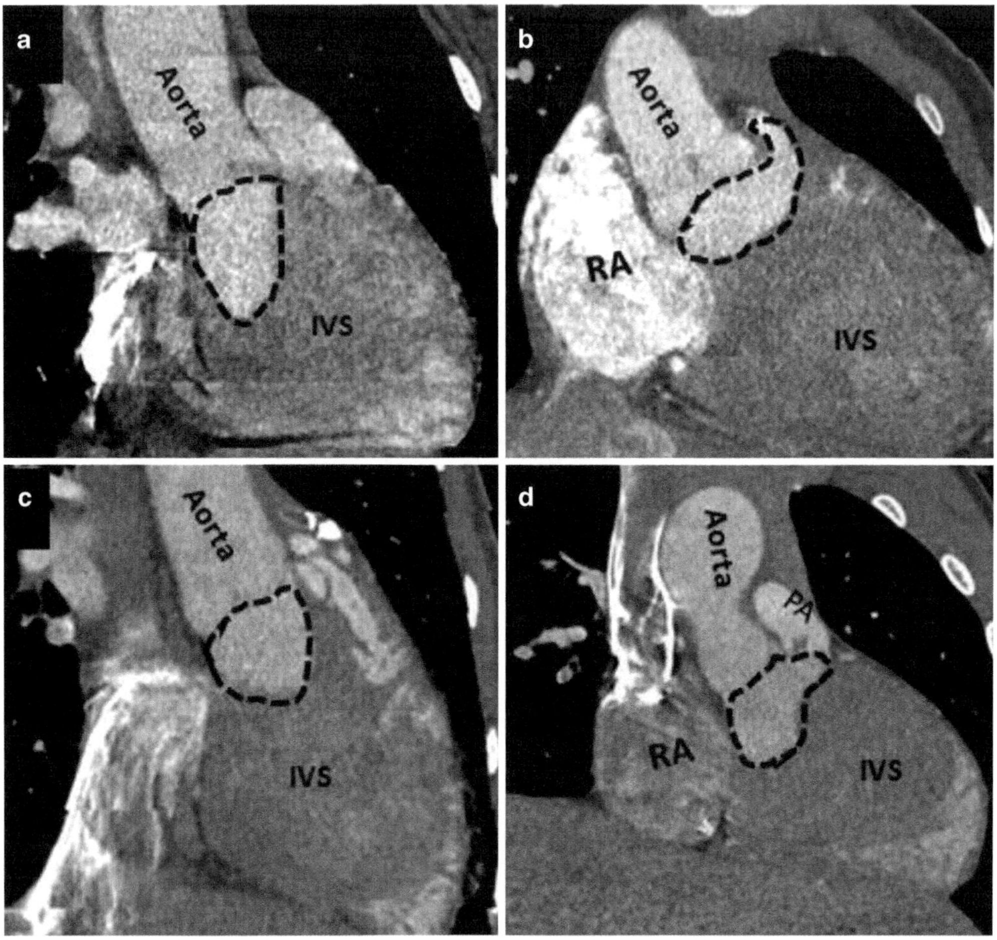

Fig. 12.17 Oblique coronal images through the IVS showing different types of perimembranous VSD (dotted lines). Perimembranous VSD with inlet extension (**a**), outlet extension (**b**), trabecular extension (**c**) and inlet and outlet extension (**d**) are shown in dotted lines

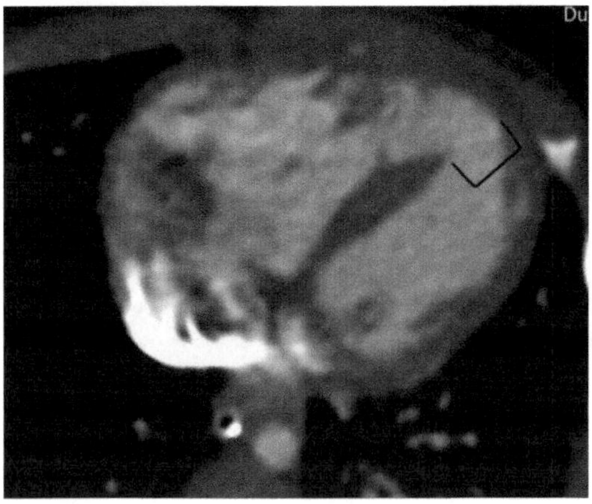

Fig. 12.18 CECT through heart showing an apical muscular VSD (square bracket)

It can be:

- Apical (distal to moderator band) (Fig. 12.18).
- Anterior (anterior to the septal band).
- Midmuscular (posterior to septal band).
- Posterior (beneath the septal leaflet of the tricuspid valve). This may be difficult to distinguish from and inlet muscular VSD [13].

Multiple muscular VSDs can also be seen giving rise to the "swiss cheese" appearance of the septum (Fig. 12.19).

Apical VSDs may be difficult to visualize on echocardiogram.

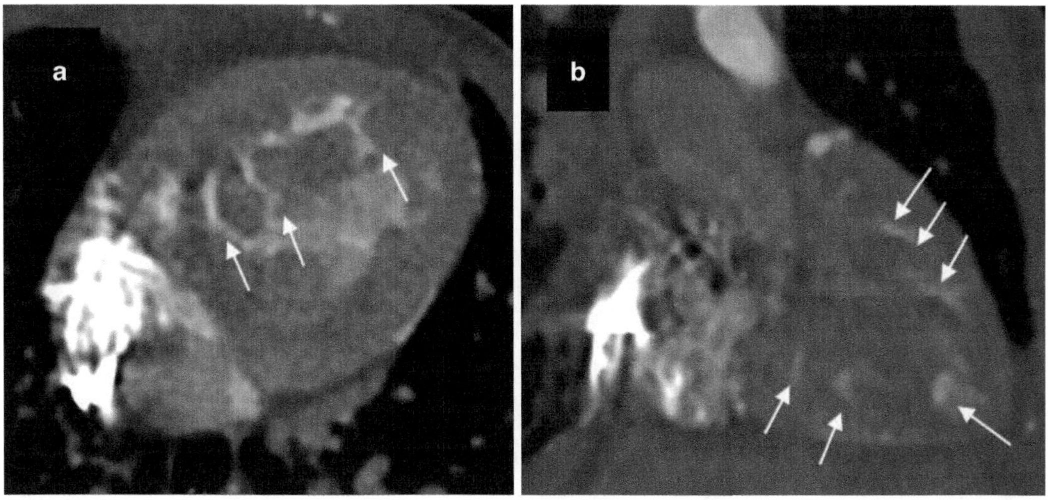

Fig. 12.19 Axial (**a**) and oblique coronal CECT (**b**) images through the interventricular septum showing multiple small muscular VSDs—"Swiss cheese septum"

12.3.7.3 **Inlet VSD** (Fig. 12.20)

Also called type 3 defects and they can be perimembranous or muscular inlet VSDs (Table 12.2). These can occur in isolation but are more commonly a part of the atrio-ventricular septal defects where they can be associated with defects in the atrial septum and atrio-ventricular valves.

Perimembranous inlet VSD is located postero-inferior to the area of fibrous continuity between AV valve and an arterial valve, posterior and superior to the tricuspid annulus, at the level of the crux of the heart, where tricuspid and mitral valves meet, with no muscular rim between the AV valves and the defect. AV valve can straddle the VSD. The AV conduction band runs along the postero-inferior rim of this defect. Therefore, during surgery, sutures should be placed away from the postero-inferior rim, to avoid heart block.

Muscular inlet VSD is in a similar location, but is completely bordered by muscle and is not contiguous with the AV valve. The AV conduction band runs close to the superior border of muscular inlet VSD, but not along its border [12].

12.3.7.4 **Outlet VSD** (Fig. 12.21)

Synonyms include infundibular, conal or conoventricular, supracristal, subpulmonary, or doubly committed subarterial or type I defects.

They can be further classified into three main types—perimembranous outlet, muscular outlet and juxta-arterial doubly committed defects with muscular or fibrous postero-inferior rim with subtypes (Table 12.2) [12]. Outlet VSDs are located between the anterosuperior and postero-inferior limbs of the septal band.

Outlet perimembranous VSDs are adjacent to the anterior leaflet of the tricuspid valve (in distinction central perimembranous defects are adjacent to the septal leaflet). The AV conduction pathway is again adjacent the postero-inferior rim of outlet perimembranous VSD and is prone to injury during surgery, but is away from the rim in muscular and juxta-arterial outlet VSDs [12].

In juxta-arterial outlet VSDs, fibrous continuity between the aortic and pulmonary valves forms the cranial border, while the muscular outlet VSDs are completely bordered by muscle and are not contiguous with AV septum or aortic or pulmonary valves [12].

12.3.8 Clinical Presentation

Clinical features depend on the degree of shunt, associated anomalies and complications.

Small restrictive VSDs can be asymptomatic, while large VSDs with significant shunts can pres-

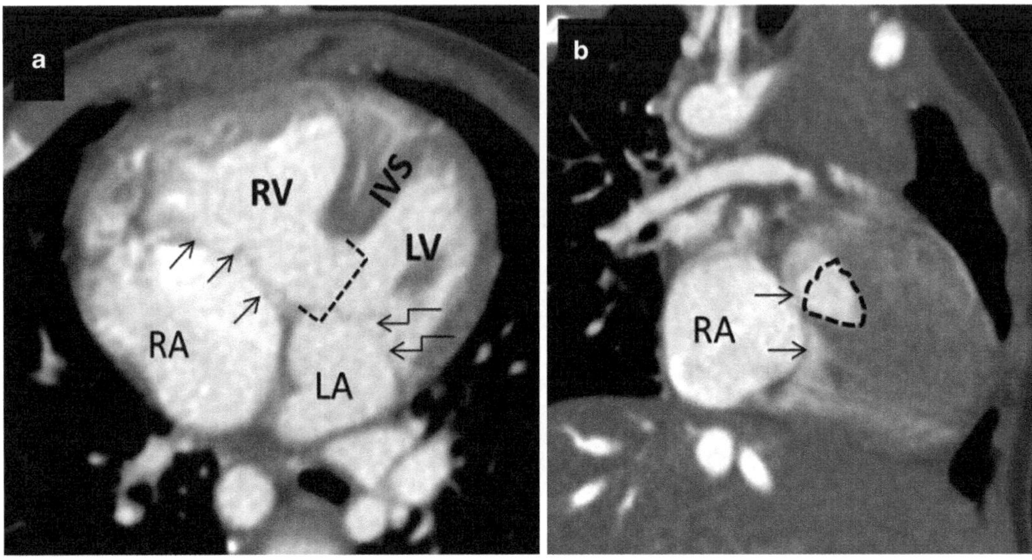

Fig. 12.20 Perimembranous inlet VSD. Axial (**a**) and oblique coronal CECT (**b**) images through the interventricular septum, showing the inlet VSD (dotted lines), at the level where the tricuspid (thin short arrows) and mitral valves (elbow arrows) meet, with no muscular rim between the AV valves and the defect. Note also the posterior and superior relation of the VSD to the tricuspid valve. *RA* right atrium; *LA* left atrium; *RV* right ventricle; *LV* left ventricle; *IVS* interventricular septum. Multiple other associated anomalies were present which are not labeled and not fully depicted on these images.

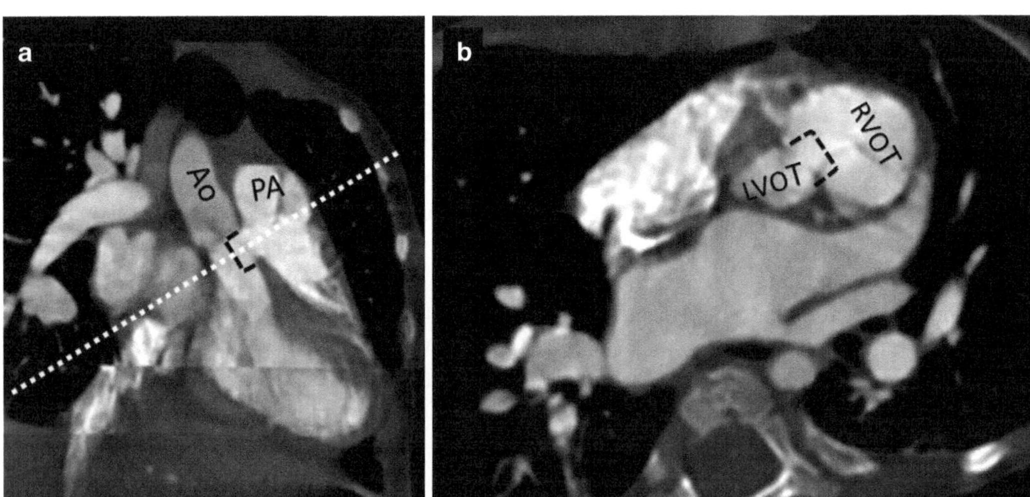

Fig. 12.21 Outlet VSD. Oblique coronal (**a**) and oblique axial images (**b**) with **b** being along the plane of the dotted white line in **a**, showing an outlet VSD (square bracket in **a**, **b**)

ent with LV volume overload and failure. They can also present with pulmonary hypertension or Eisenmenger syndrome or with complications like infective endocarditis.

12.3.9 Treatment

VSD closure is recommended in adults with VSD with significant shunts (Q_p:Q_s ≥ 1.5) with features left ventricular volume overload, provided pulmonary artery pressure is less than 50% of systemic and pulmonary vascular resistance is less than a third of the systemic [14].

Other indications for closure include complications like associated aortic regurgitation or a history of infective endocarditis.

VSD closure is contraindicated in adults with severe pulmonary hypertension and pulmonary artery pressure and vascular resistance more than two-thirds of systemic or if there is a right to left shunt [14].

Practical Tips

1. VSDs are classified according to their location and margins which can be identified on imaging by seeing the relationship of the defect to surrounding structures like AV valve, semilunar valves, crista supraventricularis and by looking for muscular rim.
2. CT/MRI can demonstrate lesions like apical VSD which are difficult to identify on echocardiogram.
3. Clinical manifestations of VSD depend on the degree of shunting which can be non-invasively measured using phase-contrast MRI.
4. Surgical closure of VSD is not recommended if there is severe pulmonary hypertension and shunt reversal.

12.4 Atrio-Ventricular Septal Defect (AVSD)

Synonyms

Endocardial cushion defects, AV canal defects, atrio-ventricular communis.

12.4.1 Introduction

AVSD includes a spectrum of abnormalities with defects in the atrio-ventricular septum and atrio-ventricular valves, resulting from abnormal development of superior and inferior endocardial cushions and their abnormal fusion with atrial and ventricular septums.

12.4.2 Classification [15] (Table 12.3)

Complete AVSD can be further divided based on:

(i) The type of bridging leaflet into the Rastelli types
(ii) Proportion of the AV valve related to each ventricle, as balanced or unbalanced

Rastelli types of complete AVSD:

- Type A—Superior bridging leaflet is divided and attached to the crest of the IVS. It is the most common type.

Table 12.3 Types of AVSD

Type of AVSD	ASD	VSD	AV valve	Comments
Incomplete or partial	Ostium primum	No	Separate AV orifices, cleft in left AV valve	Some people use thc term partial AVSD if there is an inlet VSD without ostium primum ASD.
Complete	Ostium primum	Non-restrictive large inlet VSD	Common AV valve orifice	
Transitional or intermediate	Ostium primum	Often restrictive small inlet VSD	Separate AV orifices with abnormal AV valve.	Fusion of the superior (or anterior) and inferior (or posterior) bridging leaflet results in two separate orifices.

- Type B—Straddling chordae extending from the left superior bridging leaflet to RV papillary muscles. It is rare and can be associated with single ventricle.
- Type C—Free-floating undivided superior bridging leaflet which is not attached to the crest. It can be associated with conotruncal anomalies.

Balanced Versus Unbalanced AVSD
In severely unbalanced AVSD, the common AV valve predominantly opens into one of the ventricles resulting in hypoplasia of the other ventricle. Single-ventricle palliative surgeries like Fontan procedure may be the only management option in severely unbalanced AVSD.

12.4.3 Associations

There is a strong association with Down's syndrome. AVSD constitutes 30–40% of cardiac abnormalities in patients with Down's syndrome [16]. Other described associations include left SVC, parachute mitral valve with single papillary muscle, double orifice left AV valve, patent ductus arteriosus, conotruncal anomalies like tetralogy of Fallot or double outlet right ventricle and heterotaxy syndromes.

12.4.4 Pathophysiology

One of the main abnormalities in AVSD is the left to right shunt which results in similar pathophysiology like other left to right shunts, with increased pulmonary blood flow, which results in an increase in pulmonary vascular resistance, development of pulmonary hypertension and ultimately shunt reversal or Eisenmenger syndrome.

In addition, in AVSD, AV valvular regurgitation causes significant hemodynamic disturbances with ventricular volume overload and failure.

12.4.5 Clinical Presentation

Presentation varies according to whether there is incomplete or complete AVSD and associated anomalies. Incomplete AVSD may remain asymptomatic for decades similar to ASD, while complete AVSDs present earlier in infancy with many having features of congestive heart failure.

12.4.6 Imaging Findings (Fig. 12.22)

Transthoracic and transesophageal echocardiograms are again the mainstay in the evaluation of AVSD.

CT and MRI can also demonstrate the ostium primum ASD as a defect in the antero-inferior portion of inter-atrial septum close to the AV valves. In complete AVSD, inlet VSD is also seen as a defect in the interventricular septum, located posterior to the tricuspid annulus, at the level where tricuspid and mitral valves meet. Single AV valve which can straddle the VSD, leaflets of the AV valve and chordal attachments can all be visualized on CT and MRI, in addition to depicting the valve motion, ventricular volumes and function.

Normally, the aorta is wedged between the mitral and tricuspid valves. In AVSD, the common AV valve results in unwedging of the aorta, which results in an elongated left ventricular outlet (i.e. apex to aortic root is longer than apex to AV valve). This gives the characteristic "gooseneck" appearance described on catheter angiograms.

12.4.7 Treatment

Primary complete surgical repair early in life (<6 months of age) is recommended to prevent the development of pulmonary hypertension. Single, double or modified single patch repair of ASD, VSD and separation of the AV valves is performed [17].

Severely unbalanced AVSDs may not be amenable for complete repair and may undergo palliative procedures like modified Fontan

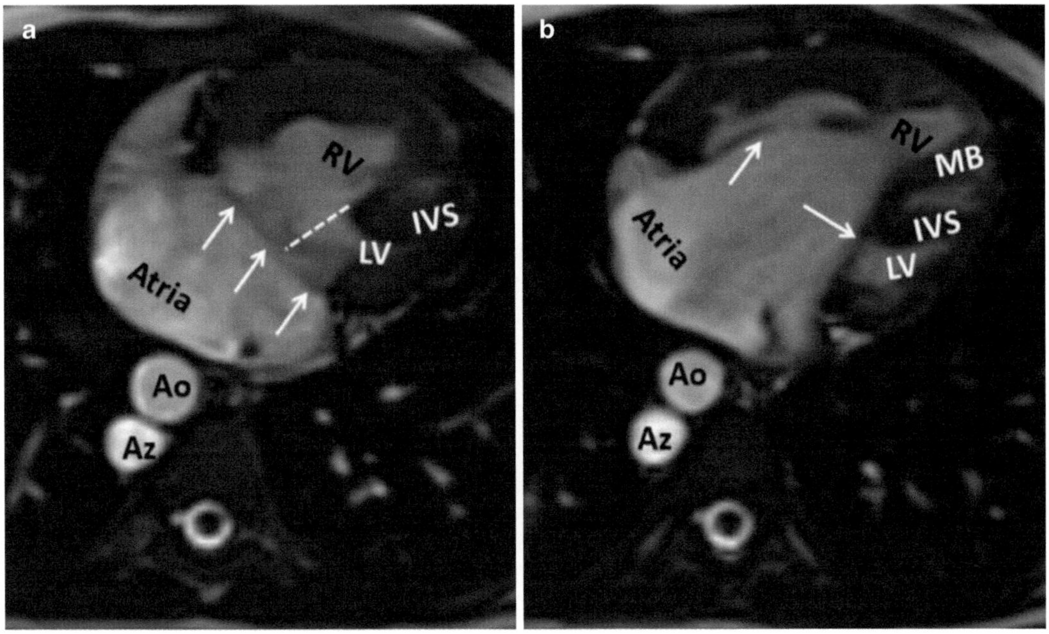

Fig. 12.22 Unbalanced complete AVSD. Still images from SSFP cine images through the heart in axial plane in systole (**a**) and diastole (**b**), showing a single atrium with absent inter-atrial septum, single AV valve (arrows) which opens predominantly into the right ventricle (RV) and a large inlet VSD (dashed line). Left ventricle (LV) is small and hypoplastic. The patient also had heterotaxy with left isomerism, bilateral left-sided bronchus, azygous continuation of IVC (Az), right-sided aortic arch and descending thoracic aorta (Ao). There was also DORV, double SVC, pulmonary stenosis (not shown). *MB* moderator band; *IVS* interventricular septum

approach, similar to patients with single ventricle cardiac defects.

Practical Tips

1. Combination of ostium primum ASD, single AV valve and inlet VSD constitutes the complete atrio-ventricular septal defect.
2. In complete AVSD, look at the configuration of the superior and inferior bridging leaflets (for Rastelli classification) and also whether the AV orifice opens equally to both ventricles (balanced) or more towards any one of the ventricles (unbalanced).

12.5 Patent Ductus Arteriosus (PDA)

12.5.1 Introduction

Ductus arteriosus is a vessel that connects the proximal descending thoracic aorta to the roof of the main pulmonary artery, close to the origin of the left pulmonary artery. Ductus arteriosus helps in bypassing the lungs by directing flow from the pulmonary artery to the aorta as the blood is oxygenated by the placenta in foetus. Normally, it spontaneously closes within 24–48 h of birth due to increased oxygen tension and reduced prostaglandin E2 and prostacyclin I2 level [18]. The levels of prostaglandin E2 and prostacyclin I2 are high in foetus due to production by the placenta and decreased metabolism in the lungs [19].

The failure of closure of ductus arteriosus beyond the neonatal period is abnormal. Isolated patent ductus arteriosus forms 10–12% of all congenital cardiac anomalies [20]. Patent ductus arteriosus may be obligatory for survival in complex cardiac abnormalities such as pulmonary atresia and tricuspid atresia where pulmonary circulation is dependent on PDA, D-Transposition of great vessels where mixing of pulmonary and systemic circulation is important for circulation and hypoplastic left heart syndrome, severe aortic stenosis, interruption of the aorta and severe coarctation of aorta where systemic circulation is dependent on the patency of ductus arteriosus [21].

12.5.2 Embryology

Ductus arterosius is formed by the distal portion of the left sixth primitive aortic arch (Fig. 12.23), connecting the left pulmonary artery to the left dorsal aorta. The distal portion of the right sixth arch normally degenerates. The proximal portion of the left sixth arch forms the main and left pulmonary artery. The proximal portion of the right sixth arch forms the right pulmonary artery. This development is complete by 8 weeks of life.

12.5.3 Morphology

Patent Ductus Arteriosus (PDA) classification system on the basis of angiogram appearance by Krichenko [22] (Fig. 12.24):

- *Type A*—conical duct with well-defined aortic ampulla and constriction near the pulmonary artery end.
- *Type B*—large duct with window-like structure which is very short in length.
- *Type C*—tubular duct without any constriction.
- *Type D*—complex duct with multiple constrictions.
- *Type E*—elongated duct with constriction remote from the edge of the trachea (as viewed on lateral angiography).

12.5.4 Pathophysiology

In foetus, ductus arteriosus allows right to left shunting of blood with low oxygen concentration from the right ventricle via the main pulmonary artery to the proximal descending thoracic aorta which subsequently flows to the placenta for oxygenation. The patency of ductus arteriosus is controlled by oxygen tension and circulating

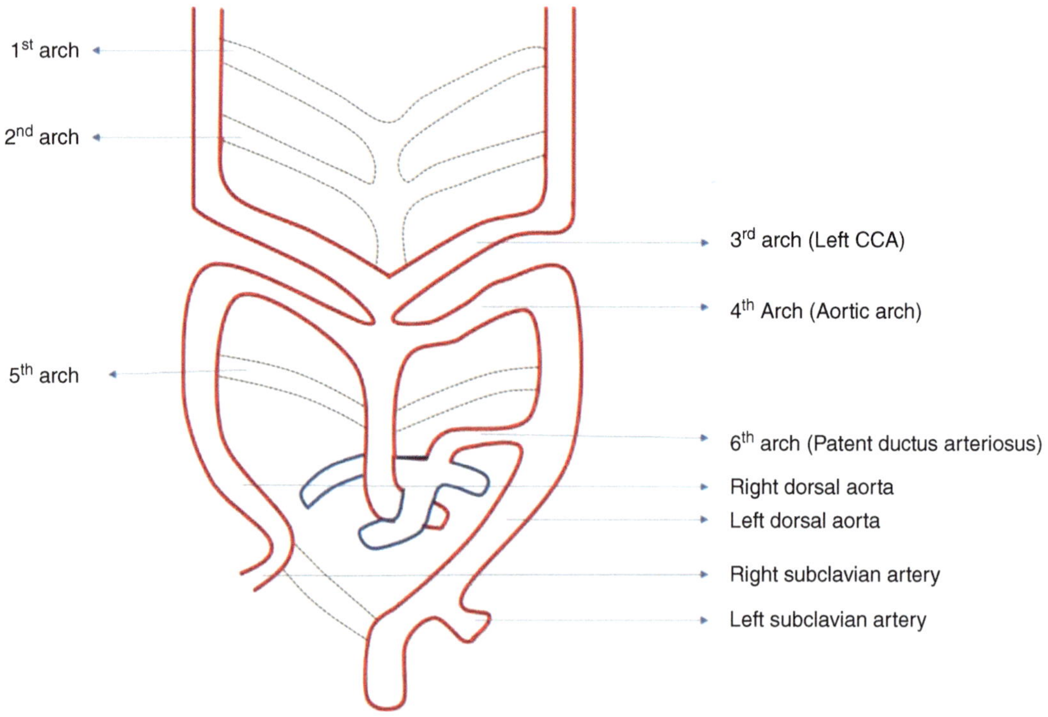

Fig. 12.23 Embryology of patent ductus arteriosus (see text for details)

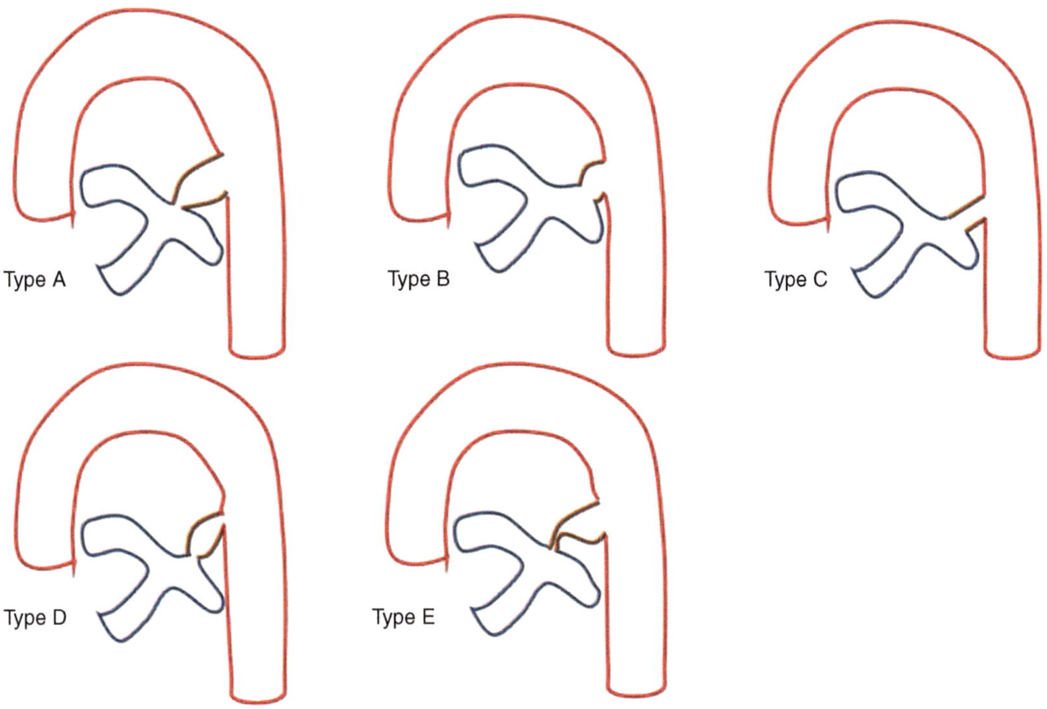

Fig. 12.24 Line diagram showing the different types of PDA as described by Krichenko (see text for details)

prostanoids from the metabolism of arachidonic acid by COX. Among all prostanoids, PGE2 produces the maximum vasodilation. After birth, the level of prostanoids reduces as the source is the placenta. Moreover, functional lungs have increased metabolism and this reduces the level of circulating prostaglandin E2 and prostacyclin I2 level. As the ductus constricts, flow is obstructed through the vasa vasorum leading to cell death and remodeling into ligamentum arteriosum [23].

The hemodynamics of patent ductus arteriosus (PDA) depends on the amount of shunting which in turn depends on the resistance and pressure gradient between the aorta and pulmonary artery. Left to right shunting results in an increase in pulmonary flow, increase in pulmonary fluid and dyspnea. Increased pulmonary flow leads to increased flow to the left heart. The diastolic pressure in the aorta decreases due to flow to PDA. Exposure of the pulmonary artery to high-pressure system results in increased pulmonary artery resistance. When pulmonary artery pressure exceeds systemic pressure, ductal shunting reverses from left to right side which is called Eisenmenger's syndrome [19]. A minority of patent ductus arteriosus are subclinical and well-tolerated into adulthood.

12.5.5 Clinical Features

As per the clinical severity, PDA is graded into silent, small, moderate, large and Eisenmenger types based on the presence and absence of murmur, wide pulse pressure, dilatation of the left ventricle and pulmonary arterial hypertension. If none of these are present, it is a silent type. If there is a continuous murmur and the rest of the findings are absent, it is a small PDA. If all the four findings are present, it is a moderate PDA. If the typical continuous murmur is absent and only systolic murmur is present along with other findings, it is a large PDA. The most severe is Eisenmenger syndrome with right to left shunt, cyanosis of feet more than arms and severe pulmonary arterial hypertension [18].

12.5.6 Imaging Findings

Chest Radiograph (CXR)—If the PDA shunt is small, CXR may be normal. The most common findings on CXR are dilatation of pulmonary artery and complications such as pulmonary arterial hypertension and cardiomegaly. These findings can be seen in any cause of left to right shunt. The most specific sign is the presence of two parallel lines due to mural calcification of the ductus called "railroad track" sign which is rarely seen [24, 25]. Calcification in the aortopulmonary window may indicate a calcified ligamentum arteriosus or calcified patent ductus arteriosus.

Echocardiography is the first modality of choice to detect PDA and the amount of shunting. The cardiac chambers, cardiac function and pulmonary artery hypertension can be assessed with ease.

Multidetector CT with intravenous contrast gives detailed size and morphology and the presence of calcification of the PDA. The ductus may be long or short or tortuous or straight with or without constrictions. The ductus may show calcification. Oblique sagittal reformatted images (Fig. 12.25) best demonstrate PDA along with the long axis views of the main pulmonary artery and descending thoracic aorta. The presence of other congenital abnormalities can also be assessed on MDCT (Fig. 12.26). The morphology and calcification have management implications.

MRI gives a good assessment of the size and morphology of PDA and the presence of other cardiac and vascular abnormalities like MDCT. MRI has the advantage of the absence of ionizing radiation and also there is no need for intravenous contrast medium. Stack of steady-state free precession imaging (Fig. 12.27) through ventricles and phase-contrast imaging through mid-ascending aorta and mid main pulmonary artery help to assess ventricular function and flow across shunt accurately (see the last section of the

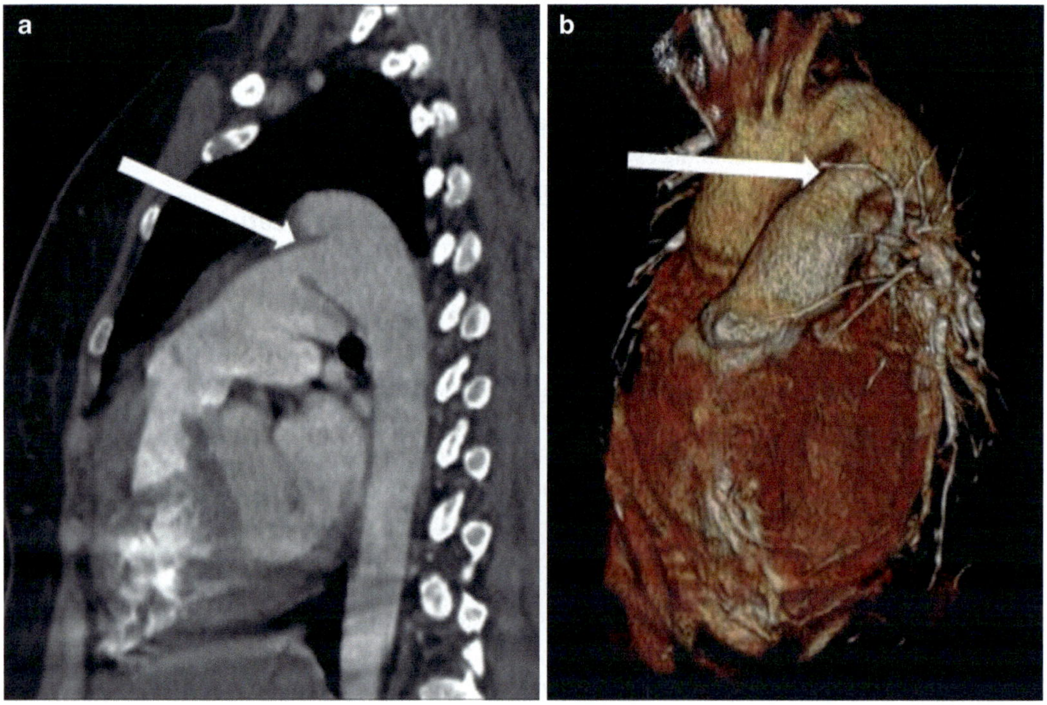

Fig. 12.25 Sagittal reformatted image (**a**) and volume-rendered (**b**) MDCT images of an adult who presented with pulmonary arterial hypertension showing previously undiagnosed patent ductus arteriosus (long thin arrow)

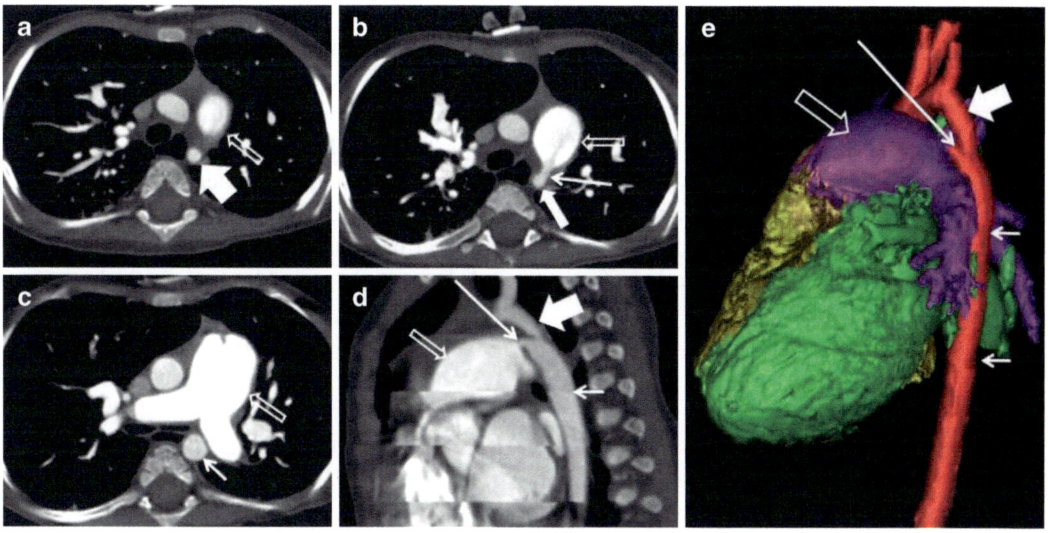

Fig. 12.26 MDCT axial images (**a**–**c**), sagittal (**d**) and 3D (**e**) reconstructed images showing patent ductus arteriosus (long thin arrow) and its negative jet on B (indicating flow from the aorta to the pulmonary artery; left to right shunt), juxta-ductal coarctation of the aorta (short thick arrow). Short thin arrow shows descending thoracic aorta and short open arrow shows dilated main pulmonary artery

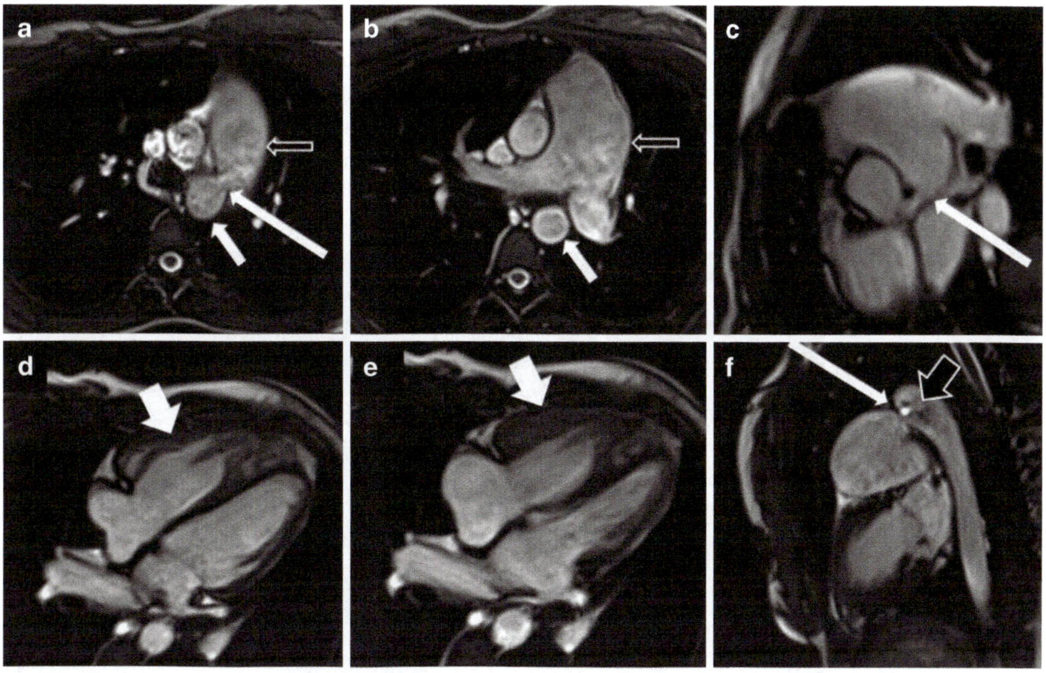

Fig. 12.27 SSFP images in axial (**a**, **b**), short axis (**c**), four-chamber—end-diastolic (**d**) and end-systolic (**e**) and oblique sagittal views (**f**) showing patent ductus arteriosus (long thin arrow) and its jet (short black arrow). Short thin arrow shows descending thoracic aorta and short open arrow shows dilated main pulmonary artery. RV hypertrophy is shown by short thick white arrow

chapter for assessment of shunt volume and degree). Calcification of the ductus is not easily identified on MRI.

Practical Tips

1. Oblique sagittal images on CT and MRI best demonstrate the morphology of the PDA.
2. CT and MRI help in the evaluation of other associated anomalies.

12.5.7 Treatment

Definitive treatment is the closure of PDA. Closure is possible only if irreversible pulmonary hypertension has not developed.

Indications for closure include:

1. Symptomatic patients with significant left to right shunting.
2. Asymptomatic patient with significant left to right shunting that results in left heart enlargement. Left to right shunting of more than 1.7 usually warrants closure.

The closure of incidentally discovered PDA in children and young adults may be reasonable as there is a risk of endarteritis. The role of closure in incidentally discovered PDA in older adults is not certain.

Transcatheter closure of small and medium PDAs with occlusion devices and coils gives excellent results. The treatment of choice of large PDA is surgical closure [19, 20]. A heavily calcified duct or a duct with morphological types D and E are not suitable for surgical closure. Surgical closure is a high risk for those above 60 years.

12.6 MRI Quantification of Shunts [26, 27]

Measurement of shunt volume can be performed non-invasively by two MR imaging methods, the volumetric and flow quantification technique:

- The volumetric method is based on assessing the right and left ventricular stroke volumes on gradient-echo cine imaging in the short-axis plane with the difference between them used to calculate the shunt volume.
- Shunt calculations can also be done using phase-contrast velocity encoded MRI to measure flow through the aorta and pulmonary

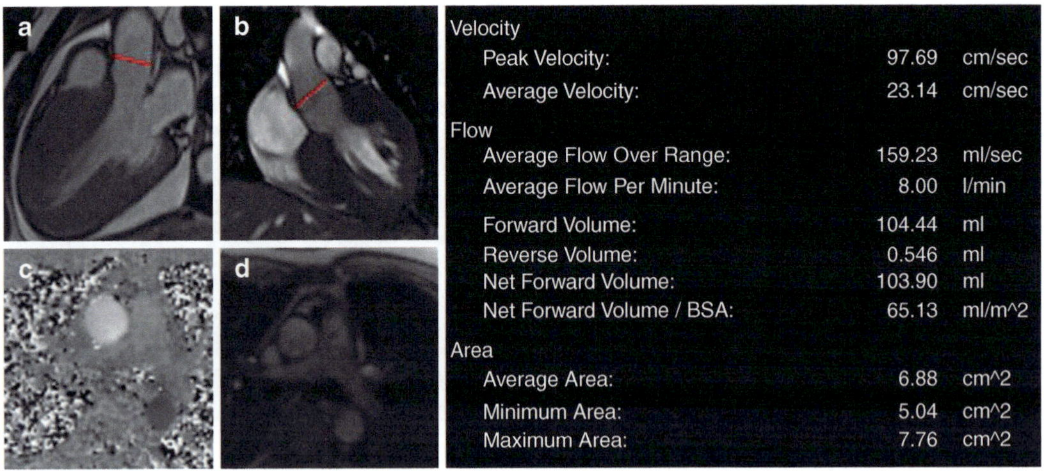

Fig. 12.28 Phase-contrast imaging through the ascending aorta. LVOT views (**a, b**) showing the expected location of planning the PC imaging. Phase (**c**) and magnitude (**d**) images obtained with PC imaging and chart showing the velocities and calculated flow

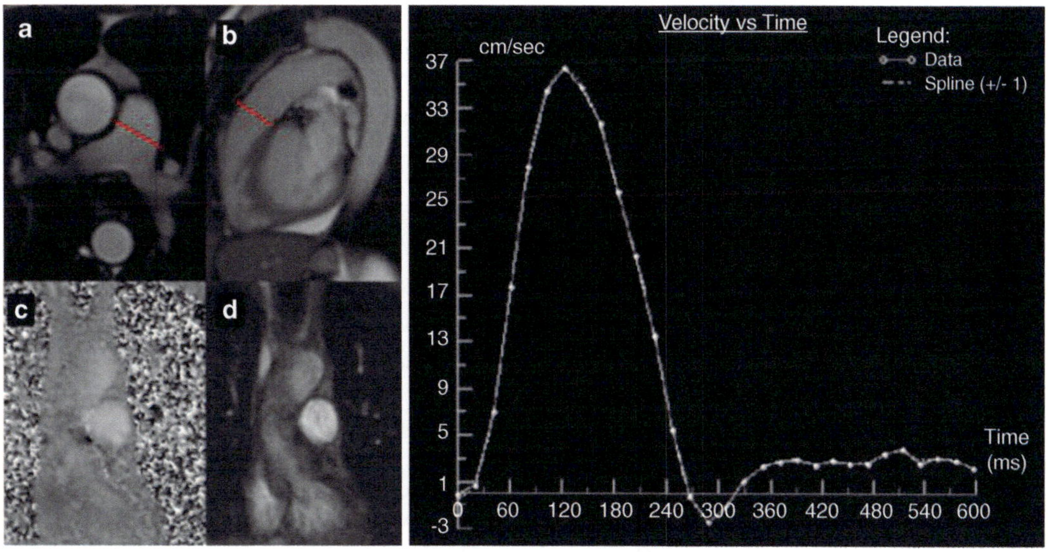

Fig. 12.29 Phase-contrast imaging through the main pulmonary artery. Axial and RVOT views (**a**, **b**) showing the expected location of planning the PC imaging. Phase (**c**) and magnitude (**d**) images obtained with PC imaging and graph showing the velocities. Area under the curve will give the volume of flow

Table 12.4 Basics of Q_p/Q_s

Qp/Qs > 1	Qp/Qs < 1
L to R shunt	R to L shunt
PO_2 normal	Low PO_2
Pulmonary overcirculation	Cyanosis
(Can eventually lead to pulmonary HT and Eisenmenger syndrome when Qp/Qs becomes <1)	

artery (Figs. 12.28 and 12.29) and calculating the difference or directly measuring the flow through the shunts (Table 12.4).

The values obtained by velocity-encoded MRI measurements of flow in the proximal great vessels are comparable to the assessment of shunt by cardiac catheterization.

Please see the chapter on phase-contrast MRI for details of how to perform these studies.

Calculations

Q_p is used to denote pulmonary flow.

Q_s is used to denote systemic flow.

Flow-through ascending aorta can be denoted as Q_{Ao} and through the main pulmonary artery as Q_{MPA}.

Q_p

In ASD and VSD, $Q_p = Q_{MPA}$.

In PDA, $Q_p = Q_{Ao} = Q_{MPA}$ + flow in PDA

Other ways to calculate Q_p in case of PDA are:

(i) By adding the flow in the right and left pulmonary arteries beyond the shunt ($Q_{RPA} + Q_{LPA}$).
(ii) Adding flow in all pulmonary veins.

Q_s

In ASD and VSD, $Q_s = Q_{Ao}$.

In PDA, $Q_s = Q_{MPA} = Q_{Ao}$ − flow in PDA.

Q_s can also be got by adding flow in descending aorta and SVC.

12.6.1 Calculating Shunt Across Atrial Septal Defect (Fig. 12.30)

In ASD, as the shunt is pre-tricuspid and occurs in diastole, there is volume overload in the right ventricle (RV), resulting in RV stroke volume (RV SV) being more than left ventricular (LV) stroke volume (LV SV). Further Q_{MPA} is the same

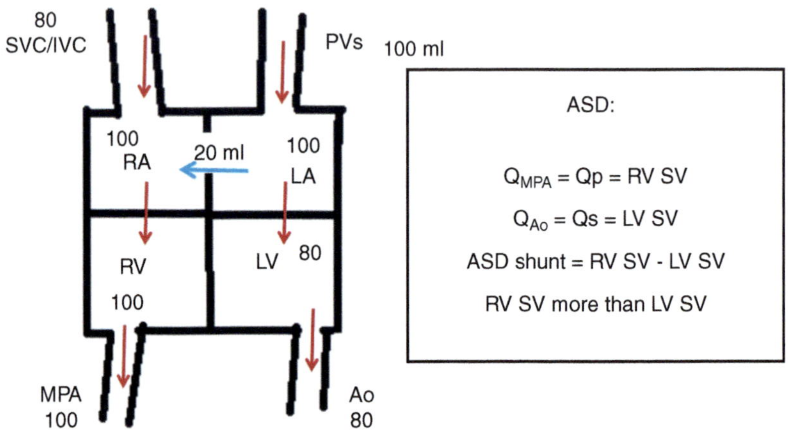

Fig. 12.30 Line diagram using hypothetical numbers to demonstrate the hemodynamics and shunt calculation in ASD

as RV SV and is also the Q_p. Similarly, Q_{Ao} is the same as LV SV and is also the Q_s.

Q_p/Q_s can be calculated by Q_{MPA}/Q_{Ao} or RV SV/LV SV.

Shunt volume can be calculated by subtracting Q_{Ao} from Q_{MPA} or LV SV from RV SV.

Shunt volume = $Q_{MPA} - Q_{Ao}$ or RV SV – LV SV.

Direct flow quantification by performing phase-contrast imaging perpendicular to the jet across the ASD has also been tried but needs more expertise. To get the phase-contrast en face image of the ASD, orthogonal images of the atrial septum in short axis and four-chamber views acquired in end-systole are used to get double oblique through the plane. Planning from end-systolic image frame maximizes the ASD flow and reduces errors due to septal motion. VENC is kept low at 50–100 cm/sec to identify low-velocity jets and low TE of about 3 ms to reduce phase offset errors.

Ostium secundum type ASD of about 10–20 mm in diameter typically results in a Q_P:Q_s of between 1.5 and 2.5:1.0. Whereas sinus venosus ASD with an anomalous pulmonary vein draining to the SVC is typically associated with a larger Q_p:Q_s, i.e. at least 2.5:1.0.

12.6.2 Calculating Shunt Across Ventricular Septal Defect (Fig. 12.31)

In VSD, as the shunt is post-tricuspid and occurs in systole, the shunted blood flows directly into the MPA without causing volume overload of the RV. Hence, LV SV will not be the same as Q_{Ao}, instead, LV SV will be the same as Q_{MPA}. Q_{Ao} will be LV SV minus the shunt volume. Similarly, Q_{MPA} includes both RV SV and the shunt volume. LV SV will be more than the RV SV. Further, Q_{MPA} which is the same as LV SV is also the Q_p. Again, Q_{Ao} is the same as RV SV and is also the Q_s.

Q_p/Q_s can be calculated by Q_{MPA}/Q_{Ao} or LV SV/RV SV.

Shunt volume can be calculated by subtracting Q_{Ao} from Q_{MPA} or RV SV from LV SV.

Shunt volume = $Q_{MPA} - Q_{Ao}$ or LV SV – RV SV.

12.6.3 Calculating Shunt Across Patent Ductus Arteriosus (Fig. 12.32)

In PDA, the shunt occurs beyond the level of the ascending aorta and proximal main pulmonary artery where the Q_{Ao} and Q_{MPA} are measured. So, the actual systemic flow Q_s is less than the Q_{Ao} by the shunt volume and actual pulmonary flow Q_p is more than the Q_{MPA} by the shunt volume. Using these two, it can be derived that Q_p is the same as Q_{Ao} and Q_s is the same as Q_{MPA}. All the LV SV flows to aorta. So, LV SV is the same as Q_{Ao} and similarly, QMPA is the same as RV SV.

LV SV will be more than the RV SV.

Q_p/Q_s can be calculated by Q_{Ao}/Q_{MPA} or LV SV/RV SV.

Shunt volume can be calculated by subtracting Q_{MPA} from Q_{Ao} or RV SV from LV SV.

Shunt volume = $Q_{Ao} - Q_{MPA}$ or LV SV – RV SV.

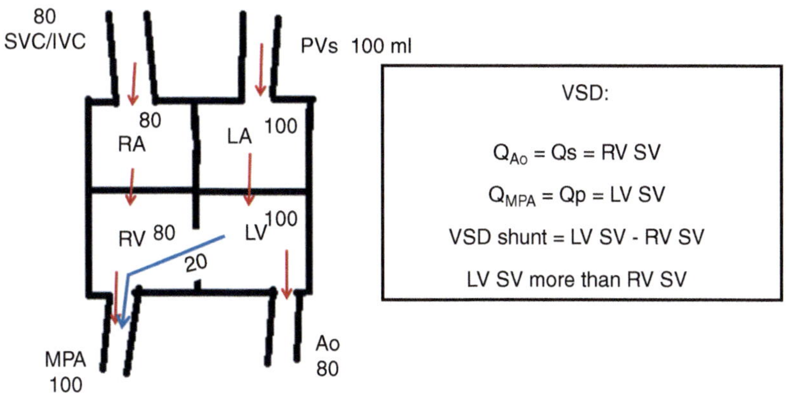

Fig. 12.31 Line diagram using hypothetical numbers to demonstrate the hemodynamics and shunt calculation in VSD

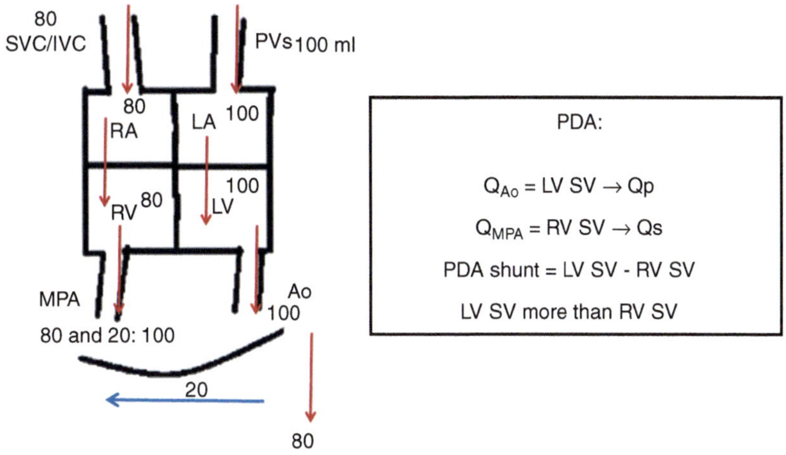

Fig. 12.32 Line diagram using hypothetical numbers to demonstrate the hemodynamics and shunt calculation in PDA

Aorto-pulmonary shunting can also be calculated by subtracting systemic venous return from Q_{Ao} [Q_{Ao} − (SVC + IVC)]. Here, as descending aortic flow at the level of the diaphragm can be used to equate to IVC and SVC flow should be measured superior to the drainage of the azygous vein into SVC (Flow in descending aorta comes back via the IVC and azygous system, so if SVC flow is measured inferior to azygous–SVC junction, azygous flow will be accounted for twice).

12.6.4 Illustrative Examples

Example 12.1

Acyanotic patient	Is there a shunt?
RV SV = 100 ml	Is it L to R or R to L?
Q_{MPA} = 100 ml	What type?
LV SV = 60 ml	If yes, what is shunt volume?
Q_{Ao} = 60 ml	What is Q_p/Q_s?

Answer 12.1

Acyanotic patient	Is there a shunt—*yes* Is it L to R or R to L—*L to R*
RV SV = 100 ml	What type? *ASD*
Q_{MPA} = 100 ml	If yes, what is shunt volume? *40 ml*
LV SV = 60 ml	What is Q_p/Q_s
Q_{Ao} = 60 ml	100/60 = *1.66*

Example 12.2

Acyanotic patient	Is there a shunt?
RV SV = 60 ml	Is it L to R or R to L?
Q_{MPA} = 100 ml	What type?
LV SV = 100 ml	If yes, what is shunt volume?
Q_{Ao} = 60 ml	What is Q_p/Q_s?

Answer 12.2

Acyanotic patient	Is there a shunt?—*yes* *L to R*
RV SV = 60 ml	What type? *VSD*
Q_{MPA} = 100 ml	If yes, what is shunt volume? *40 ml*
LV SV = 100 ml	What is Q_p/Q_s?
Q_{Ao} = 60 ml	100/60 = *1.66*

Example 12.3

Acyanotic patient	Is there a shunt?
RV SV = 60 ml	Is it L to R or R to L?
Q_{MPA} = 60 ml	What type?
LV SV = 100 ml	If yes, what is shunt volume?
Q_{Ao} = 100 ml	What is Q_p/Q_s?

Answer 12.3

Acyanotic patient	Is there a shunt?—*yes*
RV SV = 60 ml	*L to R*
Q_{MPA} = 60 ml	What type? *PDA*
LV SV = 100 ml	If yes, what is shunt volume? *40 ml*
Q_{Ao} = 100 ml	What is Q_p/Q_s – 100/60 = *1.66*

Here, Q_{MPA}/Q_{Ao} is less than 1 which could suggest a right to left shunt. But as the patient is acyanotic, it cannot be a right to left shunt. Instead, this indicates that the shunt is at the arterial level, like a PDA, i.e. Q_{MPA} is the Q_s and Q_{Ao} is the Q_p.

The above methods are useful in simple shunts without associated valvular regurgitations.

References

1. van der Linde D, Konings EE, Slager MA, et al. Birth prevalence of congenital heart disease worldwide: a systematic review and meta-analysis. J Am Coll Cardiol. 2011;58(21):2241–7.
2. Webb G, Gatzoulis MA. Atrial septal defects in the adult: recent progress and overview. Circulation. 2006;114:1645–53.
3. Van Praagh S, Carrera ME, Sanders SP, Mayer JE, Van Praagh R. Sinus venosus defects: unroofing of the right pulmonary veins - anatomic and echocardiographic findings and surgical treatment. Am Heart J. 1994;128(2):365–79.
4. Hara H, Virmani R, Ladich E, et al. Patent foramen ovale: current pathology, pathophysiology and clinical status. J Am Coll Cardiol. 2005;46(9):1768–76.
5. Funabashi N, Maeda F, Nakamura K, Suzuki K, Mita Y, Matsuo K, et al. Channel-like appearance of a patent foramen ovale with left to right shunt demonstrated by 64-slice computed tomography. Int J Cardiol. 2007;119:119–21.
6. Kim YJ, Hur J, Shim CY, Lee HJ, Ha JW, Choe KO, et al. Patent foramen ovale: diagnosis with multidetector CT – comparison with trans-esophageal echocardiography. Radiology. 2009;250:61–7.
7. Fyler DC. Ventricular septal defect. In: Fyler DC, editor. Nadas' pediatric cardiology. Philadelphia, PA: Hanley & Delfus; 1992. p. 435–57.
8. Fyler DC. Trends. In: Fyler DC, editor. Nadas' pediatric cardiology. Philadelphia, PA: Hanley & Delfus; 1992. p. 273–80.
9. Devi VS. Inderbir Singh's human embryology. 11th ed. New Delhi: Jaypee Publishers; 2018. p. 237–9.
10. Rajiah P, Kanne JP. Computed tomography of septal defects. J Cardiovasc Comput Tomogr. 2010;4(4):231–45.
11. Zhang J, Ko JM, Guileyardo JM, Roberts WC. A review of spontaneous closure of ventricular septal defect. Proc (Bayl Univ Med Cent). 2015;28(4):516–20. https://doi.org/10.1080/08998280.2015.11929329.
12. Lopez L, Houyel L, Colan SD, Anderson RH, Béland MJ, et al. Classification of ventricular septal defects for the eleventh iteration of the International Classification of Diseases - striving for consensus: a report from the International Society for Nomenclature of Paediatric and Congenital Heart Disease. Ann Thorac Surg. 2018;106:1578–89.
13. Kirklin JK, Castaneda AR, Keane JF, Fellows KE, Norwood WI. Surgical management of multiple ventricular septal defects. J Thorac Cardiovasc Surg. 1980;80:485–93.
14. Stout KK, Daniels CJ, Aboulhosn JA, Bozkurt B, Broberg CS, et al. AHA/ACC guideline for the management of adults with congenital heart disease: executive summary: a report of the American College of Cardiology/American Heart Association task force on clinical practice guidelines. J Am Coll Cardiol. 2019 Apr 2;73(12):1494–563.
15. Jacobs JP, Burke RP, Quintessenza JA, et al. Congenital heart surgery nomenclature and database project: atrioventricular canal defect. Ann Thorac Surg. 2000;69(4 suppl):S36–43.
16. Spicer RL. Cardiovascular disease in Down's syndrome. Pediatr Clin N Am. 1984;31:1331.
17. Backer CL, Stewart RD, Mavroudis C. What is the best technique for repair of complete atrioventricular canal? Semin Thorac Cardiovasc Surg. 2007;19(3):249–57.
18. Wiyono SA, Witsenburg M, de Jaegere PP, Roos-Hesselink JW. Patent ductus arteriosus in adults: case report and review illustrating the spectrum of the disease. Neth Heart J. 2008;16(7–8):255–9. https://doi.org/10.1007/bf03086157.
19. Schneider DJ, Moore JW. Patent ductus arteriosus. Circulation. 2006;114:1873–82.
20. Goitein O, Fuhrman CR, Lacomis JM. Incidental finding on MDCT of patent ductus arteriosus: use of CT and MRI to assess clinical importance. Am J Roentgenol. 2005;184(6):1924–193.
21. Cucerea M, Simon M, Moldovan E, Ungureanu M, Marian R, Suciu L. Congenital heart disease requiring maintenance of Ductus Arteriosus in critically ill newborns admitted at a tertiary neonatal intensive care unit. J Crit Care Med (Targu Mures). 2016;2(4):185–91.
22. Krichenko A, et al. Angiographic classification of the isolated, persistently patent ductus arteriosus and implications for percutaneous catheter occlusion. Am J Cardiol. 1989;63(12):877–80.
23. Levin M, McCurnin D, Seidner SR, Yoder B, Waleh N, Goldbarg S, et al. Postnatal constriction, ATP

depletion, and cell death in the mature and immature ductus arteriosus. Am J Physiol Regul Integr Comp Physiol. 2006 Feb;290(2):R359–64.

24. Mak MS, Ong CC, Tay EL, Teo LL. Clinics in diagnostic imaging (155). Incidental PDA with secondary pulmonary arterial hypertension. Singap Med J. 2014;55(9):462–7.
25. Keats TE, Steinbach HL. Patent ductus arteriosus; a critical evaluation of its roentgen signs. Radiology. 1955 Apr;64(4):528–37.
26. Rajiah P, Kanne JP. Cardiac MRI: Part 1, cardiovascular shunts. AJR Am J Roentgenol. 2011;197:W603–20.
27. Daniel G, Devos H, Kilner PJ. Calculations of cardiovascular shunts and regurgitation using magnetic resonance ventricular volume and aortic and pulmonary flow measurements. Eur Radiol. 2010;20:410–21.

13 Ebstein Anomaly

Ashita Barthur and Salil Bhargava

13.1 Introduction

Ebstein anomaly is a cardiomyopathy of the right ventricular myocardium. The primary pathology in this disease is the failure of delamination of the tricuspid valve leaflets occurring to varying degrees resulting in an entire spectrum of tricuspid valve abnormalities. This, in turn, leads to tricuspid regurgitation, dilation of the right atrium and ventricle, and right heart failure. The disease has the most variable presentation of any congenital heart disease (depending on anatomic severity), ranging from heart failure in a severely cyanotic neonate to incidental detection in an adult.

Electronic Supplementary Material The online version of this chapter (https://doi.org/10.1007/978-981-15-6755-1_13) contains supplementary material, which is available to authorized users.

A. Barthur (✉)
Department of Radiology, Sri Jayadeva Institute of Cardiovascular Sciences and Research, Bangalore, India

S. Bhargava
Department of Radiology, Sir Ganga Ram Hospital, New Delhi, India

13.2 Epidemiology and Risk Factors

The prevalence of Ebstein anomaly is approximately 1 in 20,000 live births (<1% of all congenital heart defects). There appears to be no gender predilection [1–3].

The disease is sporadic with increased risk in families with a history of congenital heart disease, with increasing maternal age, maternal benzodiazepine use, and twins. Maternal lithium therapy is associated with increased risk of the disease in the offspring as lithium blocks the Wnt/beta-catenin pathway, which signals the endothelial–mesenchymal transformation and AV valve development [4, 5].

Ebstein anomaly is genetically heterogeneous with microdeletions in 1p36 and 8p23.1 being most common. Candidate genes include the GATA4 gene (in patients with del 8p23.1), NKX2.5 (based on published patients with isolated Ebstein anomaly), and a hypothetical gene (in patients with del 1p36) [6].

Mutation of the gene MYH7 is significantly associated with the development of left ventricular non-compaction in patients with Ebstein anomaly, and this subset of patients, when identified on imaging, may require genetic and familial testing [7].

R. Rajeshkannan et al. (eds.), *CT and MRI in Congenital Heart Diseases*,
https://doi.org/10.1007/978-981-15-6755-1_13

13.3 Embryology

The endocardial cells of the atrioventricular canal undergo endothelial to mesenchymal transformation to form the atrioventricular cushions. The valves are formed by the fusion and maturation of AV cushions. They are still attached to the myocardium and have to be separated from the myocardium by a process called delamination. This process occurs from distal (toward the apex) to proximal (toward the atrioventricular junction). After completion, the hinge point of myocardial attachment of the valve leaflets is at the level of the "True" or "anatomical" tricuspid annulus (Atrioventricular junction). In a patient with Ebstein anomaly, there is a failure of delamination with incomplete separation of the valve leaflets from the underlying myocardium. This results in short valve leaflets and an apical shift of the hinge point of myocardial attachment into the right ventricle [8]. This apically shifted hinge point is referred to as the "Functional" tricuspid annulus (Fig. 13.1). Valve leaflets show variable degrees of involvement. The order of involvement is Septal > Posterior > Anterior.

13.4 Pathological Anatomy

Morphological abnormalities in Ebstein anomaly [9–11]:

1. *Failure of delamination and adherence of the proximal segments of the septal and posterior tricuspid leaflets to the underlying ventricular wall.* The free edge of the tricuspid valve leaflets may be directly attached to the endocardium by short thick chordae tendineae, muscular bands, or show complete linear attachment. The leaflets themselves are dysplastic and may be fenestrated.
2. *Large, redundant, and sail-like anterior leaflet.* More commonly, it is attached at the anatomical or true annulus. It is typically large, redundant, and sail-like in its lateral aspect near the RVOT and the medial margin of the leaflet near the inlet may be tethered and thick.
3. *Apical displacement of the functional tricuspid annulus.* The maximum displacement is at the commissure of the posterior and septal leaflets. In Ebstein anomaly, the apical displacement of the posterior and septal leaflets with respect to the mitral valve is >8 mm/m^2 (Fig. 13.2). (Please note that in structurally normal hearts, there is an apical displacement of the tricuspid valve with respect to the mitral valve of <8 mm/m^2.)
4. *Two parts to the right ventricle* (Fig. 13.1):
   (a) *Atrialized right ventricle (aRV).* It is the inlet portion of the right ventricle above the level of the displaced valve (between the true tricuspid annulus and the

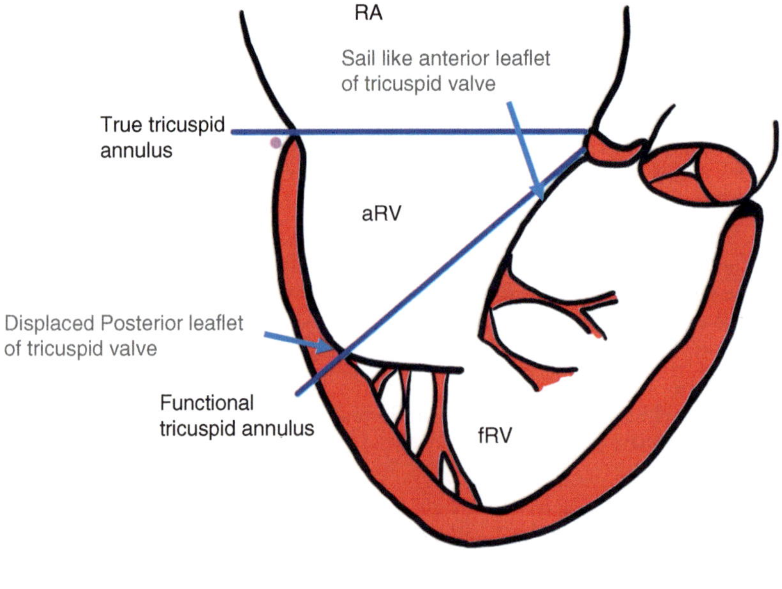

Fig. 13.1 Illustration of an Ebstein heart in the RV two-chamber or RV inflow–outflow view showing inferior and anterior displacement of the posterior leaflet toward the RVOT. This level marks the functional tricuspid annulus which divides the right ventricle into a smooth atrialized right ventricle (aRV) and a trabeculated functional right ventricle (fRV). The fRV and the RVOT appear dilated

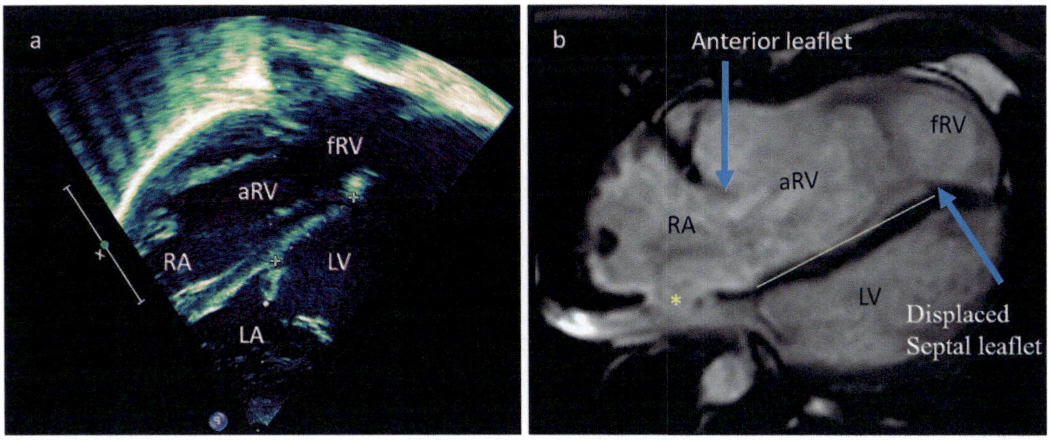

Fig. 13.2 (**a**) 2D TTE in the apical 4 chamber view showing apical displacement of the septal leaflet of the tricuspid valve. (**b**) CMR: Still image of Cine Steady State Free Precission (SSFP) in the four-chamber view showing apical displacement of the tricuspid leaflet in a different patient. Note the presence of an ASD (yellow asterisk)

functional annulus) that gets incorporated into the right atrium. The aRV progressively dilates due to tricuspid regurgitation and can account for more than half the RV volume in severe cases. The atrialized portion of the right ventricle is a thin-walled venous reservoir devoid of myocardium with ineffective contractions similar to Uhl's malformation of the right ventricle.

(b) *Functional RV (fRV).* It consists of the trabeculated and outlet portions of the right ventricle. The right ventricular apex and the outflow tract are responsible for a large portion of the right ventricular function in Ebstein anomaly. Two-thirds of cases will show a dilated right ventricle with dilation of both the aRV and fRV. In extreme cases, it may dilate to an extent that it causes compression of the left ventricle.

5. *Dilation of the True tricuspid annulus.* This occurs secondary to the atrialization of the right ventricle. The right coronary artery is a marker for the level of the true tricuspid annulus on computed tomography (CT) or cardiac magnetic resonance imaging (CMR).
6. *Abnormality in conduction pathway.* The site of developmental abnormality is in close relation to the AV node. There is a discontinuity of the central fibrous body from the AV septal ring with direct muscular connections with an associated apical displacement of the septal leaflet. It creates a potential for the formation of accessory AV conduction pathways [9, 12]. The central fibrous body may be compressed/malformed, and the right bundle may be abnormal or be fibrosed [13, 14].

The Ebstein spectrum ranges from a minimal displacement of the septal and posterior leaflets to significant displacement, tethering, and severe tricuspid regurgitation (Fig. 13.3). Rarely an imperforate membrane or muscular shelf-like projection (Fig. 13.3b) can be seen between the aRV and fRV (Videos 13.1, 13.2, 13.3, 13.4, and 13.5).

13.5 Associated Abnormalities

- *Atrial septal defect (ASD):* In 80–94% of patients, an ostium secundum ASD/patent foramen ovale (PFO) is present (Fig. 13.2). The right to left shunting increases with increased right atrial pressures (during exercise or increasing disease severity) and is responsible for moderately impaired arterial oxygen saturation and paradoxical embolization (stroke or brain abscess) [15–19]
- Partial atrioventricular canal [20]
- Ventricular septal defect (VSD) [20–22]
- Pulmonary atresia with an intact ventricular septum [22, 23]
- Tetralogy of Fallot [24]
- Hypoplastic pulmonary arteries [20]

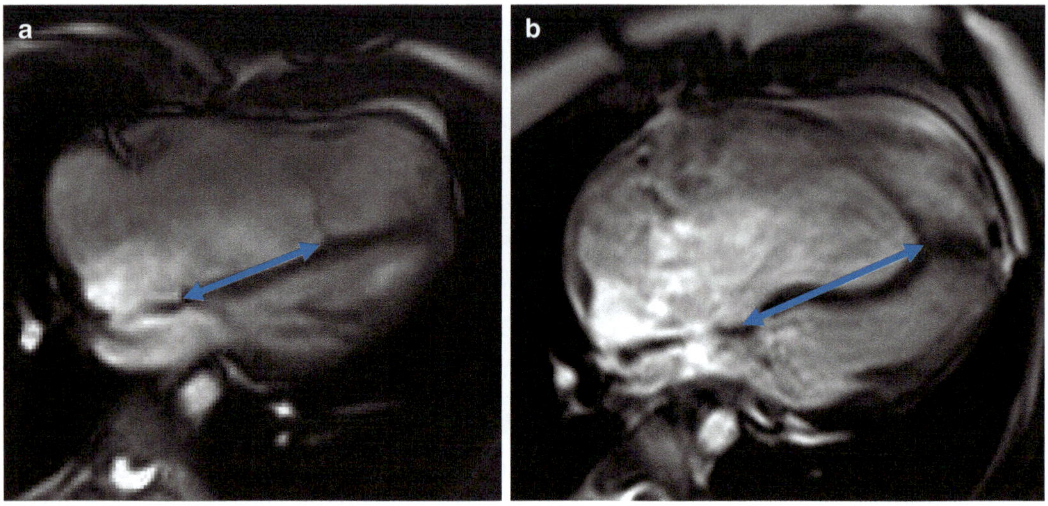

Fig. 13.3 (**a**, **b**) CMR images in the four-chamber view showing increasing degrees of apical displacement of the septal leaflet as demonstrated by the blue arrows

- Pulmonary stenosis [22, 25]
- Hypertensive pulmonary vascular disease [26]
- Patent ductus arteriosus [20]
- Parachute mitral valve, cleft anterior leaflet of the mitral valve, mitral valve prolapse [20, 22]
- Left ventricular outflow obstruction [26]
- Left ventricular non-compaction [27]
- Coarctation of aorta [28, 29]
- Corrected transposition of the great arteries [30–32]
- Subaortic stenosis [33]
- Congenital deaf-mutism [34]

13.6 Pathophysiology

Hemodynamic issues in Ebstein anomaly depend on the severity of the disease, which is in turn determined by the severity of displacement of the tricuspid valve and tricuspid regurgitation. In its mild form, the tricuspid valve function is close to normal. Whereas in the moderate to severe forms, each atrial contraction propels blood into the aRV, and subsequently, each ventricular contraction propels the blood back into the right atrium. This phenomenon becomes pronounced in Ebstein patients with significant tricuspid regurgitation (Fig. 13.4). Consequently, there is right atrial dilatation leading to an increased right atrial pressure. Raised right atrial pressure results in a right-to-left shunt across the ASD/PFO. This mixing of blood at the atrial level leads to arterial desaturation and pulmonary oligemia [35].

Despite altered cardiac hemodynamics, even those with severe Ebstein anomaly often reach adulthood, however, with a significantly shortened lifespan. Almost a quarter of deaths are due to arrhythmia and almost half die of heart failure [36]. Arrhythmia itself can cause heart failure or be a result of heart failure [37].

The right atrial enlargement makes it susceptible to atrial fibrillation and flutter. Additionally, up to one-third of Ebstein patients have an accessory conduction pathway [38]. The above two factors are responsible for a potentially fatal combination of atrial fibrillation turning into ventricular fibrillation leading to sudden cardiac death [39].

Myocardial fibrosis, shown to be a part of the pathophysiology, may be initiated by volume or pressure overload, inflammation, ischemia, cyanosis, or genetic predisposition [37, 40, 41]. The insult stimulates myofibroblasts that synthesize collagen precursors and metalloproteinase. Metalloproteinase determines myocardial elasticity and stiffness [40]. These proteins have been confirmed histopathologically in Ebstein patients [42].

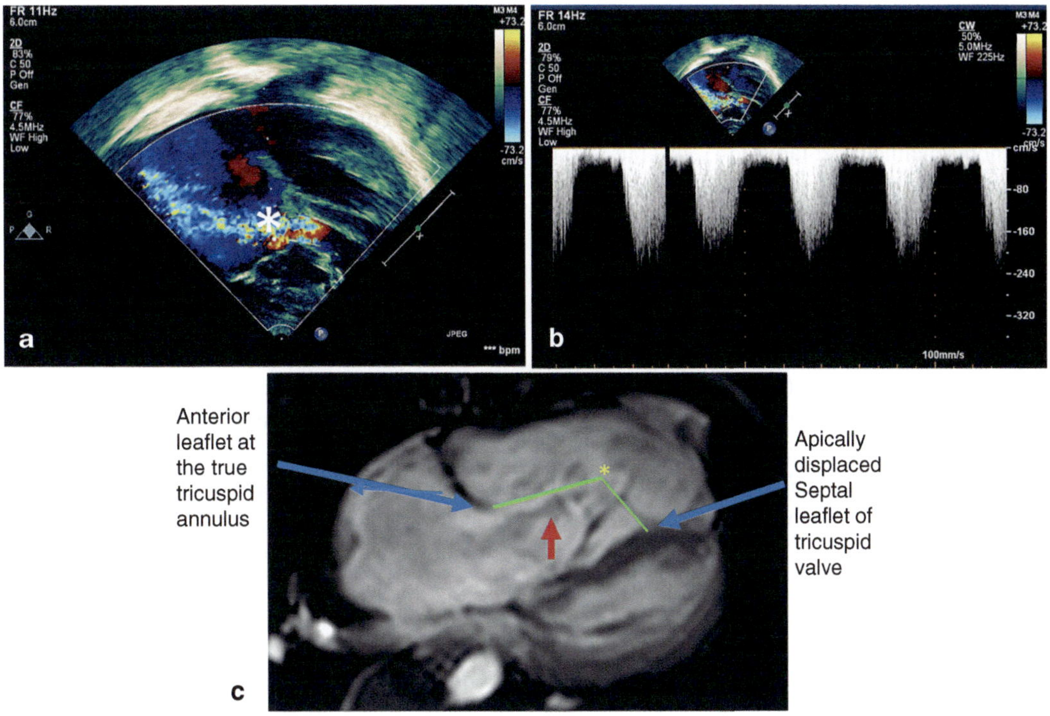

Fig. 13.4 Color Doppler interrogation (**a**) and pulse wave Doppler interrogation (**b**) of the tricuspid valve demonstrating severe tricuspid regurgitation. (**c**) CMR in the four-chamber view shows a dephasing jet of tricuspid regurgitation (small red arrow) arising from the point of coaptation of the valve leaflets (yellow asterisk)

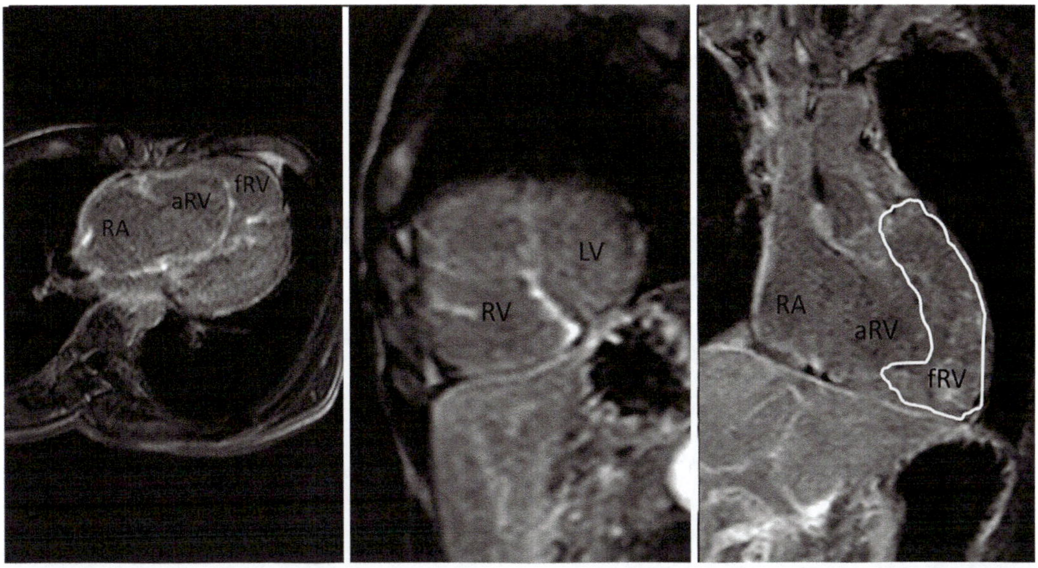

Fig. 13.5 Late gadolinium enhancement images demonstrating diffuse enhancement of the fRV, aRV, and Right atrium (RA) suggestive of fibrosis. There is also nonischemic pattern of enhancement in the lateral wall of LV

CMR, with the help of late gadolinium enhancement, helps detect myocardial inflammation, fibrosis, and injury (Fig. 13.5). Its clinical usefulness has been shown not only in ischemic and nonischemic heart failure [41, 43] but also in congenital heart disease [19, 44–46].

13.7 Classifications

Carpentier et al. [47] divided patients with Ebstein anomaly into four types (Type A–D). It is a relatively simple classification system that refers primarily to the size of the myocardium (Table 13.1).

Celermajer et al. [25] developed the GOSE score (Great Ormond Street Ebstein Echocardiographic score) for Ebstein anomaly in neonates. Measurements are made in the apical four-chamber view. GOSE score = Area of (RA + aRV)/ area of (fRV + LA + LV) (Fig. 13.6). It is frequently used for echocardiographic evaluation of the neonate (Fig. 13.6). Neonates with a score > 1.5 showed a mortality of 100%, while those less than 1.5 had a mortality of 15%. Cyanotic neonates with a score of >1 showed 100% mortality [48] (Table 13.2).

Dearani and Danielson [20] proposed a more detailed classification based on intraoperative findings (Table 13.3).

13.8 Clinical Presentation

Clinical presentations vary based on the anatomic severity of the disease. The most common presentations at different ages are mentioned below as a percentage [49]:

- Fetus: Diagnosed by an abnormal ultrasound in pregnancy (86%). Severe forms can lead to cardiomegaly, hydrops, and arrhythmias.
- Neonate: Cyanosis (74%), marked cardiomegaly, tricuspid regurgitation, and heart failure

Table 13.1 Carpentier classification

Carpentier classification	Right ventricle	Anterior leaflet	
Type A	Adequate fRV (small aRV)	Normal anterior leaflet	Moderate displacement of septal and posterior
Type B	Small fRV (Large aRV)	Freely mobile	
Type C	Small fRV (Large aRV)	Severely restricted ± RVOT obstruction	
Type D	Near-complete atrialization		

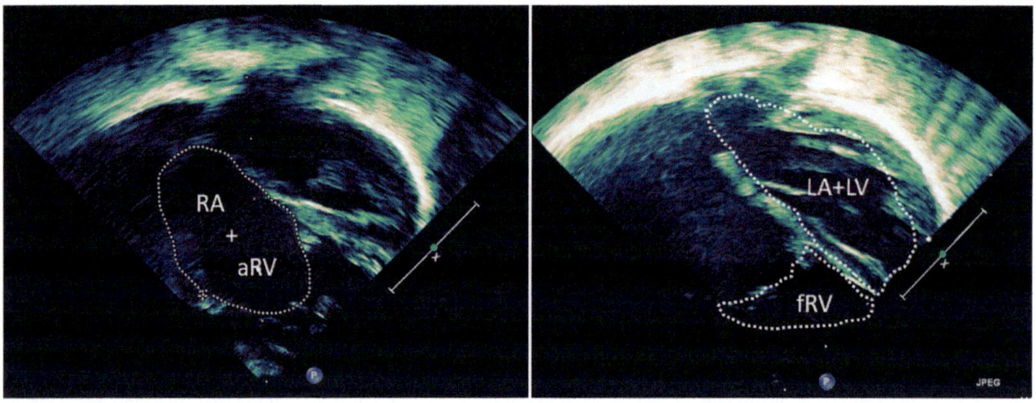

Fig. 13.6 2D Transthoracic echocardiography in the apical four-chamber view demonstrating calculation of the GOSE Score

- Infants: Right heart failure (43%)
- Children: Incidental murmur (63%)
- Adolescent and adult: Arrhythmia (42%)

Children, adolescents, and adults may be symptomatic with progressive right-sided heart failure with exertional dyspnea, fatigue, decreasing exercise tolerance, cyanosis, and palpitations. Less severe forms may be detected on an investigation for a paradoxical embolism (stroke/TIA/brain abscess).

13.9 Approach to Diagnosis and Evaluation

1. 2DTTE: Helps in diagnosis, initial anatomic evaluation, and follow-up of Ebstein anomaly.
2. CMR: Allows direct visualization of anatomical detail and is akin to echocardiography for functional assessment. The information by CMR is complementary to echocardiography. It aids in the quantification of right ventricular size and function and visualization of tricuspid valve anatomy. It is useful before and as follow-up after surgical intervention and in patients with nondiagnostic echocardiography
3. CT: Allows direct visualization of anatomical detail. However, radiation exposure is the main disadvantage. CT should be considered only in cases where other modalities were inadequate or could not be performed. Sometimes the presence of a coexistent defect such as the presence of pulmonary atresia may warrant a CT for better evaluation of the associated pathology.
4. Cardiopulmonary exercise testing with measurement of oxygen consumption: It is beneficial in asymptomatic or patients with few symptoms to assess functional limitation. It is helpful to evaluate exercise capacity, the response of heart rate and blood pressure to exercise, and exercise-induced desaturation and arrhythmias.
5. A baseline electrocardiogram (ECG) and during exercise and annual 24-hour Holter monitoring: These investigations are a part of routine assessment of arrhythmia in patients with Ebstein anomaly. An electrophysiologic study (EPS), however, is reserved for patients with tachyarrhythmias, preexcitation on ECG, or as a preoperative workup.
6. Cardiac catheterization: It helps in the hemodynamic assessment of patients with conflicting results of clinical and noninvasive tests,

Table 13.2 GOSE score

Grades	GOSE score
Grade 1	<0.5
Grade 2	0.5–0.99
Grade 3	1–1.49
Grade 4	>1.5

Table 13.3 Dearani and Danielson classification based on intraoperative findings

Dearani classification	Right ventricle	Anterior leaflet	Septal and posterior leaflets
Type I	Small to large aRV	Large and mobile (>50% delamination)	Displaced, displaced and dysplastic or absent
Type II	aRV moderate to large	Leading edge is mobile. Small and displaced apically in a spiral	Small and displaced apically in a spiral
Type III	aRV is large	Large or small with hyphenated or linear attachment of leading edge. Restricted motion with shortened, tethered, and fused chordae. Few papillary muscles insert directly.	Displaced, dysplastic, and nonreconstructable. Fenestrations common
Type IV	Near-complete atrialization	Severely deformed and displaced into the RVOT. Few or no chordae with direct insertion of papillary muscles. Leading edge has hyphenated or linear attachment.	Septal leaflet in the form of a ridge of fibrous tissue

suspicious for pulmonary artery hypertension or stenosis, and as pre-procedural evaluation for a palliative Glenn shunt.

13.10 Imaging Tests

13.10.1 Chest Radiograph (CXR)

CXR is usually performed as a part of routine evaluation. However, a CXR is not required for the diagnosis of Ebstein anomaly [50]. CXR findings largely depend upon the severity of the disease [51]. In severe cases, there is massive cardiomegaly with a small ascending aorta and a normal or oligemic pulmonary vascularity. It is described as a box-shaped heart on a frontal chest radiograph. The enlarged right atrium constitutes the right heart border. The dilated right atrium and dilated and superiorly displaced right ventricular outflow tract results in an elevated right ventricular apex and a straight or convex the left heart border (Fig. 13.7).

Differential diagnoses include other congenital heart defect resulting in right heart enlargement such as left to right shunts, pulmonary stenosis, myocardial abnormalities like Uhl's anomaly, Gerbode's defect, and massive pericardial effusion. CXR may be normal in patients with mild disease.

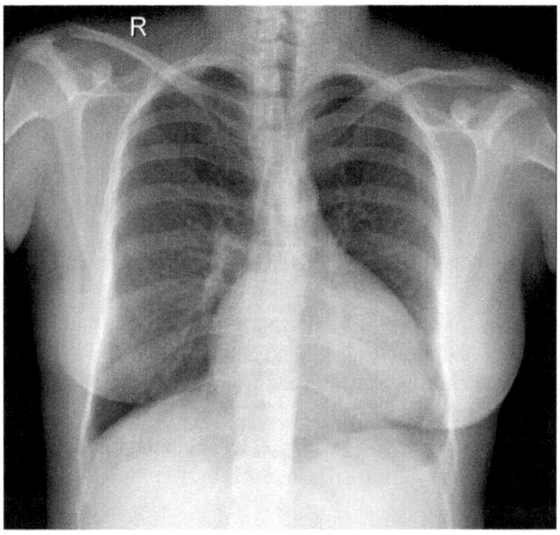

Fig. 13.7 Chest radiograph PA view showing the classic box-shaped heart of Ebstein anomaly

13.10.2 Echocardiography

A transthoracic two-dimensional echocardiography (2DTTE) performed comprehensively with color Doppler interrogation is the primary tool for diagnosing Ebstein anomaly. 2DTTE helps confirm the diagnosis, assess the severity of the disease, and identify associated cardiac defects. The most useful orientation is the four-chamber view, in which the degree of mobility of the anterior leaflet, displacement of the septal leaflet, and severity of the tricuspid regurgitation and fRV are assessed. However, all echocardiographic views are essential to assess the severity of the tricuspid valve regurgitation. Three-dimensional echocardiography (3DTTE) is being used with increasing frequency to supplement standard two-dimensional images for analysis of tricuspid valve anatomy [51]. Most important echocardiographic findings are listed below [52, 53]:

1. Critical diagnostic finding: Apical displacement of the septal leaflet of the tricuspid valve compared with the position of the anterior leaflet of the mitral valve indexed by body surface area ($\geq$8 mm/m^2) on the apical four-chamber view. The degree of displacement marks the spectrum of clinical manifestations.
2. Variable extent of the failure of the delamination of each of the three leaflets. Valve morphology of the anterior and septal leaflets are best assessed by echocardiography. Mobility, length, and attachment of valve leaflets to the underlying myocardium can be ascertained.
3. Tricuspid regurgitation: The TR jet is commonly a low-velocity jet as the pulmonary pressures are normal. The origin of the TR jet is from the coaptation surfaces of the most anteriorly or apically displaced valve leaflets. The jet can be challenging to assess either due to its laminar nature or unexpected direction, e.g., inferiorly in a valve that is displaced into the RVOT. In Ebstein anomaly, TR quantification is complex. A vena contracta width (the narrowest part of the regurgitant jet just distal to the site of regurgitation) >0.7 cm and systolic flow reversal in the hepatic veins, which are the criteria in non-Ebstein adults, are often

not present in Ebstein patients. This phenomenon is secondary to the large compliant right atrium and the atrialized right ventricle [54–56]. In an Ebstein heart, a significant leaflet coaptation gap on 2DTTE with a large regurgitant jet on Doppler interrogation is the best indicator of severe regurgitation.

4. Increased right heart volume: caused by an enlarged aRV and volume overload of fRV.
5. Associated congenital lesions:
   (a) ASD or PFO: Shunting is usually bidirectional. Saline-contrast echocardiography offers as a sensitive test to detect right-to-left intracardiac shunting, especially in a poor acoustic window.
   (b) Left-sided cardiac lesions (left ventricular systolic and diastolic dysfunction, mitral valve prolapse, bicuspid aortic valve).

GOSE Score (Celermajer Index) Refer sect. 13.7 The prognosis is worse if the ratio increases [25, 57, 58].

Intrauterine Diagnosis of Ebstein Anomaly It can be made by fetal echocardiography [59].

13.10.2.1 Transesophageal Echocardiogram (TEE)

It may provide additional information when the 2DTTE is technically insufficient to identify both structural and functional abnormalities [60].

13.10.3 CT

CMR has mostly replaced CT due to the advantage of combined anatomical and functional information without radiation exposure. CT has the advantage of multiplanar reconstruction, which allows reconstruction into true cardiac planes and oblique planes along the axis of the tricuspid valve. These views help determine the degree of apical displacement of the septal and posterior tricuspid valve leaflets relative to the atrioventricular junction. The thickening of these leaflets may be appreciated. The aRV and fRV can be differentiated. The thinned-out myocardium in the aRV can be made out compared with the more conspicuous myocardium in the fRV. Other than anatomical information on a prospectively gated scan, functional information can be obtained with CT using retrospective gating at the cost of a higher radiation dose.

13.10.3.1 Indications for CT

a. Presence of associated congenital cardiac anomalies that require CT for surgical planning (Fig. 13.8).
b. The patient is unstable or has support devices and is unlikely to tolerate the scan time required for a CMR examination.
c. CMR availability or expertise is lacking.

13.10.4 CMR

CMR provides complementary information to echocardiography. CMR is the gold standard for the assessment of ventricular volumes and function. In Ebstein anomaly, the main advantage of CMR is its ability to accurately assess the right ventricular size and function without geometric assumptions. Figure 13.9 demonstrates the method of contouring the right ventricle in Ebstein anomaly. The valve may not be visible in its entirety on each section of the end-diastole and end-systole images. To overcome this issue and to introduce uniformity in the method of contouring, a straight line is drawn joining the point of attachment of the anterior leaflet to the right ventricular free wall to the displaced septal attachment along the interventricular septum. This line is used to demarcate the distal extent of the aRV [61].

CMR is useful to assess tricuspid valve displacement and is superior to echocardiography in assessing the posterior leaflet of the tricuspid valve (Fig. 13.10) [62–64]. CMR can depict anatomy and function, including the pulmonary arteries and tricuspid valve in a single study [65, 66]. Therefore, it is recommended to perform pre- and post-operative CMR for all non-general anesthesia patients with Ebstein anomaly and for selected patients who do require general anesthesia for scanning [51].

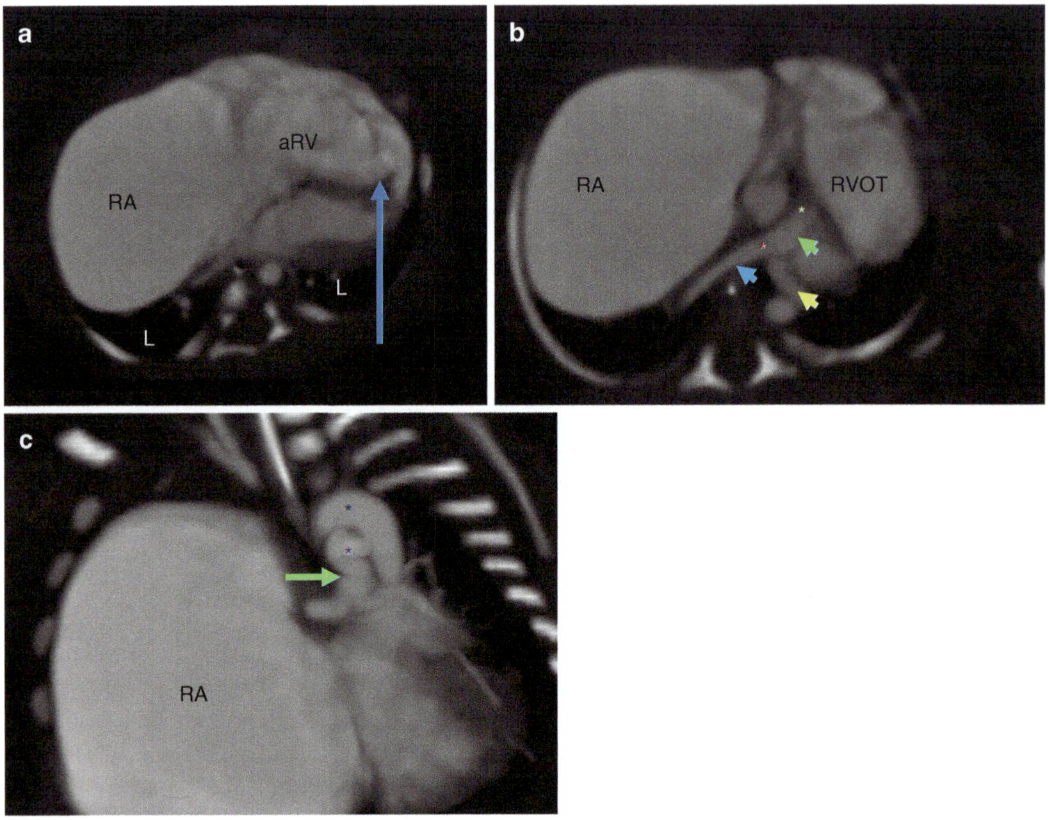

Fig. 13.8 CT pulmonary angiography images of a neonate with Ebstein anomaly and pulmonary atresia. A. The right atrium is grossly dilated (RA) causing a reduction in the available space for lung (L) expansion. The blue arrow in (**a**) represents the displaced septal attachment of the tricuspid valve. (**b**) Atretic pulmonary valve (yellow asterisk). Good sized main pulmonary artery (green arrow) and confluent branch pulmonary arteries (red asterisk); Good sized right pulmonary (blue arrow) and left pulmonary arteries (yellow arrow). (**c**) Oblique MIP reconstruction showing aortic arch (blue asterisk), the PDA in its usual location (purple asterisk) supplying the main pulmonary artery (green arrow)

CMR has shown variability in right ventricular volume calculation in Ebstein patients due to unusual tricuspid valve and right ventricular morphology and lack of standardized CMR imaging protocols. This variability leads to considerable inter-center variability in volumetric measurements [67]. Additionally, in the presence of severe TR, RVEF may overestimate true right ventricular contractility. Therefore, it makes it hard to determine postoperative right ventricular function after tricuspid valve repair or replacement. Right ventricular function is generally depressed immediately after tricuspid valve repair or replacement and may or may not recover over time with right ventricular remodeling. The presence of support devices or arrhythmias limits the use of this technique in sick patients. Additionally, CMR may miss small shunts and underestimate the degree of tricuspid regurgitation [62].

CMR can be performed using a 1.5–3 T scanner. Young and old patients tolerate CMR well. Critically ill neonates can be imaged in as few as 15 min without adverse sequelae [68]. Anatomical sequences include 2D non-cine sequences such as spin-echo sequences and magnetic resonance angiography and respiratory triggered and cardiac gated 3D whole heart DIXON sequence. Functional sequences include cine and velocity encoded imaging sequences [69–71]. A comprehensive CMR protocol involving anatomical and functional sequences will provide for a robust presurgical assessment (Refer to CMR protocol).

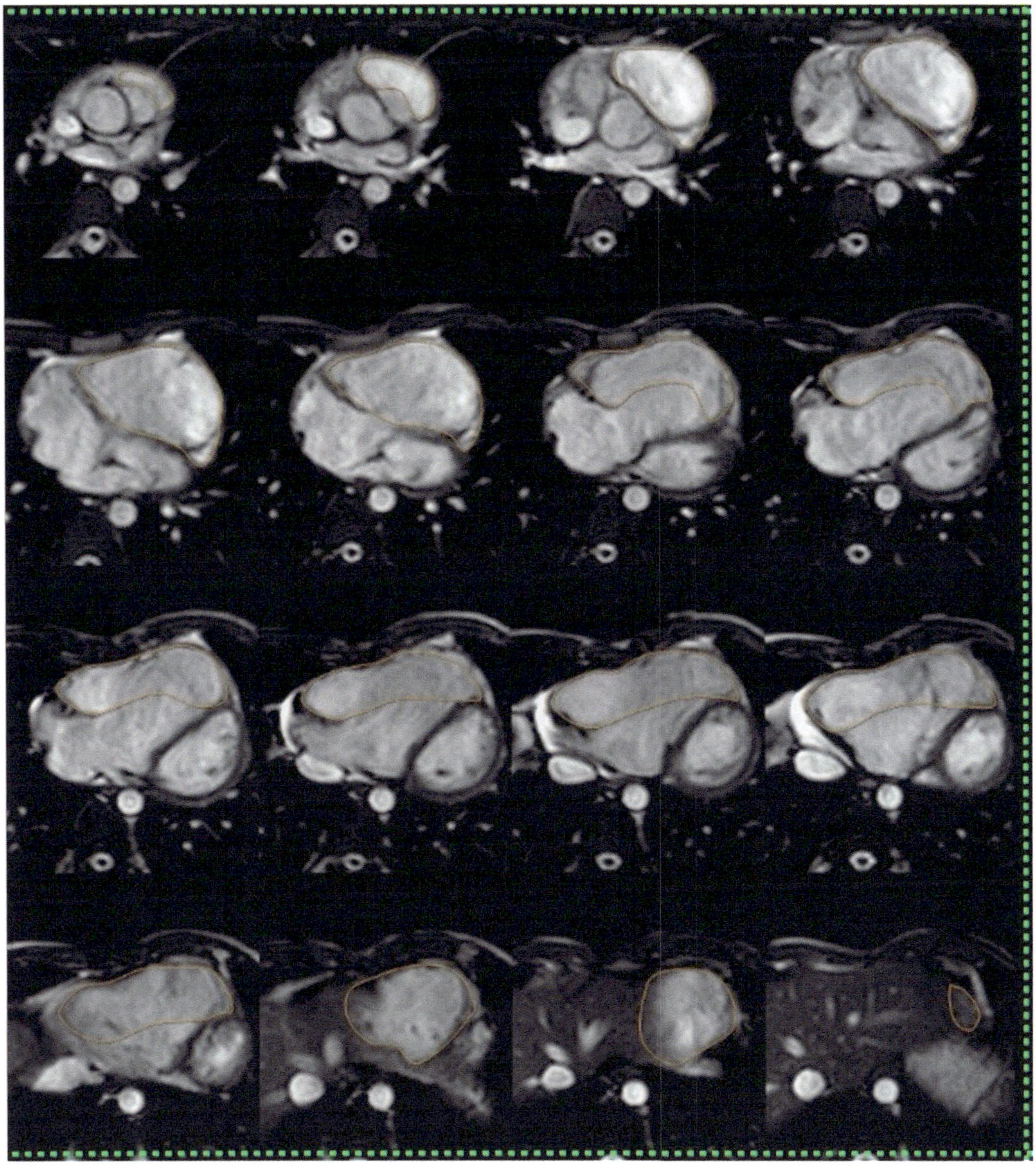

Fig. 13.9 CMR images in axial view demonstrating contouring of the fRV for right ventricular volume calculation

13.10.5 CMR Protocol

Localizers

1. Axial HASTE black blood imaging
2. Cine bSSFP: Axial sequence covering both atria and ventricles and pulmonary arteries
   Two-chamber left, two-chamber right, four-chamber, and short-axis views
   Left ventricular and right ventricular outflow tracts
   Optional: extended four-chamber covering both ventricles
3. Gadolinium magnetic resonance angiography
4. 3D whole-heart Dixon imaging
5. Late gadolinium imaging in short axis, four-chamber, two-chamber, and three-chamber views

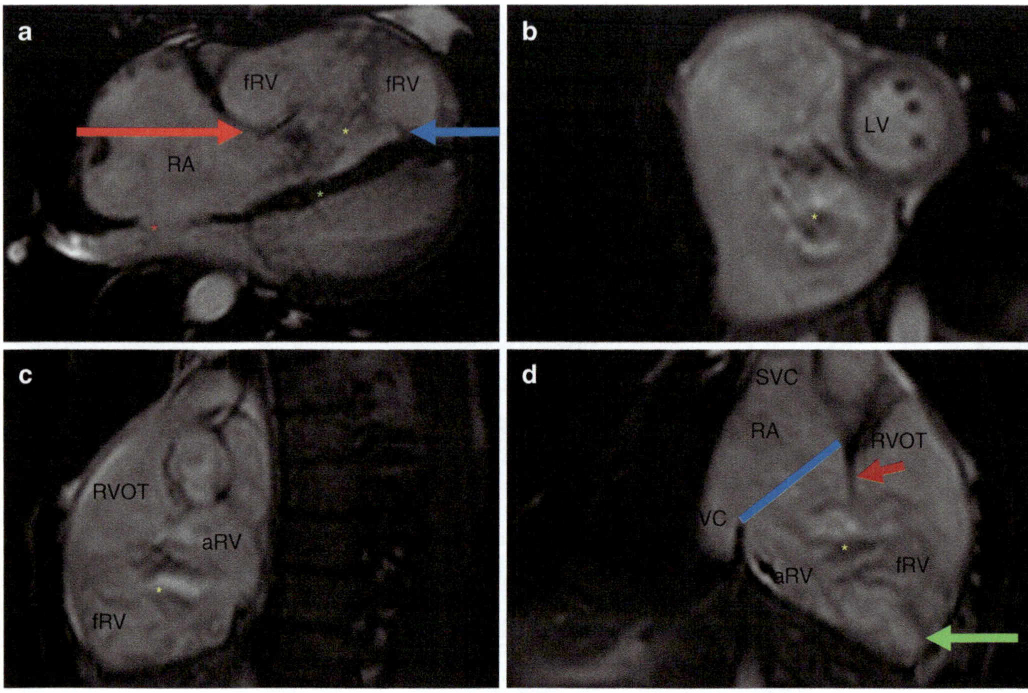

Fig. 13.10 CMR images (**a**) four-chamber view showing apical displacement of the tricuspid valve (blue arrow), sail-like anterior leaflet (red arrow), tricuspid regurgitation (yellow asterisk), fRV, smooth dyskinetic septum of the aRV (green asterisk), and ASD (red asterisk). (**b**) Short-axis view: Note that the tricuspid valve orifice is difficult to see on a true short-axis view due to derangement in the valve orientation in Ebstein anomaly. This image shows TR jet (yellow asterisk) at the level of the mid-LV. (**c**) RVOT view showing the anterior and inferiorly displaced leaflets with tricuspid regurgitation arising at the point of coaptation of the valve leaflets. (**d**) RV two-chamber view showing the anteriorly and inferior displaced posterior leaflet (green arrow) and the anterior leaflet (red arrow) at the true anatomical annulus (blue line). Note that all views are necessary to evaluate the tricuspid leaflets and to understand the orientation of the functional tricuspid annulus

6. Flow measurements: Aorta and pulmonary artery. Optional: Atrioventricular valves, SVC, descending aorta, and branch pulmonary arteries

13.10.6 Preoperative CMR Imaging Checklist

1. Ventricular volumes, function, and flows:
   (a) Right ventricular volumes and function
   (b) Atrialized right ventricular volumes
   (c) Functional right ventricular volumes
   (d) Left ventricular volumes and function, LV outflow tract
   (e) Pulmonary and Aortic flows
   (f) Q_p:Q_s
2. TR fraction and Tricuspid valve assessment:
   (a) Severity of tricuspid regurgitation (fRV stroke volume—Pulmonary artery forward flow).
   (b) RVOT for any obstruction.
   (c) Pulmonary valvar abnormalities
   (d) Anatomical assessment of the septal, anterosuperior, and posteroinferior leaflets
   (e) Tethering of leaflets and the amount of mobile leaflet available for refashioning the tricuspid valve
3. Atrial septal defect:
   (a) Size and flow quantification of ASD
4. Myocardial abnormalities:
   (a) Cine images to look for structural abnormalities due to tethering or other congenital myocardial abnormalities such as septal crypts
   (b) Late gadolinium enhancement for fibrosis
5. Associated abnormalities:
   (a) Branch pulmonary arteries

(b) VSD
(c) Systemic and pulmonary venous connections.
(d) Non-compaction

13.10.7 Postoperative CMR Imaging Checklist

1. Ventricular volumes and function:
   (a) Right ventricular volumes and function
   (b) Right ventricular volumes and function
2. Right ventricular outflow trace to look for obstruction
3. Tricuspid valve:
   (a) To assess competency post repair
4. Postoperative changes:
   (a) Plication of the right atrium
   (b) Annuloplasty
   (c) Closure of ASD, for residual fenestration
5. Tissue characterization with late gadolinium enhancement:
   (a) Fibrosis/infarct

Key Reporting Elements

- Tricuspid valve septal leaflet offset from the mitral attachment
- The posteroinferior leaflet offset
- Tricuspid valve regurgitation fraction
- Size and function of the functional right ventricle
- Size of the right atrium
- Size and function of the left ventricle
- RVOT obstruction, if any
- Branch pulmonary arteries
- Pulmonary and systemic veins
- PFO/ASD/VSD: Q_p/Q_s
- Delayed enhancement
- Postoperative complications: residual tricuspid regurgitation and RV/LV failure

13.11 Treatment

13.11.1 Prenatal

Prenatal diagnosis can be made 16–20 weeks of gestation. Most fetuses tolerate pregnancy well as the left ventricular function is normal. However, progression to fetal hydrops can occur and is associated with a very poor prognosis. Severe cardiac enlargement compromises pulmonary development and may lead to neonatal respiratory distress.

RVOT anatomic obstruction or functional pulmonary atresia indicates that the fetus will require postnatal ductal flow to support pulmonary circulation. The need for neonatal surgical intervention is higher in those with extreme right heart dilation and/or RV outflow obstruction. While the risk of neonatal surgery is high even in the most experienced centers, the prognosis for those that survive neonatal operation is quite favorable.

13.11.2 Neonates

Medical therapy is the preferred line of management, with an effort to delay surgery into childhood. However, the inability to wean the child from the ventilator and persistent metabolic dysfunction generally indicate failure of medical therapy and the need for surgerical intervention.

Indications for surgery include severe cyanosis, GOSE score of 3 or 4 with mild cyanosis, cardiothoracic ratio of >80%, and severe TR.

(a) Neonates with RVOT Obstruction

- Single ventricle palliation/Starnes procedure: The tricuspid orifice is closed using a pericardial patch with a widening of the ASD and placing a systemic to pulmonary artery shunt. This procedure now includes the fenestration of the pericardial patch to allow for RV decompression and involution. This approach is considered in the presence of RVOT obstruction or other anomalies. There is an operative survival of 80% with this procedure. Subsequent bidirectional cavo-pulmonary shunt and modified Fontan is performed. Late results are comparable with other single ventricle anomalies.
- Ebstein with pulmonary atresia and mild TR (anatomical RVOT obstruction): Modified BT shunt and a reduction right atrioplasty (to allow for the normal expansion and development of the lungs)
- Ebstein with pulmonary regurgitation and severe tricuspid regurgitation (functional

RVOT obstruction): Modified BT shunt with pulmonary artery ligation and reduction right atrioplasty.

(b) Neonates with Ebstein Without RVOT Obstruction

- Biventricular repair: This is usually a monocusp repair performed using the anterior leaflet. Early mortality remains high for this operation (approximately 25%). Intermediate results of survivors appear to be promising.
- Single ventricle palliation

13.11.3 Children, Adolescents, and Adults

Indications:

(a) NYHA class III or IV
(b) NYHA class I or II with a cardiothoracic ratio of 0.65
(c) Significantly cyanotic (arterial oxygen saturation < 90%), polycythemic (Hb level > 16 g/dL)
(d) History of paradoxical embolus
(e) Refractory atrial or ventricular arrhythmia
(f) Deteriorating exercise capacity
(g) Progressive right ventricular dilatation or reduction of right ventricular systolic function

Biventricular repair: After infancy, a biventricular repair is the preferred choice. Tricuspid valve repair, right ventricular plication (plication refers to the folding over and suturing of the wall of the right ventricle to reduce the RV volume and to bring the leaflets closer to the true annulus), right atrioplasty (reducing the right atrial volume), closure or subtotal closure of ASD, and correction of any associated anomalies are performed as routine.

One and a half ventricle repair: If there are advanced signs of right heart failure with significant RV enlargement or dysfunction, a bidirectional cavo-pulmonary shunt is added to decompress the right ventricle and increase preload to the left ventricle.

Tricuspid repair and replacement: Tricuspid valve repair is preferred to replacement. Various techniques have been described for tricuspid valve replacement; however, the closest to anatomic reconstruction is the cone repair described by da Silva et al. (Fig. 13.11).

Arrhythmia surgery: Anti-arrhythmia procedures including a right atrial maze, left atrial maze, cavo-tricuspid isthmus ablation pulmonary vein isolation may be performed as indicated.

Heart transplantation: This is the last resort when the right and left ventricular functions are severely impaired with LVEF < 25%.

13.12 Ebsteinoid Malformation of Left AV Valve in L-TGA

L-transposition of great arteries (L-TGA) is characterized by situs solitus, atrioventricular, and ventriculoarterial discordance. In this condition, right atrium empties systemic venous blood into right-sided morphological LV and then into the pulmonary artery and the left atrium drains the pulmonary venous blood into left-sided morphological RV and then into the aorta. Since the AV valves always correspond to the morphological ventricle, the tricuspid valve is located on the left side in L-TGA. Ebstein malformation of such left-sided AV valve is called as Ebsteinoid malformation to differentiate it from classic Ebstein anomaly discussed earlier in D-looped heart (Fig. 13.12). These children develop symptoms early in life due to associated lesions like VSD and pulmonary outflow tract obstruction. Compared to the concordant AV connection, Ebsteinoid patients with discordant connection show relatively less RV enlargement [72]. Reduced blood flow into ascending aorta leads to abnormal aortic development [73]. Chest radiograph shows left atrial enlargement with straightening of left superior mediastinum caused by the ascending aorta arising from the anterior and leftward aortic valve (Fig. 13.13) (Videos 13.6, 13.7, 13.8, 13.9, 13.10, 13.11, 13.12, 13.13, and 13.14).

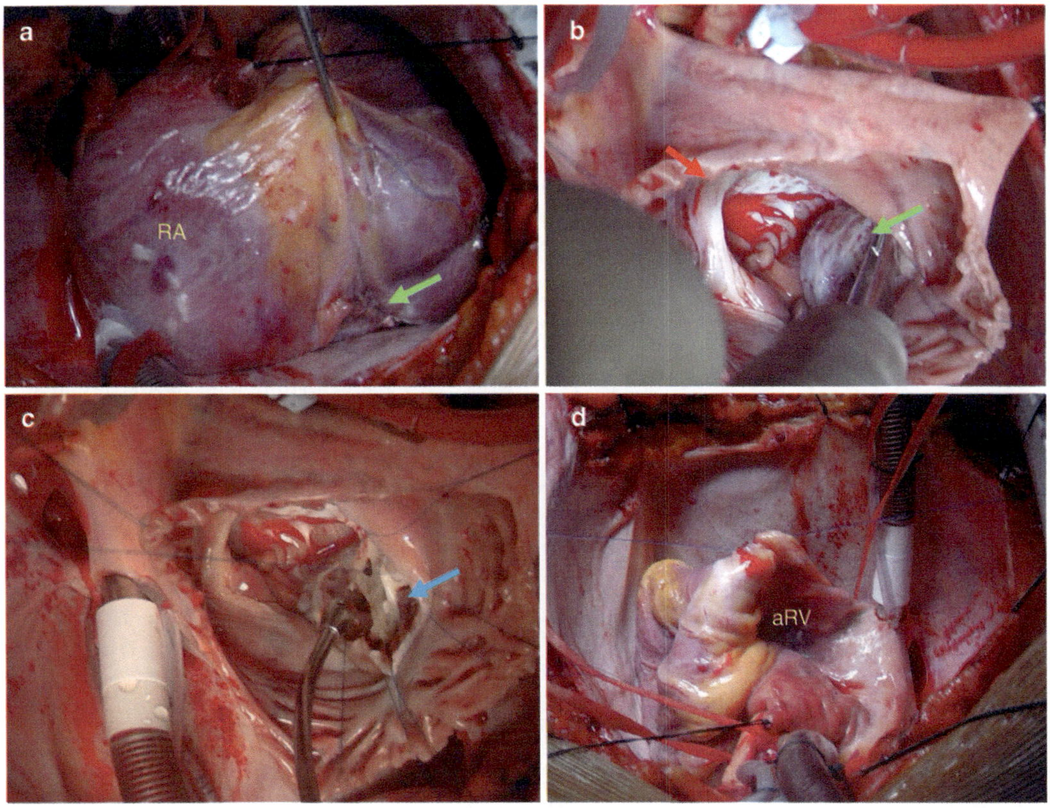

Fig. 13.11 Intraoperative images of Cone repair for Ebstein anomaly (**a**). External appearance of the Ebstein heart with green arrow showing the line of plication of the right ventricle. (**b**) Viewing the displaced septal and posterior leaflets (green arrow) with respect to the true tricuspid annulus (red arrow). (**c**) Line of surgical delamination (blue arrow) separating and mobilizing the leaflet tissue proximally toward the true annulus. (**d**) External appearance showing a collapsed atrialized part of the RV. Courtesy of images: Dr. Raja Joshi. Sir Ganga Ram hospital, New Delhi

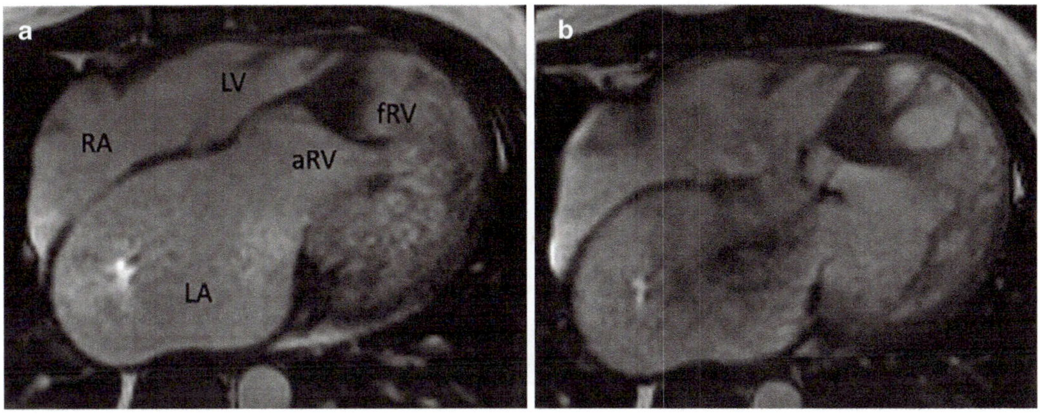

Fig. 13.12 CMR images of Ebsteinoid malformation of left AV valve in a patient with L-TGA taken during diastole (**a**) and systole (**b**) showing apically displaced tricuspid valve in to the left-sided morphological RV (Ref to Videos 13.6, 13.7, 13.8, 13.9, 13.10, 13.11, 13.12, 13.13, and 13.14)

13.13 Differential Diagnosis

Endomyocardial fibrosis (EMF) can mimic Ebstein anomaly on echo due to apical displacement of the tricuspid valve with severe regurgitation and huge dilatation of RA [74]. Demonstration of RV apical mass obliterating the cavity and endocardial calcification help in the diagnosis of EMF. Diffuse endocardial delayed enhancement and trilayer appearance are characteristic of EMF (Figs. 13.14 and 13.15).

Other conditions that mimic Ebstein anomaly are tricuspid valve dysplasia, tricuspid prolapse, RV dysplasia, endocarditis, and annular dilatation secondary to free pulmonary regurgitation [75].

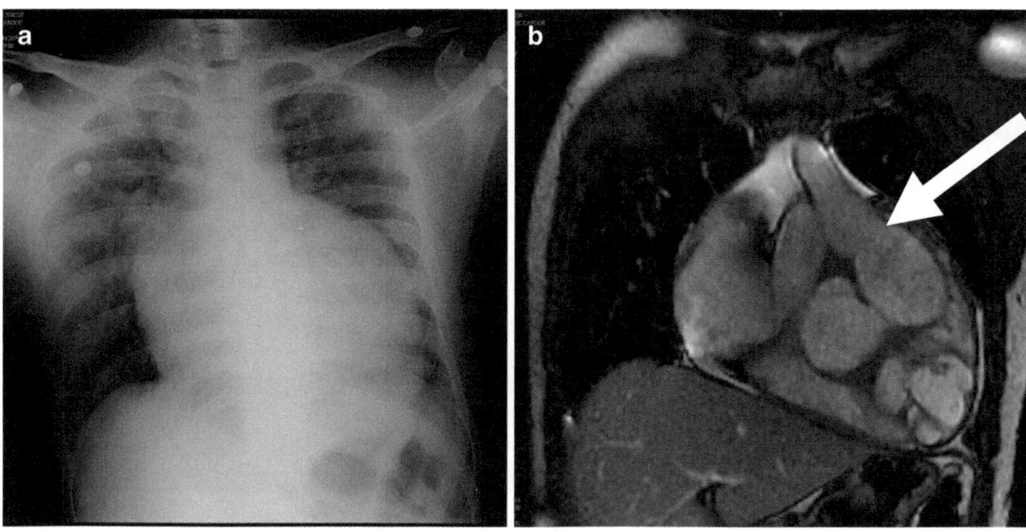

Fig. 13.13 Ebsteinoid malformation of left AV valve. Chest radiograph (**a**) with correlation coronal MRI (**b**) shows left atrial enlargement with straightening of left superior mediastinum caused by the ascending aorta (arrow) arising from the anterior and leftward aortic valve

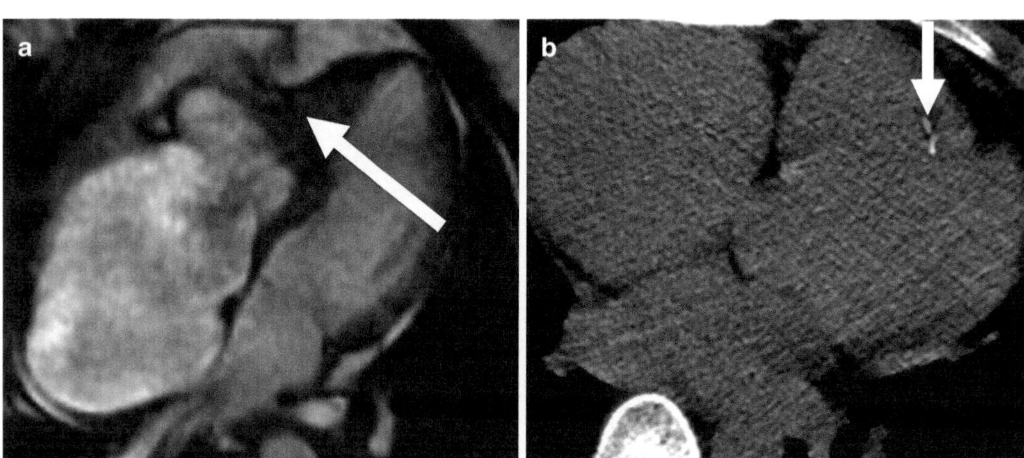

Fig. 13.14 Endomyocardial fibrosis with apically displaced tricuspid valve with atrial dilatation mimicking Ebstein anomaly. Presence of mass obliterating the RV apex (arrow in **a**) and endocardial calcification on CT scan (arrow in **b**) help in making correct diagnosis. (**c**) Late gadolinium enhancement (LGE) MRI shows diffuse endocardial enhancement

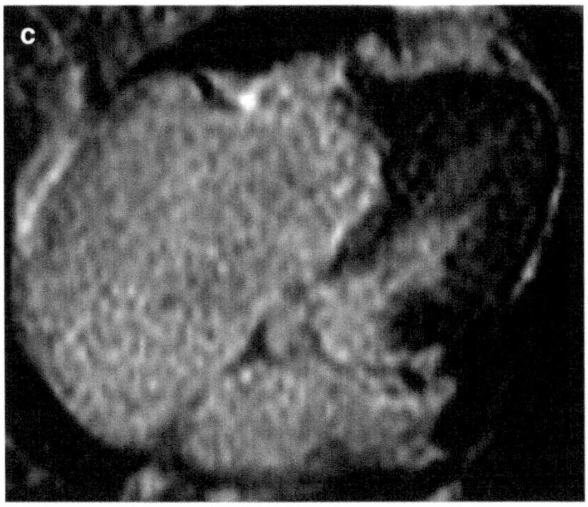

Fig. 13.14 (continued)

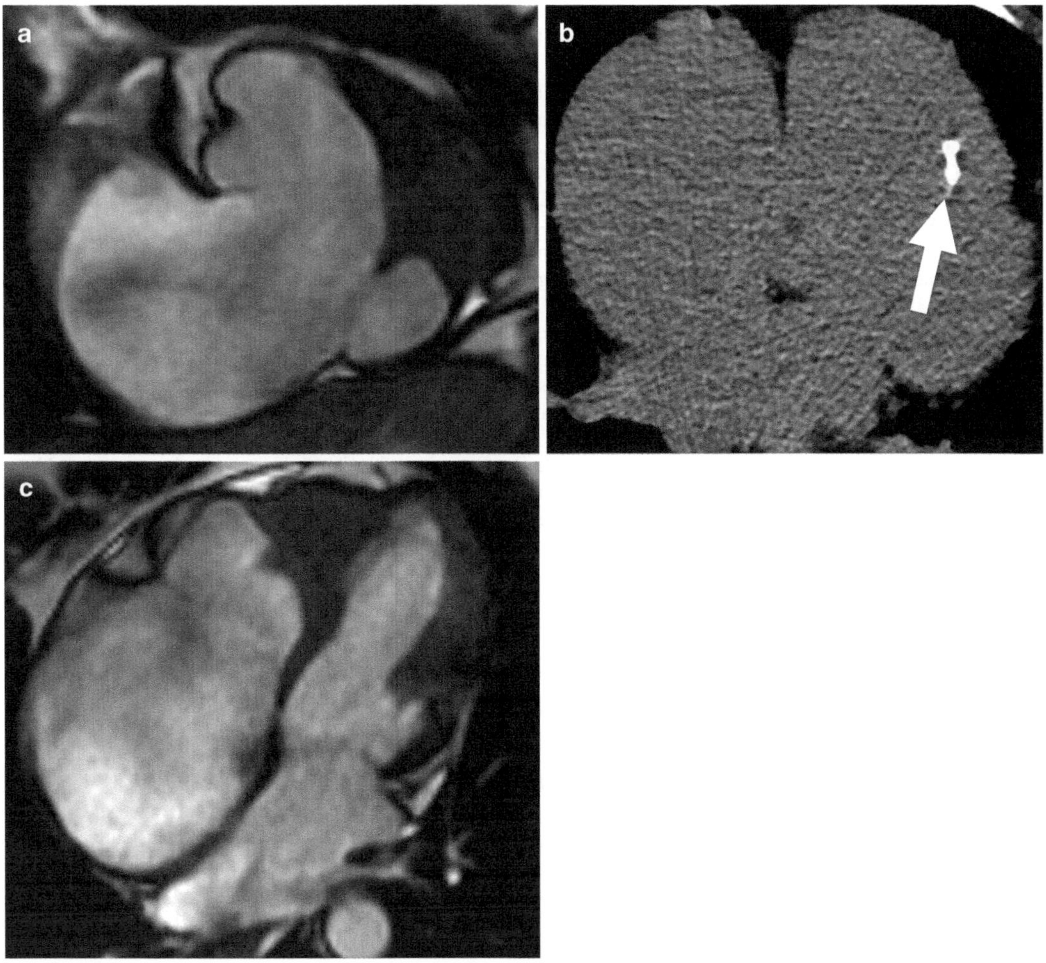

Fig. 13.15 Endomyocardial fibrosis with apically displaced tricuspid valve and atrial dilatation mimicking Ebstein anomaly. RV two-chamber (**a**) and four-chamber (**c**) cine images show mass obliterating the RV apex. (**b**) Dense endocardial calcification is seen on CT scan (arrow in **b**)

Acknowledgment Figures 13.12 to 13.15, Video files 13.1, 13.2, 13.3, 13.4, 13.5, 13.6, 13.7, 13.8, 13.9, 13.10, 13.11, 13.12, 13.13, and 13.14 are provided by Dr. Ramiah Rajeshkannan, Amrita Institute of Medical Sciences, Kochi, India.

References

1. Correa-Villaseñor A, Ferencz C, Neill CA, Wilson PD, Boughman JA. Ebstein's malformation of the tricuspid valve: genetic and environmental factors. The Baltimore-Washington Infant Study Group. Teratology. 1994;50(2):137–47.
2. Lupo PJ, Langlois PH, Mitchell LE. Epidemiology of Ebstein anomaly: prevalence and patterns in Texas, 1999-2005. Am J Med Genet Part A. 2011 May;155(5):1007–14.
3. Pradat P, Francannet C, Harris JA, Robert E. The epidemiology of cardiovascular defects, part I: a study based on data from three large registries of congenital malformations. Pediatr Cardiol. 2019;24(3):195–221.
4. Hurlstone AFL, Haramis APG, Wienholds E, Begthel H, Korving J, Van Eeden F, et al. The Wnt/β-catenin pathway regulates cardiac valve formation. Nature. 2003 Oct 9;425(6958):633–7.
5. Liebner S, Cattelino A, Gallini R, Rudini N, Iurlaro M, Piccolo S, et al. β-Catenin is required for endothelial-mesenchymal transformation during heart cushion development in the mouse. J Cell Biol. 2004 Aug 2;166(3):359–67.
6. Digilio MC, Bernardini L, Lepri F, Giuffrida MG, Guida V, Baban A, et al. Ebstein anomaly: genetic heterogeneity and association with microdeletions 1p36 and 8p23.1. Am J Med Genet Part A. 2011 Sep;155(9):2196–202.
7. Postma AV, Van Engelen K, Van De Meerakker J, Rahman T, Probst S, Baars MJH, et al. Mutations in the sarcomere gene MYH7 in Ebstein anomaly. Circ Cardiovasc Genet. 2011 Feb;4(1):43–50.
8. Kanani M, Moorman AFM, Cook AC, Webb S, Brown NA, Lamers WH, et al. Development of the atrioventricular valves: clinicomorphological correlations. Ann Thorac Surg. 2005;79(5):1797–804.
9. Edwards WD. Embryology and pathologic features of Ebstein's anomaly. Prog Pediatr Cardiol. 1993;2(1):5–15.
10. Jost CHA, Connolly HM, Dearani JA, Edwards WD, Danielson GK. Congenital heart disease for the adult cardiologist. Ebstein's Anomaly. 2007;115:277–85.
11. Boston US, Dearani JA, O'Leary PW, Driscoll DJ, Danielson GK. Tricuspid valve repair for Ebstein's anomaly in young children: a 30-year experience. Ann Thorac Surg. 2006 Feb;81(2):690–6.
12. Frescura C, Angelini A, Daliento L, Thiene G. Morphological aspects of Ebstein's anomaly in adults. Thorac Cardiovasc Surg. 2000;48(4):203–8.
13. Lev M, Liberthson RR, Joseph RH, Seten CE, Eckner FA, Kunske RD, et al. The pathologic anatomy of Ebstein's disease. Arch Pathol. 1970 Oct;90(4):334–43.
14. Anderson KR, Zuberbuhler JR, Anderson RH, Becker AE, Lie JT. Morphologic spectrum of Ebstein's anomaly of the heart. A review. Mayo Clin Proc. 1979;54(3):174–80.
15. Danielson GK, Driscoll DJ, Mair DD, Warnes CA, Oliver WC. Operative treatment of Ebstein's anomaly. J Thorac Cardiovasc Surg. 1992 Nov;104(5):1195–202.
16. Brickner ME, Hillis LD, Lange RA. Congenital heart disease in adults. Second of two parts. N Engl J Med. 2000 Feb 3;342(5):334–42.
17. Driscoll DJ, Mottram CD, Danielson GK. Spectrum of exercise intolerance in 45 patients with Ebstein's anomaly and observations on exercise tolerance in 11 patients after surgical repair. J Am Coll Cardiol. 1988;11(4):831–6.
18. Attenhofer Jost CH, Connolly HM, Scott CG, Burkhart HM, Ammash NM, Dearani JA. Increased risk of possible paradoxical embolic events in adults with Ebstein anomaly and severe tricuspid regurgitation. Congenit Heart Dis. 2014 Jan;9(1):30–7.
19. Broberg CS, Prasad SK, Carr C, Babu-Narayan SV, Dimopoulos K, Gatzoulis MA. Myocardial fibrosis in Eisenmenger syndrome: a descriptive cohort study exploring associations of late gadolinium enhancement with clinical status and survival. J Cardiovasc Magn Reson. 2014 May;14:16(1).
20. Dearani JA, Danielson GK. Congenital heart surgery nomenclature and database project: Ebstein's anomaly and tricuspid valve disease. Ann Thorac Surg. 2000;69(4 Suppl):S106–17.
21. Cromme-dukhuis AH, Hamer JPM. Two-dimensional colour-coded echocardiography in Ebstein's anomaly. Eur Heart J. 1990;11(12):1113–5.
22. Gültekin F, Baskin E, Gökalp A, Dogan K. A pregnant woman with Ebstein's anomaly. A case report. Mater Med Pol. 2019;26(4):149–51.
23. Park IS, Nakanishi T, Nakazawa M, Takanashi Y, Imai Y, Momma K. Radiofrequency pulmonary valvotomy using a new 2-French catheter. Cathet Cardiovasc Diagn. 1998;45(1):37–42.
24. Sahai S, Kothari SS, Wasir HS. Tetralogy of Fallot with Ebstein's anomaly of the tricuspid valve. Indian Heart J. 2019;46(1):53–4.
25. Celermajer DS, Cullen S, Sullivan ID, Spiegelhalter DJ, Wyse RKH, Deanfield JE. Outcome in neonates with Ebstein's anomaly. J Am Coll Cardiol. 1992;19(5):1041–6.
26. Fukuda T, Suzuki T, Sato M, Morikawa M. Complete atrioventricular septal defect and Ebstein's anomaly. Pediatr Cardiol. 1999 May;20(3):232–5.
27. Attenhofer Jost CH, Connolly HM, O'Leary PW, Warnes CA, Tajik AJ, Seward JB. Left heart lesions in patients with Ebstein anomaly. Mayo Clin Proc. 2005;80:361–8.
28. Salkar HR, Salkar RG, Sengupta PP. Ebstein's anomaly with coarctation of the aorta—an unusual association. Indian Heart J. 2019;48(3):283–4.

29. Ebaid M, Azeka E, Ikari NM, Sosa EA, Marcial MB, Atik E. Ebstein's anomaly with coarctation of the aorta. An unusual association. Arq Bras Cardiol. 1999 Aug;73(2):219–24.
30. Silverman NH, Gerlis LM, Horowitz ES, Ho SY, Neches WH, Anderson RH. Pathologic elucidation of the echocardiographic features of Ebstein's malformation of the morphologically tricuspid valve in discordant atrioventricular connections. Am J Cardiol. 1995 Dec 15;76(17):1277–83.
31. Yesil M, Bayata S, Postaci N, Aksoy I. New onset complete heart block and corrected transposition of great arteries in the seventh decade. Pacing Clin Electrophysiol. 1997;20(1):134–5.
32. Brugada J, Valls V, Freixa R, Gonzalez E, Herreros B, Matas M, et al. Radiofrequency ablation of a posteroseptal atrioventricular accessory pathway in a left-sided tricuspid ring with Ebsteinlike anomaly in a patient with congenitally corrected transposition of the great arteries. Pacing Clin Electrophysiol. 2000;23(1):133–6.
33. Isobe M, Tanaka M, Sekiguchi M. Subaortic stenosis due to accessory tissue of the mitral valve associated with Ebstein's anomaly in an adult. Int J Cardiol. 1996 Dec 13;57(3):286–8.
34. Khan IA, Cohen RA. Ebstein's anomaly of the tricuspid valve associated with congenital deafmutism. Int J Cardiol. 1999 Aug 31;70(3):219–21.
35. Voges I, Al-Mallah MH, Scognamiglio G, Di Salvo G. Right heart-pulmonary circulation unit in congenital heart diseases. Heart Failure Clin. 2018;14:283–95.
36. Attenhofer Jost CH, Connolly HM, Dearani JA, Edwards WD, Danielson GK. Ebstein's anomaly. Circulation. 2007 Jan 16;115(2):277–85.
37. Khairy P, van Hare GF, Balaji S, Berul CI, Cecchin F, Cohen MI, et al. PACES/HRS expert consensus statement on the recognition and management of arrhythmias in adult congenital heart disease. Can J Cardiol. 2014 Oct 1;30(10):e1–63.
38. Roten L, Lukac P, De Groot N, Nielsen JC, Szili-Torok T, Jensen HK, et al. Catheter ablation of arrhythmias in Ebstein's anomaly: a multicenter study. J Cardiovasc Electrophysiol. 2011 Dec;22(12):1391–6.
39. Hebe J. Ebstein's anomaly in adults. Arrhythmias: diagnosis and therapeutic approach. Thorac Cardiovasc Surg. 2000;48(4):214–9.
40. Segura AM, Frazier OH, Buja LM. Fibrosis and heart failure. Heart Fail Rev. 2014 Mar;19(2):173–85.
41. Stirrat J, White JA. The prognostic role of late gadolinium enhancement magnetic resonance imaging in patients with cardiomyopathy. Can J Cardiol. 2013;29:329–36.
42. Daliento L, Angelini A, Ho SY, Frescura C, Turrini P, Baratella MC, et al. Angiographic and morphologic features of the left ventricle in Ebstein's malformation. Am J Cardiol. 1997 Oct 15;80(8):1051–9.
43. Ikeda Y, Inomata T, Iida Y, Iwamoto-Ishida M, Nabeta T, Ishii S, et al. Time course of left ventricular reverse remodeling in response to pharmacotherapy: clinical implication for heart failure prognosis in patients with idiopathic dilated cardiomyopathy. Heart Vessels. 2016 Apr;31(4):545–54.
44. Babu-Narayan SV, Goktekin O, Moon JC, Broberg CS, Pantely GA, Pennell DJ, et al. Late gadolinium enhancement cardiovascular magnetic resonance of the systemic right ventricle in adults with previous atrial redirection surgery for transposition of the great arteries. Circulation. 2005 Apr 26;111(16):2091–8.
45. Babu-narayan SV, Kilner PJ, Li W, Moon JC, Goktekin O, Davlouros PA, et al. Ventricular fibrosis suggested by cardiovascular magnetic resonance in adults with repaired tetralogy of Fallot and its relationship to adverse markers of clinical outcome. Circulation. 2015;113(3):405–14.
46. Rathod RH, Prakash A, Powell AJ, Geva T. Myocardial fibrosis identified by cardiac magnetic resonance late gadolinium enhancement is associated with adverse ventricular mechanics and ventricular tachycardia late after Fontan operation. J Am Coll Cardiol. 2010;55(16):1721–8.
47. Carpentier A, Chauvaud S, Macé L, Relland J, Mihaileanu S, Marino JP, et al. A new reconstructive operation for Ebstein's anomaly of the tricuspid valve. J Thorac Cardiovasc Surg. 1988 Jul;96(1):92–101.
48. Yetman AT, Freedom RM, BW MC. Outcome in cyanotic neonates with Ebstein's anomaly. Am J Cardiol. 1998 Mar 15;81(6):749–54.
49. Celermajer DS, Bull C, Till JA, Cullen S, Vassillikos VP, Sullivan ID, et al. Ebstein's anomaly: presentation and outcome from fetus to adult. J Am Coll Cardiol. 1994;23(1):170–6.
50. Warnes CA, Williams RG, Bashore TM, Child JS, Connolly HM, Dearani JA, del Nido P, Fasules JW, Graham TP, Hijazi ZM, Hunt SA, King ME, Landzberg MJ, Miner PD, Radford MJ, Walsh EP, Webb GD, Smith SC, Jacobs AK, Adams CD, Anderson JL, Antman EM, Buller YC, Warnes CA, Williams RG, Bashore TM, Child JS, Connolly HM, et al. ACC/AHA 2008 guidelines for the management of adults with congenital heart disease. A report of the American College of Cardiology/American Heart Association Task Force on Practice Guidelines. J Am Coll Cardiol. 2008 Dec 2;52(23):e210–5.
51. Dearani JA, Mora BN, Nelson TJ, Haile DT, O'Leary PW. Ebstein anomaly review: what's now, what's next? Expert Rev Cardiovasc Ther. 2015;13(10):1101–9.
52. Shiina A, Seward JB, Edwards WD, Hagler DJ, Tajik AJ. Two-dimensional echocardiographic spectrum of Ebstein's anomaly: detailed anatomic assessment. J Am Coll Cardiol. 1984;3(2):356–70.
53. Gussenhoven EJ, Stewart PA, Becker AE, Essed CE, Ligtvoet KM, De Villeneuve VH. "Offsetting" of the septal tricuspid leaflet in normal hearts and in hearts with Ebstein's anomaly. Anatomic and echographic correlation. Am J Cardiol. 1984 Jul 1;54(1):172–6.
54. Bonow RO, Carabello BA, Chatterjee K, de Leon AC, Faxon DP, Freed MD, et al. 2008 Focused update incorporated into the ACC/AHA 2006 guidelines for the management of patients with valvular heart disease: a report of the American College of Cardiology/

American Heart Association Task Force on Practice Guidelines (Writing Committee to Revise the 1998 Guidelines for the Management of Patients With Valvular Heart Disease). Endorsed by the Society of Cardiovascular Anesthesiologists, Society for Cardiovascular Angiography and Interventions, and Society of Thoracic Surgeons. Circulation. 2008 Oct;118(15):e523–661.
55. Zoghbi WA, Enriquez-Sarano M, Foster E, Grayburn PA, Kraft CD, Levine RA, et al. Recommendations for evaluation of the severity of native Valvular regurgitation with two-dimensional and Doppler echocardiography. J Am Soc Echocardiogr. 2003;16(7):777–802.
56. Graham TP, Driscoll DJ, Gersony WM, Newburger JW, Rocchini A, Towbin JA. Task force 2: congenital heart disease. J Am Coll Cardiol. 2005;45:1326–33.
57. Knott-Craig CJ, Goldberg SP, Kirklin JK. Surgical strategy to prevent cardiac injury during reoperation in infants. J Cardiothorac Surg. 2008 Feb;28:3(1).
58. Knott-Craig CJ, Goldberg SP, Overholt ED, Colvin EV, Kirklin JK. Repair of neonates and young infants with Ebstein's anomaly and related disorders. Ann Thorac Surg. 2007;84(2):587–92.
59. Freud LR, Escobar-Diaz MC, Kalish BT, Komarlu R, Puchalski MD, Jaeggi ET, et al. Outcomes and predictors of perinatal mortality in fetuses with Ebstein anomaly or tricuspid valve dysplasia in the current era: a multicenter study. Circulation. 2015 Aug 11;132(6):481–9.
60. Stout KK, Daniels CJ, Aboulhosn JA, Bozkurt B, Broberg CS, Colman JM, et al. 2018 AHA/ACC guideline for the management of adults with congenital heart disease: a report of the American College of Cardiology/American Heart Association task force on clinical practice guidelines. Circulation. 2019;139:698–800.
61. Yalonetsky S, Tobler D, Greutmann M, Crean AM, Wintersperger BJ, Nguyen ET, et al. Cardiac magnetic resonance imaging and the assessment of Ebstein anomaly in adults. Am J Cardiol. 2011 Mar 1;107(5):767–73.
62. Jost CHA, Edmister WD, Julsrud PR, Dearani JA, Tepe MS, Warnes CA, et al. Prospective comparison of echocardiography versus cardiac magnetic resonance imaging in patients with Ebstein's anomaly. Int J Cardiovasc Imaging. 2012 Jun;28(5):1147–59.
63. Cawley PJ, Maki JH, Otto CM. Cardiovascular magnetic resonance imaging for valvular heart disease. Technique and validation. Circulation. 2009 Jan 27;119(3):468–78.
64. Kilner PJ, Geva T, Kaemmerer H, Trindade PT, Schwitter J, Webb GD. Recommendations for cardiovascular magnetic resonance in adults with congenital heart disease from the respective working groups of the European Society of Cardiology. Eur Heart J. 2010;31:794–805.
65. Mũoz-Castellanos L, Espinola-Zavaleta N, Kuri-Nivón M, Keirns C. Ebstein's anomaly: anatomo-echocardiographic correlation. Cardiovasc Ultrasound. 2007;5:43.
66. Vettukattil JJ, Bharucha T, Anderson RH. Defining Ebstein's malformation using three-dimensional echocardiography. Interact Cardiovasc Thorac Surg. 2007 Dec;6(6):685–90.
67. Alfakih K, Plein S, Bloomer T, Jones T, Ridgway J, Sivananthan M. Comparison of right ventricular volume measurements between axial and short axis orientation using steady-state free precession magnetic resonance imaging. J Magn Reson Imaging. 2003 Jul 1;18(1):25–32.
68. Kastler B, Livolsi A, Zhu H, Roy E, Zollner G, Dietemann JL. Potential role of MR imaging in the diagnostic management of Ebstein anomaly in a newborn. J Comput Assist Tomogr. 1990;14(5):825–7.
69. Choi YH, Park JH, Choe YH, Yoo SJ. MR imaging of Ebstein's anomaly of the tricuspid valve. Am J Roentgenol. 1994 Sep;163(3):539–43.
70. Eustace S, Kruskal JB, Hartnell GG. Ebstein's anomaly presenting in adulthood: the role of cine magnetic resonance imaging in diagnosis. Clin Radiol. 1994 Oct;49(10):690–2.
71. Bonello B, Kilner PJ. Review of the role of cardiovascular magnetic resonance in congenital heart disease, with a focus on right ventricle assessment. Arch Cardiovasc Dis. 2012;105:605–13.
72. Otero-Coto E, Perez-Martinez V, Palacios V, Caffarena JM. Ebstein's anomaly of the left-sided atrioventricular (AV) valve in AV discordance. Thorac Cardiovasc Surg. 1980 Oct;28(5):364–7.
73. Celermajer DS, Cullen S, Deanfield JE, Sullivan ID. Congenitally corrected transposition and Ebstein's anomaly of the systemic atrioventricular valve: association with aortic arch obstruction. J Am Coll Cardiol. 1991;18(4):1056–8.
74. Agarwal R, Sahayaraj A, Sankar M, Cherian KM. Endomyocardial fibrosis mimicking Ebstein's anomaly: a diagnostic challenge. Tex Heart Inst J. 2009;36(3):250–1.
75. Ammash NM, Warnes CA, Connolly HM, Danielson GK, Seward JB. Mimics of Ebstein's anomaly. Am Heart J. 1997 Sep;134(3):508–13.

14 Pre- and Postoperative Imaging in Tetralogy of Fallot

Shruthi Kalyan, Subhajit Das, and Vimal Raj

14.1 Definition

Tetralogy of Fallot (TOF) is a group of congenital heart malformations that has four major components [1]:

1. Right ventricular outflow tract obstruction (RVOTO)
2. Ventricular septal defect (VSD)
3. Overriding of the aorta
4. Right ventricular hypertrophy

14.2 Introduction

TOF is the most common cyanotic Congenital Heart Disease (CHD). The clinical manifestation and prognosis of the disease may vary based on the degree of severity of these four components of the disease. The cause for TOF is thought to be multifactorial. Associated chromosomal anomalies including Trisomy of 21, 18, 13 and microdeletions of chromosome 22q11.2 have been noted [2]. Embryologically, TOF is attributed to failure of fusion of conal and ventricular septa with anterior malalignment of the conal septum leading to the classic tetrad of findings [3, 4]. Another variant of TOF is also well described as "Pentalogy of Fallot"; this describes TOF plus atrial septal defect (ASD).

14.3 Pathophysiology

The main abnormality in TOF is the RVOTO and VSD. The RVOT obstruction causes increased pressure within the right ventricle (RV) leading to RV hypertrophy. As the pressure increases there is shunting of deoxygenated blood from RV to the left ventricle (LV). The overriding of VSD (straddling across the septum) also contributes to the passage of deoxygenated blood into the systemic circulation, which presents as cyanosis. The severity of cyanosis/systemic hypoxia hence is a marker of severity of RVOTO. RVOT obstruction may happen at various levels: infundibulum, valvular, or supravalvular (pulmonary arteries) (Fig. 14.1). Varying severity of obstruction may also be seen from mild stenosis to the total absence of the valve or the pulmonary arteries (atresia). In some patients, cyanosis may not be apparent due to mild stenosis, the so-called

Electronic supplementary material The online version of this chapter (https://doi.org/10.1007/978-981-15-6755-1_14) contains supplementary material, which is available to authorized users.

S. Kalyan
Star Hospitals, Hyderabad, India

S. Das
Rabindranath Tagore International Institute of Cardiac Sciences, Kolkata, India

V. Raj (✉)
Department of Cardiothoracic Imaging, Narayana Hrudayalaya, Bangalore, Karnataka, India

R. Rajeshkannan et al. (eds.), *CT and MRI in Congenital Heart Diseases*,
https://doi.org/10.1007/978-981-15-6755-1_14

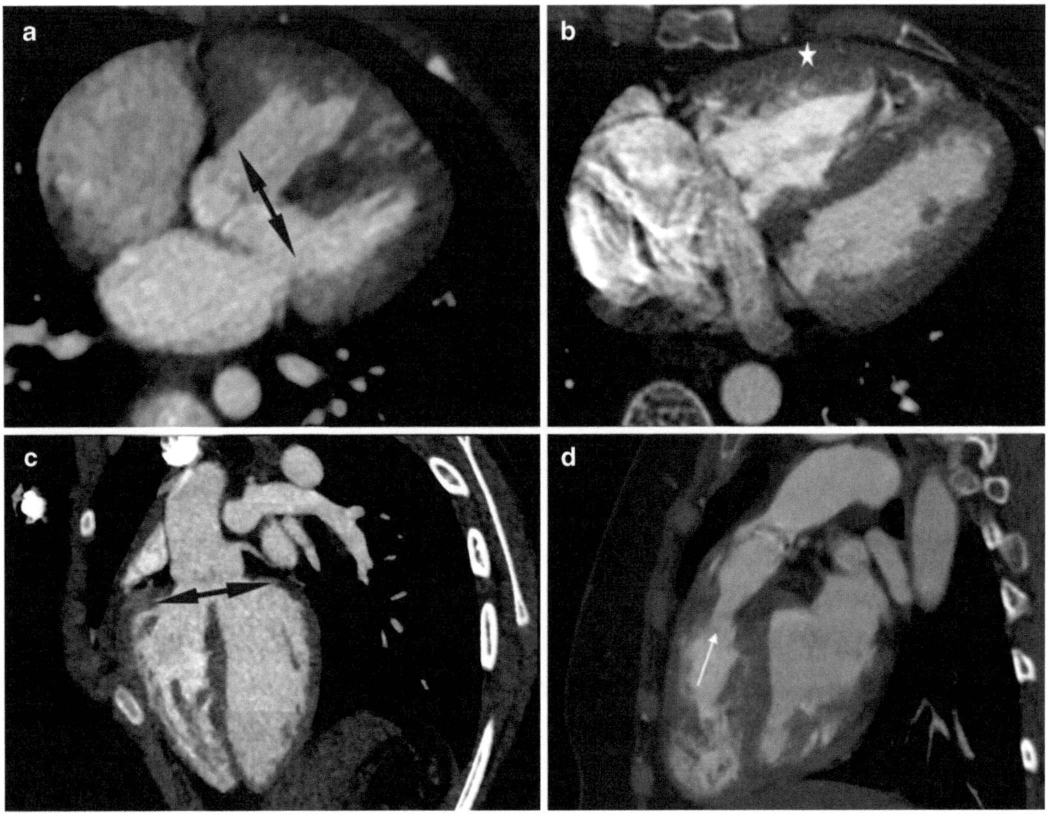

Fig. 14.1 MDCT images of a patient with Tetralogy of Fallot (TOF). Axial (**a**, **b**), LVOT (**c**), and RVOT (**d**) images showing VSD (double black arrow), overriding of the aorta of the VSD (**c**), Infundibular (white arrow) and valvular stenosis. There is also RV hypertrophy (star) with some dilatation of RV

"pink tetralogy." Patients can have obstruction at multiple levels of RVOT, which needs to be clearly determined to ensure appropriate therapy.

In the absence of normal pulmonary arterial supply, the lungs derive blood supply from various sources such as Patent Ductus Arteriosus (PDA), aortopulmonary/pleuro-pulmonary collaterals, and bronchial arteries. These vascular channels also have a significant bearing on the management of the patients and need to be adequately imaged.

PDA It is a vascular channel that extends from the undersurface of the aortic arch or proximal descending aorta to the pulmonary artery. In cases of pulmonary atresia, PDA becomes an essential source of pulmonary blood flow ("duct-dependent circulation") (Fig. 14.2).

Major Aortopulmonary Collaterals (MAPCAs) These are primitive intersegmental arteries that have failed to involute. These extend from the aorta or its major branches and supply the lungs. These can be broadly classified as direct or indirect (on the basis of origin) and protected or unprotected (based on the presence or absence of stenosis). MAPCAs and bronchial artery differentiation can be made on the basis that bronchial arteries often provide mediastinal branches and, in some cases, branch to the spinal cord. MAPCAs often anastomose with the intrapulmonary arteries at or near the pulmonary hilum.

Various combinations and associations are possible in TOF and have been well described. These include:

- TOF with pulmonary atresia (PA) with or without MAPCAs/ PDA
- TOF with absent pulmonary valve

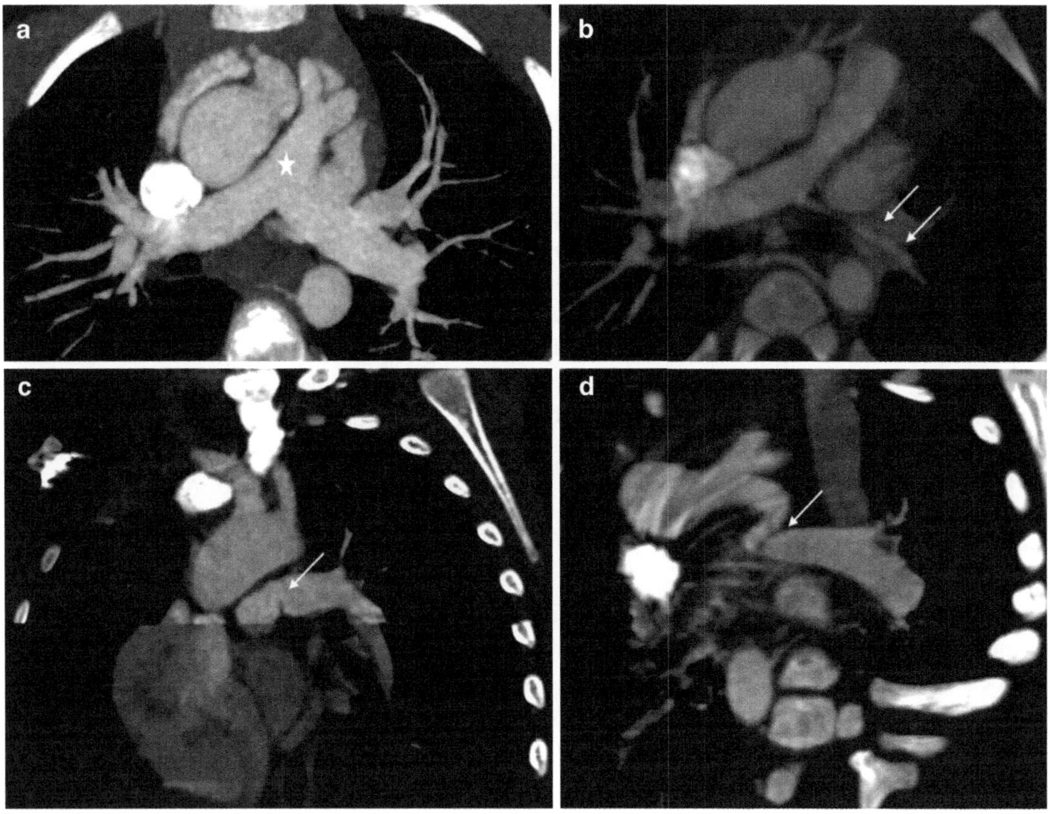

Fig. 14.2 MDCT MPR images showing various pulmonary artery anatomies. (**a**) Showing good-sized confluent branch pulmonary arteries (star). (**b**) Showing diffusely small LPA with confluent branch pulmonary arteries (white arrows). (**c**) Showing mild proximal LPA stenosis with good-caliber vessel distally (white arrow). (**d**) Showing LPA being formed by PDA with focal stenosis in the distal PDA (white arrow)

- TOF with double outlet right ventricle (DORV) where both aorta and pulmonary artery arise from RV
- TOF with ASD—Pentalogy of Fallot
- TOF with right aortic arch
- TOF with coronary artery anomalies
- TOF with anomalous pulmonary venous return

14.4 Management of TOF

Pulmonary outflow obstruction with VSD results in reduced pulmonary circulation, right to left shunt with subsequent cyanosis. The severity of cyanosis determines the time for initial surgical correction while pulmonary anatomy determines the type of procedure [5]. Most patients undergo planned elective surgical repair between 3 and 6 months of age, although few may require earlier correction in case of severe cyanosis.

14.4.1 Single-Stage Repair

One-stage, complete surgical repair is the surgery of choice at most centers. A complete surgical repair of TOF involves VSD closure with a pericardial patch and relief of any pulmonary outflow tract obstruction. The surgical technique will depend on the level and degree of pulmonary obstruction [6]. In pulmonary stenosis, a longitudinal incision is performed through the main PA, pulmonary annulus into the RV infundibulum, and reconstructed with a trans-annular patch. In patients with an adequate size pulmonary annulus, a pulmonary valvuloplasty may be performed along with enlargement of the main pulmonary artery, infundibular resection, and VSD closure [7]. In pulmonary atresia with good-sized branch PAs, an RV–PA conduit is the choice with the closure of VSD. In patients with anomalous coronary anatomy with major coronary crossing anterior to RVOT, infundibular resection cannot be made. An RV–PA conduit is hence employed. In patients with pulmonary atresia and MAPCAs, unifocalization is performed wherein collaterals are attached to the right ventricle through a conduit/homograft.

14.4.2 Multi-stage Repair

Multi-stage repair involves a palliative systemic to pulmonary artery shunt, such as Modified Blalock–Taussig [8] (BT shunt) followed by a definitive repair later. The shunt helps to increase the pulmonary blood flow and size of the pulmonary arteries.

14.4.3 Natural History Post Surgery

Most patients with complete cardiac repair have an uneventful postoperative recovery. Nearly 90% of children who undergo corrective surgery survive into adulthood [9]. These patients are usually asymptomatic in the early years with long-term morbidity related to abnormal RV hemodynamics. Pulmonary regurgitation (PR) and pulmonary restenosis are the most common complications of TOF repair, which eventually lead to chronic RV overload and subsequent RV dilatation and failure [7]. Pulmonary valve replacement (PVR) is the treatment of choice in the setting of RV dysfunction and PR; however, the timing of this procedure is debatable [10, 11]. Early repair at the asymptomatic stage to prevent RV failure has to be weighed against the need for repeat surgery in the future because of the finite life span of the bio-prosthetic valve [12, 13].

14.5 Imaging Techniques

14.5.1 Chest Radiograph

Chest radiograph (CXR) is often the primary investigation in children with suspected CHD. In TOF, CXR has a classical description of a "boot-shaped heart" attributed to RV hypertrophy and RVOT obstruction/narrowing. This may not be apparent in the early stages of the disease wherein CXR is useful in assessing the cardiac/visceral situs and also estimate the pulmonary vasculature (oligemia/plethora/normal). It is also useful in looking at the aortic arch and pulmonary complications associated with TOF.

14.5.2 Echocardiography

Transthoracic echocardiography (TTE) is the mainstay of imaging in TOF both pre- and postoperatively but can have a limited role in assessing extracardiac vascular structures [5]. TTE is very good at assessing the valves, ventricular function, and the septum. It is, however, significantly operator-dependent and interpretation may be limited in patients with poor acoustic windows. Coronary anatomy, pulmonary venous return, MAPCAs, and RV size are some of the parameters where cross-sectional imaging provides more accurate and reproducible data.

14.5.3 Cardiac Catheterization

For many decades, catheter angiography has been considered as a definite test and is routinely performed preoperatively. Surgical planning, accurate assessment of vasculature (especially MAPCAs), and hemodynamic data relating to pulmonary blood flow are the robust data provided by catheter angiography. It is an invasive technique often requiring sedation/anesthesia with long procedure times. The focus has now shifted to limiting the use of catheter studies only for hemodynamic data, which may have a significant effect on the surgical planning. The growing role of CMR and CTA as the preferred adjunctive tests to echocardiography is related to a simultaneous proportional decline in the use of invasive angiography [14]. Over the last few years, hybrid procedures are being performed integrating Magnetic Resonance (MR) imaging with invasive angiography to reduce radiation exposure and avoid repeated sedation of the child.

14.5.4 Computed Tomography Angiography (CTA)

Multidetector Computed Tomography (MDCT) angiography offers a fast and reliable supplement to TTE in the assessment of patients with TOF. With recent technical advances in the field of MDCT, the scan duration and amount of radiation exposure have seen a steady decline. Scanners with 64 or more rows of detectors are preferred for scanning children to obtain the best results. MDCT is very good in confirming the presence or absence of pulmonary arteries and localizing any peripheral stenosis, which is often not well seen on TTE. The origin, course, and segmental supply of MAPCAs can be very well depicted with MDCT. Surgical planning is significantly aided by the anatomical knowledge of coronaries, PDA, and coarctation provided by MDCT.

Cardiac CTA protocols**:** MDCT imaging parameters will vary from one unit to other (due to different scanners) and from one patient to the other (due to clinical indication). At the outset, a scanner with larger coverage per rotation (for example 256 slice scanner has 8 cm coverage per rotation vs 128 slice scanner has 4 cm coverage per rotation) and better temporal resolution (assessed by the rotation speed of the scanner or dual source) is preferred. Exposure parameters (kV and mas) are altered according to the size of the patient with the help of iterative technology and automated dose regulation to keep radiation dose at its minimum.

Conscious oral/intravenous sedation is often sufficient in most patients with older children not requiring any sedation. Peripheral venous access is secured via a 22 or 20G needle (both upper and lower limb are suitable). Contrast injection rate varies from 0.8 to 3 ml/s based on the age of the patient and the venous access. Contrast volume of up to 1 ml per kilo of body weight is sufficient. Contrast injection is followed by a saline chase of equal volume (up to 20 ml) at the same rate of injection of contrast to get the best results [15]. The timing of study is determined by using the bolus-tracking technique and the scan is started after the contrast reaches the RV or the pulmonary artery.

ECG gating of study helps in reducing cardiac motion-related artifacts. This is especially useful in assessing coronary arteries and aortic root in various pathologies. However, there is increased radiation exposure and hence many units use it only in specific cases. The decision of gating will also depend on the MDCT scanner at hand with radiation exposure not being a major burden in some scanners. Some of the older versions of the scanners cannot perform gating at higher heart rates and pre-procedure preparation may be required to bring down the resting heart rate of the patient. Often, a dual run protocol is utilized wherein one run gets optimal opacification of the pulmonary arteries and the right heart chambers while the second run depicts the pulmonary and systemic veins and the aorta better. The entire thoracic cavity and upper abdomen (upto bottom of the kidneys) should be covered for comprehensive assessment.

Post-processing of images by curved planar reconstruction, maximum intensity projection (MIP), minimum intensity projection, and volume-rendering technique (VRT) are used for the purpose of creating representative images. These are useful in surgical planning, communicating the anatomical problems to the patient, and getting their consent for further management.

The main disadvantage of MDCT is radiation exposure and the use of iodinated contrast injection, especially since some of the patients require multiple follow-ups. Lack of functional/hemodynamic data is the other drawback compared to TTE/MR imaging and catheter angiography.

14.5.5 Cardiac MR (CMR)

CMR gives anatomic and functional information without exposing the patient to ionizing radiation or the risk of an adverse reaction to iodinated contrast material. CMR is considered gold standard in functional and volumetric assessment of the ventricles. Phase-contrast (PC) MR can provide valuable data to quantify flow, its direction and also assess the severity of stenosis. It is also possible to accurately quantify the pulmonary (Q_p) and systemic flow (Q_s), thereby quantifying the shunt and helping in making critical clinical decisions. Contrast-enhanced MR angiography (MRA) is particularly useful for the assessment of smaller or deeper vascular structures that may not be readily seen on TTE. CMR is also preferred in patients who would require regular follow-up and extensive hemodynamic data for surgical planning. Patients who have undergone intracardiac repair (ICR) for TOF often need regular CMR scans to assess RV volumes, function, and degree of pulmonary regurgitation.

Cardiac MR Protocol Conscious sedation or general anesthesia is often required in children below the age of 6 to perform CMR. Imaging can be performed during breath-hold or free breathing. CMR examinations can take a long time, hence pre-planning is of essence to ensure appropriate data is acquired. Standard CMR protocols for assessment of patients with TOF comprises a mixture of anatomical, cine (functional), MRA, PC, and in selected cases delayed enhancement sequences [16]. Static black blood/white blood images are acquired in multiple planes to determine the anatomy and planning of the study. Cine images are performed in various long axis (two-chamber, three-chamber, four-chamber, LVOT/RVOT), short-axis, and axial planes to assess for function, ventricular volumes, and valvular competency. PC images are acquired at the level of the ascending aorta, MPA, RPA, and LPA to assess the Q_p, Q_s, and also differential flow in the lungs. MRA is reserved to assess vascular structures that are not readily visible in cine and static images. Delayed enhancement imaging can demonstrate myocardial fibrosis, which can have significant prognostic information.

14.6 Preoperative Imaging of TOF

It is important to have a standardized protocol for clinical and imaging assessment of patients with TOF. Based on the availability of resources and competency, different institutes may have different assessment algorithms. Invariably, all patients have a CXR followed by TTE, which may provide all the necessary information. Use of MDCT/CMR is routine in some centers while others use these modalities preoperatively only as a problem-solving tool. Catheter angiography use is restricted to cases that require hemodynamic data (pulmonary arterial pressures/pulmonary vascular resistance, etc.) prior to management decision.

Primary focus of preoperative imaging in TOF include:

- Characterization of the primary lesion—RVOT obstruction and VSD
- Pulmonary arterial anatomy
- Associated anomalies involving aorta/collaterals, PDA, pulmonary veins, coronary arteries, etc.
- Functional status

14.6.1 Characterization of Primary Lesion

14.6.1.1 Right Ventricle Outflow Tract Obstruction (RVOTO)

Right ventricular outflow obstruction can happen at one or multiple levels simultaneously (infundibulum, valvular, or supravalvular). The severity of obstruction can also vary from minor stenosis to the total absence of the valve or the vessel. Dynamic examination with TTE, CMR, ECG-gated CT is useful for this. TTE is the mainstay in this assessment and very accurate in the assessment of the subvalvular and valvular anatomy. Hypertrophied muscle bundles in infundibulum (subvalvular) are very well depicted by TTE and

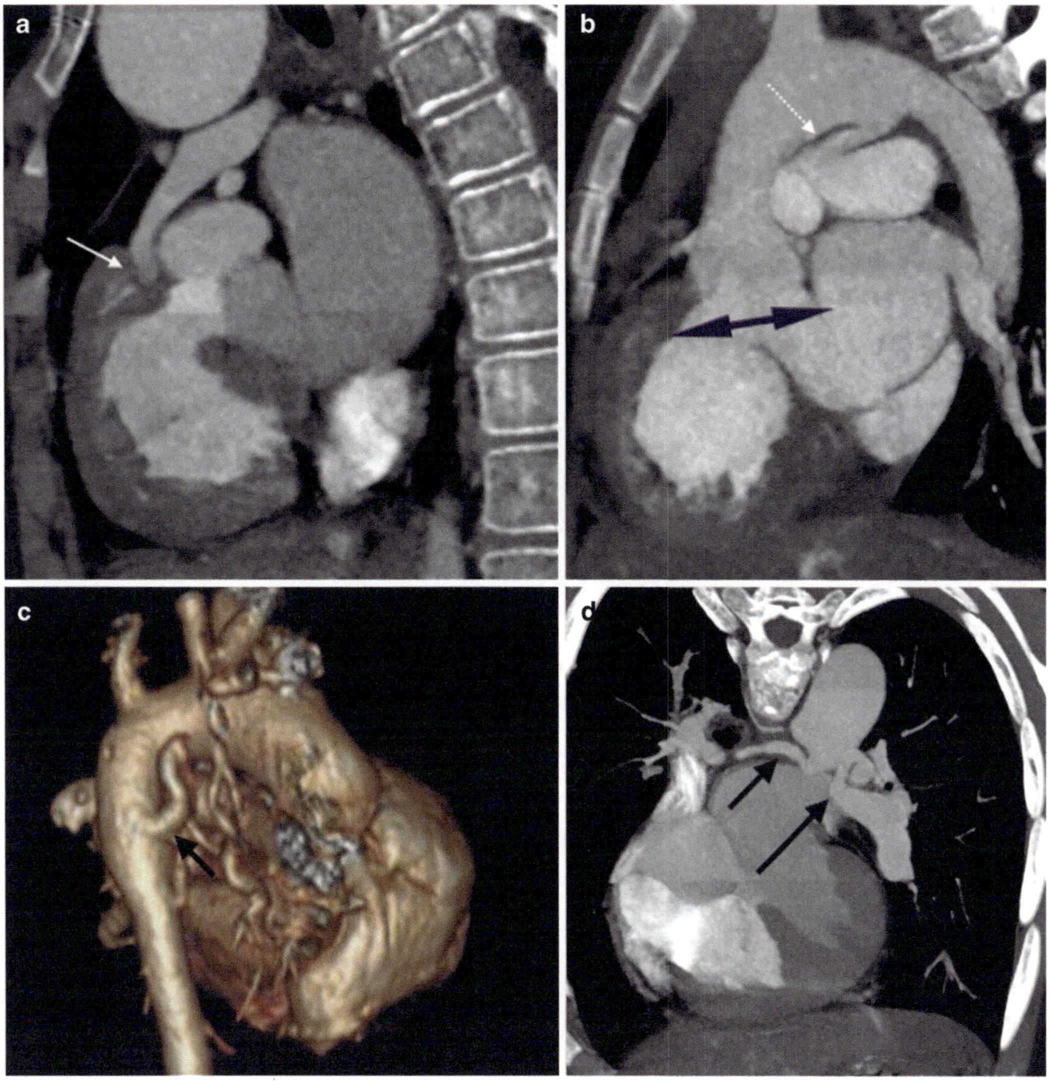

Fig. 14.3 MDCT images in a patient with membranous pulmonary atresia (**a** white arrow) and VSD with overriding of the aorta (double black arrow). Other sources of pulmonary arterial supply depicted are a PDA (dotted arrow in **b**) and MAPCAs (black arrows) in (**c**, **d**)

it is also possible to assess the degree of narrowing.

In pulmonary atresia, there is an absence of pulmonary valve with or without the absence of the pulmonary arteries. In membranous pulmonary atresia, there is an absence of the valve with the presence of the main pulmonary artery and its branches (Fig. 14.3). In long segment pulmonary atresia, there is an absence of the valve and the pulmonary arteries to varying degrees. TTE is often not able to clearly define the degree and extent of pulmonary arterial stenosis/atresia and MDCT/CMR are useful. RVOT stenting in patients with RVOTO is gaining popularity as a palliative alternative to modified BT shunts (Fig. 14.4). This improves blood supply to the lungs and helps in the growth of native pulmonary arteries so total correction can be performed at a later stage. MDCT and CMR are essential in providing accurate dimensions of the RVOT in the planning of this procedure.

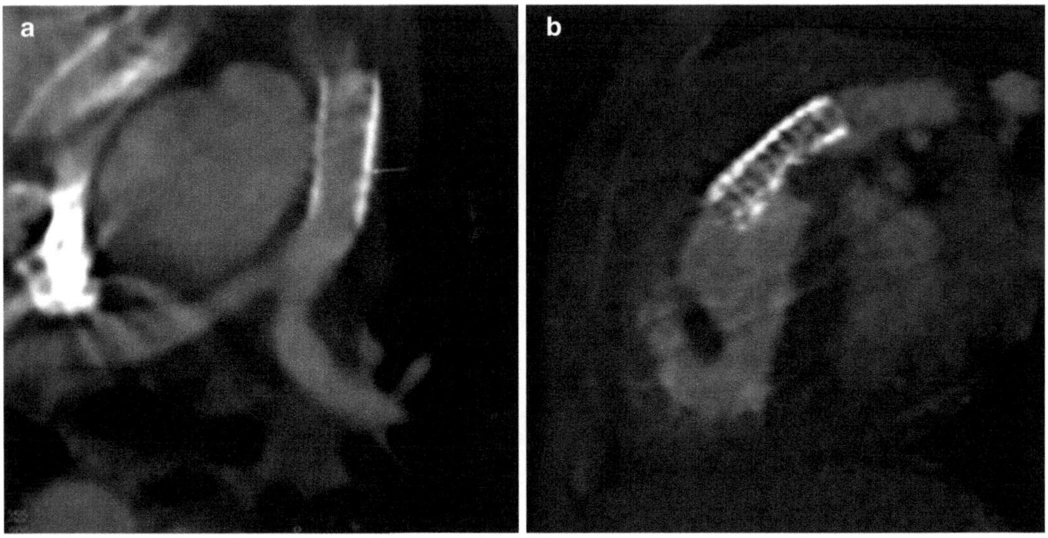

Fig. 14.4 MDCT MPR images showing a patient with patent RVOT stent (arrow) with confluent branch pulmonary arteries

In some variants of TOF, there is an absence of normal pulmonary valve (absent pulmonary valve) with some strand-like tissue replacing it. This is best seen with TTE and CMR while MDCT may not be able to show this well. These patients often have grossly enlarged main pulmonary artery.

14.6.1.2 Ventricular Septal Defect

The size and location of the VSD is easily and accurately assessed with TTE. This is usually sub-aortic in nature and involves the membranous portion of the interventricular septum. MDCT and CMR can also demonstrate the VSD and assess the size of the VSD (Fig. 14.5). CMR can provide extra information with regards to the amount of shunting, but this is often not required in true TOF. Sub-aortic nature of the VSD means that there is overriding of VSD by the aorta (aorta getting supply from both ventricles).

DORV (Double Outlet Right Ventricle) is a variant of TOF wherein; the aorta and the pulmonary arteries arise from the RV. On imaging, this can be ascertained by seeing the loss of aortomitral continuity (aortic and mitral valve are normally coupled through a fibrous sheet) meaning aorta is arising from RV. The aortic overriding of VSD of more than 60% toward the RV is also suggestive of DORV.

VSD closure by the pericardial patch is achieved if the aorta is "routable" to LV (blood from LV can be directed to aorta after VSD closure). In some cases, the size/location of VSD and orientation/position of aorta make it impossible to close the VSD and divert LV blood to the aorta (non-routable VSD). In such cases, the surgical procedure will need to be modified.

3D modeling of MDCT/CMR data can also be used for surgical planning in complex cases. Some patients with TOF may also have additional VSDs in the muscular septum, these are easily assessed with TTE itself.

14.6.2 Pulmonary Arteries

Analysis of the pulmonary artery anatomy is the most important aspect of diagnostic imaging of patients with TOF. Surgical management varies based on pulmonary arterial anatomy and the presence/absence of other sources of vascular supply to the lungs (Fig. 14.2). Cross-sectional imaging is better at ascertaining these compared to TTE. The assessment should include:

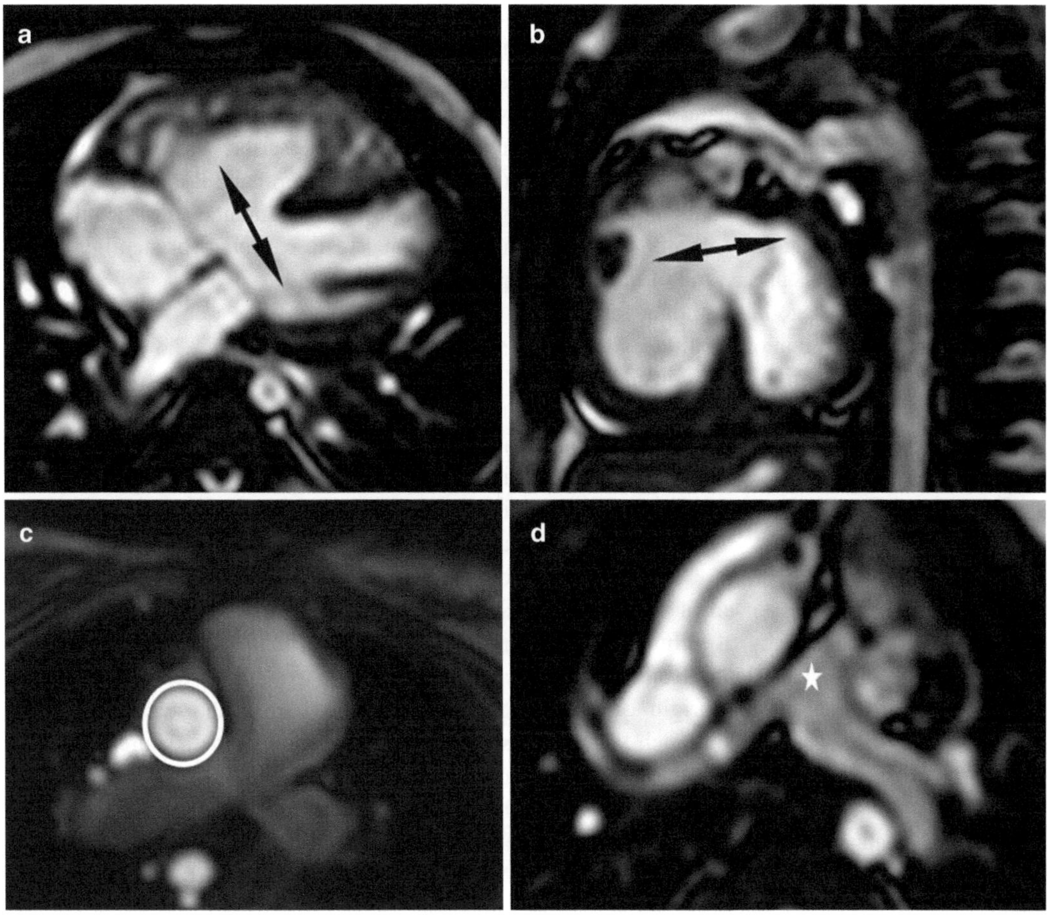

Fig. 14.5 CMR images of a patient with TOF showing the VSD with overriding of the aorta (**a**, **b**) with double black arrow and confluent (star) branch pulmonary arteries with smallish RPA (**d**). Phase-contrast flow images to assess flow at the level of the aorta (**c**)

- Presence or absence of native main and branch pulmonary arteries
- Presence of confluence of pulmonary arteries (i.e., right and left pulmonary arteries are connected to each other)
- Size of main and branch pulmonary arteries especially at the hila and any stenosis
- Source of blood to the native pulmonary arteries

The location and severity of pulmonary stenosis is important to depict. Focal areas of narrowing can often be dealt with augmentation plasty during surgery or palliatively managed with angioplasty. In a patient with non-confluent pulmonary arteries or long segment of pulmonary stenosis/atresia, the surgical correction is modified. Pulmonary artery sizes can be compared with age and body surface area matched normal controls by giving "Z" score. This can be determined from many freely available online sources. Few other indices are also available to assess the size of the pulmonary arteries and their suitability for surgical correction. Two such indices (primarily described in catheter angiography) can also be utilized in cross-section imaging:

- *McGoon ratio*

McGoon ratio is calculated by dividing the sum of the diameters of the distal right pulmonary artery and distal left pulmonary artery (LPA) divided by the diameter of aorta just above the diaphragm. Lower the ratio, smaller the branch pulmonary arteries. An average value of 2.1 is noted in normal subjects and a ratio of more than 1.7 is considered as a good candidate for complete surgical correction in our institute. Children with a ratio of less than 1.2 are considered for staged repair [17]. Patients with a ratio of 1.2–1.7 are discussed and surgical decision is based on a combination of parameters.

- *Nakata index*

Nakata index is widely used in preoperative assessment of the adequacy of pulmonary vascular bed [18]. It is calculated from the PAs immediately proximal to the origin of upper lobe branches of the respective branch Pas. The sum of the cross-sectional area of RPA and LPA is divided by body surface area (BSA) of the patient. A Nakata index of >150 is acceptable for complete repair without prior palliative shunt.

In pulmonary atresia or severe pulmonary stenosis, the main and/or branch pulmonary arteries/lungs may derive their blood supply from other sources. It is important to map the source of supply to each pulmonary artery and also different parts of the lungs. The following sources should be looked at:

- *PDA*

PDA, if present, is an important source of pulmonary blood supply. In some cases of pulmonary atresia, PDA is often the only source of pulmonary blood supply (duct dependent supply). In the left aortic arch, PDA often connects to LPA and in the right arch to the RPA (Fig. 14.2). There is often a focal area of stenosis in the branch pulmonary artery at the junction with PDA. This may restrict the flow to the lungs and can be corrected by PDA stenting. There is growing evidence supporting the use of PDA stenting as an alternative for other aortopulmonary shunts such as modified BT shunt [19]. In such cases, it is important to describe the PDA anatomy (length, size at the aorta and PA and point of origin in relation to arch branches) in detail so the interventional team can plan for stenting appropriately (Fig. 14.3).

- *MAPCAs*

It is important to clearly delineate the total number of MAPCAs, their origin, course, proximity to structures like veins and airways, and intrapulmonary connections. The size of collaterals can also be described as—Large (>2 mm in diameter), Medium (1–2 mm in diameter), and small (<1 mm in diameter). Stenosis occurs in most MAPCAs, particularly at the aortic origin and pulmonary anastomotic sites (Fig. 14.3). In cases of pulmonary atresia and severe pulmonary stenosis, MAPCAs are the main source of supply to the lungs, and unifocalization procedure may be required as part of surgical repair. Catheter angiography is often used in collaboration with MDCT to assess these as part of surgical planning (Fig. 14.3).

- Collaterals may also be seen from bronchial/subclavian/coronary arteries and also pleuroparenchymal collaterals. MDCT is excellent in assessing these collaterals [7]. Before doing major corrective surgery in patients, it is important to know the adequacy of the pulmonary blood supply in each bronchopulmonary segment. If both MAPCAs and native pulmonary arteries supply a bronchopulmonary segment, ligations of MAPCAs do not affect lung arborization. If a bronchopulmonary segment is exclusively supplied by MAPCAs, then that segment needs to be unifocalized.

14.6.2.1 Aortic Anatomy

- Left aortic arch is the most common anatomy encountered in patients with TOF. Patients may have aberrant origin and course of the

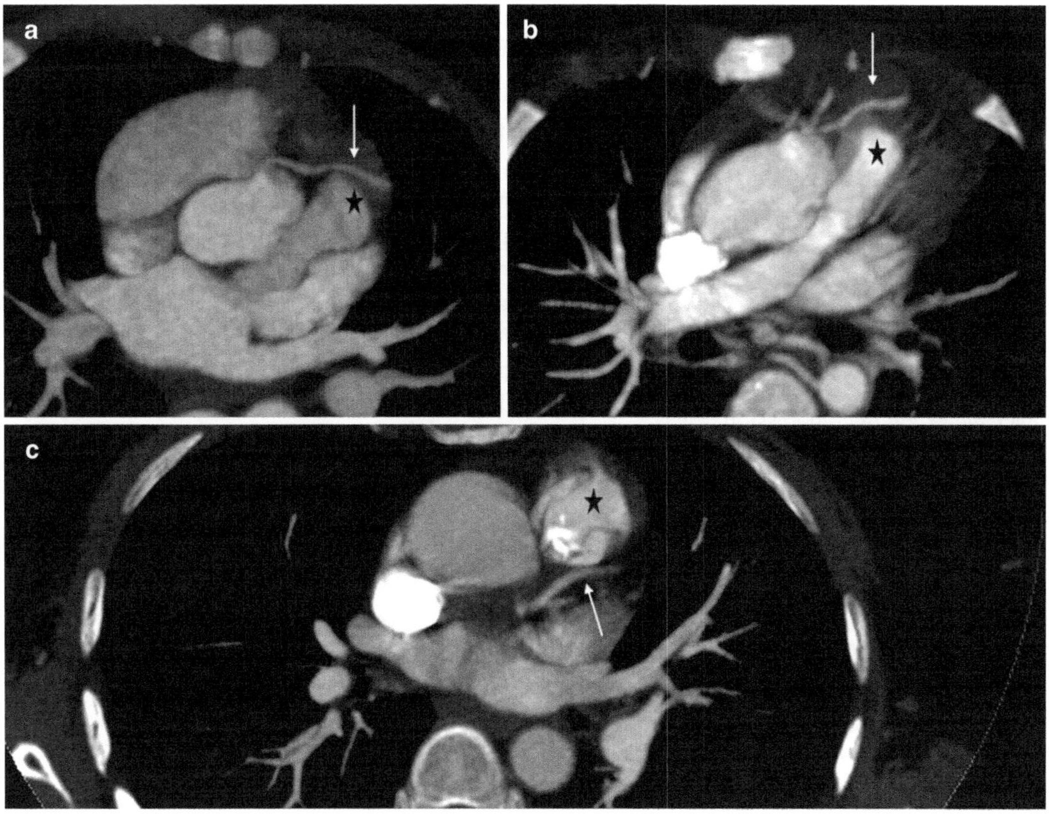

Fig. 14.6 MDCT images showing coronary anatomy in relation to the RVOT (black arrow). Major coronary crossing (LAD) is seen crossing anterior to RVOT (white arrow in **a**, **b**). Normal anatomy of the LAD in image (**c**)

right subclavian artery, which may cause some compression of the esophagus and could contribute to a vascular loop. Right-sided aortic arch may also be seen in patients with TOF (Fig. 14.5). Coarctation of aorta, double aortic arch, or even truncus abnormalities may be seen. In older children or adolescents, there is often dilatation of the aortic root. The left/right aortic arch anatomies are important to plan for aortopulmonary shunts and also PDA stents.

14.6.2.2 Coronary Anatomy

The incidence of coronary artery anomalies in TOF is reported to be 2–10% [20]. Common coronary anomalies associated with TOF are anomalous origin of the left anterior descending artery (LAD) from the right coronary artery (RCA) coursing anterior to the infundibulum of the RV. The second-most common anomaly is that of a single coronary ostium. When undiagnosed, these vessels are at a significant risk of surgical injury during right ventriculotomy or RVOT repair (Fig. 14.6).

14.6.2.3 Atrial Septal Defects

Atrial septal defects (ASD) may also be seen in patients with TOF and TTE is often best at depicting this. The presence, location, and size of the defect may have an impact on surgical planning.

14.6.2.4 Pulmonary Venous Return

Anomalous pulmonary venous return may also be seen in patients with TOF. This is one anomaly that is often not accurately mapped with TTE and hence cross-sectional imaging is preferred.

14.6.2.5 Airway Compression

Pulmonary artery dilatation can compress airways as seen in TOF with absent pulmonary valve or with post-stenotic dilatation. The lower trachea, right and left main bronchus can be affected. Tracheomalacia and bronchomalacia are the end result of prolonged extrinsic compression. Airway compression can result in frequent upper respiratory infections, wheezing, pneumonia, atelectasis, and hyperinflation. Extrinsic compression can easily mimic foreign body aspiration and pneumonia. MDCT or CMR can help in localizing the level and extent of compression.

14.7 Postoperative Imaging in TOF

Imaging plays an important role in the assessment of patients who have undergone TOF repair (single-stage or multi-stage). TTE remains the first modality for the assessment of these patients. Regular follow-up with CMR is also findings its place in clinical protocols for assessing patients who undergo ICR.

14.7.1 Imaging Post BT Shunt

Modified BT shunt using prosthetic material is performed in patients with small-sized pulmonary arteries as a two-staged correction or as a palliative procedure. The shunt could get stenosed or obstructed (Fig. 14.7) or there could be pseudo-aneurysm at the anastomotic sites [8]. TTE may often not be able to see some of these shunts and cross-sectional imaging is better. The growth of the native pulmonary arteries can also be assessed at the same time.

14.7.2 Imaging Post Intracardiac Repair (ICR)

Pulmonary regurgitation (PR) following ICR is almost universal with over 80% of patients developing PR that eventually contributes to

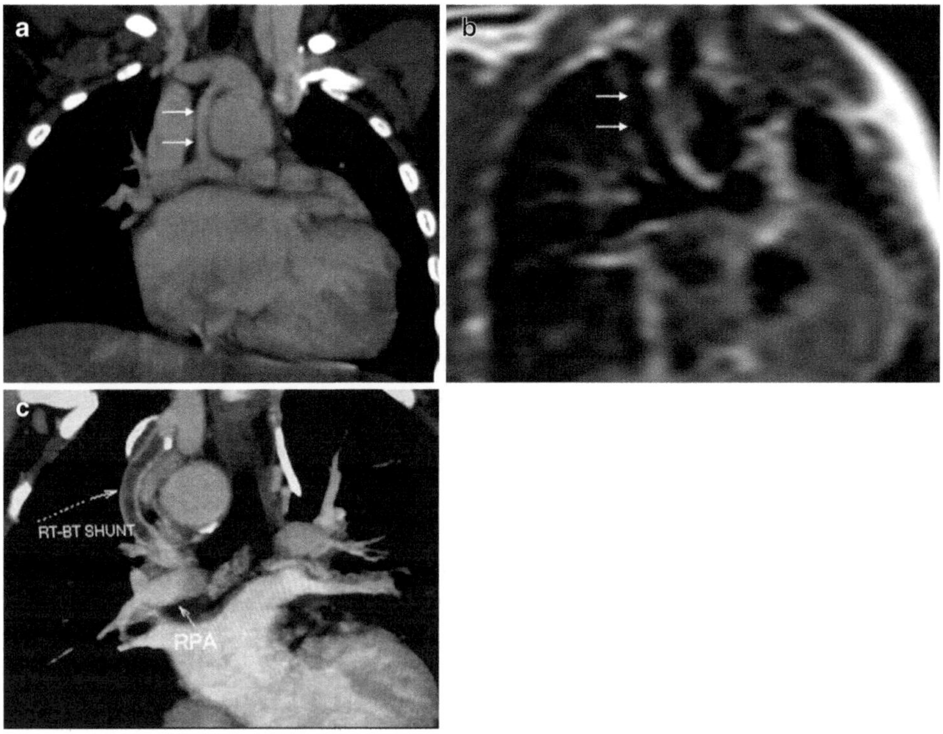

Fig. 14.7 MDCT (**a**/**c**) and CMR (**b**) images in patients post modified BT shunt (arrows) showing patent stents in (**a**, **b**) and thrombosed in (**c**)

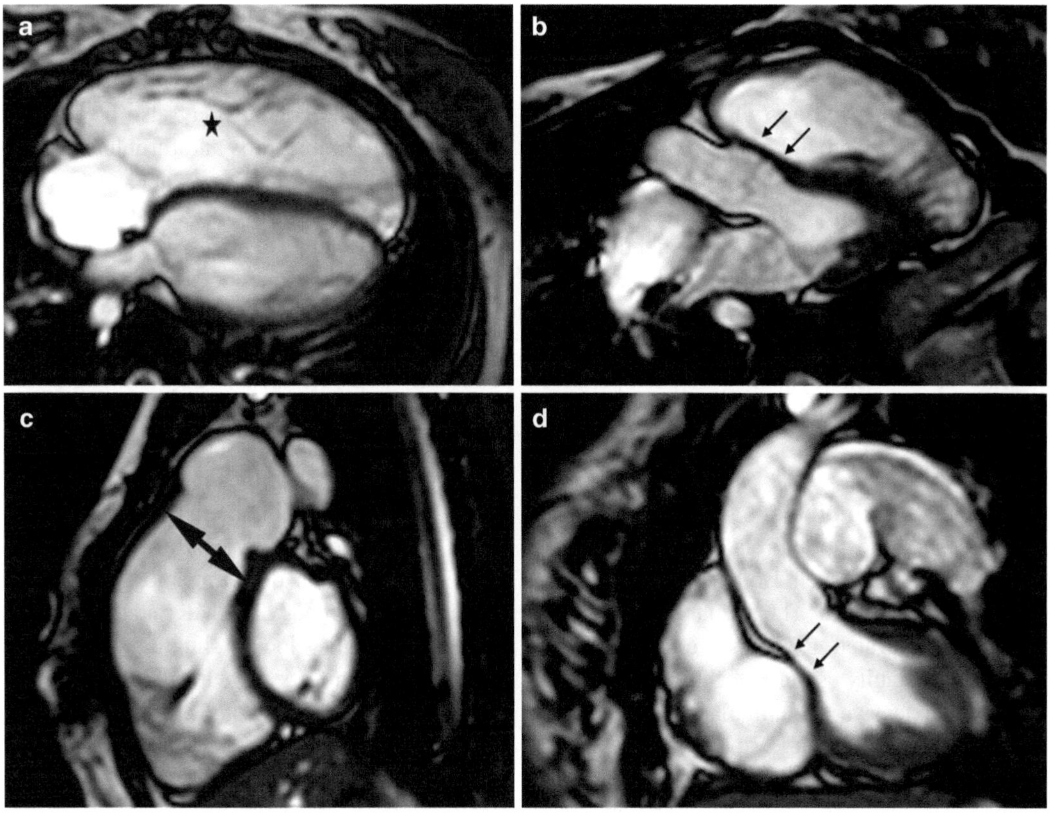

Fig. 14.8 CMR images in a patient post ICR for TOF. (**a**) Shows a dilated RV (black arrow) and (**c**) demonstrates dilated RVOT (double black arrow) secondary to a trans-annular patch. Pericardial VSD patch is intact (black arrows in **b**, **d**)

RV dilatation and dysfunction. PR has a tendency to increase with age [21]. Pulmonary valve replacement (PVR) has a proven effect on improving the functional status of RV and reducing the RV dimensions [22, 23]. CMR is the imaging modality of choice to assess RV function and volumes [24] (Fig. 14.8). Phase-contrast imaging allows accurate assessment of velocity, direction, and volume of flow that helps in quantifying PR [25]. Pulmonary arterial assessment is also important to ensure no residual or recurrent stenosis is present. As mentioned previously, the timing of PVR is debatable with two different schools of thought. One such recommendation by Geva et al. [21] suggests the following parameters for PVR.

Moderate or severe PR (PR fraction ≥25%) with asymptomatic patient, two or more of the following criteria:

- RVEDVi (indexed RV end diastolic volume) > 150 mL/m^2
- RVESVi (indexed RV end systolic volume) >80 mL/m^2
- LV ejection fraction (LVEF) < 55%; RVEF <47%
- Large RVOT aneurysm
- QRS duration on ECG > 140 ms
- Sustained tachyarrhythmia related to right heart volume load

For symptomatic patients, only one quantitative criterion in addition to PR.

Other complications that one may encounter post ICR include:

Tricuspid Regurgitation (TR) The prevalence of moderate to severe TR is approximately 10% [26]. TR is usually functional as a result of progressive RV dilatation and subsequent annular dilatation of the tricuspid valve. The quantification of the TR can be made by phase-contrast studies alone or in combination of RV volumetric data and pulmonary Q flows. Quantification of TR and its role in RV hemodynamics in postoperative cases of TOF lacks validity due to a lack of robust data [26].

Pulmonary Infundibular Aneurysm RVOT aneurysms are most often related to the integrity of the transannular patch. Both true and pseudoaneurysms can be seen. The primary contributing factors are elevated RV pressure from RVOT obstruction, faulty suture technique, trauma, infection, extensive infundibular muscle resection, and ischemic insult [27]. The size of RVOT is best assessed with CT and MRI. True aneurysm is an indication for late interventions, whereas false aneurysm is usually an emergency due to chances of rupture.

Residual Stenosis of the Pulmonary Arteries or Infundibulum After TOF repair, RVOT obstruction/pulmonary artery stenosis can be encountered. Stenosis may be present from the RVOT level to distal pulmonary level and can aggravate the RV dysfunction in the presence of PR [28]. CMR phase contrast studies can detect peak velocity and estimate gradient across the stenotic area. Assessment of the individual branch pulmonary arteries can also be made with the phase contrast studies and provide differential perfusion of the lungs.

Conduit Calcifications and Stenosis Different types of conduits are available for repair of TOF; these include homografts, stented xenografts, and stentless xenografts. Usually, there are no immediate postoperative complications, but delayed postoperative obstruction invariably develops due to patient prosthesis mismatch, conduit kinking, distal anastomotic stenosis, extensive intimal proliferation, and calcification or extrinsic sternal compression. The conduit may also be complicated by graft endocarditis and thrombus formation. MDCT or CMR can easily detect the cause, level, and degree of conduit stenosis. CMR has the added advantage of assessing RV function and PR, which can further deteriorate in the presence of conduit obstruction [29].

Residual VSD Residual VSD, although rare is one of the complications following ICR. Immediate surgical intervention is needed in hemodynamically significant VSD and close follow-up is required in others to detect any evidence of an increase in size and shunt. Although TTE is sufficient in detecting most VSD, they can also be identified with CMR and the shunt be quantified. High-velocity shunting through a small VSD manifests as a local loss of signal intensity or a signal void on SSFP images [26].

Aortic Root Dilatation and Aortic Regurgitation Progressive aortic root dilatation along with aortic regurgitation can be seen. It predisposes to dissection and rupture and may require aortic valve and/or aortic root surgery. This is more often described in adults than in the pediatric population. It is secondary to chronic volume overload of the ascending aorta [29]. Progressive dilatation of the aortic root of more than 5.5 cm is an indication for aortic root surgery. Thus, meticulous follow-up of the aortic root after TOF repair is recommended [29].

Left Ventricular Dysfunction CMR can accurately detect LV dysfunction, even in the presence of RV volume overload where echocardiographic assessment can be suboptimal. LV dysfunction is a rare complication but recently, it is described as a strongest predictor of poor clinical status. Proposed mechanisms include akinesia resulting from the VSD patch, septal fibrosis, chronic volume loading from early palliative shunt creation, abnormal septal motion, and myocardial injury at the time of repair [26].

Specific Learning Points

- The four components of TOF are RVOT obstruction, VSD, aorta-overriding VSD with RV hypertrophy.
- TTE is the mainstay in diagnostic imaging of patients with TOF with reducing use of catheter angiography.
- Preoperative assessment of pulmonary arterial confluence, their size, and areas of stenosis is essential and indices such as McGoon's/Nakata are important in every case of TOF.
- All sources of pulmonary arterial flow need to be mapped in every case of TOF.
- Any major coronary artery crossing anterior to RVOT will alter surgical procedure.
- CMR is preferred imaging modality post ICR to assess RV volumes, function, and pulmonary regurgitation.
- MDCT is useful in planning for RVOT and/or PDA stenting as part of a staged repair of patients with TOF.

14.8 Conclusion

TOF is the most common cyanotic CHD and can have varied presentations and associations. TTE remains the mainstay of imaging patients with known or suspected TOF. MDCT and CMR provide vital information, often not available on TTE, and have an important role in imaging both pre- and postoperative patients with TOF. Combinations of different imaging modalities have to be employed to ensure optimal assessment of all patients with TOF. In our practice, MDCT is used in almost every patient prior to surgery to ensure optimal assessment of all cardiac and extracardiac structures. CMR has also become a standard test in regular follow-up patients in the postoperative period.

References

1. Becker AE, Connor M, Anderson RH. Tetralogy of Fallot: a morphometric and geometric study. Am J Cardiol. 1975;35(3):402–12. https://doi.org/10.1016/0002-9149(75)90034-x.
2. Bailliard F, Anderson RH. Tetralogy of Fallot. Orphanet J Rare Dis. 2009;4:2. https://doi.org/10.1186/1750-1172-4-2.
3. Van Praagh R, Van Praagh S. The anatomy of common aorticopulmonary trunk (truncus arteriosus communis) and its embryologic implications. A study of 57 necropsy cases. Am J Cardiol. 1965;16(3):406–25. https://doi.org/10.1016/0002-9149(65)90732-0.
4. Van Praagh R. The first Stella van Praagh memorial lecture: the history and anatomy of tetralogy of Fallot. Semin Thorac Cardiovasc Surg Pediatr Card Surg Annu. 2009;2009:19–38. https://doi.org/10.1053/j.pcsu.2009.01.004.
5. Jonas RA. Early primary repair of tetralogy of Fallot. Semin Thorac Cardiovasc Surg Pediatr Card Surg Annu. 2009;2009:39–47. https://doi.org/10.1053/j.pcsu.2009.01.021.
6. Gartner RD, Sutton NJ, Weinstein S, et al. MRI and computed tomography of cardiac and pulmonary complications of tetralogy of Fallot in adults. J Thorac Imaging. 2010;25(2):183–90. https://doi.org/10.1097/RTI.0b013e31819d14fe.
7. Castaneda AR, Freed MD, Williams RG, et al. Repair of tetralogy of Fallot in infancy. Early and late results. J Thorac Cardiovasc Surg. 1977;74(3):372–81.
8. Patel DL, Rana YR, Sheth MM, et al. MSCT imaging of various shunts and grafts in post operative cases of congenital heart diseases. Int J Res Med Sci. 2019;7(3):860. https://doi.org/10.18203/2320-6012.ijrms20190937.
9. Huehnergarth KV, Gurvitz M, Stout KK, et al. Repaired tetralogy of Fallot in the adult: monitoring and management. Heart. 2008;94(12):1663–9. https://doi.org/10.1136/hrt.2008.147249.
10. Burchill LJ, Wald RM, Harris L, et al. Pulmonary valve replacement in adults with repaired tetralogy of Fallot. Semin Thorac Cardiovasc Surg Pediatr Card Surg Annu. 2011;14(1):92–7. https://doi.org/10.1053/j.pcsu.2011.01.016.
11. Vliegen HW, van Straten A, de Roos A, et al. Magnetic resonance imaging to assess the hemodynamic effects of pulmonary valve replacement in adults late after repair of tetralogy of Fallot. Circulation. 2002;106(13):1703–7. https://doi.org/10.1161/01.cir.0000030995.59403.f8.
12. Lim C, Lee JY, Kim WH, et al. Early replacement of pulmonary valve after repair of tetralogy: is it really beneficial? Eur J Cardio Thorac Surg. 2004;25(5):728–34. https://doi.org/10.1016/j.ejcts.2004.01.036.
13. Therrien J, Siu SC, McLaughlin PR, et al. Pulmonary valve replacement in adults late after repair of tetralogy of Fallot: are we operating too late? J Am Coll Cardiol. 2000;36(5):1670–5. https://doi.org/10.1016/s0735-1097(00)00930-x.
14. Han BK, Lesser AM, Vezmar M, et al. Cardiovascular imaging trends in congenital heart disease: a single center experience. J Cardiovasc Comput Tomogr. 2013;7(6):361–6. https://doi.org/10.1016/j.jcct.2013.11.002.
15. Stinn B, Stolzmann P, Fornaro J, et al. Technical principles of computed tomography in patients with congenital heart disease. Insights Imaging. 2011;2(3):349–56. https://doi.org/10.1007/s13244-011-0088-1.

16. Fratz S, Chung T, Greil GF, et al. Guidelines and protocols for cardiovascular magnetic resonance in children and adults with congenital heart disease: SCMR expert consensus group on congenital heart disease. J Cardiovasc Magn Reson. 2013;15:51. https://doi.org/10.1186/1532-429X-15-51.
17. Piehler JM, Danielson GK, McGoon DC, et al. Management of pulmonary atresia with ventricular septal defect and hypoplastic pulmonary arteries by right ventricular outflow construction. J Thorac Cardiovasc Surg. 1980;80(4):552–67.
18. Nakata S, Imai Y, Takanashi Y, et al. A new method for the quantitative standardization of cross-sectional areas of the pulmonary arteries in congenital heart diseases with decreased pulmonary blood flow. J Thorac Cardiovasc Surg. 1984;88(4):610–9.
19. Glatz AC, Petit CJ, Goldstein BH, et al. Comparison between patent Ductus Arteriosus stent and modified Blalock-Taussig shunt as palliation for infants with ductal-dependent pulmonary blood flow: insights from the congenital catheterization research collaborative. Circulation. 2018;137(6):589–601. https://doi.org/10.1161/CIRCULATIONAHA.117.029987.
20. Dabizzi RP, Teodori G, Barletta GA, et al. Associated coronary and cardiac anomalies in the tetralogy of Fallot. An angiographic study. Eur Heart J. 1990;11(8):692–704. https://doi.org/10.1093/oxfordjournals.eurheartj.a059784.
21. Geva T. Repaired tetralogy of Fallot: the roles of cardiovascular magnetic resonance in evaluating pathophysiology and for pulmonary valve replacement decision support. J Cardiovasc Magn Reson. 2011;13:9. https://doi.org/10.1186/1532-429X-13-9.
22. Nollert G, Fischlein T, Bouterwek S, et al. Long-term survival in patients with repair of tetralogy of Fallot: 36-year follow-up of 490 survivors of the first year after surgical repair. J Am Coll Cardiol. 1997;30(5):1374–83. https://doi.org/10.1016/s0735-1097(97)00318-5.
23. Eyskens B, Reybrouck T, Bogaert J, et al. Homograft insertion for pulmonary regurgitation after repair of tetralogy of Fallot improves cardiorespiratory exercise performance. Am J Cardiol. 2000;85(2):221–5. https://doi.org/10.1016/s0002-9149(99)00640-2.
24. Geva T, Sandweiss BM, Gauvreau K, et al. Factors associated with impaired clinical status in long-term survivors of tetralogy of Fallot repair evaluated by magnetic resonance imaging. J Am Coll Cardiol. 2004;43(6):1068–74. https://doi.org/10.1016/j.jacc.2003.10.045.
25. Helbing WA, Niezen RA, Le Cessie S, et al. Right ventricular diastolic function in children with pulmonary regurgitation after repair of tetralogy of Fallot: volumetric evaluation by magnetic resonance velocity mapping. J Am Coll Cardiol. 1996;28(7):1827–35. https://doi.org/10.1016/S0735-1097(96)00387-7.
26. Norton KI, Tong C, Glass RB, et al. Cardiac MR imaging assessment following tetralogy of Fallot repair. Radiographics. 2006;26(1):197–211. https://doi.org/10.1148/rg.261055064.
27. Davlouros PA, Kilner PJ, Hornung TS, et al. Right ventricular function in adults with repaired tetralogy of Fallot assessed with cardiovascular magnetic resonance imaging: detrimental role of right ventricular outflow aneurysms or akinesia and adverse right-to-left ventricular interaction. J Am Coll Cardiol. 2002;40(11):2044–52. https://doi.org/10.1016/s0735-1097(02)02566-4.
28. Tulevski II, Hirsch A, Dodge-Khatami A, et al. Effect of pulmonary valve regurgitation on right ventricular function in patients with chronic right ventricular pressure overload. Am J Cardiol. 2003;92(1):113–6. https://doi.org/10.1016/s0002-9149(03)00484-3.
29. Vaujois L, Gorincour G, Alison M, et al. Imaging of postoperative tetralogy of Fallot repair. Diagn Interv Imaging. 2016;97(5):549–60. https://doi.org/10.1016/j.diii.2016.02.007.

Double Outlet Right Ventricle: Morphology and Function

15

Megha M. Sheth, Yashpal Rana, and Ramiah Rajeshkannan

15.1 Introduction

Conotruncal anomalies represent congenital heart defects resulting from abnormality of formation and/or separation of the outflow tracts of the heart and great vessels. Double outlet right ventricle (DORV) is a type of conotruncal anomaly and includes a wide spectrum of anatomic malformations characterized by the origin of both the aorta and pulmonary arterial trunks entirely or predominately from the morphological right ventricle (RV) [1, 2]. DORV accounts for approximately 1% of all congenital heart disease (CHD).

When an arterial valve or valves override(s) the ventricular septum through a VSD, a "50% rule" is applied [3]. *According to this rule, an overriding arterial trunk is considered as arising from the RV when more than half of the circumference of its valve belongs to the RV.*

As we know that there are three major anatomical segments of heart—i.e., visceroatrial situs, atrioventricular connection, and ventriculo-arterial connections. As the term "DORV" describes a form of ventriculoarterial connection, it can occur with any combination of visceroatrial situs and atrioventricular connection, making it an extremely heterogeneous group.

This results in different clinical manifestations and requires a comprehensive diagnostic approach and different surgical management options.

Although echocardiography is considered as an initial imaging modality of choice, it is limited in the reliable assessment because of operator dependency, a small field of view and acoustic window, poor assessment of extracardiac complex vascular anatomy. Catheter angiography is an invasive technique that has several disadvantages including the overlap of adjacent cardiovascular structures and relatively poor depiction of complex intracardiac anatomy. Cross-sectional imaging with Multislice CT (MSCT) or Magnetic Resonance Imaging (MRI) help overcome the limitations of echocardiography and conventional angiography with the ability of simultaneously depicting the systemic and the pulmonary vascular systems. Imaging specialists should be well versed with the complex morphology and physiology of DORV, as well as with various palliative and corrective surgical procedures performed in these patients.

Electronic Supplementary Material The online version of this chapter (https://doi.org/10.1007/978-981-15-6755-1_15) contains supplementary material, which is available to authorized users.

M. M. Sheth (✉) · Y. Rana
U.N. Mehta Institute of Cardiology and Research Centre, Ahmedabad, Gujarat, India

R. Rajeshkannan
Department of Radiology, Amrita School of Medicine, Amrita Institute of Medical Sciences and Research Centre, Amrita Vishwa Vidyapeetham, Kochi, Kerala, India

R. Rajeshkannan et al. (eds.), *CT and MRI in Congenital Heart Diseases*,
https://doi.org/10.1007/978-981-15-6755-1_15

15.2 History

The earliest description of this condition was done in 1793 by Mr. John Abernethy (1764–1831) of London [4]. In 1949, Taussig and Bing reported a case with the aorta arising entirely from the right ventricle and the pulmonary orifice overlaying the ventricular septum through a VSD [5]. Calhoun Witham introduced the specific term "double outlet right ventricle" in 1957 [6].

15.3 Embryology

DORV results from an aberration in the formation of the primary outlet of the heart, i.e., conotruncus, during embryonic development. Chromosomal anomalies such as 22q11.2 deletion syndrome, trisomy 13, trisomy 18, and CHARGE syndrome have been found to be associated with DORV.

15.4 Pathophysiology

The hemodynamic physiology of DORV is extremely complex, VSD being the only source of egress from the left ventricle. The complexity and clinical manifestations revolve around factors like the relationship of the VSD to the arterial valves, size of the VSD, presence or absence of outflow tracts—aortic or pulmonary obstruction and associated anomalies. In the presence of a subaortic VSD, saturated LV blood tends to be directed predominantly to the aorta without significant mixing of RV unsaturated blood. Severe pulmonary stenosis can lead to right to left shunt.

When the VSD is subpulmonary, the aorta is perfused preferentially with deoxygenated systemic venous blood with physiology similar to transposition. The degree of systemic hypoxia is dependent on the adequacy of mixing between blood in the systemic and pulmonary circuits.

The most common mode of presentation is cyanosis usually due to pulmonary outflow obstruction. Tachypnea or difficulty in breathing, poor feeding, slow weight gain, recurrent respiratory tract infections, and failure to thrive are also common. Children without pulmonary obstruction are prone to develop pulmonary arterial hypertension (PAH).

15.5 CT and MR Imaging Techniques

15.5.1 MSCT

Scan Technique Few specific modifications are required from a routine scan. Two runs are recommended to diagnose any abnormal venous drainage—though this depends upon the scanner and institution protocol. ECG-gated scan is preferable to demonstrate complex intracardiac anatomy. Saline chasing bolus to be avoided to get good opacification of the right side of the heart.

All image data should be evaluated using various image reformatting techniques including curved multi-planar reconstruction (c-MPR), maximum intensity projection (MIP), and 3D volume-rendering technique (VRT) to get all the clinically relevant information.

Practical Tips It is important to examine source images as well apart from reconstructed images; as some information might be missed by interpreting only reconstructed images.

Preoperative MSCT with 3D Volume-Rendered (VR) imaging in DORV accurately depicts the following parameters [7]:

- Type of VSD and its relationship to the semilunar valves
- Size of the VSD in relation to the diameter of the pulmonary artery and aorta
- Distance between the VSD and aortic valve
- Distance between the VSD and pulmonary valve

All the above measurements are to be taken and reported, along with routability of the aorta, which is better assessed with MRI.

The morphologic structure and patency of the outflow tracts and presence and severity of subpulmonic obstruction can be well demonstrated on MSCT [8]. Any coexistent anomalies and the state of the extracardiac vascular anatomy can also be evaluated on MSCT. 3D printed heart models with contrast-enhanced CT/MRI in the recent era is revolutionizing surgical outcome [9].

MSCT has proved to be an invaluable diagnostic and decision-making tool as a complement to echocardiography and increasingly as a substitute for invasive angiography in the management of DORV.

15.5.2 MRI Techniques

Cardiac MRI is very useful in preoperative evaluation of complex DORV especially in older children with poor echo windows as well as in postoperative assessment. Recommended MRI protocol include the following sequences:

- Black blood sequences: Spin echo sequences in short-axis, four-chamber, and axial views for evaluation of gross cardiac and extracardiac anatomy, VSD, and pulmonary artery sizes, etc.
- Cine imaging stacks in the four-chamber view, short-axis view, vertical long-axis view, and both ventricular outflow tract view for evaluation of ventricular function, diagnosis of valvular regurgitation and to assess the dynamic relationship between VSD to aorta route. Selected angulated views to image the ventricular septum "en face" has also used.
- Contrast-enhanced Magnetic Resonance angiography (MRA) and respiratory triggered ECG-gated 3D SSFP sequence for evaluation of great vessels and intracardiac anatomy including coronary artery course. The 3D dataset can be used for creating 3D print models.
- Phase-contrast imaging of the main pulmonary artery and the aorta to quantify left-to-right shunts (Q_P:Q_S) and to assess the possible hemodynamic significance of stenosis.

While calculating ventricular volumes, it is important to note that intraventricular baffling or tunneling compromises the RV volume as a part of the RV is incorporated into the LV outflow tract. Therefore, the RV volume needs to be assessed after subtracting the estimated volume of LV to aorta pathway.

Despite the great capabilities of MR imaging for anatomic and functional assessment of the heart, it is time-consuming and may require a lengthy period of patient sedation; hence its use in seriously ill or uncooperative children is often limited. On the other hand, MSCT offers the advantages of short acquisition times and widespread availability.

15.6 Morphology of DORV

To understand the pathophysiology of DORV, it is important to know the morphology of the ventricular outflow tracts.

What is aorto-mitral fibrous continuity?

- The morphologic left ventricle shows fibrous continuity between the aortic and mitral valves. It is well seen on CT scan as a hypodense linear structure between aortic and mitral valves (Fig. 15.1).
- In the morphological right ventricle, there is a muscular structure (ventriculo-infundibular fold) between the pulmonary and tricuspid valves that manifests as discontinuity between the valves (Fig. 15.2).

So if aorto-mitral fibrous continuity is present, then aorta arises from left ventricle and loss of

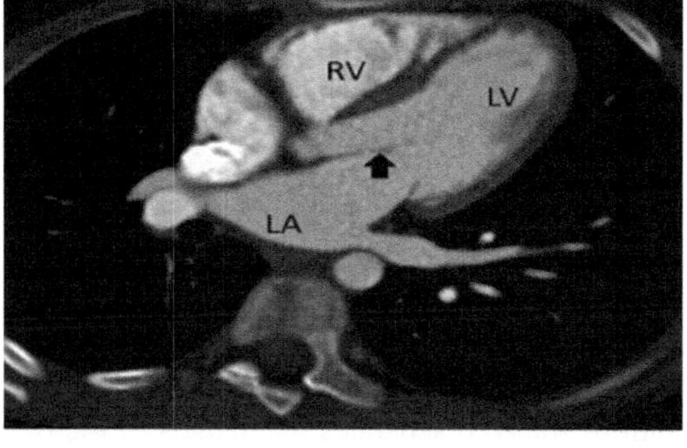

Fig. 15.1 Black arrow shows the aorto-mitral fibrous continuity between aortic and mitral valves

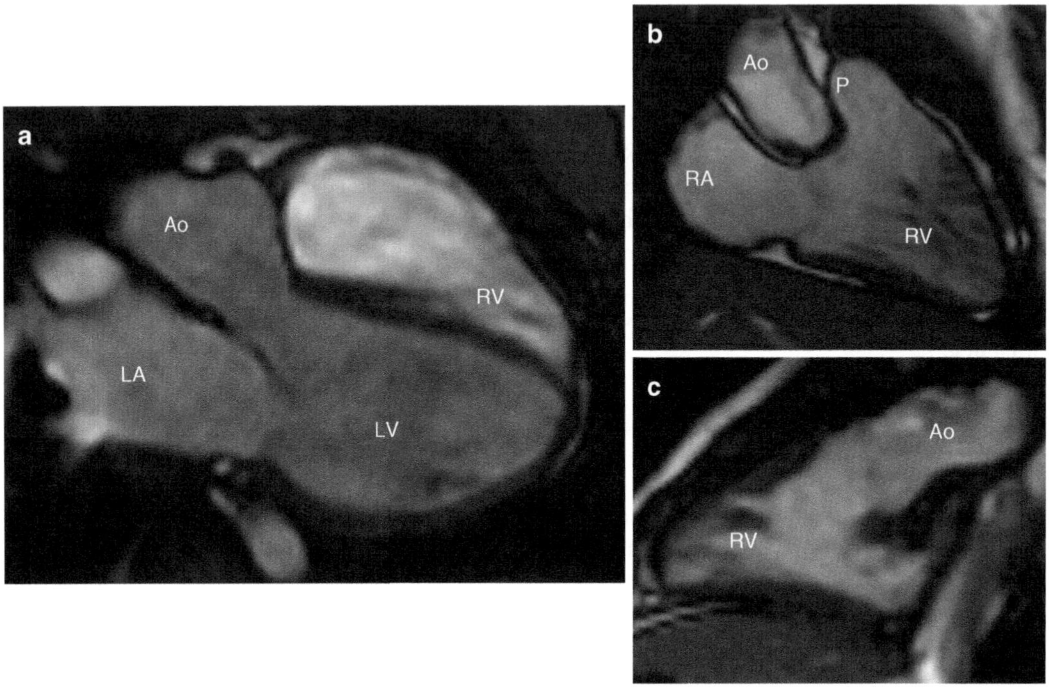

Fig. 15.2 SSFP MRI cine image of LVOT (**a**) shows the normal aorta-mitral fibrous continuity. RVOT view in a normal heart (**b**) and DORV case (**c**) show absent fibrous continuity between the right AV valve and semilunar valve. *Ao* aorta; *LA* left atrium; *LV* left ventricle; *P* pulmonary valve; *RA* right atrium; *RV* right ventricle

aorto-mitral fibrous continuity with subaortic conus is seen in DORV. The conal musculature is usually seen below both great arteries in DORV.

What Is Pulmonary Conus? The pulmonary conus (also known as infundibulum) is a conical muscular pouch formed from the upper and left angle of the right ventricle that supports the leaflets of arterial valve.

The ventriculo-infundibular fold is a muscular structure that is interposed between the leaflets of an atrioventricular and an arterial valve, thereby separates the inlet of the ventricle from its outlet. It is an important landmark for the surgeon as cutting through this muscular fold takes the surgeon outside the heart, and into the transverse pericardial sinus.

The outlet septum, or conal septum, is a muscle that is interposed between the two ventricular outflow tracts. It separates the leaflets of the two arterial valves.

When considering the intracardiac anatomy in DORV, the hearts having both great arteries arising from the right ventricle are not a single spectrum of pathology. More often, there are two infundibular tracts giving rise to both great vessels.

The great arteries can have normal spiraling relationship (subaortic VSD) or be parallel to each other. In most DORV with subpulmonic VSD, the aorta and pulmonary artery are side by side, with D-malposed aorta (aorta on right side). Other less common great arterial relationship includes right and anterior aorta, aorta directly anterior to the pulmonary artery and rarely left and anterior aorta (L malposition) [10].

Almost three-fourths of patients with DORV have some degree of pulmonary stenosis due to narrowing between the outlet septum and the free wall of its infundibulum. Subaortic outflow tract obstruction with or without obstructive lesions of the aortic arch is common in DORV with a subpulmonary VSD. There are multiple distinct groups of cases showing very different intracardiac anatomy.

Different types of VSD are encountered in DORV, based on the relationship of the VSD (subaortic, doubly committed, subpulmonary, or noncommitted) with the great arteries [11]. When the VSD is under the aorta, it is called as subaortic VSD. When the VSD is under the pulmonary artery, it is called as subpulmonic VSD [12]. When the VSD is under both of the great arteries, it is called doubly committed and when the VSD is not near the aorta or the pulmonary artery it is called noncommitted or remote VSD. Schematic diagrams depicting various types of VSD in DORV are shown in Fig. 15.3.

Subaortic VSD is the most common type, followed by subpulmonic VSD, noncommitted VSD, and doubly committed VSD [13–17].

Practical Tips To identify the type of VSD, align the plane along the septum and then view the VSD enface (Fig. 15.4). This is important as the surgeon usually approaches the VSD from the RV side.

15.7 Common Variants of DORV (Summarized in Table 15.1)

15.7.1 Tetralogy of Fallot (TOF)-Like Variant (Figs. 15.5, 15.6, and 15.7)

Tetralogy of Fallot is characterized by anterior, leftward, and superior displacement of the infundibular septum that causes a malaligned VSD, narrowing of the pulmonary outflow tract, overriding of the aortic valve and right ventricular

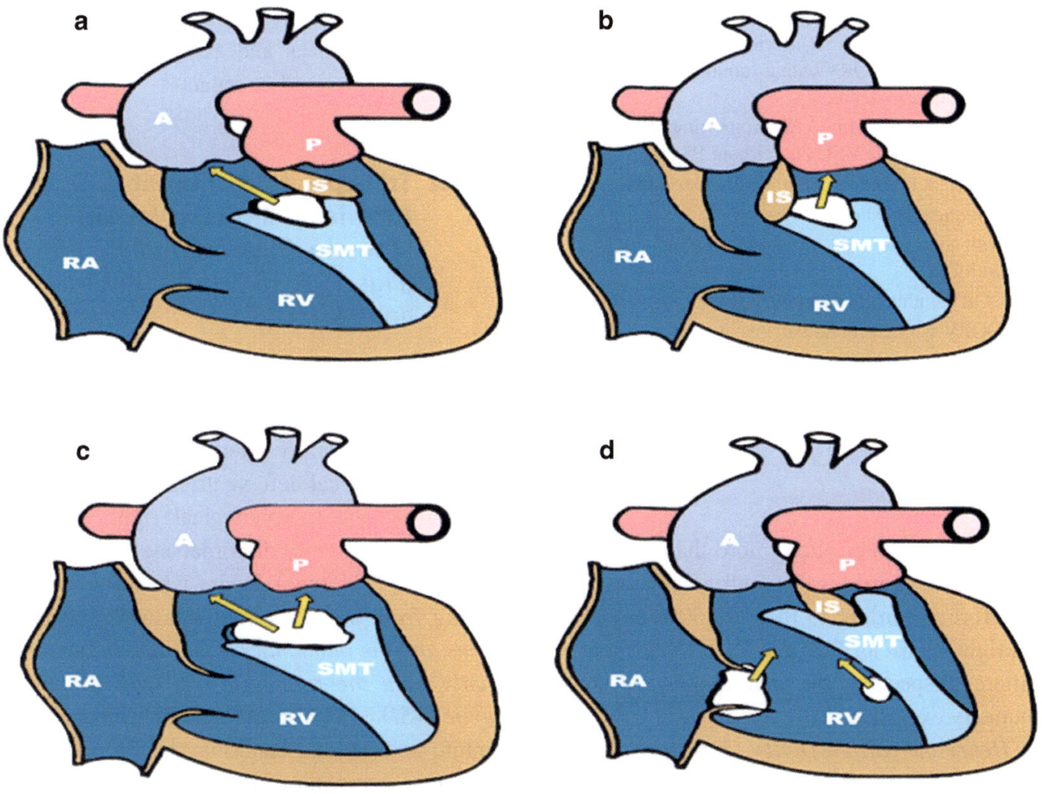

Fig. 15.3 Schematic diagrams depicting various types of VSD. (**a**) Subaortic VSD, (**b**) Subpulmonic VSD, (**c**) Doubly committed VSD, (**d**) Noncommitted VSD. *A* aorta; *P* pulmonary trunk; *RA* right atrium; *RV* right ventricle; *SMT* Septo-Marginal Trabeculae; *IS* infundibular septum

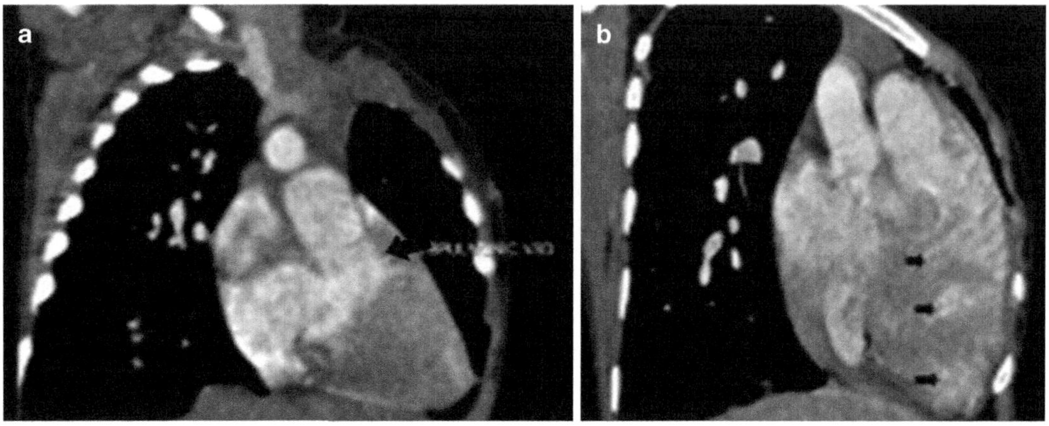

Fig. 15.4 Enface view of the interventricular septum (**a**) showing a subpulmonic VSD (Black arrow) and (**b**) showing multiple mid muscular VSDs (short black arrows)—"*Swiss cheese appearance*"

Table 15.1 Variants of DORV

Common variants
(a) Tetralogy of Fallot (TOF)-like variant consisting of DORV with a subaortic VSD and pulmonary stenosis (PS)
(b) Transposition of great arteries (TGA)-like variant consisting of DORV with a subpulmonic VSD (Taussig–Bing anomaly)
(c) A variant resembling VSD, consisting of DORV with a subaortic VSD but without PS
(d) A variant resembling a univentricular heart
Less frequent variants
(e) with subaortic VSD, aorta left to pulmonary trunk with PS
(f) DORV with noncommitted VSD
(g) DORV with discordant atrioventricular connection
(h) DORV with ambiguous atrioventricular connection
(i) DORV with mirror image atrial arrangement with any of the above combination
(j) DORV without VSD

hypertrophy. Quiet often, more than 50% of the aortic valve overrides the ventricular septum and therefore according to the rule 50% belongs to the right ventricle. TOF and DORV represent two different aspects of the abnormality and are not mutually exclusive.

Hence the variant DORV (TOF type) wherein apart from all the features of TOF, aortic overriding is more than 50% into the right ventricle.

In these subtypes, the VSD is subaortic or doubly committed, with the aorta spiraling from right to left relative to the pulmonary trunk. These children present with clinical features similar to TOF and have progressively worsening cyanosis. Surgical treatment involves the placement of an intraventricular patch to direct left ventricular blood to the aorta and relief of pulmonary obstruction (intracardiac repair).

15.7.2 Transposition of Great Arteries (TGA)-Like Variant (Taussig–Bing Anomaly) (Figs. 15.8, 15.9, 15.10, 15.11, and 15.12)

Transposition of the great arteries (TGA) is another form of ventriculoarterial connection in which the pulmonary arterial trunk arises from the morphological left ventricle and the aorta arises from the morphological right ventricle, i.e., ventriculoarterial discordance.

DORV (TGA type) occurs when the aorta is arising from the right ventricle with subaortic conus and the pulmonary artery arises predominantly from the right ventricle with a subpulmonic VSD. Hypertrophy of the infundibular septum and parietal band may lead to subaortic obstruction and may also be associated with coarctation of the aorta.

The children are cyanosed in the newborn period and are prone to develop early pulmo-

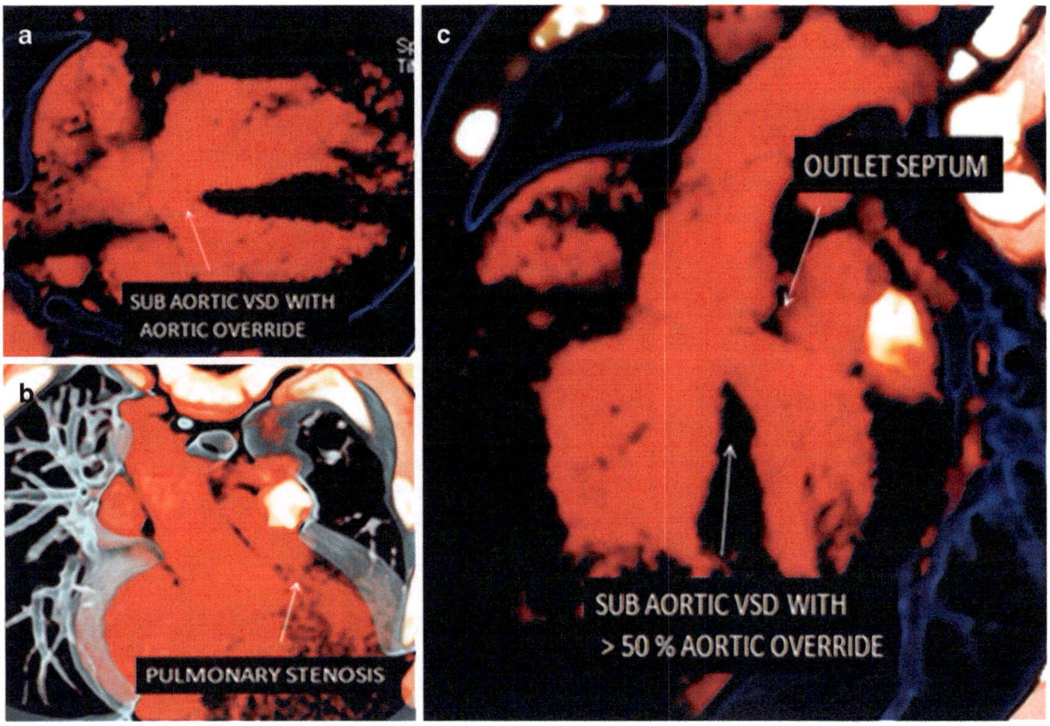

Fig. 15.5 TOF-like variant—DORV with subaortic VSD and PS. VRT thin images showing (**a**) subaortic VSD, (**b**) pulmonary stenosis, (**c**) >50% aortic override

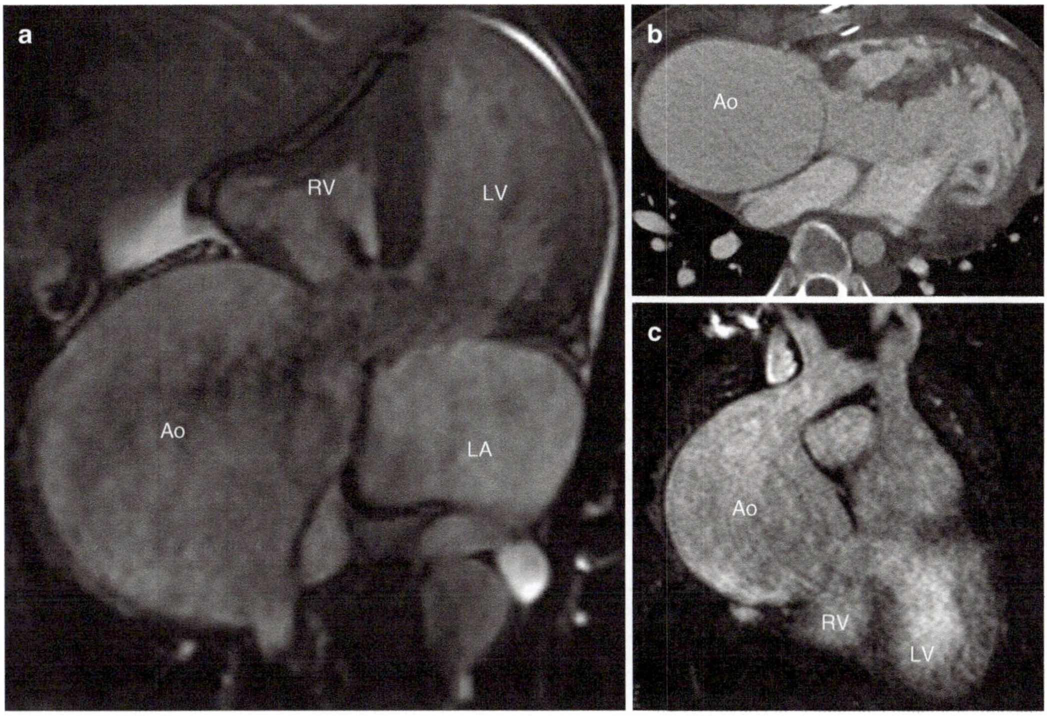

Fig. 15.6 A 28-year-old male with DORV. Oblique axial SSFP (**a**), oblique axial CT (**b**) and coronal MRA (**c**) show DORV, subaortic VSD, aneurysmally dilated ascending aorta, aortic stenosis, and severe aortic regurgitation. *Ao* aorta; *LA* left atrium; *LV* left ventricle; *RV* right ventricle (Ref to Videos 15.1, 15.2, 15.3, 15.4, and 15.5)

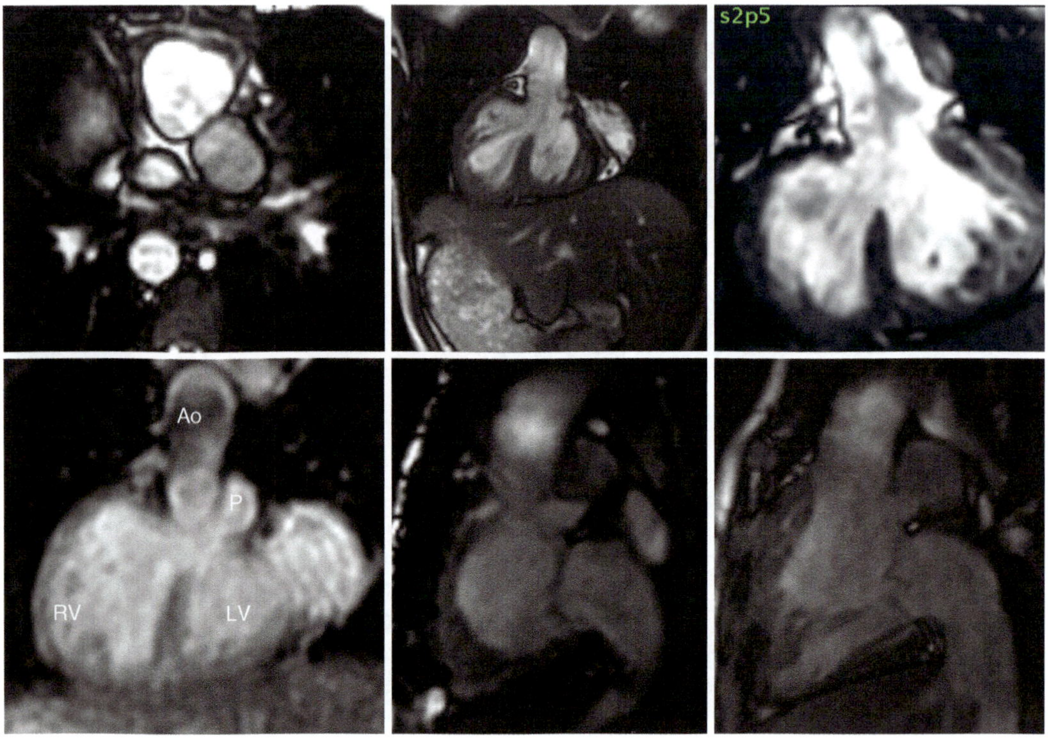

Fig. 15.7 A 17-year-old girl with DORV, situs inversus, dextrocardia, and d-malposed great arteries. VSD is doubly committed, but predominantly committed to the aorta with pulmonary stenosis (Ref to Videos 15.6, 15.7, 15.8, 15.9, 15.10, 15.11, and 15.12)

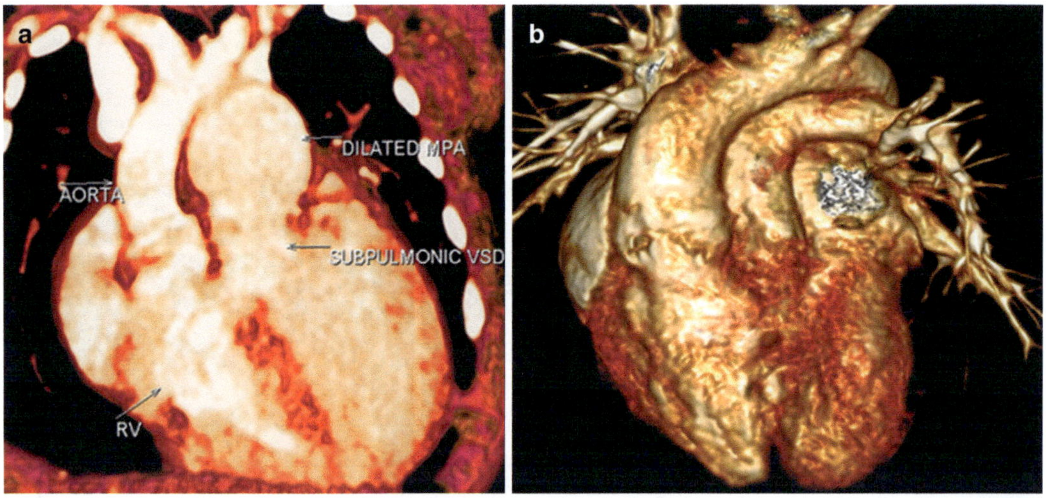

Fig. 15.8 TGA-like variant—DORV with a subpulmonic VSD (Taussig–Bing anomaly). (**a**) VRT thin image, (**b**) 3D VRT image showing DORV with a subpulmonic VSD

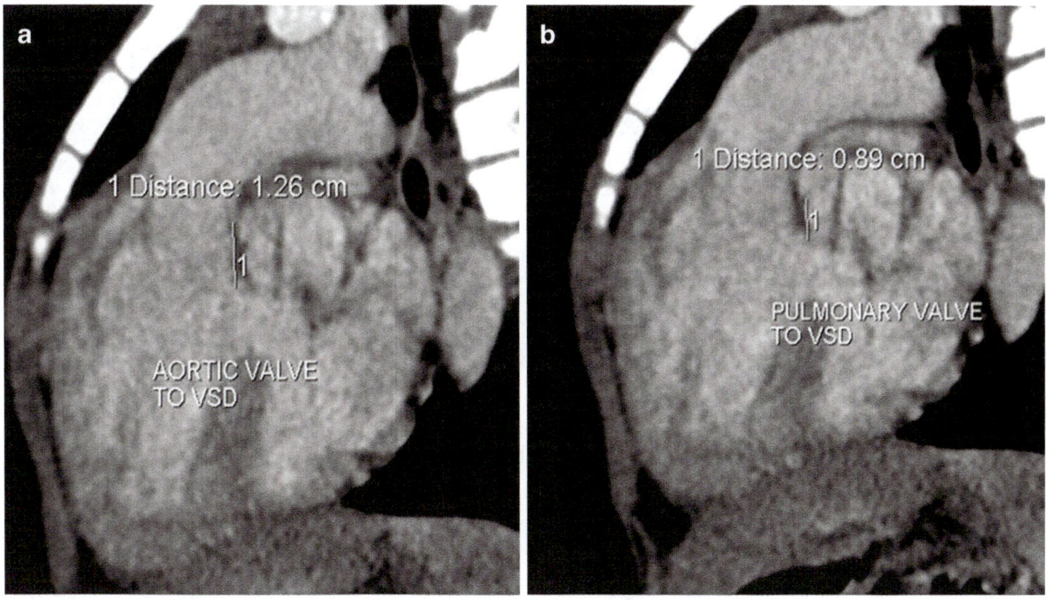

Fig. 15.9 DORV with subpulmonic VSD and PS. Coronal oblique images showing (**a**) aortic annulus to the upper border of VSD distance, (**b**) pulmonary annulus to upper border of VSD distance

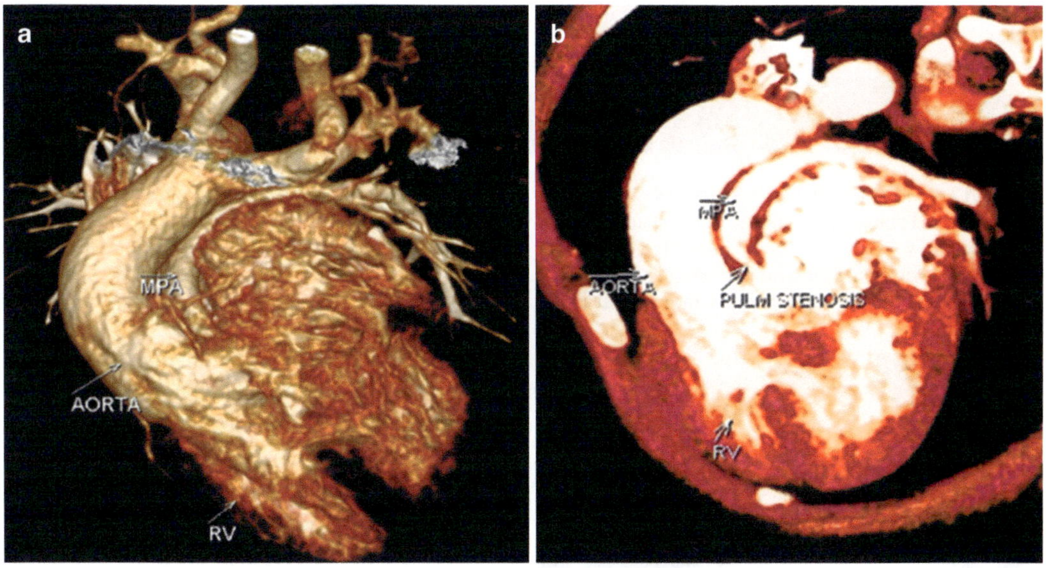

Fig. 15.10 DORV with subpulmonic and noncommitted mid-muscular VSDs. (**a**) 3D VRT, (**b**) VRT thin image

nary hypertension. It is treated by placing a patch to connect the LV to the pulmonary artery and an "Arterial Switch" operation (as for TGA) may be done so that the left ventricle is connected to the aorta and the RV to the pulmonary circulation.

15.7.3 Variant Resembling VSD (Fig. 15.13)

In this variant of DORV, the VSD is usually subaortic or doubly committed and no pulmonary stenosis. These children may not have cya-

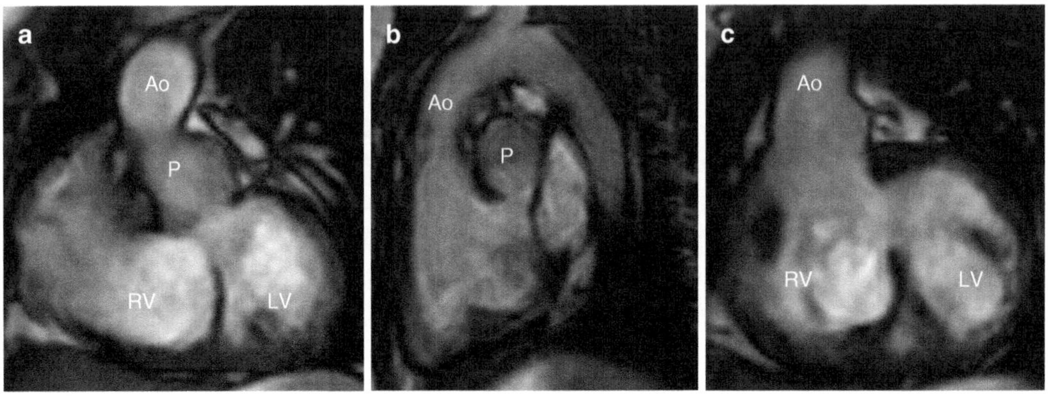

Fig. 15.11 A 11-year-old girl with TGA type of DORV. Pulmonary trunk (P) overriding the large conoventricular VSD (**a**), aorta (Ao) is directly anterior to the pulmonary artery (**b**). LV to aorta appears routable through the VSD (**c**)

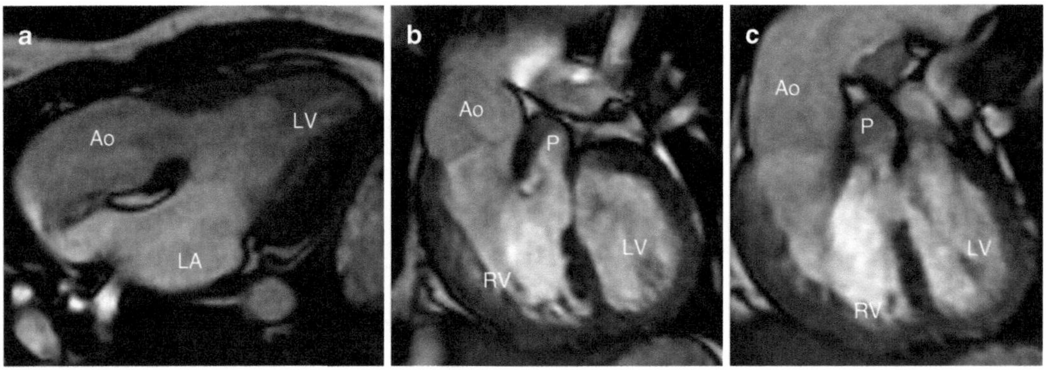

Fig. 15.12 A 17-year-old female with DORV, subpulmonary VSD, and pulmonary stenosis. Three chamber SSFP (**a**) and outflow SSFP MRI (**b**, **c**) show a large conoventricular VSD with some superior inlet extension. Long LV to aorta route with tricuspid and subaortic conal tissue along the pathway. Tricuspid valve also attached to subaortic conal septum. *Ao* aorta; *LA* left atrium; *LV* left ventricle; *P* pulmonary artery; *RV* right ventricle (Ref to Videos 15.13, 15.14, 15.15, 15.16, 15.17, 15.18, and 15.19)

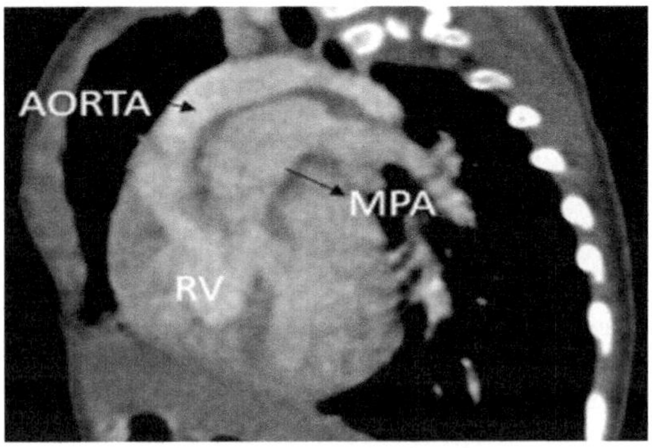

Fig. 15.13 Variant resembling VSD-DORV with subpulmonic VSD but without pulmonary stenosis

nosis, but develop early pulmonary arterial hypertension as there is increased flow to the pulmonary circulation. Repair involves the placement of an intraventricular patch to direct left ventricular blood to the aorta.

15.7.4 Variant Resembling a Univentricular Heart (Figs. 15.14, 15.15, and 15.16)

In this variant of DORV, there is a single dominant ventricle of RV morphology with aplastic/hypoplastic LV and both great vessels arising from the dominant ventricle of RV morphology.

This is also found to be associated with AV cushion defects and double inlet of dominant RV.

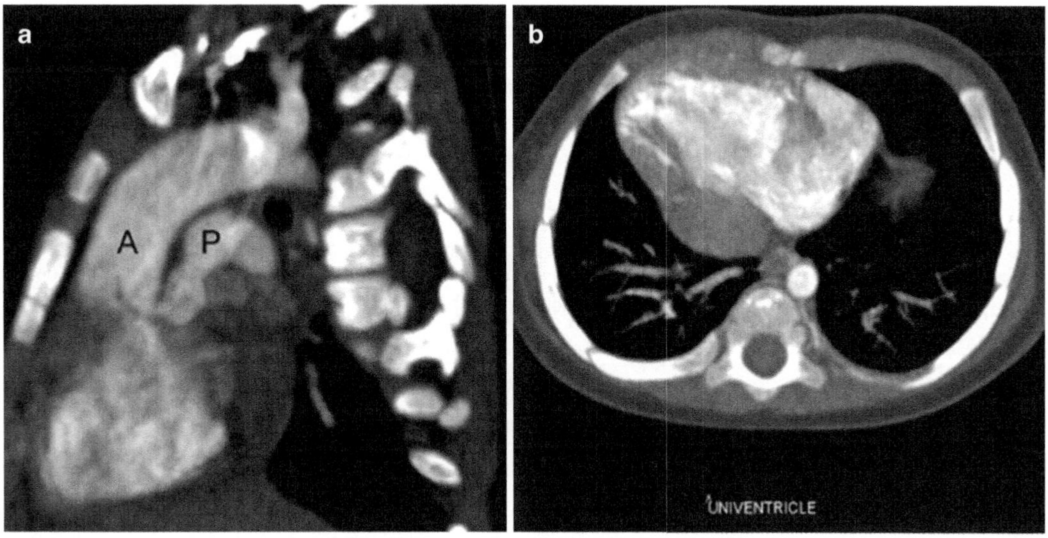

Fig. 15.14 DORV variant with univentricular morphology. (**a**) Sagittal oblique MIP image, (**b**) Axial oblique MPR image. *A* aorta; *P* pulmonary trunk

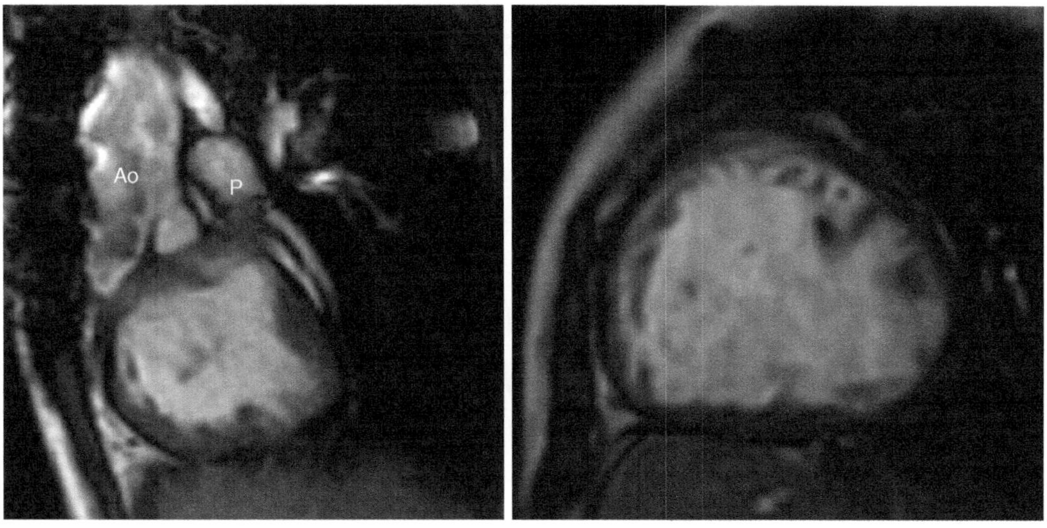

Fig. 15.15 A 10-year-old girl with single ventricle and DORV. *Ao* aorta; *P* pulmonary artery

15.8 Less Frequent Variants of DORV

15.8.1 DORV with Subaortic VSD, Aorta Left to Pulmonary Trunk with PS (Figs. 15.17 and 15.18)

The key point in diagnosing this variant is that, despite the aorta being left-sided, the heart exhibits usual atrial arrangement with concordant AV connections. So, this entity is an exception to loop rule. In these cases, VSD is usually subaortic, so it is considered amenable for corrective surgery. Great arteries are parallelly arranged [18].

15.8.2 DORV with Noncommitted VSD (Fig. 15.19)

When the distance between VSD and the two arterial valves was greater than the diameter of the aortic valve, it is termed a noncommitted VSD [19].

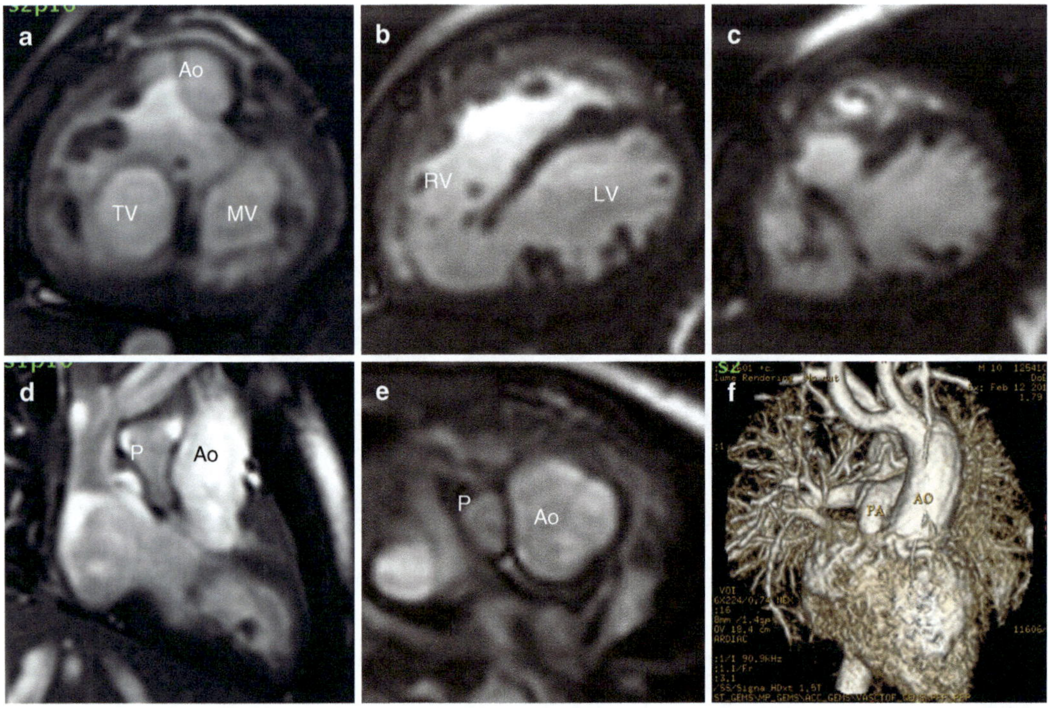

Fig. 15.16 A 10-year-old boy with DORV and multiple VSD at conoventricular (**a**), posterior (**b**), and apical muscular (**c**) regions. L-malposed aorta with severe pulmonary stenosis (**d–f**). The complex intracardiac anatomy with multiple large VSDs and severe pulmonary stenosis make him unsuitable for biventricular repair. So he was recommended to undergo single ventricle Fontan pathway of palliation. *Ao* aorta; *LV* left ventricle; *MV* mitral valve; *P* pulmonary artery; *RV* right ventricle; *TV* tricuspid valve

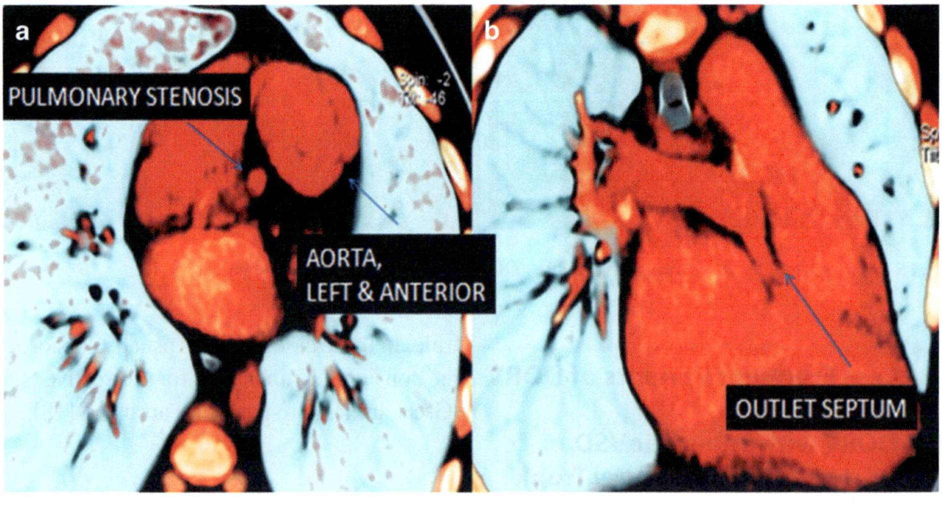

Fig. 15.17 DORV with subaortic VSD, aorta left to pulmonary trunk with PS. (**a**) VRT thin image showing aorta left to the pulmonary trunk, (**b**) VRT thin image showing PS and outlet septum

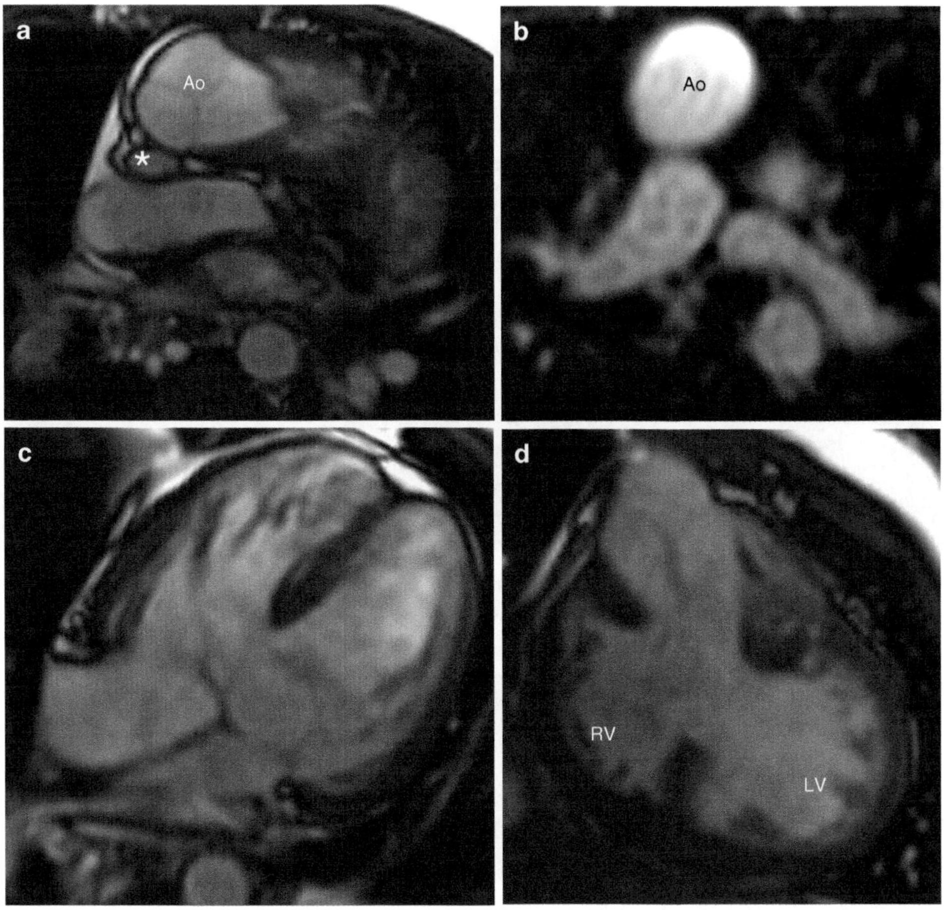

Fig. 15.18 A 12-year-old boy with DORV L-malposed aorta (Ao), severe pulmonary stenosis (*), nonconfluent pulmonary arteries (**b**), large inlet VSD (**c**) with conoventricular extension. LV appears routable to aorta across the VSD with a long patch (**d**)

The remoteness of the VSD from the arterial valves is determined by the location of the VSD within the septum and also by the extent of the muscular infundibulum.

As already explained earlier, the VSD is the only egress of the left ventricle in DORV. Hence, its small size implies left ventricular outflow tract obstruction [20, 21]. The VSD is considered restrictive when the diameter of the defect is smaller than the diameter of the aortic valve [22]. A restrictive VSD is seen in approximately 10% of DORV cases, most commonly occurring in the variety with a noncommitted VSD [23].

15.8.3 DORV with Discordant Atrioventricular Connection (Figs. 15.20 and 15.21)

This variant mimics congenitally corrected TGA (CCTGA) as the right atrium connects to the anatomic left ventricle, left atrium connects to the anatomic right ventricle, but both great arteries arise completely from the anatomic right ventricle [24]. These two entities were thought to differ only in the grade of overriding of the posterior pulmonary artery. There is a higher incidence of dextrocardia and L-malposed great arteries.

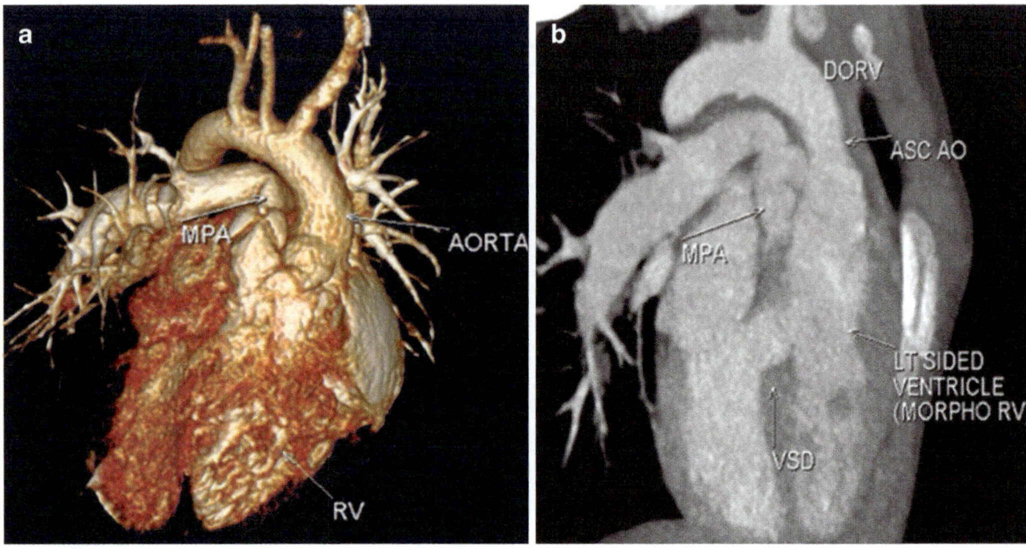

Fig. 15.19 DORV with discordant atrioventricular connection (Aorta left to the pulmonary trunk) and noncommitted VSD. (**a**) 3D VRT image, (**b**) coronal oblique MIP image

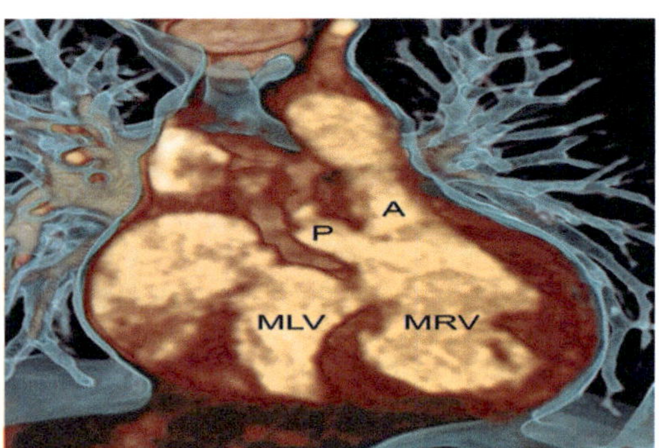

Fig. 15.20 Coronal oblique VRT thin image showing DORV with discordant atrioventricular connection (L-loop ventricle) and L-malposed aorta (aorta left to pulmonary trunk). *A* aorta; *P* pulmonary trunk; *MRV* morphological right ventricle; *MLV* morphological left ventricle

DORV with AV discordance is more prone to present with VSD and subvalvular pulmonary stenosis, while those with CCTGA have a greater likelihood of presenting with tricuspid regurgitation and atrioventricular block.

15.8.4 DORV with Mirror-Image Atrial Arrangement (Fig. 15.22)

In situs inversus, the internal organs including atria show mirror image arrangement. Along with mirror-imaged atrial arrangement, any of the previously mentioned DORV variations may occur.

15.8.5 DORV with Isomeric Atrial Appendages (Ambiguous AV Connection)

Double outlet right ventricle is frequent in the presence of isomeric atrial appendages, being particularly common in the overall group of patients having isomeric right appendages. When DORV occurs in the setting of heterotaxy, other associated abnormalities including pulmonary venous anomalies are to be assessed (Figs. 15.23 and 15.24).

15.8.6 DORV Without VSD

Very rarely DORV occurs with an intact ventricular septum [20]. This variety is usually associated with severe hypoplasia/atresia of the mitral valve and left ventricle. Most of the reported cases show findings suggesting spontaneous closure of the restrictive VSD postnatally or during fetal life [20].

Practical Tips Why is it important to differentiate all the subtypes of DORV?—Because each type of DORV is managed in different ways.

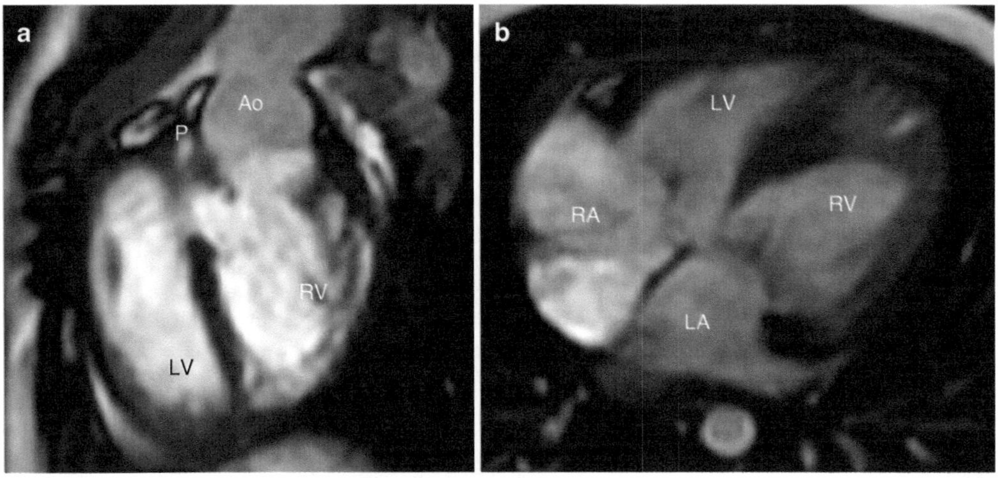

Fig. 15.21 An 8-year-old child with DORV and AV discordance (L loop ventricle). Outflow view (**a**) and four-chamber MRI (**b**) show both great arteries are arising from the left-sided morphological RV. *Ao* aorta; *LA* left atrium; *LV* left ventricle; *P* pulmonary artery; *RA* right atrium; *RV* right ventricle (Ref to Videos 15.20, 15.21, 15.22, 15.23, and 15.24)

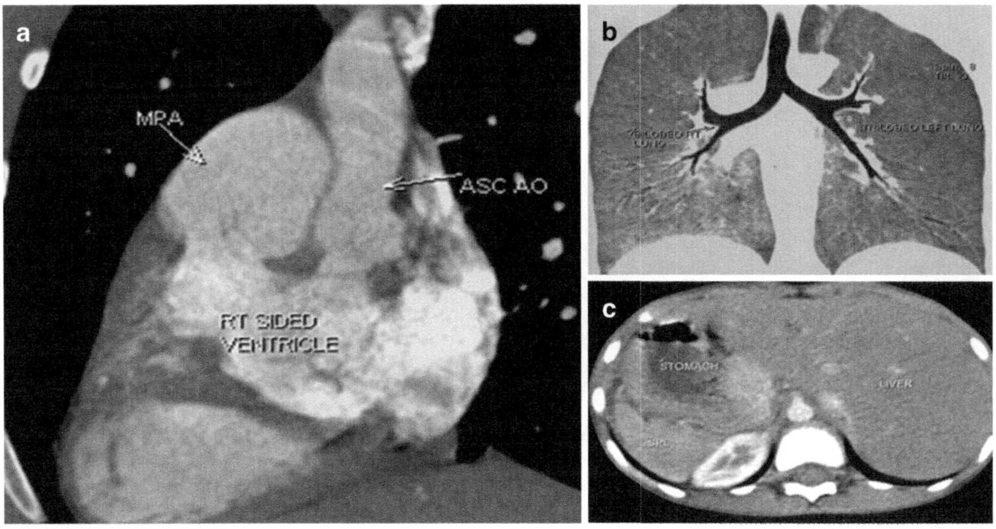

Fig. 15.22 DORV with situs inversus. (**a**) Coronal oblique MIP image showing DORV, (**b**) Coronal MinIP image showing inverted bronchial branching pattern, (**c**) axial MPR image showing spleen and stomach on the right side while liver on left side

15.9 Associated Other Cardiac Anomalies

Commonly observed associated cardiac anomalies are endocardial cushion defects or atrioventricular canal defects (AVCD) (Fig. 15.25), coarctation of the aorta (Fig. 15.26), transposition of great arteries, abnormal pulmonary venous drainage (Fig. 15.27), juxtaposition of atrial appendages (Fig. 15.28), aortopulmonary window (Fig. 15.29), coronary anomaly (Fig. 15.30), right side aortic arch, double aortic arch (Fig. 15.31), and mitral valve problems. Extracardiac anomalies, such as heterotaxy (polysplenia, asplenia, situs ambiguous) and intestinal malrotation, are frequent.

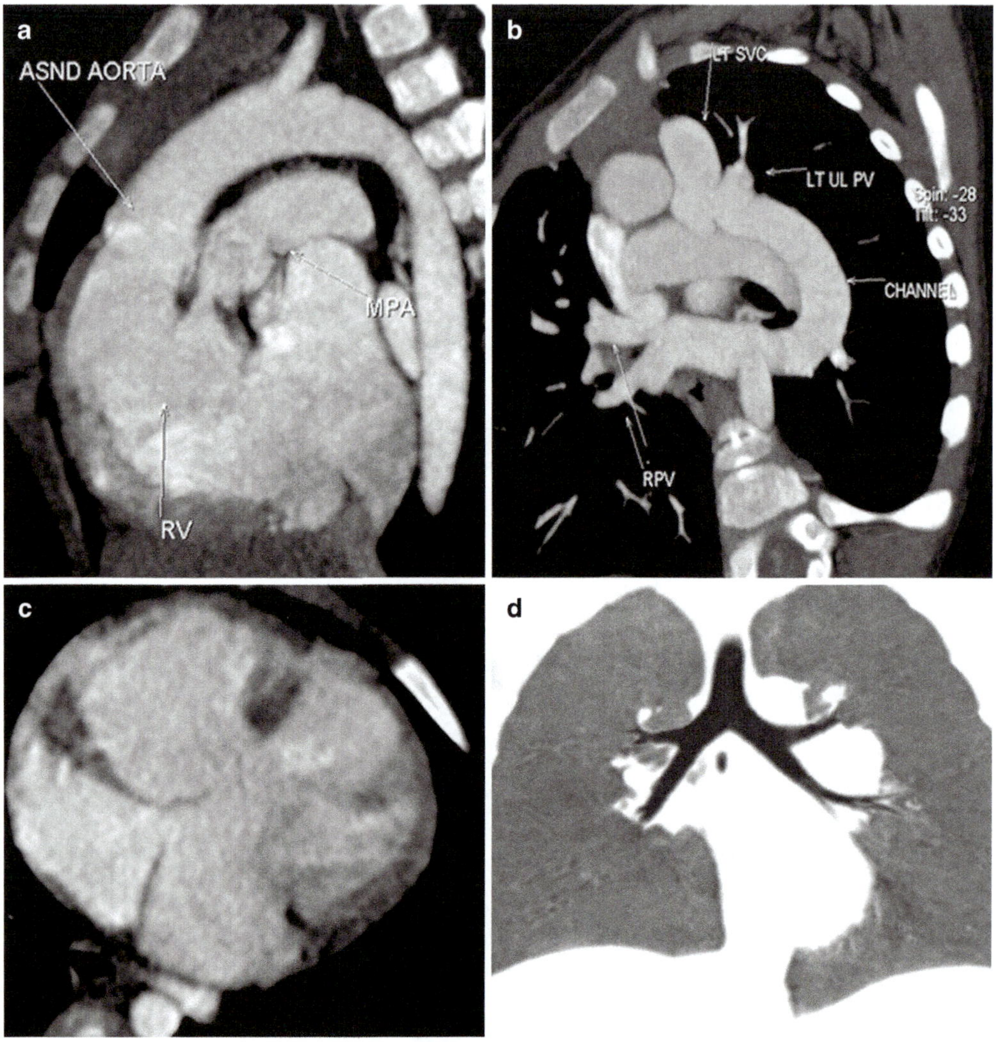

Fig. 15.23 DORV with complete AVCD, TAPVC, and right isomerism (**a**) Coronal oblique MIP image showing DORV, (**b**) coronal oblique MIP image showing supracardiac TAPVC, (**c**) axial MPR image showing complete AVCD—atrioventricular canal defect, (**d**) coronal MinIP image showing bilateral eparterial bronchi

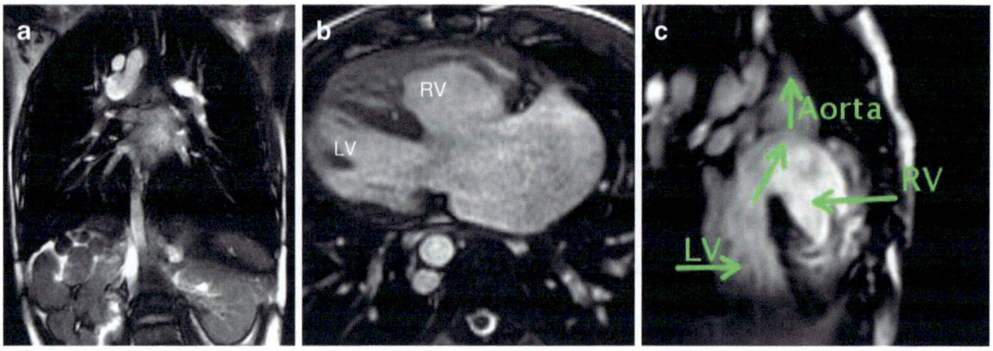

Fig. 15.24 A 12-year-old child with left isomerism (polysplenia, both side hyparterial bronchi) (**a**), dextrocardia, complete AV canal defect (**b**). Both great arteries are arising from the left-sided morphological RV with clear LV to aorta route (**c**) (Ref to Videos 15.25, 15.26, 15.27, 15.28, 15.29, 15.30, 15.31, and 15.32)

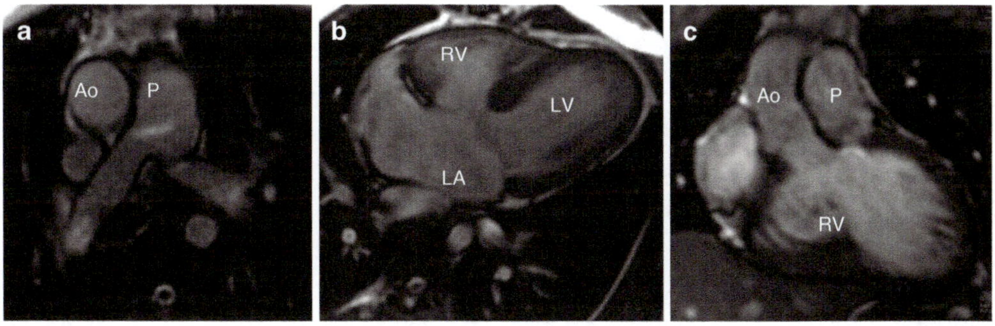

Fig. 15.25 A 39-year-old patient with DORV, D-malposed aorta (**a**), common atrium, Common AV valve, hypoplastic RV (**b**), both great arteries come from RV with severe infundibular pulmonary stenosis (**c**). *Ao* aorta; *LA* left atrium; *LV* left ventricle; *P* pulmonary artery; *RV* right ventricle

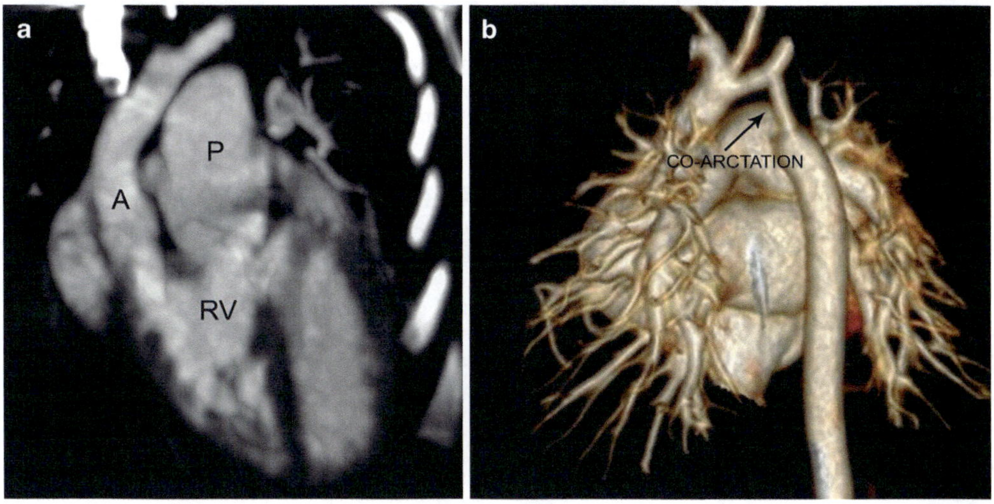

Fig. 15.26 DORV with juxta-ductal coarctation of aorta (**a**) coronal oblique MIP image, (**b**) 3D VRT image. *A* aorta; *P* pulmonary trunk; *RV* right ventricle

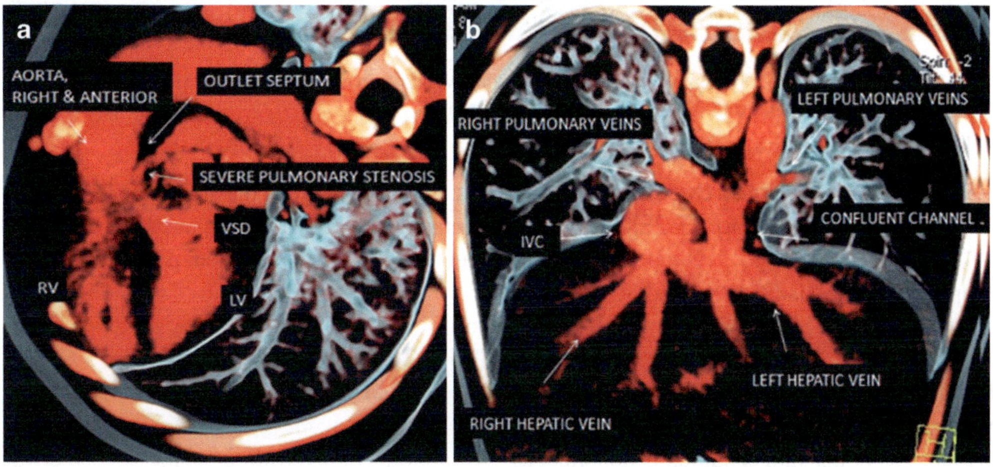

Fig. 15.27 DORV with infracardiac TAPVC (**a**) VRT thin image showing DORVwith PS, (**b**) VRT thin image showing Infracardiac TAPVC

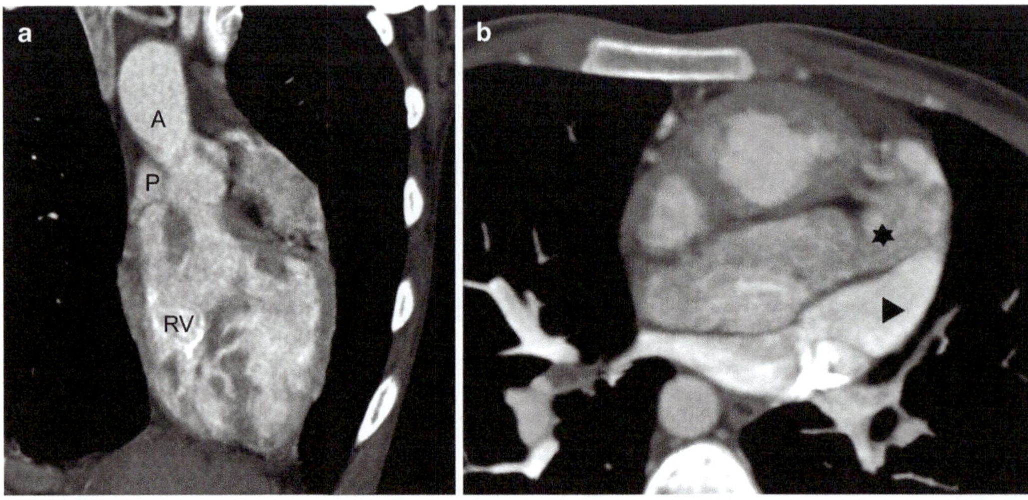

Fig. 15.28 DORV with L-juxtaposed both atrial appendages (**a**) coronal oblique MIP image showing DORV, (**b**) axial MPR image showing L-juxtaposed both atrial appendages. *A* aorta; *P* pulmonary trunk. Star mark denotes right atrial appendage. Arrowhead mark denotes left atrial appendage

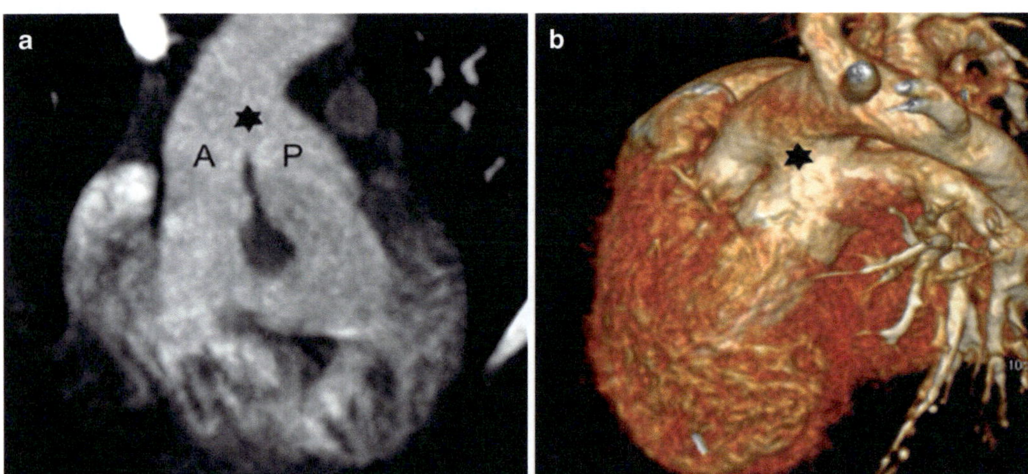

Fig. 15.29 DORV with type-I proximal AP (aortopulmonary) window. (**a**) Coronal oblique MIP image, (**b**) 3D VRT image. *A* aorta; *P* pulmonary trunk. Star mark denotes AP window

15.9.1 Juxtaposition of the Atrial Appendages (Fig. 15.28)

Juxtaposition is a condition where the whole or part of the appendage of one atrium is displaced to the other. The left juxtaposition of the right atrial appendage is much more common than the right juxtaposition [25].

Awareness of this rare condition is important as the unusual atrial anatomy may complicate the surgical procedure when the atrial septal defect needs to be closed or when intra-atrial rerouting of the pulmonary or systemic venous pathways is required.

15.9.2 Abnormalities of the Atrioventricular Valves

Straddling or overriding of the tricuspid valve, mitral valve, or both valves is not frequent.

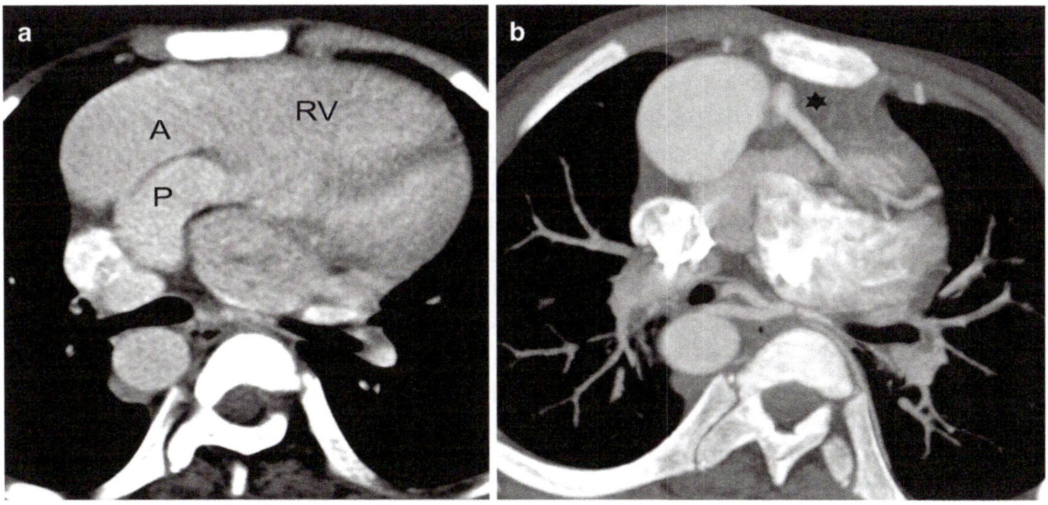

Fig. 15.30 DORV with coronary anomaly (**a**) Axial oblique MIP image showing DORV, (**b**) axial oblique MIP image showing coronary crossing RVOT. *A* aorta; *P* pulmonary trunk; *RV* right ventricle. Star mark denotes coronary crossing RVOT

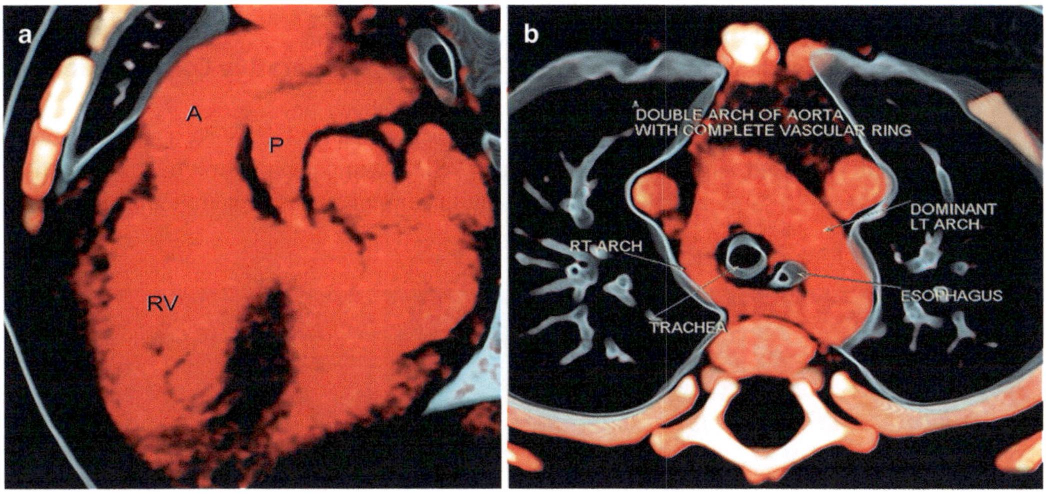

Fig. 15.31 DORV with a double aortic arch. (**a**) VRT thin image showing DORV with PS, (**b**) VRT thin image showing double aortic arch encircling trachea and esophagus

15.10 3D Printing in DORV

DORV with two ventricles and remote VSD still represents a significant therapeutic challenge [26]. The critical aspect of baffling the left ventricular outflow through the VSD to the aorta is sometimes challenging to assess completely on the basis of information obtained from conventional echocardiography. Recently, virtual 3D heart models generated from cardiac MR or CT datasets have been used to delineate the intracardiac anatomy in complex DORV [27, 28].

15.11 Surgical Repair [29–33]

The ideal surgery is biventricular repair by connecting the morphological left ventricle (LV) to the aorta through the VSD and the morphological RV to the pulmonary artery, that leaves the patient with functioning right and left ventricles. The orientation of the VSD is critical for selecting the appropriate surgical approach to avoid obstructing a newly created subaortic or subpulmonary outflow channel. In addition to VSD and its relation to great arteries, outflow tract obstruction, chordal attachments of atrioventricular valves, and the distance between the tricuspid and pulmonary valve will also determine the surgical approach (Figs. 15.32, 15.33, and 15.34).

Indications for single ventricle pathway surgery (Fontan correction) includes hypoplasia of one of the ventricle (Fig. 15.35), substantial straddling of an atrioventricular valve, significant atresia of the mitral valve, large AV canal defect, and extremely unroutable VSD [34].

Various common surgical strategies depending on the DORV variant are as shown in Table 15.2.

15.11.1 LV to Aorta Routability

The goal of surgical correction is to connect ventricle to the great artery, without compromising AV valve function, without outflow obstruction, without compromising ventricular volume and function and avoiding injury to the conduction pathway. Advanced echo, MRI, and 3D models are very useful to achieve the goal. The following parameters are checked to assess the routability:

- Type of VSD
- Conal septum—prominent/hypoplastic, deviation and outflow obstruction
- AV valve anatomy—complete AV canal defect, straddling/overriding, attachment of leaflet to conal septum
- VSD to semilunar valve distance
- Tricuspid to pulmonary valve distance

15.11.2 Postoperative Complications

Complications after DORV repair include residual VSD, ventricular outflow tract obstruction, semilunar valve stenosis/regurgitation, homograft

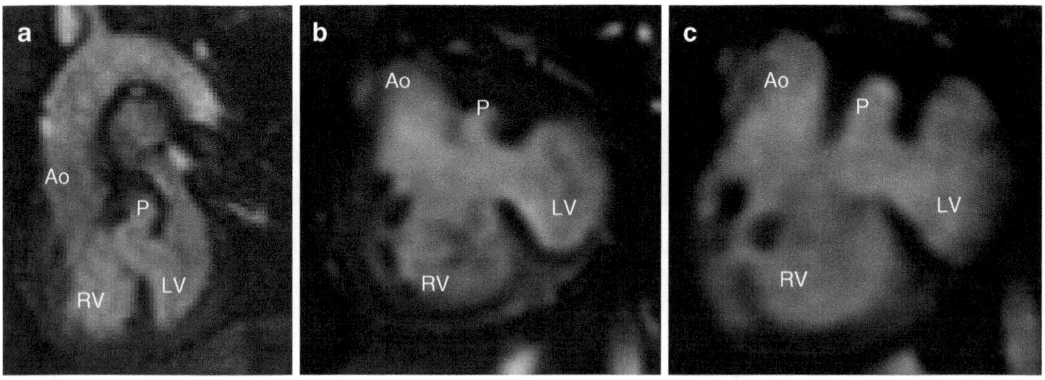

Fig. 15.32 A 6-year-old boy with DORV. Outflow view (**a**) and basal short axis view (**b**, **c**) show DORV, severe PS, Large CV VSD with inlet extension, two good size ventricles, and function. VSD is routable to the aorta with about 1 cm subaortic conus to be excised. Surgery was performed with the routing of VSD to aorta, infundibular and conal septum resection and Rastelli procedure. He developed complete heart block 25 days after surgery and managed with a permanent pacemaker. *Ao* aorta; *LV* left ventricle; *P* pulmonary artery; *RV* right ventricle (Ref to Videos 15.33, 15.34, 15.35, and 15.36)

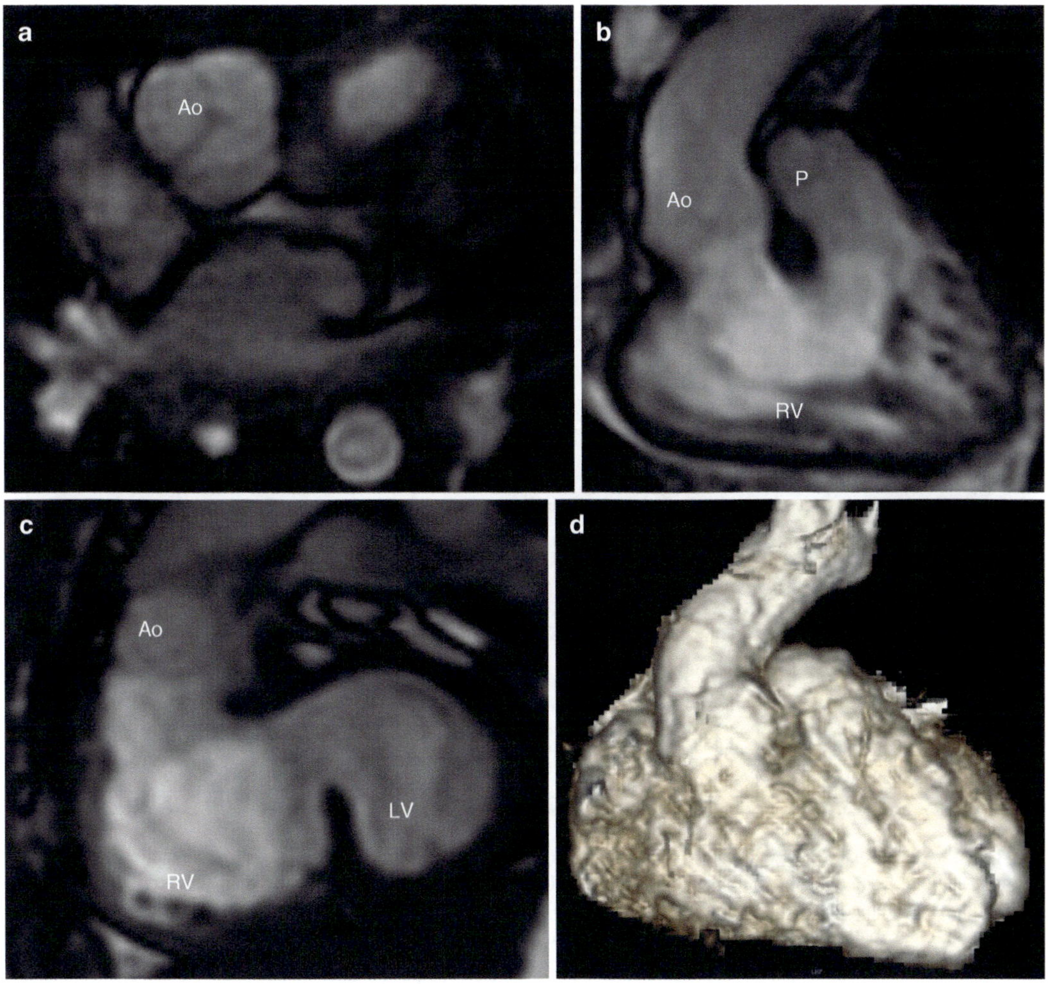

Fig. 15.33 An 8-year-old boy with DORV. Axial (**a**), outflow views (**b**, **c**) and MRA VRT (**d**) show DORV and large VSD—predominantly inlet in location, extending into subaortic/conoventricular region with most of the LV–Aorta route occupied by tricuspid valve tissue (**c**). Severely hypertrophied conal septum (**a**, **c**). Side-by-side great arteries (rightward Aorta, leftward PA) (**a**, **d**). He underwent successful surgery by tunneling of VSD to the aorta using e-PTFE patch, transatrial resection of the conal septum, and tricuspid valve repair. *Ao* aorta; *LV* left ventricle; *P* pulmonary artery; *RV* right ventricle (Ref to Videos 15.37, 15.38, 15.39, 15.40, 15.41, 15.42, 15.43, and 15.44)

stenosis, homograft obstruction, and coronary artery abnormalities after arterial switch (Figs. 15.36, 15.37, and 15.38). Injury to bundle of His which may run along the margin of VSD can lead to conduction abnormality including complete heart block.

15.12 Double Outlet Left Ventricle (DOLV)

In contrast to the double outlet right ventricle, DOLV is a rarity. Both great arteries arise from the left ventricle with bilaterally deficient

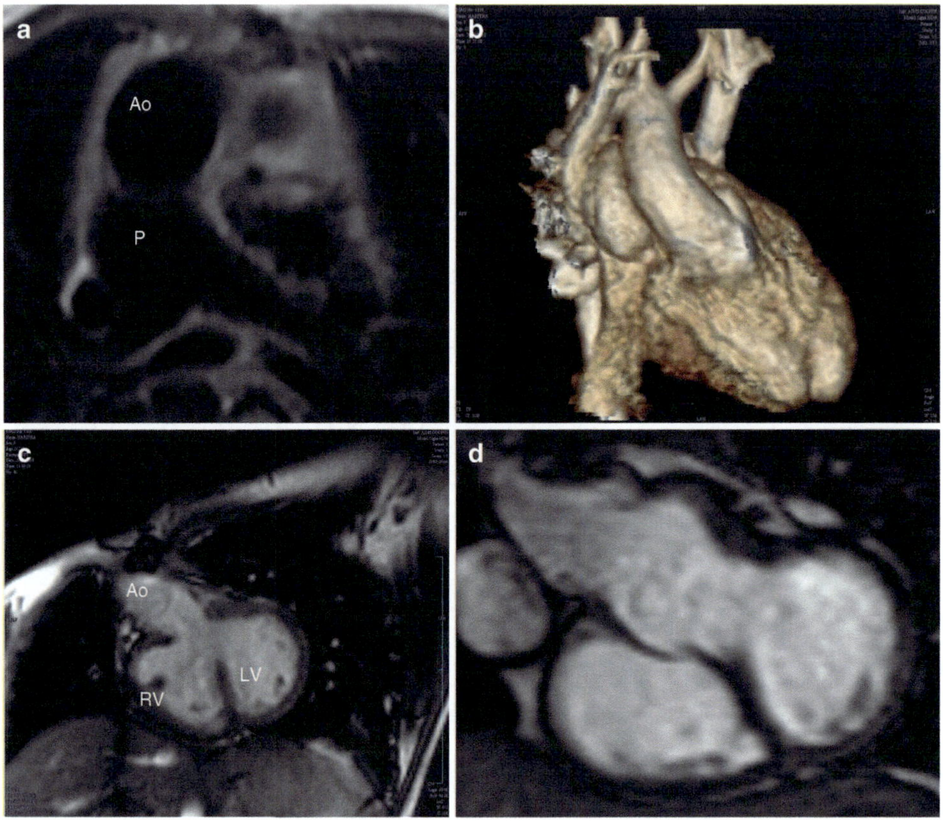

Fig. 15.34 A 12-year-old girl with DORV (Taussig–Bing anomaly), single large conoventricular subpulmonic VSD with mild inlet extension, dilated L-malposed aorta (**a**, **b**). There is a clear path between the LV and the aorta (routable VSD). Prominent subaortic conus and part of the Tricuspid Valve comes in path, but probably not enough to preclude VSD routing (**c**). She underwent routing of the VSD to the aorta using two GoreTex patches, infundibular resection, MPA division, and RV-PA conduit. Postoperative MRI (**d**) shows widely patent LV to aorta tunnel. *Ao* aorta; *LV* left ventricle; *P* pulmonary artery; *RV* right ventricle (Ref to Videos 15.45, 15.46, 15.47, 15.48, 15.49, 15.50, 15.51, 15.52, 15.53, and 15.54)

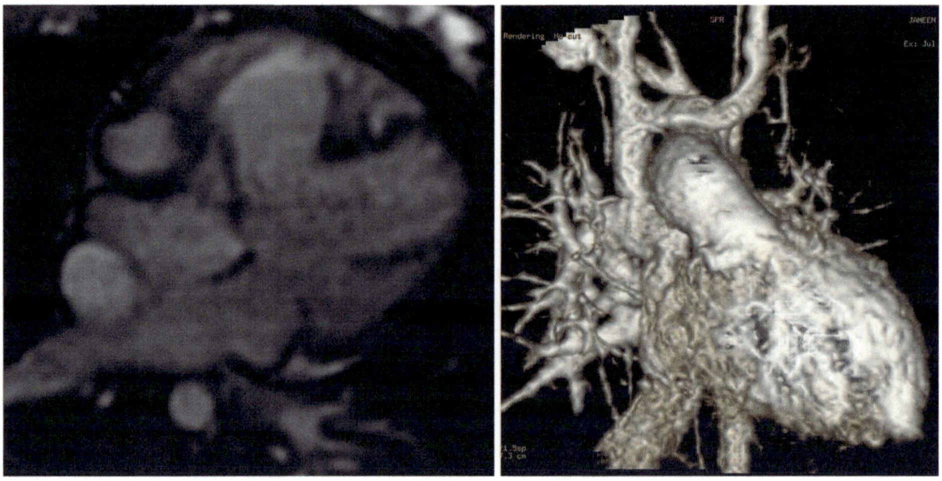

Fig. 15.35 A case of DORV underwent Fontan surgery because of inadequate RV size for biventricular repair (Ref to Videos 15.55, 15.56, 15.57, and 15.58)

Table 15.2 Management strategies based on variant of DORV

Type	Management
VSD type	VSD closure with LV to aorta routing within the first 6 months
TOF type	VSD closure with LV to aorta routing and relief of pulmonary obstruction in the age of 4 to 12 months
TGA type	Early corrective surgery with arterial switch, VSD closure – Alternatively Rastelli procedure—baffling of the LV to aortic valve and placement of a conduit from RV to pulmonary trunk
Single ventricle type	Fontan surgery

infundibulums. A high frequency of obstruction in the pulmonary outflow tract is found when the VSD is subaortic (Fig. 15.39). DOLV occurs most commonly in the form of atrial situs solitus with atrioventricular (AV) concordance but is often associated with cardiac anomalies such as a VSD, an atrial septal defect, pulmonary stenosis, right ventricular hypoplasia, patent ductus arteriosus, and tricuspid atresia [35, 36].

15.13 Conclusion

DORV is an extremely heterogeneous group of malformations that require a comprehensive diagnostic approach for tailored surgical man-

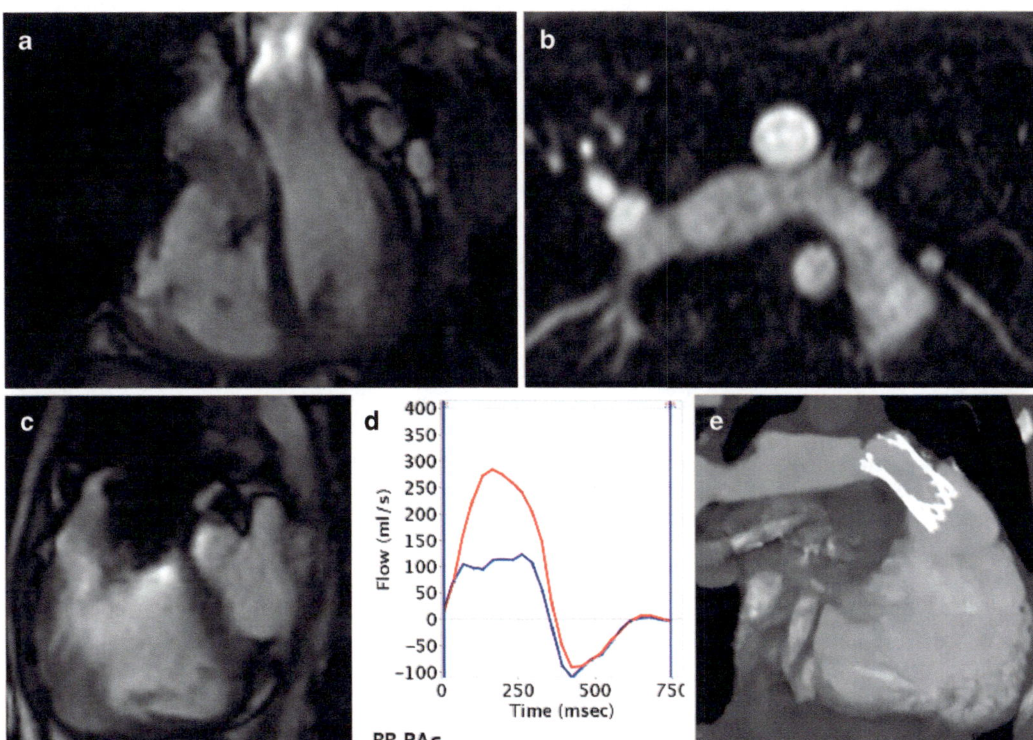

Fig. 15.36 Follow-up case of DORV underwent multiple staged procedures leading to intracardiac repair, RV to PA conduit, and RVOT stenting. CMR show a patent VSD patch without any residual VSD (outflow view-**a**), confluent unobstructed branch pulmonary arteries (MRA-**b**), significant pulmonary regurgitation (PC flow curve-**d**) (calculates as about 40%). RV to PA conduit stent cause severe artifact on MRI (**c**) and better evaluated by CT (**e**)

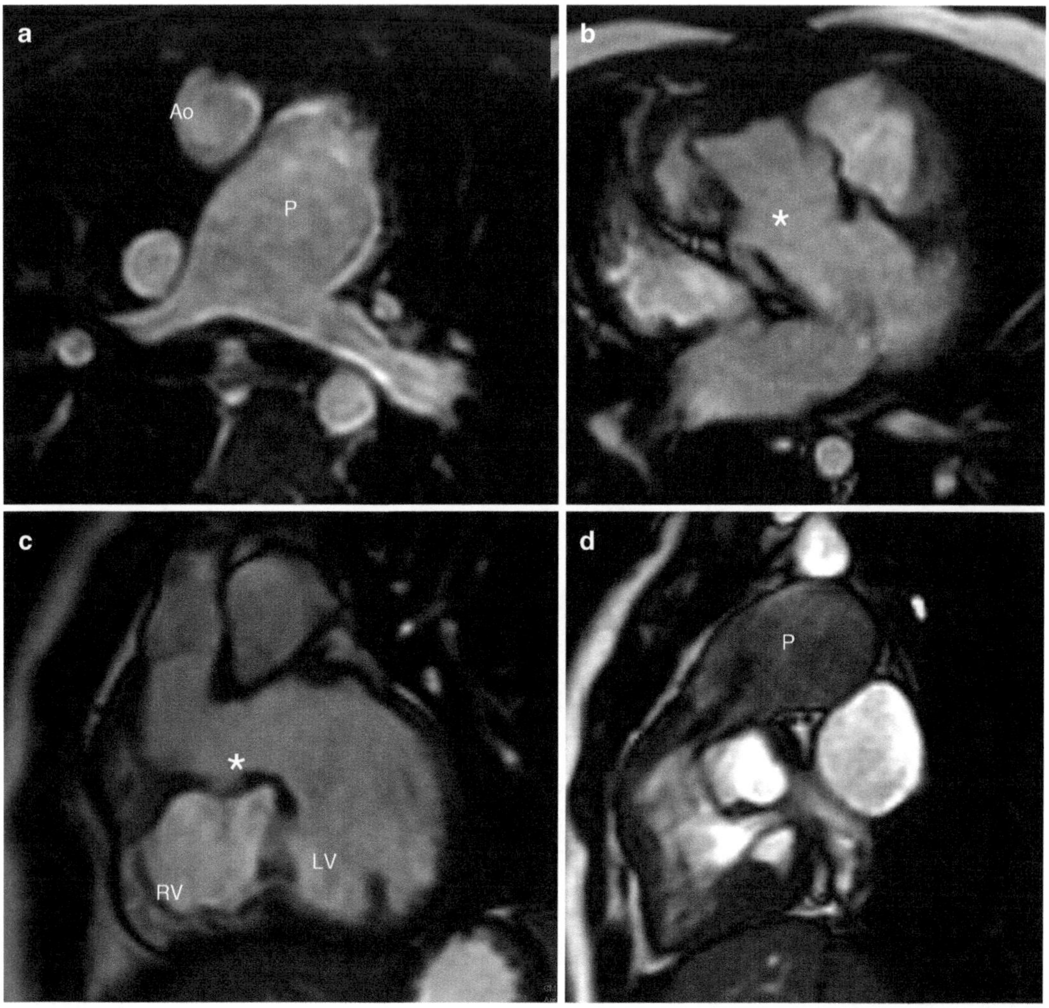

Fig. 15.37 A patient with DORV, large inlet VSD, moderate size CV-VSD underwent multiple e-PTFE patches. Postoperative MRI shows confluent branch pulmonary arteries (**a**), widely patent LV to aorta tunnel (* in **b**, **c**), subpulmonic obstruction (**d**) and dilated MPA. *Ao* aorta; *LV* left ventricle; *P* pulmonary artery; *RV* right ventricle

agement. DORV with subaortic VSD and pulmonary stenosis resembles that of TOF. Taussig–Bing type of DORV is treated similarly to TGA. The location of VSD, as seen from the side of the right ventricle, needs to be described. Other essential anatomic information analyzed include: atrial arrangements, atrioventricular connection, AV valve morphology including the attachment of subvalvular apparatus, ventriculoarterial connection, morphology of outflow tract obstruction, the relationship of great arteries, and other associated anomalies.

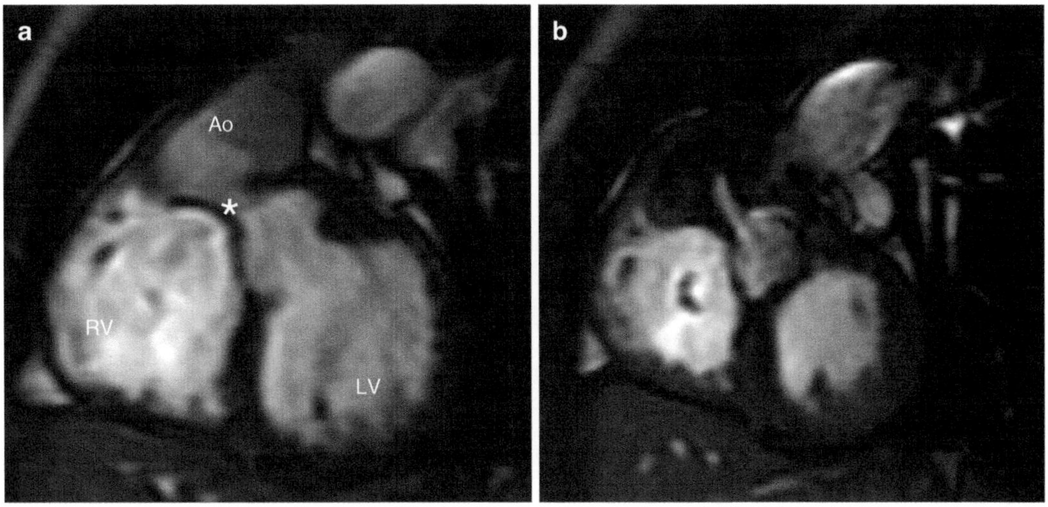

Fig. 15.38 A 10-year-old child status post DORV repair (Complex Kawashima intraventricular tunneling with fenestrated VSD closure). Short-axis cine images during diastole (**a**) and systole (**b**) show subvalvular aortic stenosis (*) in the LV–Aorta tunnel resulting from the indentation of the VSD patch and the presence of subaortic conal tissue. *Ao* aorta; *LV* left ventricle; *RV* right ventricle (Ref to Videos 15.59, 15.60, 15.61, 15.62, 15.53, and 15.64)

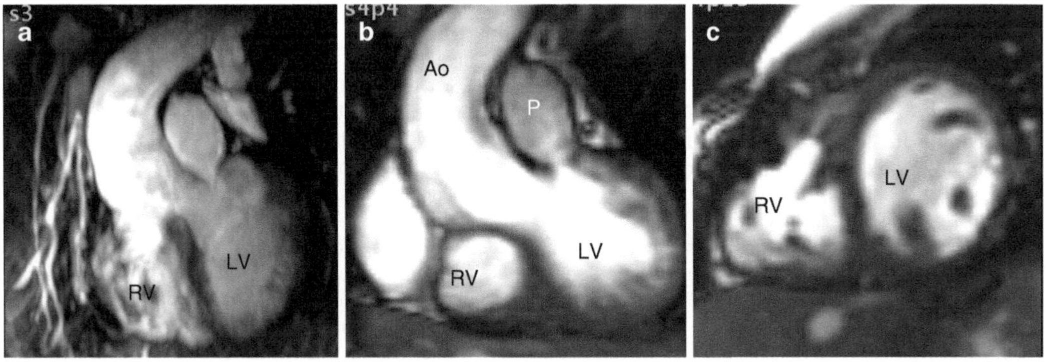

Fig. 15.39 A 5-year-old boy, outflow views (**a**, **b**) and short axis MRI (**c**) showing DOLV (PA from LV, Aorta overriding the ventricles), large conoventricular VSD (**a**) with inlet extension, severe pulmonary stenosis (**a**, **b**), relatively small RV (**c**). Since the post-tunneling estimated RV volume was low, he underwent Fontan surgery. *Ao* aorta; *LV* left ventricle; *P* pulmonary artery; *RV* right ventricle

References

1. Walters HL III, Mavroudis C, Tchervenkov CI, Jacobs JP, Lacour-Gayet F, Jacobs ML. Congenital heart surgery nomenclature and database project: double outlet right ventricle. Ann Thorac Surg. 2000;69:S249–63.
2. Lev M, Bharati S, Meng L, Liberthson RR, Paul MH, Idriss F. A concept of double outlet right ventricle. J Thorac Cardiovasc Surg. 1972;64:271–81.
3. Wilcox BR, Ho SY, Macartney FJ, Becker AE, Gerlis LM, Anderson RH. Surgical anatomy of double outlet right ventricle with situs solitus and atrioventricular concordance. J Thorac Cardiovasc Surg. 1981;92:405–17.
4. Abernethy J. Surgical and physiological essays. Part II. London: James Evans, Pater-Noster-Row; 1793. p. 157–65.
5. Taussig HB, Bing RJ. Complete transposition of the aorta and a levoposition of the pulmonary artery. Am Heart J. 1949;37:551–9.
6. Witham AC. Double outlet right ventricle. A partial transposition complex. Am Heart J. 1957;53:928–39.

7. Chen SJ, Lin MT, Liu KL, Chang CI, Chen HY, et al. Usefulness of 3D reconstructed computed tomography imaging for double outlet right ventricle. J Formos Med Assoc. 2008;107(5):371–80.
8. Shi K, Yang Z, Chen J, Zhang G, Xu H, et al. Assessment of double outlet right ventricle associated with multiple malformations in pediatric patients using retrospective ECG-gated dual-source computed tomography. PLoS One. 2015;10(6):e0130987.
9. Yoo SJ, Spray T, Austin EH 3rd, Yun TJ, van Arsdell GS. Hands-on surgical training of congenital heart surgery using 3-dimensional print models. J Thorac Cardiovasc Surg. 2017;153:1530–40. https://doi.org/10.1016/j.jtcvs.2016.12.054.
10. Guo W, Lin ML, Gu ZQ, et al. Double outlet right ventricle, a clinical-roentgenologic-pathologic study of 28 consecutive patients. Chest. 1984;85:526–32.
11. Van Praagh R, Geva T, Kreutzer J. Ventricular septal defects: how shall we describe, name, and classify them? J Am Coll Cardiol. 1989;14:1298–9.
12. Sebastian L, Erwin O, Lars H, et al. Pre- and postoperative evaluation of congenital heart disease in children and adults with 64-section CT. Radiographics. 2007;27:829–46.
13. Aoki M, Forbess JM, Jonas RA, Mayer RE, Castaneda AR. Results of biventricular repair for double outlet right ventricle. Thorac Cardiovasc Surg. 1984;107:338–50.
14. Kleinert S, Sano T, Weintraoub RG, Karl TR, Wilkinson JL. Anatomic features and surgical strategies in double outlet right ventricle. Circulaion. 1997;96:1233–9.
15. Belli E, Serraf A, Lacour Gayet F, Inamo J, Houyet L, Bruniaux J, Planché C. Surgical treatment of subaortic stenosis after biventricular repair of double outlet right ventricle. J Thorac Cardiovasc Surg. 1996;122:1570–80.
16. Brown JW, Ruzmetov M, Okada Y, Vijay P, Turrentine MW. Surgical results in patients with double outlet right ventricle: a 20 year experience. Ann Thorac Surg. 2001;72:630–5.
17. Bradley T, Karamlou T, Kulik A, Mitrovic B, Vigneswara T, Jaffer S, Glasgow PD, Williams WG, VanArsdell G, McCrindle BW. Determinants of repair type, reintervention, and mortality in 393 children with double outlet right ventricle. J Thorac Cardiovasc Surg. 2007;134:969–73.
18. Lincoln C, Anderson RH, Shinebourne EA, English TAH, Wilkinson JL. Double outlet right ventricle with l-malposition of the aorta. Br Heart J. 1975;37:453–63.
19. Belli E, Serraf A, Lacour-Gayet F, Hubler M, Zoghby J, Houyel L, Planche C. Double outlet right ventricle with non-committed ventricular septal defect. Eur J Cardiothorac Surg. 1999;15:747–52.
20. Edwards JE, James JW, Dushane JW. Congenital malformation of the heart; origin of transposed great vessels from the right ventricle associated with atresia of the left ventricular outlet, double orifice of the mitral valve and single coronary artery. Lab Investig. 1952;1:197–207.
21. Lavoie R, Sestier F, Gilbert G, Chameides L, Van Praagh R, Grondin P. Double outlet right ventricle with left ventricular outflow tract obstruction due to small ventricular septal defect. Am Heart J. 1971;82:290–9.
22. Mazzucco A, Faggian G, Stellin G, Bortolotti U, Livi U, Rizzoli G, Gallucci V. Surgical management of double-outlet right ventricle. J Thorac Cardiovasc Surg. 1985;90:29–34.
23. Belli E, Serraf A, Lacour-Gayet F, et al. Double-outlet right ventricle with non-committed ventricular septal defect. Eur J Cardiothorac Surg. 1999;15:747–52.
24. Tabry IF, Mcgoon DC, Danielson GK, et al. Surgical management of double outlet right ventricle associated with atrioventricular discordance. J Thorac Cardiovasc Surg. 1978;76:336–44.
25. Anjos RT, Ho SY, Anderson RH. Surgical implications of juxtaposition of the atrial appendages. A review of forty-nine autopsied hearts. J Thorac Cardiovasc Surg. 1990;99:897–904.
26. Lacour-Gayet F. Biventricular repair of double outlet right ventricle with noncommitted ventricular septal defect. Semin Thorac Cardiovasc Surg Pediatr Card Surg Annu. 2002;5:163–72.
27. Farooqi KM, Uppu SC, Nguyen K. Application of virtual three-dimensional models for simultaneous visualization of intracardiac anatomic relationships in double outlet right ventricle. Pediatr Cardiol. 2016;37(1):90–8.
28. Yim D, Dragulescu A, Ide H, et al. Essential modifiers of double outlet right ventricle - revisit with endocardial surface images and 3-dimensional print models. Circ Cardiovasc Imaging. 2018;11:e006891.
29. Harvey JC, Sondheimer HM, William WG, et al. Repair of double outlet right ventricle. J Thoracic Cardiovasc Surg. 1977;73:611–5.
30. Brown JW, Ruzmetov M, Okada Y, Vijay P, Turrentine MW. Surgical results in patients with double outlet right ventricle: a 20-year experience. AnnThorac Surg. 2001;72(5):1630–5.
31. Wetter J, Sinzobahamvya N, Blaschczok HC, et al. Results of arterial switch operation for primary total correction of the Taussig-Bing anomaly. Ann Thorac Surg. 2004;77(1):41–6. discussion 47
32. Belli E, Serraf A, Lacour-Gayet F, et al. Surgical treatment of subaortic stenosis after biventricular repair of double-outlet right ventricle. J Thorac Cardiovasc Surg. 1996;112(6):1570–8.
33. Lacour-Gayet F, Haun C, Ntalakoura K, Belli E, Houyel L, Marcsek P, et al. Biventricular repair of

double outlet right ventricle with non-committed ventricular septal defect (VSD) by VSD rerouting to the pulmonary artery and arterial switch. Eur J Cardiothorac Surg. 2002;21:1042–8.
34. Delius RE, Rademecker MA, de Level MR, et al. Is a high risk biventricular repair always preferable to conversion to a single ventricle repair? J Thorac Cardiovasc Surg. 1996;112:1561–9.
35. Bharati S, Lev M, Stewart R, McAllister H, Kirklin J. The morphologic spectrum of double outlet left ventricle and its surgical significance. Circulation. 1978;58:558–65.
36. Galal O, Hatle L, Al HZ. Changes of management in a patient with double outlet left ventricle. Cardiol Young. 1999;9:602–5.

Pre- and Postoperative Imaging in Transposition of Great Arteries

16

T. R. Kapilamoorthy and Ramiah Rajeshkannan

16.1 Introduction

In transposition of the great arteries (TGA), the position of the aorta and the pulmonary artery is reversed.

It is classified as follows:

1. Complete-TGA (CTGA) in which there is atrioventricular concordance with ventriculo-arterial discordance. Aorta lies anterior and to the right (D-transposed aorta) of the main pulmonary artery (MPA).
   It is sub-classified as:
   (a) Simple transposition (without associated defects) 50%
   (b) Complex transposition (with VSD 25%, LVOT obstruction 25%)
2. Congenitally Corrected TGA (CCTGA) in which both atrioventricular and ventriculoarterial discordance are seen. The right ventricle acts as the systemic ventricle pumping into the aorta and the left ventricle pumps the systemic venous return into the pulmonary artery. Here aorta lies anterior and to the left of MPA (L-transposed aorta)

Electronic Supplementary Material The online version of this chapter (https://doi.org/10.1007/978-981-15-6755-1_16) contains supplementary material, which is available to authorized users.

T. R. Kapilamoorthy (✉)
Department of Imaging Sciences and Interventional Radiology, Sree Chitra Tirunal Institute for Medical Sciences and Technology, Trivandrum, Kerala, India

R. Rajeshkannan
Department of Radiology, Amrita School of Medicine, Amrita Institute of Medical Sciences and Research Centre, Amrita Vishwa Vidyapeetham, Kochi, Kerala, India

16.2 Embryology

The exact events during maldevelopment are not known. The most accepted version is the migration and subsequent inversion of conus. In normal cases, the subaortic conus is resorbed and there is migration of subpulmonic conus anteriorly toward RV. In TGA, the subpulmonary conus disappears and the subaortic conus migrates forward toward the RV and thus aorta gets connected to RV. The pulmonary artery is posterior and gets connected to LV with a fibrous continuity of pulmonary and mitral valve [1, 2].

16.3 Morphology

By Van Praag segmental anatomy [3], CTGA is designated as Situs solitus (S), Dextro ventricular loop (D), Rightward (D) and anterior aorta (Figs. 16.1, 16.2, and 16.3). In one third of cases aorta is to the left and anterior. In situs inversus CTGA become (I, L, L). The aorta and pulmonary artery cross each other in normal cases. But in TGA, they run parallel and do not cross.

R. Rajeshkannan et al. (eds.), *CT and MRI in Congenital Heart Diseases*,
https://doi.org/10.1007/978-981-15-6755-1_16

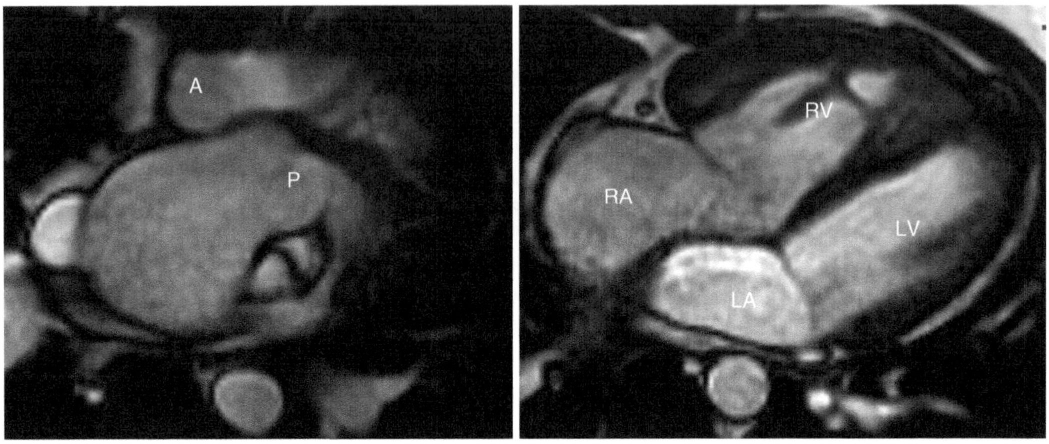

Fig. 16.1 A case of complete TGA. MRI shows aorta placed on the right and anterior to the pulmonary artery (D transposed aorta) with D loop ventricle (RV is right of LV). *A* ascending aorta; *LA* left atrium; *LV* left ventricle; *P* pulmonary trunk; *RA* right atrium; *RV* right ventricle

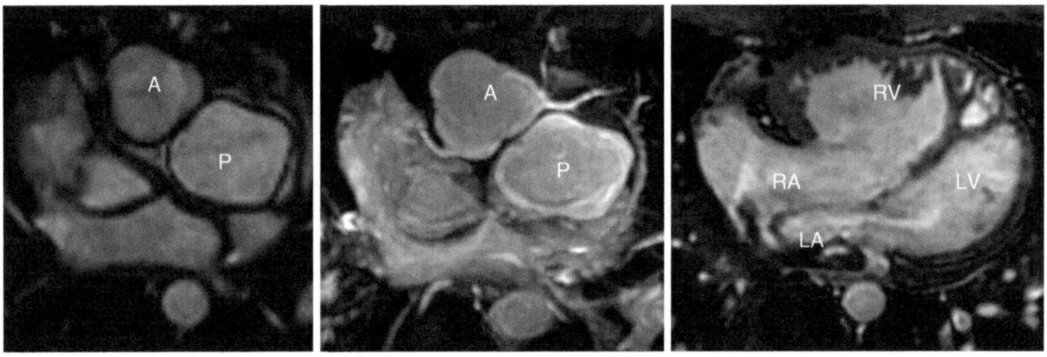

Fig. 16.2 A case of CTGA, peri-membranous VSD, Regressed LV. Status post Sennings + VSD closure at 4 months of age. Note the normal coronary arteries arising from the facing sinuses. *A* ascending aorta; *LA* left atrium; *LV* left ventricle; *P* pulmonary trunk; *RA* right atrium; *RV* right ventricle (Ref to Videos 16.1, 16.2, 16.3, 16.4, 16.5, 16.6, 16.7, and 16.8)

CCTGA is designated as situs solitus (S), levo-ventricular loop (L), and leftward (L) and anterior aorta (Figs. 16.4, 16.5, and 16.6). In situs inversus it becomes (I, D, D) (Videos 16.17, 16.18, 16.19, 16.20, 16.21, 16.22, 16.23, and 16.24).

Ventricles are usually arranged in a side-by-side manner, but they also can have a superoinferior relationship with the right ventricle placed above the left ventricle (Figs. 16.7 and 16.8) [4].

16.3.1 Coronary Arteries in TGA [5, 6]

Analysis of location and number of coronary artery origins is an important step in decision-making for the appropriate surgery. ECG-gated CT study with optimal phase selection helps in identifying coronary origins and course clearly. Post-processing evaluation can be performed using dedicated workstations. Axial, curved multiplanar reconstructions (MPR), maximum intensity projection (MIP), and volume-rendered technique (VRT) are used for proper assessment of coronaries.

In TGA, the coronaries originate from the two aortic sinuses facing the pulmonary artery. Variations do occur, the most common being that of the left anterior descending artery and circumflex arteries (Figs. 16.9 and 16.10) (Videos 16.38, 16.39, 16.40, 16.41, and 16.42)

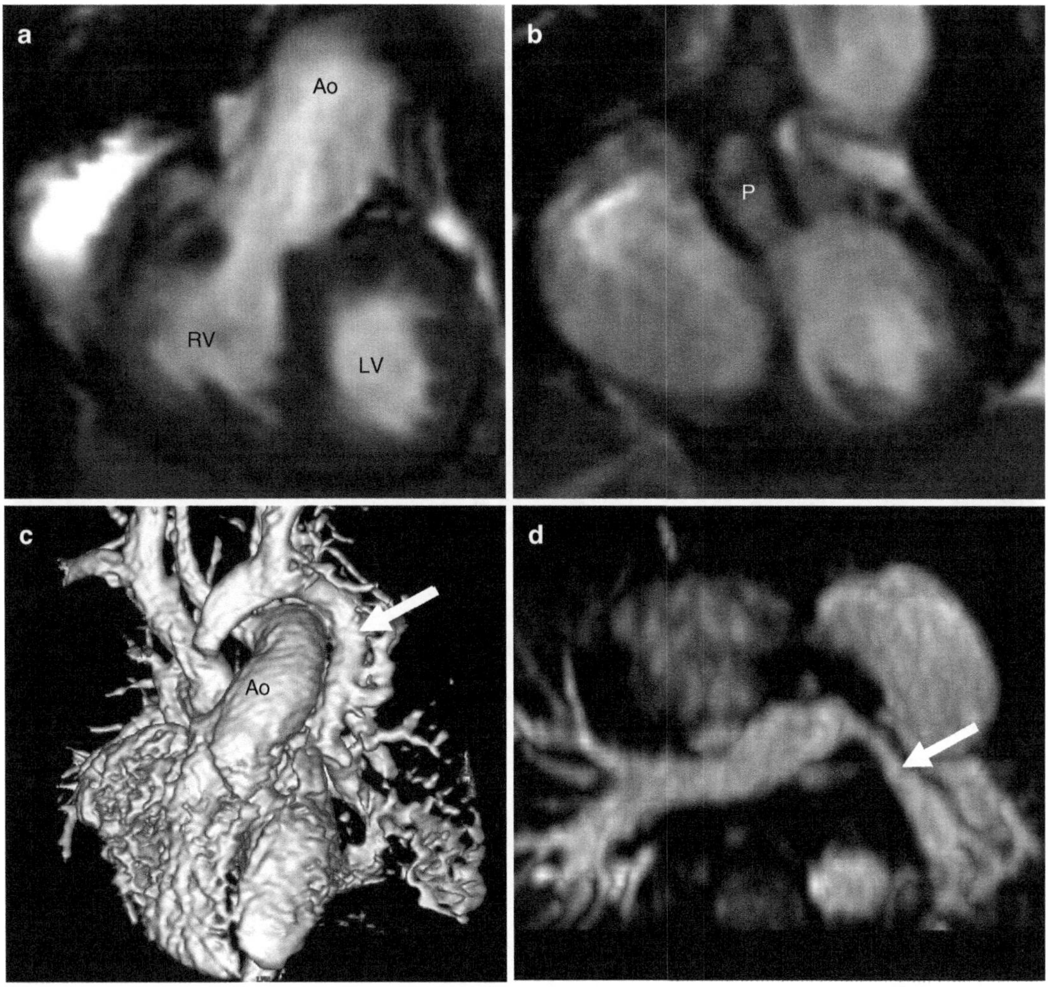

Fig. 16.3 Comprehensive assessment of a case of D-TGA by CMR. Images show adequate sized D loop ventricles, aorta (Ao) arising predominantly from the right ventricle (RV), pulmonary trunk (P) from the left ventricle (LV), anomalous drainage of the left upper pulmonary vein into the left innominate vein (arrow in **c**), confluent pulmonary arteries with tight left pulmonary stenosis (arrow in **d**)

16.4 Differential Diagnosis

The closest mimicker of TGA is double outlet RV(DORV). In this condition, more than 50% of the aorta and pulmonary artery arise from RV. In TGA, aorta arises exclusively from the RV and pulmonary artery from LV. In DORV, there are bilateral coni separating the outlet valves from inlet valves. In TGA, there is fibrous continuity between the mitral valve and pulmonary valve [7].

Anatomically corrected malposition of great arteries is an abnormal arrangement in which both arterial trunks arise from appropriate ventricles but in abnormal relationships to each other with parallel great arteries [8]. Bilateral subarterial infundibulum is seen in 50% of cases. As opposed to TGA, there is no ventriculoarterial discordance (Fig. 16.11).

16.5 Pathophysiology

The parallel circuit of CTGA is compatible with life, only if accompanied by a communication between the two circuits like ASD/VSD/PDA with a mixing of blood. Progressive cyanosis

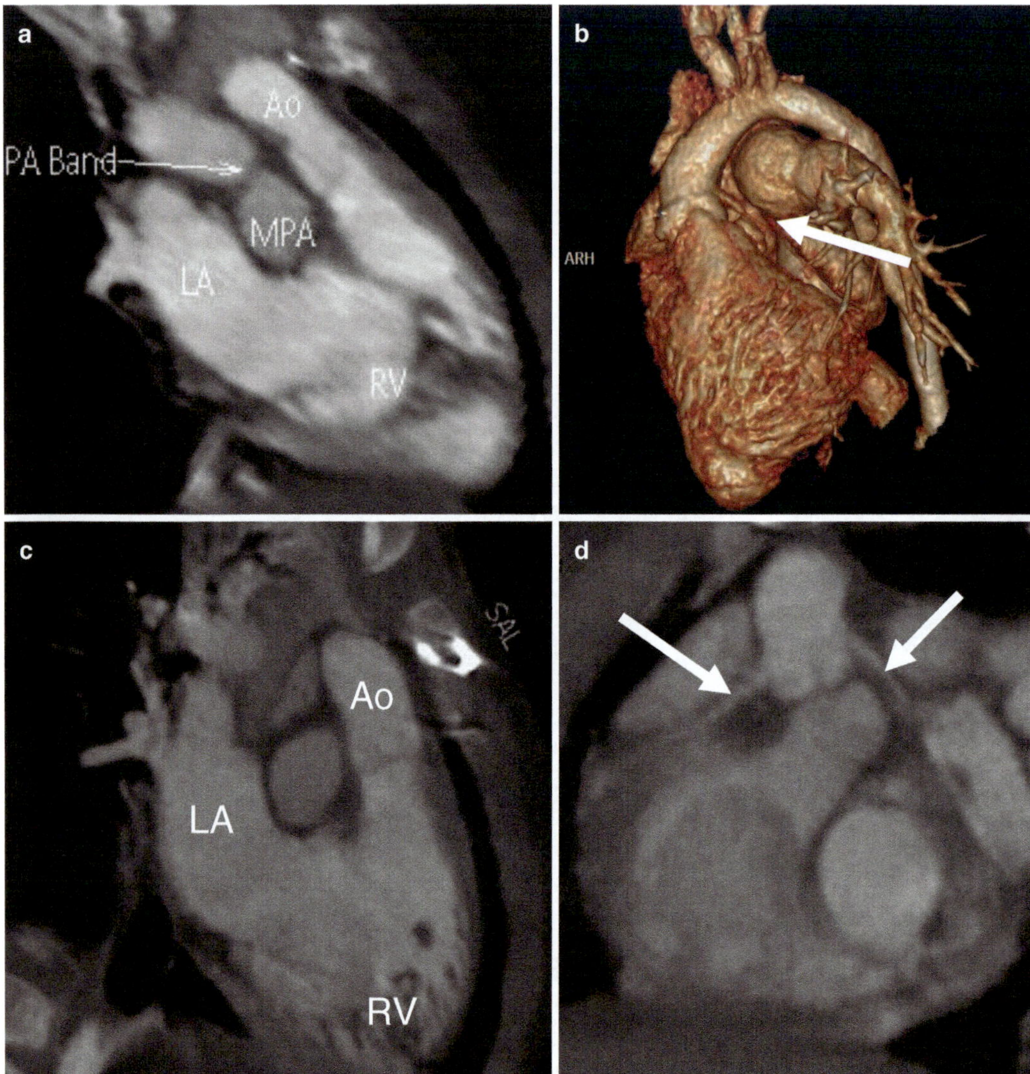

Fig. 16.4 A 3-year-old child with CCTGA with PA band (arrow in B). Note both side proximal coronary arteries (arrows in D). *Ao* ascending aorta; *LA* left atrium; *MPA* pulmonary trunk; *RV* right ventricle

develops early in life with intact ventricular septum. In complex transposition, there is rapid development of pulmonary vascular obstructive disease. In 30% of TGA cases under 2 years, there is evidence of precapillary bronchopulmonary anastomosis angiographically which accelerates the pulmonary vascular disease.

16.6 Clinical Aspects

In a typical scenario, if a cyanosed large baby is born to a diabetic mother, one has to suspect TGA. Usually, there is cardiomegaly with increased pulmonary blood flow and no murmur [9].

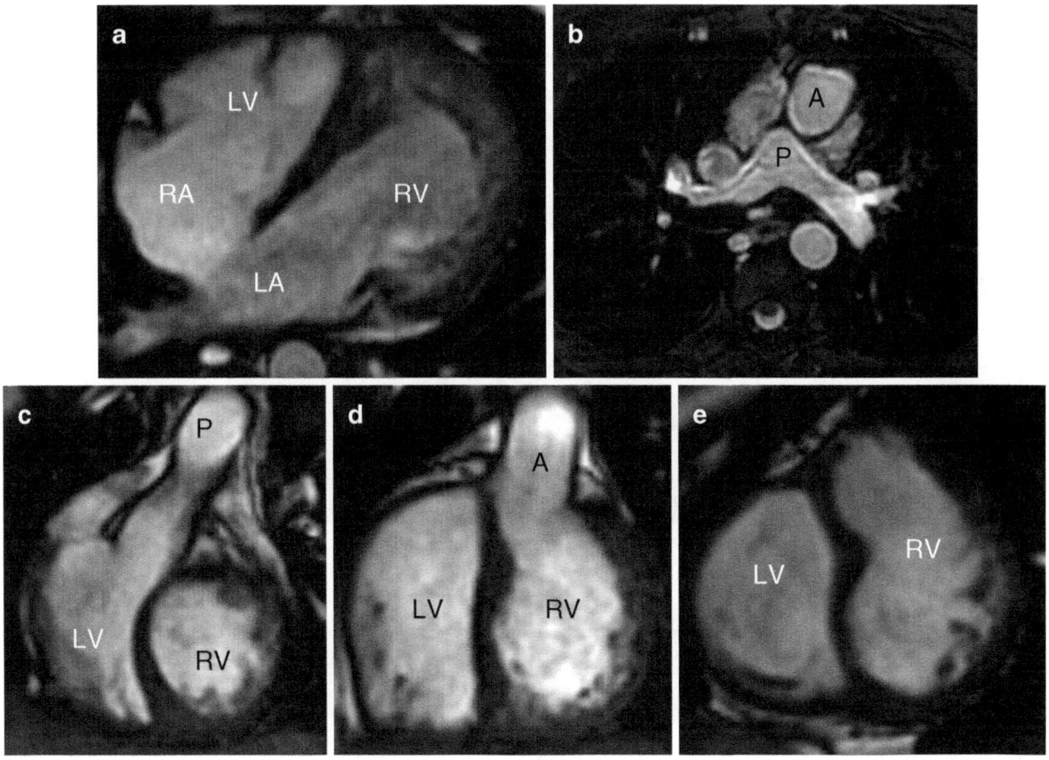

Fig. 16.5 An 18-year-old boy with LTGA with intact ventricular septum showing thin-walled regressed LV without pulmonary stenosis. *A* ascending aorta; *LA* left atrium; *LV* left ventricle; *P* pulmonary trunk; *RA* right atrium; *RV* right ventricle (Ref to Videos 16.9, 16.10, 16.11, 16.12, 16.13, 16.14, 16.15, and 16.16)

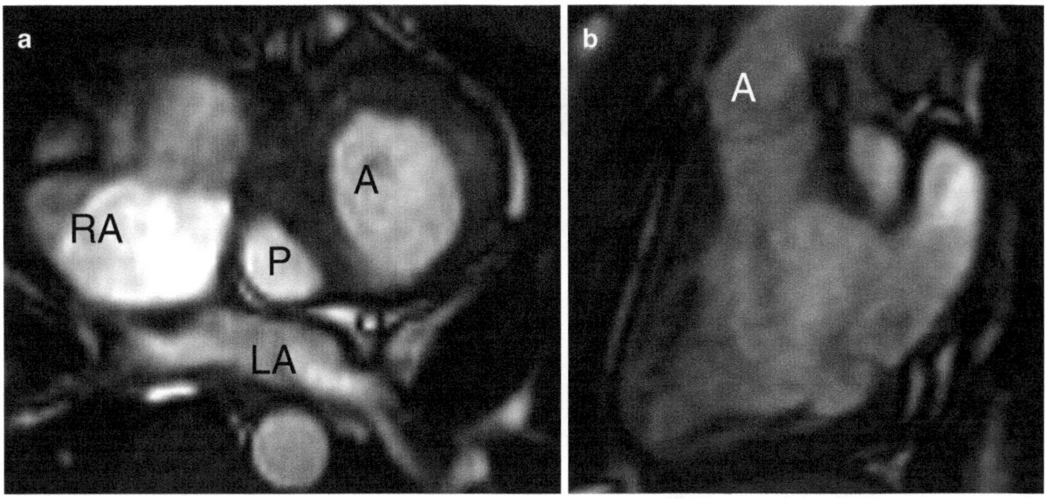

Fig. 16.6 A case of LTGA VSD with pulmonary stenosis. Axial view (**a**) shows L posed aorta with subaortic conus. RV inflow outflow view (**b**) shows discontinuity between the tricuspid valve and aortic valve. LV outflow view (**c**) shows severe valvar and supravalvar pulmonary stenosis. Outflow view perpendicular to interventricular septum (**d**) shows large conal tissue along the LV to aorta pathway. *A* ascending aorta; *LA* left atrium; *LV* left ventricle; *P* pulmonary trunk; *RA* right atrium; *RV* right ventricle

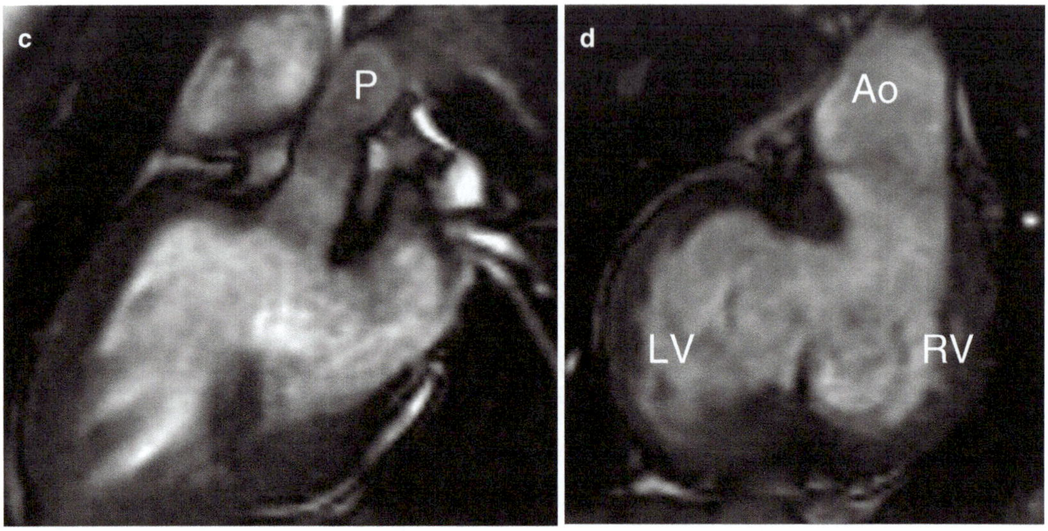

Fig. 16.6 (continued)

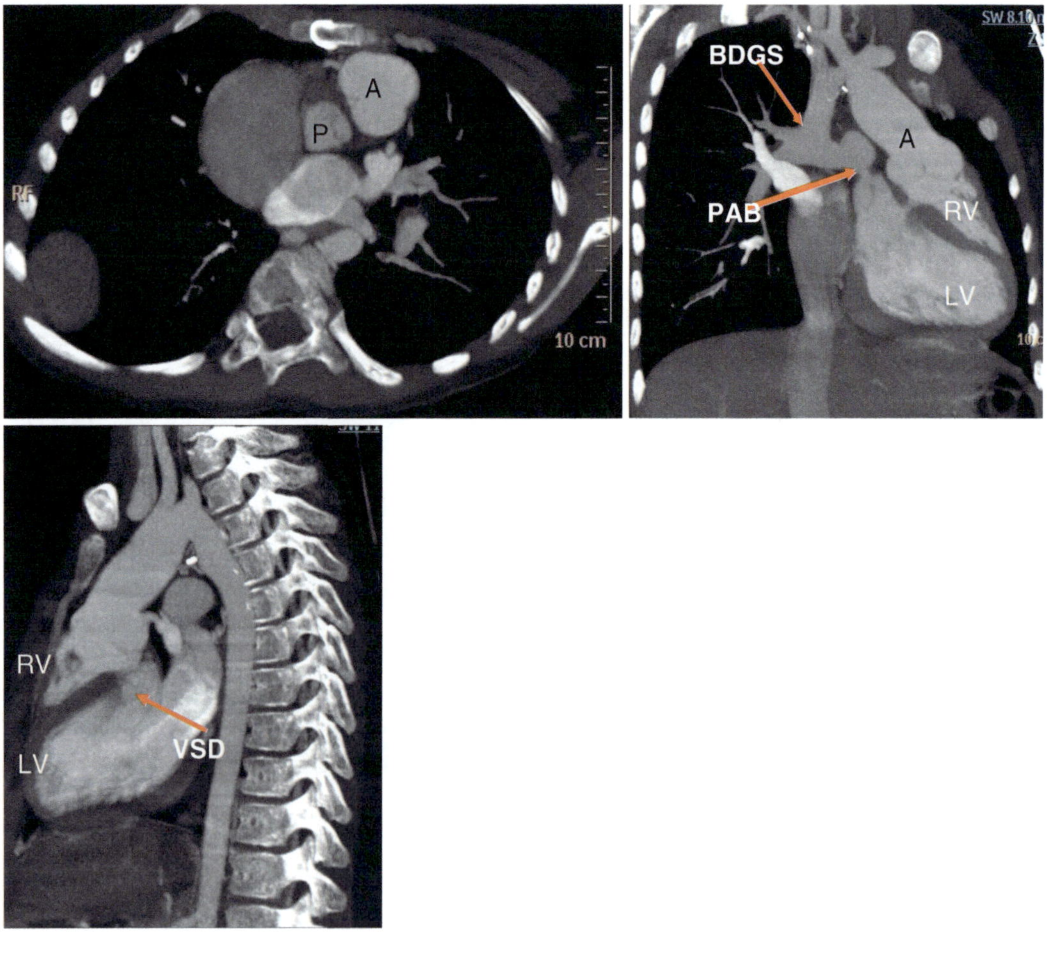

Fig. 16.7 A 10-year-old child with supero-inferior ventricles with TGA had PA banding at 14 weeks of life and BDGS at 1 year. *A* ascending aorta; *BDGS* bidirectional Glenn shunt; *LV* left ventricle; *P* pulmonary trunk; *PAB* PA band; *RV* right ventricle

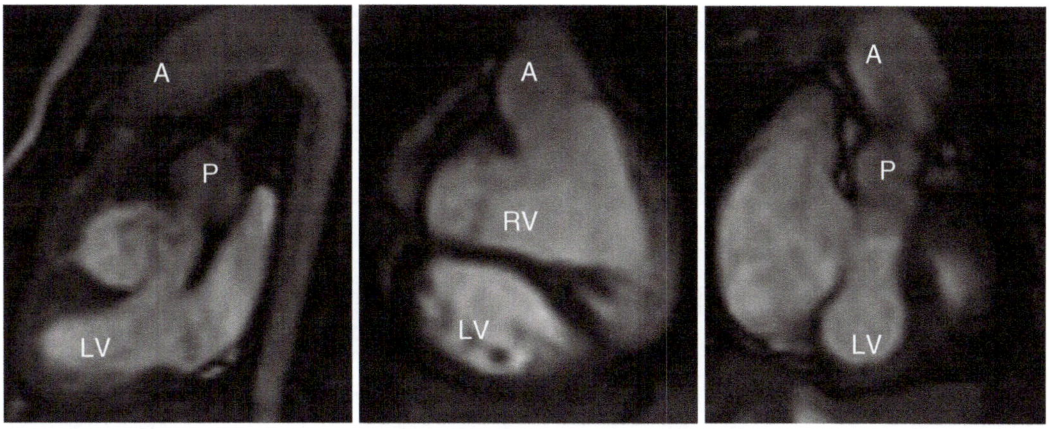

Fig. 16.8 A case of crisscross heart with superoinferiorly related ventricles and transposition of great arteries. Aorta (A) arises from the superior right ventricle (RV) and pulmonary artery (P) from the inferior left ventricle (LV). L, posed aorta, Severe subvalvar PS due to deviated coal septum, large conoventricular VSD with significant inlet extension (Ref to Videos 16.25, 16.26, 16.27, 16.28, 16.29, 16.30, 16.31, 16.32, 16.33, 16.34, 16.35, 16.36, and 16.37)

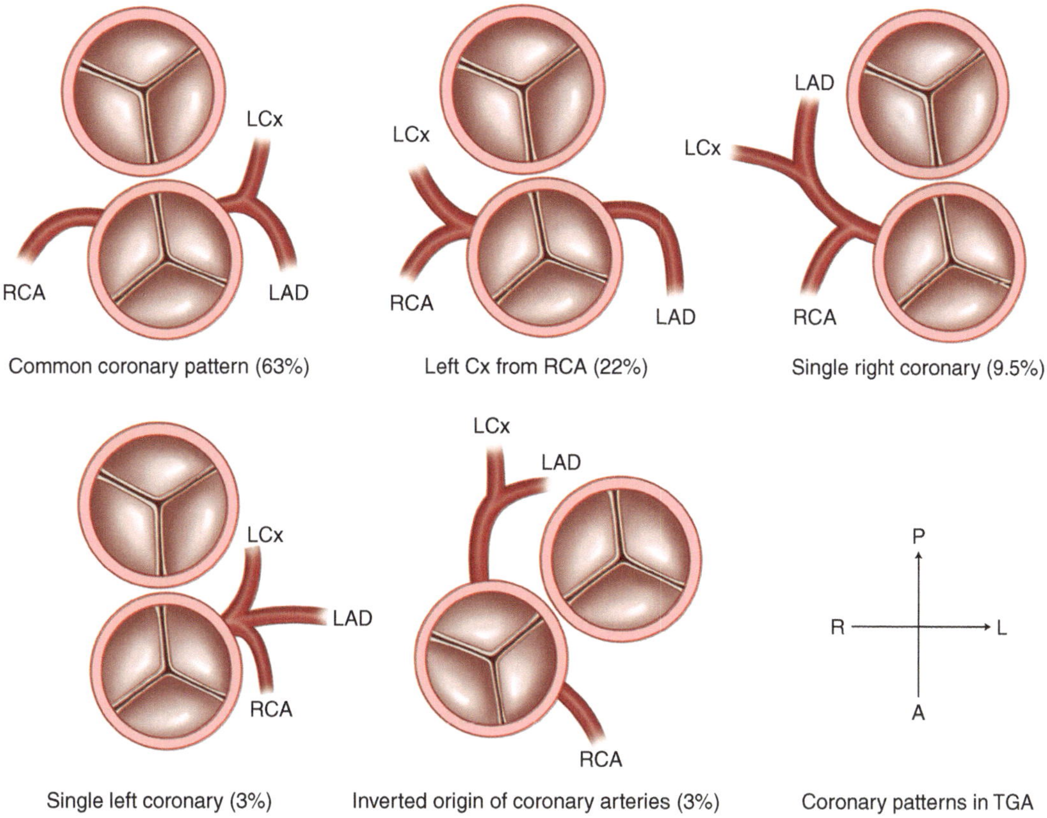

Fig. 16.9 Coronary patterns in TGA

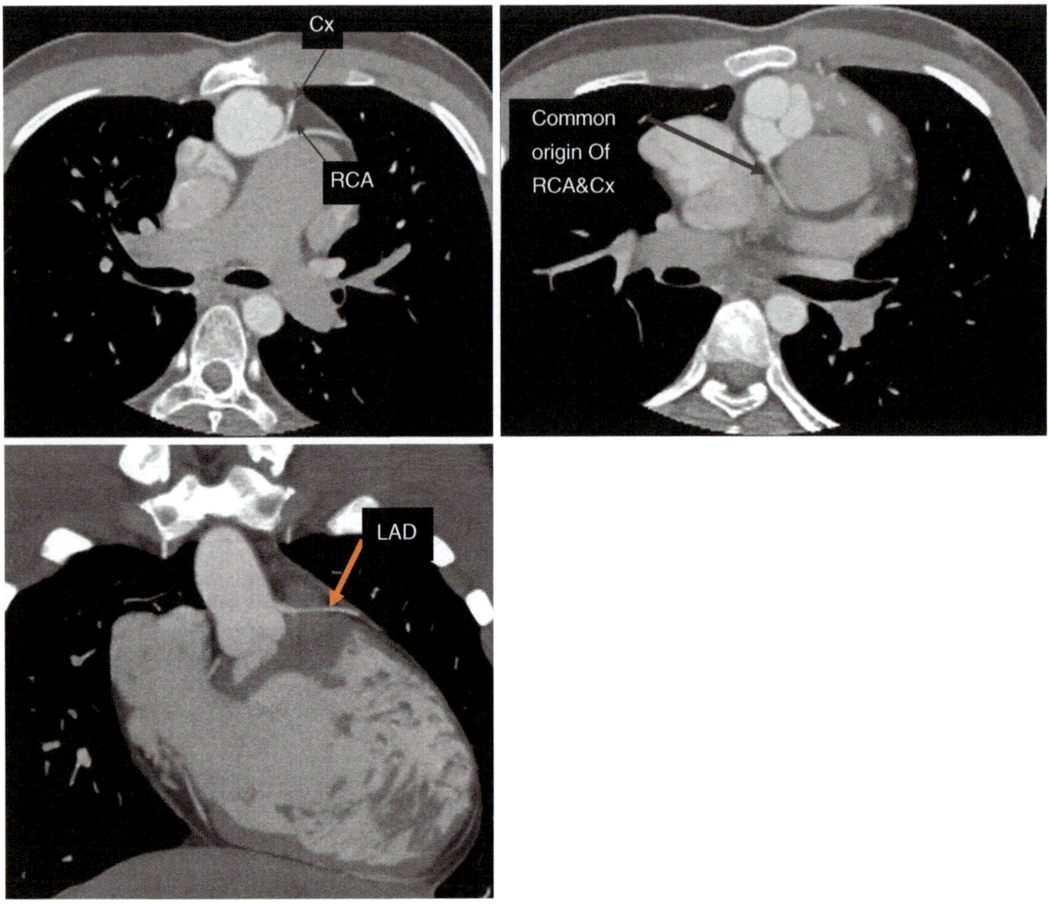

Fig. 16.10 Left-sided cusp of aorta gives rise to LMCA and courses to left as LAD. Posterior cusp gives rise to RCA and LCX, arising from a common origin

16.7 Management of TGA

Newborn with small or restrictive PDA is dealt with by Prostaglandin infusion along with treatment of heart failure. In the case of a small ASD, balloon atrial septostomy (Rashkind) is done.

16.7.1 Surgical Options

Surgical correction for TGA can be done at three different levels [10].

(i) Arterial level

Jatene arterial switch operation (ASO): It is done for TGA in the first 2 weeks of life. It consists of the division of great arteries and isolation of coronary ostia and anastomosing with the neo-aortic root. The pulmonary trunk is taken in front of the aortic trunk by the Lecompte maneuver. The ASO has largely replaced the atrial switch surgery when feasible.

(ii) Atrial level: Mustard/Senning atrial switch procedure

It is palliative and is considered in cases where the time window for the arterial switch has passed (beyond 4 weeks). Also, it is done when relative contraindications of the ASO exist, e.g., when coronary arteries are difficult to transfer. In atrial switch surgery, all pulmonary venous blood is redirected to morphological RV (systemic ventricle) and the systemic venous blood to LV. The Mustard operation uses pericardial or a

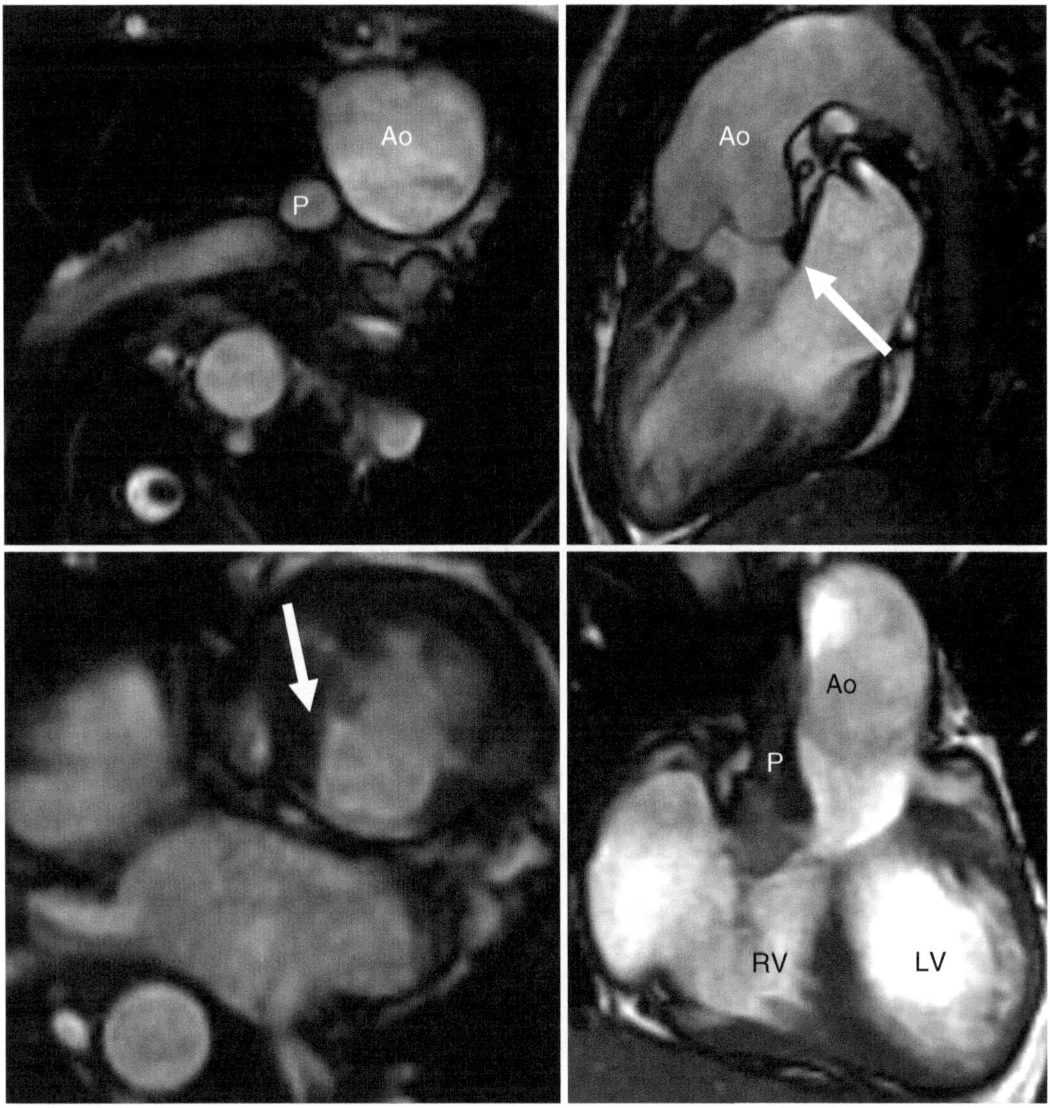

Fig. 16.11 A case of anatomically corrected malposition of great arteries. Images show L posed aorta, subarterial conal tissue (arrow) below both great arteries, but no ventriculo-arterial (VA) discordance. *Ao* aorta; *LV* left ventricle; *P* pulmonary trunk; *RV* right ventricle

prosthetic baffle and Senning operation uses atrial septal flap and the RA free wall to redirect the systemic venous return.

(iii) Ventricular level: Rastelli procedure for TGA with VSD and pulmonary stenosis [11, 12]

Rastelli procedure is done for patients with TGA having left ventricular outflow tract obstruction (which precludes doing an arterial switch operation). The procedure consists of three steps:

1. The main pulmonary artery is ligated above the annulus.
2. Systemic blood is diverted using a conduit through the VSD to the aorta to make the left ventricle to function as the systemic ventricle.

3. A second external conduit is then placed between the right ventricle and the main pulmonary artery.

Restoration of the normal cardiac anatomy with minimal postoperative complications is the current standard of care in congenital heart disease surgery. In this respect, double switch surgery and Nikaidoh procedure gain importance.

Double switch surgery Here systemic and pulmonary blood flow is redirected at atrial level (Senning) along with an arterial switch which entirely corrects the hemodynamics by the appropriate chambers

Nikaidoh Procedure This is an alternative to patients in whom the Rastelli procedure is not feasible, e.g., with multiple/small VSD well away from LVOT, mitral-tricuspid straddling, etc. Here aorta tethered by the coronary arteries is moved posteriorly into the LVOT position. Left ventricular outflow is reconstructed by repositioning of the aortic root and closure of the ventricular septal defect by a patch. The distal segment of the main pulmonary artery is transfixed to the aorta and the right ventricular tract is reconstructed with a pericardial patch.

16.8 Expected Complications of Surgery

Arterial Switch Operation (ASO)

(a) Coronary artery obstruction, which may lead to myocardial ischemia, infarction, and even death, is a serious but rare complication.
(b) Supravalvular pulmonary stenosis at the anastomotic site is the most common cause of repeat surgery.
(c) Neo-aortic root dilatation with valvular regurgitation and supravalvular neo-aortic stenosis are rare.
(d) Origin stenosis of left and right branch pulmonary arteries secondary to tension created by switch or due to differential growth.

Mustard/Senning Atrial Switch Procedure

- Superior vena cava (SVC) baffle obstruction
- Baffle leak
- Arrhythmias (atrial and ventricular)
- Tricuspid valve insufficiency
- RV (systemic ventricular) dysfunction/failure

Rastelli Operation

- Conduit needs replacement as the child grows.
- Conduit obstruction and complete heart block.
- LVOT obstruction occurs at the level of VSD/intraventricular tunnels.

16.9 Imaging in TGA

Chest Skiagram

Heart is egg shaped with a narrow pedicle. The full extend of pedicle is best seen in lateral view. This clinches the diagnosis in plain x-ray. There is associated increased pulmonary blood flow.

Cardiac CT Angiography

Technique: MDCT with a minimum of 64 slice is used. All efforts to reduce radiation dose is done. For non-gated acquisition, use 80 kV for children weighing less than 25 kg. Retrospective gating is reserved only for demonstration of coronary artery and avoid multiphase examinations. Contrast is injected with a dual-head pressure injector and a volume of 1–2 ml/kg is used. A saline chase avoids streak artifact of contrast (Fig. 16.12).

The following points are noted (apart from morphology) in TGA cases which aid in planning surgery:

- Number of coronary arteries: Two coronaries needed for arterial switch [13].
- Assessment of aortic valve plane (Figs. 16.13 and 16.14).
- Sizeable aortic sinus: Size of the aorta to the pulmonary artery needs to be similar.
- Location of VSD: If VSD size is more than aortic sinus, then biventricular repair will be difficult.
- AV valve ratio: Mitral to tricuspid valve ratio should be greater than 2:3.

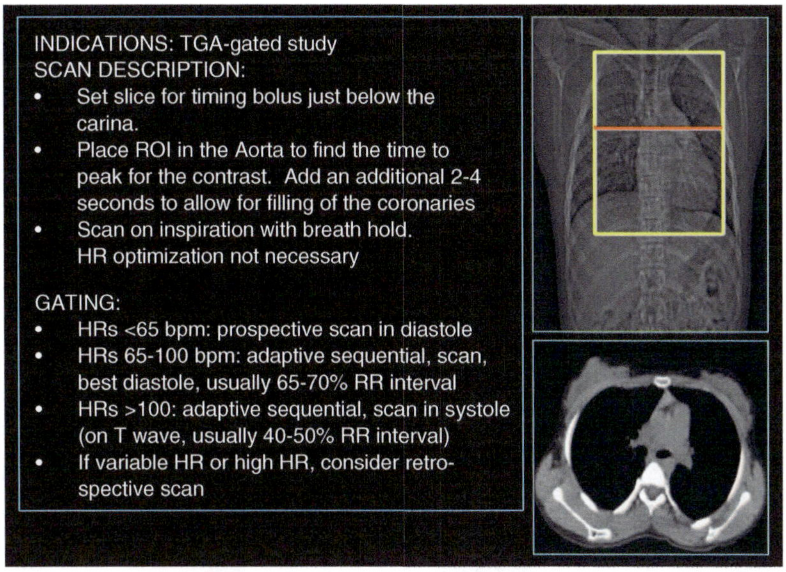

Fig. 16.12 TGA: CT protocols for ECG-gated study

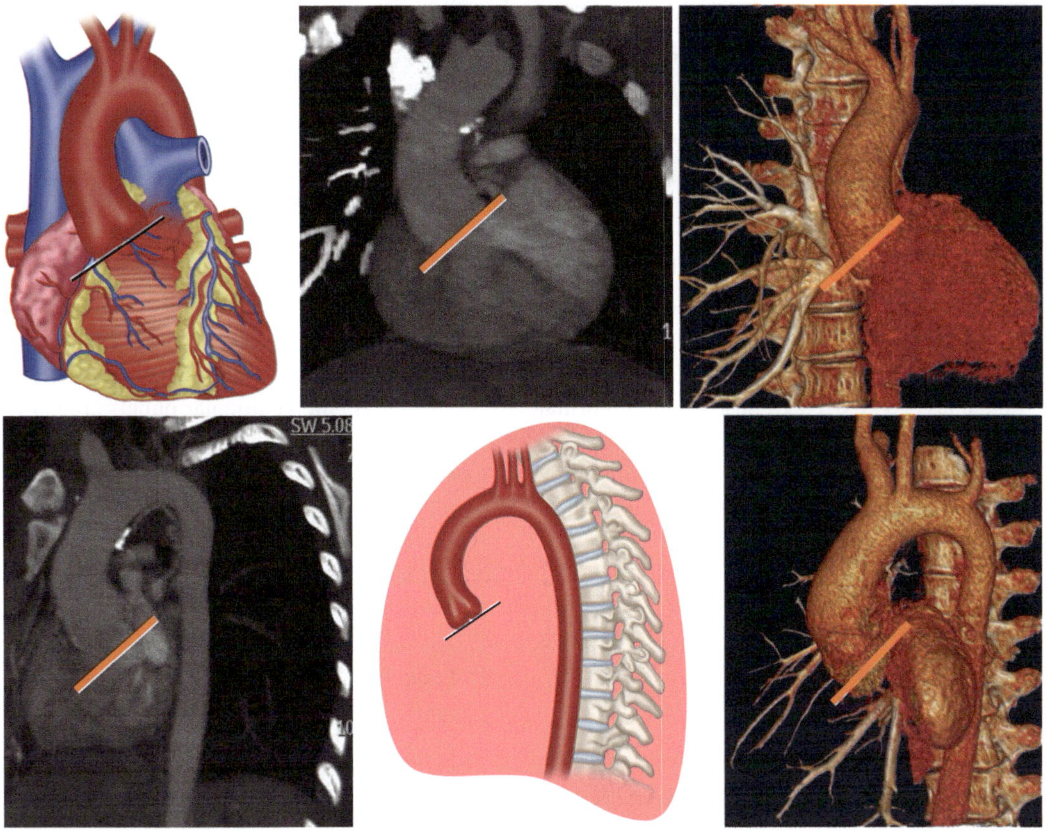

Fig. 16.13 Normal tilt of aortic valve plane

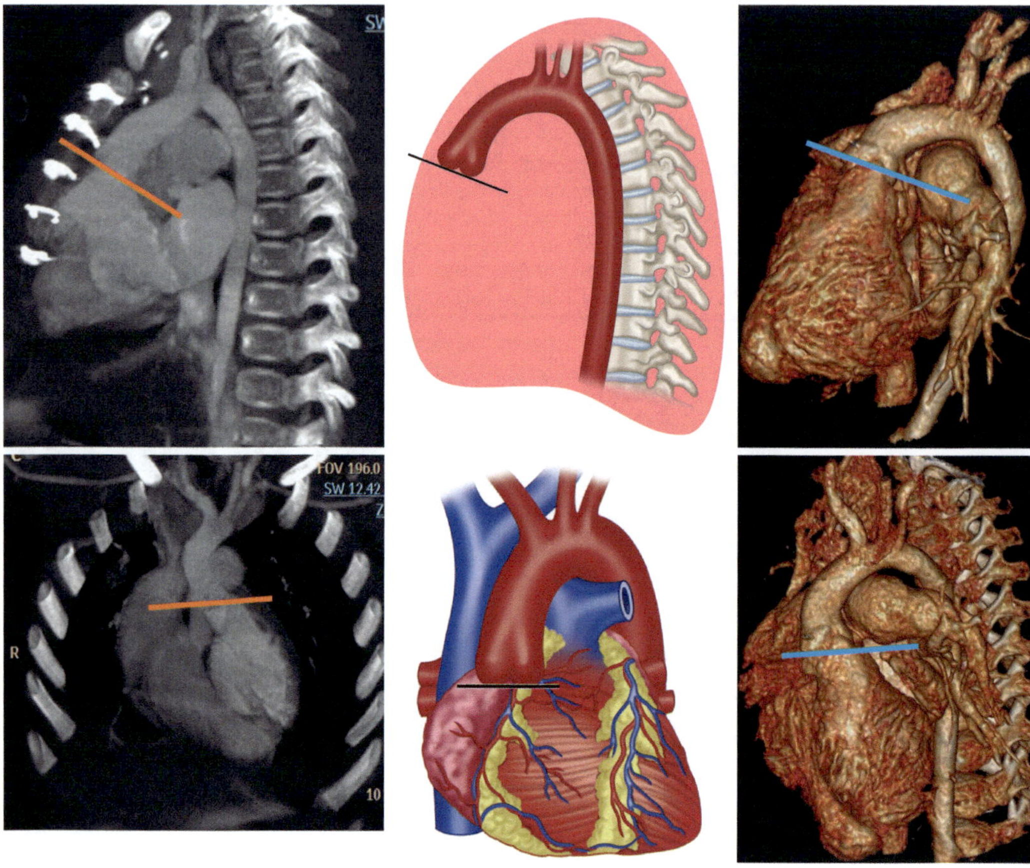

Fig. 16.14 The normal tilt of the aortic valve plane is altered and the aortic valve plane is displaced forward and anteriorly in TGA

- Additional requisites for biventricular repair includes good-sized ventricle, with normal biventricular function and a small VSD.
- Associated abnormalities like pulmonary artery stenosis, major aortopulmonary collateral (MAPCA), and RV aneurysm (Figs. 16.15, 16.16, and 16.17).

CT angiography is also useful in assessing postoperative cases to look at the status of baffles, conduits, and stents (Fig. 16.18).

Cardiac MRI

Complete Transposition of the Great Arteries:

- Axial, coronal, and sagittal sections are taken routinely. Cine images are taken as and when necessary.
- The ventricular chambers have normal relationships. As the ventricular outlets are parallel, the entire septum and arterial valves are seen in the coronal plane.

Congenitally Corrected Transposition of the Great Arteries:

(i) Assess A-V and V-A connections.
(ii) Look for VSD—(usually inlet) and associated AV valve straddling if present. Identify any outflow tract obstruction.
(iii) Integrity of tricuspid valve—Ebstein's malformation (Fig. 16.19).
(iv) Other associated anomalies like dextrocardia, aortic arch hypoplasia/coarctation [14].

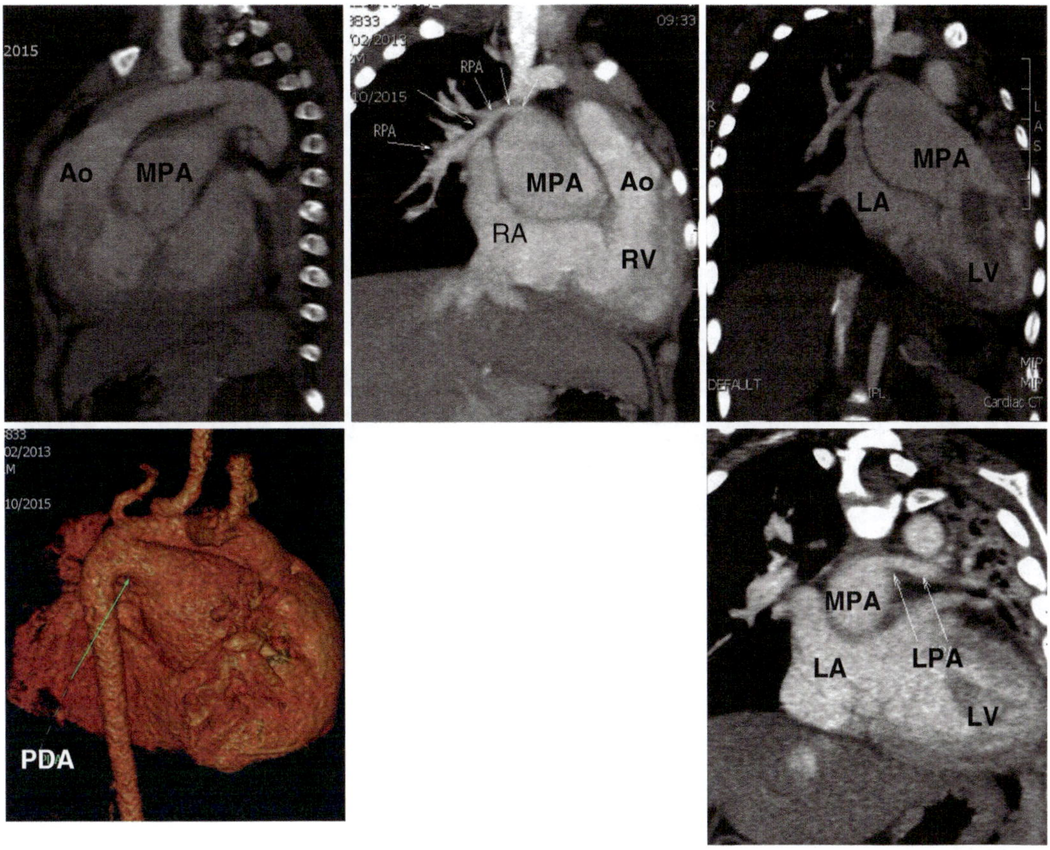

Fig. 16.15 A 2-year-old child with D-TGA and peripheral pulmonary stenosis. *Ao* aorta; *LA* left atrium; *LPA* left pulmonary artery; *LV* left ventricle; *MPA* main pulmonary artery; *PDA* patent ductus arteriosus; *RV* right ventricle

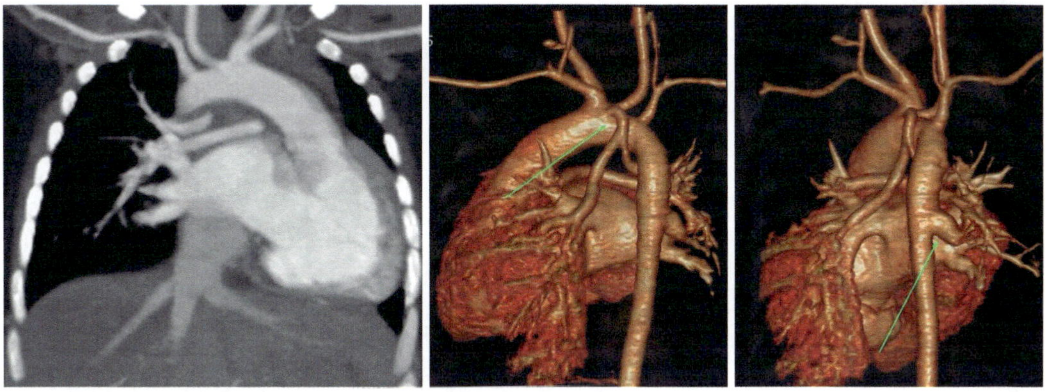

Fig. 16.16 CCTGA with pulmonary atresia and MAPCAs (arrows)

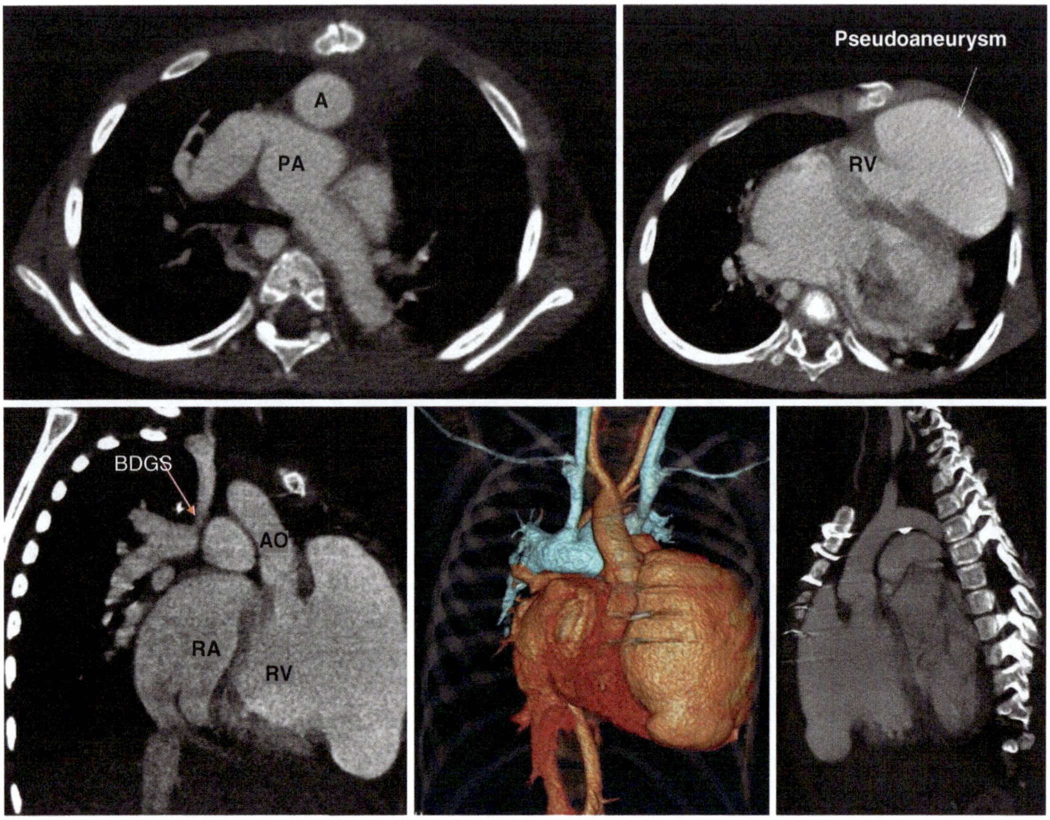

Fig. 16.17 D-TGA: Pseudoaneurysm from RV (Arrow); Bilateral functioning BDGS; RA enlargement. *A* ascending aorta; *LA* left atrium; *P* pulmonary trunk; *RA* right atrium; *RV* right ventricle

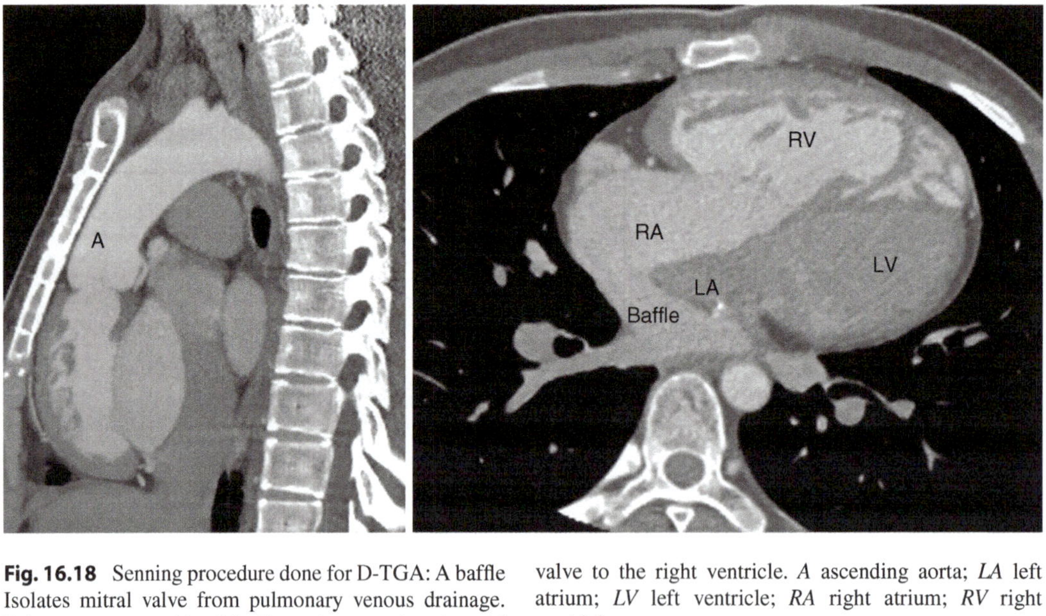

Fig. 16.18 Senning procedure done for D-TGA: A baffle Isolates mitral valve from pulmonary venous drainage. Pulmonary venous blood is diverted across the tricuspid valve to the right ventricle. *A* ascending aorta; *LA* left atrium; *LV* left ventricle; *RA* right atrium; *RV* right ventricle

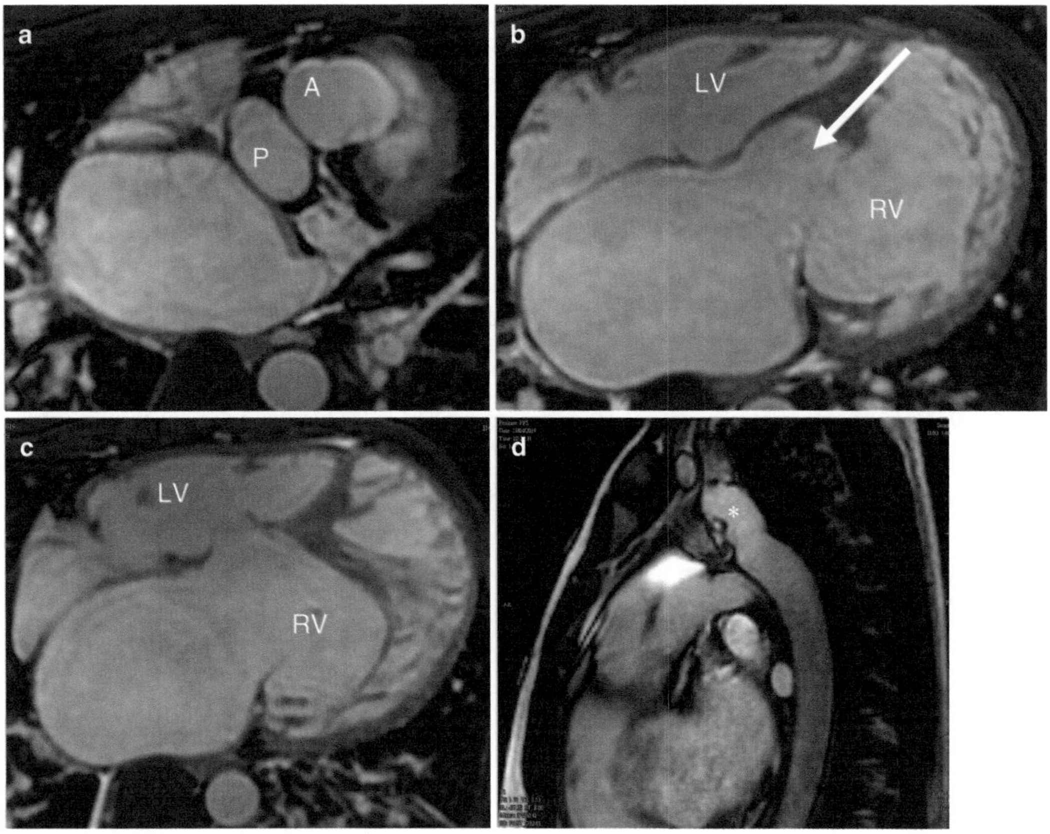

Fig. 16.19 Ebsteinoid malformation of left AV valve in a patient with LTGA showing apically displaced tricuspid valve (arrow in **b**) on the left-sided morphological RV. Note the narrowing of the aorta (*) in **d**. *A* ascending aorta; *LA* left atrium; *LV* left ventricle; *P* pulmonary trunk; *RA* right atrium; *RV* right ventricle

16.10 Postoperative evaluation [15]

16.10.1 Senning and Mustard Repair

To evaluate post-atrial switch by cine MRI, in addition to routine planes, three other views are taken namely (Figs. 16.20, 16.21, 16.22, and 16.23):

(i) Systemic venous baffle view (oblique coronal)
(ii) Pulmonary venous baffle view (oblique axial)
(iii) Ventricular outflow tract views (oblique sagittal)
(iv) TRICKS MR angiography—to assess the sequential filling of the chambers and to demonstrate baffle leak

The following points are to be clarified in an MRI scan:

(i) Ventricular function, volumes and RV mass, valvular leak especially tricuspid valve.
(ii) Patency of systemic and pulmonary venous pathways and degree of obstruction if any (Fig. 16.24).
(iii) The degree of obstruction in the above pathways can be quantified with in-plane phase-contrast (PC) MRI—velocity more than 100 cm/s suggests significant obstruction. Continuous flow pattern without phasic variation also suggests significant obstruction (Fig. 16.25). Diastolic flow reversal in the ipsilateral artery (without pulmonary regurgitation) and continuous flow in the

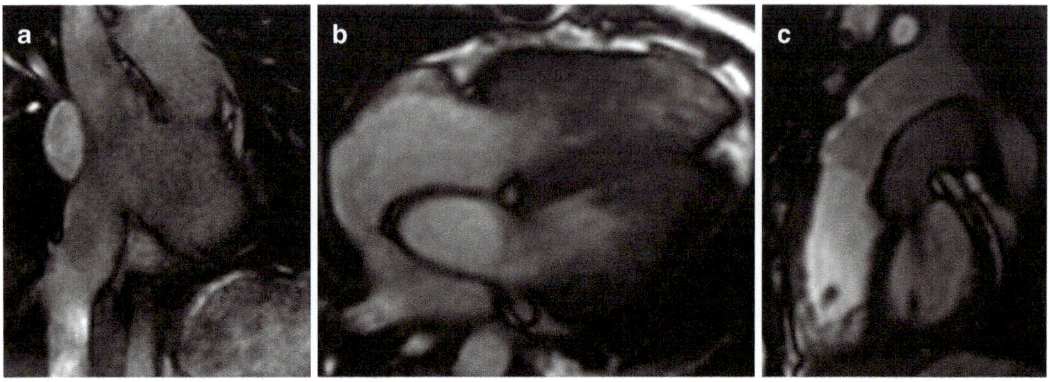

Fig. 16.20 Three unique views taken to evaluate post atrial redirection surgery. (**a**) Shows systemic venous baffle with SVC and IVC venous blood redirected into the mitral valve. (**b**) Shows pulmonary venous baffle redirecting the flow to the tricuspid valve. (**c**) Shows a parallel outflow view to demonstrate pulmonary obstruction. (Ref to Videos 16.43, 16.44, 16.45, 16.46, 16.47, 16.48, 16.49, 16.50, 16.51, and 16.52)

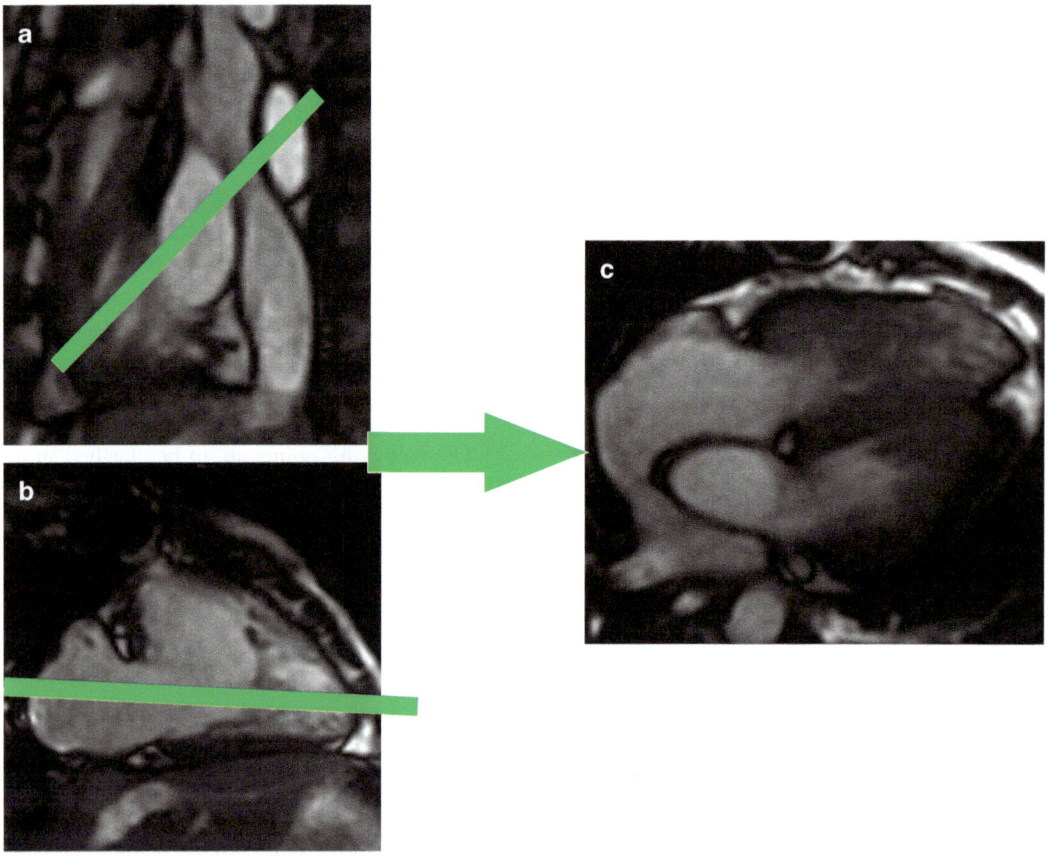

Fig. 16.21 Planning for pulmonary venous baffle. On true sagittal image (**a**), the plane should go through dumbbell shape pulmonary venous baffle. On RV two-chamber view (**b**), plan like four-chamber view

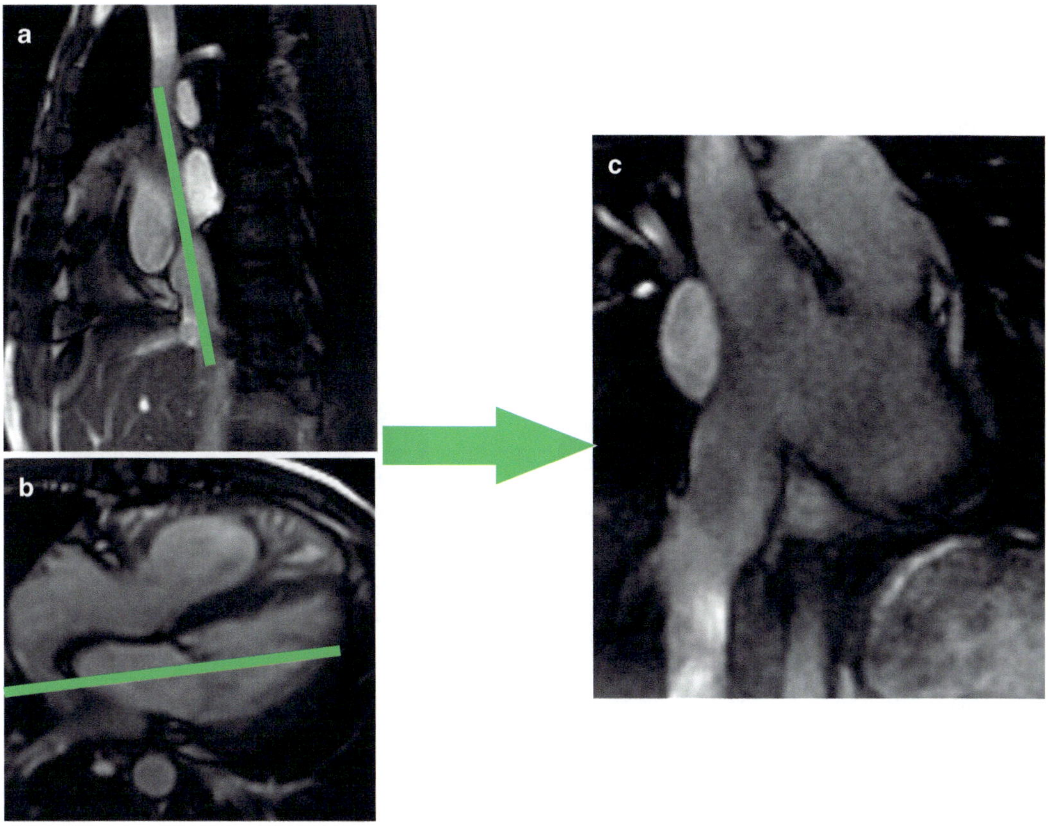

Fig. 16.22 Planning for systemic venous baffle. On true sagittal image (**a**), the scan plane will go through SVC and IVC. On true axial image (**b**), it will go through the mitral valve

contralateral pulmonary artery may be seen in severe pulmonary venous baffle obstruction [16].

(iv) Atrial baffles leak if any with a degree of leak.

(v) Look for secondary azygous vein dilatation if there is baffle obstruction. Using PC MRI flow direction in the dilated azygos vein, the site of obstruction can be suspected. Upward flow may suggest IVC baffle obstruction and downward flow suggests SVC baffle stenosis.

(vi) Assess the ventricular volumes, mass especially in cases of increased systemic pressures.

(vii) Perform LGE to assess ventricular fibrosis/scar.

Practical Pearls

Findings to be assessed in each view of post-Sennings surgery:

- Systemic venous baffle view—obstruction/leak
- Pulmonary venous baffle view—obstruction/leak
- Outflow view—LVOT obstruction and pulmonary stenosis, aortic regurgitation

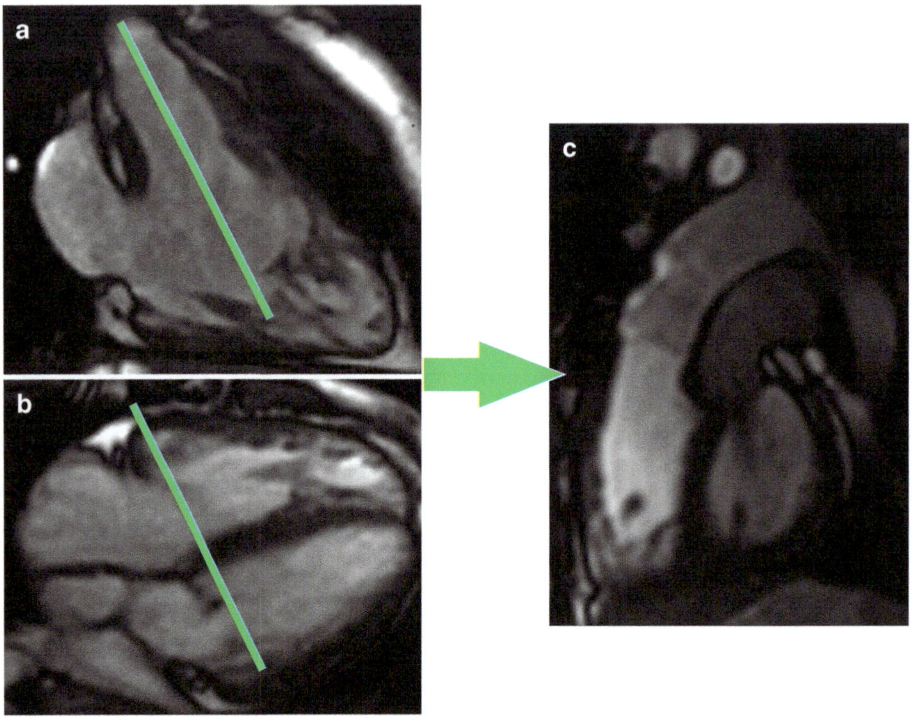

Fig. 16.23 Planning for ventricular outflow view. From RV three-chamber view (**a**), the scan plane extends along the long axis of aorta. On the four-chamber view (**b**), it will pass perpendicular to interventricular septum

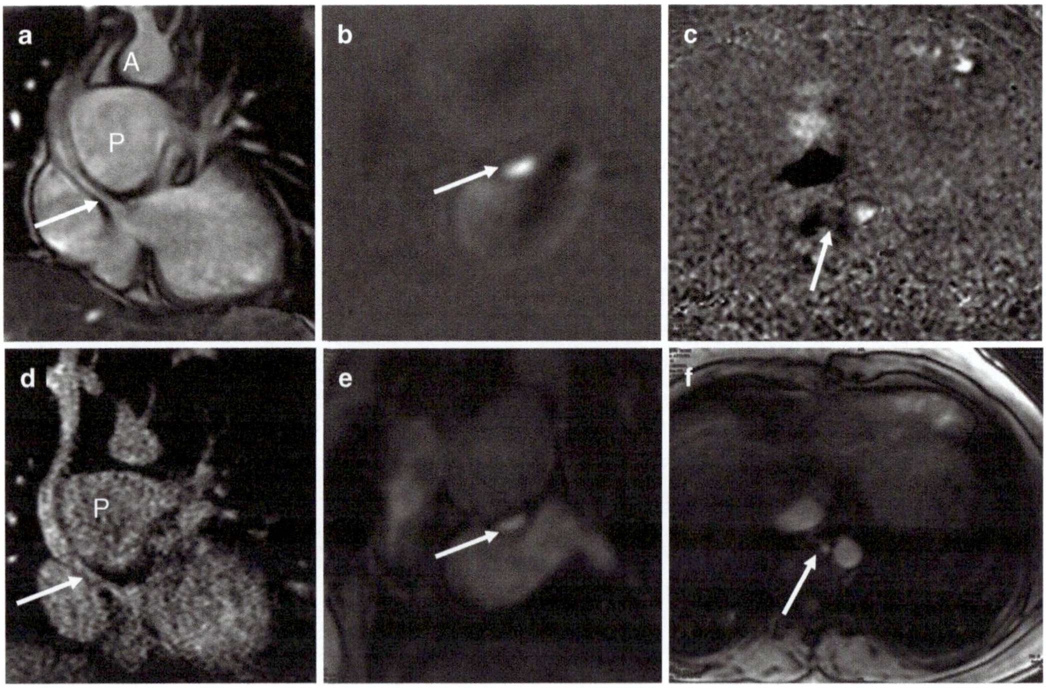

Fig. 16.24 Status post Senning surgery. Coronal oblique SSFP (**a**), MRA (**d**) show SVC baffle obstruction (arrow in **a**, **d**) due to dilated MPA. Phase-contrast MRI through the obstruction (arrow in **b**, **e**) shows low-velocity jet. Normal caudocranial azygos flow noted (arrow in **c**, **f**) suggesting low level stenosis

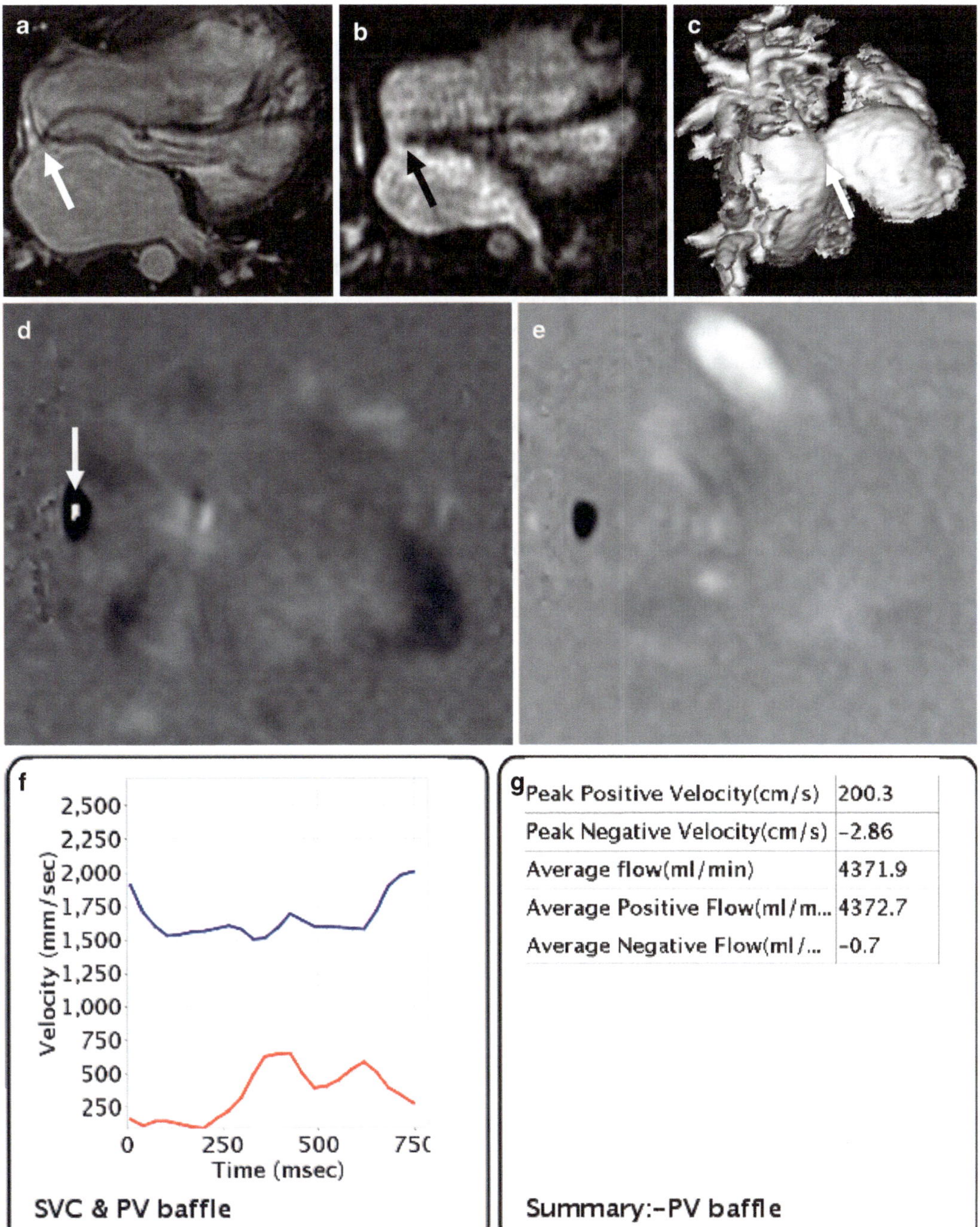

Fig. 16.25 Pulmonary venous baffle obstruction following atrial switch operation. (**a**) SSFP cine image demonstrates the stenotic jet. Axial MIP (**b**) and VRT (**c**) MRA show tight stenosis at pulmonary venous baffle. (**d**) Phase-contrast MRI shows aliasing artifact (arrow) at 150 cm/s and corrected at 200 cm/s (**e**). (**f**) shows the continuous flow pattern (blue tracing) in the pulmonary venous baffle compared to normal phasic variation in the SVC baffle (red tracing). Peak velocity recorded at pulmonary venous baffle was 200 cm/s suggesting significant stenosis

- Four-chamber view—RV dilatation, tricuspid regurgitation
- Short-axis view—biventricular function
- Multislice stack axial, coronal and sagittal—overview of all

16.10.2 Arterial Switch Operation

(i) Look for any RVOT obstruction and neo-pulmonary valve/aortic valve stenosis or supravalvar surgical suture site stenosis.
(ii) Right ventricular dysfunction lead to secondary tricuspid annular dilatation and valve regurgitation. MRI can be used to measure regurgitant fraction and RV volumes.
(iii) Look for any branch distortion of pulmonary arteries following the Le Compte procedure (Fig. 16.26). Quantify proportional flow in branch PAs.
(iv) Studies have shown that detection of branch pulmonary artery stenosis in ASO patients by CMR is accurate and superior to the information obtained by echocardiography [17].
(v) Look for dilatation of ascending aorta at the site of coronary button transfer (Fig. 16.27).
(vi) Look for ventricular function, volumes, and RV mass.
(vii) Assess coronary arteries—ostial stenosis, proximal kinking, and subsequent ventricular dysfunction or infarction. There are two principal CMR techniques to diagnose inducible coronary artery ischemia: (1) Contrast-enhanced stress perfusion study using vasodilator stress agents like adenosine and (2) evaluation for inducible regional wall motion abnormalities using dobutamine stress MRI [18].

16.10.3 Rastelli Operation

(i) Look for RV-PA conduit—stenosis and valve regurgitation if present (Fig. 16.28).
(ii) Look for branch pulmonary arteries stenosis.
(iii) Look for LVOT obstruction—ostium secondum VSD and/or VSD tunnel becoming restrictive.
(iv) Look for the integrity of the VSD patch.
(v) Assess ventricular function, volumes, and mass.

16.10.4 Double Switch Surgery

The standard surgical approach to CCTGA is basically to treat the individual-associated abnormalities, such as repair of AV valve, relief of pulmonary stenosis by repair or conduit (Videos 16.56, 16.57, 16.58, and 16.59), and closure of a ventricular septal defect [19]. In spite of correcting these associated anomalies, the right ventricle may fail after a standard surgery because it supports the systemic circulation.

More recent surgical approaches for CCTGA have focused on the so-called "anatomic" repairs by double switch procedure which return the LV to the systemic circulation and may, therefore, result in improved long-term prognosis [20]. The double switch operation consists of:

1. Senning atrial baffle procedure—To redirect systemic and pulmonary venous blood flow at the atrial level.
2. Arterial switch procedure—To redirect LV blood to aorta and RV blood to the pulmonary artery.

When CCTGA is associated with a ventricular septal defect and pulmonary outflow tract obstruction, an atrial switch operation can be combined with a Rastelli-type of operation, which is called an Ilbawi operation (Figs. 16.29 and 16.30) (Videos 16.60, 16.61, 16.62, 16.63, 16.64, 16.65, and 16.66) [21, 22].

16.10.5 Nikaidoh Procedure

This complex procedure is also known as aortic translocation. It is performed to avoid late obstruction of the baffled LV outflow tract that can occur after the Rastelli operation. The Nikaidoh procedure involves the division of the small posterior pulmonary annulus and

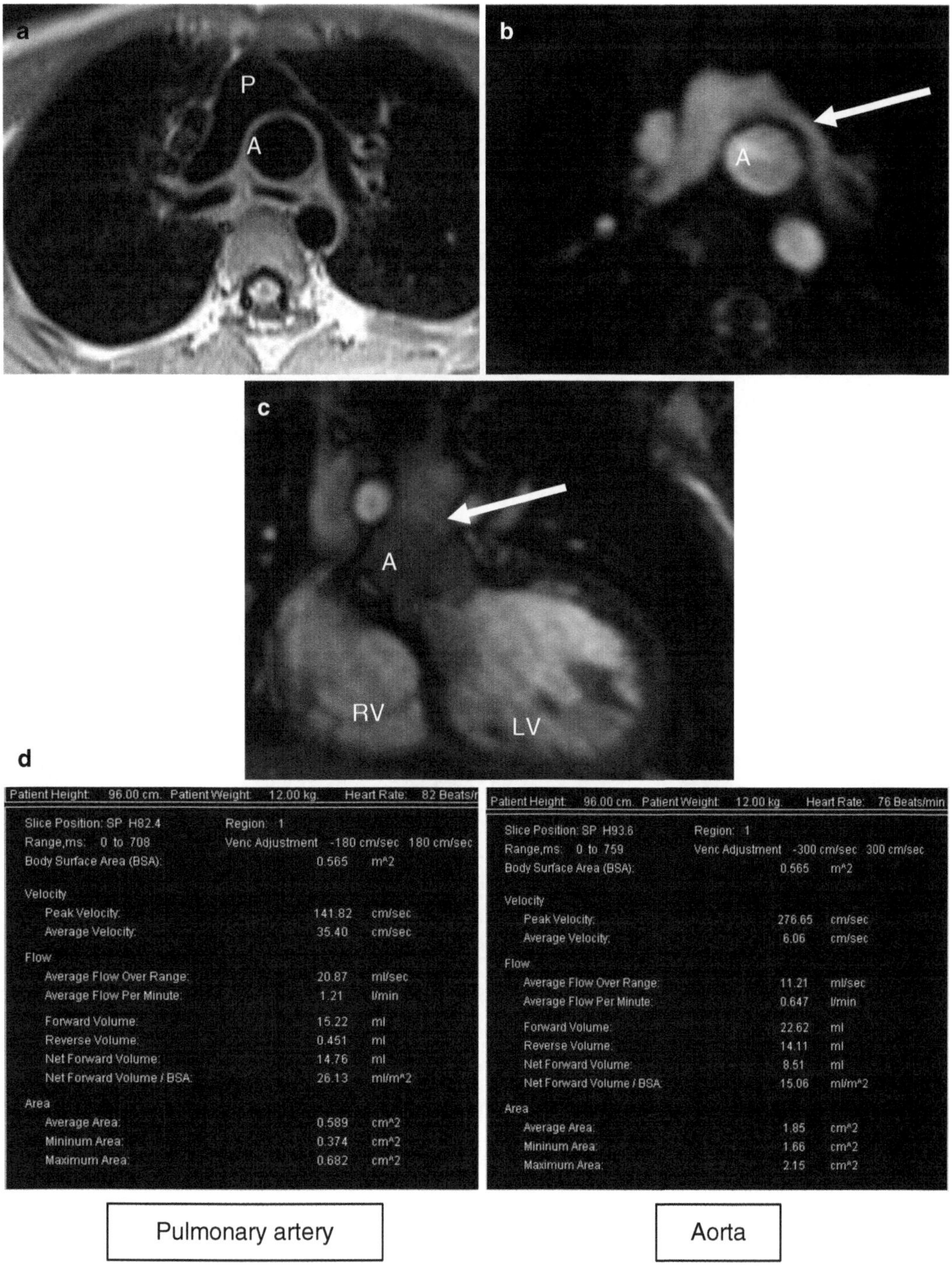

Fig. 16.26 A 3-year-old child with D-TGA, VSD-closure, post arterial switch (Lecompte maneuver), now having diffuse LPA stenosis (arrow in **b**) and narrowing of the aorta (arrow in **c**). (**d**) Phase-contrast flow assessment shows: neo-aortic flow = PSV 2.7 m/s, Volume—0.65 L/min, AR—60%. Neo PA flow = PSV 1.41 m/s, Volume—1.2 L/min. No PR. *A* ascending aorta; *LV* left ventricle; *P* pulmonary trunk; *RV* right ventricle (Ref to Videos 16.53, 16.54, and 16.55)

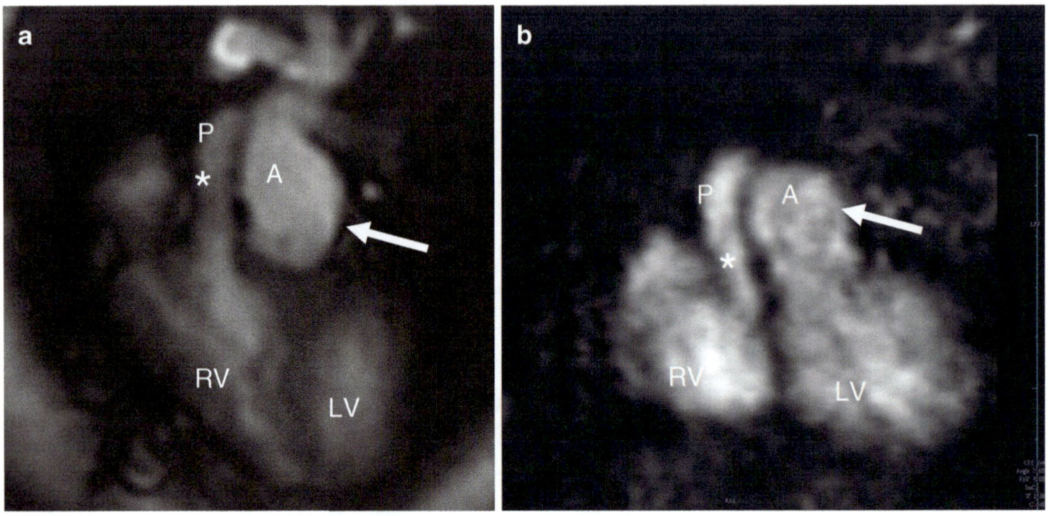

Fig. 16.27 Outflow views of SSFP (**a**) and MRA (**b**) after arterial switch surgery show right ventricular outflow obstruction (*) and neo-aortic root dilatation (arrow). *A* ascending aorta; *LV* left ventricle; *P* pulmonary trunk; *RV* right ventricle

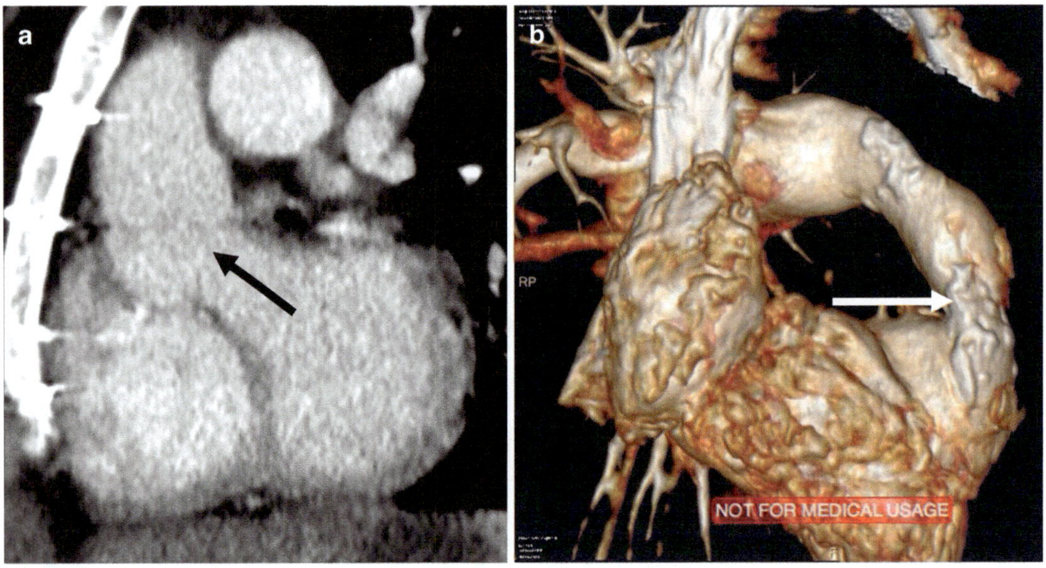

Fig. 16.28 A case of CTGA with VSD and pulmonary stenosis—status post intraventricular tunneling and Rastelli surgery. CT shows widely patent LV to aorta tunnel (arrow in **a**) and RV to PA conduit stenosis (arrow in **b**)

mobilization of the aortic root, which is moved to the open pulmonary annulus, thus bringing it closer to the left ventricle. The coronary artery translocation may be needed to avoid kinking, and the VSD is closed with a patch. A conduit is placed from the right ventricle to the pulmonary artery. The benefit of the Nikaidoh procedure is that it potentially avoids the development of subaortic obstruction seen with Rastelli surgery [23, 24].

A residual VSD is common after the Nikaidoh procedure because of the complex baffle positioning (Videos 16.67, 16.68, 16.69, 16.70, 16.71, 16.72, 16.73, and 16.74).

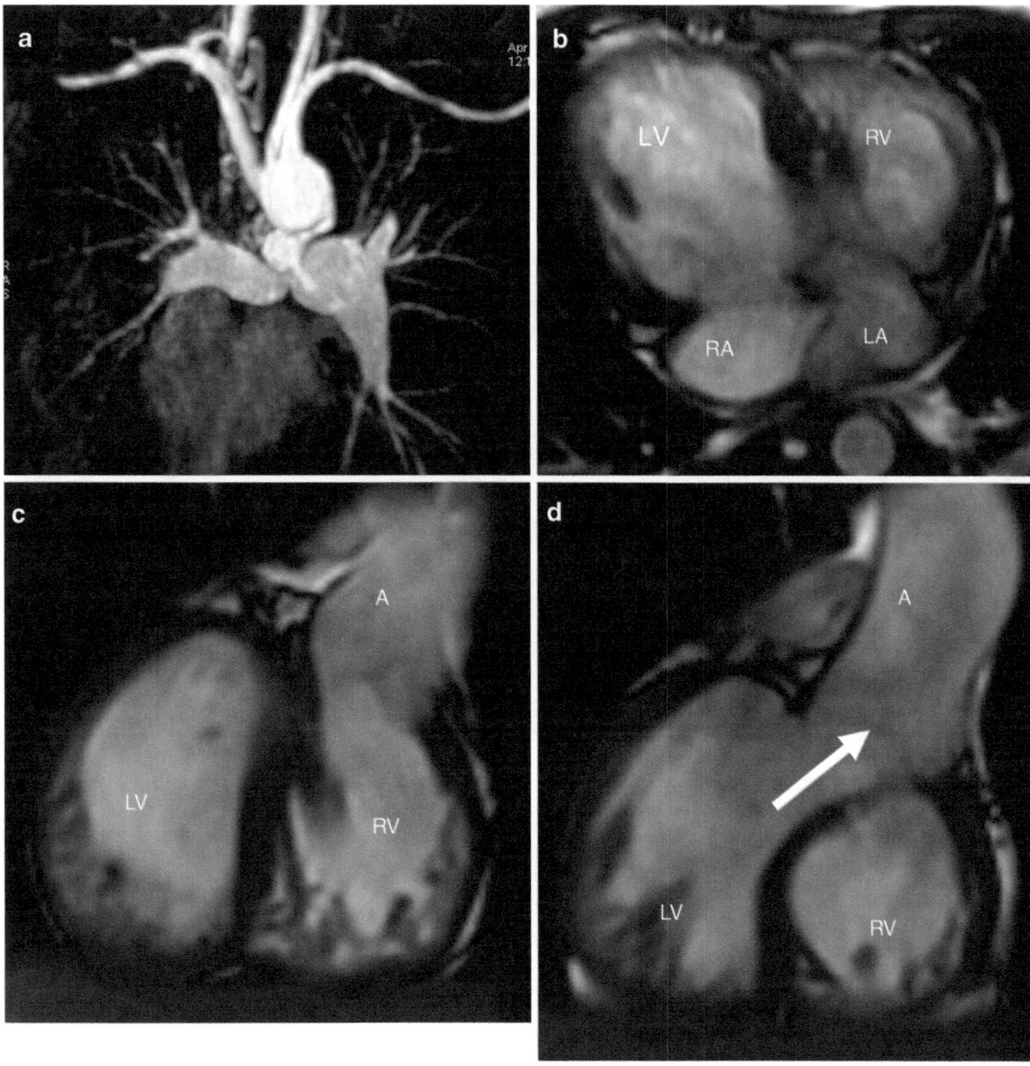

Fig. 16.29 A case of congenitally corrected TGA with pulmonary atresia. MRA reconstructed image (**a**) shows the confluent pulmonary arteries supplied by a stenotic PDA. Axial SSFP (**b**) shows mesocardia with L loop ventricles and atrioventricular discordance. Outflow views show the aorta arising from left-sided RV (**c**) with clear LV to aorta pathway through VSD (arrow in **d**). *A* ascending aorta; *LA* left atrium; *LV* left ventricle; *RA* right atrium; *RV* right ventricle (Ref to Videos 16.60, 16.61, 16.62, 16.63, 16.64, 16.65, and 16.66)

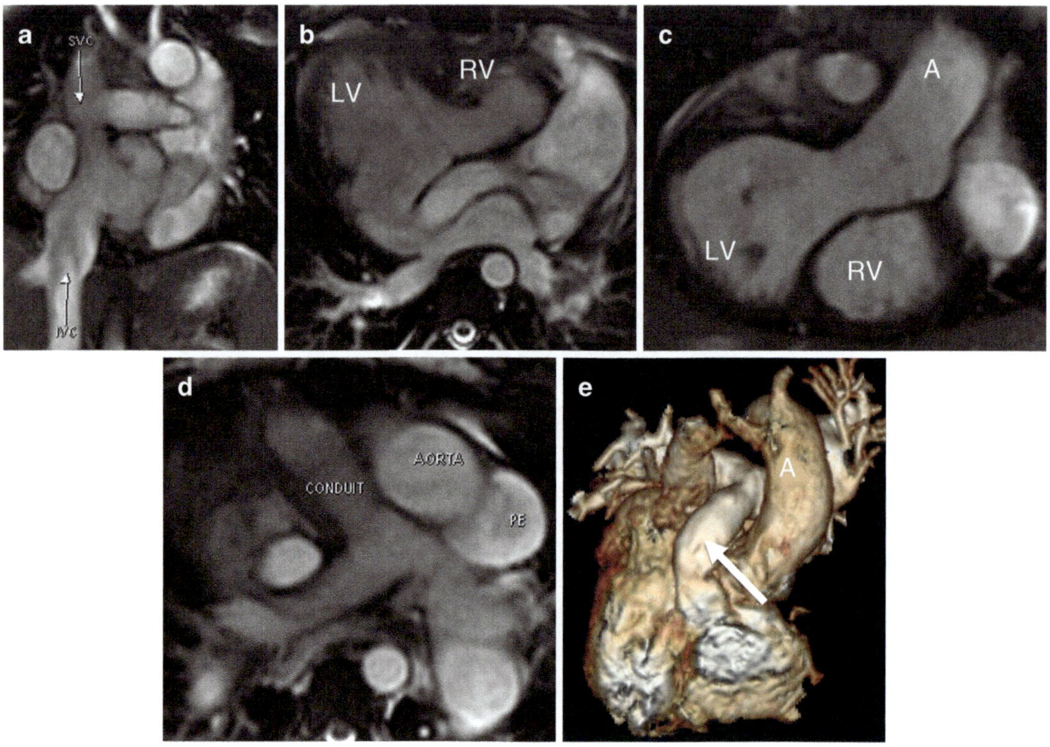

Fig. 16.30 Double switch for the patient shown in Fig. 16.29. Both SVC and IVC blood is redirected to left-sided RV (**a**). (**b**) Shows the pulmonary venous blood redirected to right-sided LV. (**c**) Demonstrate the LV to aorta tunnel with closure of VSD. (**d**, **e**) Show RV to PA conduit (arrow in **e**). *A* ascending aorta; *LV* left ventricle; *P* pulmonary trunk; *RV* right ventricle (Ref to Videos 16.60, 16.61, 16.62, 16.63, 16.64, 16.65, and 16.66)

16.11 Comparison Between Cardiac CT Versus Cardiac MRI

The examination time is prolonged in MRI with associated general anesthesia. Hence, in critically ill children, CT scan is preferred with shorter examination time and anesthesia. Also, postoperative cases with sternal wires, pacemakers precludes the clear delineation of coronary artery and retrosternal structures by MRI in which case CT scan is preferred. Presently MRI scan is also is capable of showing the retrosternal anatomy well [25]. Functional assessment like flow quantification, valve assessment, RV volume, is best carried out in MRI. The mediastinum, lungs, and airways are best assessed by CT scan (See Table 16.1)

Practical Tips

1. Just as in any other cardiac imaging, understand the need for imaging. Echocardiography remains the mainstay in the diagnosis of TGA. Routability of VSD when in doubt or when flow quantification and valve assessment is required, then MRI is the modality of choice.
2. Postoperative evaluation in Mustard/Senning surgeries are best done by MRI. This includes baffle anatomy, ventricular function, flow in AV valves and semilunar valves, and evidence of ischemia in delayed contrast enhancement.

Table 16.1 Comparison between cardiac CT and cardiac MRI in TGA

Parameters	Cardiac CT	Cardiac MRI
Examination time	Very short	Prolonged
Require for general anesthesia	Optional	Mandatory
Spatial resolution (mm)	0.4–0.6	1.0–2.0
Temporal resolution (ms)	90–180	20–50
Intracardiac anatomy	Inferior	Superior
Mediastinum, lungs and airways, calcification	Superior	Inferior

References

1. Robert H, Anderson SW, Brown NA, et al. Development of the heart: formation of the ventricular outflow tracts, arterial valves, and intrapericardial arterial trunks. Heart. 2003;89:1110–8.
2. Lin C-J, Lin C-Y, Chen C-H, et al. Partitioning the heart: mechanisms of cardiac septation and valve development. Development. 2012;139:3277–99.
3. Van Praagh R. The importance of segmental situs in the diagnosis of congenital heart disease. Semin Roemgenol. 1985;20(3):254–71.
4. Freedom RM, Culham G, Rowe RD. The criss-cross heart and superoinferior ventricular heart, an angiographic study. Am J Cardiol. 1978;42:620–8.
5. Yacoub M, Radley-Smith R. Anatomy of the coronary arteries in transposition of the great arteries and methods for their transfer in anatomical correction. Thorax. 1978;33:418–24.
6. da Cruz EM. Paediatric and congenital cardiology, cardiac surgery and intensive care, vol. 4. New York: Springer; 2014.
7. Chan FP, Ho VB, Reddy GP. Transposition of great arteries: cardiovascular imaging. St. Louis: Elsevier/Saunders; 2011.
8. Cavalle-Garrido T, Bernasconi A, Perrin D, Anderson RH. Hearts with concordant ventriculoarterial connections but parallel arterial trunks. Heart. 2007;93:100–6.
9. Anderson RH, et al. Paediatric cardiology. London: Churchill Livingstone; 1987.
10. Castafieda AR, et al. Cardiac surgery of the neonate and infant. Philadelphia: WB Saunders; 1994.
11. Rastelli GC, McGoon DC, Wallace RB. Anatomic correction of transposition of the great arteries with ventricular septal defect and subpulmonary stenosis. J Thorac Cardiovasc Surg. 1969;58(4):545–52.
12. Bautista-Hernandez V, Marx GR, Bacha EA, del Nido PJ. Aortic root translocation plus arterial switch for transposition of the great arteries with left ventricular outflow tract obstruction: intermediate-term results. J Am Coll Cardiol. 2007;49(4):485–90.
13. Young PM, Gerber TC, Williamson EE, et al. Normal, variant, and anomalous configurations of the coronary vasculature. AJR. 2011;197:816–26.
14. Lundstrom U, Bull C, Wyse RKH, Somerville J. The natural and unnatural history of congenitally corrected transposition. Am J Cardiol. 1990;65:1222–9.
15. Gaca AM, Jaggers JJ, Dudley LT, Bisset GS. Repair of congenital heart disease: a primer—part 1 and 2. Radiology. 2008;247(3):617–31.
16. Matthews CE, Hussain T, Miles C, et al. Left-sided pulmonary venous pathway obstruction after mustard operation. Congenit Heart Dis. 2013;8(1):66–70.
17. Blakenberg F, Rhee J, Hardy C, Helton G, Higgins SS, Higgins CB. MRI vs echocardiography in the evaluation of the Jatene procedure. J Comput Assist Tomogr. 1994;18:749–54.
18. Tobler D, Motwani M, Wald RM, Roche SL, Verocai F, Iwanochko RM, et al. Evaluation of a comprehensive cardiovascular magnetic resonance protocol in young adults late after the arterial switch operation for d-transposition of the great arteries. J Cardiovasc Magn Reson. 2014;16:98.
19. Hornung TS, Calder L. Congenital heart disease: congenitally corrected transposition of the great arteries. Heart. 2010;96:1154–61. https://doi.org/10.1136/hrt.2008.150532.
20. Imai Y, Sawatari K, Hoshino S, Ishihara K, Nakazawa M, Momma K. Ventricular function after anatomic repair in patients with atrioventricular discordance. J Thorac Cardiovasc Surg. 1994;107(5):1272–83.
21. Ilbawi MN, DeLeon SY, Backer CL, et al. An alternative approach to the surgical management of physiologically corrected transposition with ventricular septal defect and pulmonary stenosis or atresia. J Thorac Cardiovasc Surg. 1990;100(3):410–5.
22. Hörer J, Haas F, Cleuziou J, et al. Intermediate-term results of the Senning or Mustard procedures combined with the Rastelli operation for patients with discordant atrioventricular connections associated with discordant ventriculoarterial connections or double outlet right ventricle. Cardiol Young. 2007;17(2):158–65.
23. Nikaidoh H. Aortic translocation and biventricular outflow tract reconstruction. A new surgical repair for transposition of the great arteries associated with ventricular septal defect and pulmonary stenosis. J Thorac Cardiovasc Surg. 1984;88:365–72.
24. Cohen MS, Eidem BW, Cetta F, et al. Multimodality imaging guidelines of patients with transposition of the great arteries: a report from the American Society of Echocardiography Developed in Collaboration with the Society for Cardiovascular Magnetic Resonance and the Society of Cardiovascular Computed Tomography. J Am Soc Echocardiogr. 2016;29:571–621.
25. Zahr RA, Gooty V, et al. Feasibility of real-time cine cardiac magnetic resonance imaging to predict the presence of significant retrosternal adhesions prior to redo-sternotomy. J Cardiovasc Magn Reson. 2019;21:67.

17 Imaging of Single Ventricle

Johann Christopher, Sudeep Verma, and Ramiah Rajeshkannan

17.1 Introduction

In a broad sense, any congenital heart condition with only one functional ventricular chamber can be included under the term single ventricle. Nearly 10% of the congenital heart defect belong to the group of functionally univentricular heart. Most often it refers to an interventricular septum being absent or rudimentary. It can be either a double inlet or double outlet type of ventricle with restricted or unprotected pulmonary blood flow. There is a wide array of diseases that are included under the banner of single ventricle including tricuspid atresia, mitral atresia and double inlet ventricles. All the lesions where atrioventricular (AV) connection is completely or predominantly committed to a single ventricular connection is generally referred to as a univentricular or single ventricle heart.

The operational viewpoint is that only one ventricular chamber is available for the support of the circulation. Most of these conditions are treated with multistage shunt surgeries. In the initial neonatal period, the shunt has to be high pressure (systemic arterial to pulmonary artery) later a low pressure (superior systemic bidirectional Glenn (BDG)) source is connected to pulmonary arteries. In the later stage, there is a complete systemic venous to pulmonary circulation (Fontan). This modification was initially discovered in the 1960s and has undergone multiple modifications to get to its present state today.

17.2 Evolution of Concept of Single Ventricle

The concept of univentricular heart has changed from a heart with only one ventricle committed to an atrium to any heart where the ventricles are unable to sustain in series separate pulmonary and systemic circulations. This definition now also includes lesions like mitral or tricuspid atresia, severe pulmonary/aortic stenosis with hypoplastic ventricle, large intracardiac tumours, severe Ebsteins with large atrialised RV and small functional RV which were traditionally not included in univentricular heart, and now referred to as functionally univentricular heart [1]. In functionally univentricular hearts, systemic circulation is supported by only one ventricle, and the other ventricle if present is nonfunctional by virtue of its small size and inadequate function. It is generally agreed that the atrioventricular (AV) connection is central in defining the univentricular heart.

Electronic Supplementary Material The online version of this chapter (https://doi.org/10.1007/978-981-15-6755-1_17) contains supplementary material, which is available to authorized users.

J. Christopher (✉) · S. Verma
CARE Hospitals, Hyderabad, India

R. Rajeshkannan
Department of Radiology, Amrita School of Medicine, Amrita Institute of Medical Sciences and Research Centre, Amrita Vishwa Vidyapeetham, Kochi, Kerala, India

R. Rajeshkannan et al. (eds.), *CT and MRI in Congenital Heart Diseases*,
https://doi.org/10.1007/978-981-15-6755-1_17

A "single ventricle" was characterised as lacking two well-developed ventricles, which thereby excluded hearts with inadequate septum but well-formed ventricles. Disorder of lateralisation (Heterotaxy syndromes) is the disorder where single ventricles are often seen.

17.3 Classification

17.3.1 True Univentricular Heart

Heart with one large and one hypoplastic ventricular chamber. Such hearts are usually the consequence of univentricular AV connection—double inlet left ventricle (DILV), double inlet right ventricle (DIRV), double inlet ventricle of indeterminate anatomy or absent AV connection (Figs. 17.1, 17.2, and 17.3).

17.3.2 Functionally Univentricular Heart

Normal AV and VA connection and presence of both inflow and outflow portion, but one of the chambers is unable to sustain the pulmonary or systemic circulation, e.g. pulmonary atresia-intact ventricular septum (Fig. 17.4), aortic atresia, severe aortic/pulmonary stenosis with small respective ventricles, a severe form of Ebstein, large intraventricular tumour.

17.4 Physiology of Univentricular Hearts

Physiology of the univentricular heart depends on such key determinants as an obstruction to outflow, inflow and/or flow across the atrial septum; systemic and pulmonary venous return; pulmonary vascular resistance; and AV valve regurgitation.

In the presence of systemic or pulmonary circulation obstruction—ratio of flow into the unobstructed circulation and obstructed vascular bed depends upon the relative resistance across both vascular beds [2, 3].

Systemic circulation obstruction: In significant PDA dependent circulation with R to L shunt and flow depends upon the resistance in both vascular beds. Patients present with shock, acidosis and poor pulses (e.g. Mitral atresia).

Pulmonary circulation obstruction: In significant PDA dependent L to R shunt with a presentation more with cyanosis and later acidosis (e.g. pulmonary atresia-intact ventricular septum, hypoplastic right heart syndrome).

Pulmonary venous obstruction: Presents in two ways. First direct obstruction to the pulmonary venous outflow in the form of venous stenosis with or without total anomalous pulmonary venous connection (TAPVC). Secondly, obstruction at the AV valve level as seen with mitral stenosis/atresia with restrictive ASD.

Systemic venous obstruction: Restrictive ASD (e.g. Tricuspid atresia) in the absence of unob-

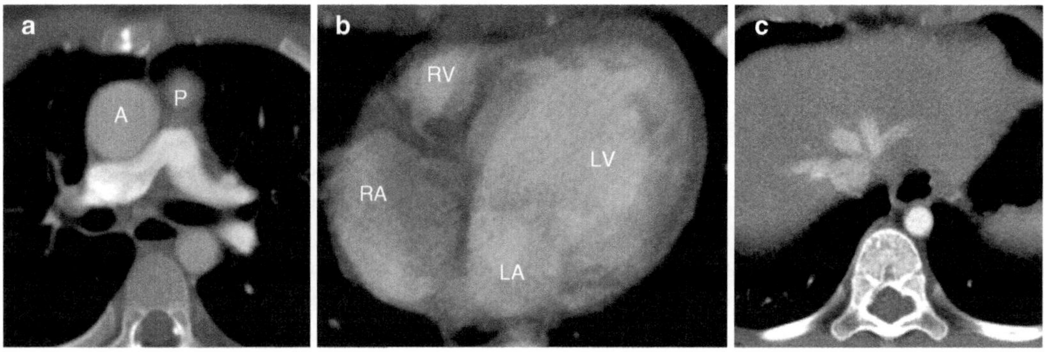

Fig. 17.1 A 4-year-old boy with tricuspid atresia, status post BDGS for pre-Fontan assessment. CT shows confluent branch pulmonary arteries (**a**), absent right AV connection (**b**), normal hepatic vein and IVC drainage (**c**). *A* ascending aorta; *LA* left atrium; *LV* left ventricle; *P* pulmonary trunk; *RA* right atrium; *RV* right ventricle

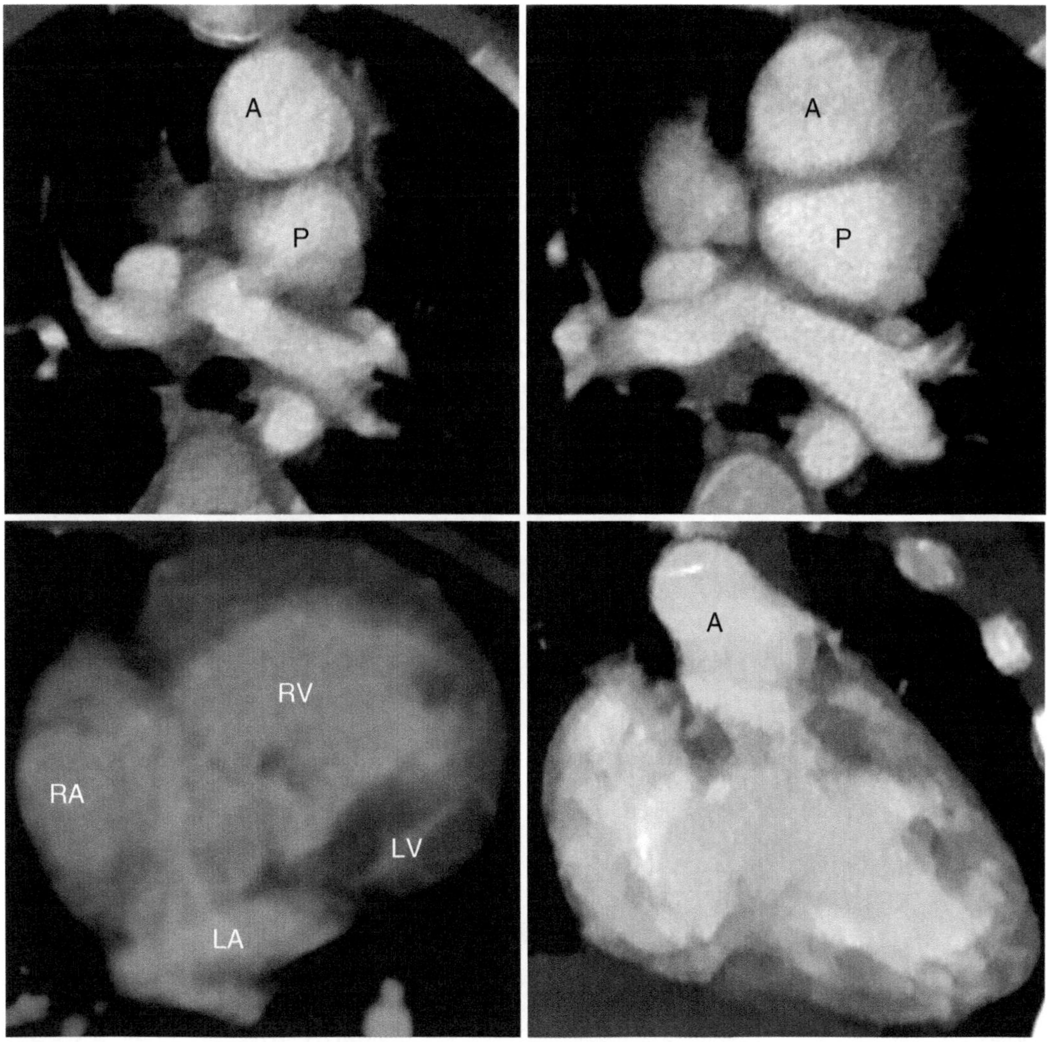

Fig. 17.2 A 13-month-old child with mitral atresia, DORV, D-posed aorta, subaortic conus s/p PA band and atrial septectomy at 1 month of age for pre-Glenn evaluation. CT showed normal aorta with good size confluent branch pulmonary arteries. *A* ascending aorta; *LA* left atrium; *LV* left ventricle; *P* pulmonary trunk; *RA* right atrium; *RV* right ventricle

structed systemic/pulmonary flow obstruction presents more with pulmonary congestion and high output failure. In the presence of significant AV valve regurgitation (AVVR) and decreased ventricular function, features of heart failure are more pronounced.

Bulboventricular foramen (BVF) is the interventricular communication through which the main ventricular chamber feeds blood to the rudimentary outflow chamber. A restrictive VSD/BVF also compromises flow to the vessel arising from the outflow chamber (Fig. 17.5). Functional AV valve without AVVR and preserved ventricular function along with the above-mentioned resistances at pulmonary and systemic beds and unrestrictive ASD are important for optimal physiology of univentricular heart. The absence of ventricular interdependence in the univentricular heart causes abnormal systolic and diastolic function irrespective of the morphology of a single ventricle [4, 5]. Patients with univentricular hearts characteristically have a complete admixture of systemic and

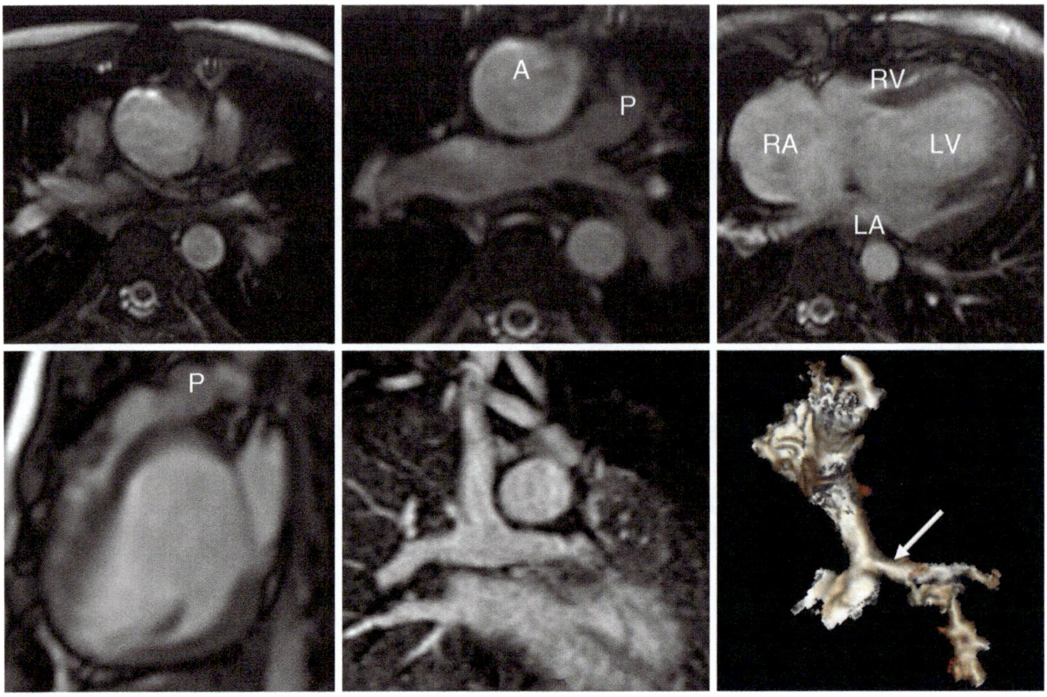

Fig. 17.3 A 13-year-old boy with DILV (S, D, S), ventriculoarterial concordance, functional BDGS and diffuse LPA stenosis (arrow) with reduced flow in LPA compared to RPA on phase-contrast flow study (not shown). *A* ascending aorta; *LA* left atrium; *LV* left ventricle; *P* pulmonary trunk; *RA* right atrium; *RV* right ventricle (Ref to Videos 17.1, 17.2, and 17.3)

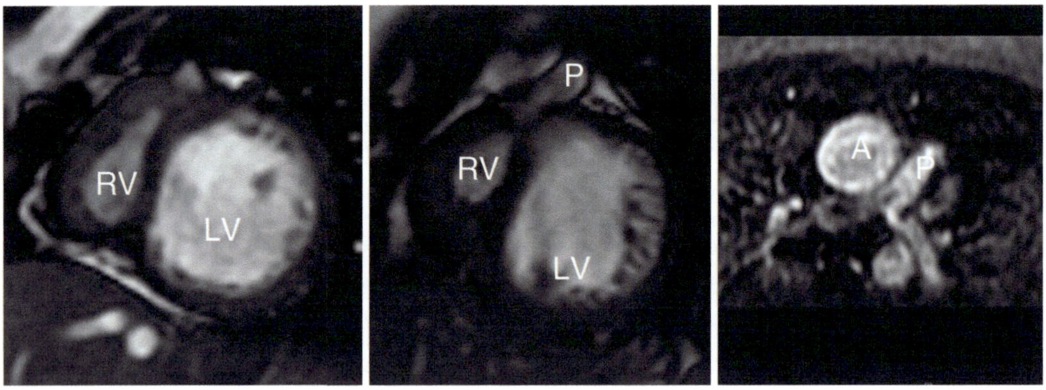

Fig. 17.4 A case of pulmonary atresia with intact ventricular septum with hypoplastic right ventricle (RV). *A* ascending aorta; *LV* left ventricle; *P* pulmonary trunk; *RV* right ventricle

pulmonary venous circulations at the ventricular level. If one assumes a pulmonary venous oxygen saturation of 96% and normal systemic blood flow, the arterial oxygen saturation reflects total pulmonary blood flow. As a rule of thumb, values ≥85% and <75% signify increased and decreased pulmonary blood flow, respectively.

In short, six variables responsible for physiological derangements of the univentricular heart are:

1. The inherent mechanics of single ventricle
2. The mechanics of morphological RV/LV
3. The morphology and functional state of the AV valve

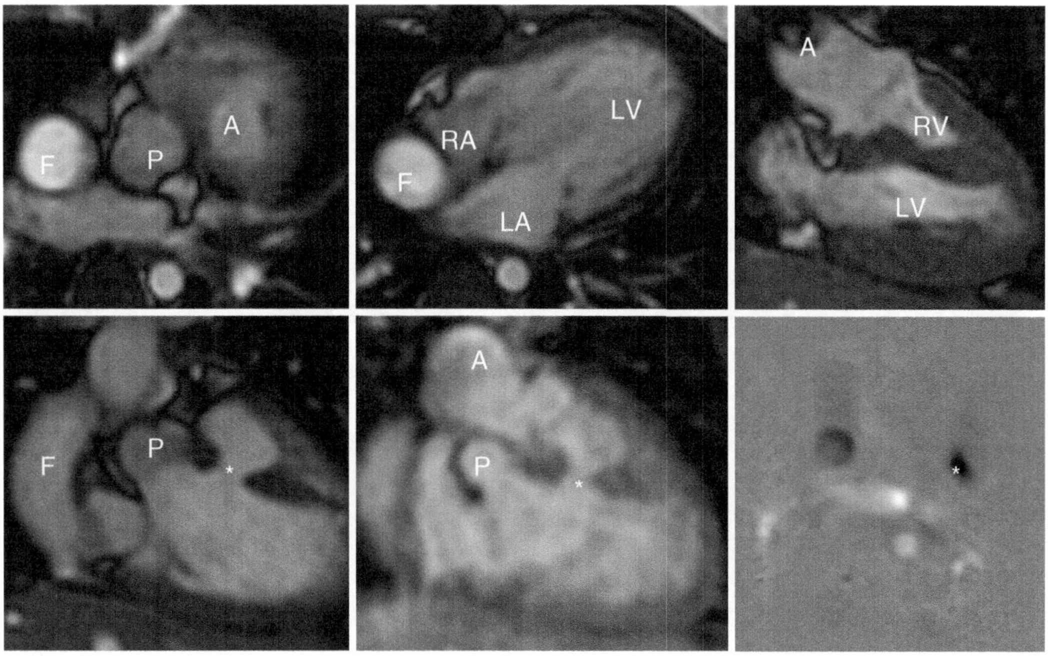

Fig. 17.5 A 11-year-old girl with DILV (S, L, L), status post extracardiac Fontan surgery to assess aortic outflow obstruction. MRI showed unobstructed Fontan and Glenn circuit, hypoplastic leftward and superior RV giving rise to L-posed aorta, obstructive bulboventricular foramen (BVF) (*). Underwent successful enlargement of BVF. *A* ascending aorta; *F* Fontan conduit; *LV* left ventricle; *P* ligated pulmonary trunk; *RV* right ventricle (Ref to Videos 17.4, 17.5, 17.6, and 17.7)

4. Degree of mixing within the single ventricle
5. The pulmonary vascular resistance (PVR)
6. Presence and degree of pulmonary stenosis [4–9]

17.5 Pattern/Arrangement of Univentricular Heart

Double inlet ventricle is the classic form of single or common ventricle where both AV valves communicate into a single chamber. Basic classification of double inlet ventricle is:

- Type A: Double inlet LV—most common form of single ventricle
- Type B: Double inlet RV
- Type C: Double inlet ventricle of mixed morphology (absence of ventricular septum)
- Type D: Double inlet ventricle of indeterminate or undifferentiated morphology [10]

17.5.1 Univentricular Hearts That Are Morphological LV

The outlet chamber (RV) is anterosuperior and either to the right or left side (Fig. 17.6).

Noninverted: outlet chamber in the right anterosuperior position

Inverted: outlet chamber in left anterosuperior position

Aorta discordantly from the small outlet chamber and PA trunk from the single morphological LV causing malposed great arteries [11].

Subgroups of DILV based on great artery relationship are:

- I: Normally related great arteries (NRGA)—Holmes heart
- II: Right and anterior aorta
- III: Left and anterior aorta
- IV: Left and posterior aorta (inverted) [10]

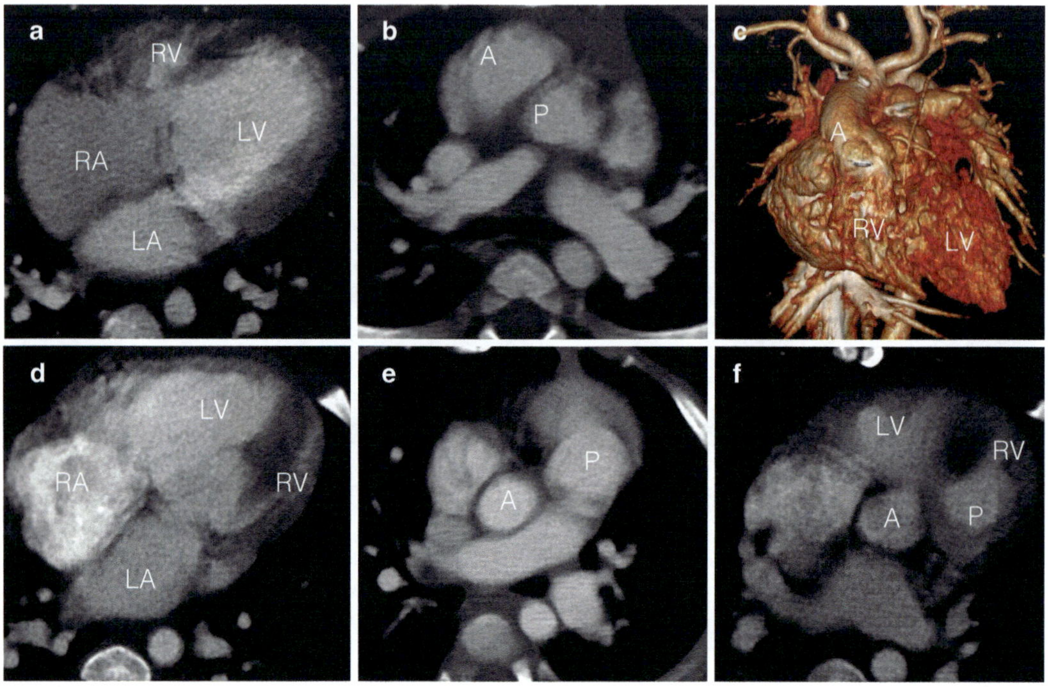

Fig. 17.6 Varying morphology of DILV. (**a**–**c**) Show DILV (S, D, D), hypoplastic RV located right and anterior, D-malposed aorta and ventriculoarterial discordance (TGA). (**d**–**f**) Show DILV, atrioventricular discordance, L loop ventricle, hypoplastic RV located left and posterior with double outlet RV. *A* ascending aorta; *LA* left atrium; *LV* left ventricle; *P* pulmonary trunk; *RA* right atrium; *RV* right ventricle

17.5.2 Univentricular Heart with Morphological Right Ventricle

There is a right ventricular morphology and incorporates within its mass an LV remnant or trabecular pouch that varies in size. This trabecular pouch occupies a lateral, posterior or inferior position within the ventricular mass and may or may not communicate with the cavity. Both arteries are arising from RV giving rise to double outlet right ventricle (DORV) arrangement. BVF represents embryological communication between the main chamber and outlet chamber. Outlet foramen is used mostly to refer to the orifice between a single LV and the outlet chamber. Restrictive outlet foramen can be present at birth or can be acquired later causing subaortic stenosis [11, 12]. PA trunk, when it arises from a single morphological ventricle, the accompanying pulmonary stenosis is either subpulmonary or has a bicuspid pulmonary valve. Pulmonary stenosis in Holmes heart results from the restriction of blood flow. The term hypoplastic left heart syndrome (HLHS) describes a spectrum of cardiac abnormalities characterised by hypoplasia of left ventricle associated with severe stenosis/atresia of mitral/aortic valve and hypoplasia of ascending and arch of the aorta.

Single inlet ventricle: the main denominator of a single inlet ventricle is a single AV connection to one ventricular chamber. It can include all forms of univentricular AV connection resulting from atresia or absence of either the right or left AV valve. Mitral/tricuspid atresia are the typical examples of such as in both the conditions one of the AV valves is atretic with a hypoplastic/rudimentary chamber.

Common inlet ventricle: communication of both atria to a single ventricle chamber by common AV valve. Typically seen in heterotaxy syndromes. As with unbalanced AV canal defects, the main or larger chamber as determined by the predominant commitment of the common AV valve may be LV (type A Vaan Praag), RV (type B) or a ventricle with undifferentiated myocardium (type D).

17.6 Epidemiology and Natural History

Male-to-female ratio in the univentricular heart is between 2: 1 and 4:1 [13]. Recurrence rate in siblings is rare [14]. The most common type of single ventricle is HLHS with high cardiovascular malformations risk of 19–33% in siblings [15, 16]. Tricuspid atresia is the second common type of single ventricle present in 2.9% and 1.4% of congenital heart disease autopsy and clinical series, respectively [17]. DILV comprises 1% of all CHD [18]. Although genetic determinants of other forms of the univentricular heart have not been extensively elaborated, several subtypes that include DILV, single inlet, common inlet and complex single ventricle heterotaxy syndromes are thought to be polygenic in nature, with recurrence and transmission risks far below that expected from Mendelian inheritance [16]. The risk to siblings and offspring of affected individuals is similar and generally in the order of 2–5% [19–21]. Patients with unrepaired univentricular hearts have a poor prognosis. In the largest series of unoperated patients, Moodie et al. reported that 70% with well-formed single left ventricles died before age 16, with an annual attrition rate of 4.8% [22]. The natural history is even bleaker for patients with univentricular hearts of right ventricular morphology, with 50% survival 4 years after diagnosis [22]. The most common causes of mortality were arrhythmias, congestive heart failure and sudden unexplained death.

17.7 Fontan Circulation

In the management of single ventricle physiology, the crux and endgame management is the creation of the Fontan circulation. It is the direction of systemic venous blood to the lungs and the pulmonary venous blood to the aorta. It is a staged procedure where the upper systemic blood

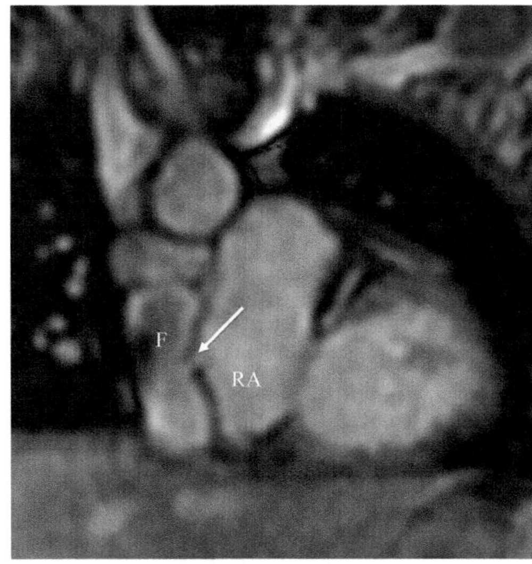

Fig. 17.7 Coronal oblique 3D SSFP image shows fenestration (arrow) connecting the Fontan conduit (F) and right atrium (RA)

is directed to the pulmonary circuit (Bidirectional Glenn) initially followed by the lower systemic blood to the pulmonary circuit (Fontan). A fenestration can be made between the higher-pressure systemic venous pathway and the lower-pressure atrium as a "safety pop-off" route when the systemic venous pressure is expected to raise especially during the post-operative period (Fig. 17.7). Blood passing through the fenestration will bypass the pulmonary vascular bed. The fenestrations tend to close spontaneously and, if spontaneous closure does not occur, the fenestration can be closed by placing an occlusive device during catheterisation when indicated.

There are significant disadvantages to this approach including failing systemic ventricle, arrhythmias, AV valve leakage, thrombosis of the circuit, pulmonary thromboembolism and stroke, hepatic fibrosis, progressive cyanosis due to shunt, and lymphatic dysfunction leading to protein-losing enteropathy, chylous effusions and plastic bronchitis (Fig. 17.8). The potential complications entail an organised approach to cardiac imaging evaluation to ensure successful outcomes.

Prior to bidirectional Glenn, additional surgery may not be needed (e.g. tricuspid atresia, normally related great arteries and ventricular

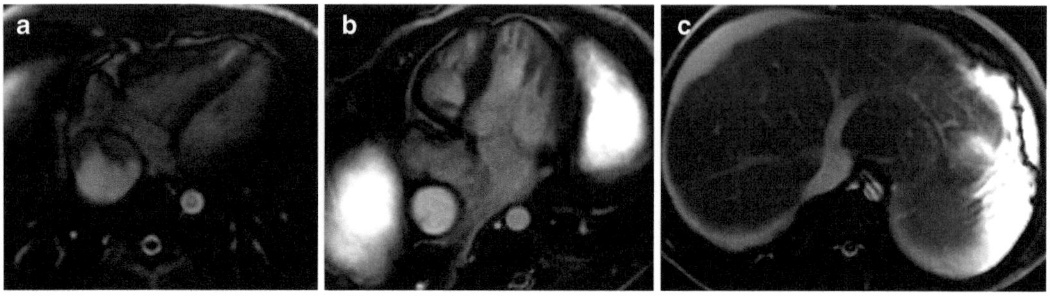

Fig. 17.8 Complications of Fontan circulation. (**a**) Shows clot inside the Fontan conduit. (**b**, **c**) Show ascites and cirrhotic liver in a case of failing Fontan

septal defect) if adequate but restricted pulmonary blood flow is present with good aortic flow. Patients with hypoplastic left heart syndrome, however, need immediate surgery (Norwood stage I) in the neonatal period. The Norwood procedure consists of:

1. Atrial septectomy to provide unrestricted blood flow across the interatrial septum.
2. Anastomosis of MPA to hypoplastic ascending aorta (Damus–Kaye–Stansel (DKS) surgery) to provide systemic blood flow.
3. Systemic to pulmonary artery shunt (BT shunt) to provide pulmonary blood flow.

A right ventricular to pulmonary artery conduit (Sano procedure) has recently been substituted for the systemic to pulmonary artery shunt.

17.8 Imaging of the Single Ventricle

Imaging is based on three broad categories:

1. Detection of obstruction of surgically altered venous and arterial channels for blood flow
2. Detection of new collateral flow and valve regurgitation
3. Assessment of early myocardial dysfunction

The tools to evaluate these issues are essentially the ECG, chest radiography, echocardiography, cardiac CTA and cardiac MRI.

17.8.1 ECG

It is always abnormal, due to heterogeneity of the univentricular heart. The ECG pattern is highly variable.

Single morphological LV: QRS axis inferior and to the right, posterior AV node hypoplastic without His bundle. There is a well-developed anterior accessory AV node present [23].

Non-inverted outflow chamber: left axis, superior Q in V5–V6.

Inverted outflow chamber: right axis, inferior, PR prolongation, no left precordial leads Q [23].

Depending upon the increased or decreased flow, P waves show changes. With right isomerism wandering pacemaker is seen while in left isomerism in absence of recognisable sinus node slow atrial or junctional escape rates are seen.

In DILV AV conduction is usually abnormal with prolonged PR interval or high-degree AV block [24].

In patients with tricuspid atresia, the PR interval is usually normal with tall and broad P-waves. Left axis deviation is characteristic [25].

17.8.2 X-Ray

The key diagnostic feature of X-ray is the location of the outlet chamber. Outlet chambers form the localised convexity at the upper part of the left heart border giving rise to the aorta with convexity to the left or vertically. In Holmes heart, this convexity is very distinctly convex and gives rise to PA [26, 27]. With the exception of Holmes heart, great arteries are transposed and this posteromedial PA may give rise to a waterfall appearance [26, 27]. Unlike TGA with a biventricular heart, thymic shadow absence is not a feature of a univentricular heart with transposition. Cardiomegaly presents due to volume overload of the single ventricle in the presence of increased pulmonary blood flow. LA enlargement is seen best in lateral film. While in a single ventricle with PS, cardiomegaly is not seen but the outflow chamber is seen at the left upper border with convexity or vertical shadow of the aorta [26, 27]. In the presence of pulmonary atresia, an inverted outlet chamber box-like cardiac silhouette is seen. Univentricular right ventricle heart giving rise to both great arteries with aorta anterior and PA posterior has features similar to DORV with narrow pedicle. As a result, aortic convexity in such a heart is usually towards the right. PS is more common than increased blood flow as a result heart size is usually not increased with normal or reduced pulmonary vascularity [28].

17.8.3 **Echocardigraphy** (Figs. 17.9, 17.10, 17.11, and 17.12)

17.8.3.1 Approach

A notable contribution was done by authors like Van Praagh and De la Cruz, who emphasised the importance of delineating deformed heart into three segments like atrial, ventricular and arterial components, along with Anderson and co-

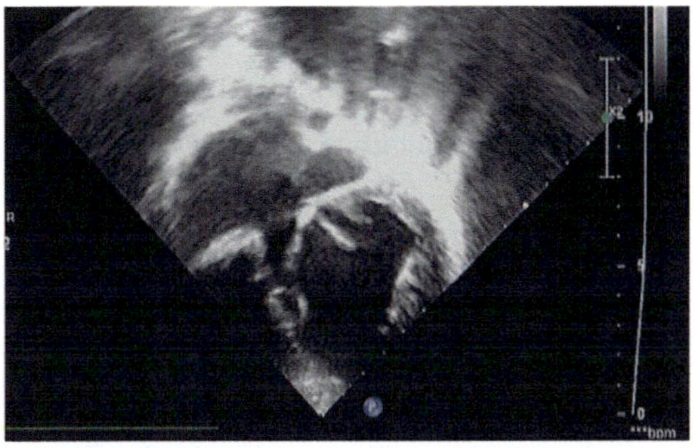

Fig. 17.9 ECHO image of DILV

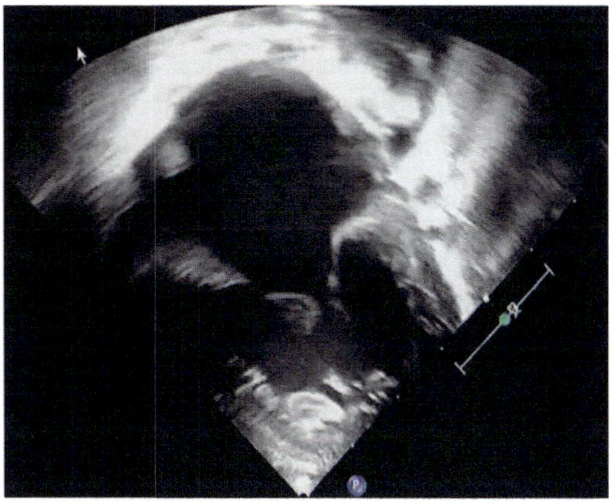

Fig. 17.10 ECHO image of single ventricle of indeterminate morphology with single AV valve

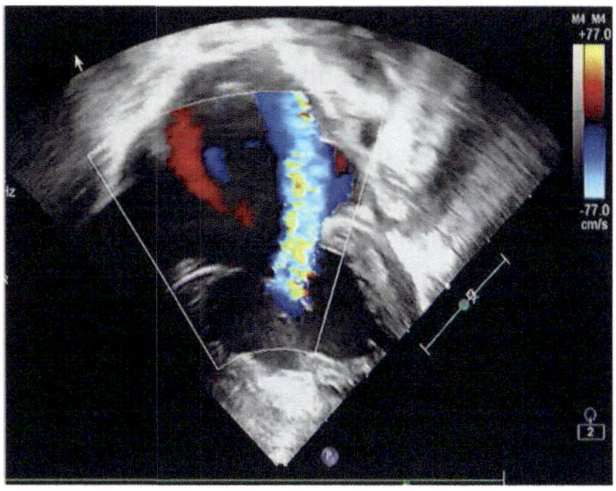

Fig. 17.11 ECHO image of severe AVVR in single ventricle

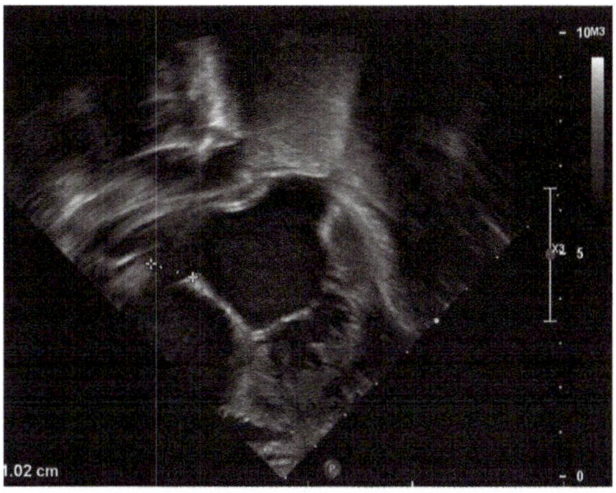

Fig. 17.12 ECHO image of Tricuspid atresia

workers who further refined evaluation to include systemic categorisation and clinical application.

In addition to these three components, AV valves and semilunar valves which lie in between are also to be considered. While performing echocardiogram segmental sequential approach has to be followed where the evaluation starts by determining situs after looking at the great vessels (aorta, IVC) in relation to each other at a lower thoracic and abdominal level along with the position of the liver, stomach and hepatic veins. Usually, abdominal situs goes in hand with atrial situs, with some notable exceptions.

Ventricular determination: to identify the morphology of the ventricle remains the main challenge for the single ventricular heart.

LV: relatively smooth appearance with numerous fine, mesh-like apical trabeculations. In a single ventricle, in addition to this main point, any ventricle with absent to atretic infundibulum with direct arterial communication or exit only through a VSD is considered to be left ventricle.

RV: Irregular, surface with few but coarse trabeculations. Presence of infundibulum in the chamber giving rise to artery is referred to as the right ventricle. This applies to the main chamber as well as for the hypoplastic outlet chamber.

17.8.3.2 AV Valve

The rule which applies to the normal heart like TV goes with RV, MV goes with LV does not apply to the univentricular heart, hence valve nomenclature should be referred to as right or left. Equal or more than 50% annular commitment to a ventricular chamber establishes the valve connection to that ventricular chamber. Convention dictates that if >75% of a common AV valve annulus empties into one ventricular chamber, a common inlet connection is present.

17.8.3.3 Great Arteries

It is the same as of normal heart—whether VA concordance is present or not it depends upon the determination of ventricular morphology. In 80–90% cases, the ventricular chamber that receives the atrioventricular connections is a morphologic LV that incorporates at its base an outflow chamber that is devoid of sinus or inlet component. This outlet chamber is devoid or virtually devoid of trabeculae and that is remote from the crux of the heart. In 10–25% cases, the main chamber to receive the AV connections has right ventricular morphology and incorporates within its mass an LV remnant or trabecular pouch that varies in size and formation. This trabecular pouch occupies a lateral, posterior or inferior position within the ventricular mass and may or may not communicate with the cavity. In less than 10% of cases, the single ventricle has indeterminate morphologic features and incorporates neither an outlet chamber nor a trabecular pouch. Given the variability of intracardiac anatomy in a suspected single ventricle condition observation and scanning from as many transducer positions as possible is mandatory and it is useful to image by sweeping the transducer and imaging in multiple views.

Echocardiography is one of the main tools for the initial assessment of the single ventricle and subsequently after palliation. In order to detect obstructed systemic flow, the subxiphoid view should be used for imaging the IVC as it courses superiorly to its pulmonary connection. Imaging of the length of SVC has to be done from the suprasternal notch and the high right parasternal position. Spontaneous echo contrast (SEC) can also be visualised in the SVC which may be a precursor to thrombosis. The cavopulmonary channels should be evaluated with colour flow mapping and spectral Doppler. High atrial pressure impedes transpulmonary flow, and without the support of a right ventricular pump, the Fontan circulation has minimal potential to overcome this. Thus, high atrial pressure is generally poorly tolerated in the Fontan.

Doppler techniques for assessing the severity of atrioventricular valve regurgitation should be applied [29] including observation of width of the vena contract, the size of the regurgitant signal by flow mapping and the presence or absence of flow reversal in the pulmonary veins. Careful measurement of a well-aligned spectral Doppler ventricular inflow signal provides an estimate of a diastolic transvalvular gradient, which could compromise the Fontan physiology. The aortic valve can sometimes be congenitally deformed in a single ventricle with subsequent dysfunction. Many single ventricles have associated hypoplasia of the aortic arch, ascending aorta, aortic valve, or subaortic ventricular outflow tract and in these circumstances, reconstruction of the aortic arch is necessary prior to the Fontan operation. When there is aortic valve atresia, a Norwood operation is done, in which the pulmonary valve and proximal pulmonary artery are incorporated into an aortic arch reconstruction. The Norwood operation and the Damus–Kaye–Stansel (DKS) operation commonly performed for subaortic obstruction in a single ventricle set the nidus for aortic obstruction in the future. Ventricular outflow obstruction or valve regurgitation can elevate end-diastolic pressure and consequently atrial pressure, which is poorly tolerated in the Fontan patient. Detailed examination of the semilunar valves is warranted, with assessment of annular and subaortic dimensions and observation for anatomic thickening and prolapse or restriction of mobility. The reconstructed aorta should be measured at the Sinuses of Valsalva, sinotubular junction and the ascending aorta for pathological dilation, which could be associated with aortic valve dysfunction [30]. Doppler parameters for the assessment of semilunar valve regurgitation or stenosis should be applied.

Systemic venous collateral connections to the pulmonary venous side of the circulation (veno-atrial collaterals) can develop and enlarge gradually after Fontan, promoting progressive cyanosis [31]. ECHO is not a sensitive investigation to detect collaterals; however, the presence of collaterals from continuous low-velocity mediastinal signals are noted on a low Nyquist colour flow map from the high parasternal or suprasternal transducer positions. Agitated saline contrast injection in an upper extremity resulting in prompt opacification of the atrium adds supportive evidence for these collaterals but reveals little anatomic detail and no quantitation of shunt volume. Aortopulmonary arterial collateral connections are also common in Fontan circulation and result in volume loading of the single ventricle [32]. They produce high-velocity, arterial pattern Doppler flow signals in the mediastinum, but the course, size, number and precise points of termination in the pulmonary arterial tree generally cannot be determined with precision.

Deterioration of ventricular performance in the palliated univentricular heart has major potential for adverse clinical consequences. Diastolic dysfunction is common in the failing single ventricle. The effectiveness of the Fontan circulation to overcome this and augment cardiac output by preloading the failing ventricle is limited by the lack of a ventricular pump on the pulmonary arterial side of the circulation. The Fontan circulation is particularly vulnerable to low cardiac output state when the ventricle fails. Thus, even when ventricular systolic function appears to be preserved, diastolic dysfunction can have adverse clinical consequences for the palliated single ventricle. Unfortunately, some single ventricles are anatomic right ventricles and are poorly suited to sustain good systolic and diastolic function in the long term. Even anatomic left ventricles, subjected to multiple episodes of cardiopulmonary bypass and/or circulatory arrest during staged surgical palliation, are also at high risk for late dysfunction.

Quantitation of ventricular function is challenging in a single ventricle, especially with unreliable ventricular geometry [33]. The common technique is to estimate ejection fraction using the biplane Simpson's method [30]. Pulmonary venous flow patterns and atrioventricular valve diastolic deceleration time should be evaluated as potential indicators of diastolic function in single ventricle. Echo indices to measure diastolic dysfunction include pulmonary venous flow patterns, AV valve deceleration time, diastolic filling time, peak filling rate, time to peak filling, isovolumic relaxation interval, E wave deceleration times and E:A velocity ratio [34]. Tissue Doppler and deformation imaging add to the strength of the assessment [35].

Palliation of many forms of single ventricle requires repair of aortic coarctation or more extensive aortic arch reconstruction [36]. This can promote ventricular hypertrophy, and ultimately deterioration of diastolic and systolic ventricular function. The aortic arch must, therefore, be imaged carefully for anatomic narrowing throughout its length, but especially at the distal end. In the descending aorta, high-velocity systolic flow and prominent continuation of prograde flow into diastole (diastolic runoff) are hallmarks of obstruction. Suprasternal, high left parasternal transducer and subxiphoid views are the best to image this.

Atrial septum resection is done fairly early in the course of work up to Fontan and is usually incomplete, and obstruction can be present. Pulmonary venous hypertension can result, which impedes forward flow through the pulmonary circulation. 2D imaging of the atrial septal remnant with colour flow mapping and spectral recordings of interatrial flow from the subxiphoid transducer position usually results in early detection.

Fenestration may develop leaks causing cyanosis [37]. The subxiphoid views are usually adequate to recognise small gaps in the barrier between the Fontan and atrial proper. Mean gradients in the range of 4–8 mm Hg are usually recorded. TEE may be required if the image quality is insufficient.

Echocardiography is an excellent frontline non-invasive imaging tool for the initial detection and assessment of single ventricle physiology. It is however limited in poor acoustic windows and in the assessment of Fontan complications for which higher investigations have to be used.

17.8.4 Cardiac MRI (Figs. 17.13, 17.14, 17.15, and 17.16)

Cardiovascular MRI is the most commonly used non-invasive advanced imaging modality in congenital heart disease. However, deep sedation or general anaesthesia is required in young children, scan times are relatively long, and gadolinium is used in many patients for angiography. It is an extremely useful add on tool in the evaluation of Fontan. It is a complementary imaging modality to echocardiography and overcomes the limitations of poor acoustic windows, which become increasingly common as patients approach adulthood [38]. Unlike CT or X-ray angiography, CMR uses no ionising radiation, which is a great advantage for younger patients with congenital heart disease for whom medical radiation exposures carry a greater lifetime risk for cancer than adults [39, 40]. Anaesthesia poses an increased risk for patients with complex congenital heart disease undergoing MRI evaluation, and there is concern that repeated anaesthesia exposure of young patients may have adverse neurological effects [41]. Gadolinium deposits have been found in brain tissue after repeated dosing in both children and adult patients, the significance of which is not yet known [42]. Risk assessment of non-invasive modalities should include assessment of risk from anaesthesia and iodinated or gadolinium-based contrast exposure in addition to radiation exposure and vascular-access requirements.

MRI compatible pacemakers are generally the norm these days; hence, pacemakers are no longer a significant contraindication for MRI imaging [43, 44]. Patients with palliated single ventricle physiology undergo catheterisation procedures to place occluding devices, endovascular coils, vascular stents and percutaneous valves. These implants contain a variable amount of ferromagnetic material that causes inhomogeneity artefacts limiting CMR diagnostic imaging. Image reduction up to one-third has been reported [45].

CMR offers high spatial resolution vascular and cardiac anatomic information usually acquired as a contiguous stack of images in a prescribed geometric plane or as a single 3D data set that can be reformatted and manipulated in any dimension.

CMR is generally considered the reference standard for the assessment of ventricular size and function [46]. Ventricular size and indices of systolic function are clinically important parameters in the follow-up of patients after the Fontan operation. Ventricular volumes are measured by the manual tracing of endocardial and epicardial borders on a contiguous stack of short-axis images at end-diastole and end-systole. Simpson's method is then applied to calculate ventricular volumes, ejection fraction, stroke volume, mass and mass:volume ratio.

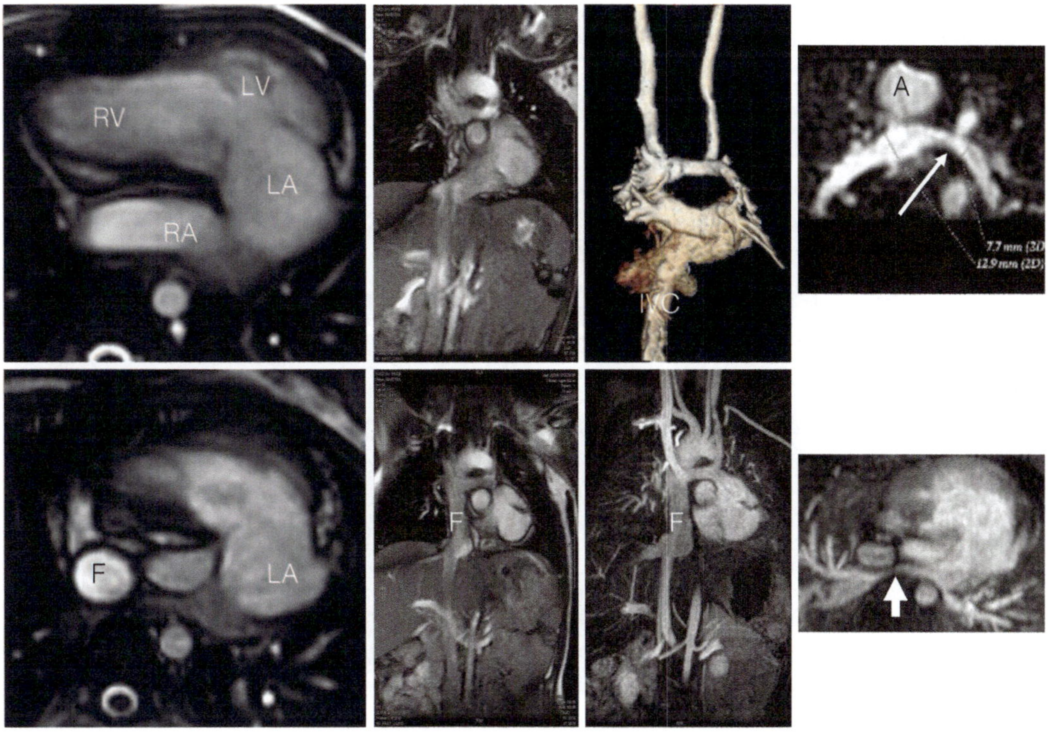

Fig. 17.13 A 11-year-old girl with tricuspid atresia. Pre-Fontan MRI (upper row) shows mesocardia, absent right AV connection, widely patent BDGS, confluent pulmonary arteries mild diffuse LPA stenosis (long arrow), IVC and hepatic veins open to RA. Post-operative MRI (lower row) shows patent extracardiac Fontan circuit with compression of right pulmonary vein by the conduit (short arrow). *A* ascending aorta; *F* Fontan conduit; *LA* left atrium; *LV* left ventricle; *RA* right atrium; *RV* right ventricle (Ref to Videos 17.8, 17.9, 17.10, 17.11, 17.12, 17.13, 17.14, 17.15, and 17.16)

The end-diastolic volume index in echo is significantly underestimated compared to CMR [47]. A higher CMR-derived EDVi was independently associated with death and transplant [48]. Interobserver variability is also lower in CMR compared to Echo.

Thrombi in the Fontan pathway are quite common, found in up to one-third of all patients [49]. In addition to high spatial resolution and 3D imaging of these structures, CMR offers unique tools for the evaluation of these pathways. By performing an early post gadolinium inversion recovery echo pulse sequence with a long inversion time, the thrombus will appear black compared with the surrounding blood pool and myocardium. The evaluation of pulmonary embolism (PE) is a special function of CMR and overcomes some of the disadvantages of other techniques like CT and V/Q scan.

Myocardial fibrosis detection is also a unique property of CMR by using a late post gadolinium inversion recovery echo pulse sequence. Histological studies have validated the correlation of late gadolinium enhancement (LGE) with the presence and extent of myocardial fibrosis [50]. LGE is seen in one-third of all Fontan patients [51]. The extent of LGE is associated with lower ejection fraction, increased EDVi, increased mass and a higher frequency of non-sustained ventricular tachycardia.

Aortopulmonary collaterals (APCs) are vascular connections between the systemic and pulmonary circulations which pose numerous physiological implications including ventricular volume overload and an increased incidence of pleural effusion. APCs are common in patients with functional single ventricles. The flow is quantified well by CMR flow measurements [32].

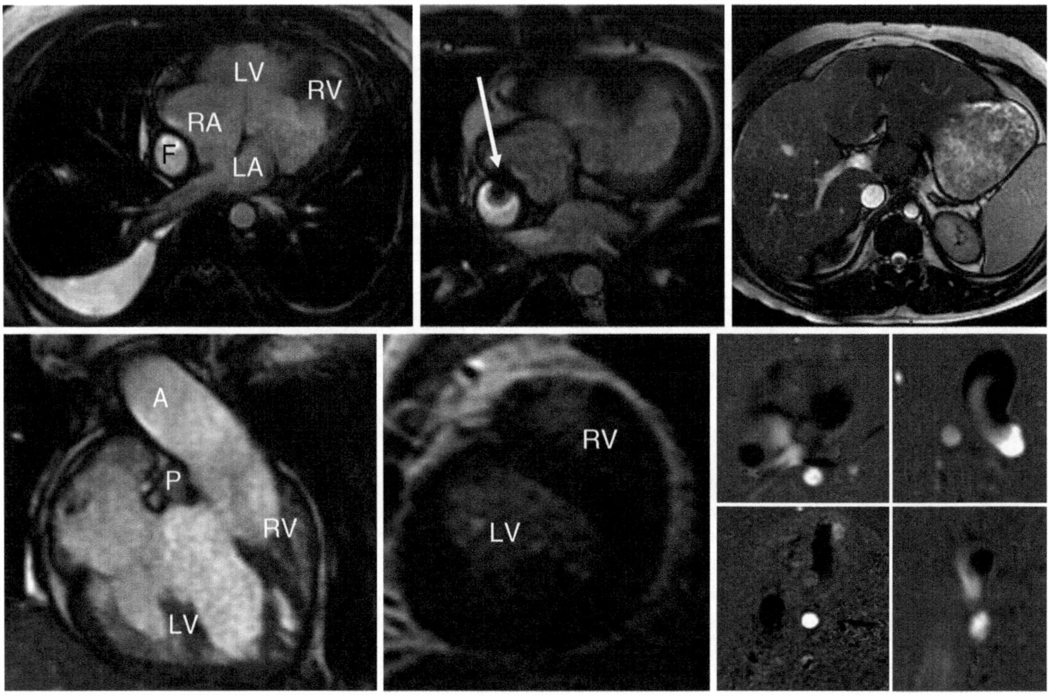

Fig. 17.14 A 15-year-old boy with SLL, single ventricle (LV morphology), inverted right and anterior rudimentary RV, L-Posed aorta, Confluent PAs S/P fenestrated extracardiac Fontan at 6 years of age. Underwent Fontan fenestration closure at 9 years of age for systemic desaturation. Later he developed Protein Losing Enteropathy with anasarca. So refenestration with stenting was done. CMR was used for a comprehensive assessment of morphology, function, flow and late gadolinium enhancement. *A* ascending aorta; *F* Fontan conduit; *LA* left atrium; *LV* left ventricle; *P* pulmonary trunk; *RA* right atrium; *RV* right ventricle

Total APC flow can be calculated by subtracting the sum of right and left pulmonary arterial flows from the sum of the individual pulmonary vein flows. In some cases, APC flow represents one-third of the total systemic output and they are associated with increased EDVi and older age at the time of Fontan surgery.

CMR also allows for the assessment of flow in any direction. When flow is acquired in all directions within a 3D dataset, it is termed 4D flow. Computational fluid dynamics (CFD) is a branch of fluid mechanics used to describe how velocity, pressure and geometries of a moving fluid are related to each other. Applications of 4D flow and CFD offer the ability to measure and visualise complex flow patterns, which are important in the Fontan circulation. [52] There is data to suggest that some of the exercise intolerance seen in patients after the Fontan operation may be due to inefficiencies of the geometry and flow dynamics of the total cavopulmonary connection.

17.8.5 Cardiac CT (Figs. 17.16, 17.17, 17.18, 17.19, and 17.20)

Cardiac CT is used in situations where CMR is contraindicated or unsuccessful. It can help in providing information in challenging situations. CT has excellent spatial resolution and very short procedure times. Fast data acquisition with a substantial reduction in radiation exposure is achievable in the newer dual-source CT scanners using low-dose protocols. ECG-gated cine CT allows measurements of ventricular size and function. CT has been shown to be accurate for the evaluation of anatomy and function for most indications of congenital heart disease (CHD) [53].

For post-Fontan assessment by CTA, it is preferable to use a dual-injection technique using an upper extremity vein and a dorsal foot vein in order to opacify both upper and lower extremity circulation.

An early arterial scan is needed to identify AP collaterals. But streaming artefact from unopacified hepatic and renal veins can confuse with the diagnosis of shunt thrombosis. A 1-minute delayed scan usually provides adequate contrast opacification of the intrathoracic vasculature with only minor inhomogeneity. The 3-minute delayed scan provides the most homogeneous contrast opacification for the detection of a thrombus in the Fontan pathway.

High-resolution CT (HRCT) and CT angiogram are very useful to assess pulmonary complications after the Fontan procedure. Due to the absence of pulsatile blood flow and underfilling of the pulmonary vascular bed, patients with Fontan circulation are at increased risk for the formation of pulmonary arteriovenous malformations (AVMs). CT can be used to diagnose these pulmonary AVMs and thromboembolic compli-

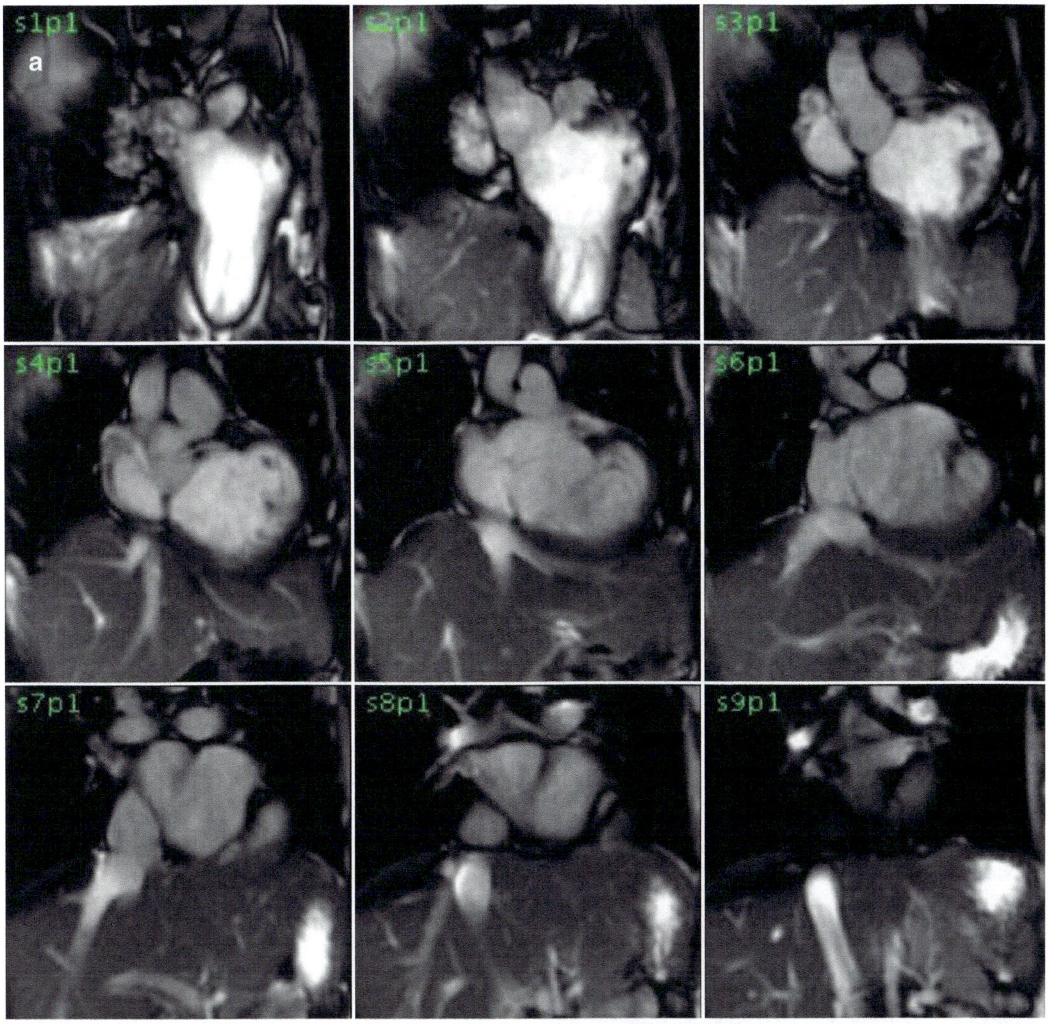

Fig. 17.15 A 15-year-old boy, herneated single ventricle, common AV valve, D-posed great arteries, Severe pulmonary stenosis with confluent pulmonary arteries. Underwent BDGS at 7 years of age. Cardiac MRI was used for a comprehensive assessment of morphology, function and flows. *A* coronal stack cine; *B* axial stack cine; *C* sagittal cine (Ref to Videos 17.17, 17.18, 17.19, 17.20, 17.21, and 17.22)

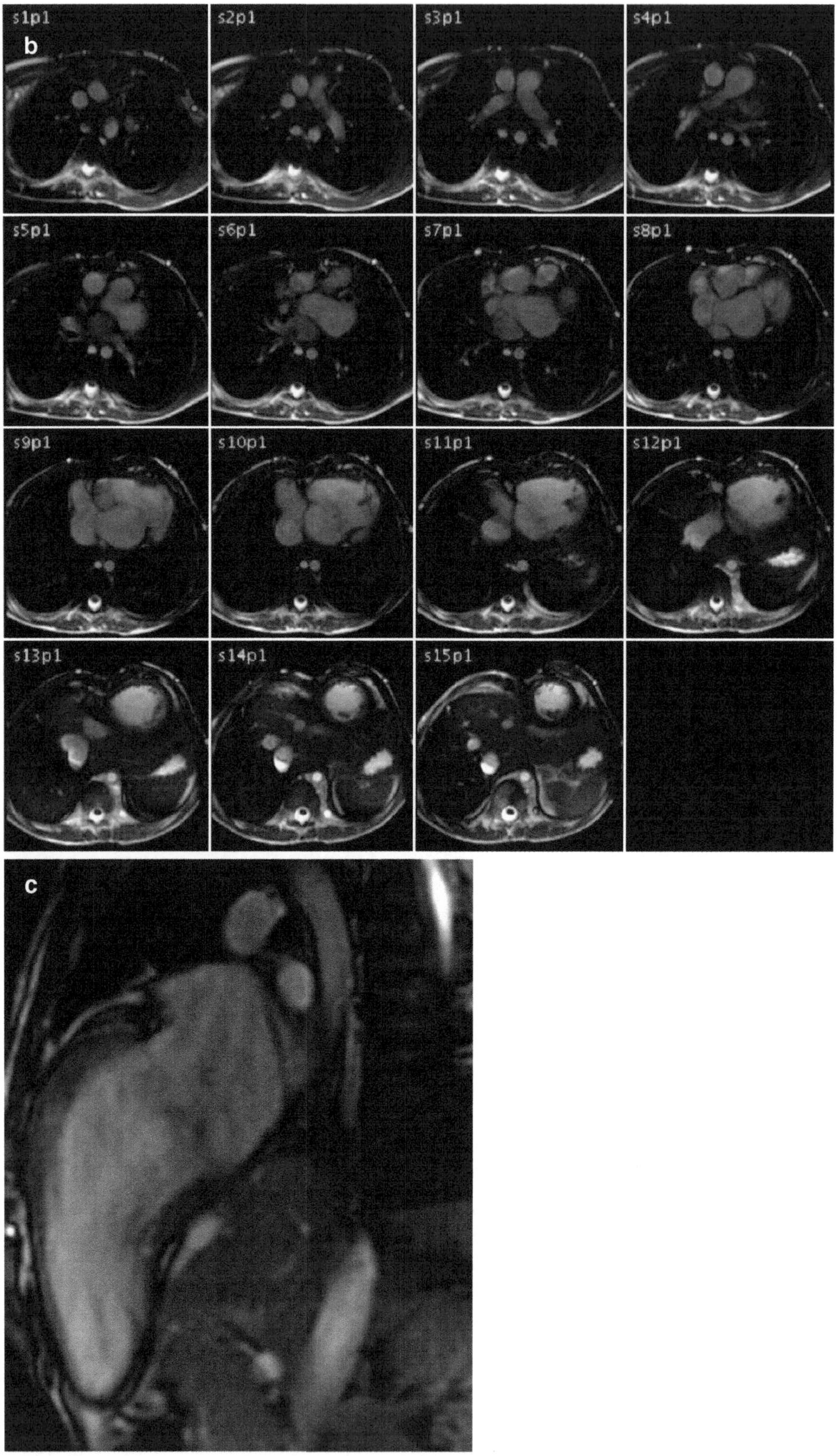

Fig. 17.15 (continued)

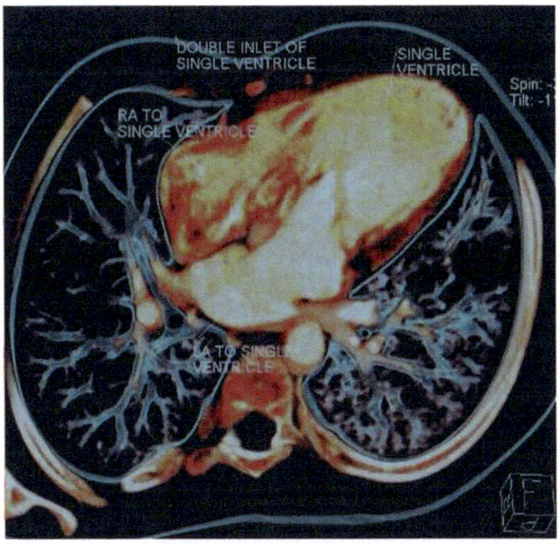

Fig. 17.16 CT VRT image of double inlet single ventricle

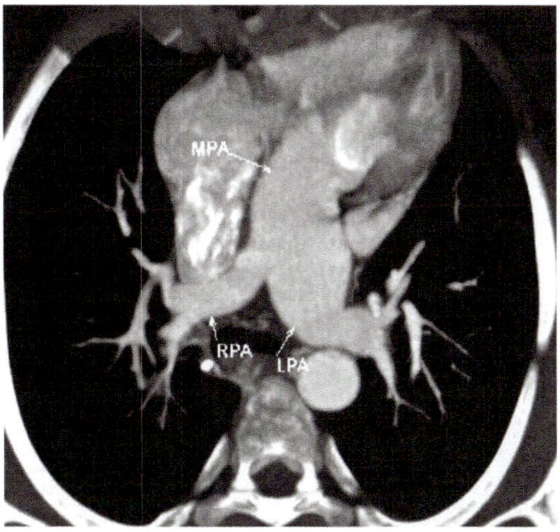

Fig. 17.17 CT MIP image of a dilated pulmonary artery arising from the single ventricle

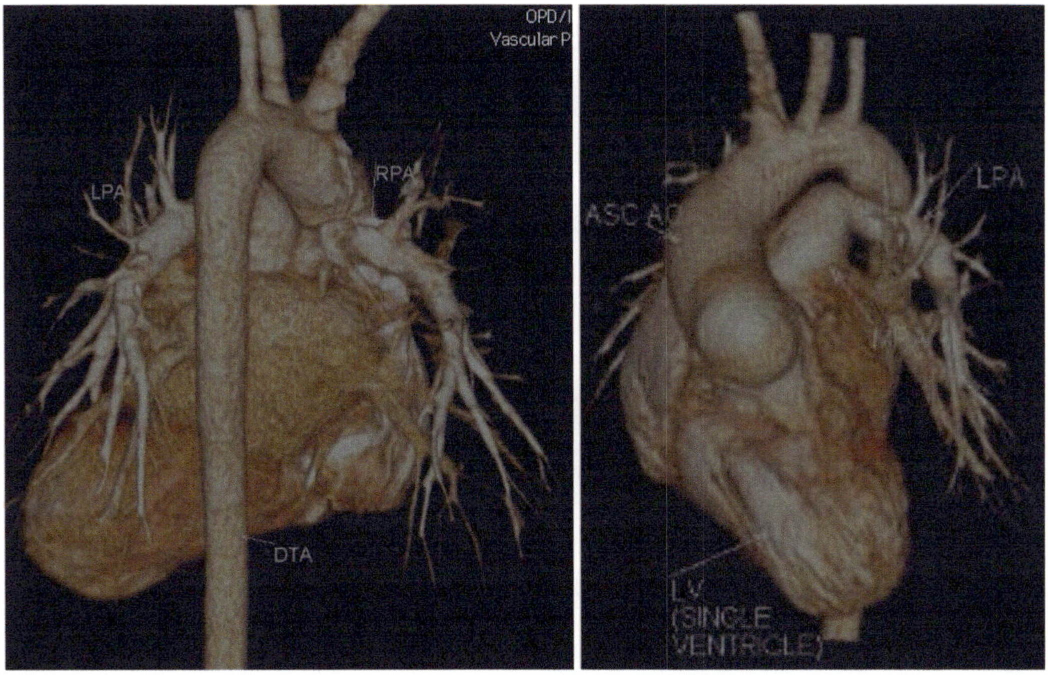

Fig. 17.18 CT VRT image of a single ventricle case shows dilated ascending aorta and left descending thoracic aorta

cations. CT also has the advantage of picking up AP collaterals and venovenous collaterals.

High intrathoracic lymphatic pressure or obstruction of lymphatic flow may lead to the development of lymphoalveolar fistula and bronchial casts, producing a rare complication known as plastic bronchitis. The CT scan allows visualisation of impacted casts within the major airways with associated distal atelectasis and consolidation. CT can be used to guide bronchoscopy and to monitor treatment responses, and thereby may improve clinical outcomes [54].

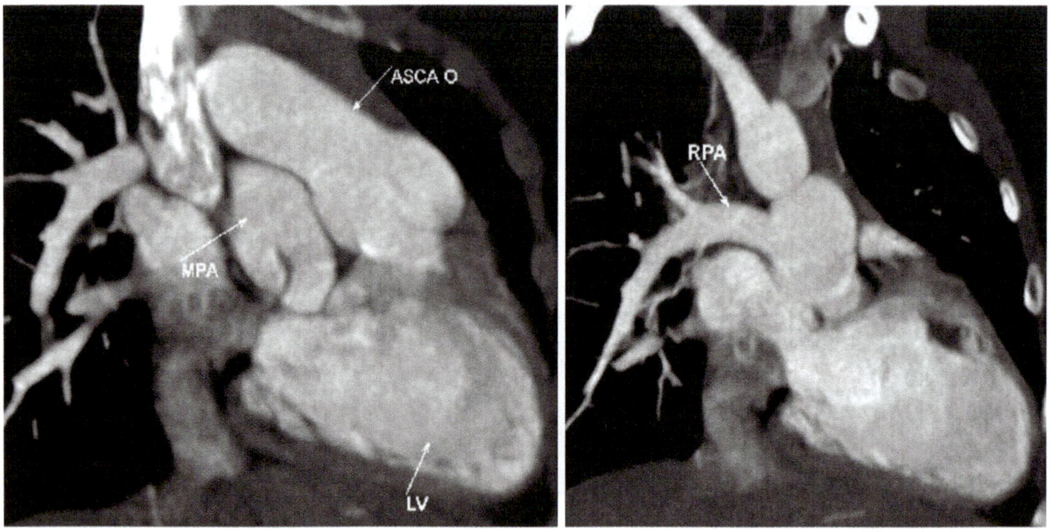

Fig. 17.19 CT MIP image of a dilated MPA and RPA arising from the single ventricle

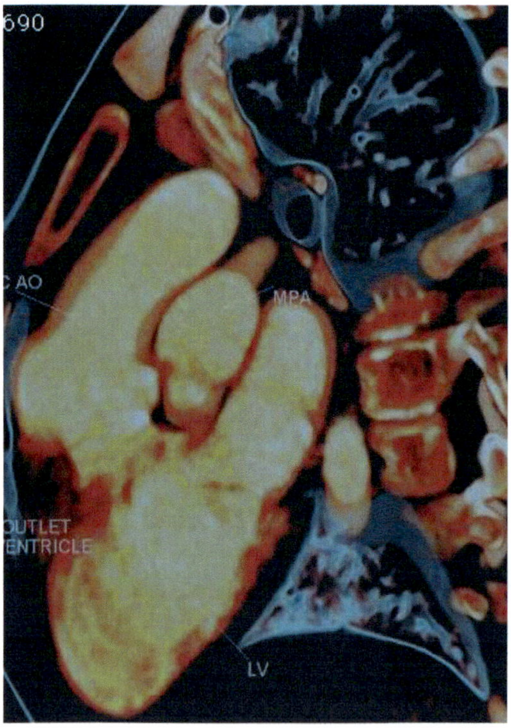

Fig. 17.20 CT VRT image of a double outlet single ventricle

17.8.5.1 Scanning Protocol

The treating physician and anesthesiologist decide the sedation policy, free-breathing versus intubation, IV site and gauge. Imaging is performed by using a 128 slice and above scanner for best results and acceptable radiation. The radiation dose is kept to a minimum by reducing the kilovoltage and tube current appropriately. The acceptable protocol is: children weighing less than 10 kg, 10–19 kg and 20–30 kg, 80 kV and 80 mAs, 80 kV and 100 mAs, and 100 kV and 120 mAs, respectively. Prior to scanning, the pitch is set automatically by the scanner software. A bolus of iodinated contrast material (350 mg/mL, Omnipaque; GE Healthcare) at a dose of 1.5 ml/kg with a dual-head power injector at a rate of 1.5–2.0 ml/s for a 22-gauge cannula, 3.0 ml/s for a 20-gauge cannula and 4.0–5.0 ml/s for an 18-gauge cannula followed by a 10–20 ml of saline flush at the same rate to that of the contrast injection is administered. For timing purposes, an automated bolus-tracking software is used, starting the scan automatically 6 s after contrast agent density in the descending aorta reaches a predefined threshold of 130 HU. The entire volume of the heart and pulmonary arteries are covered during one breath-hold in approximately 5 s with simultaneous recording of the ECG trace. Patients are scanned in the supine position. Cardiac CT is performed from the thoracic inlet level to L1–L2. When there is suspicion of anomalous pulmonary venous drainage, the scan can be extended down to the lower border of the liver.

17.8.5.2 Image Analysis

All image data are evaluated using a 3D post-processing workstation. Various image reformatting techniques including curved planar reconstruction, maximum intensity projection (MIP), minimum intensity projection, and volume-rendering technique (VRT) are used to get all the clinically relevant information. Curved planar reformatting and MIP are primarily used to evaluate curved structures such as the pulmonary arteries and major aortopulmonary collateral arteries (MAPCAs). Minimum intensity projection is used to evaluate the airway and lung parenchyma. For 3D reformatting of the complex anatomy, VRT is used. Thin-section multiplanar reformatting is used for quantitative analysis of the structure in question.

CT is a robust alternative diagnostic modality for the diagnosis of functional univentricular heart disease. In a significant number of patients, cardiac CT is able to provide additional information on extracardiac findings such as hypoplastic aortic arch, infracardiac type total anomalous pulmonary venous return and hypoplastic left lung. For highly select indications, the risk profile may sometimes be in favour of using cardiac CT compared with other diagnostic methods when risks from anaesthesia are considered. Univentricular heart patients are exposed to relatively high cumulative radiation levels during staged palliation [55]. These results show that the radiation dose from CT varies considerably depending on the type of scanner used and the aggressiveness of dose reduction. The standard diagnostic protocol at a majority of centres remains invasive catheterisation before surgical palliation, despite data showing a favourable risk profile for non-invasive evaluation [56]. Non-invasive assessment before surgical palliation has shown similar operative outcomes compared with invasive catheterisation involving lower risk as measured by radiation exposure, vascular access complications, length of anaesthesia and adverse events [57].

Cardiac CT is an alternative imaging modality that can be used as part of the non-invasive imaging modality when cardiac MRI is considered to pose a high risk or when there is an imaging artefact [58]. When anaesthesia is needed, a single breath-hold is required for data acquisition and the length of anaesthesia will be relatively short. Cardiac CT can diagnose accurately and be performed with low radiation exposure in patients with functional univentricular heart disease. The aorta, pulmonary artery and lung can be evaluated completely and simultaneously as well. Cardiac CT is an effective advanced non-invasive imaging modality for a comprehensive evaluation of the functional univentricular heart patients, particularly if cardiac MRI poses a high risk or is contraindicated.

17.8.6 Cardiac Catheterisation

It has been used primarily as a diagnostic tool in the past prior to good sequences available on cardiac MRI; however, in recent time, it has been adapted to include specific palliative interventions to deal with some of the common complications of the Fontan circulation. Echocardiography and CMR have an important role in the assessment and planning of any intervention. Angiography is used as a guide to confirm the non-invasive finding during the procedure. Catheterisation is only utilised for patients in whom intervention is likely considered on the basis of echocardiography or clinical examination, and for patients with poor ventricular function and severe valve regurgitation in whom haemodynamics are considered relevant to clinical management. Some experts now propose a non-invasive algorithm for evaluation before surgical palliation in patients with single ventricle heart disease considered to be at a low risk for requiring intervention [59].

17.9 Common Conditions Producing Univentricular Heart

17.9.1 Tricuspid Atresia

It is characterised by the complete absence of connection between the right atrium and right ventricle with hypoplastic right ventricle

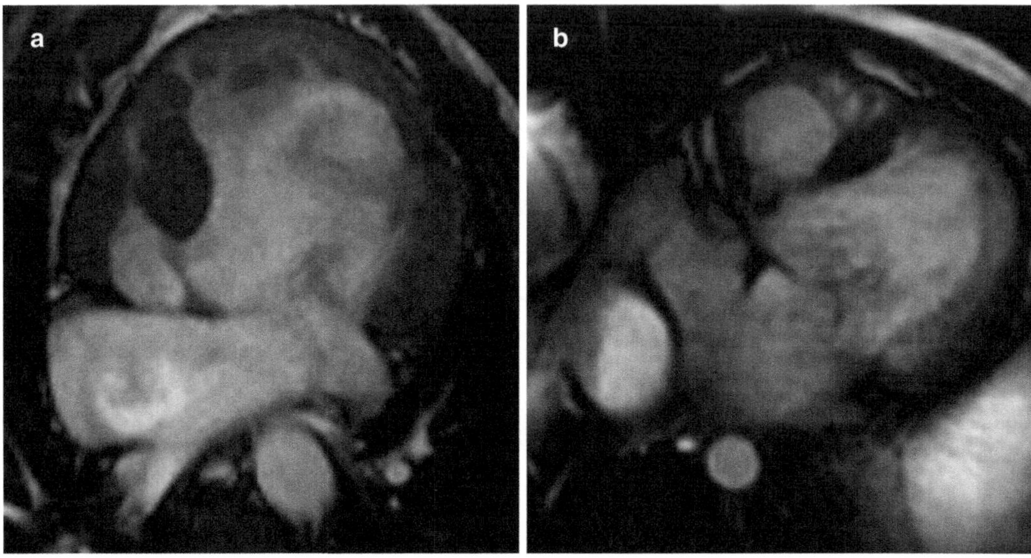

Fig. 17.21 Two different cases of tricuspid atresia: Imperforate tricuspid valve (**a**) (Ref to Video 17.23) and complete absence of right AV connection by fibrofatty muscular tissue (**b**)

(Figs. 17.21 and 17.22). Tricuspid atresia may range from an imperforate membrane (rare) to the total absence of the valve with the area replaced by fibrofatty muscular tissue. Classic fatty wedge is seen in the right AV groove on axial or long-axis four-chamber views. An unrestrictive atrial septal defect (ASD) is the only outlet for the RA in the native form. The left atrium and the mitral valve are dilated since they receive both the pulmonary and the systemic venous returns. The right ventricle is generally poorly developed and a VSD is the only possible intracardiac outlet to the PA with the dominant single and frequently dilated LV supporting both circulations. The incomplete right ventricle is carried on the anterosuperior shoulder of the ventricular mass, almost always with its trabecular component to the right. In two-third of cases, the VA connection is concordant, with the LV connected to the aorta and hypoplastic RV to the PA with a restrictive VSD and pulmonary and subpulmonary stenoses leading to profound cyanosis. Transposition of great arteries are seen in one-third of cases [60].

17.9.2 Double Inlet Left Ventricle (DILV)

DILV occurs when both AV valves are connected to the dominant left ventricle with the hypoplastic right ventricle (Figs. 17.23 and 17.24). Commonly it is associated with ventriculoarterial discordance so that the aorta arises from the smaller right ventricle. The left ventricle pumps the blood through the bulboventricular foramen (VSD) into the aorta and pulmonary artery arises directly from the left ventricle. If the DILV is associated with concordant ventriculoarterial connection and normally related great arteries then it is called as Holmes heart. Other rare forms include right-sided RV with ventriculo-arterial discordance and double outlet ventricle [61].

The bulboventricular foramen has a tendency to become obstructive over time. In the setting of discordant ventriculoarterial connections, such a reduction in the size produces subaortic obstruction but results in subpulmonary obstruction when it is the pulmonary trunk which arises from the incomplete right ventricle. DILV needs to differentiated from an unbalanced AV canal defect (AVCD). In

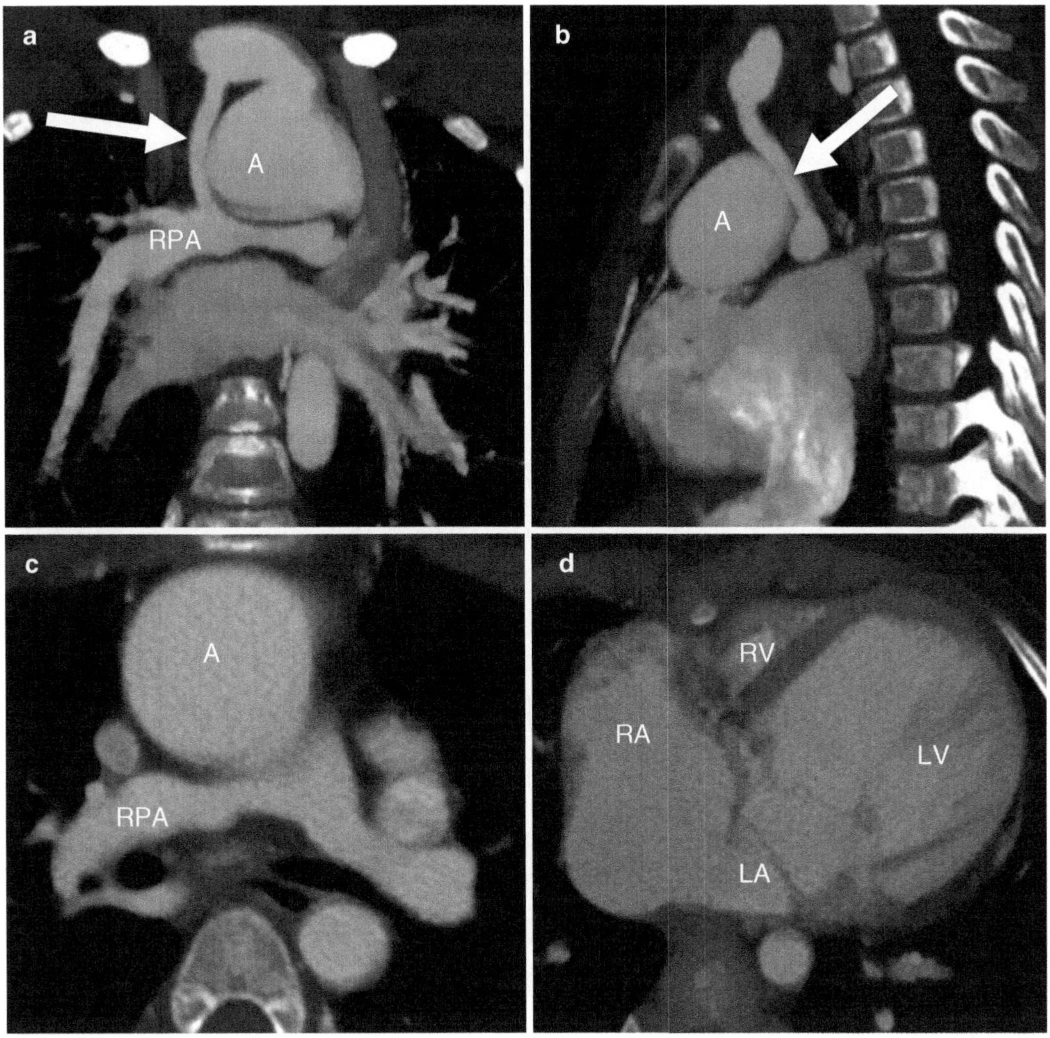

Fig. 17.22 A 4-year-old girl with tricuspid atresia, pulmonary atresia S/P BT shunt at 10 months. CT showed unobstructed BT shunt flows (arrow), right pulmonary stenosis (RPA) stenosis, Nakata index: 421 mm^2/m^2, McGoon ratio of 2. double SVC. Later she successfully underwent RPA plasty and bilateral BDGS. *A* ascending aorta; *LA* left atrium; *LV* left ventricle; *RA* right atrium; *RPA* right pulmonary artery; *RV* right ventricle

DILV, both AV valves points towards the dominant ventricle, whereas in AVCD they point towards their corresponding ventricular apices.

17.9.3 Hypoplastic Left Heart Syndrome

Hypoplastic left heart syndrome (HLHS) is a complex combination of cardiac malformations that probably results from multiple developmental errors in the early stages of cardiogenesis characterised by hypoplasia or atresia of the aortic/mitral valves and hypoplasia of the left ventricle/ascending aorta and coarctation of the aorta (Fig. 17.25). HLHS is the most common form of single ventricle. However, because of its complex nature, different surgical approach and prognosis, often it is described as a separate entity by many authors [62].

If the mitral valve is atretic left atrial blood is shunted across an interatrial communication

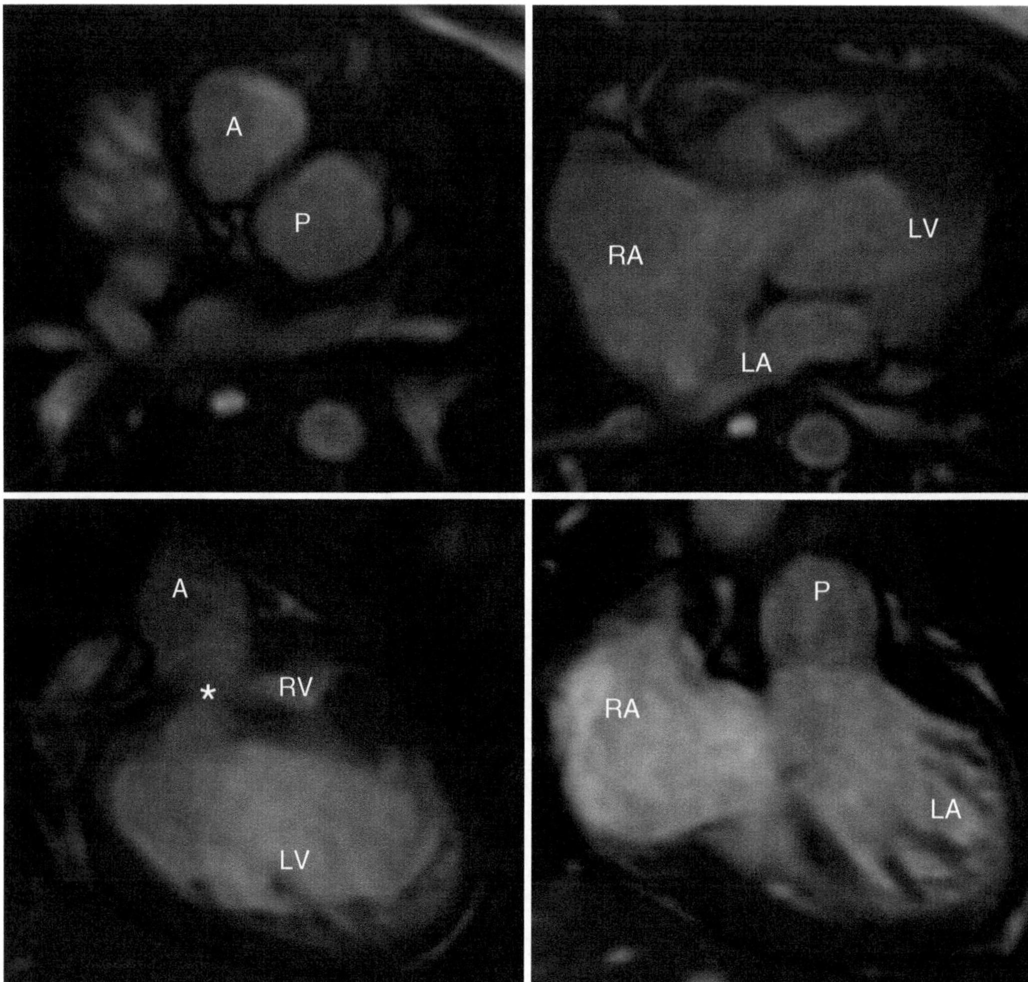

Fig. 17.23 A 15-year-old girl with D-malposed aorta and DILV. Aorta arises from hypoplastic anterosuperior RV. *A* ascending aorta; *LA* left atrium; *LV* left ventricle; *P* pulmonary trunk; *RA* right atrium; *RV* right ventricle; * bulboventricular foramen (Ref to Videos 17.24, 17.25, 17.26, 17.27, 17.28, 17.29, 17.30, and 17.31)

into the right side of the heart. If the mitral valve is stenotic, blood can enter into the left ventricle and then enter the ascending aorta via a stenotic aortic valve. If the aortic valve is atretic, the ascending aorta will be hypoplastic with retrograde flow to coronary arteries via a patent ductus arteriosus.

Norwood et al. described a multistage palliative surgical procedure for relief of HLHS [63]. It has three stages aimed to make the right ventricle as the systemic pumping chamber and divert all systemic veins directly into pulmonary arteries. Figures 17.26, 17.27 and 17.28 demonstrate CT findings of three stages of surgery in the child shown in Fig. 17.25.

Stage I: It is done at the neonatal period consisting of atrial septectomy, anastomosis of the main pulmonary artery to the aorta and a modified BT shunt. Additional procedures done during this stage include ductal ligation and coarctation repair if needed.

Stage II: The bidirectional Glenn shunt (BDGS) or hemi-Fontan procedure, is typically performed at 3–6 months of age when pulmonary

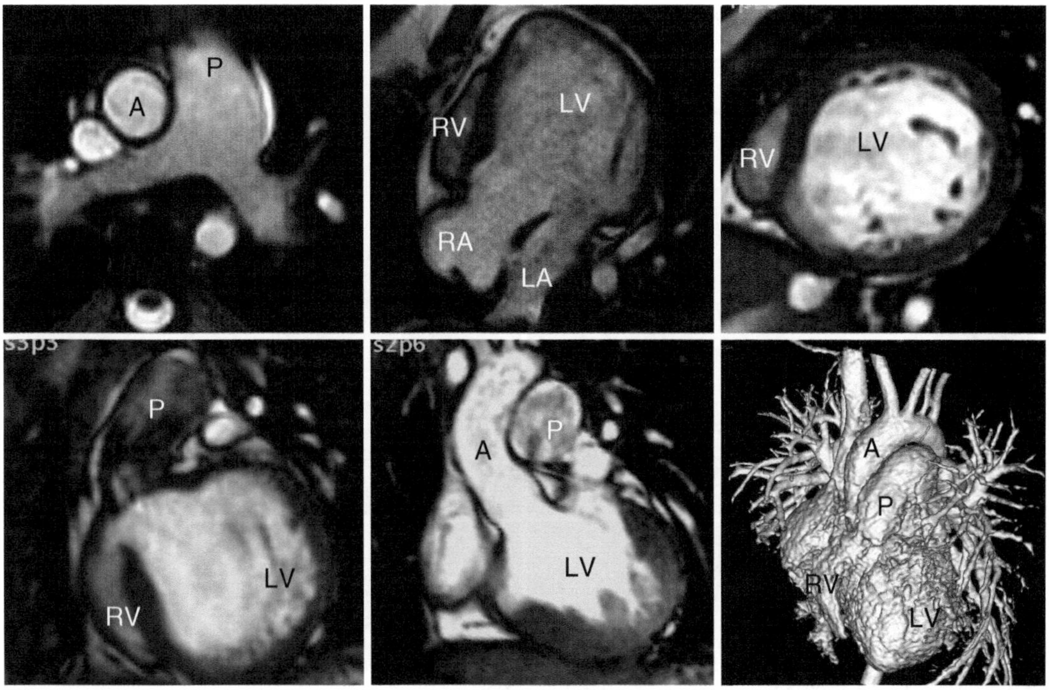

Fig. 17.24 A 13-year-old girl s, d, s DILV, single ventricle, normally related great arteries (Holmes heart), MPA from hypoplastic rudimentary right-sided RV. Unobstructed aortic outflow. Moderate to severe subvalvar pulmonary stenosis—mainly dynamic, at the level of the bulboventricular foramen and the subvalvar RVOT. *A* ascending aorta; *LA* left atrium; *LV* left ventricle; *P* pulmonary trunk; *RA* right atrium; *RV* right ventricle (Ref to Videos 17.32, 17.33, 17.34, 17.35, 17.36, 17.37, 17.38, and 17.39)

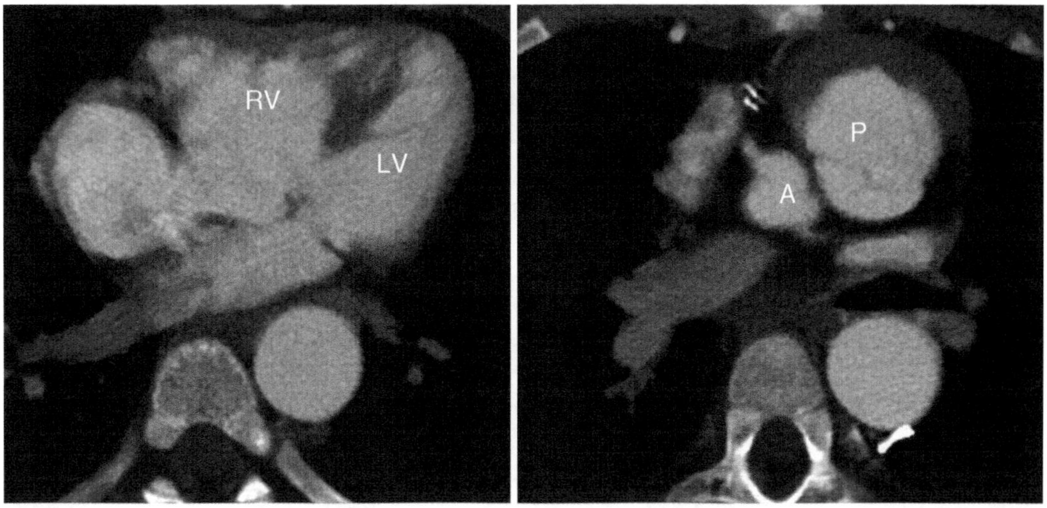

Fig. 17.25 A case of HLHS with aortic atresia and hypoplastic ascending aorta. *A* ascending aorta; *LV* left ventricle; *P* pulmonary trunk; *RV* right ventricle

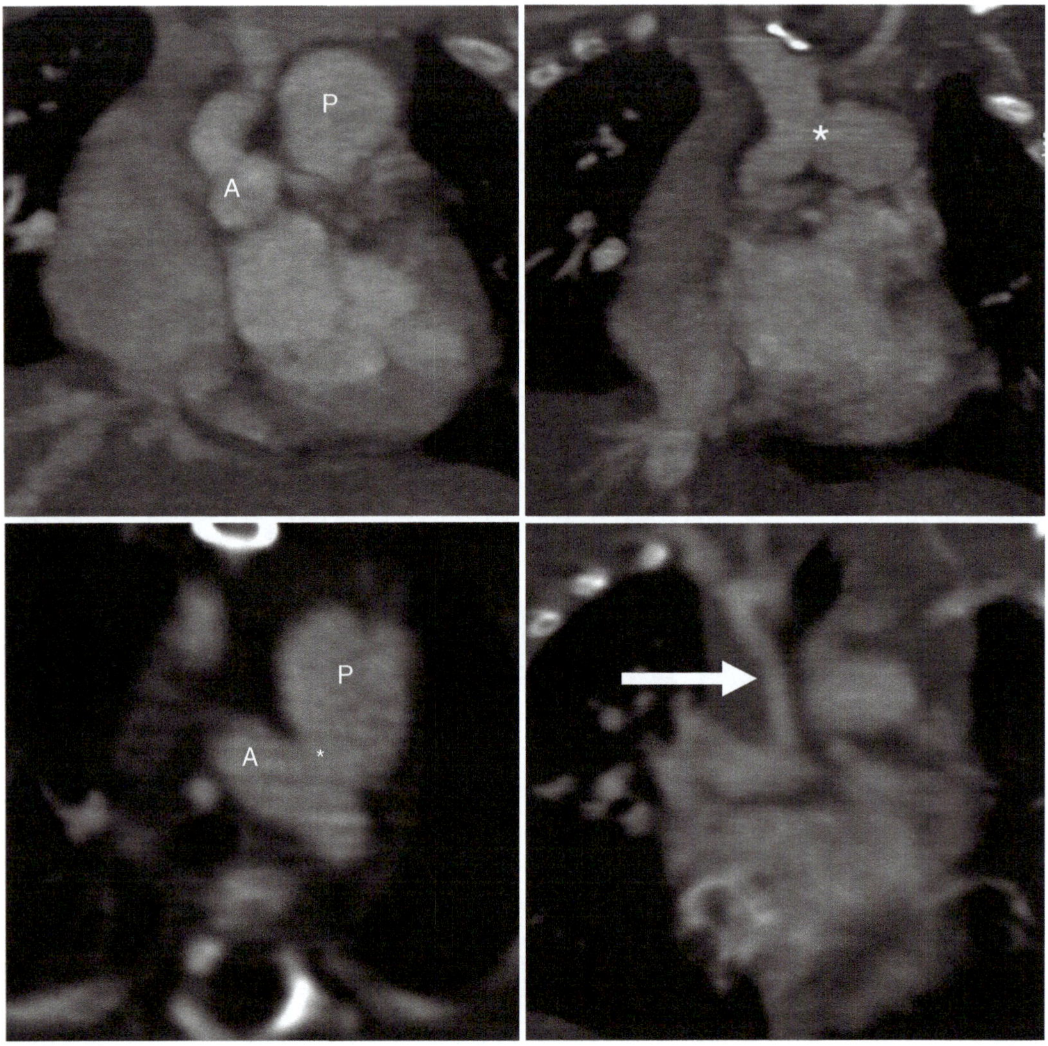

Fig. 17.26 Post-Norwood procedure stage I in neonate for HLHS with aortic atresia and hypoplastic arch. Note the patent DKS anastomosis (*) and BT shunt (arrow). *A* ascending aorta; *P* pulmonary trunk

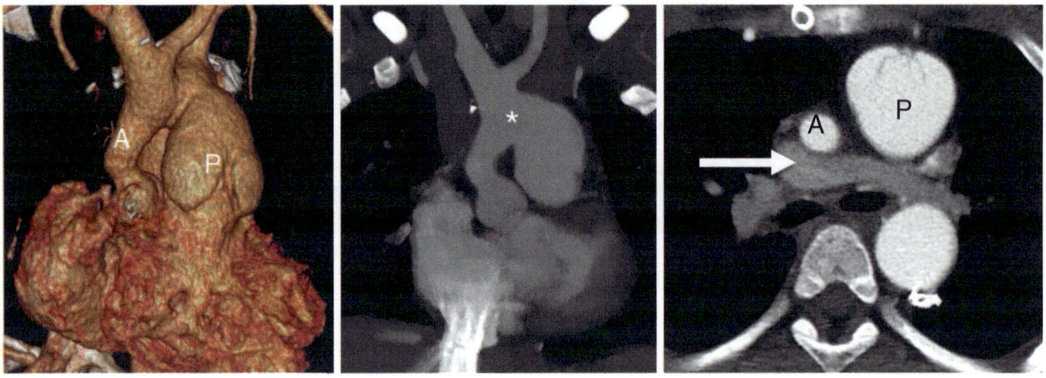

Fig. 17.27 Post BDGS + AV valve repair + Atrial septectomy with balloon dilatation of residual coarctation at 5 years of age. *A* ascending aorta; *P* pulmonary trunk; * DKS anastomosis

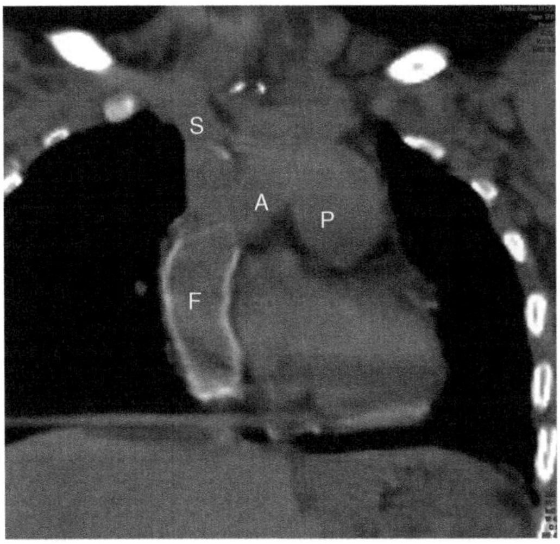

Fig. 17.28 Status post extracardiac fenestrated Fontan completion. *A* ascending aorta; *F* Fontan conduit; *P* pulmonary trunk; *S* SVC

arterial resistance has decreased to normal levels. BDGS consists of dissection of the superior vena cava at its junction with the atrium and end-to-side anastomosis of the dissected superior vena cava to the ipsilateral pulmonary artery.

Stage III: It is performed at 2–4 years of age, is a Fontan procedure. This is performed to direct the remaining hepatic veins and the inferior vena cava to the pulmonary arteries.

17.10 Conclusion

Single ventricle assessment and management is complex. Physicians involved in the management of these patients have to anticipate a wide array of problems unique to the peculiar Fontan circulation and treat them accordingly. Clinical surveillance must be anatomically comprehensive enough to encompass a wide variety of structural problems, yet physiologically focused to elucidate the specific haemodynamic deficiencies each patient presents. Echocardiography and CMR are well-suited imaging tools in the evaluation of the Fontan circulation. A thorough knowledge of the inherent problems in the Fontan circulation and the understanding of the shortcomings of various non-invasive imaging tools will allow a comprehensive assessment of these patients in a structured manner by cardiac imaging physicians.

References

1. Frescural C, Thienal G. The new concept of univentricular connection. Front Pediatr. 2014;2:62.
2. Nelson DP, Schwartz SM, Chang AC. Neonatal physiology of the functionally univentricular heart. Cardiol Young. 2004;14(Suppl 1):52–60.
3. Rahimtoola SH, Ongley PA, Swan HJ. The hemodynamics of common (or single) ventricle. Circulation. 1966;34:14–23.
4. Fogel MA, Weinberg PM, Gupt Fellows KE, Hoffman EA. A study in ventricular-ventricular interaction. Single right ventricles compared with systemic right ventricles in a dual chamber circulation. Circulation. 1995;92:219–30.
5. Fogel MA, Weinbery PM, Gupta KB, et al. Mechanic of the single left ventricle: a study in ventricular-ventricular interaction II. Circulation. 1998;98:330–8.
6. Damiano RJ Jr, La FP, Cox JL, Lowe JE, Santamore WP. Significant left ventricle contribution to right ventricular systolic function. Am J Physiol. 1991;261:H1514–24.
7. Williams RV, Ritter S, Tani LY, Pagoto LT, Munich LL. Quantitative assessment of ventricular function in children with single ventricle using the Doppler myocardial performance index. Am J Cardiol. 2000;86:1106–10.
8. Piran S, Veldtman G, Sir S, Webb GD, Liu PP. Heart failure and ventricular dysfunction in patients wth single or systemic right ventricles. Circulation. 2002;105:1189–94.
9. Macartney FJ, Patridge JB, Scott O, Deverall PB. Common or single ventricle. An angiocardiographic and hemodynamic study of 42 patients. Circulation. 1976;53:543–54.
10. Van Praagh R, Vaan Praagh S, Vlad P, et al. Diagnosis of the anatomic types of single or common ventricle. Am J Cardiol. 1965;15:345–66.
11. Van Praagh R, Ongley PA, Swan HJ. Anatomic types of single or common ventricle in man. Morphologic and geometric asserts of 60 necropsied cases. Am J Cardiol. 1964;13:367–86.
12. Bevilacqua M, Sanders SP, Van PS, Colan SD, Parness I. Double inlet single left ventricle. Echocardiographic anatomy with emphasis on the morphology of the atrioventricular valves and ventricular septal defect. J Am Coll Cardiol. 1919;18:559–68.
13. Hallermann FJ, Davis GD, Ritter DG, Kincaid OW. Roentgenographic features of common ventricle. Radiology. 1966;87:409–23.
14. Shapiro SR, Ruckman RN, Kapur S, et al. Single ventricle with truncus arteriosus in siblings. Am Heart J. 1981;102:456–9.

15. Loffredo CA, Chokkalingam A, Sill AM, Boughman JA, Clark EB, Scheel J, Brenner JI. Prevalence of congenital cardiovascular malformations among relatives of infants with hypoplastic left heart, coarctation of the aorta, and d-transposition of the great arteries. Am J Med Genet A. 2004;124:225–30.
16. Gill HK, Splitt M, Sharland GK, Simpson JM. Patterns of recurrence of congenital heart disease: an analysis of 6, 640 consecutive pregnancies evaluated by detailed fetal echocardiography. J Am Coll Cardiol. 2003;42:923–9.
17. Rao PS. Tricuspid atresia. Curr Treat Options Cardiovasc Med. 2000;2:507–20.
18. Franklin RC, Spiegelhalter DJ, Anderson RH, Macartney FJ, Rossi Filho RI, Douglas JM, Rigby ML, Deanfield JE. Double-inlet ventricle presenting in infancy: I: survival without definitive repair. J Thorac Cardiovasc Surg. 1991;101:767–76.
19. Weigel TJ, Driscoll DJ, Michels VV. Occurrence of congenital heart defects in siblings of patients with univentricular heart and tricuspid atresia. Am J Cardiol. 1989;64:768–71.
20. Burn J, Brennan P, Little J, Holloway S, Coffey R, Somerville J, Dennis NR, Allan L, Arnold R, Deanfield JE, Godman M, Houston A, Keeton B, Oakley C, Scott O, Silove E, Wilkinson J, Pembrey M, Hunter AS. Recurrence risks in offspring of adults with major heart defects: results from first cohort of British collaborative study. Lancet. 1998;351:311–6.
21. Shapiro SR, Ruckman RN, Kapur S, Chandra R, Galioto FM, Perry LW, Scott LP 3rd. Single ventricle with truncus arteriosus in siblings. Am Heart J. 1981;102(3 Pt 1):456–9.
22. Moodie DS, Ritter DG, Tajik AJ, O'Fallon WM. Long-term follow-up in the unoperated univentricular heart. Am J Cardiol. 1984;53:1124–8.
23. Davachi F, Moller JH. The electrocardiogram and vectorcardiogram in single ventricle. Anatomic correlations. Am J Cardiol. 1974;33:95–106.
24. Shaher RM. The electrocardiogram in single ventricle. Br Heart J. 1963;25:465–73.
25. Neill CA, Brink AJ. Left axis deviation in tricuspid atresia and single ventricle: the electrocardiogram in 36 autopsied cases. Circulation. 1955;12:612–9.
26. Carey LS, Ruttenberg HD. Roentgenographic features of common ventricle with inversions of the infundibulum: corrected transposition with rudimentary left ventricle. Am J Roentgenol Radium Ther Nucl Med. 1964;92:652–68.
27. Elliot LP, Gedugaudas E. The roentgenologic findings in common ventricle with transposition of the great vessels. Radiology. 1964;82:850–65.
28. Shinebourne EA, Lau KC, Calcaterra G, Anderson RH. Univentricular heart of right ventricular type: clinical, angiographic and electocardiographic features. Am J Cardiol. 1980;46:439–45.
29. Kutty S, Colen TM, Smallhorn JF. Three-dimensional echocardiography in the assessment of congenital mitral valve disease. J Am Soc Echocardiogr. 2014;27:142–54.
30. Lopez L, Colan SD, Frommelt PC, et al. Recommendations for quantification methods during the performance of a pediatric echocardiogram: a report from the Pediatric Measurements Writing Group of the American Society of Echocardiography Pediatric and Congenital Heart Disease Council. J Am Soc Echocardiogr. 2010;23:465–95.
31. Heinemann M, Breuer J, Steger V, et al. Incidence and impact of systemic venous collateral development after Glenn and Fontan procedures. Thorac Cardiovasc Surg. 2001;49:172–8.
32. Grosse-Wortmann L, Al-Otay A, Yoo SJ. Aortopulmonary collaterals after bidirectional cavopulmonary connection or Fontan completion: quantification with MRI. Circ Cardiovasc Imaging. 2009;2:219–25.
33. Akagi T, Benson LN, Williams WG, et al. Regional ventricular wall motion abnormalities in tricuspid atresia after the Fontan procedure. J Am Coll Cardiol. 1993;22:1182–8.
34. Cheung YF, Penny DJ, Redington AN. Serial assessment of left ventricular diastolic function after Fontan procedure. Heart. 2000;83:420–4.
35. Li SJ, Wong SJ, Cheung YF. Atrial and ventricular mechanics in patients after Fontan-type procedures: atriopulmonary connection versus extracardiac conduit. J Am Soc Echocardiogr. 2014;27:666–74.
36. Larrazabal LA, Selamet Tierney ES, Brown DW, et al. Ventricular function deteriorates with recurrent coarctation in hypoplastic left heart syndrome. Ann Thorac Surg. 2008;86:869–74. discussion 869–874
37. Lemler MS, Scott WA, Leonard SR, et al. Fenestration improves clinical outcome of the fontan procedure: a prospective, randomized study. Circulation. 2002;105:207–12.
38. Fratz S, Chung T, Greil GF, et al. Guidelines and protocols for cardiovascular magnetic resonance in children and adults with congenital heart disease: SCMR expert consensus group on congenital heart disease. J Cardiovasc Magn Reson. 2013;15:51.
39. Ait-Ali L, Andreassi MG, Foffa I, et al. Cumulative patient effective dose and acute radiation-induced chromosomal DNA damage in children with congenital heart disease. Heart. 2010;96:269–74.
40. Glatz AC, Purrington KS, Klinger A, et al. Cumulative exposure to medical radiation for children requiring surgery for congenital heart disease. J Pediatr. 2014;164:789–94.
41. Ramamoorthy C, Haberkern CM, Bhananker SM, et al. Anesthesia related cardiac arrest in children with heart disease: data from the Pediatric Perioperative Cardiac Arrest (POCA) registry. Anesth Analg. 2010;110:1376–82.
42. Miller JH, Hu HH, Pokorney A, Cornejo P, Towbin R. MRI brain signal intensity changes of a child during the course of 35 gadolinium contrast examinations. Pediatrics. 2015;136:1637–40.
43. Levine GN, Gomes AS, Arai AE, American Heart Association Committee on Diagnostic and Interventional Cardiac Catheterization;

American Heart Association Council on Clinical Cardiology; American Heart Association Council on Cardiovascular Radiology and Intervention, et al. Safety of magnetic resonance imaging in children. Heart. 2015;10:1–10.
44. Martin ET, Coman JA, Shellock FG, et al. Magnetic resonance imaging and cardiac pacemaker safety at 1.5-Tesla. J Am Coll Cardiol. 2004;43:1315–24.
45. Garg R, Powell AJ, Sena L, et al. Effects of metallic implants on magnetic resonance imaging evaluation of Fontan palliation. Am J Cardiol. 2005;95:688–91.
46. Kilner PJ, Geva T, Kaemmerer H, et al. Recommendations for cardiovascular magnetic resonance in adults with congenital heart disease from the respective working groups of the European Society of Cardiology. Eur Heart J. 2010;31:794–805.
47. Margossian R, Schwartz ML, Prakash A, et al. Pediatric Heart Network Investigators. Comparison of echocardiographic and cardiac magnetic resonance imaging measurements of functional single ventricular volumes, mass, and ejection fraction (from the Pediatric Heart Network Fontan Cross-Sectional Study). Am J Cardiol. 2009;104:419–28.
48. Rathod RH, Prakash A, Kim YY, et al. Cardiac magnetic resonance parameters predict transplantation-free survival in patients with fontan circulation. Circ Cardiovasc Imaging. 2014;7:502–9.
49. Monagle P, Cochrane A, Roberts R, et al. Fontan Anticoagulation Study Group. A multicenter, randomized trial comparing heparin/warfarin and acetylsalicylic acid as primary thromboprophylaxis for 2 years after the Fontan procedure in children. J Am Coll Cardiol. 2011;58:645–51.
50. Kehr E, Sono M, Chugh SS, et al. Gadolinium-enhanced magnetic resonance imaging for detection and quantification of fibrosis in human myocardium in vitro. Int J Cardiovasc Imaging. 2008;24:61–8.
51. Rathod RH, Prakash A, Powell AJ, et al. Myocardial fibrosis identified by cardiac magnetic resonance late gadolinium enhancement is associated with adverse ventricular mechanics and ventricular tachycardia late after Fontan operation. J Am Coll Cardiol. 2010;55:1721–8.
52. Haggerty CM, Restrepo M, Tang E, et al. Fontan hemodynamics from 100 patient-specific cardiac magnetic resonance studies: a computational fluid dynamics analysis. J Thorac Cardiovasc Surg. 2014;148:1481–9.
53. Han BK, Rigsby CK, Hlavacek A, et al. Computed tomography imaging in patients with congenital heart disease part I: rationale and utility. An expert consensus document of the Society of Cardiovascular Computed Tomography (SCCT): endorsed by the Society of Pediatric Radiology (SPR) and the North American Society of Cardiac Imaging (NASCI). J Cardiovasc Comput Tomogr. 2013;7:338–53.
54. Fredenburg TB, Johnson TR, Cohen MD. The Fontan procedure: anatomy, complications, and manifestations of failure. Radiographics. 2011;31:453–63.
55. Downing TE, McDonnell A, Zhu X, et al. Cumulative medical radiation exposure throughout staged palliation of single ventricle congenital heart disease. Pediatr Cardiol. 2015;36:190–5.
56. Feinstein JA, Benson DW, Dubin AM, Cohen MS, Maxey DM, Mahle WT, et al. Hypoplastic left heart syndrome: current considerations and expectations. J Am Coll Cardiol. 2012;59(1 Suppl):S1–42.
57. Brown DW, Gauvreau K, Powell AJ, et al. Cardiac magnetic resonance versus routine cardiac catheterization before bidirectional glenn anastomosis in infants with functional single ventricle: a prospective randomized trial. Circulation. 2007;116:2718–25.
58. Han BK, Lesser JR. CT imaging in congenital heart disease: an approach to imaging and interpreting complex lesions after surgical intervention for tetralogy of Fallot, transposition of the great arteries, and single ventricle heart disease. J Cardiovasc Comput Tomogr. 2013;7:338–53.
59. Fogel MA. Is routine cardiac catheterization necessary in the management of patients with single ventricles across staged Fontan reconstruction? No! Pediatr Cardiol. 2005;26:154–8.
60. Frescura C, Thiene G. The new concept of univentricular heart. Frontiers Paediatr. 2014;2:1–17. https://doi.org/10.3389/fped.2014.00062.
61. Uemura H, Ho SY, Adachi I, Yagihara T. Morphologic spectrum of ventriculoarterial connection in hearts with double inlet left ventricle: implications for surgical procedures. Ann Thorac Surg. 2008;86:1321–7.
62. Dianna ME, Bardo MD, Frankel DG, Kimberly E, et al. Hypoplastic left heart syndrome. Radiographics. 2001;21:705–17.
63. Norwood WI. Hypoplastic left heart syndrome. Ann Thorac Surg. 1991;52:688–95.

18 CT and MR Imaging in Post-operative CHD

Priya Jagia and Mumun Sinha

18.1 Introduction

With an increasing number of patients reaching adulthood following surgical repair or palliation of congenital heart defects (CHDs), their regular follow-up assumes importance. For identifying complications, planning procedures and for prognostication, imaging in the form of either cardiac magnetic resonance (CMR) or cardiac computed tomography angiography (CTA) has assumed an important role. Two dimensional and Doppler echocardiography, despite being inexpensive and readily available, has its own limitations in the assessment of complicated post-operative anatomy of conduits and shunts, small residual defects and pulmonary venous drainage to name a few. Echocardiography is also limited by its poor acoustic window for evaluation of right ventricular and outflow tract anatomy and function and the operator dependence of the technique further amplifies the need for cross-sectional imaging [1]. The two imaging modalities (CTA and CMR) available are not only valuable for the anatomical and functional evaluation of post-operative CHDs but also identify the late post-operative sequelae and intra-/extracardiac complications of the palliative and therapeutic procedures. They also act as a guide to early intervention, prognostication and decision-making process. Though the two modalities are complementary and supplementary to echocardiography, CMR has definite advantages over cardiac CTA in the evaluation of post-operative CHDs given its superiority for the evaluation of ventricular and valvular function, assessment of the functional significance of stenosis and diagnosis and haemodynamic evaluation of small residual/recurrent septal defects. The need for multiple imaging follow-ups also tips the balance in favour of CMR, it being a radiation-free modality. However, some centres may still prefer CTA because of its availability, lower cost and faster scan times.

P. Jagia (✉) · M. Sinha
Department of Cardiovascular Radiology and Endovascular Interventions, All India Institute of Medical Sciences, New Delhi, India

18.2 Suggested Imaging Protocol

18.2.1 CMR Protocol

May include some or all of these:

(i) Localisers
(ii) Spin echo sequences: T2 weighted fat saturated and T1 weighted sequences short axis and four-chamber views for evaluation of gross cardiac and extracardiac anatomy, pulmonary artery (PA) sizes, pleural, pericardial effusions, etc.
(iii) Cine imaging stacks in the four-chamber view, short-axis view, vertical long-axis

R. Rajeshkannan et al. (eds.), *CT and MRI in Congenital Heart Diseases*,
https://doi.org/10.1007/978-981-15-6755-1_18

view and right ventricular outflow tract (RVOT) view for evaluation of ventricular function, focal dyskinesias/regional wall motion abnormalities, diagnosis of valvular/conduit regurgitation (seen as dephasing jets). Any stenosis can be evaluated in various cardiac phases to assess for its possible haemodynamic/physiological significance.

(iv) Contrast-enhanced Magnetic Resonance angiography (MRA) or Time-resolved MR (TWIST: Time-resolved Angiography with Interleaved Stochastic Trajectories) Angiography for evaluation of great vessels and central/peripheral pulmonary stenosis.

(v) Phase-sensitive inversion recovery (PSIR) images in similar views as cine imaging at 5 and 15 min following contrast administration for evaluation of myocardial fibrosis.

(vi) Phase-contrast imaging of the main pulmonary artery and the aorta (true axials of these major arteries) to quantify residual left-to-right shunts (Q_p:Q_s) and assess the possible haemodynamic significance of a stenosis.

Though almost all sutures, clips and plugs are MR compatible, metallic artefacts can hinder optimal anatomic and functional evaluation. In such cases, using spin-echo sequences, lower echo times, small voxel sizes, thinner slices and signal averaging over multiple breath-holds can, to some extent, mitigate the problem.

For post-contrast scans, intravenous gadolinium is administered in the dose of 0.2 mmol/kg body weight.

With free-breathing acquisition techniques, imaging times have considerably reduced and general anaesthesia (GA) is no longer an absolute requirement. For neonates, infants and small children, a short GA or sedation usually suffices. Acquisition times are short and acquisition is generally smooth in slightly older and co-operative children after adequate counselling.

18.2.2 CTA Protocol

Non-ionic iodinated contrast (1.0–1.5 ml/kg) is administered via a peripheral intravenous line using a power injector at rates varying from 3.5 to 4.5 ml/s. Manual triggering is advised after assessment of optimal contrast enhancement in view of the complexity and multiplicity of residual shunts and likely presence of stenosis and obstructions. The data set is acquired at a lower tube potential (80 kV), using automatic tube current modulation (Care Dose). For calculation of ventricular function on CTA, acquisition could be retrospectively gated and this gives a multiphasic evaluation of an entire cardiac cycle.

For post-processing of images, optimal images are obtained in both systole and diastole with a thickness of 0.75 mm and soft tissue reconstruction. Advanced dose reduction techniques such as anatomy-based tube current modulation (Care Dose), low kV, high pitch and use of ECG-guided current modulation where the tube current is reduced to 4% of its nominal value during the non-diagnostic phases of the cardiac cycle, allow for performance of very low dose scans in paediatric patients [2].

For optimal evaluation of Glenn shunt, it is advisable to inject contrast in a vein contralateral to the side of the cavopulmonary anastomosis so as to avoid streak artefacts potentially obscuring the circuit [3]. Additional delayed acquisition is required to optimally opacify the circuit for correct evaluation and for ruling out partial thrombosis. For bilateral Glenn, a lower limb intravenous injection and delayed acquisition avoids both streak artefacts and artefacts from contrast mixing with unopacified blood simulating the appearance of a thrombus. Similarly, efforts should be made to correctly image the inferior cavopulmonary anastomosis in the Fontan circuit.

18.3 Common Surgical Procedures Used for Palliation and Correction of CHDs and Their Imaging Findings

For correct evaluation post-operative CHDs, a thorough understanding of the surgical procedures, their expected anatomy and function is imperative.

18.4 Palliative Procedures

Systemic arterial-to-pulmonary artery shunts are common palliative surgical procedures performed. Their rationale is to increase the delivery of systemic blood to the lungs, thereby increasing blood oxygenation and decreasing cyanosis. They also help in enlarging the pulmonary arteries for a later stage repair. These arterial shunts are done for patients of cyanotic CHD with pulmonary stenosis/atresia or functionally single ventricles. The most commonly performed arterial shunt is the modified Blalock–Taussig (BT) shunt in which a graft is used to connect the subclavian and ipsilateral pulmonary arteries (side-to-side anastomosis), causing minimal distortion of the arterial anatomy (Fig. 18.1). Potts and Waterston-Cooley shunts between the pulmonary artery and descending and ascending aorta, respectively, have now become obsolete and are rarely seen [4]. Another shunt which is also sometimes seen during CHD follow-ups is the central shunt in which a prosthetic graft is placed to connect the ascending aorta and main pulmonary artery (Fig. 18.2). This is done for hypoplastic central pulmonary arteries (Table 18.1).

In some CHD patients, there is only one functional ventricle. These CHDs are characterised by atresia of an atrioventricular or semilunar valve (tricuspid atresia, mitral atresia, pulmonary atresia with intact ventricular septum, right or left ventricular hypoplasia, selected cases of Ebstein anomaly). These single ventricle type CHDs result in the mixing of the systemic and pulmonary venous blood causing cyanosis. Also, the single ventricle is chronically overloaded as it has to support both the systemic and pulmonary circulations. The ventricular function and valvular regurgitation in such cases deteriorate with time.

The rationale of palliation in such cases is to separate the systemic and pulmonary circuits by passively channelling the systemic venous return to pulmonary arteries (PAs). This avoids mixing and reduces the volume load on the single ventricle. Such palliation however comes at the cost of higher central venous pressure.

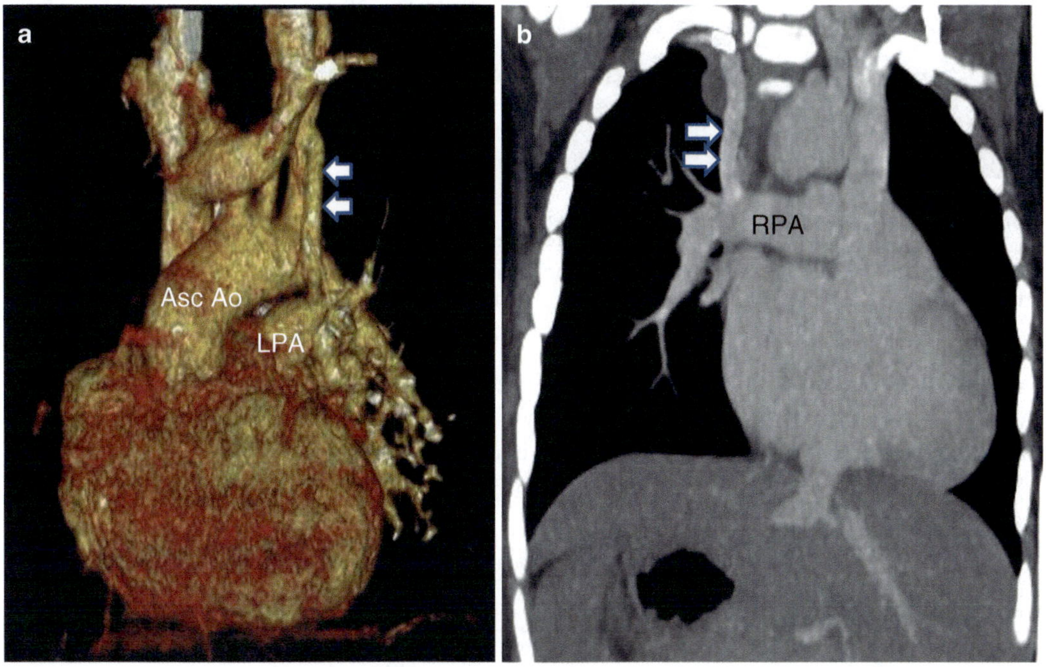

Fig. 18.1 Cardiac CTA volume-rendered image (**a**) shows a patent left-sided Blalock–Taussig (BT) shunt (white solid arrows) connecting the left subclavian artery and left pulmonary artery (LPA). Cardiac CTA maximum intensity projection image in the coronal plane (**b**) shows a patent right-sided BT shunt (white solid arrows)

Glenn originally described a unidirectional anastomosis between the transected distal end of the right pulmonary artery and the side of the superior vena cava (SVC) [5]. The SVC was ligated distal to the anastomotic site. This procedure is currently used in its modified form and is a bidirectional end-to-side anastomosis between SVC and the right pulmonary artery and provides bidirectional non-pulsatile flow to both the lungs (Figs. 18.3 and 18.4). The azygous vein is also ligated to prevent blood egressing from the SVC. The shunt diverts upper body systemic venous blood directly to the lungs improving oxygenation, cyanosis and the workload of the single ventricle. Improvement in cyanosis is partial since the deoxygenated inferior vena cava (IVC) blood continues to reach the systemic circulation. However, it provides excellent long-

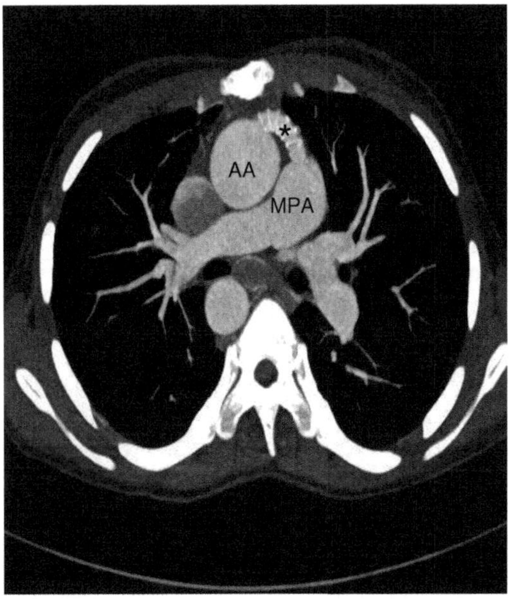

Fig. 18.2 Cardiac CTA maximum intensity projection image in the axial plane shows a patent central shunt (*) between the Ascending aorta (AA) and Main pulmonary artery (MPA)

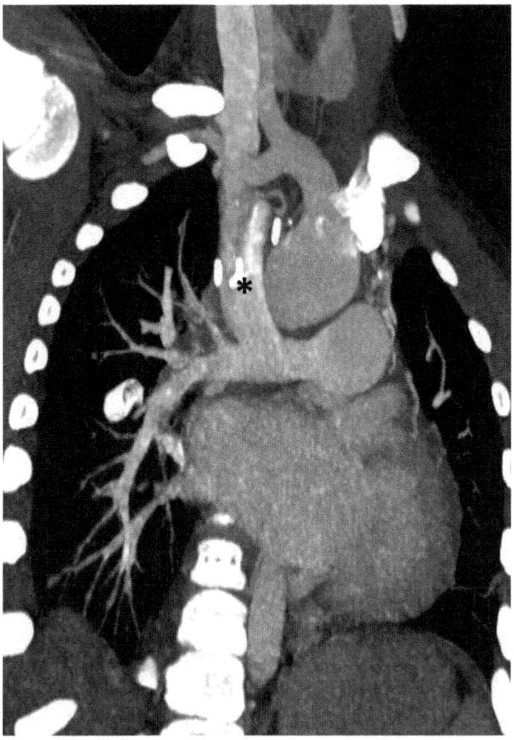

Fig. 18.3 Cardiac CTA maximum intensity projection image in the oblique coronal plane shows a patent Glenn shunt (*)

Table 18.1 Staged palliation of CHDs with functionally single ventricle

Palliative surgery for functionally single ventricle	Timing	Rationale
Stage 1: Systemic-pulmonary shunt or RV to PA conduit in hypoplastic left ventricles (shunt should be restrictive to minimise pulmonary flow, PVR and ventricular volume overload)	Less than 6 months	(i) Provide just enough pulmonary blood for adequate oxygen delivery. (ii) Growth of pulmonary artery to allow low PVR.
Stage 2: Superior cavopulmonary connection (BDG) or Hemi-Fontan	2–6 months	(i) To ensure low-pressure pulmonary blood flow. (ii) Reduced ventricular volume overload.
Stage 3: Completion Fontan	1–5 years	(i) Entire systemic venous blood is routed to PA. (ii) Fenestration in the baffle decompresses systemic venous pressure and increases preload on systemic ventricle.

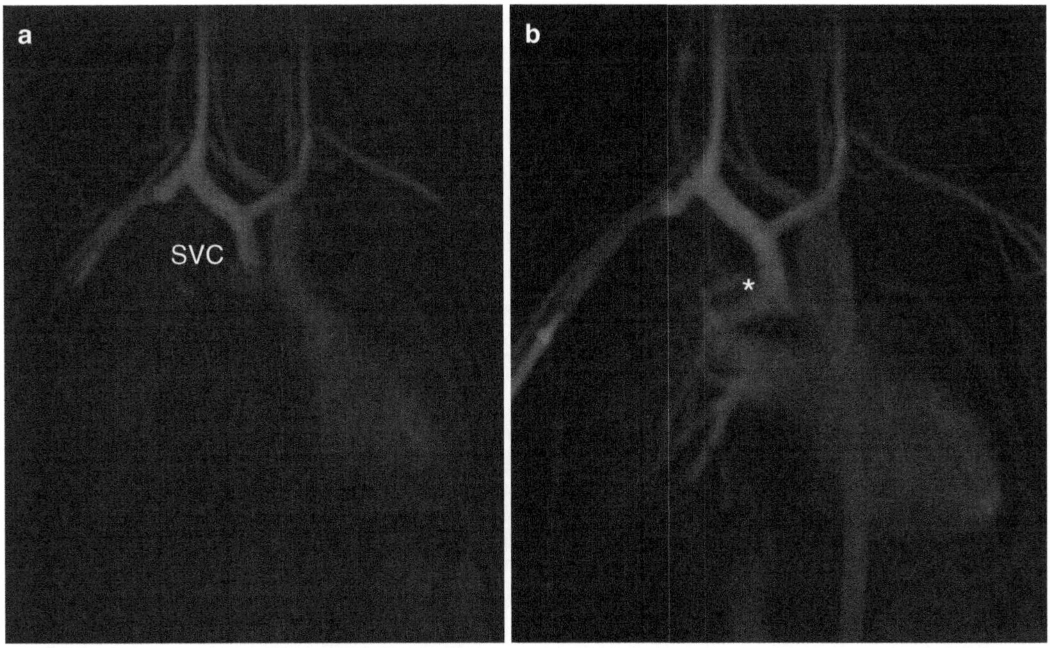

Fig. 18.4 Coronal maximum intensity projection MRA TWIST images with peripheral intravenous injection of contrast via the right upper limb in a patient of Glenn shunt show early contrast opacification of the right subclavian vein, brachiocephalic vein and superior vena cava (**a**), progressive opacification of the superior vena cava and superior vena cava to right pulmonary artery anastomosis (*) (**b**)

term palliation in complex CHDs with low pulmonary flow and resistance (mean PA pressure less than 15 mm of Hg and pulmonary vascular resistance (PVR) less than 2 units/m^2). In many cases (high-risk Fontan candidates), Glenn shunt is considered final palliation.

In many cases, surgeons may leave the additional antegrade pulmonary flow to improve branch PA growth, to further improve oxygenation and reduce the chances of pulmonary arteriovenous malformations [6–8]. This, however, comes at the cost of persistent effusions and chylothorax due to higher central venous pressure [9, 10]. With various studies associating reduced survival to additional antegrade flow, the current trend is to occlude antegrade ventricle to PA flow.

The surgery prior to Fontan can be a restrictive synthetic conduit (3–4 mm internal diameter) between a systemic central vessel and a proximal PA (arterial shunts described initially) or a conduit between the right ventricle and the left PA. Both these allow the pulmonary arteries to grow to allow a low pulmonary resistance. This is followed later by the *bidirectional Glenn (BDG)* to the proximal right PA usually after ligating the systemic to pulmonary shunt. This staging prior to Fontan allows for adaptation.

The selected patients for Fontan should be in sinus rhythm, have adequately sized PAs, low PVR and good ventricular function. The absence of any one of these selection criteria increases the risk of a poor outcome [11].

A *Fontan circulation* usually performed at 1–5 years of age is a surgically created total cavopulmonary connection (TCPC) to divert the entire systemic deoxygenated blood in the SVC and IVC to the PAs circumventing the heart, thus saving it from volume overload and functional deterioration (Fig. 18.5). The connection can be either an intraatrial tunnel or an extracardiac conduit. A fenestration may be intentionally made to decompress the systemic venous pressure and increase the preload in the post-operative period. This is important in patients with suboptimal PVR.

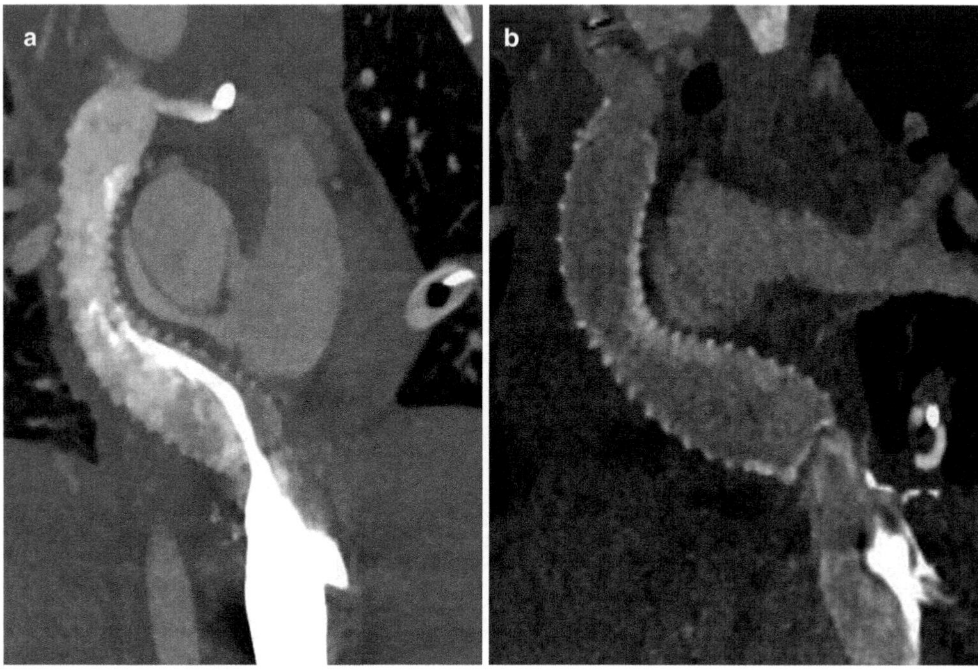

Fig. 18.5 Cardiac CTA early (**a**) and late (**b**) contrast-enhanced images in the oblique coronal plane with injection of contrast via the lower limb peripheral vein in a patient of Fontan circulation. Early contrast-enhanced images show streak artefacts obscuring the inferior anastomotic site

18.4.1 Other Palliative Procedures

In the Rastelli procedure, performed for double outlet right ventricles (DORV) and transposition of great arteries (TGA) with pulmonary outflow obstruction, an extracardiac conduit is used to establish continuity between the right ventricle and main pulmonary artery and the VSD is enlarged, if necessary, to prevent left ventricular outflow tract obstruction (Fig. 18.6). A prosthetic tunnel is created from the left ventricle to aorta through the ventricular septal defect (VSD) [12].

Another palliative procedure, pulmonary artery banding may be done to train the left ventricle (LV) in neonates with TGA without a VSD who are not repaired in the neonatal period. It can also be used to train the LV in patients with l-TGA who may be candidates for an arterial switch procedure. It involves encircling the main PA with a ring of prosthetic material. PA banding is also performed in patients with congenital heart diseases and excessive pulmonary blood flow to protect the pulmonary vasculature from hypertrophy and irreversible pulmonary hypertension.

18.5 Corrective Surgeries for Common CHDs

18.5.1 Tetralogy of Fallot (TOF)

The rationale for the total correction of TOF includes closure of the VSD using a pericardial or synthetic patch and augmenting the right ventricular outflow tract (RVOT). Infundibulectomy (resection of the muscle band RVOT causing moderate stenosis) is performed when the pulmonary valve annulus is adequate and can be preserved. For the pulmonary valve, a commissurotomy can be performed to increase its diameter. A pericardial/Gore-Tex patch is then sewn along the margin of the defect. This increases the RVOT diameter. Branch pulmonary stenosis (PS) can be similarly dealt with. The major disadvantage of this procedure is the obligatory pulmonary regurgitation (PR) afterward. A right ventricle to pulmonary artery extracardiac conduit is generally performed in the presence of pulmonary atresia or when a major coronary artery crosses the right ventricular outflow tract (anomalous prepulmonic course) (Fig. 18.6).

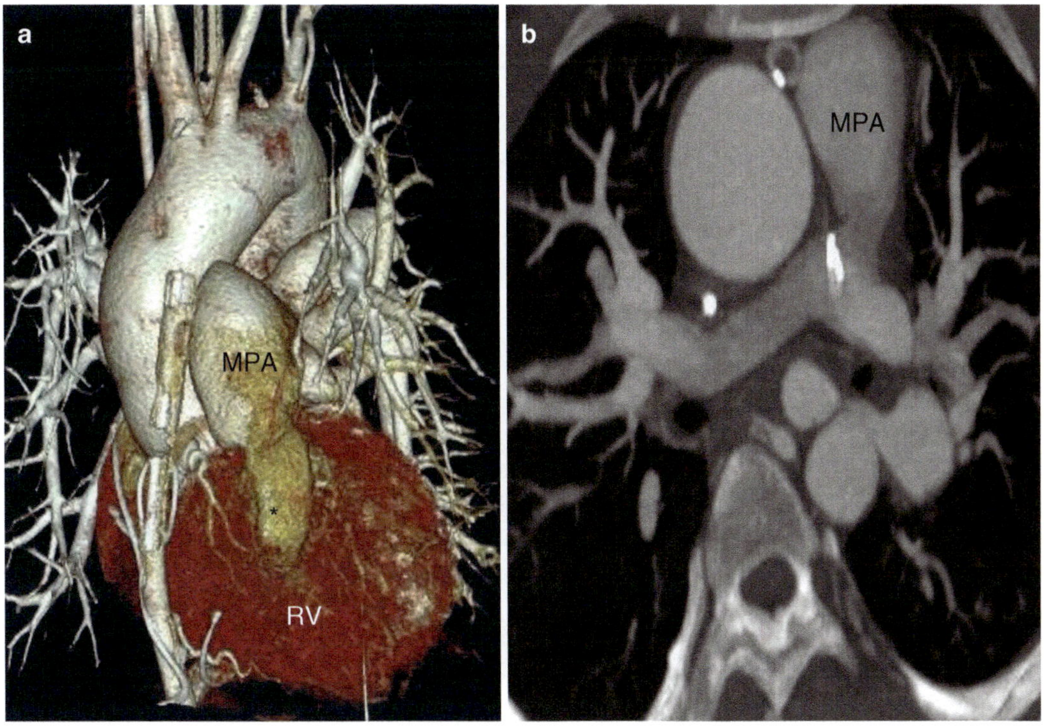

Fig. 18.6 Cardiac CTA volume-rendered image (**a**) and maximum intensity projection image in the axial plane (**b**) in a patient of tetralogy of Fallot with patent right ventricle (RV) to main pulmonary artery (MPA) conduit (*)

18.5.2 Transposition of Great Arteries (TGA)

Physiological correction of d-TGA involves atrial switch where systemic venous blood from the superior vena cava (SVC) and inferior vena cava (IVC) is redirected to the left ventricle. Pulmonary venous blood from the pulmonary veins is redirected to the right ventricle through intraatrial baffle using atrial (*Senning procedure*) or artificial pericardial tissue (Mustard procedure).

The *Jatene arterial switch operation* involves switching the main PA and the aorta and relocating the ostia of the coronary arteries to the neoaorta [13]. The *Lecompte procedure* is also performed, whereby the main pulmonary artery bifurcation is placed anterior to the ascending aorta [14] (Fig. 18.7).

In *Damus–Kaye–Stansel* (DKS) procedure performed for cases d-TGA with subaortic stenosis, the main PA is transected just proximal to bifurcation and the proximal PA is anastomosed to side of ascending aorta forming a channel from the left ventricle to the aorta via the proximal PA, thus bypassing the subaortic stenosis. An external conduit is then placed between the RV and the main PA to establish pulmonary flow [15].

The patients with congenitally corrected TGA undergo an atrial correction procedure and an arterial switch, or an atrial switch and a Rastelli-type repair. These procedures are more commonly performed in children of several months to years of age.

18.5.3 Double Outlet Right Ventricle (DORV)

A TOF-type DORV requires a surgery similar to corrective repair of TOF. DORV, TGA type (subpulmonary VSDs—Taussig–Bing)—can be managed by either of these: (1) patch tunnelling of the VSD to the pulmonary artery combined with an atrial switch; (2) tunnelling of the VSD to the pulmonary artery, DKS aortopulmonary connection with valved extra cardiac RV to PA conduit;

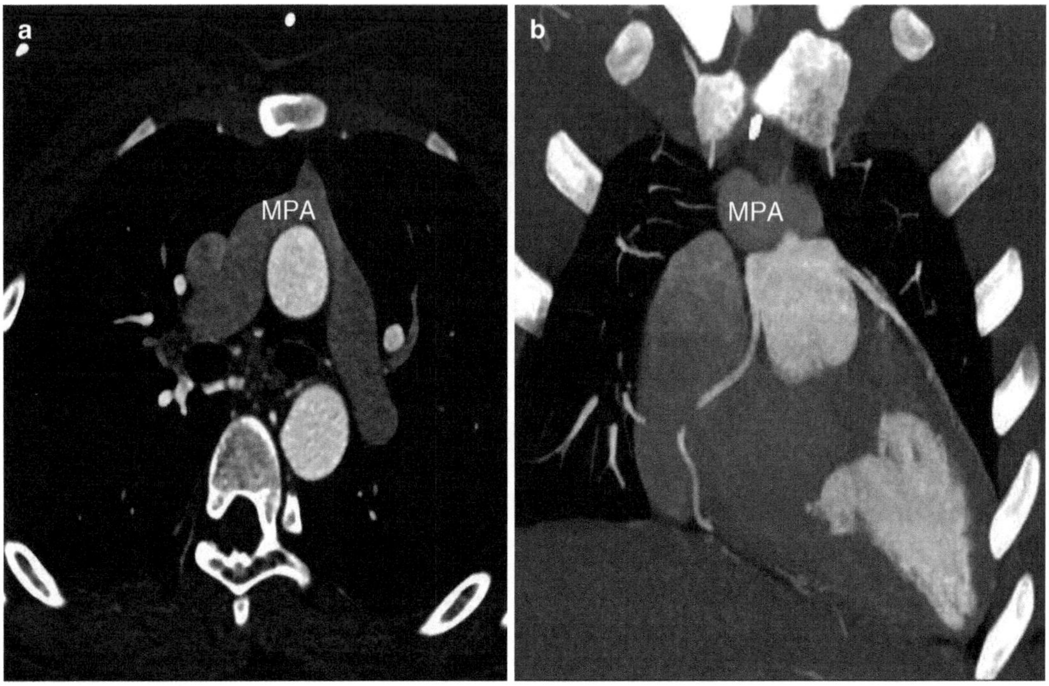

Fig. 18.7 Cardiac CTA images in the axial (**a**) and oblique coronal (**b**) planes in a patient of Jatene arterial switch and Le compte manoeuvre show the main pulmonary artery (MPA) anterior to the neoaorta

(3) direct tunnelling of the VSD to the aorta (*Kawashima repair*); (4) tunnelling of the VSD to the pulmonary artery combined with an arterial switch procedure; (5) VSD closure to the aorta with the placement of an RV to PA conduit; (6) tunnelling of the VSD to the aorta with translocation of the pulmonary artery (Lecompte) or aortic translocation and biventricular outflow tract reconstruction (*Nikaidoh procedure*).

18.5.4 Coarctation of Aorta

The surgical treatment of coarctation, preferred in infants, involves resection and end-to-end anastomosis or interposition graft or subclavian patch aortoplasty or extra-anatomic bypass. Associated arch or long segment thoracic aortic hypoplasia requires long segment extra-anatomic bypass grafts. Endovascular treatment involves the use of balloon angioplasty with/without covered or uncovered stents. Uncovered stents are used in patients without pseudoaneurysm.

18.6 Imaging of Complications of Palliative Shunts

The imaging evaluation of systemic arterial-to-pulmonary artery shunts includes CTA or Magnetic resonance angiography (MRA). Some centres prefer CTA because of its wider availability, excellent spatial resolution and multiplanar reconstruction capability. This however comes at the cost of increased radiation doses (especially important as these patients require multiple imaging follow-ups).

Anatomical distortion, shunt and subclavian artery stenosis, obstruction, anastomotic site and shunt pseudoaneurysm can be diagnosed and characterised on both modalities, CMR being a better technique for visualising shunt patency and quantifying the increase in the size of the pulmonary arteries after the procedure. CTA is an easily available modality for the same (Figs. 18.8 and 18.9). CMR also helps in the assessment of left ventricular dysfunction secondary to volume overload seen with arterial shunts [16]. A seroma,

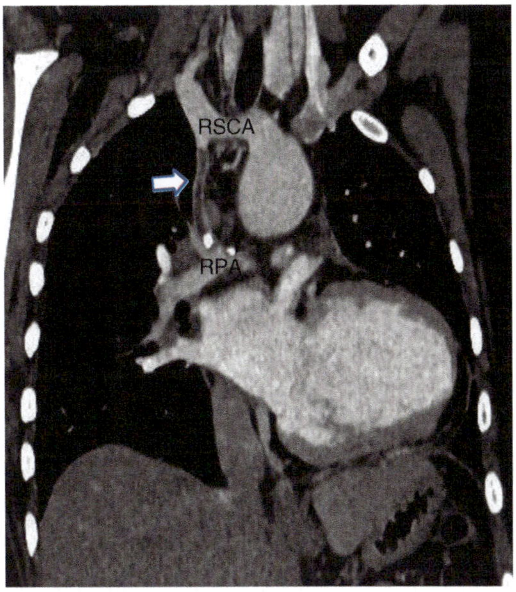

Fig. 18.8 Cardiac CTA image in the oblique coronal plane show thrombosis of the right-sided Blalock–Taussig shunt (white solid arrow)

formed due to fluid seepage across the BT shunt graft, is an uncommon complication. Its presence is suggested on follow-up radiographs and its confirmation may require further imaging (Fig. 18.10). Attenuation of the lesion on CT or its signal intensity on CMR help differentiate it from close differential diagnoses (hematoma/abscess) [17].

The disadvantages of central shunt can be excessive pulmonary flow or distortion of PAs with patient growth.

In functionally single ventricles, the goals of Stage 1 palliation or a Glenn shunt are to provide unobstructed, but limited systemic blood flow through undistorted pulmonary arteries. The pulmonary venous return should also be unobstructed and there should be minimal atrioventricular valve regurgitation.

An elevated SVC pressure after Glenn shunt can be secondary to any aetiology which increases the PA pressure (thrombosis, distorted central

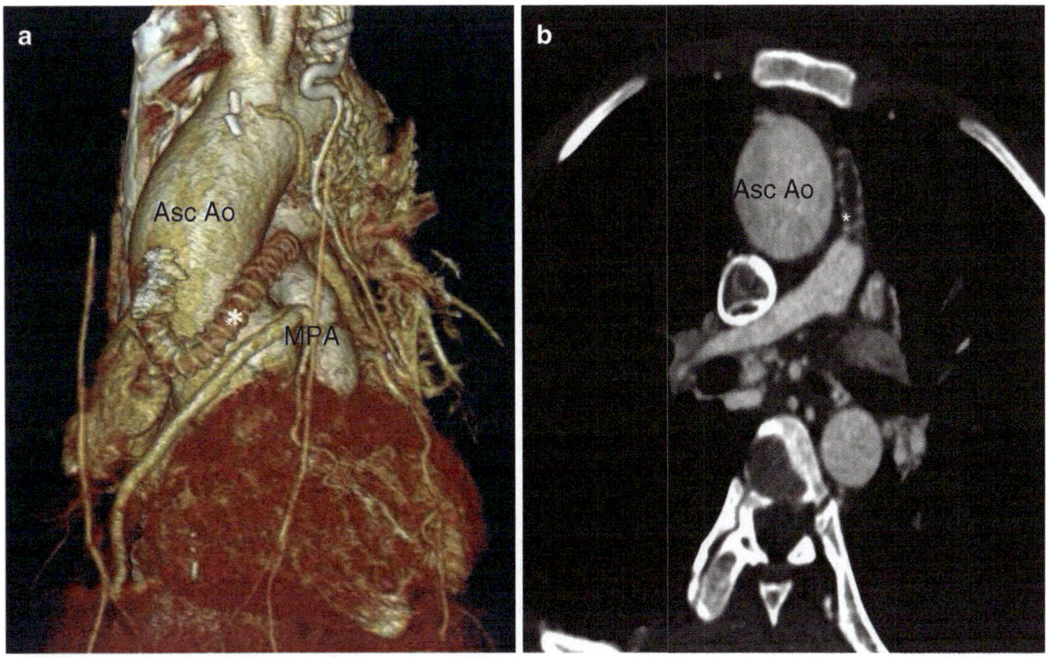

Fig. 18.9 Cardiac CTA volume-rendered image shows a central shunt (*) connecting the ascending aorta (Asc Ao) and main pulmonary artery (MPA). Maximum intensity projection image in the axial plane shows a thrombosed central shunt (*) between the Ascending aorta (AA) and Main pulmonary artery (MPA)

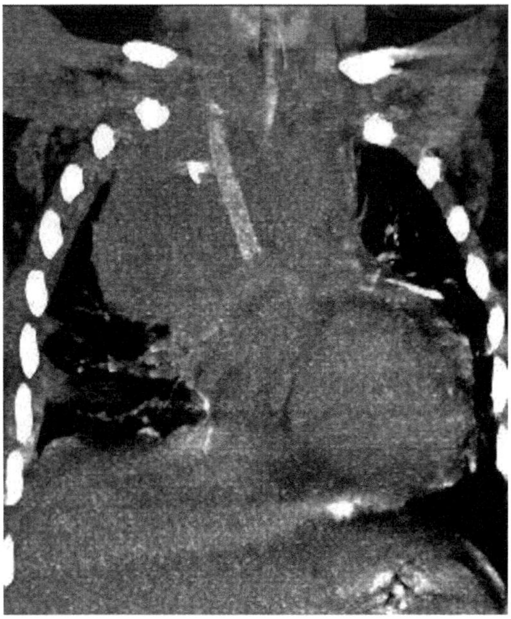

Fig. 18.10 Seroma non-contrast CT image in the coronal plane in a patient of BT shunt shows a well-defined hypodense collection adjacent to the BT shunt. No intralesional hyperdensities, calcification or air seen

PA, central/peripheral PS). Since significant elevations of central venous pressure may limit cerebral blood flow, pressures more than 18 mm Hg are an indication to investigate for such causes. Persistent pleural effusions are the result of low cardiac output due to a combination of reduced post-operative preload, systolic and diastolic dysfunction (Fig. 18.11). In such cases, it is pertinent to inquire about obstructions to systemic blood flow which increase afterload, atrioventricular (AV) regurgitation which causes post-capillary hypertension and pulmonary vein (PV) stenosis which also causes post-capillary hypertension.

Mediastinal venovenous collaterals are a manifestation of raised venous pressures [18] (Fig. 18.12). The majority of collaterals originate from the brachiocephalic vein or its junction with SVC and drain into IVC or its tributaries leading to return of systemic venous blood into the systemic circulation without oxygenation thus increasing cyanosis. Dilated azygos vein may be an indirect evidence of elevated PA pressure

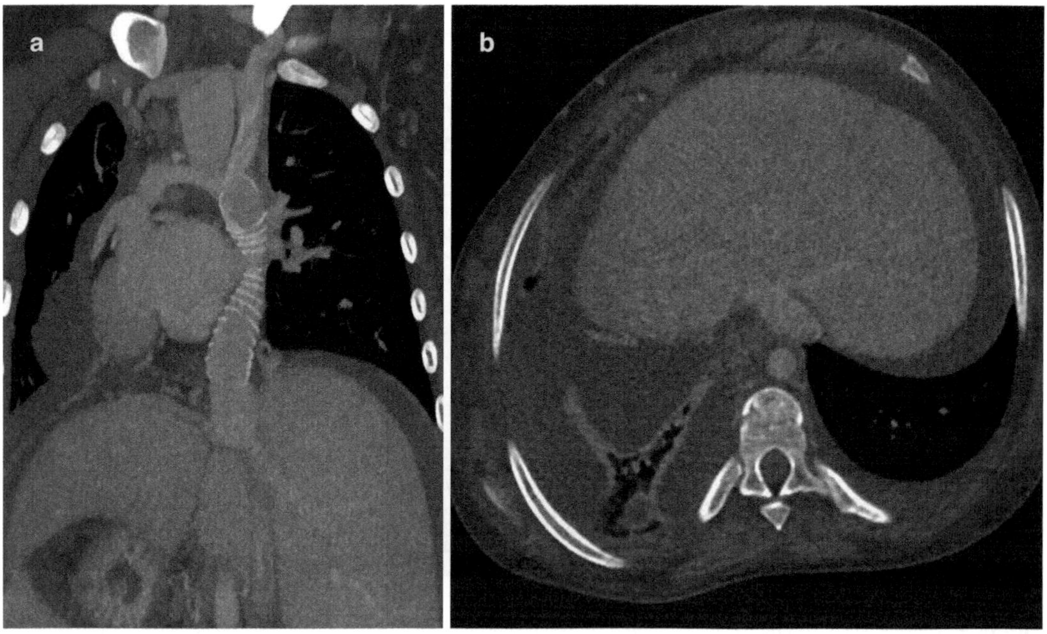

Fig. 18.11 Cardiac CTA maximum intensity projection images in the coronal plane (**a**) and axial plane (**b**) in a patient of patent Fontan circuit show bilateral pleural effusion and ascites

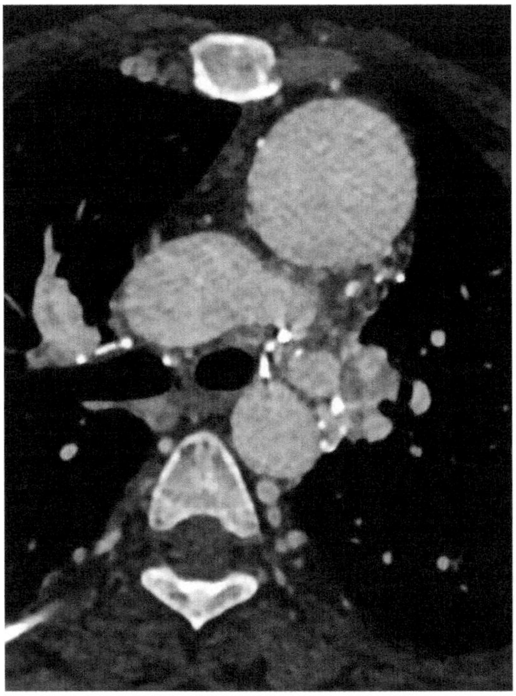

Fig. 18.12 Cardiac CTA image in the axial plane shows venous collaterals in the mediastinum

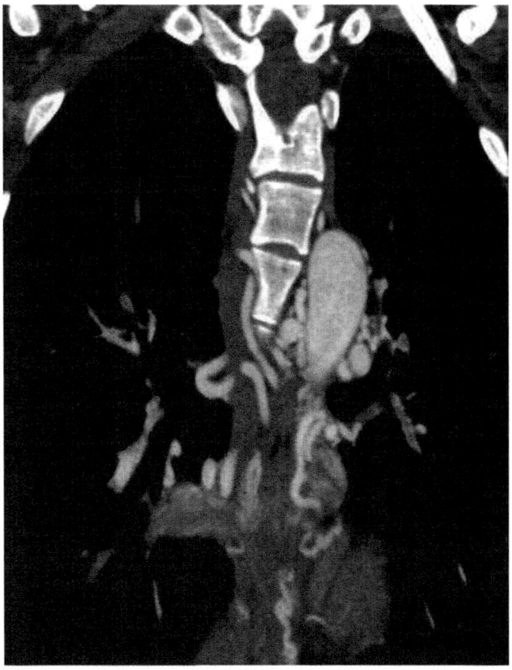

Fig. 18.13 Cardiac CTA image in the coronal plane shows multiple significant aortopulmonary collaterals (white arrow) from the descending aorta

leading to venovenous collaterals. These collaterals can be successfully embolised when diagnosed (on contrast-enhanced cross-sectional imaging techniques) and indicated.

The development of aortopulmonary collateral vessels after the BDG shunt is well known (Fig. 18.13). These collaterals elevate the systemic venous pressure by competitive flow. Significant aortopulmonary collaterals are also a culprit for hemoptysis, increased incidence of pleural effusions and prolonged hospital stay. Triedman et al. found that the patients who underwent BDG were more likely to have aortopulmonary collaterals (65% of BDG patients) than those who underwent Fontan surgery (35% of Fontan patients) [19].

Pulmonary arteriovenous malformations (AVMs) have an incidence between 25 and 37% in patients of Glenn and likely result from endothelial dysfunction due to chronic non-pulsatile pulmonary flow or absence of unidentified factor produced by the liver [20] (Fig. 18.14). They diminish

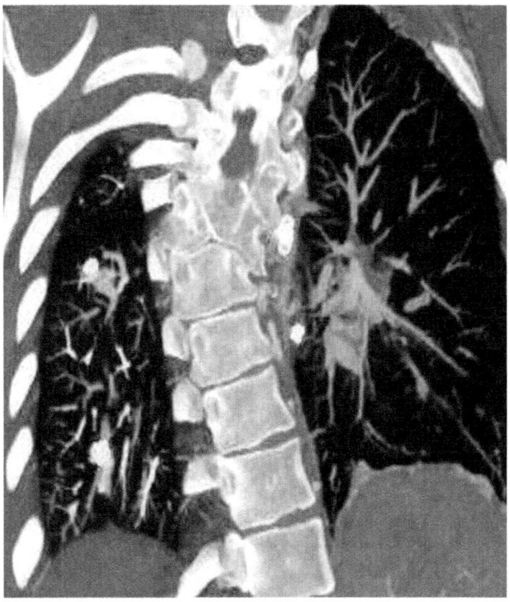

Fig. 18.14 Cardiac CTA images in the oblique coronal plane in a patient of Glenn shunt show recanalised arteriovenous malformations in the right lung

Table 18.2 Complications of Glenn shunt and their appropriate imaging

Complication	Aetiology	Preferred cross-sectional imaging modality
Elevated central venous pressure	(i) Development of PA stenosis/thrombosis. (ii) Development of shunt thrombosis.	CMR with MRA > cardiac CTA as it aides additional imaging of PAs and shunt using cine and phase-contrast sequences essential for assessment of haemodynamic significance of borderline stenosis.
Persistent or new pleural effusion	(i) Reduction in post-operative preload. (ii) Development of systolic and/or diastolic dysfunction. (iii) Development or recanalisation of aortopulmonary collaterals. (iv) Elevation of venous pressures.	CMR > cardiac CTA for evaluation of cardiac/valvular function.
Mediastinal venovenous collaterals	Elevation of venous pressures.	CMR with MRA > cardiac CTA.
Aortopulmonary collaterals	New or recanalisation	MRA = CTA MR, however, provides radiation-free assessment, permitting multiple imaging follow-ups.
Pulmonary AVMs	(i) Development of endothelial dysfunction due to chronic non-pulsatile pulmonary flow. (ii) Absence of unidentified factor produced by liver.	CTA > MRA because of better spatial resolution.

or disappear completely after Fontan completion at the cost of elevation in hepatic venous pressure. CTA and CMR are complementary and supplement invasive angiography and contrast echocardiography (Table 18.2).

A Fontan circuit is a tricky procedure as its take-up or acceptance in a patient is dependent on the delicate match between preload and afterload. Some patients develop a state of low cardiac output, pleural effusion and other signs of failure of Fontan circulation owing to a sudden reduction in preload to the hypertrophied ventricle and preload-afterload mismatch. A preoperative McGoon ratio of more than 1.8 is used to carefully select patients, as those with a ratio of less than 1.8 are at increased risk of death and Fontan dysfunction. Other complications of Fontan circulation include thromboembolic events related to atrial dilatation, arrhythmias, valvular regurgitation, stenosis of the cavopulmonary anastomosis or pulmonary arteries, ventricular dysfunction, ischemic complications due to surgical coronary artery lesions, and protein-losing enteropathy [21]. High intrathoracic lymphatic pressure or obstruction of lymphatic flow may lead to the development of lymphoalveolar fistula and bronchial casts, producing a rare complication known as plastic bronchitis.

Though CTA is routinely advised for assessment of circuit anatomy, thrombosis and coronary lesions, the haemodynamics of the circuits mandate the need for delayed acquisitions for optimal contrast opacification which come at the cost of increased radiation exposure. CMR is the modality of choice for haemodynamic evaluation, assessment of the significance of stenoses, AV regurgitation, calculation of cardiac function and identification of fibrosis.

In the Rastelli procedure, post-operative degeneration and stenosis of the extracardiac conduit (with or without regurgitation) is almost inevitable (Fig. 18.15). Left ventricular dysfunction is also common. Less common complications are: right ventricular dysfunction secondary to conduit dysfunction, obstruction of the tunnel from the left ventricle to the aortic valve and branch pulmonary artery stenosis. Extracardiac conduit patency, haemodynamic changes, ventricular function and valvular regurgitation can be effectively evaluated with CMR.

PA banding can result in dilatation of the proximal portion of the PA, with resultant valve regurgi-

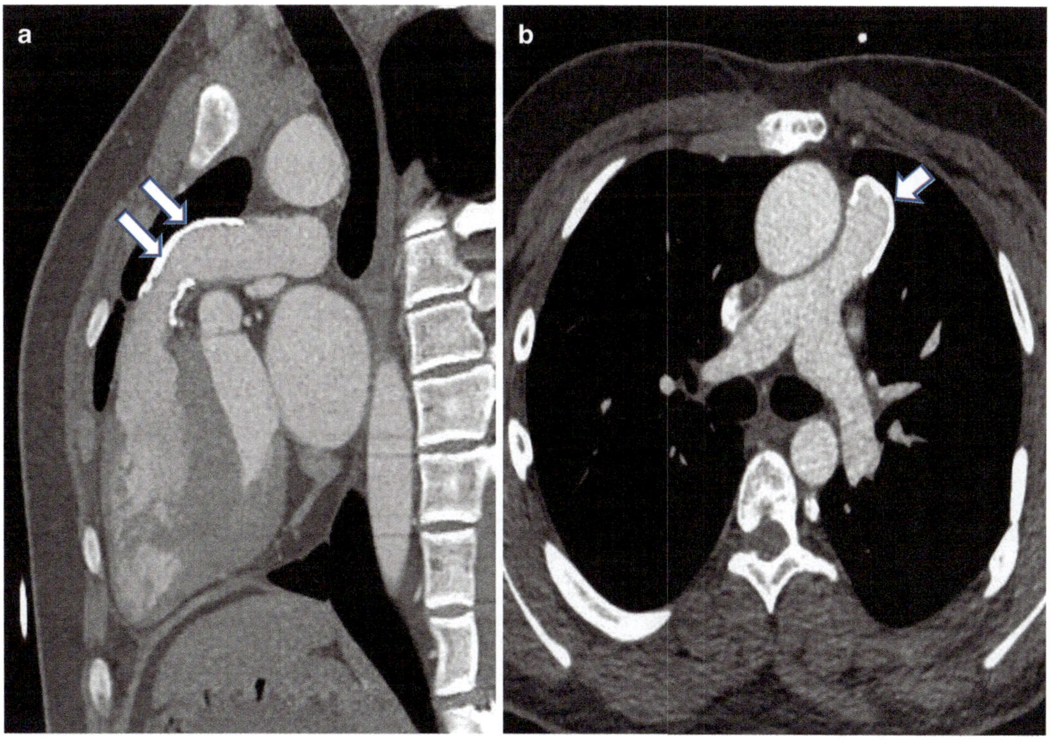

Fig. 18.15 Cardiac CTA images in the oblique sagittal plane (**a**) and axial plane (**b**) show calcific degeneration of the right ventricular to pulmonary artery conduit (white solid arrows)

tation, pulmonary valve injury (when the band is placed too close to the pulmonary valve), erosion of the band with secondary stenosis or pseudoaneurysm, pulmonary artery stenosis (particularly right pulmonary stenosis if the band migrates distally) [22]. CTA provides anatomical characterisation, relationship to surrounding structures and appearance of the pulmonary vascular tree (Fig. 18.16). CMR is paramount in the evaluation of mass and function of the pulmonary ventricle.

18.7 Imaging of Complications of Repaired CHDs

18.7.1 Tetralogy of Fallot (TOF) and TOF-Type Double Outlet Right Ventricle (DORV)

CMR is the investigation of choice for the evaluation of repaired TOF and DORV. Residual RVOT stenosis (the commonest late complication post-infundibulectomy) is diagnosed in suspected cases by visualising the narrowing of RVOT (which persists even during diastole) [23]. CMR can help in its quantification. Right ventricular outflow patch dyskinesia/aneurysm can occur secondary to RV dysfunction. Varying degree of tricuspid regurgitation (TR) is associated with the obligatory PR in patients after transannular patch repair (Figs. 18.17 and 18.18). Recurrent/residual ventricular septal defect also requires MR quantification of Q_p/Q_s which is not possible on CTA. Also, small defects in distorted post-operative anatomies are better imaged on CMR. Progressive left ventricular dysfunction is a poor prognostic marker in these patients. This is assessed best on CMR, including subclinical dysfunction utilising tagging and strain imaging. A myocardial infarction secondary to vascular injury is visualised on CMR, though the anomalous course of coronary and its relationship to surrounding structures is best diagnosed on CTA.

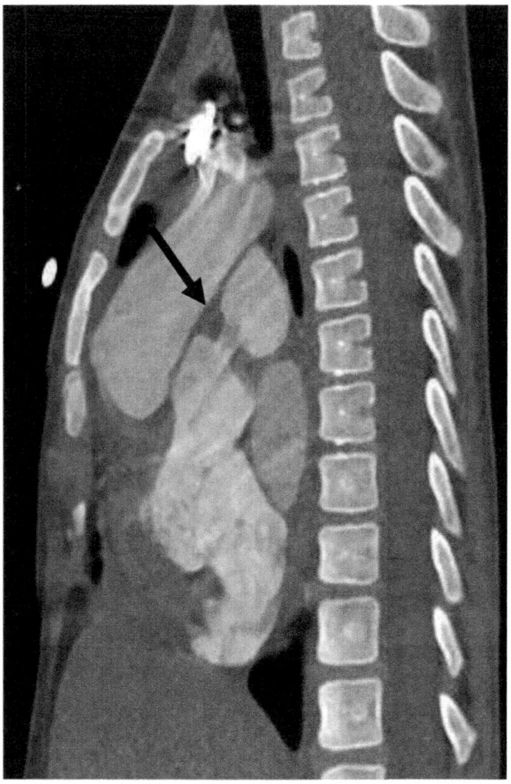

Fig. 18.16 Cardiac CTA image in the sagittal plane shows a hypodense ring (PA band) encircling the main pulmonary artery in the patient of transposition of great arteries without ventricular septal defect

Regarding PR, there are definite CMR criteria for decision-making for pulmonary valve replacement [24] (Fig. 18.19).

Residual main pulmonary and missed branch pulmonary stenosis are culprits for RV dysfunction and PR. These require a combination of both

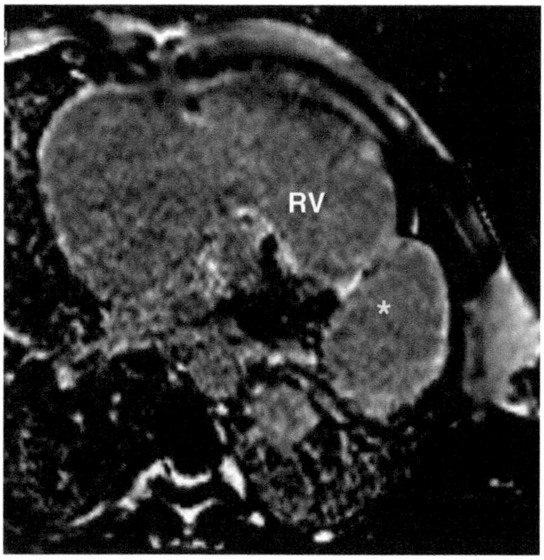

Fig. 18.18 Same case as Fig. 18.17—CMR phase-sensitive inversion recovery images show late gadolinium enhancement in the right ventricle (RV) and right ventricular outflow tract outpouching (*)

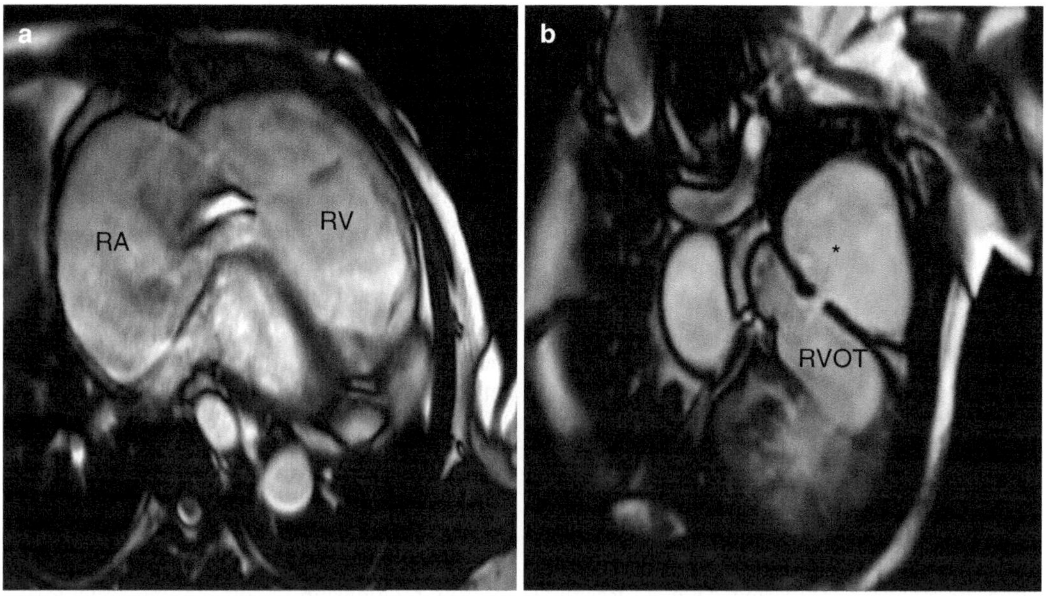

Fig. 18.17 CMR-gated cine images in the four-chamber plane (a) show a dilated right atrium (RA) and right ventricle with a dephasing jet of tricuspid regurgitation. Coronal images show a narrow neck saccular outpouching (*) arising from the right ventricular outflow tract (RVOT) suggesting a pseudoaneurysm

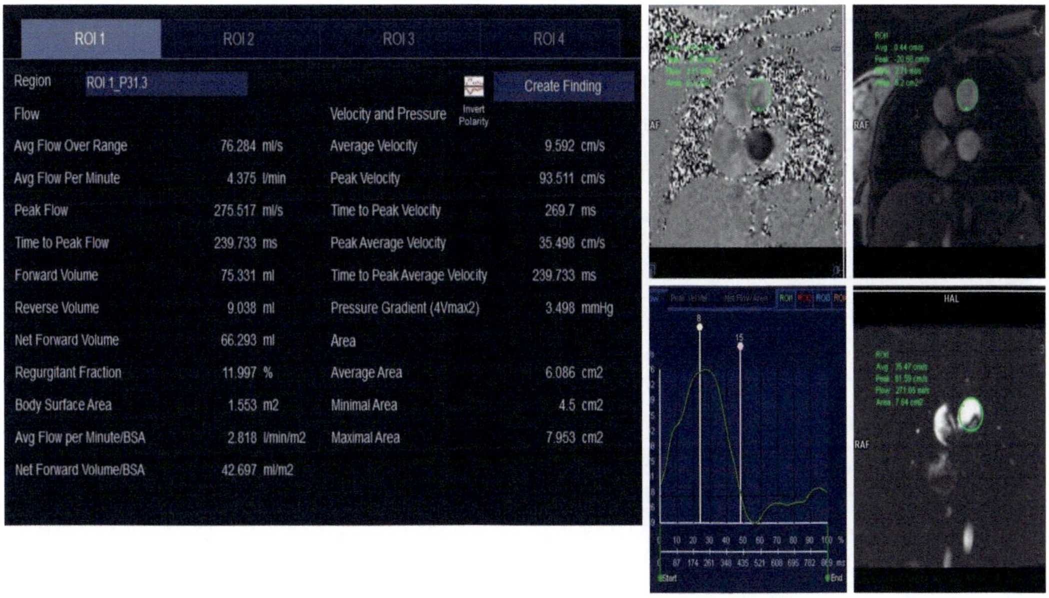

Fig. 18.19 Through plane phase-contrast images of the main pulmonary artery just above the pulmonary valve allow calculation of the flows and pulmonary regurgitant fraction

anatomical and functional imaging. TWIST on CMR can provide both, though has a poor spatial resolution (Fig. 18.20).

18.7.2 Transposition of Great Arteries (TGA) and TGA-Type Double Outlet Right Ventricle (DORV)

A common complication of atrial switch procedure is baffle and vena cava stenosis or obstruction [25]. Obstruction is more common in the superior than in the inferior conduit. The patency of the venous pathway can be effectively evaluated on CMR. Small baffle leaks are more common than obstruction (Fig. 18.21). They are usually small and haemodynamically insignificant but the risk for paradoxical embolism increases. There is progressive right (systemic) ventricular hypertrophy and dilatation with secondary tricuspid valve insufficiency and ultimately right (systemic) ventricular failure. This often occurs in the second or third decades of life when transplantation is the only solution. Late gadolinium-enhanced imaging can be used to detect fibrosis of the systemic ventricle, a finding that is associated with ventricular dysfunction, poor functional tolerance, arrhythmia, and progressive deterioration (Fig. 18.22).

A Jatene arterial switch requires serial imaging for quantitative evaluation of the function of the ventricles, ischemic complications (due to coronary artery translocation) and evaluation of the outflow tracts for obstruction and insufficiency (Fig. 18.23) [26]. In patients in whom the presence of coronary ischemia is suspected, conventional catheter coronary angiography is probably the imaging modality of choice.

The pulmonary arteries need assessment for central and peripheral stenosis related to inadequate growth. Dilatation of neoaorta is invariable, and despite neoaortic root dilatation, haemodynamically significant aortic valve regurgitation is uncommon. Infrequently, a neoaorta aneurysm bulges into the pulmonary bifurcation during systole. The anatomic and functional significance of such obstructions can be more accurately assessed with MR imaging.

The development of left ventricular dysfunction is a rare complication of a double-switch procedure.

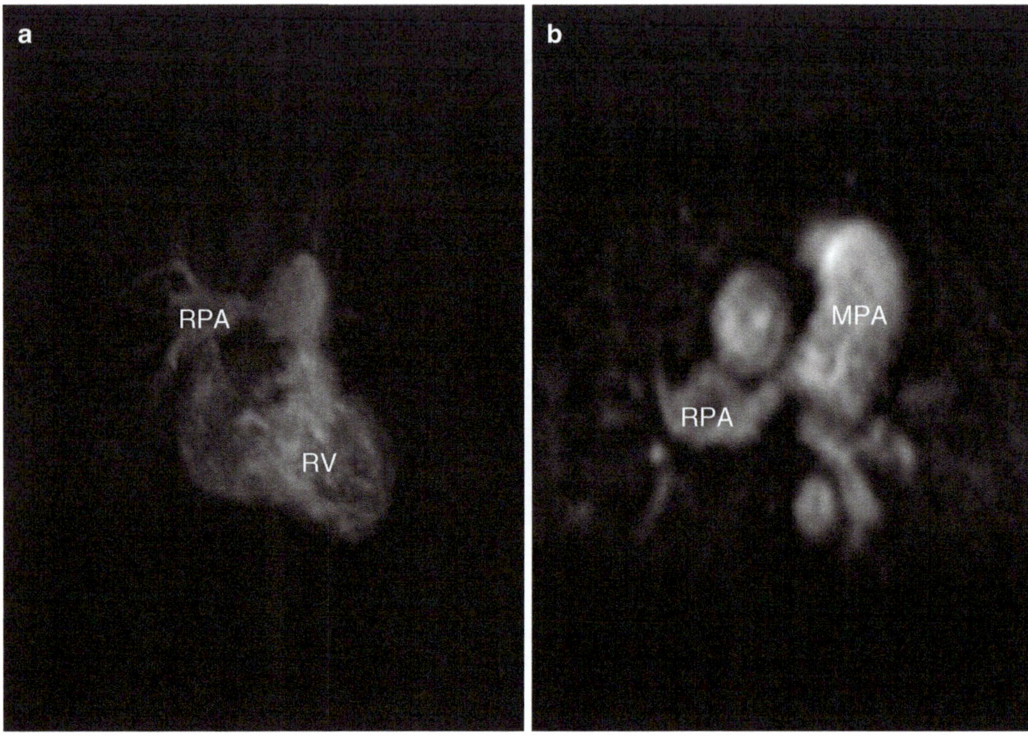

Fig. 18.20 Post-contrast MRA TWIST images in the coronal (**a**) and axial plane (**b**) in a patient of post-operative TOF show significant ostial stenosis of the right pulmonary artery (RPA)

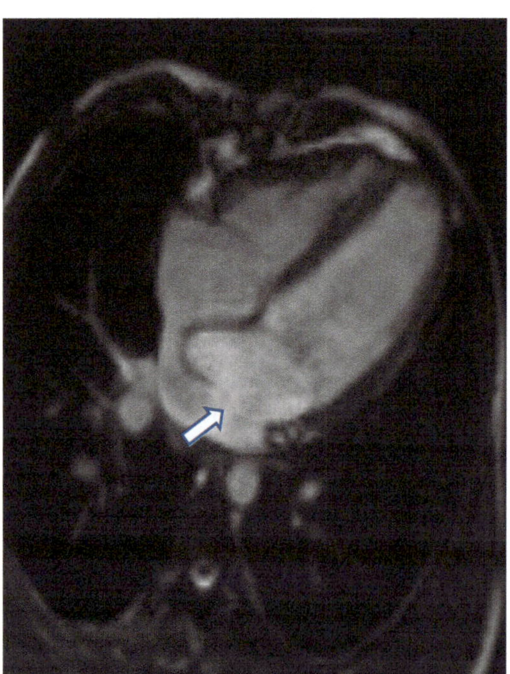

Fig. 18.21 Post-op Senning-CMR gated cine four-chamber image showing break in the continuity of the intraatrial baffle (white solid arrows) with baffle leak

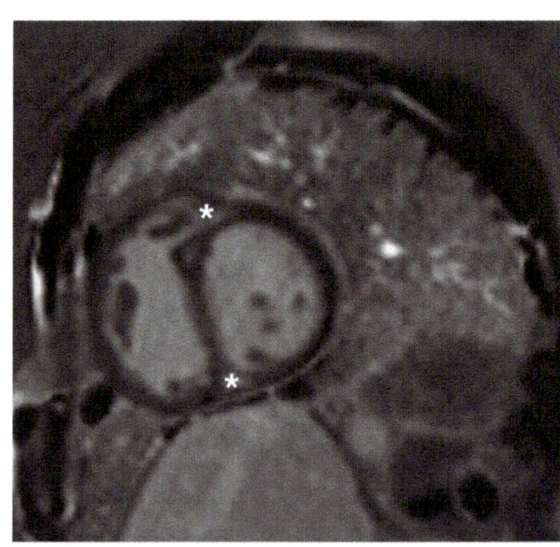

Fig. 18.22 Short-axis LGE images show enhancement at the superior and inferior RV insertion points (*) suggestive of fibrosis

Post DKS, CMR helps in the quantitative evaluation of right and left ventricular function, conduit and outflow tract obstruction and insufficiency.

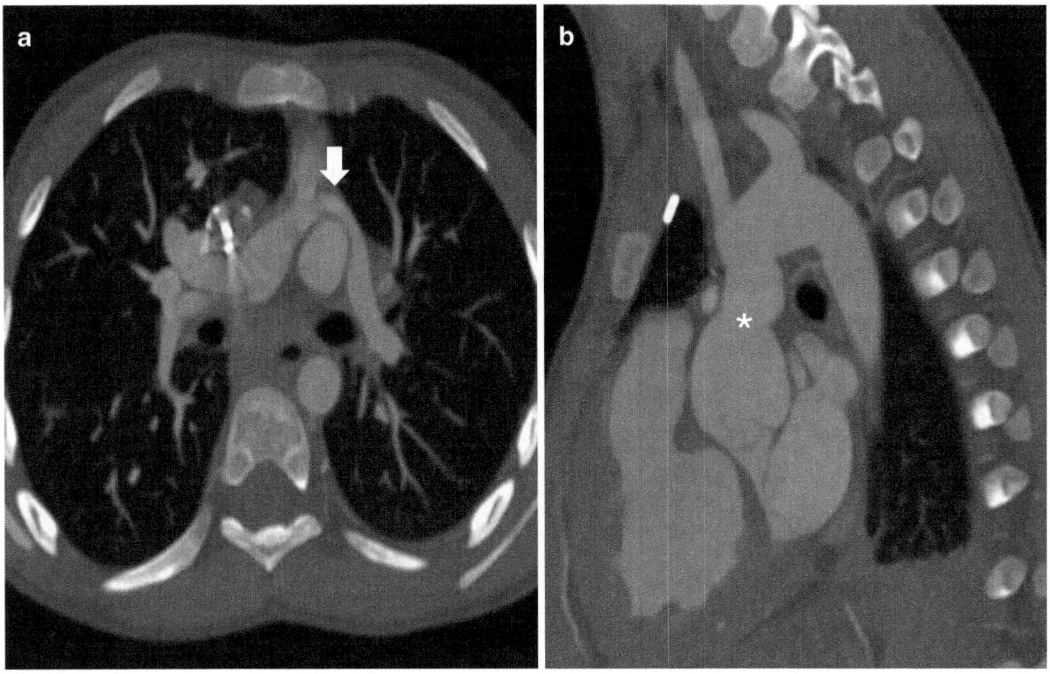

Fig. 18.23 Cardiac CTA images in the axial (**a**) and oblique sagittal (**b**) planes in a patient of Jatene arterial switch and Le compte manoeuvre show the main pulmonary artery (MPA) anterior to the neoaorta. There is significant ostial stenosis of the left pulmonary artery (white solid arrow) and short segment mild narrowing of the ascending aorta (*)

18.7.3 Coarctation of Aorta

Contrast-enhanced MRA provides anatomical characterisation of pre- or post-surgical coarctation with respect to the site, length, associated arch/thoracic/abdominal aortic abnormalities, patent ductus and collateralisation. In addition, CMR assesses biventricular and valvular function, myocardial mass, fibrosis, associated intracardiac defects (including VSD and bicuspid aortic valve). Phase-contrast images are important for the calculation of gradients across the aortic valve as well as the coarcted segment which is important for assessing the haemodynamic significance of native and recurrent/residual coarctation. The amount of flow in the aorta just below the level of diaphragm minus flow volume just distal to the stenosed segment gives the exact volume of collateral flow. Though contrast-enhanced MRA provides excellent anatomical detail of the aorta and collaterals, cine images of the aorta (both transverse and longitudinal axes) and phase-contrast imaging for calculation of gradients are sufficient for diagnosis, treatment planning and assessment of re-coarctation. Time-resolved, velocity-encoded 3D phase-contrast MRI (4D flow MRI) is another non-invasive method of assessment of pressure gradients which has shown excellent correlation with invasive catheter measurements [27, 28]. In light of these advantages, CMR with MRA has definite advantages over CTA. These patients also require multiple follow-ups and cumulative radiation doses from CTA are a major disadvantage. Gated CTA can provide a similar anatomic assessment of aortic, intracardiac, thoracic and extrathoracic abnormalities including calculation of biventricular function but fails in the detection of myocardial fibrosis and in the calculation of gradients.

18.8 Conclusion

CMR and MRA when available, are the modalities of choice for the appropriate radiation-free evaluation of post-operative CHDs, as these provide comprehensive morphoanatomical and functional characterisation. MRA with routine cine images are sufficient for anatomical information of native vessels as well as shunts/conduits. By quantitatively assessing the haemodynamics, they aid decision-making for re-interventions (valve replacements, angioplasties, closure of residual defects, etc.). Cardiac function and fibrosis which are prognostic markers are best evaluated on CMR.

References

1. Opfer E, Shah S. Advances in pediatric cardiovascular imaging. Mo Med. 2018;115(4):354–60.
2. Litmanovich DE, Tack DM, Shahrzad M, Bankier AA. Dose reduction in cardiothoracic CT: review of currently available methods. Radiographics. 2014 Oct;34(6):1469–89.
3. Sonavane SK, Milner DM, Singh SP, Abdel Aal AK, Shahir KS, Chaturvedi A. Comprehensive imaging review of the superior vena cava. Radiographics. 2015 Nov-Dec;35(7):1873–92.
4. Rodríguez E, Soler R, Fernández R, Raposo I. Postoperative imaging in cyanotic congenital heart diseases: part 1. Normal findings. AJR Am J Roentgenol. 2007 Dec;189(6):1353–60.
5. Glenn WW. Circulatory bypass of the right side of the heart. IV. Shunt between superior vena cava and distal right pulmonary artery; report of clinical application. N Engl J Med. 1958 Jul 17;259(3):117–20.
6. Caspi J, Pettitt TW, Ferguson TB, Stopa AR, Sandhu SK. Effects of controlled antegrade pulmonary blood flow on cardiac function after bidirectional cavopulmonary anastomosis. Ann Thorac Surg. 2003;76:1917–22.
7. Calvaruso DF, Rubino A, Ocello S, Salviato N, Guardì D, Petruccelli DF, Cipriani A, Fattouch K, Agati S, Mignosa C, Zannini L, Marcelletti CF. Bidirectional Glenn and antegrade pulmonary blood flow: temporary or definitive palliation? Ann Thorac Surg. 2008 Apr;85(4):1389–95.
8. van Slooten Y, Elzenga NJ, Waterbolk TW, van Melle JP, Berger RMF, Ebels T. The effect of additional pulmonary blood flow on timing of the total cavopulmonary connection. Ann Thorac Surg. 2012;93:2028–34.
9. McElhinney DB, Marianeschi SM, Reddy VM. Additional pulmonary blood flow with the bidirectional Glenn anastomosis: does it make a difference? Ann Thorac Surg. 1998;66:668–72.
10. Ferns SJ, El Zein C, Multani K, Sajan I, Subramanian S, Polimenakos AC, Ilbawi MN. Is additional pulsatile pulmonary blood flow beneficial to patients with bidirectional Glenn? J Thorac Cardiovasc Surg. 2013 Feb;145(2):451–4.
11. Gewillig M, Brown SC. The Fontan circulation after 45 years: update in physiology. Heart. 2016 Jul 15;102(14):1081–6.
12. Naito Y, Fujita T, Tomino T, Koh Y, Isobe F, Manabe H, Kamiya T. Rastelli operation as one stage anatomical correction for infants with complete transposition of the great arteries and ventricular septal defect. Jpn J Surg. 1985 Jan;15(1):36–42.
13. Schidlow DN, Jenkins KJ, Gauvreau K, Croti UA, Giang DTC, Konda RK, Novick WM, Sandoval NF, Castañeda A. Transposition of the great arteries in the developing world: surgery and outcomes. J Am Coll Cardiol. 2017 Jan 3;69(1):43–51.
14. Kim YJ, Song H, Lee JR, Rho JR, Suh KP. Lecompte procedure for complete transposition of the great arteries with ventricular septal defect and pulmonary stenosis. Ann Thorac Surg. 1994 Apr;57(4):876–9.
15. Rosenblum J, Anvari F, Alsoufi B. The Damus-Kaye-Stansel 0peration: management of systemic ventricular outflow tract obstruction. Multimed Man Cardiothorac Surg. 2018 Feb;13:2018.
16. Ntsinjana HN, Hughes ML, Taylor AM. The role of cardiovascular magnetic resonance in pediatric congenital heart disease. J Cardiovasc Magn Reson. 2011 Sep 21;13:51.
17. LeBlanc J, Albus R, Williams WG, Moes CA, Wilson G, Freedom RM, Trusler GA. Serous fluid leakage: a complication following the modified Blalock Taussig shunt. J Thorac Cardiovasc Surg. 1984 Aug;88(2):259–62.
18. Heinemann M, Breuer J, Steger V, Steil E, Sieverding L, Ziemer G. Incidence and impact of systemic venous collateral development after Glenn and Fontan procedures. Thorac Cardiovasc Surg. 2001 Jun;49(3):172–8.
19. Triedman JK, Bridges ND, Mayer JE Jr, Lock JE. Prevalence and risk factors for aortopulmonary collateral vessels after Fontan and bidirectional Glenn procedures. J Am Coll Cardiol. 1993 Jul;22(1):207–15.
20. Ashrafian H, Swan L. The mechanism of formation of pulmonary arteriovenous malformations associated with the classic Glenn shunt (superior cavopulmonary anastomosis). Heart. 2002 Dec;88(6):639.
21. Fredenburg TB, Johnson TR, Cohen MD. The Fontan procedure: anatomy, complications, and manifestations of failure. Radiographics. 2011 Mar-Apr;31(2):453–63.
22. Pinho P, Von Oppell UO, Brink J, Hewitson J. Pulmonary artery banding: adequacy and long-term outcome. Eur J Cardiothorac Surg. 1997 Jan;11(1):105–11.
23. Ho KW, Tan RS, Wong KY, Tan TH, Shankar S, Tan JL. Late complications following tetralogy of Fallot repair: the need for long-term follow-up. Ann Acad Med Singap. 2007 Nov;36(11):947–53.
24. Geva T. Indications for pulmonary valve replacement in repaired tetralogy of fallot: the quest continues. Circulation. 2013 Oct 22;128(17):1855–7.

25. Reddy V, Sharma S, Cobanoglu A. Atrial switch (Senning procedure) in the era of the arterial switch operation: current indications and results. Eur J Cardiothorac Surg. 1996;10(7):546–50.
26. Vargo P, Mavroudis C, Stewart RD, Backer CL. Late complications following the arterial switch operation. World J Pediatr Congenit Heart Surg. 2011 Jan;2(1):37–42.
27. Goubergrits L, Riesenkampff E, Yevtushenko P, Schaller J, Kertzscher U, Hennemuth A, Berger F, Schubert S, Kuehne T. MRI-based computational fluid dynamics for diagnosis and treatment prediction: clinical validation study in patients with coarctation of aorta. J Magn Reson Imaging. 2015 Apr;41(4):909–16.
28. Rengier F, Delles M, Eichhorn J, Azad YJ, von Tengg-Kobligk H, Ley-Zaporozhan J, Dillmann R, Kauczor HU, Unterhinninghofen R, Ley S. Noninvasive pressure difference mapping derived from 4D flow MRI in patients with unrepaired and repaired aortic coarctation. Cardiovasc Diagn Ther. 2014 Apr;4(2):97–103.

Valvular Heart Disease

19

Jahnavi Gaduputi,
Bhavana Nagabhushana Reddy,
D. Prashanth Reddy, and Sanjaya Viswamitra

19.1 Introduction

Valvular heart disease (VHD) is common worldwide and is estimated to account for as many as 20% of cardiac surgeries performed in the developed countries. It may be congenital in origin or secondary to another disease process [1, 2].

Among the multiple available modalities, Doppler echocardiography is the most frequently used tool for evaluating VHD in a comprehensive manner allowing correct assessment of both valve morphology and function [3]. Cardiovascular evaluation is required to determine the valve involvement, effect in flow dynamics such as stenosis/regurgitation, associated hemodynamic complications due to pressure or volume overload, and extracardiac association. Cardiac imaging is used as a surveillance tool to monitor the progression of VHD, to assess the preoperative risk, optimal time for intervention, and postoperative follow-up [4].

Electronic Supplementary Material The online version of this chapter (https://doi.org/10.1007/978-981-15-6755-1_19) contains supplementary material, which is available to authorized users.

J. Gaduputi (✉) · B. N. Reddy · D. P. Reddy · S. Viswamitra
Department of Radiology, Sri Sathya Sai Institute of Higher Medical Sciences,
Whitefield, Bengaluru, Karnataka, India
e-mail: jahnavi.i@sssihms.org.in

Although Doppler echocardiography is the primary imaging modality in the evaluation of VHD, cardiac magnetic resonance imaging (CMR) with unlimited planes, superior image quality, higher accuracy, and reproducibility has emerged as an important tool for a comprehensive assessment of VHD. This is especially true when echocardiography is limited in patients with poor acoustic windows and by operator competence [5]. This review describes the optimal use of CMR in valve disease.

Figure 19.1 described the overall assessment needed in the diagnosis and management of VHD patients.

19.1.1 MRI Assessment of Valve Morphology

The two atrioventricular (AV) and two semilunar (SL) ventriculoarterial cardiac valves ensure a sequential unidirectional forward flow through the cardiac cycle. The atrioventricular valves are mitral and tricuspid valves having large asymmetrical leaflets, while the semilunar ventriculoarterial valves are aortic and pulmonary valves having symmetrical cusps. The AV and SL valves differ in their support structure.

The AV valves have specialized sub-valvular supporting structures, consisting of the valvular annulus, chordae tendineae, and papillary muscles which attach the free edge of the

R. Rajeshkannan et al. (eds.), *CT and MRI in Congenital Heart Diseases*,
https://doi.org/10.1007/978-981-15-6755-1_19

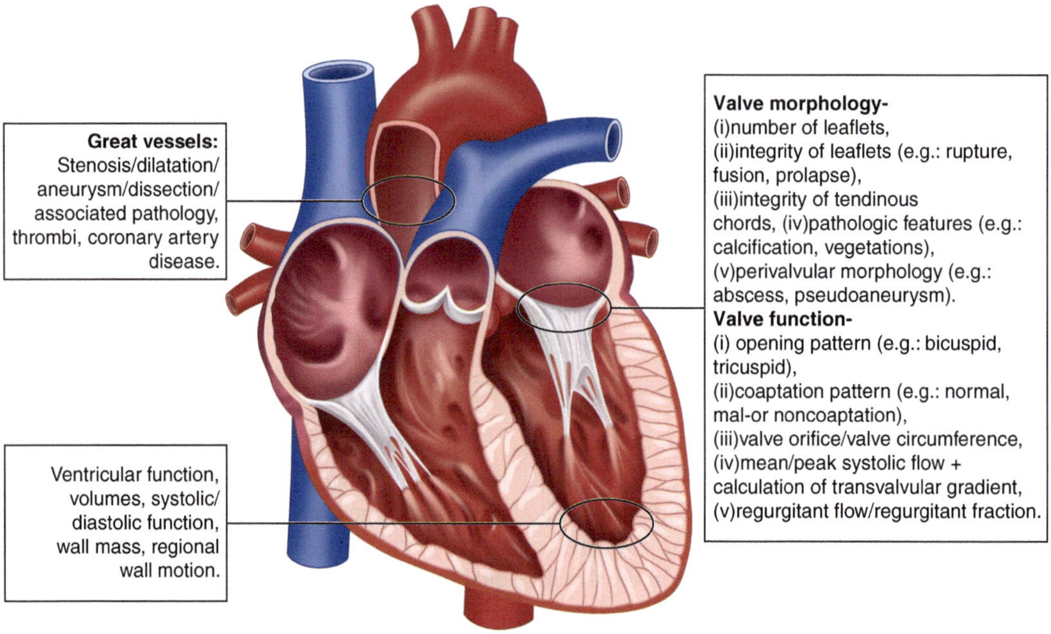

Fig. 19.1 Information needed in the diagnosis and management of VHD patients

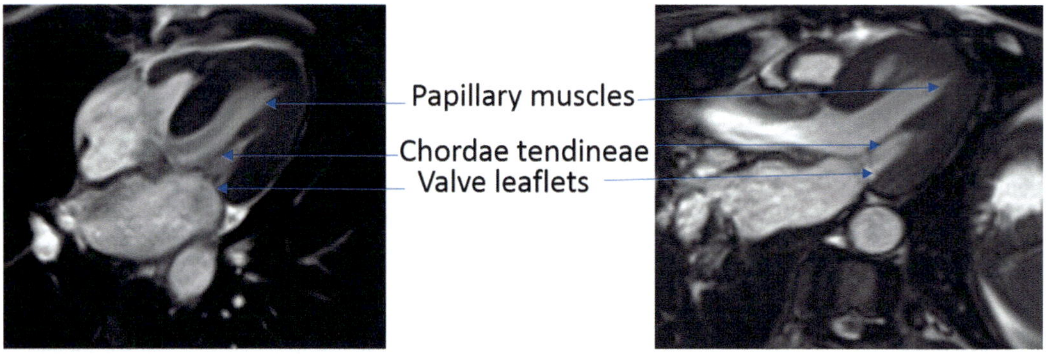

Fig. 19.2 Horizontal long axis/four-chamber and three-chamber images showing the chordae tendineae forming the subvalvular apparatus

leaflets to the inner ventricular walls (Fig. 19.2). The valvular annulus of the AV valves/annulus fibrosa is continuous with the cardiac fibrous skeleton. The aortic root contains crown-shaped aortic valve annulus, the sino-tubular junction, and the sinus of Valsalva with coronary ostia. The continuity of triangular fibrous tissue from the non-coronary aortic cusp left coronary aortic cusp to the anterior leaflet of the mitral valve is termed aortomitral continuity. The aortic root is designed such that the systolic vortices/eddy currents forming in the sinuses promote coronary flow and reduce stress on aortic leaflets [6–8].

While non-coaptation of the valve leaflets leads to backward flow, the narrowing of valvular/subvalvular/supravalvular regions hinders the forward flow of the blood. Non-coaptation of the valve can be the result of a valvular abnormality or an abnormality in the supporting subvalvular

Table 19.1 CMR pulse sequences for valvular heart disease

b-SSFP cine.	Spoiled gradient echo cine.	Phase contrast with velocity encoding.	Turbo spin echo (T1, T2, with or without fat saturation)
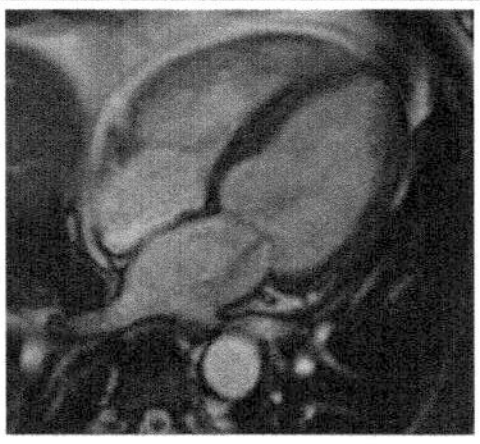	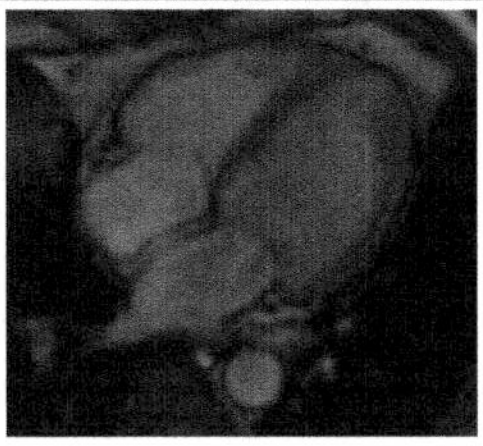	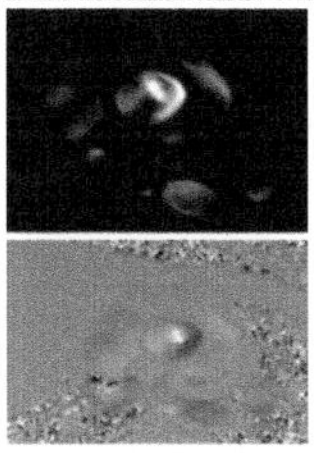	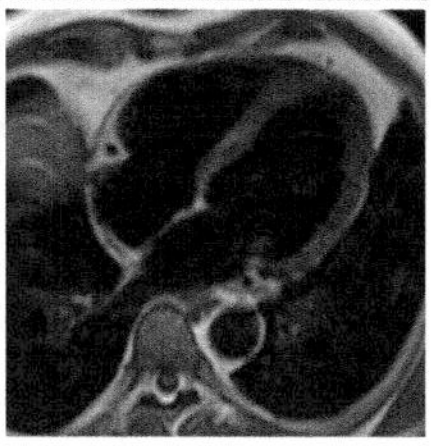
Valve anatomy and motion	Valve anatomy and motion	Flow volumetry—Flow velocity, forward and regurgitant volumes. (Magnitude image on the top. Phase contrast image at the bottom).	Valve mass characterization.
Ventricular volumes and function	Turbulent jet visualization.		
Turbulent jet visualization (Note the turbulent mitral regurgitation jet).	Prosthetic valve assessment.		

apparatus or dilatation of the annulus. These are described in the respective subsections.

Of the many sequences that are available for assessment of valve morphology, ECG-gated balanced-steady-state free precession (b-SSFP) pulse sequence is the mainstay of cine CMR imaging. Cine SSFP has a high contrast between blood pool and surrounding structures with high signal-to-noise ratio and is commonly used to visualize valve morphology and motion (Table 19.1). This sequence also provides an excellent assessment of supporting structures of the valves. Cine SSFP image is acquired as an ECG-gated image over several cardiac cycles and each slice can be obtained within a single breath-hold lasting for 5–8 s. The b-SSFP cine images acquired parallel to the valve can accurately visualize the valve morphology. Echocardiography uses complicated formulae to calculate the valve area, while CMR can do direct planimetry of the orifice area.

The spoiled gradient-echo sequences with longer echo times are occasionally useful, especially in the evaluation of turbulent jets and prosthetic valves [5, 8, 9]. T1, T2 sequences help in the characterization of valvular masses. The turbo spine echo sequences used previously were black-blood images that provide

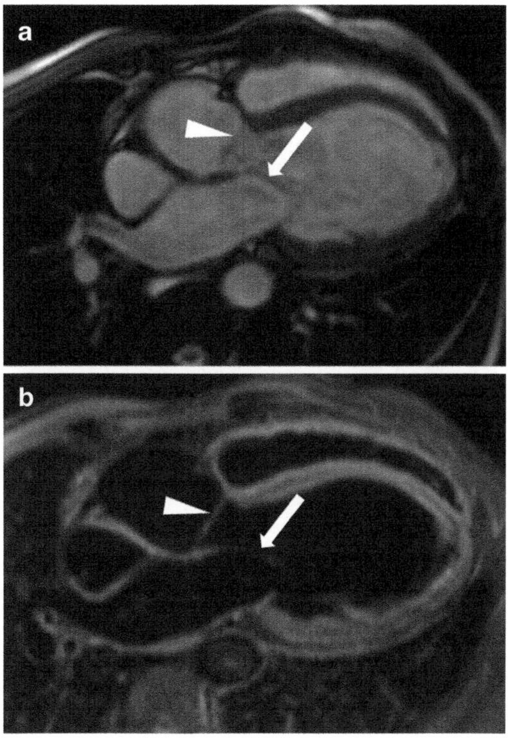

Fig. 19.3 Valvular morphology on “bright blood” and “dark blood” MRI on a three-chamber view in diastole demonstrating the aortic (arrowhead) and mitral (arrow) valves. (**a**) The valve leaflets appear as low-signal intensity structures surrounded by bright blood. (**b**) The valve leaflets appear as high-signal intensity structures surrounded by the dark blood

poor contrast resolution between the myocardium and blood. These have been replaced by b-SSFP images (Fig. 19.3).

19.1.2 Flow Mechanics and Valve Mathematics

19.1.2.1 Normal Flow Patterns

Flow is the movement of particles across a plane. In this chapter, flow refers to blood flow across valves during the cardiac cycle and varies with systole and diastole. "Laminar flow" is defined as uniform velocity in parallel lines. Movement of blood within the heart and in the blood vessel is composed of multiple concentric laminae, each of the lamina having uniform velocity. The advancing edge of the laminar flow can be "flat" or "curved" depending upon the velocities in each lamina (Fig. 19.4). According to Poiseuille's law of resistance, if the flow of the fluid in a channel encounters negligible resistance, the velocity of flow is the same in all laminae, giving a flat velocity profile. However, the flow of viscous fluid has the least velocity in the peripheral lamina and highest velocity in the central lamina, producing a curved/parabolic velocity profile. Although for most calculations, the blood flow within the heart and in proximal great vessels is considered to have a flat—velocity profile, it is important to understand that the highest velocity is present in the center of the jet.

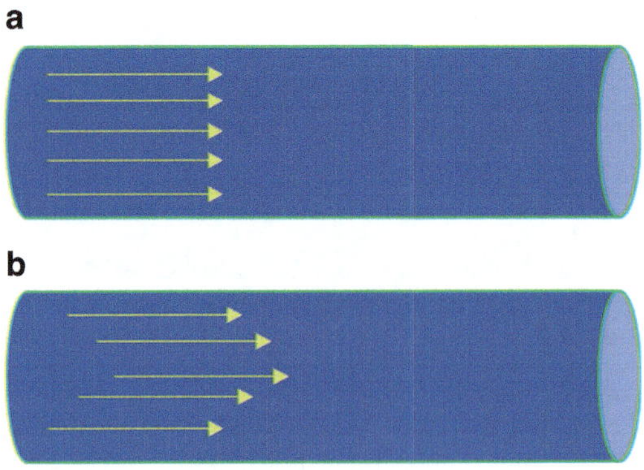

Fig. 19.4 Schematic images representing the flat flow (**a**) and curved flow (**b**) profiles

Continuity Equation

By the principle of continuity of flow in fluid dynamics, the stroke volume proximal to the valve and the stroke volume of the blood traversing the valve is considered equal.

$$\text{Stroke volume proximal} = \text{Stroke volume valve.} \tag{19.1}$$

The volume of the blood (V) that passes through a given area can be calculated as a product of the valve orifice area (VOA) and velocity-time integral (VTI). VTI represents the distance traversed by a given volume of blood depending upon its velocity and time (Fig. 19.5).

$$V\left(\text{cm}^3\right) = \text{VOA}\left(\text{cm}^2\right) \times \text{VTI}\left(\text{cm}\right). \tag{19.2}$$

This is one of the echocardiographic methods to back-calculate the area of a stenotic valve based on the measurement of the flow distal to it and the volume. Forward volume can be measured proximal to the valve and used in the measurement based on the continuity equation.

Thus, VOA (valve area) calculation: VOA = V/VTI.

CMR valve measurements aim to get thin slices across at the valve orifice and use planimetry.

The next equation correlates flow as velocity (v) and pressure gradient. Flow across a normal valve or any area of a vessel is proportional to the pressure gradient (ΔP) across the area, given by the simplified, modified Bernoulli equation as:

$$\varnothing P = 4v^2. \tag{19.3}$$

Think of this as a showerhead. When only the central hole is open the pressure of water on your head is much greater than when all the orifices of the showerhead are open. Figure 19.5 describing the continuity equation also shows the effective pressure gradient change with the smaller column from a "stenotic valve." The stenotic valve will have a faster flow to accommodate the same volume over time and the pressure gradients will also be increased. CMR and Echo both use the velocity to calculate the pressure gradient across the valve.

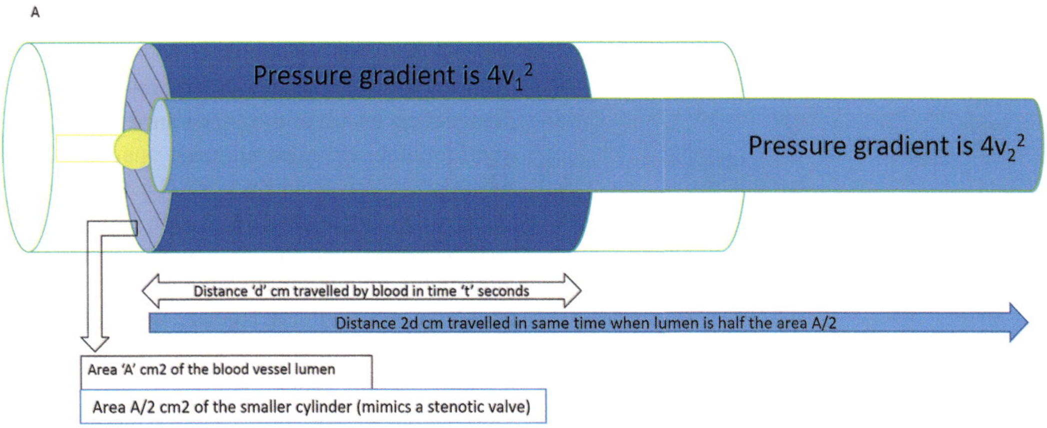

Fig. 19.5 Graphic/pictorial depiction of cross-sectional area and VTI and pressure gradient. VTI: calculated length of the cylinder representing the volume of flow across the plane. Notice that the cylinder has to be longer to accommodate that same volume of fluid that flows across the smaller orifice (narrow light blue cylinder) as compared to the larger orifice (shaded dark blue cylinder with a yellow dot). $4v^2$: The pressure gradient is naturally smaller for the slower v1 velocity as compared to the v2 velocity. The analogy that the pressure from a shower head with all holes open (larger area) is smaller than the pressure from all the water through only the central hole (smaller area)

Vena Contracta This is another term that echocardiographers use frequently. Imagine flow from one chamber through a small valve opening into a larger chamber. Based on the continuity equation above, one can visualize the speed increasing as the flow converges to the valve and then expanding and decreasing on the other side. This is true for normal, stenotic, and regurgitant flows. As the name indicates, the vena contracta is the narrowest part of the converging flow not necessarily turbulence, and can occur at or near the valve (Fig. 19.6). Echo uses the width of this in calculating flows. CMR can image this with in-plane phase-contrast imaging.

19.1.2.2 Abnormal Flow Patterns

Proximal flow patterns: As discussed above, the flow from a chamber converges to the valve and is narrowest at the vena contracta. As described, one can visualize these as represented by small spheres of isovelocity that increase to spheres of higher velocity as they converge to an abnormal valve (Fig. 19.6). The velocities with stenosis or regurgitation can be much higher than the range measured for normal valves and lead to color aliasing. Echo describes the interface of this aliasing as a proximal isovelocity surface area (PISA). This proximal flow profile varies in shape from semi-elliptical in atrioventricular valve pathologies to flat morphology in semilunar valves.

Flow pattern at the orifice: There is the formation of high velocity, laminar jet at the valve orifice. However, the narrowest part of the tapered jet, i.e., vena contracta, is distal to the narrowing at the orifice itself.

Distal flow disturbance: The downstream flow, distal to the valvular orifice, is disorganized containing different flow velocity in multiple directions. The length of this downstream disturbance is dependent on the valvular orifice area and the severity of stenosis (Fig. 19.6) [10–12].

It is necessary for the CMR imager to understand the terms that Echo uses and how the flow is measured on Echo. The CMR imager is advised to spend some time in the echo lab and appreciate the correlation of CMR and Echo, since the full details of Echo evaluation is beyond the scope of this chapter. This helps the CMR imager discuss the findings on CMR with the cardiologist.

19.1.3 MRI Techniques to Evaluate Valvular Function

Measurement of flow on cardiac imaging is done by phase-contrast technique (PC). PC is similar to Doppler imaging on many fronts. Both evaluate variation of flow based on velocity and time

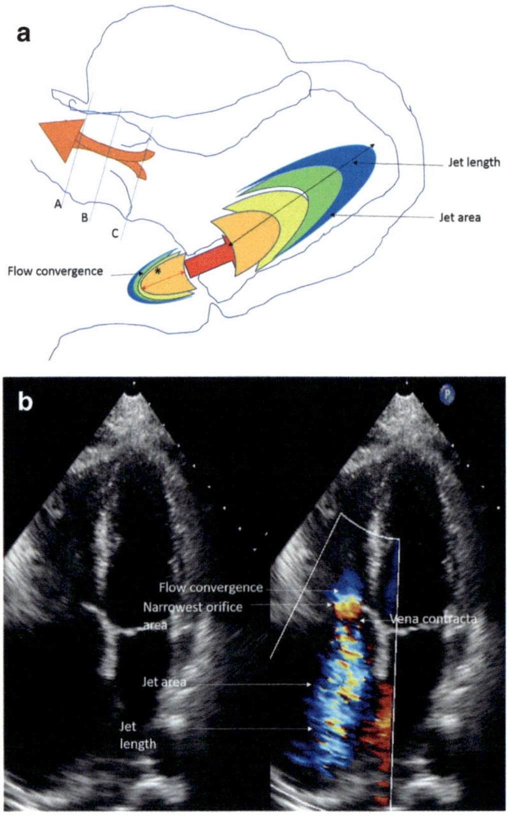

Fig. 19.6 Graphic image demonstrating various components of a regurgitant jet. (**a**) Three-chamber heart diagram. Color coded to show the various isovelocity components within the flow across the mitral valve. PISA calculation uses the innermost velocity radius where aliasing occurs, which is the Orange region * marked above. PISA radius is depicted by a red bidirectional arrow. Also shows the change in jet diameter size as it passes through the aortic valve. Vena contracta is the narrowest portion of the flow. (**b**) In the diagram below of flow through the aortic valve. Note that the narrowest portion need not be at the valve orifice and is often a few mm from the orifice in the direction of flow. (**b**) Apical four-chamber echocardiographic image showing tricuspid regurgitation. PISA identifies the various iso velocity profiles and areas ONLY along the proximal region

across valves. CMR differs in that it requires multiple imaging sequences and techniques, for example, cine SSFP for morphology and PC for flow. Echo Doppler has the versatility of switching on or off Doppler to acquire the information. CMR is consistent in its planes of imaging while echo is dependent on the skill of the operator. Echo has the superior temporal resolution of 20 ms compared to CMR, which averages around 40 ms (range of 25–50 ms) [5].

Stenosis and regurgitation describe flow across abnormal valves. The flow is turbulent (non-laminar) or accelerated or reversed. Most imagers are aware of the appearance of such patterns of flow on color Doppler imaging. CMR images are grayscale images. The flow can be depicted as bright or dark jets on cine gradient and SSFP images. In stenosis, bright jets have more cohesive laminar flow while the dark component of the jet is from loss of coherent flow and turbulence. Regurgitant flow is the most commonly dark line since it is in the opposite direction to static or slow-flowing blood and similar to turbulence.

As discussed above, although echo velocity measurements are very accurate, echo uses multiple surrogates and assumptions to identify the actual volume of abnormal flow. CMR has the advantage of accurate and reproducible volume measurements using the Simpsons method of summing the products of all the volumes of the individual slice (area × slice thickness). CMR correlates well with Echo in measuring flow. In the absence of septal defects, the blood flow from a chamber can only be distributed across the inlet and outlet valves. Thus, correlating the stroke volume with actual flow across a valve allows CMR to quantify flow more accurately and in complex multivalve situations.

In normal individuals, the output of the left ventricle (LV) and the right ventricle (RV) obtained by quantification of the through-plane flow in the proximal ascending aorta and the pulmonary trunk has a 1:1 ratio. Differences in the ratio can be caused by left-to-right or right-to-left shunt or by valvular dysfunction.

The imaging assessment of valvular function includes the assessment of the valvular anatomy (as discussed earlier in this chapter), the severity of regurgitation/stenosis, and consequent ventricular changes due to volume or pressure overload.

19.1.3.1 Qualitative Assessment of Valve Function

The regurgitant or stenotic jet can be qualitatively assessed on the appearance of the jet. The visual assessment of turbulent flow jets across stenotic or regurgitant valves is feasible on b-SSFP and spoiled gradient echo cine images. The jets appear as areas of signal void due to spin dephasing in moving protons [5, 9].

The SSFP flow-related signal loss occurs where voxels span a range of velocities, in the shear layers that happen to surround the more coherent jet core. The width of the jet origin and/or the vena contracta in regurgitant jets provide useful information as milder the leaks, narrower the jets.

The cine images of the flow assist in planning the placement of subsequent velocity-encoded images. However, the signal loss seen on SSFP images is diminished by the balanced gradients as compared to GRE images. Hence in the assessment of the degree of regurgitation, SSFP imaging can underestimate the degree of flow disturbance. Narrow jets are difficult to visualize due to the lack of shear layers at the edge of the jet. Additionally, the direction of the jet can be such that it is not in the plane of the imaging.

In this regard, spoiled gradient echo sequences are more sensitive than SSFP sequences for evaluating the presence and magnitude of turbulent jets [5, 9], due to longer echo time in GRE and the nonuse of balanced pulse gradients.

The visual assessment is at best a rough and approximate guide to the degree of regurgitation or stenosis.

19.1.3.2 Quantitative Assessment of Valve Function

One of the unique advantages of CMR is its ability to quantify flow directly using through-plane PC velocity encoding (VENC) without relying on calculation from complex equations, like echo or invasive catheterization.

The principle of PC is based on the differences between moving and stationary protons when exposed to two gradients that are exactly opposite of each other (bipolar) but applied consecutively in the timing of the pulse. The stationary protons are exposed to the same gradient not having changed location. The moving protons, however, are exposed to different first and reversal gradient strength proportional to the velocity of the protons having moved to a different location. This is termed as “phase shift.” The faster the flow, the greater the phase shift. The strength of the equal and opposite gradients and the duration determines the fastest velocity that can be measured and is termed the VENC of the velocity encoding gradient. The phase shifts experienced by the stationary tissue are eliminated by the application of a bipolar gradient. The phase difference persisting after the application of bipolar gradients is used for the calculation of flow velocities [13–16]. The velocity encoding requires preprogramming a maximum velocity. This can be achieved by setting the VENC manually or by using a VENC scout on the phase-contrast sequence and adjusted to avoid aliasing. This programmed highest velocity is assumed to have a phase shift of 180 degrees. If the sampled jet contains a higher velocity than the programmed maximum velocity, the velocity is misregistered leading to aliasing (Fig. 19.7).

For example, if the VENC is set at 100 cm/s and the jet has a maximum velocity of 150 cm/s, the phase shift of 150 cm/s is assigned as −270 degree (180-degree phase shift for 100 cm/s with an additional 90-degree phase shift for the next 50 cm/s). This aliased high velocity is registered as the flow in the opposite direction and assigned an inverted signal in the velocity images [13]. Hence the accuracy of VENC depends upon how close the programmed maximum velocity is to the true maximum velocity within the jet [17].

The directional information is represented as positive or “white” in the direction of phase-encoding and negative or “black” in the opposite direction, similar to the “red” and “blue” color-coding on color Doppler. The net phase of moving protons is proportional to the velocity of blood and can be displayed as a phase map, where different velocities are represented by different signal intensities [5], where stationary objects with a phase-shift of zero appear gray and mottled having no velocity (Fig. 19.6).

This concept can be expanded further by adding flow encoding bipolar gradients in all three spatial dimensions to measure 3D flow which can be analyzed with respect to time, leading to 4D flow (time-resolved 3D flow quantification) with the ability to visualize various 3D patterns of flow [18, 19].

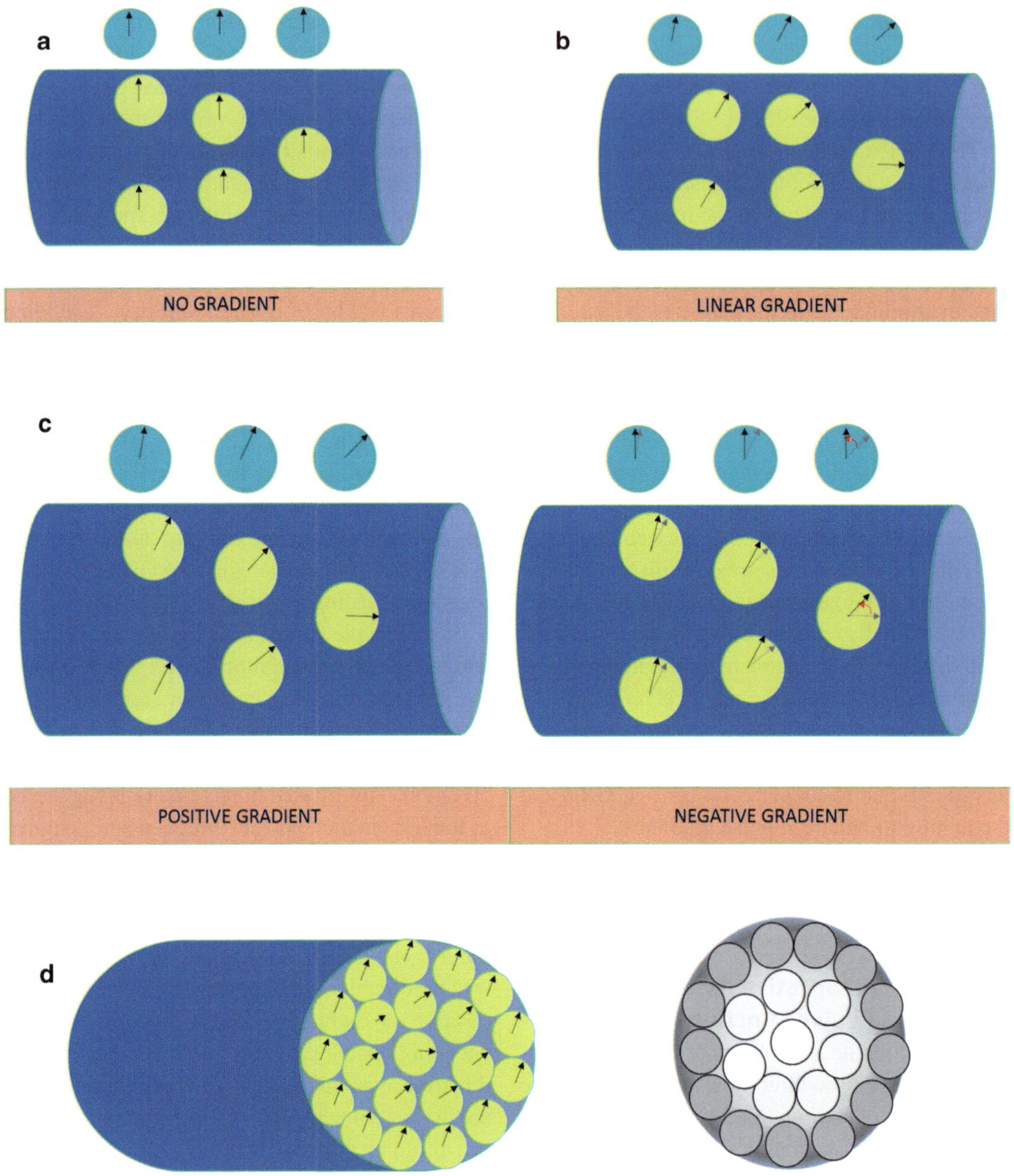

Fig. 19.7 Graphic image showing the dephasing of stationary and moving spins in absence of gradient (**a**), in the presence of linear-gradient (**b**) and on the application of bipolar gradients (**c**). (**d**) Represents en-face view of the vessel with different phase shifts proportional to the velocity in the curved profile laminar flow and the grayscale velocity map calculated based on the phase shift

In through-plane maps, the flow is derived by integrating the velocity of each pixel and its area over time. The region of interest is traced on these images for each frame of the cardiac cycle. The phase-contrast flow measurements can be retrospectively ECG gated or prospectively triggered and obtained with either free-breathing or breath-hold techniques. In prospective gating, data acquired for a fixed time interval with the R wave serving as the trigger for the start of acquisition. The data acquisition is paused at the end of each cardiac cycle. This time interval is called "arrhythmia rejection window." The flow in the late diastolic phase is not measured in this acquisition [13].

Though the shorter breath-hold acquisitions do not account for the physiological effects of breathing on cardiac filling, they are useful in patients with dyspnea. Free-breathing techniques account for physiological effects of breath-holding; however, these have a longer sampling time and require temporal averaging of flow measurements. They also have the advantage of having improved temporal resolution. The imaging plane should be perpendicular to the valve with the velocity vectors of most voxels perpendicular to the imaging plane.

The best position for flow measurements is not exactly at the level of the valve, but just proximal or distal to the valve annulus. Correction for the motion of the valve annulus through the imaging plane during the cardiac cycle can be obtained with a slice-tracking technique if available [9].

$$\text{Flow volume}\left(\text{cm}^3/\text{s}\right) = \left(\text{Velocity within each pixel}\left(\text{cm/s}\right)\right) \times \left(\text{area}\left(\text{cm}^2\right)\right)$$

CMR flow—velocity maps generate two sets of images, the magnitude images, which delineate the anatomy of the vessel, absolute velocity being studied and structures surrounding it and the phase velocity maps in which velocities are encoded based on direction within each pixel.

Velocities can also be assessed with either "through-plane" or "in-plane" phase-contrast sequences. The in-plane sequences can demonstrate the origin and direction of a jet and can be useful for visualizing the site of stenosis and measuring velocity along the course of a jet or can assist in planning the subsequent perpendicular or "through-plane" slice. Till recently, the flow could only be accurately measured on through-plane evaluation. In-plane sequences are prone to partial volume effects as the width of the stenotic jets (2–4 mm) is smaller than 5–7 mm slice thickness of the image.

In-plane sequences continue to be less accurate for measuring peak velocity in a stenotic lesion, due to the partial volume effects, presence of several velocities within a single voxel and averaging of the phase shift [6]. In fast-changing jet velocities, CMR can underestimate true peak velocity, especially when velocities are above 3.5–4 m/s [20, 21] due to either the signal loss from turbulence, phase shift errors due to fast acceleration, or intravoxel dephasing [22]. This limitation can be partially rectified by using ultrashort echo-time sequences (~2 ms) [21].

While echocardiography measures velocity integral—VTI, CMR measures flow integral, which gives the total forward volume through the plane. PISA and VTI calculations are based on in-plane flow, the PC VENC imaging is based on through-plane flow. Table 19.2 shows the differences between the in-plane and through-plane PC VENC imaging.

One of the limitations of PC MRI is an underestimation of peak velocity in jets with high flow velocities of short duration which can occur at flows greater than 3.5 m/s. Also, the retrospective ECG-gated phase-contrast flow mapping averages flow information over multiple cardiac cycles hence is prone to errors in patients with arrhythmias. In such cases, real-time phase-contrast flow imaging may be performed without ECG gating.

As a rule of thumb, the peak velocity of the ascending aorta varies from 100–160 cm/s and VENC for the first measurement is set at 150–200 cm/s, while the peak velocity of the main pulmonary artery varies from 60 to 120 cm/s with VENC for the first measurement set at 120–180 cm/s [13].

Table 19.2 Comparison of in-plane and through-plane PC VENC imaging

"In-plane" PC VENC images	"Through-plane" PC VENC images
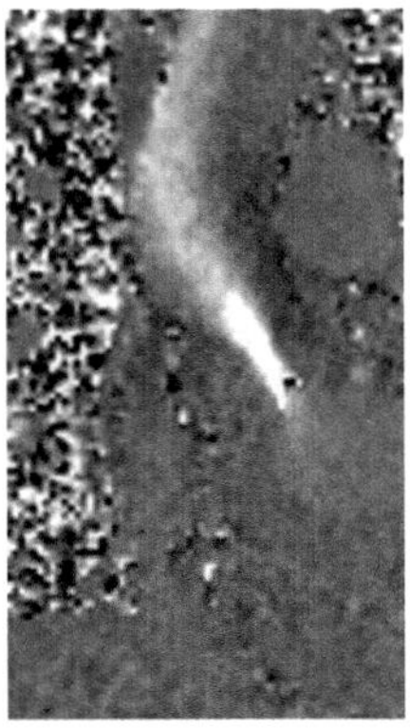	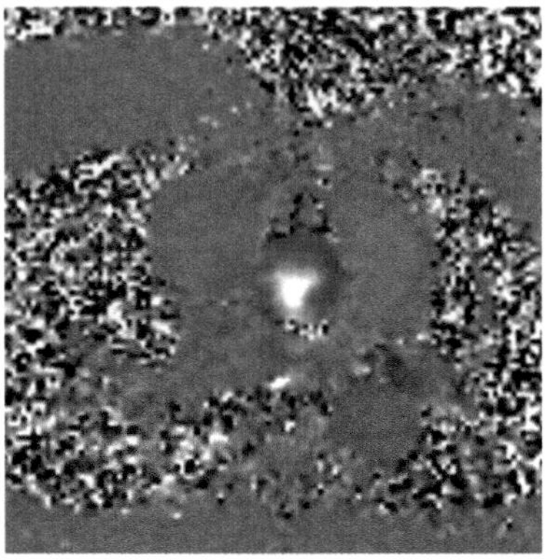
Imaged parallel to the flow	Imaged perpendicular to the flow
Flow measurement difficult	Flow measurement easy
More prone to partial voluming-underestimation of peak velocity in stenotic jets Can help plan "through-plane" images	Less prone to partial voluming

Potential Pitfalls of Flow Quantification Using Phase-Contrast Imaging

- In the absence of valvular regurgitations and intracardiac shunts, the flow through the pulmonary artery (Q_p) is assumed to be equal to the flow through the aorta (Q_s), i.e., $Q_p = Q_s$. However, there can be small differences in these Q_p, Q_s values. A difference of <5% is considered acceptable [13, 23].
- The accuracy of the flow measurements obtained by PC VENC imaging depends upon the positioning of the imaging slice. In through-plane imaging, the slice has to be perpendicular to the jet. An angle difference of ±15% is acceptable, as up to this level, the flow measurements are proportional to an increase in area [13].
- In the aorta, the through-plane imaging slice is commonly placed perpendicular to and close to the sino-tubular junction. The aortic compliance at this level can lead to underestimation of regurgitant flow volumes. Placement of through-plane imaging slice at a sino-tubular junction can pick up the normal reverse flow to the coronary arteries as regurgitation. This coronary artery flow is approximately 6% of the forward flow. These errors can be overcome by placing the imaging slice between the aortic annulus and coronary artery origins [23].
- Another source for error is the systolic apical movement of the aortic valve plane, causing an increased gap between the valvular orifice and the imaging slice, leading to underestimation of the peak velocity and regurgitant volumes [9].
- VENC set too high can lead to increase noise and reduced temporal resolution. This reduces the accuracy of flow quantification for velocities >3.5 m/s [24].
- VENC set too high or low can lead to aliasing [13].

Interpretation of Phase-Contrast Flow Maps

The CMR imager should be familiar with the flow maps derived from the PC VENC imaging. These may differ from vendor to vendor. Typical ones are flow–time, velocity–time, peak velocity–time, and net flow–time graphs. It is also recommended that the CMR imager compare the values from the flow maps to the stroke volumes. Figure 19.8 shows various steps required to obtain PC VENC images.

The flow–time, velocity–time curves are represented as a graph with the flow (ml/s) or velocity (cm/s) plotted on *Y*-axis and time (s) plotted in *X*-axis using multiple reconstructed frames per cardiac cycle.

The graphs obtained in the normal aorta, aortic stenosis, and regurgitation are explained below.

Figure 19.9 describes the various flow–time, velocity–time, and net flow–time graphs obtained from velocity encoded phase-contrast imaging through the aorta and main pulmonary artery.

Figure 19.10 describes the various flow–time, velocity–time, and net flow–time graphs obtained from velocity encoded phase-contrast imaging in aortic stenosis.

Figure 19.11 describes the various flow–time, velocity–time, and net flow–time graphs obtained from velocity encoded phase-contrast imaging in aortic regurgitation.

19.2 Merits and Limitations of Echocardiography and CMR

CMR provides more accurate measurements than transthoracic echocardiography, due to the geometric assumptions and complex formulae used for volume and area calculations. CMR with its ability to visualize the entire ventricular cavity and volumetric analysis using modified Simpson's technique has more accuracy than echocardiography.

Echocardiography overestimates ejection fraction with a higher interstudy and interobserver variability, compared to CMR. 3D Echocardiography with better visualization of endocardial borders is comparable to

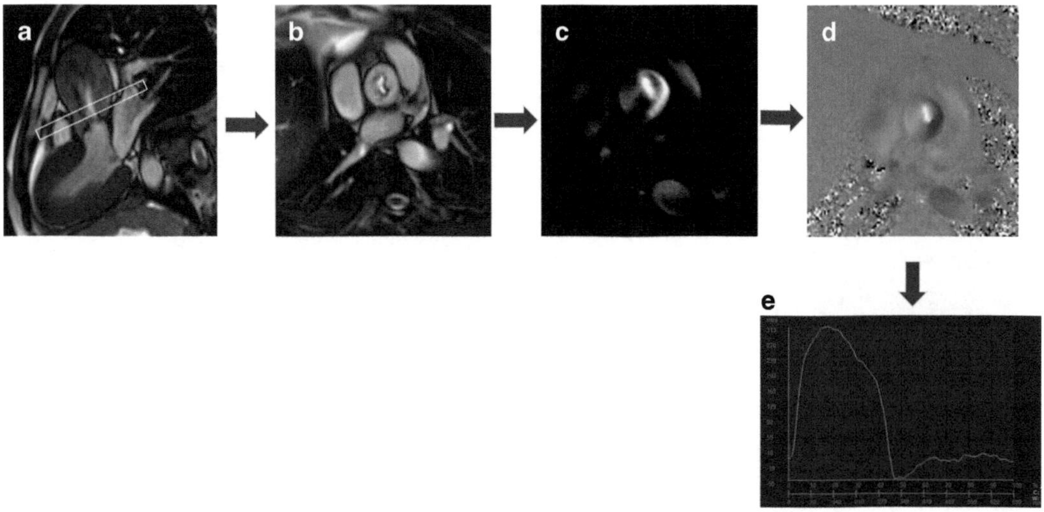

Fig. 19.8 Steps to obtain flow quantification in MRI. The stenotic/regurgitant jet is localized on cine b-SSFP images (**a**). An axial plane of the vessel is obtained perpendicular to the jet (**b**). This plane is used for PC imaging. After selecting an appropriate VENC, magnitude (**c**) and velocity images (**d**) obtained by PC sequence are analyzed by post-processing software to obtain flow, velocity, and net flow data (**e**)

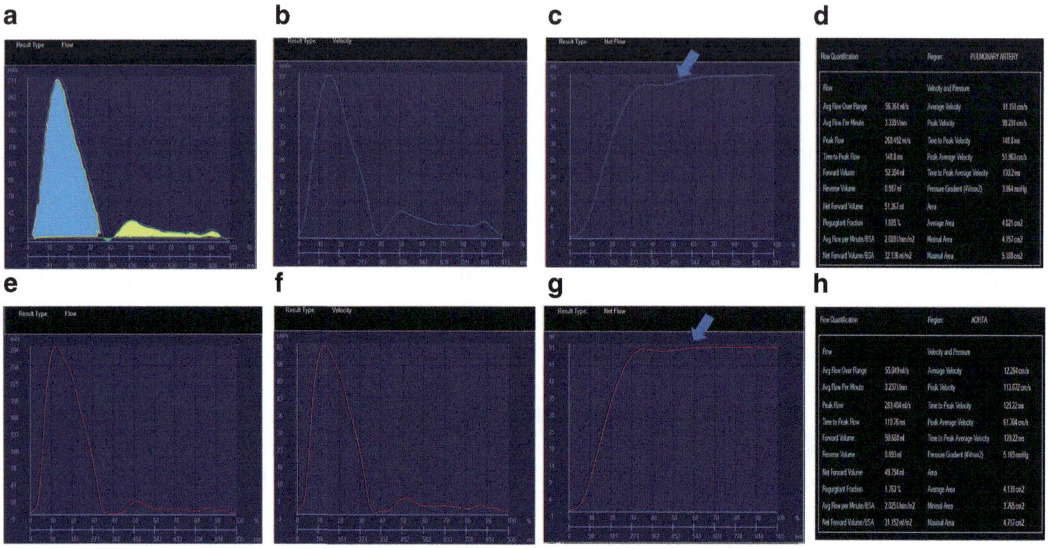

Fig. 19.9 The normal flow–time, velocity–time, and net flow–time curves obtained from the pulmonary artery (Top: **a**–**d**) and aorta (Bottom: **e**–**h**). The blue area represents the early systolic forward flow, green areas represents a minimal diastolic reversal on the closure of semilunar valves and the yellow area represents the late diastolic forward flow. The stroke volume = blue + green + yellow. The net forward flow = blue + yellow. The regurgitant flow = green. Also note the steady plateau of the late net flow–time curve (blue arrow)

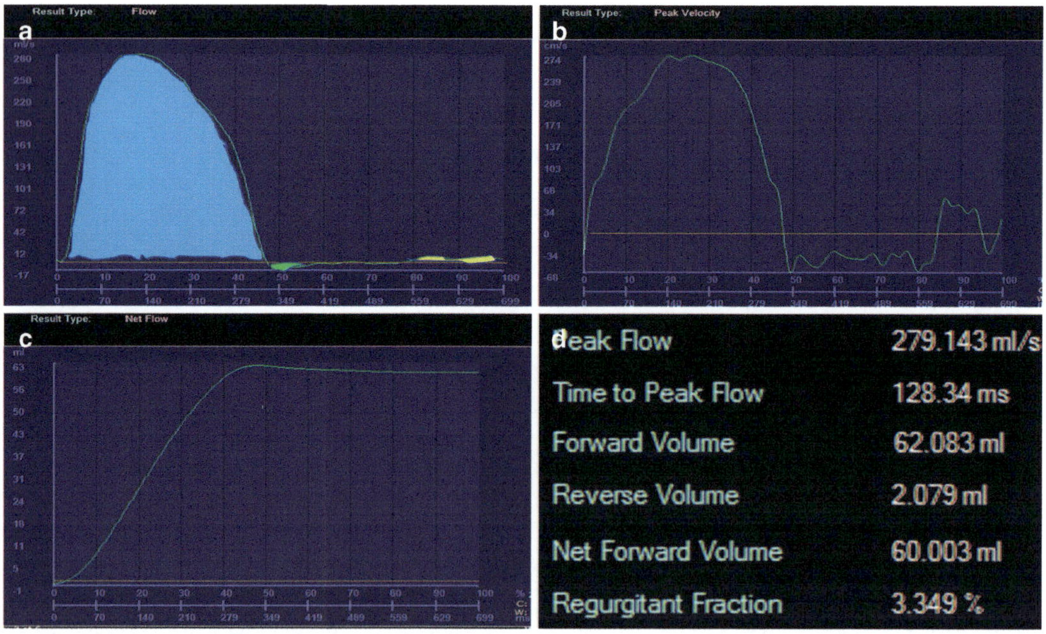

Fig. 19.10 The flow–time curve (**a**), peak velocity–time curve (**b**), net flow curve (**c**) and flow quantification analysis (**d**) in aortic stenosis demonstrating a rapid early high-velocity flow with a peak velocity of 279 cm/s. The blue area represents the early high volume systolic forward flow, green areas represents a minimal diastolic reversal on the closure of semilunar valves, and the yellow area represents the late diastolic forward flow. The stroke volume = blue + green + yellow. The net forward flow = blue + yellow. The regurgitant flow = green

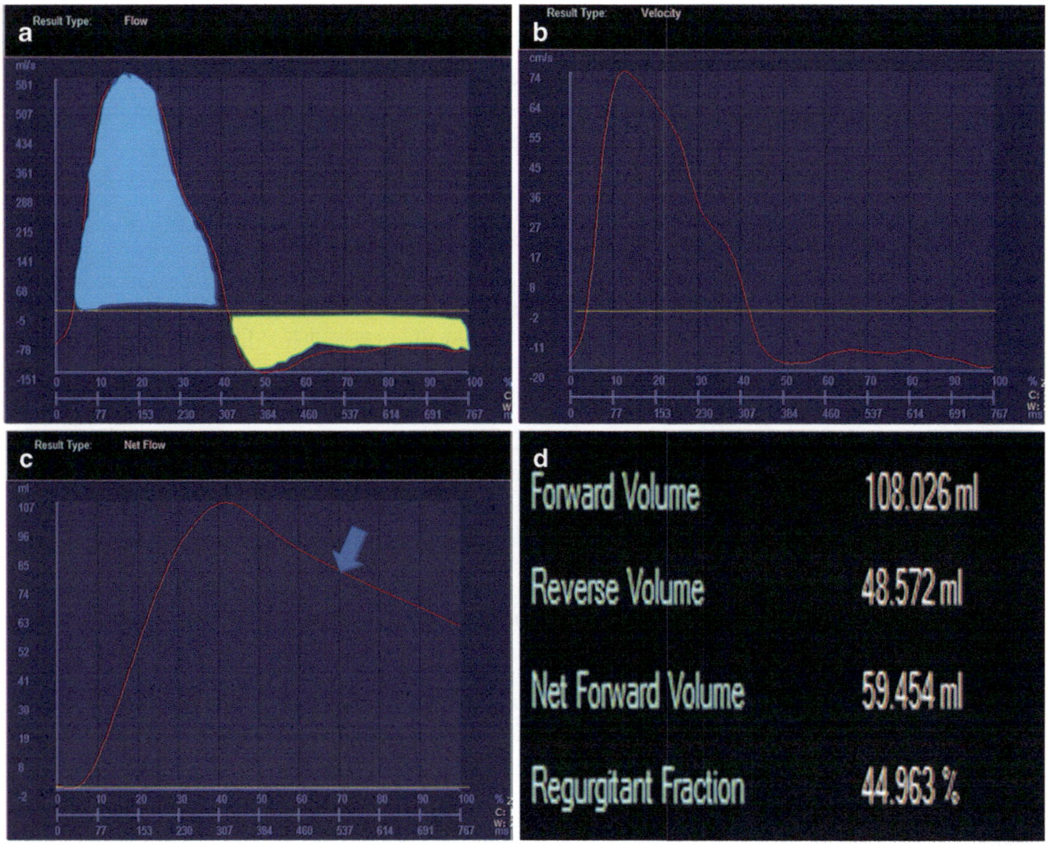

Fig. 19.11 The flow–time curve (**a**), velocity–time curve (**b**), net flow curve (**c**) and flow quantification analysis (**d**) in aortic regurgitation demonstrating an early forward flow with peak velocity quantified as 149 cm/s, followed by flow reversal. The curve above the yellow line indicates the forward flow and curve below indicates the regurgitant flow (note the negative flow and velocity values on *Y*-axis) with a regurgitant fraction of 40%. The blue area represents the early systolic forward flow and the yellow area represents the regurgitant flow. The stroke volume = blue + yellow. The net forward flow = blue. The regurgitant flow = yellow. Also note the decline of the net flow–time curve due to regurgitation (arrow in **c**)

CMR. However, CMR is superior to 3D echo in the measurement of ventricular mass, due to difficulty in assessing the epicardial border on echo. However, CMR is still the better choice for volumetric evaluation of the right ventricle [25–27].

Compared to CMR, echocardiography can overestimate the regurgitant jets due to PISA errors or underestimate eccentrically located jets [28–31].

Table 19.3 describes various merits and limitations of echocardiography.

Table 19.4 describes various merits and limitations of CMR.

19.3 Role of CT in the Assessment of VHD

Though not routinely used for assessment of VHD, multidetector computed tomography (MDCT) plays an important role in the assessment of calcification of native valve leaflets and annulus for preoperative risk assessment of annular rupture in patients undergoing transvalvular aortic/mitral valve replacement (Fig. 19.12). MDCT is also used to assess postoperative complications such as a perivalvular leak, assessment of the prosthetic valve compli-

Table 19.3 Merits and limitations of echocardiography

Merits of transthoracic echocardiography	Limitations of transthoracic echocardiography
Widely available, cost-effective, and portable.	Operator dependent.
Good temporal resolution of 20–30 ms for 2D imaging and 40–50 ms for color Doppler imaging.	Poor acoustic window in some patients.
Unlimited imaging planes.	Inadequate/inaccurate acquisition windows for LVOT, RV, RVOT, and MPA.
Reliable estimations of transvalvular pressure gradients.	The elliptical shape of LVOT and the presence of calcification can lead to underestimation of LVOT diameter. Even minor measurement errors will be magnified as the measurement will be squared in calculations.
Easy estimation of dynamic flow changes on Valsalva maneuver	Malalignment of the echo probe compared to the jet direction.
Good patient compliance.	Several geometric assumptions such as circular outflow tract and laminar flow profile may not hold true.
It can be performed in an emergency, postoperative period.	Errors in PISA measurement lead to an overestimation of regurgitant jets.
It can be performed in patients with poor breath-holding capacity.	Difficulty in identify the regurgitant orifice, irregular jets that are eccentrically.
It can be performed in pregnant women and children.	Directed, fan-shaped/crescentic morphology, non-hemispheric shell.
Non-ionizing radiation.	The regurgitant jet may not be static throughout the systole, especially in mitral prolapse, leading to wrong PISA measurement.

Table 19.4 Merits and limitations of CMR

Merits of CMR	Limitations of CMR
Large field of view. Good spatial resolution with a temporal resolution of 25–45 ms. Excellent visualization of cardiovascular anatomy. Flow quantification without geometric assumptions. Precise calculation of ventricular volumes and mass. Tissue characterization. Good inter- and intraobserver reproducibility Evaluation of pericardium and extracardiac structures. Evaluation and characterization of tumors.	Limited access, costly, and non-portable. CMR cannot be performed in medically unstable, claustrophobic, morbidly obese individuals (exceeding the weight limit of the MRI machine or chest circumference > 70 cm). Motion artifacts due to inadequate breath-holding or due to arrhythmias. Susceptibility artifacts in prosthetic valves, implanted devices, and stents. Contraindicated in MRI non-compatible metallic devices. E.g., aneurysm clips/pacemakers/implanted cardiac devices/catheters/cochlear implants/retained metallic foreign bodies.

cations as discussed further in the chapter [32, 33]. The full scope of CT is beyond the scope of this chapter.

The rest of the chapter will deal with individual valve abnormalities. The format is divided into a brief review of the pathology affecting the valve, the measurement of valve, and quantification of the flow. The reader is referred to the multiple tables in the chapter that describe the current classification of the flow abnormalities.

19.4 Aortic Valve

19.4.1 Aortic Stenosis

Aortic stenosis (AS) is the most common valve disease requiring surgery in the developed world [34]. The most common cause of AS is the fibrocalcific degeneration of the aortic valve seen in the elderly. Other causes are congenital bicuspid valve (Fig. 19.13) or acquired, e.g., rheumatic heart disease. Besides valvular stenosis, narrow-

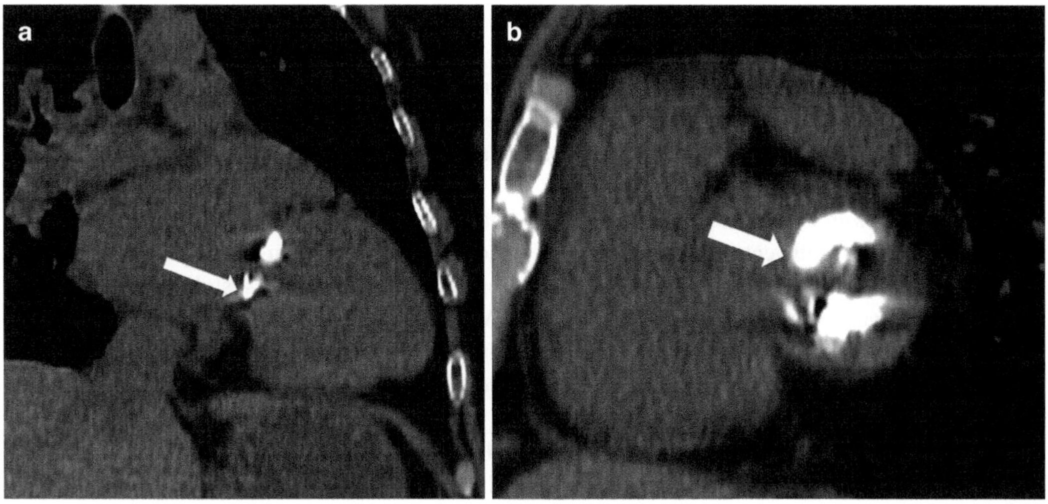

Fig. 19.12 A 38-year-old woman with chronic rheumatic heart disease. The oblique sagittal and axial images of non-contrast computed tomography, similar to the vertical long axis and axial view of the mitral valve plane demonstrating dense calcification of mitral valve leaflets and annulus

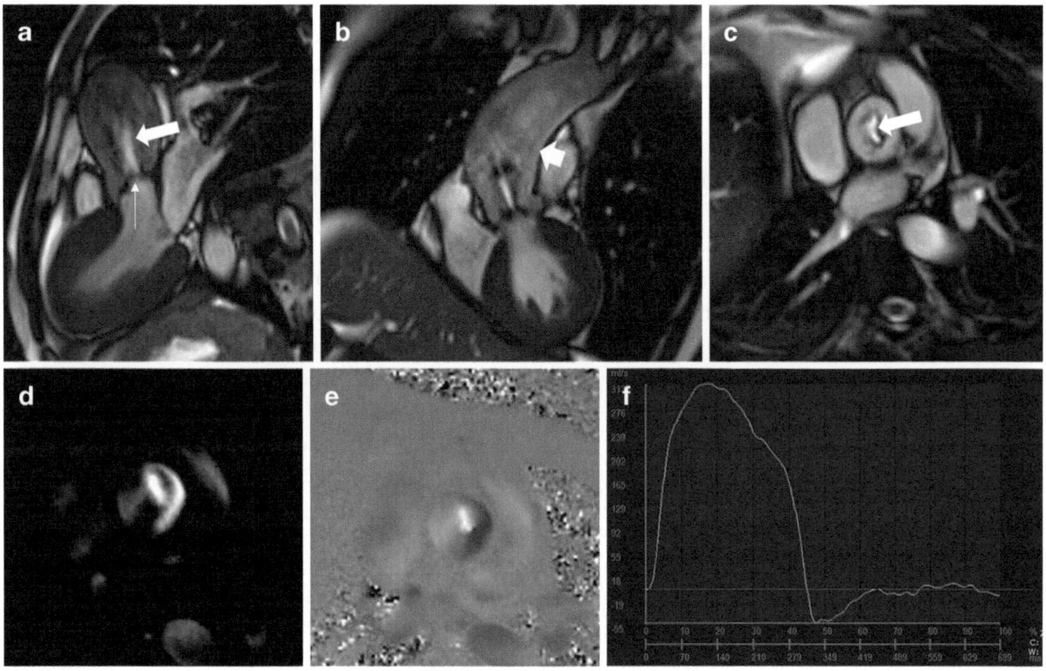

Fig. 19.13 A 43-year-old woman with a congenital bicuspid aortic valve with aortic stenosis. Standard left ventricular outflow tract (LVOT) view (**a**) and "coronal" LVOT view (**b**), acquired perpendicular to the standard LVOT view through the valve tips demonstrating domed leaflets (thin arrow) with restricted tips and a high-velocity jet. Short-axis cine imaging (**c**), magnitude (**d**), and phase-contrast velocity mapping (**e**) perpendicular through aortic valve demonstrating aortic stenosis with peak velocity–time curves (**f**) with a peak velocity of 274 cm/s. Also note the dilatation of the ascending aorta (arrow in **b**)

ing of the subvalvular or supravalvular regions may also cause AS.

The subvalvular aortic stenosis is rare and can occur by a variety of anatomic and dynamic causes, such as a subvalvular membrane, thick fibromuscular ridge, abnormal mitral valve cords, misaligned VSD with a posterior deviation of the outlet septum into the left ventricular outflow tract, idiopathic hypertrophic cardiomyopathy [35].

The supravalvular aortic stenosis is extremely rare, can be the result of morphological variations in the ascending aorta, with a hypoplastic aortic root, membrane in the aortic root, or diffuse hypoplasia of the ascending aorta. Supravalvular aortic stenosis can occur as a part of William's syndrome [2, 36, 37].

The CMR assessment of aortic stenosis includes an accurate anatomical assessment of the valve, aortic root, quantification of LV mass, volume, function, and measurement of the stenotic jet velocity [9] (Videos 19.1 to 19.7).

Box 19.1 describes the acquisition planning in aortic stenosis.

Valve Planimetry

The valvular orifice area can be measured directly or indirectly.

Direct planimetry: Direct planimetry correlates well with the aortic valve areas measured on transesophageal echocardiography, cardiac catheterization, and direct measurement of autopsy specimens [38–41]. However, the direct planimetry is suboptimal in cases with heavily calcified valves due to signal void and stenotic jet turbulence [8, 17].

Indirect planimetry: As mentioned previously, while echo calculates the valve area indirectly by the continuity equation and by using the velocity time integral (VTI) for systolic forward flow in LVOT(VTI_{LVOT}) and the aortic valve (VTI_{Ao}), planimetry is the method of choice for aortic valve area [5, 9].

Flow Quantification

The peak velocity measured in VENC may be underestimated due to the small width of high-velocity jets, lower temporal resolution, and artifacts from turbulent jets [5, 9, 17]. Real-time optimization of flow parameters at the time of imaging should thus be considered for every patient.

19.4.1.1 Ventricular Mass, Function, and Tissue Characterization

CMR can comprehensively evaluate not only the stenosis but the effects on the myocardium. Due to pressure overload in aortic stenosis, there is left ventricular hypertrophy and an increase in ventricular mass with altered LV contraction. Interstitial myocardial fibrosis occurring in AS may be focal or diffuse. Late gadolinium enhancement (LGE) in AS may demonstrate focal patchy mid-myocardial enhancement. Diffuse myocardial fibrosis in AS will increase extracellular volume fraction and native T1 relaxation times [42–44]. Myocardial tagging may demonstrate altered myocardial contractility and relaxation patterns with long and delayed diastolic untwisting [45–47].

19.4.1.2 Aortic Root Evaluation

CMR can evaluate the size of the aortic annulus in post-stenotic aortic root dilatation associated with the bicuspid aortic valve. 4D flow studies demonstrate helical and chaotic flow patterns in these cases [48, 49].

Table 19.5 describes the 2014 ACC AHA guidelines for the staging of valvular aortic stenosis.

Box 19.1 Acquisition planning in aortic stenosis

Acquisition planning in aortic stenosis.
Standard LVOT SSFP cine view.
"Coronal" LVOT SSFP cine view.
Short axis stack—to calculate LV and RV volumes
Axial stack SSFP cine perpendicular to aortic valve—by acquiring multiple thin (4–5 mm) slices with no slice gap, placed parallel to the valve tips in systole.
In-plane velocity mapping in LVOT view—to identify the area of the jet with maximal velocity (vena contracta).
Through-plane velocity mapping perpendicular to the area of maximum velocity, with velocity encoding (VENC) set manually (or by using a VENC scout) on the phase-contrast sequence and adjusted to avoid aliasing.
LGE—assesses the presence and extent of myocardial replacement fibrosis.
Aortic root evaluation

Table 19.5 2014 ACC/AHA guidelines for staging of valvular aortic stenosis

	Grade A	Grade B	Grade C	Grade D
	At risk of AS	Progressive AS	Asymptomatic severe AS	Symptomatic severe AS
Valve hemodynamics	Aortic $V_{max} < 2$ m/s	Mild AS: Aortic V_{max}. 2.0–2.9 m/s or mean $\Delta P < 20$ mmHg Moderate AS: Aortic V_{max}. 3.0–3.9 m/s or mean ΔP 20–39 mmHg	C1-aortic $V_{max} \geq 4$ m/s Mean $\Delta P \geq 40$ mmHg AVA typically is ≤ 1.0 cm^2 (or AVAi ≤ 0.6 cm^2/m^2) Very severe AS is an aortic $V_{max} \geq 5$ m/s or mean $\Delta P \geq 60$ mmHg C2-aortic $V_{max} \geq 4$ m/s or mean $\Delta P \geq 40$ mmHg AVA typically ≤ 1.0 cm^2 (or AVAi ≤ 0.6 cm^2/m^2)	D1-aortic $V_{max} \geq 4$ m/s or mean $\Delta P \geq 40$ mmHg AVA typically ≤ 1.0 cm^2 (or AVAi ≤ 0.6 cm^2/m^2) D2-AVA ≤ 1.0 cm^2 with resting aortic $V_{max} < 4$ m/s or mean $\Delta P < 40$ mmHg Dobutamine stress echo shows AVA ≤ 1.0 cm^2 with $V_{max} \geq 4$ m/s at any flow rate. D2-AVA ≤ 1.0 cm^2 with aortic $V_{max} < 4$ m/s or mean $\Delta P < 40$ mmHg indexed AVA ≤ 0.6 cm^2/m^2 and Stroke volume index < 35 mL/m^2 Measured when patient is normotensive (systolic BP < 140 mmHg)
Valve anatomy	Bicuspid aortic valve (or other congenital valve anomalies) Aortic valve sclerosis	Mild-moderate leaflet calcification of a bicuspid or trileaflet valve with some reduction in systolic motion or Rheumatic valve changes with commissural fusion	C1-severe leaflet calcification or congenital stenosis with severely reduced leaflet opening. C2-severe leaflet calcification or congenital stenosis with severely reduced leaflet opening	D1-severe leaflet calcification or congenital stenosis with severely reduced leaflet opening. D2-Evere leaflet calcification with severely reduced leaflet motion. D3-severe leaflet calcification with severely reduced leaflet motion
Hemodynamic consequences		Early LV diastolic dysfunction may be present. Normal LVEF	C1-LV diastolic dysfunction Mild LV hypertrophy Normal LVEF C2-LVEF < 50%	D1-LV diastolic dysfunction LV hypertrophy pulmonary hypertension may be present D2-LV diastolic dysfunction LV hypertrophy LVEF < 50% D3-increased LV relative wall thickness Small LV chamber with low stroke volume Restrictive diastolic filling LVEF $\geq$ 50%

AVA aortic valve area; *AVAi* aortic valve area indexed to body surface area; *BP* blood pressure; *LVEF* left ventricular ejection fraction; ΔP pressure gradient; V_{max} maximum aortic velocity

Table 19.6 2014 ACC/AHA summary of recommendations for AS: timing of intervention

Indicated	Patients with severe AS (stage C or D) when undergoing other cardiac surgery
Recommended	Symptomatic patients with severe high-gradient AS who have symptoms by history or on exercise testing (stage D1). Asymptomatic patients with severe AS (stage C2) and LVEF < 50%. Patients with severe AS (stage C or D) when undergoing other cardiac surgery.
Reasonable	Asymptomatic patients with very severe AS (stage C1, aortic velocity 5.0 m/s) and low surgical risk. Asymptomatic patients (stage C1) with severe AS and decreased exercise tolerance or an exercise fall in BP Symptomatic patients with low-flow/low-gradient severe AS with reduced LVEF (stage D2) with a low-dose dobutamine stress study that shows an aortic velocity 4.0 m/s (or mean pressure gradient 40 mm Hg) with a valve area $\leq$1.0 cm^2 at any dobutamine dose Symptomatic patients who have low-flow/low-gradient severe AS (stage D3) who are normotensive and have an LVEF 50% if clinical, hemodynamic, and anatomic data support valve obstruction as the most likely cause of symptoms. Patients with moderate AS (stage B) (aortic velocity 3.0–3.9 m/s) who are undergoing other cardiac surgery.
May be considered	Asymptomatic patients with severe AS (stage C1) and rapid disease progression and low surgical risk.

AVR aortic valve replacement by either surgical or transcatheter approach

Table 19.6 describes the 2014 ACC/AHA summary of recommendations for the timing of intervention in aortic stenosis.

19.4.2 Aortic Regurgitation

Aortic regurgitation can be caused by various conditions which result in abnormalities of the cusps, annulus, aortic root, such as rheumatic heart disease, bicuspid valve, dilatation of the aortic root in chronic hypertension or in collagen vascular disease, like Marfan's syndrome, Ehler–Danlos syndrome, ankylosing spondylitis, or aortic dissection (Fig. 19.14). Regurgitant fraction >33% has a higher likelihood of surgery within 9 years [50].

The imager might encounter multiple difficulties in CMR quantification of AR, due to the apical movement of the aortic valve in systole leading to a gap between the valve and the imaging slice. This gap could potentially contain a portion of the regurgitant jet that might not proceed until the imaging slice, leading to an underestimation of the regurgitant volume.

Box 19.2 describes the acquisition planning in aortic regurgitation.

Valve planimetry: The valvular orifice area can be measured directly as in AS.

Flow quantification: AR can be quantified on CMR directly or indirectly:

1. Direct quantification: The direct method may be more prone to measurement errors due to the apical movement of the aortic valve. Direct measurement can be calculated using through-plane PC VENC MR imaging with the imaging slice placed close to the valve [17]. However, some authors recommend flow calculation at the annulus, sino-tubular junction, and at the level of pulmonary artery bifurcation as there may be higher regurgitant fraction at the pulmonary artery level than at the annulus [5, 51].
2. Indirect Quantification: In the indirect method, AR can be calculated as the difference between left ventricular stroke volume (LVSV) and right ventricular stroke volume (RVSV), which are the same, barring the presence of other valve dysfunction/shunts [5, 9, 17].

Valve mathematics for AR:

- AR Regurgitant volume = LVSV-RVSV = LVSV − net forward flow in aorta.
- Regurgitant fraction (%) = Regurgitant volume/Forward volume × 100

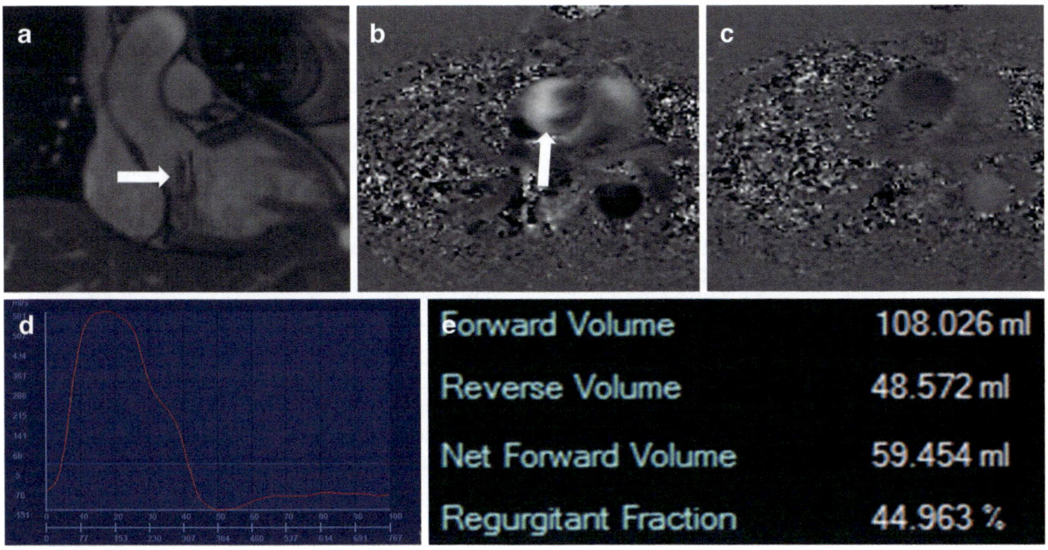

Fig. 19.14 A 38-year-old woman with moderate aortic regurgitation. Coronal SSFP (**a**) image demonstrating an eccentric aortic regurgitant jet (arrow in **a**). The phase-contrast velocity images (**b**, **c**) demonstrate forward and backward flow in (arrow in **b**) and backward flow in (**c**). The flow–time curve (**d**) obtained shows a large regurgitant flow with regurgitant fraction of 44.9% (**e**)

Box 19.2 Acquisition planning in aortic regurgitation

Acquisition planning in aortic regurgitation.
Standard LVOT SSFP cine view.
"Coronal" LVOT SSFP cine view.
Short axis stack—to calculate LV and RV volumes
Axial stack SSFP cine perpendicular to aortic valve—by acquiring multiple thin (4–5 mm) slices with no slice gap, placed parallel and close to the valve.
Through-plane velocity mapping—imaging plane placed parallel and close to the valve, with VENC set manually (or by using a VENC scout) on the phase-contrast sequence and adjusted to avoid aliasing.
Aortic root evaluation

Ventricular Mass and Function: The ventricular changes depend upon the chronicity of the AR. In acute AR, there is no time for LV to adapt to the volume changes, leading to left heart failure. In chronic AR, the LV adapts to volume overload with LV hypertrophy followed by dilatation.

Aortic root evaluation: CMR can evaluate the size of the aortic annulus, aortic root dilatation, periaortic inflammation in aortitis, flap extension in aortic dissection.

Table 19.7 describes the 2014 ACC AHA guidelines for the staging of aortic regurgitation.

Table 19.8 describes CMR classification of aortic regurgitation [52].

19.5 Mitral Valve

19.5.1 Mitral Stenosis

Rheumatic disease is the most common cause of mitral stenosis (MS) (Fig. 19.15), which causes thickening and calcification of the mitral valve resulting in commissural and chordal fusion. Nonrheumatic causes include left atrial myxoma, infective endocarditis vegetations, tumors, or thrombus, which prolapse into the valvular orifice in diastolic causing obstruction.

The echocardiography is usually the first modality in evaluating patients with mitral stenosis and is usually enough for treatment planning. CMR is useful in cases with inconsistent Doppler echocardiography findings or in patients with a poor acoustic window or in the presence of complex flow patterns. CMR with its multi-planimetric capabili-

Table 19.7 2014 ACC/AHA Guidelines for the staging of aortic regurgitation

	Grade A	Grade B	Grade C	Grade D
	At risk of AR	Progressive AR	Asymptomatic severe AR	Symptomatic severe AR
Valve hemodynamics	AR-none or trace	Mild AR Jet width < 25% of LVOT VC < 0.3 cm RV < 30 mL/beat RF < 30% ERO < 0.10 cm^2 Angiography grade 1+ Moderate AR: Jet width 25%–64% of LVOT VC 0.03–0.6 cm; RVol 30–59 mL/beat RF 30%–49%; ERO.010–0.29 cm^2 Angiography grade 2	Severe AR Jet width ≥ 65% of LVOT VC > 0.6 cm Holodiastolic flow reversal in the proximal abdominal aorta RVol ≥ 60 mL/beat RF ≥ 50% ERO ≥ 0.3 cm^2 angiography grade 3+ to 4 In addition, diagnosis of chronic severe AR requires evidence of LV dilation	Severe AR Jet width ≥ 65% of LVOT VC > 0.6 cm Holodiastolic flow reversal in the proximal abdominal aorta RVol ≥ 60 mL/beat RF ≥ 50% ERO ≥ 0.3 cm^2 Angiography grade 3+ to 4+ In addition, diagnosis of chronic severe AR requires evidence of LV dilation
Valve anatomy	Bicuspid aortic valve (or other congenital valve anomalies) Aortic valve sclerosis Diseases of the aortic sinuses or ascending aorta History of rheumatic fever or known rheumatic heart disease IE	Mild-to-moderate calcification of a trileaflet valve bicuspid aortic valve (or other congenital valve anomalies) Dilated aortic sinuses Rheumatic valve changes Previous IE	Calcific aortic valve disease Bicuspid valve (or other congenital abnormalities) Dilated aortic sinuses or ascending aorta Rheumatic valve changes IE with abnormal leaflet closure or perforation	Calcific valve disease bicuspid valve (or other congenital abnormalities) Dilated aortic sinuses or ascending aorta Rheumatic valve changes Previous IE with abnormal leaflet closure or perforation
Hemodynamic consequences	–	Normal LV systolic function Normal LV volume or mild LV dilation	C1—Normal LVEF (≥50%) Mild-moderate LV dilation (LVESD ≤ 50 mm) C2-abnormal LV systolic function with depressed LVEF (<50%) or severe LV dilatation (LVESD > 50 mm or indexed LVESD > 25 mm/m^2	Symptomatic severe AR may occur with normal systolic function (LVEF ≥ 50%) Mild-moderate LV dysfunction (LVEF 40%–50%), or severe LV dysfunction (LVEF < 40%) Moderate–severe LV dilation is present

ERO effective regurgitant orifice; *HF* heart failure; *IE* infective endocarditis; *LV* left ventricular; *LVEF* left ventricular ejection fraction; *LVESD* left ventricular end-systolic dimension; *LVOT* left ventricular outflow tract; *RF* regurgitant fraction; *RVol* regurgitant volume ties can visualize flow jet in any plane or direction. However, a major drawback for CMR in MS is the presence of atrial fibrillation [53].

Box 19.3 describes the acquisition planning in mitral stenosis.

Valve Planimetry

Direct measurement of the orifice area can be performed by imaging the mitral valve orifice, using multiple thin slices (4–5 mm) placed parallel to the mitral valve tips during diastole [54].

Flow Assessment

(i) Qualitative Assessment: Cine gradient-echo imaging evaluates the degree of MS on the basis of the size and extent of the abnormal flow jet in the left ventricle in diastole and associated anatomic findings such as valve leaflet thickening and bulging, reduced valve motion, left atrial enlargement, left atrial appendage thrombus. The signal void due to abnormal flow jet is well seen on the four-chamber view and the coronal oblique view encompassing the left atrium and the left ventricle.

Table 19.8 CMR grading of aortic regurgitation

Mild AR	Moderate AR	Moderate–severe AR	Severe AR
≤15%	16–25%	26–48%	>48%

(ii) Quantitative Assessment: The maximum velocity within the stenotic jet can be calculated with the help of through-plane PC VENC MR imaging perpendicular to the direction of flow and the pressure gradient across the valve can be calculated using simplified Bernoulli equation as described previously [53, 55].

Table 19.9 describes 2014 ACC/AHA guidelines for the staging of mitral stenosis.

19.5.2 Mitral Regurgitation

Mitral regurgitation (MR) is the result of malfunctioning of the mitral valve apparatus, consisting of valve leaflets, mitral annulus, chordae

Box 19.3 Acquisition planning in mitral stenosis

Acquisition planning in mitral stenosis
Horizontal long-axis/four-chamber view—to visualize valve morphology and motion.
Vertical long-axis/two-chamber view—to visualize valve morphology and motion.
Short axis stack—to calculate LV and RV volumes
Standard LVOT SSFP cine view.
"Coronal" LVOT SSFP cine view.
Axial stack SSFP cine perpendicular to mitral valve-by acquiring multiple thin (4–5 mm) slices with no slice gap, placed parallel to the valve tips in diastole.
Through-plane velocity mapping in the short-axis view of the mitral valve—to directly quantify MS.

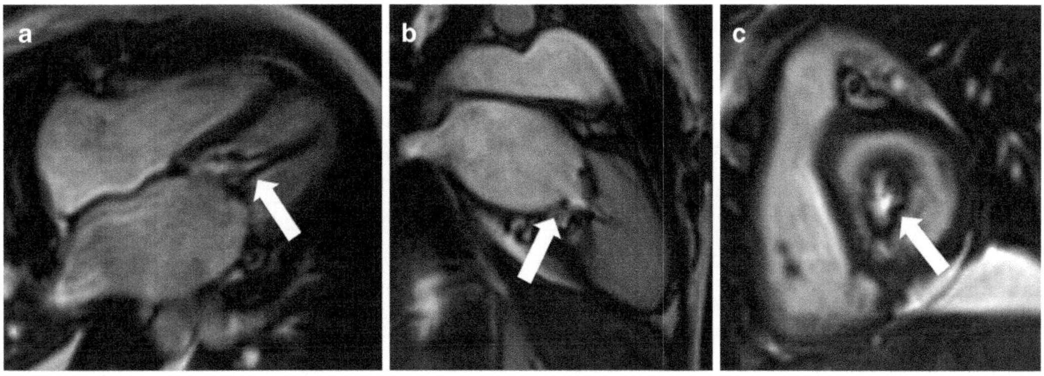

Fig. 19.15 A 40-year-old man with chronic rheumatic heart disease. The horizontal long-axis (**a**), vertical long-axis (**b**) and short-axis images (**c**) SSSP images demonstrating stenotic jet into the left ventricle with thickened chordae tendineae (arrow in **a**, **b**) and thickened valvular leaflets with reduced orifice area (arrow in **c**). Also note the dilated left atrium

Table 19.9 2014 ACC/AHA guidelines for staging of mitral stenosis

	Grade A	Grade B	Grade C	Grade D
	At risk of MS	Progressive MS	Asymptomatic severe MS	Symptomatic severe MS
Valve hemodynamics	Normal transmitral flow velocity	Increased transmitral flow velocities MVA > 1.5 cm^2 Diastolic pressure half-time < 150 ms	MVA ≤ 1.5 cm^2 (MVA ≤ 1.0 cm^2 with very severe MS) Diastolic pressure half-time ≥ 150 ms (diastolic pressure half-time ≥ 220 ms with very severe MS)	MVA ≤ 1.5 cm^2 (MVA ≤ 1.0 cm^2 with very severe MS) Diastolic pressure half-time ≥ 150 ms (diastolic pressure half-time ≥ 220 ms with very severe MS)
Valve anatomy	Mild valve doming during diastole	Rheumatic valve changes with commissural fusion and diastolic doming of the mitral valve leaflets Planimetered MVA > 1.5 cm^2	Rheumatic valve changes with commissural fusion and diastolic doming of the mitral valve leaflets Planimetered MVA ≤ 1.5 cm^2 (MVA ≤ 1.0 cm^2 with very severe MS)	Rheumatic valve changes with commissural fusion and diastolic doming of the mitral valve leaflets Planimetered MVA ≤ 1.5 cm^2
Hemodynamic consequences	None	Mild-to-moderate LA enlargement Normal pulmonary pressure at rest	Severe LA enlargement Elevated PASP >30 mmHg	Severe LA enlargement Elevated PASP >30 mmHg

LA left atrial; *LV* left ventricular; *MS* mitral stenosis; *MVA* mitral valve area; *PASP* pulmonary artery systolic pressure

tendineae, papillary muscles, and the adjacent LV wall. The common causes of MR are rheumatic heart disease, degeneration of the valve, mitral valve prolapse, endomyocardial fibrosis, myocardial infarction with rupture of the papillary muscle, dilated cardiomyopathy leading to widening of the mitral annulus (Fig. 19.16). Mitral valve prolapse is the most common cause of mitral regurgitation in developed countries and is characterized by systolic bowing of the mitral leaflet, with protrusion of >2 mm beyond the annular plane into the left atrium. Mitral valve prolapse is associated with >5 mm thickening of the leaflets. The rupture of chordae tendineae or papillary muscles can cause complete systolic eversion of the leaflets, termed as “flail valve” (Fig. 19.17) [56, 57].

Box 19.4 describes the acquisition planning in mitral regurgitation.

Valve Planimetry

The regurgitant orifice is imaged using multiple thin slices (4–5 mm) placed parallel to the mitral annulus through the mitral valve tips in systole [41].

Flow Assessment

Mitral regurgitation can be quantified on CMR directly or indirectly. In patients with regular heart rate, there is good agreement between direct and indirect methods:

(i) Direct quantification: The direct method involves only a single data acquisition and is less prone to measurement errors. However, this method is not commonly used as it difficult to measure accurately in cases with high velocity, angulated jets, and a highly mobile mitral valve. Errors due to high-velocity jets can be overcome by selecting an appropriately high-velocity window and a short TE sequence [58]. Jet angulation can be accommodated by careful placement of the imaging slice perpendicular to the predominant direction of the flow jet, thereby minimizing partial volume and angulation errors. In routine practice, the distance moved by the valve is ~ 1–1.5 cm, which can be partially accommodated by using a phase-contrast sequence with reasonable errors.

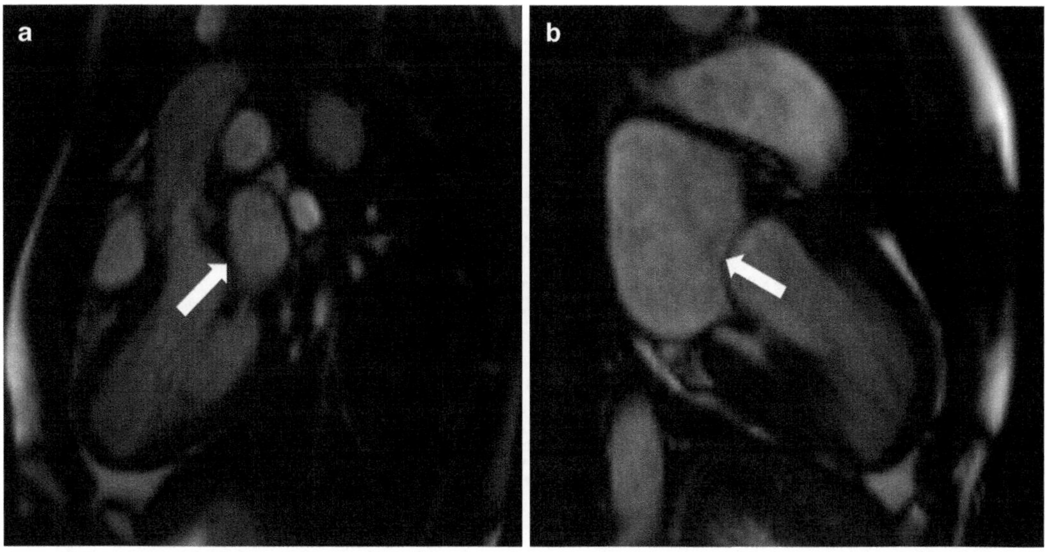

Fig. 19.16 A 28-year-old man with mitral valve prolapse. Three-chamber (**a**) and vertical long axis (**b**) SSFP images showing systolic bowing of the mitral valve leaflet (arrows in **a**, **b**)

(ii) Indirect Quantification: In the indirect method, mitral regurgitation is calculated as the difference between left ventricular stroke volume (LVSV) and forward aortic flow. In patients with mitral regurgitation and an atrial septal defect, the mitral regurgitation is calculated as the difference between the LVSV and the aortic flow, while the Q_p/Q_s is calculated as the ratio of the pulmonary artery flow to aortic flow [58–60].

$$\text{Regurgitation volume} = \text{LVSV} - \text{forward flow in aorta}$$

$$\text{Regurgitant fraction}(\%) = \text{Regurgitant volume} / \text{LVSV} \times 100$$

Figure 19.18 illustrates the calculation of regurgitation fraction in various scenarios [52].

Note: Diastolic LV dysfunction is characterized by the abnormal transmitral flow. The through-plane phase-contrast images acquired at the level of the mitral valve can calculate the transmitral flow. The PC images are obtained with the perpendicular acquisition plane at the top of the mitral valve opening. The rapid early diastolic filling of the LV caused by isovolumetric LV relaxation is represented by the larger "E" wave and late end-diastolic LV filling caused by atrial contraction is represented by smaller "A" wave (Fig. 19.19). In diastolic dysfunction, the A wave is usually larger than E wave. The pseudo normal type of diastolic dysfunction can be differentiated from normal by assessing the pulmonary venous flow and duration of end-diastolic "A" wave in the pulmonary venous flow [61].

Table 19.10 describes the 2014 ACC AHA guidelines for the staging of primary MR.

Table 19.11 describes the 2014 ACC AHA guidelines for the staging of secondary MR.

Table 19.12 describes CMR classification of aortic regurgitation [50].

19.6 Pulmonary Valve

19.6.1 Pulmonary Stenosis

Pulmonary stenosis (PS) can be congenital, e.g., TOF, congenital stenosis, Noonan syndrome, LEOPARD (Lentigines, electrocardiographic

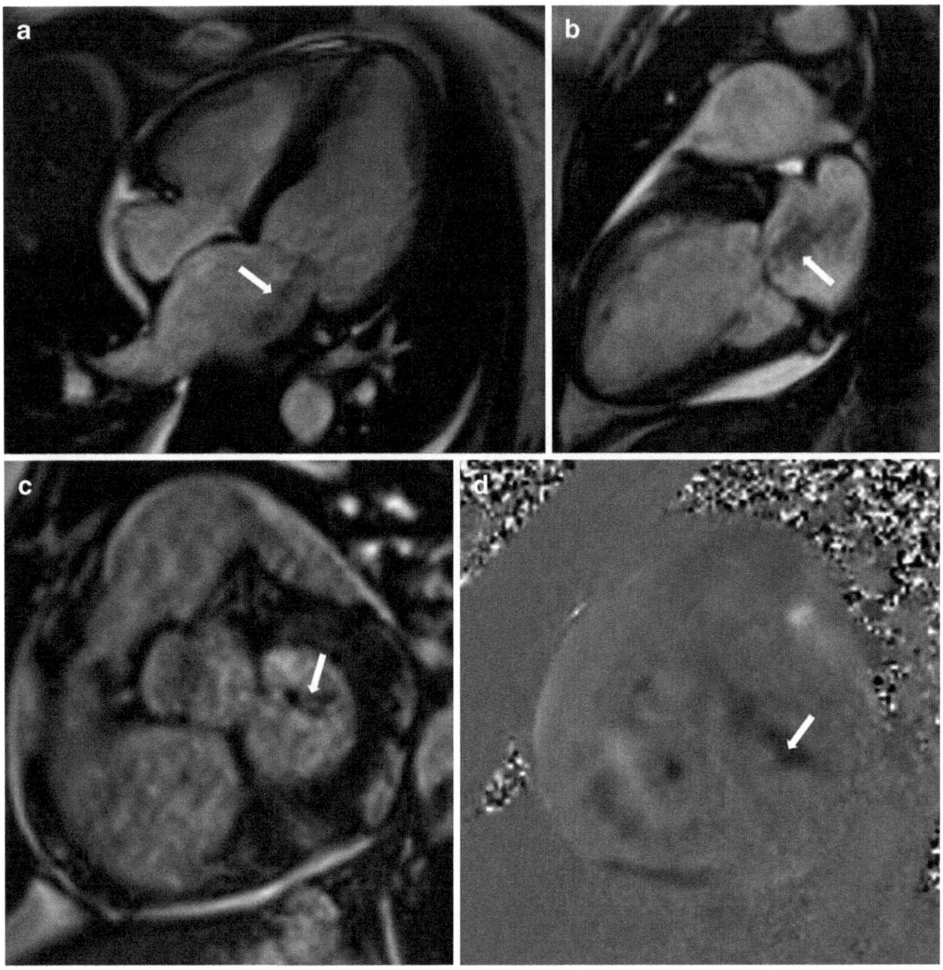

Fig. 19.17 Mitral regurgitation in a 52-year-old woman with dilated ischemic cardiomyopathy. Balanced-SSFP cine MRI in four-chamber (**a**), two-chamber view (**b**), basal short-axis view (**c**), and velocity-mapping (phase images) (**d**). The direction of the jet is eccentrically located abutting the lateral left atrial wall (arrow in **a**). Velocity mapping (systolic phase) shows a dark regurgitant jet (arrow **d**)

Box 19.4 Acquisition planning in mitral regurgitation

Acquisition planning in mitral regurgitation
Horizontal long-axis/four-chamber view—to visualize valve morphology and motion. Vertical long-axis/two-chamber view—to visualize valve morphology and motion. Short-axis stack—to calculate LV and RV volumes Standard LVOT SSFP cine view. 'Coronal' LVOT SSFP cine view. Axial stack SSFP cine perpendicular to mitral valve—by acquiring multiple thin (4–5 mm) slices with no slice gap, placed parallel to the valve tips in systole. Through-plane velocity mapping in short-axis view of the mitral valve—to directly quantify MR Through-plane velocity mapping in LVOT view above the aortic valve—to measure aortic forward flow and indirectly quantify MR.

Box 19.5 Acquisition planning in pulmonary stenosis

Acquisition planning in pulmonary stenosis
Standard RVOT view: To visualize valve morphology, motion, and planning of through-plane PC velocity mapping. Horizontal RVOT view: To visualize valve morphology and motion of RVOT in systole. Short-axis stack—to calculate LV and RV volumes and mass. Through-plane PC VENC standard RVOT view above the pulmonary valve—to quantify PS. Pulmonary artery imaging—to assess the dilatation of the main pulmonary artery. Additional assessment in TOF—assessment of VSD with Q_p:Q_s ratio.

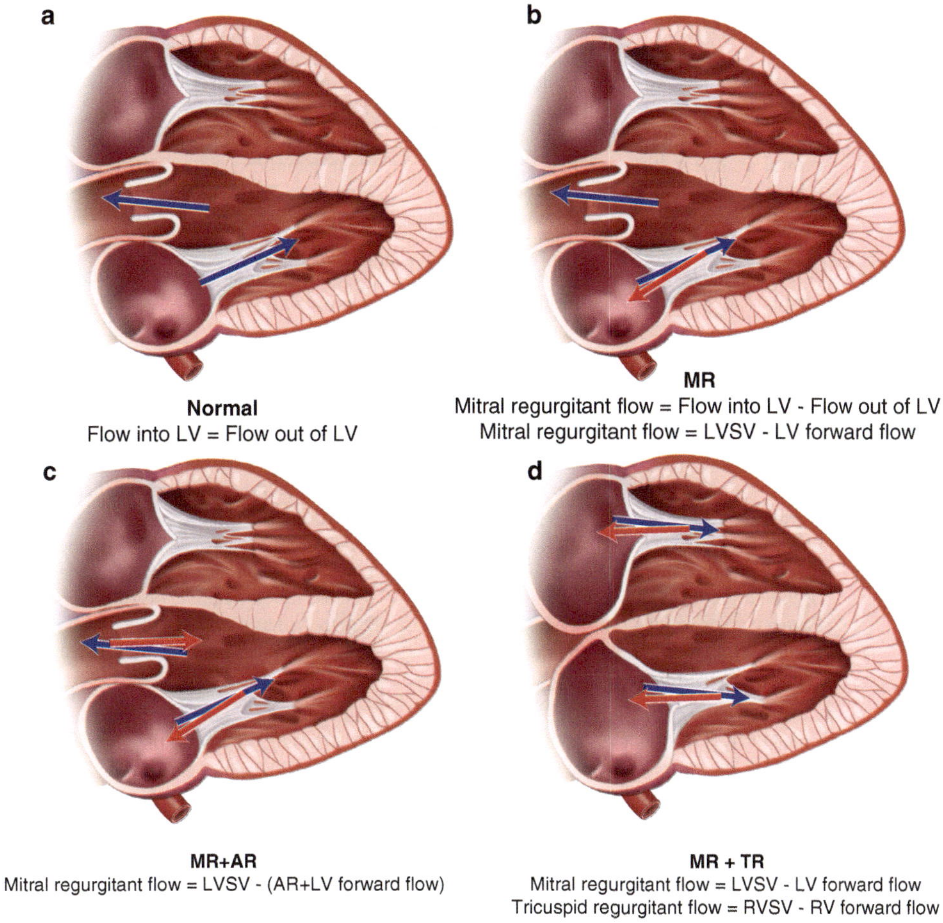

Fig. 19.18 Graphic/schematic image showing various MR quantification in multiple scenarios

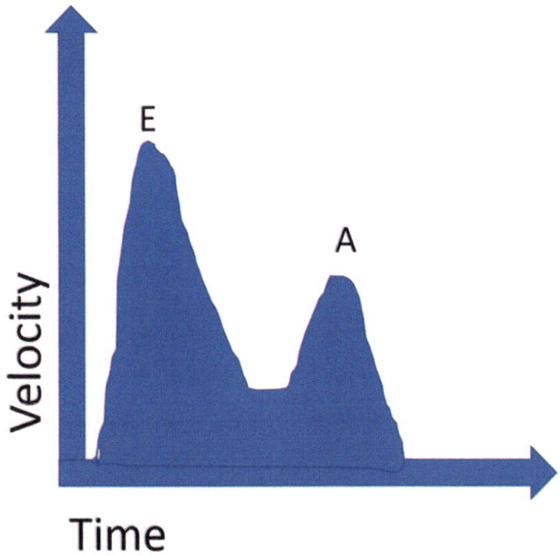

Fig. 19.19 Normal E and A waves of transmitral flow

anomalies, ocular hypertelorism, pulmonary stenosis, abnormalities of genitalia, retardation of growth, and deafness) syndrome or acquired, e.g., rheumatic heart disease, carcinoid heart disease, bacterial endocarditis. Besides valvular stenosis, narrowing of the subvalvular or supravalvular regions can also cause PS. Subvalvular obstruction may be the result of chronic pulmonary stenosis due to hypertrophy of septomarginal trabeculation with resultant "two-chambered" appearance or RVOT obstruction related to TOF (Fig. 19.20). This subvalvular stenosis is a dynamic phenomenon, with systolic obstruction due to contraction of the infundibulum. Supravalvular pulmonary stenosis is rare and may be congenital due to the main pulmonary artery membrane/stenosis or sequelae of prior surgery [62, 63].

Table 19.10 2014 ACC AHA guidelines for staging of primary MR

	Grade A	Grade B	Grade C	Grade D
	At risk of MR	Progressive MR	Asymptomatic severe MR	Symptomatic severe MR
Valve hemodynamics	No MR jet or small central jet area < 20% LA on Doppler Small vena contracta < 0.30 cm	ERO < 0.20 cm^2 Regurgitant volume < 30 mL Regurgitant fraction < 50%	ERO ≥ 0.20 cm^2 Regurgitant volume ≥ 30 mL Regurgitant fraction ≥ 50%	ERO ≥ 0.20 cm^2 Regurgitant volume ≥ 30 mL Regurgitant fraction ≥ 50%
Valve anatomy	Normal valve leaflets, chords, and annulus in a patient with coronary disease/cardiomyopathy	Regional wall motion abnormalities with mild tethering of mitral leaflet Annular dilation with mild loss of central coaptation of the mitral leaflets	Regional wall motion abnormalities and/or LV dilation with severe tethering of mitral leaflet Annular dilation with severe loss of central coaptation of the mitral leaflets	Regional wall motion abnormalities and/or LV dilation with severe tethering of mitral leaflet Annular dilation with severe loss of central coaptation of the mitral leaflets
Associated cardiac findings	Normal or mildly dilated LV size with fixed (infarction) or inducible (ischemia) RWMA Primary myocardial disease with LV dilation and systolic dysfunction	RWMA with reduced LV systolic function LV dilation and systolic dysfunction due to primary myocardial Disease	RWMA with reduced LV systolic function LV dilation and systolic dysfunction due to primary myocardial disease	RWMA with reduced LV systolic function LV dilation and systolic dysfunction due to primary myocardial disease

ERO effective regurgitant orifice; *IE* infective endocarditis; *LA* left atrium/atrial; *LV* left ventricular; *LVEF* left ventricular ejection fraction; *LVESD* left ventricular end-systolic dimension; *MR* mitral regurgitation

Table 19.11 2014 ACC AHA guidelines for staging of secondary MR

	Grade A	Grade B	Grade C	Grade D
	At risk of MR	Progressive MR	Asymptomatic severe MR	Symptomatic severe MR
Valve hemodynamics	No MR jet or small central jet area < 20% LA on Doppler Small VC < 0.30 cm	ERO <0.20 cm^2 RV <30 mL RF < 50%	ERO ≥ 0.20 cm^2 RV ≥ 30 mL RF ≥ 50%	ERO ≥ 0.20 cm^2 RV ≥ 30 mL RF ≥ 50%
Valve anatomy	Normal valve leaflets, chords, and annulus in a patient with coronary disease or cardiomyopathy	RWMA with mild tethering of mitral leaflet Annular dilation with mild loss of central coaptation of the mitral leaflets	RWMA and/or LV dilation with severe tethering of mitral leaflet Annular dilation with severe loss of central coaptation of the mitral leaflets	RWMA and/or LV dilation with severe tethering of mitral leaflet Annular dilation with severe loss of central coaptation of the mitral leaflets
Associated cardiac findings	Normal or mildly dilated LV size with fixed (infarction) or inducible (ischemia) regional wall motion abnormalities Primary myocardial disease with LV dilation and systolic dysfunction	RWMA with reduced LV systolic function LV dilation and systolic dysfunction due to primary myocardial disease	RWMA with reduced LV systolic function LV dilation and systolic dysfunction due to primary myocardial disease	RWMA with reduced LV systolic function LV dilation and systolic dysfunction due to primary myocardial disease

ERO effective regurgitant orifice; *HF* heart failure; *LA* left atrium; *LV* left ventricular; *MR* mitral regurgitation; *TTE* transthoracic echocardiogram

Table 19.12 CMR grading of mitral regurgitation

Mild MR	Moderate MR	Moderate–severe MR	Severe MR
≤15%	16–25%	26–48%	>48%

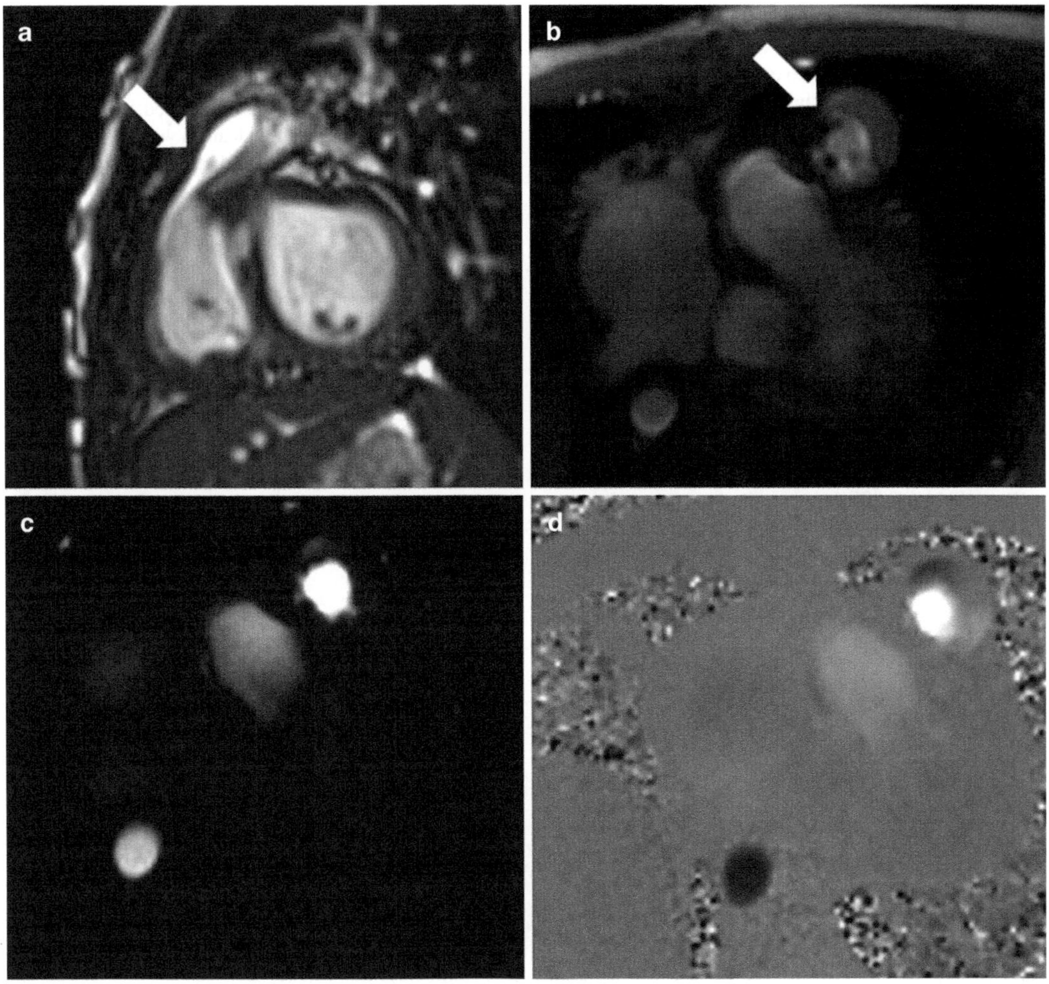

Fig 19.20 Subvalvular pulmonary stenosis in a 19-year-old man with repaired tetralogy of Fallot and bicuspid valve repair on follow-up. The standard RVOT SSFP and axial SSFP image at the level of pulmonary valve demonstrating stenotic jet arising in the subvalvular region, below the pulmonary valve (arrow in **a**) and bicuspid morphology of pulmonary valve (arrow in **b**). The magnitude and velocity images (**c, d**) show a high signal forward flow

Box 19.6 describes the acquisition planning in pulmonary stenosis.

Valve Planimetry

Direct measurement of the orifice area can be performed by placing an imaging plane at the pulmonary valve (Videos 19.8 to 19.13).

Flow Assessment Direct Quantitative Assessment: can be calculated directly using through-plane PC VENC imaging.

Table 19.13 describes the 2014 ACC/AHA guidelines for the staging of severe pulmonic stenosis.

19.6.2 Pulmonary Regurgitation

Mild pulmonary regurgitation is seen in 30% of the normal population [8]. Pulmonary regurgitation is frequent following surgical interventions such as pulmonary valvulotomy, infundibulectomy,

Box 19.6 Acquisition planning in pulmonary regurgitation

Acquisition planning in pulmonary regurgitation
Standard RVOT view: To visualize valve morphology, motion, and planning of through-plane PC velocity mapping. An ideal standard RVOT view is an oblique sagittal plane which includes the proximal main pulmonary artery and foreshortened right ventricle. The outflow tract must remain in-plane during the entire cardiac cycle. This, however, is difficult due to the significant long-axis motion of the RV. Horizontal RVOT view: To visualize valve morphology and motion of RVOT in systole. Acquiring a cine image in a more horizontal plane through the standard RVOT, perpendicular to the standard RVOT view, allows visualization of the degree of movement of the RVOT in systole and can help plan a subsequent improved RVOT view throughout the whole cardiac cycle. Short-axis stack—to calculate LV and RV volumes and mass. Standard LVOT SSFP cine view. "Coronal" LVOT SSFP cine view. Through-plane velocity mapping in standard RVOT view above the pulmonary valve—to directly quantify PR Through-plane velocity mapping in LVOT view above the aortic valve—to measure aortic forward flow and indirectly quantify PR. Pulmonary artery imaging—to assess dilatation or stenosis of main and branch pulmonary arteries.

Table 19.13 2014 ACC/AHA guidelines for staging of severe pulmonic stenosis

	Stage C, D
	Asymptomatic severe PS, symptomatic severe PS
Valve hemodynamics	$V_{max} > 4$ m/s Peak instantaneous gradient > 64 mmHg
Valve anatomy	Thickened, distorted, possibly calcified leaflets with systolic doming and/or reduced excursion Other anatomic abnormalities may be present, such as narrowed RVOT
Hemodynamic consequences	RVH Possible RV, RA enlargement Post stenotic enlargement of main PA

PA pulmonary artery; *PS* pulmonic stenosis; *RA* right atrium; *RV* right ventricle; *RVH* right ventricular hypertrophy; *RVOT* right ventricular outflow; V_{max} maximal pulmonic valve jet velocity

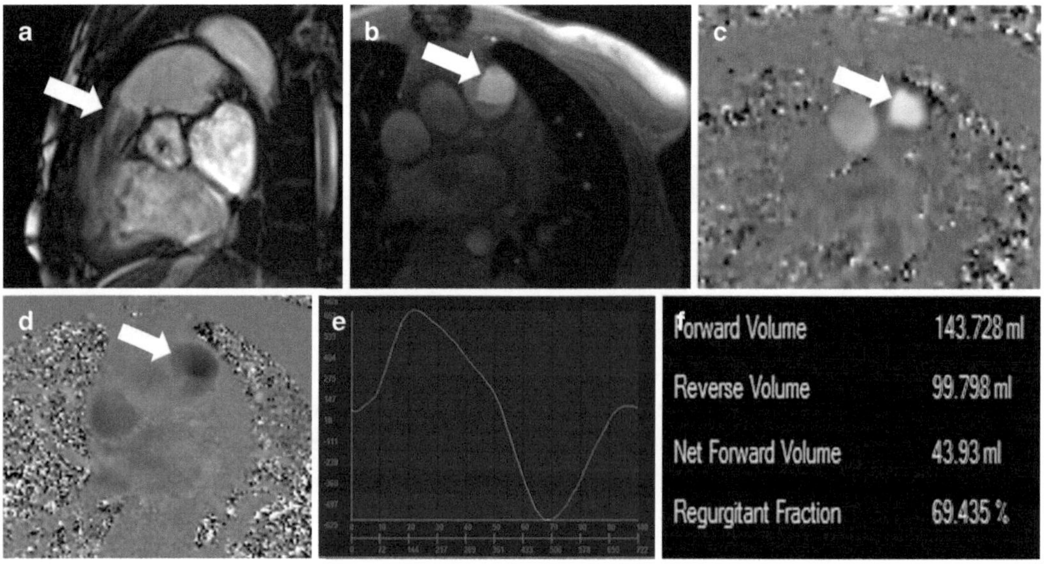

Fig. 19.21 Severe pulmonary regurgitation in a 30-year-old woman with repaired tetralogy of Fallot on follow-up. Standard b-SSFP RVOT (**a**), axial b-SSFP, and phase-contrast velocity images at the level of the pulmonary valve (**b**–**d**) demonstrating severe pulmonary regurgitation (arrow in **a**). The forward and reversal of flow are noted on phase-contrast images (arrow in **c**, **d**). The flow–time graph demonstrates forwards and reversal of flow, with a regurgitant fraction of 69% (**f**)

e.g., repair of tetralogy of Fallot, leading to enlargement of valve orifice and right ventricular outflow tract (RVOT) (TOF) (Fig. 19.21) [64]. The echocardiographic assessment of the pulmonary valve and RVOT is difficult due to their retrosternal location, leading to the suboptimal assessment of the pulmonary valve function. The volumetric assessment of the right ventricle can be difficult on echocardiography due to its unusual shape. Hence, CMR with multiple imaging planes allows accurate assessment of RV anatomy, volumes, velocity, and regurgitant fractions and plays an important role in clinical decision-making [65].

Box 19.6 describes the acquisition planning in pulmonary regurgitation.

Valve Planimetry
Direct measurement of the orifice area can be performed by placing an imaging plane at the pulmonary valve

Flow Assessment

(i) Direct Quantitative Assessment: The pulmonary regurgitation can be calculated directly using through-plane PC VENC MR imaging.
(ii) Indirect Quantitative Assessment: In the absence of other valvular leaks, PR can be indirectly calculated as the difference in LV and RV stroke volumes.

$$\text{PR Regurgitant volume} = \text{RVSV} - \text{LVSV}.$$

$$\text{Regurgitant fraction}\left(\%\right) = \text{Regurgitant volume} / \text{Forward volume} \times 100.$$

Table 19.14 describes the 2014 ACC/AHA guidelines for the staging of severe pulmonic regurgitation.

19.7 Tricuspid Valve

19.7.1 Tricuspid Stenosis

Tricuspid stenosis (TS) is rare as the tricuspid annulus is much larger than the mitral annulus [66].

Table 19.14 2014 ACC/AHA guidelines for staging of severe pulmonic regurgitation

	Stage C, D
	Asymptomatic severe PR, symptomatic severe PR
Valve hemodynamics	Color jet fills RVOT CW jet density and contour: dense laminar flow with steep deceleration slope; may terminate abruptly
Valve anatomy	Distorted or absent leaflets, annular dilation
Hemodynamic consequences	Paradoxical septal motion (volume overload pattern) RV enlargement

CW continuous wave; *PR* pulmonic regurgitation; *RV* right ventricular; *RVOT* right ventricular outflow tract

Rheumatic heart disease is the most common cause of TS. Other causes include congenital stenosis (Fig. 19.22), congenital atresia, carcinoid, infective endocarditis, and systemic lupus erythematosus.

Box 19.7 describes the acquisition planning in tricuspid stenosis.

Valve Planimetry
Direct measurement of the orifice area can be performed by imaging the tricuspid valve orifice using multiple thin slices (4–5 mm) placed parallel to the valve tips during diastole.

Flow Assessment
TS can be calculated directly using through-plane PC VEC MR imaging.

Table 19.15 describes the 2014 ACC/AHA guidelines for the staging of severe tricuspid stenosis.

19.7.2 Tricuspid Regurgitation

Tricuspid regurgitation (TR) is usually secondary to dilatation of the right ventricle and tricuspid annulus. Other causes of TR include infectious endocarditis in intravenous drug abus-

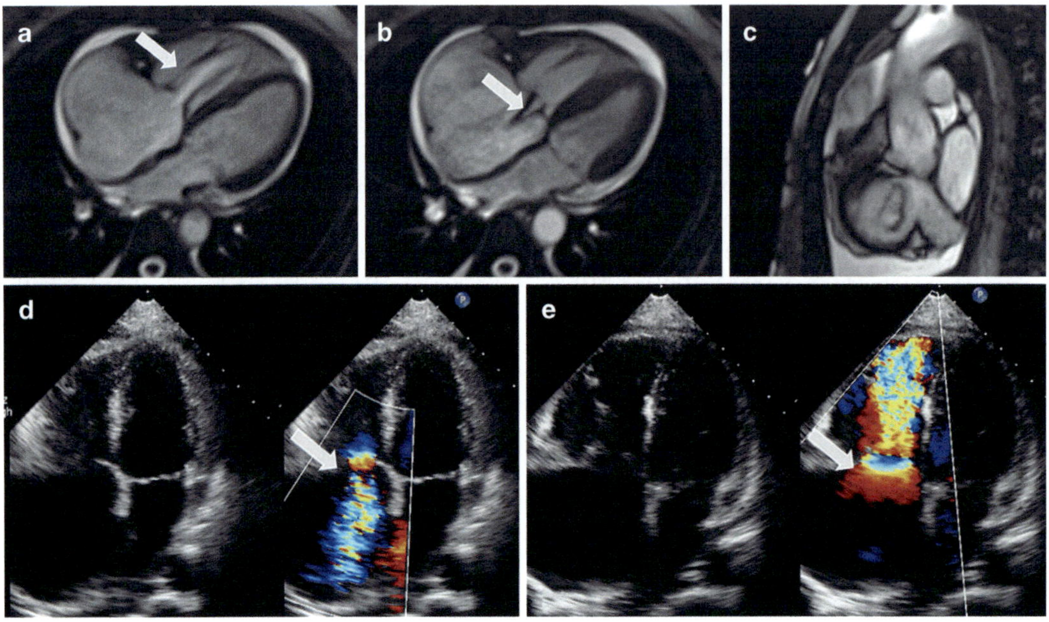

Fig. 19.22 A 35-year-old woman with thickened noncoapting tricuspid valves causing tricuspid stenosis and regurgitation. The b-SSFP horizontal long axis (**a**, **b**) demonstrate turbulent stenotic (arrow in **a**) and regurgitant jets (arrow in **b**). The axial view of the tricuspid valve demonstrates thickened leaflets. Apical four-chamber echocardiographic images (**d**, **e**) demonstrate tricuspid regurgitant and stenotic jets (arrow in **d**, **e**)

Box 19.7 Acquisition planning in tricuspid stenosis

Acquisition planning in tricuspid stenosis
Horizontal long-axis/four-chamber view—to visualize valve morphology and motion. RV two-chamber view—to visualize valve morphology and motion. Modified four-chamber view—if the stenotic jet is not well seen on standard four-chamber view. Short-axis stack—to calculate LV and RV volumes In-plane PC VENC imaging in the horizontal long axis or RV two-chamber view. Through-plane PC VENC imaging short-axis view of the tricuspid valve.

Table 19.15 2014 ACC/AHA guidelines for staging severe tricuspid stenosis

	Stage C, D
	Asymptomatic severe TS, symptomatic severe TS
Valve hemodynamics	$T\frac{1}{2} \geq 190$ ms Valve area ≤ 1.0 cm^2
Valve anatomy	Thickened, distorted, calcified leaflets
Hemodynamic consequences	RA/IVC enlargement

IVC inferior vena cava; *RA* right atrium; *T½* pressure half-time; *TS* tricuspid stenosis

ers, blunt chest trauma, and carcinoid heart disease [67, 68].

In the Ebstein anomaly, there is abnormal apical placement of the septal and mural leaflets of the tricuspid valve (Fig. 19.23). Difficulty in identifying the true right ventricle on short-axis images leads to erroneous calculations of TR, RV volumes and function. Ebstein anomaly will be discussed in chapter [68, 69].

Box 19.8 describes the acquisition planning in tricuspid regurgitation.

Valve Planimetry

Direct measurement of the orifice area can be performed by imaging the tricuspid valve orifice using multiple thin slices (4–5 mm) placed parallel to the valve tips during diastole.

Flow Assessment

TR can be calculated directly using through-plane PC VENC MR imaging.

Visualizing the regurgitant jet as a signal void is often difficult on SSFP sequences due

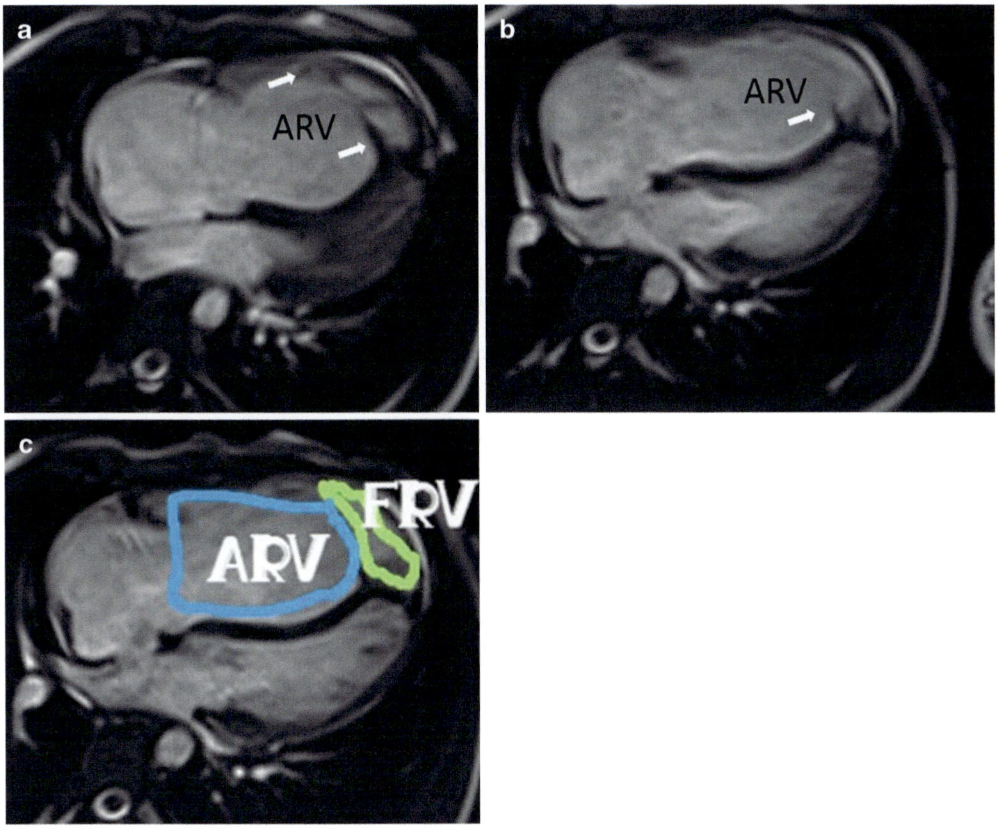

Fig. 19.23 A 10-year-old boy with Ebstein anomaly. Axial cine SSFP imaging at end-systole (**a**) and end-diastole (**b**) demonstrating abnormal apical implantation of the tricuspid valve leaflets (arrows). The atrialized right ventricle (ARV) and the functional right ventricle (FRV) depicted in (**c**)

Box 19.8 Acquisition planning in tricuspid regurgitation

Acquisition planning in tricuspid regurgitation
Horizontal long-axis/four-chamber view—to visualize valve morphology and motion.
RV two-chamber view—to visualize valve morphology and motion.
Modified four-chamber view—if the regurgitant jet is not well seen on standard four-chamber view.
Short-axis stack—to calculate LV and RV volumes
Standard and horizontal RVOT view
In-plane PC VENC imaging in the horizontal long axis or RV two-chamber view.
Through-plane PC VENC imaging short-axis view of the tricuspid valve
Through-plane PC VENC imaging in standard RVOT view above the pulmonary valve—to quantify forward flow.

to lower shear and turbulence. However, the qualitative assessment of the TR jet can be achieved with in-plane velocity mapping in a long-axis RV view or through-plane velocity mapping.

Wider jets of >7 mm vena contracta suggest more severe tricuspid regurgitation [5, 9].

Indirect Quantification: TR can be calculated using pulmonary flow measurement combined with RV stroke volume [4]:

$$\text{TR volume} = \text{RVSV} - \text{pulmonary forward flow} = \text{RVSV} - \text{LVSV}.$$

$$\text{Regurgitant fraction}\left(\%\right) = \text{TR} / \text{RVSV} \times 100\%.$$

Table 19.16 2014 ACC/AHA guidelines for staging tricuspid regurgitation

	Grade A	Grade B	Grade C	Grade D
	At risk of TS	Progressive TS	Asymptomatic severe TS	Symptomatic severe TS
Valve hemodynamics	None	Mild TR central jet area < 5.0 cm^2 CW jet density and contour: soft and parabolic Hepatic vein flow: systolic dominance Moderate TR Central jet area 5–10 cm^2 Vena contracta width < 0.70 cm CW jet density and contour: dense, variable contour Hepatic vein flow: Systolic blunting	Central jet area > 10.0 cm^2 Vena contracta width > 0.7 cm CW jet density and contour: dense, triangular with early peak Hepatic vein flow: systolic reversal	Central jet area > 10.0 cm^2 Vena contracta width > 0.70 cm CW jet density and contour: dense, triangular with early peak Hepatic vein flow: systolic reversal
Valve anatomy	Primary—mild rheumatic change Mild prolapse other (e.g., IE with vegetation, early carcinoid deposition, radiation) intra-annular RV pacemaker or ICD lead post cardiac transplant (biopsy related) Functional—Normal Early annular dilation	Primary—progressive leaflet deterioration/destruction Moderate-to-severe prolapse, limited chordal rupture Functional—early annular dilation moderate leaflet tethering	Primary—Flail or grossly distorted leaflets Functional—severe annular dilation (>40 mm or 21 mm/m^2) Marked leaflet tethering	Primary—Flail or grossly distorted leaflets Functional—severe annular dilation (>40 mm or >21 mm/m^2) Marked leaflet tethering
Hemodynamic consequences	None	Mild TR RV/RA/IVC size normal Moderate TR No RV enlargement No or mild RA enlargement No or mild IVC enlargement with normal respirophasic variation Normal RA pressure	RV/RA/IVC dilated with decreased IVC respirophasic variation Elevated RA pressure with "c-V" wave Diastolic interventricular septal flattening may be present	RV/RA/IVC dilated with decreased IVC respirophasic variation Elevated RA pressure with "c-V" wave Diastolic interventricular septal flattening Reduced RV systolic function in the late phase

CW continuous wave; *ICD* implantable cardioverter-defibrillator; *IE* infective endocarditis; *IVC* inferior vena cava; *RA* right atrium; *RV* right ventricle; *TR* tricuspid regurgitation

Table 19.16 describes the 2014 ACC/AHA guidelines for the staging of tricuspid regurgitation.

19.8 Prosthetic Valves

Prosthetic valves (PV) evaluation includes the assessment of morphology, function, thrombosis, infective endocarditis, paravalvular, and sewing complications. Echocardiography is the primary imaging modality used in the assessment of PV. While both CMR and CT can complement and add to echocardiographic evaluation, CT is mainly used in structural assessment and associated complications, CMR can evaluate and quantify valvular dysfunction (Fig. 19.24) [69–71].

Box 19.9 describes the acquisition planning for imaging of prosthetic valves.

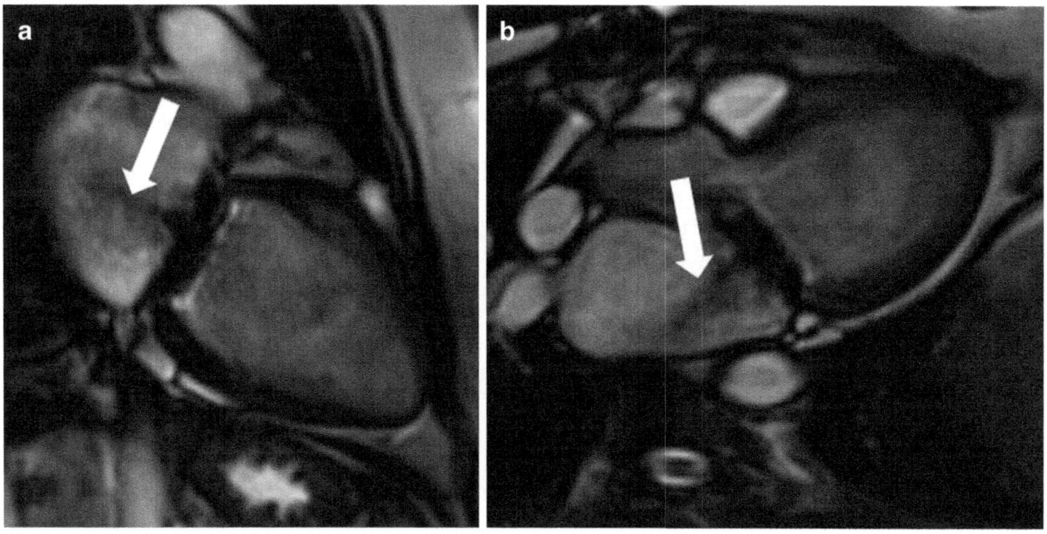

Fig. 19.24 A 58-year-old man with a prosthetic mitral valve. The vertical long-axis (**a**) and three-chamber SSFP images demonstrating mitral regurgitation jet (arrows in **a**, **b**)

Box 19.9 Acquisition planning in prosthetic valve evaluation

Acquisition planning in prosthetic valve evaluation
Non-contrast CT—to detect calcification, thrombus. Contrast CT with triphasic contrast material bolus technique. Prospective ECG triggering—to assessing morphology. Retrospective ECG gating—to assess morphology and function. Delayed phase (60–90 s)—to evaluate abscess cavities and thrombus. Further evaluation of coronary arteries and retrosternal anatomy.
b-SSFP or spoiled GRE images in regular long-axis and short-axis planes across the PV. Spoiled GRE is less susceptible to artifacts. Through-plane PC VENC imaging downstream to the PV—to assess forward and regurgitant flow. LGE—tissue characterization. T1, T2, T1 map, T2 map—tissue characterization. 4D flow—to assess flow patterns.

Other Valve Pathologies

Tumors and pseudotumors can primarily arise or secondarily involve the valves, e.g., thrombi, infective endocarditis vegetation, myxoma, papillary fibroelastoma, undifferentiated sarcoma, and rhabdomyosarcoma [72]. These are discussed in detail in the chapter on cardiac mass.

19.9 Conclusion

CMR plays a central role in the assessment of cardiac valve morphology and function with the ability to accurately calculate the stenotic/regurgitant flows, biventricular mass, and volumes (Videos 19.14 to 19.19). Thus, providing a complete comprehensive picture of cardiac valvular disease, associated changes in ventricles and great vessels.

References

1. Choo WS, Steeds RP. Cardiac imaging in valvular heart disease. Br J Radiol. 2011;84:S245–57.
2. Bennett CJ, Maleszewski JJ, Araoz PA. CT and MR imaging of the aortic valve: radiologic-pathologic correlation. RadioGraphics. 2012 Sep;32(5):1399–420.
3. Masci PG, Dymarkowski S, Bogaert J. Valvular heart disease: what does cardiovascular MRI add? Eur Radiol. 2008;18(2):197–208.
4. Chambers JB, Garbi M, Nieman K, Myerson S, Pierard LA, Habib G, et al. Appropriateness criteria for the use of cardiovascular imaging in heart

valve disease in adults: a European Association of Cardiovascular Imaging report of literature review and current practice. Eur Heart J Cardiovasc Imaging. 2017;18(5):489–98.
5. Gulsin GS, Singh A, McCann GP. Cardiovascular magnetic resonance in the evaluation of heart valve disease. BMC Med Imaging. 2017;17(1):67.
6. Hai JJ, Lachman N, Syed FF, Desimone CV, Asirvatham SJ. The anatomic basis for ventricular arrhythmia in the normal heart: what the student of anatomy needs to know. Clin Anat. 2014;27(6):885–93.
7. Hinton RB, Yutzey KE. Heart valve structure and function in development and disease. Annu Rev Physiol. 2011;73:29–46.
8. Charitos EI, Sievers H-H. Anatomy of the aortic root: implications for valve-sparing surgery. Ann Cardiothorac Surg. 2013 Jan 28;2(1):53–6.
9. Myerson SG. Heart valve disease: investigation by cardiovascular magnetic resonance. J Cardiovasc Magn Reson. 2012;14(1):7.
10. Otto CM. Textbook of clinical echocardiography. New York: Elsevier; 2018.
11. Catherine MO. Valvular heart disease: a companion to Braunwald's heart disease. 4th ed. Philadelphia: Elsevier, Saunders; 2013.
12. Quiñones MA, Otto CM, Stoddard M, Waggoner A, Zoghbi WA. Recommendations for quantification of Doppler echocardiography: a report from the Doppler Quantification Task Force of the Nomenclature and Standards Committee of the American Society of Echocardiography. J Am Soc Echocardiogr. 2002;15(2):167–84.
13. Lotz J, Meier C, Leppert A, Galanski M. Cardiovascular flow measurement with phase-contrast MR imaging: basic facts and implementation. Radiographics. 2002;22(3):651–71.
14. Moran PR, Moran RA, Karstaedt N. Verification and evaluation of internal flow and motion. True magnetic resonance imaging by the phase gradient modulation method. Radiology. 1985;154(2):433–41.
15. Spritzer CE, Pelc NJ, Lee JN, Evans AJ, Sostman HD, Riederer SJ. Rapid MR imaging of blood flow with a phase-sensitive, limited-flip-angle, gradient recalled pulse sequence: preliminary experience. Radiology. 1990;176(1):255–62.
16. O'donnell M. NMR blood flow imaging using multiecho, phase contrast sequences. Med Phys. 1985;12(1):59–64.
17. Cawley PJ, Maki JH, Otto CM. Cardiovascular magnetic resonance imaging for valvular heart disease. Circulation. 2009 Jan 27;119(3):468–78.
18. Sträter A, Huber A, Rudolph J, Berndt M, Rasper M, Rummeny EJ, et al. 4D-flow MRI: technique and applications. Rofo. 2018 Nov;190(11):1025–35.
19. Azarine A, Garçon P, Stansal A, Canepa N, Angelopoulos G, Silvera S, et al. Four-dimensional flow MRI: principles and cardiovascular applications. RadioGraphics. 2019 Mar 22;39(3):632–48.
20. Sondergaard L, Thomsen C, Stahlberg F, Gymoese E, Lindvig K, Hildebrandt P, et al. Mitral and aortic valvular flow: quantification with MR phase mapping. J Magn Reson Imaging. 1992;2(3):295–302.
21. O'Brien KR, Cowan BR, Jain M, Stewart RA, Kerr AJ, Young AA. MRI phase contrast velocity and flow errors in turbulent stenotic jets. J Magn Reson Imaging. 2008;28(1):210–8.
22. Firmin DN, Nayler GL, Kilner PJ, Longmore DB. The application of phase shifts in NMR for flow measurement. Magn Reson Med. 1990;14(2):230–41.
23. Sommer G, Bremerich J, Lund G. Magnetic resonance imaging in valvular heart disease: clinical application and current role for patient management. J Magn Reson Imaging. 2012;35(6):1241–52.
24. Mathew RC, Löffler AI, Salerno M. Role of cardiac magnetic resonance imaging in valvular heart disease: diagnosis, assessment, and management. Curr Cardiol Rep. 2018 Sep 26;20(11):119.
25. Crean AM, Maredia N, Ballard G, Menezes R, Wharton G, Forster J, et al. 3D Echo systematically underestimates right ventricular volumes compared to cardiovascular magnetic resonance in adult congenital heart disease patients with moderate or severe RV dilatation. J Cardiovasc Magn Reson. 2011 Dec 8;13(1):78.
26. Marwick TH, Stefan N, Petersen Steffen E. Use of cardiac magnetic resonance and echocardiography in population-based studies. Circ Cardiovasc Imaging. 2013 Jul 1;6(4):590–6.
27. Nowosielski M, Schocke M, Mayr A, Pedarnig K, Klug G, Köhler A, et al. Comparison of wall thickening and ejection fraction by cardiovascular magnetic resonance and echocardiography in acute myocardial infarction. J Cardiovasc Magn Reson. 2009 Jul 9;11(1):22.
28. Myerson SG, d'Arcy J, Christiansen JP, Dobson LE, Mohiaddin R, Francis JM, et al. Determination of clinical outcome in mitral regurgitation with cardiovascular magnetic resonance quantification. Circulation. 2016;133(23):2287–96.
29. Park SJ, Dweck MR. Multimodality imaging for the assessment of severe aortic stenosis. J Cardiovasc Imaging. 2019 Oct;27(4):235–46.
30. Cavalcante JL, Lalude OO, Schoenhagen P, Lerakis S. Cardiovascular magnetic resonance imaging for structural and valvular heart disease interventions. JACC Cardiovasc Interv. 2016;9(5):399–425.
31. Harvey JJ, Hoey ETD, Ganeshan A. Imaging of the aortic valve with MRI and CT angiography. Clin Radiol. 2013 Dec;68(12):1192–205.
32. Blanke P, Schoepf UJ, Leipsic JA. CT in transcatheter aortic valve replacement. Radiology. 2013 Dec 1;269(3):650–69.
33. Salgado RA, Leipsic JA, Shivalkar B, Ardies L, Van Herck PL, Op de Beeck BJ, et al. Preprocedural CT evaluation of transcatheter aortic valve replacement: what the radiologist needs to know. RadioGraphics. 2014 Oct 1;34(6):1491–514.
34. Rahimtoola SH. Severe aortic stenosis with low systolic gradient: the good and bad news. Circulation. 2000;101:1892–4.

35. Devabhaktuni SR, Chakfeh E, Malik AO, Pengson JA, Rana J, Ahsan CH. Subvalvular aortic stenosis: a review of current literature. Clin Cardiol. 2018;41(1):131–6.
36. Kupic EA, Abrams HL. Supravalvular aortic stenosis. Am J Roentgenol Radium Ther Nucl Med. 1966;98(4):822–35.
37. Guner A, Havan N, Gunduz S, Akgun T, Guvendi B, Kahveci G. Evaluation of the congenital supravalvular aortic stenosis by different imaging modalities. Echocardiography. 2017;34(9):1376–8.
38. Reant P, Lederlin M, Lafitte S, Serri K, Montaudon M, Corneloup O, et al. Absolute assessment of aortic valve stenosis by planimetry using cardiovascular magnetic resonance imaging: comparison with transoesophageal echocardiography, transthoracic echocardiography, and cardiac catheterisation. Eur J Radiol. 2006;59(2):276–83.
39. John AS, Dill T, Brandt RR, Rau M, Ricken W, Bachmann G, et al. Magnetic resonance to assess the aortic valve area in aortic stenosis: how does it compare to current diagnostic standards? J Am Coll Cardiol. 2003;42(3):519–26.
40. Tanaka K, Makaryus AN, Wolff SD. Correlation of aortic valve area obtained by the velocity-encoded phase contrast continuity method to direct planimetry using cardiovascular magnetic resonance. J Cardiovasc Magn Reson. 2007;9(5):799–805.
41. Buchner S, Debl K, Schmid F-X, Luchner A, Djavidani B. Cardiovascular magnetic resonance assessment of the aortic valve stenosis: an in vivo and ex vivo study. BMC Med Imaging. 2015;15(1):34.
42. Nigri M, Azevedo CF, Rochitte CE, Schraibman V, Tarasoutchi F, Pommerantzeff PM, et al. Contrast-enhanced magnetic resonance imaging identifies focal regions of intramyocardial fibrosis in patients with severe aortic valve disease: correlation with quantitative histopathology. Am Heart J. 2009;157(2):361–8.
43. Bull S, White SK, Piechnik SK, Flett AS, Ferreira VM, Loudon M, et al. Human non-contrast T1 values and correlation with histology in diffuse fibrosis. Heart. 2013;99(13):932–7.
44. Hein S, Arnon E, Kostin S, Schönburg M, Elsässer A, Polyakova V, et al. Progression from compensated hypertrophy to failure in the pressure-overloaded human heart: structural deterioration and compensatory mechanisms. Circulation. 2003;107(7):984–91.
45. Stuber M, Scheidegger MB, Fischer SE, Nagel E, Steinemann F, Hess OM, et al. Alterations in the local myocardial motion pattern in patients suffering from pressure overload due to aortic stenosis. Circulation. 1999;100(4):361–8.
46. Nagel E, Stuber M, Burkhard B, Fischer SE, Scheidegger MB, Boesiger P, et al. Cardiac rotation and relaxation in patients with aortic valve stenosis. Eur Heart J. 2000;21(7):582–9.
47. Sandstede JJW, Beer M, Hofmann S, Lipke C, Harre K, Pabst T, et al. Changes in left and right ventricular cardiac function after valve replacement for aortic stenosis determined by cine MR imaging. J Magn Reson Imaging. 2000;12(2):240–6.
48. Bissell MM, Hess AT, Biasiolli L, Glaze SJ, Loudon M, Pitcher A, et al. Aortic dilation in bicuspid aortic valve disease: flow pattern is a major contributor and differs with valve fusion type. Circ Cardiovasc Imaging. 2013;6(4):499–507.
49. Girdauskas E, Borger MA, Secknus M-A, Girdauskas G, Kuntze T. Is aortopathy in bicuspid aortic valve disease a congenital defect or a result of abnormal hemodynamics? A critical reappraisal of a one-sided argument. Eur J Cardiothorac Surg. 2011;39(6):809–14.
50. Myerson SG, d'Arcy J, Mohiaddin R, Greenwood JP, Karamitsos TD, Francis JM, et al. Aortic regurgitation quantification using cardiovascular magnetic resonance: association with clinical outcome. Circulation. 2012;126(12):1452–60.
51. Bertelsen L, Svendsen JH, Køber L, Haugan K, Højberg S, Thomsen C, et al. Flow measurement at the aortic root - impact of location of through-plane phase contrast velocity mapping. J Cardiovasc Magn Reson. 2016 Sep 7;18(1):55.
52. Gelfand EV, Hughes S, Hauser TH, Yeon SB, Goepfert L, Kissinger KV, et al. Severity of mitral and aortic regurgitation as assessed by cardiovascular magnetic resonance: optimizing correlation with Doppler echocardiography. J Cardiovasc Magn Reson. 2006;8(3):503–7.
53. Didier D, Ratib O, Lerch R, Friedli B. Detection and quantification of valvular heart disease with dynamic cardiac MR imaging. Radiographics. 2000;20(5):1279–99.
54. Djavidani B, Debl K, Lenhart M, Seitz J, Paetzel C, Schmid FX, et al. Planimetry of mitral valve stenosis by magnetic resonance imaging. J Am Coll Cardiol. 2005;45(12):2048–53.
55. Heidenreich PA, Steffens J, Fujita N, O'Sullivan M, Caputo GR, Foster E, et al. Evaluation of mitral stenosis with velocity-encoded cine-magnetic resonance imaging. Am J Cardiol. 1995;75(5):365–9.
56. Morris MF, Maleszewski JJ, Suri RM, Burkhart HM, Foley TA, Bonnichsen CR, et al. CT and MR imaging of the mitral valve: radiologic-pathologic correlation. RadioGraphics. 2010 Oct 1;30(6):1603–20.
57. Durst R, Gilon D. Imaging of mitral valve prolapse: what can we learn from imaging about the mechanism of the disease? J Cardiovasc Dev Dis. 2015 Jul 10;2(3):165–75.
58. Myerson SG, Francis JM, Neubauer S. Direct and indirect quantification of mitral regurgitation with cardiovascular magnetic resonance, and the effect of heart rate variability. Magn Reson Mater Phys Biol Med. 2010;23(4):243–9.
59. Kilner PJ, Gatehouse PD, Firmin DN. Flow measurement by magnetic resonance: a unique asset worth optimising. J Cardiovasc Magn Reson. 2007;9(4):723–8.
60. Uretsky S, Argulian E, Narula J, Wolff SD. Use of cardiac magnetic resonance imaging in assessing mitral

regurgitation: current evidence. J Am Coll Cardiol. 2018;71(5):547–63.
61. Caudron J, Fares J, Bauer F, Dacher J-N. Evaluation of left ventricular diastolic function with cardiac MR imaging. RadioGraphics. 2011 Jan 1;31(1):239–59.
62. Saremi F, Gera A, Yen Ho S, Hijazi ZM, Sánchez-Quintana D. CT and MR imaging of the pulmonary valve. Radiographics. 2014;34(1):51–71.
63. Saremi F, Ho SY, Cabrera JA, Sánchez-Quintana D. Right ventricular outflow tract imaging with CT and MRI: part 1, morphology. Am J Roentgenol. 2013;200(1):W39–50.
64. Rebergen SA, Chin JG, Ottenkamp J, Van der Wall EE, de Roos A. Pulmonary regurgitation in the late post-operative follow-up of tetralogy of Fallot. Volumetric quantitation by nuclear magnetic resonance velocity mapping. Circulation. 1993;88(5):2257–66.
65. Vliegen HW, van Straten A, de Roos A, Roest AA, Schoof PH, Zwinderman AH, et al. Magnetic resonance imaging to assess the hemodynamic effects of pulmonary valve replacement in adults late after repair of tetralogy of Fallot. Circulation. 2002;106(13):1703–7.
66. Shah S, Jenkins T, Markowitz A, Gilkeson R, Rajiah P. Multimodal imaging of the tricuspid valve: normal appearance and pathological entities. Insights Imaging. 2016 Jun 9;7(5):649–67.
67. Panduranga P, Al-Abri S, Al-Lawati J. Intravenous drug abuse and tricuspid valve endocarditis: growing trends in the Middle East Gulf region. World J Cardiol. 2013 Nov 26;5(11):397–403.
68. Saremi F, Hassani C, Millan-Nunez V, Sánchez-Quintana D. Imaging evaluation of tricuspid valve: analysis of morphology and function with CT and MRI. Am J Roentgenol. 2015 May;204(5):W531–42.
69. Lancellotti P, Pibarot P, Chambers J, Edvardsen T, Delgado V, Dulgheru R, et al. Recommendations for the imaging assessment of prosthetic heart valves: a report from the European Association of Cardiovascular Imaging endorsed by the Chinese Society of Echocardiography, the Inter-American Society of Echocardiography, and the Brazilian Department of Cardiovascular Imaging. Eur Heart J. 2016 Jun 1;17(6):589–90.
70. Dominika S, Petr S, Tanis W, PTM MW, Tim L, van Herwerden Lex A, et al. Multimodality imaging assessment of prosthetic heart valves. Circ Cardiovasc Imaging. 2015 Sep 1;8(9):e003703.
71. Habets J, Willem PTMM, Budde RPJ. Multidetector CT angiography in evaluation of prosthetic heart valve dysfunction. RadioGraphics. 2020; https://doi.org/10.1148/rg.327125702.
72. Sparrow PJ, Kurian JB, Jones TR, Sivananthan MU. MR imaging of cardiac tumors. RadioGraphics. 2005 Sep;25(5):1255–76.

Part III

Special Topics in CHD

20 Techniques and Clinical Applications of Phase-Contrast MRI in CHD

Ramiah Rajeshkannan

20.1 Introduction

Phase-contrast magnetic resonance imaging (PC-MRI) also known as velocity-encoded cine magnetic resonance imaging (VENC-MRI) is the primary technique for blood flow measurements, qualitative and quantitative information on both flow volume and flow velocity in the great vessels [1–3].

In PC-MRI, applications of gradient pulses induce phase shifts in moving protons that are directly proportional to their velocity along the direction of the gradient. On PC-MR images, signal intensity is velocity encoded (VENC); hence, stationary protons appear gray, flow in one direction appears brighter, and flow in the opposite direction appears darker. It is a non-contrast technique that is frequently used to estimate pulmonary blood flow (*Q*p) and systemic blood flow (*Q*s) to calculate the pulmonary-to-systemic flow ratio (*Q*p:*Q*s) to determine shunt volume and fraction [4, 5]. PC-MRI allows accurate estimation of velocity profiles across a valve or any vascular structure, thereby providing quantitative measurements comparable to those provided by duplex Doppler or color Doppler ultrasonography. MR velocity mapping may be of considerable value when Doppler echocardiography results are unsatisfactory or equivocal, particularly because MR is suited for the analysis of volumetric flow and complex flow patterns [6].

In this chapter, we discuss the basics of phase-contrast MRI techniques, describe the pitfalls and limitations associated with phase-contrast imaging, provide guidelines for post-processing and data analysis, and present specific clinical applications.

20.2 Phase-Contrast MRI: Basic Concepts

PC-MRI is based on the principle that the moving protons change phase or spin angle, in proportion to their velocity. In a constant magnetic field, all protons spin with the same phase. When a gradient is applied to the magnetic field, however, the position of the protons affects their precession, resulting in spins precessing with different phases, depending upon their location within the magnetic field gradient [7]. Here two equal but opposing velocity encoding gradient pulses are applied. In stationary tissue, the net effect of two pulses cancel each other, but if the tissue moves

Electronic Supplementary Material The online version of this chapter (https://doi.org/10.1007/978-981-15-6755-1_20) contains supplementary material, which is available to authorized users.

R. Rajeshkannan (✉)
Department of Radiology, Amrita School of Medicine, Amrita Institute of Medical Sciences and Research Centre, Amrita Vishwa Vidyapeetham, Kochi, Kerala, India
e-mail: rajeshkr@aims.amrita.edu

R. Rajeshkannan et al. (eds.), *CT and MRI in Congenital Heart Diseases*,
https://doi.org/10.1007/978-981-15-6755-1_20

in between the application of the gradient pulses, they induce a phase shift accurately proportional to velocity along the gradient's direction. To eliminate the phase shifts caused by other sequence parameters, both reference and velocity-encoded scans are acquired together. Subtracting the reference phase image from the velocity-encoded phase image makes the phase-contrast image and velocity map that are used for pixel-wise calculation of all velocities.

Velocity-encoded images are generated with a gray scale display, corresponding to the range of velocities from −VENC to +VENC. On PC-MR images, signal intensity is velocity encoded; hence stationary tissue appears mid-gray (zero-value pixels), with increasing velocities in opposite directions shown brighter (positive pixels) and darker (negative pixels), with an accurate linear relationship to velocity.

The peak velocity encoding (VENC) value and its sensitivity and direction are defined by the user. Therefore, the user has to select the peak velocity expected in the vessel of interest before starting the measurement. By entering this threshold value as the encoding velocity, the amplitudes of the flow-sensitizing gradients are calculated so that the peak velocity corresponds to a phase shift of 180°. The closer the VENC is to the maximum expected velocity (ideal VENC), the more precise is the measurement.

Velocity encoding (VENC) is given in centimeters per second. It determines the highest and lowest detectable velocity encoded by a phase-contrast sequence. Therefore, a VENC of 100 cm/s describes a phase-contrast experiment with a measurable range of flow velocities of up to 100 cm/s.

Signal intensities are processed into an anatomic image or the magnitude image, and the phase information is used to calculate the velocity in each voxel in the form of a phase or velocity image. In the phase image, the stationary tissues appear mid gray color and the flowing vessel appears either white or black depending on the direction of the flow. On the phase images, the signal amplitude (brightness) of each voxel is proportional to the mean flow velocity within that voxel.

With the sequences commonly available for routine clinical use, phase-contrast measurement is not able to provide real-time velocity information. Instead, all measured velocities are averaged over a range of cardiac cycles.

Velocity can be encoded in planes that are perpendicular to the direction of flow by using slice-selective direction (through-plane velocity measurement), in planes that are parallel to the direction of flow by using phase-encoded or frequency-encoded directions (in-plane velocity measurement).

With newer 4D flow imaging, ECG synchronized 3D phase-contrast CMR using three-directional velocity encoding can be employed to detect and visualize global and local blood flow characteristics of entire targeted vascular regions [8].

20.3 Imaging Technique

20.3.1 Basic Scan Parameters

For PC-CMR flow measurements, the use of retrospective ECG-gating is preferred over prospective gating so that the entire diastolic portion of the cardiac cycle is captured [9]. The quality of the ECG-gating should be continuously monitored during the scan. If the heart rate changes significantly or there are frequent invalid triggers, the sequence should be stopped and repeated; otherwise, it will give erroneous flow results [10].

Measurements can be performed with free-breathing with multiple signal averages [2–4] or by shortening the scan time so that it can comfortably be performed within a breath-hold. The acquisition length is usually 90–120 s, with NEX (Number of Excitations) of 3. To enable the acquisition of a slice location within a breath-hold (e.g., approximately 18 heartbeats), a segmented acquisition is often used. Since physiological changes can occur with breath-holding that alter the measurements [11–13] and may confound clinical interpretation, the author recommends free-breathing acquisitions. This is especially important when assessing post-Fontan circulation where pulmonary flow is partly dependent on respiration.

The slice is prescribed in an oblique plane so that it perpendicularly intersects the vessel of interest. The velocity encoding direction should be set to the through-plane direction for the quantification of flow. The vessel of interest should be as close to the scanner's isocenter as possible to maximize gradient fidelity. This is accomplished by prescribing the plane so that the center of the image is at the same level as the vessel in the superoinferior direction.

Placement of the imaging plane in regions of turbulent flow should be avoided as such flow can lead to signal loss and inaccuracies. Similarly, positioning of the imaging plane away from ferromagnetic implanted devices is recommended as these disrupt the magnetic field gradients.

Depending on the vessel of interest 5–8 mm slice thickness is selected to achieve good SNR (signal to noise ratio) and spatial resolution [14]. For better spatial resolution, the FOV (Field of View) and matrix size is selected in such a way that at least four true pixel is available across the vessel diameter in both directions [3].

At higher heart rates, typically seen in younger children, the number of views per segment should be decreased to maintain adequate temporal resolution. The temporal resolution in PC-MRI is calculated by the equation:

$$\text{Temporal resolution} = 2 \times \text{TR} \times \text{VPS}.$$

Here TR is the repetition time and VPS is the number of *k*-space lines that are sampled for each frame within each heartbeat. In order to accommodate >20 phases per cardiac cycle, the VPS should be adjusted according to the heart rate (Table 20.1). About 20–30 phases are reconstructed per cardiac cycle to get good temporal resolution.

Table 20.1 Recommended views per segment (VPS) depending on the heart rate

Heart rate (BPM)	RR interval (ms)	VPS
<50	>1200	4
50–75	800–1200	3
75–100	600–800	2
>100	<600	1

20.3.2 Recommended Velocities

Correct VENC can be identified using velocity scout sequence if available. A review of previous echo reports will be helpful to select the right velocity. It is recommended to set the VENC at approximately 1.3–1.5 times the peak expected velocity (Table 20.2).

Phantom correction of the phase offset errors due to local non-compensated eddy currents has been shown to result in more accurate measurements of blood flow in complex congenital heart diseases [15, 16]. Immediately after the patient has been shifted from the scanner, a stationary fluid-filled phantom is placed at the position of the patient's heart, and the images are repeated using the same clinical parameters to establish a baseline of zero velocity. The patient is requested to sit in a chair with ECG cables connected. The phantom data is acquired within 15–20 min of obtaining the PC flow imaging. The size of the phantom is chosen based on patient size.

Since the presence of intravascular contrast agent does not affect the PC-MRI, it can be acquired both before and after contrast injection. Imaging parameteres for free-breathing and breath-hold PC-MRI are given in Table 20.3.

Table 20.2 Recommended velocities for different vessels

Structure of interest	VENC (cm/s)
SVC/IVC	60–90
Ascending aorta	150–200
MPA/Branch PAs	120–150
Pulmonary veins	60–90
AV valve	80–120

Table 20.3 Sequence and parameters used for phase-contrast flow measurement

Sequence parameter	Free-breathing	Breath-hold
Sequence	FastCine PC	FastCine PC
Slice thickness (mm)	5–8 mm	8–10 mm
Echo time TR/TE (ms)	5/3	5/3
Field of view (FOV) (cm)	26–32	26–32
Matrix size	256 × 160	192 × 128
Views per segment	1–4	4–8
Reconstructed frames per cardiac cycle	24–30	24–30
NEX	2–3	1
Scan time (s)	90–120	12–16 s

Practical Pearls for PC-MRI Planning

- Free-breathing sequence.
- In-plane for visual assessment and through-plane for quantification.
- Plan perpendicular to vessel using two long-axis plane. For peak velocity measurement plan perpendicular to the jet.
- Set the VENC just higher than expected velocity.
- Temporal resolution: Adjust the VPS as per heart rate.
- Need high spatial resolution for small vessels.

20.4 Planning for Specific Vessels

20.4.1 Ascending Aorta

Imaging plane is selected from two long-axis planes of the ascending aorta. Image is acquired at the level of sinotubular junction (Fig. 20.1). Imaging plane can also be selected at the level of the MPA bifurcation. The encoding velocity selected is about 150–200 cm/s.

Ascending aortic flow can be used as the total systemic flow (*Q*s) if no extracardiac shunts. It is to be noted that the coronary flow which represents about 0.5% cardiac output is not included in the *Q*s calculation.

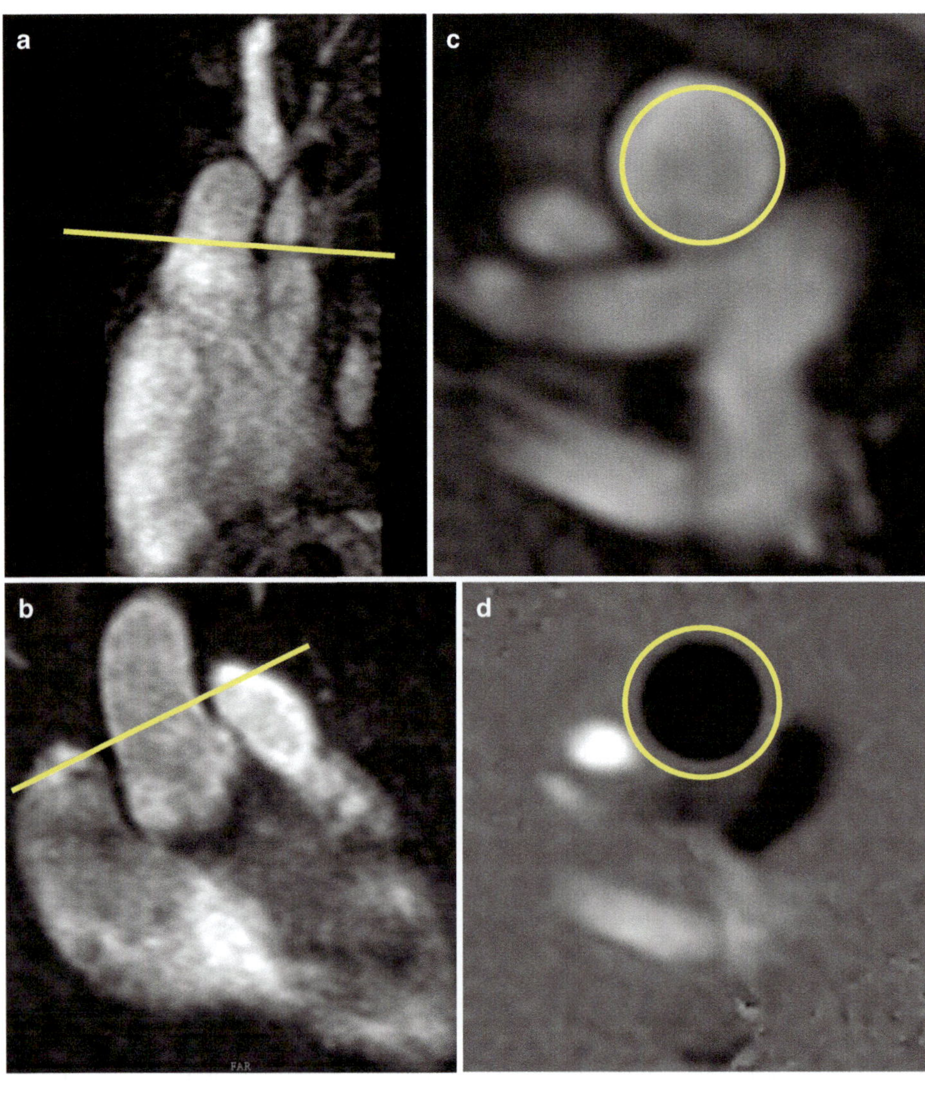

Fig. 20.1 Oblique long axis reconstructed MRA images (**a**, **b**) showing the planning for ascending aortic PC at the sinotubular junction. Magnitude image (**c**) and phase image (**d**) showing the contouring for ascending aorta

20.4.2 Main Pulmonary Artery

Imaging plane is selected from the oblique axial and sagittal planes and the point between the pulmonary valve and MPA bifurcation is selected for acquisition (Fig. 20.2). The usual VENC selected is about 120–150 cm/s. Since the distance between the pulmonary valve and the pulmonary bifurcation is usually less than 2 cm, it is very critical to plan the imaging plane correctly. Many of the pathological conditions cause distortion and dilatation of MPA, so its flow to represent the total pulmonary flow (*Q*p) is not reliable. But MPA flow map can be used for direct calculation of pulmonary regurgitation.

20.4.3 Branch Pulmonary Arteries

The encoding velocity selected is about 120–180 cm/s. The right pulmonary artery plane is selected from oblique axial and coronal images (Fig. 20.3). The imaging plane is selected between the origin and bifurcation.

Since the left pulmonary artery has a more sagittal course, the imaging plane is selected from oblique axial and sagittal images (Fig. 20.4). Generally, combined RPA plus the LPA flow is taken as the *Q*p for calculation of shunts if there are no aorta pulmonary collaterals.

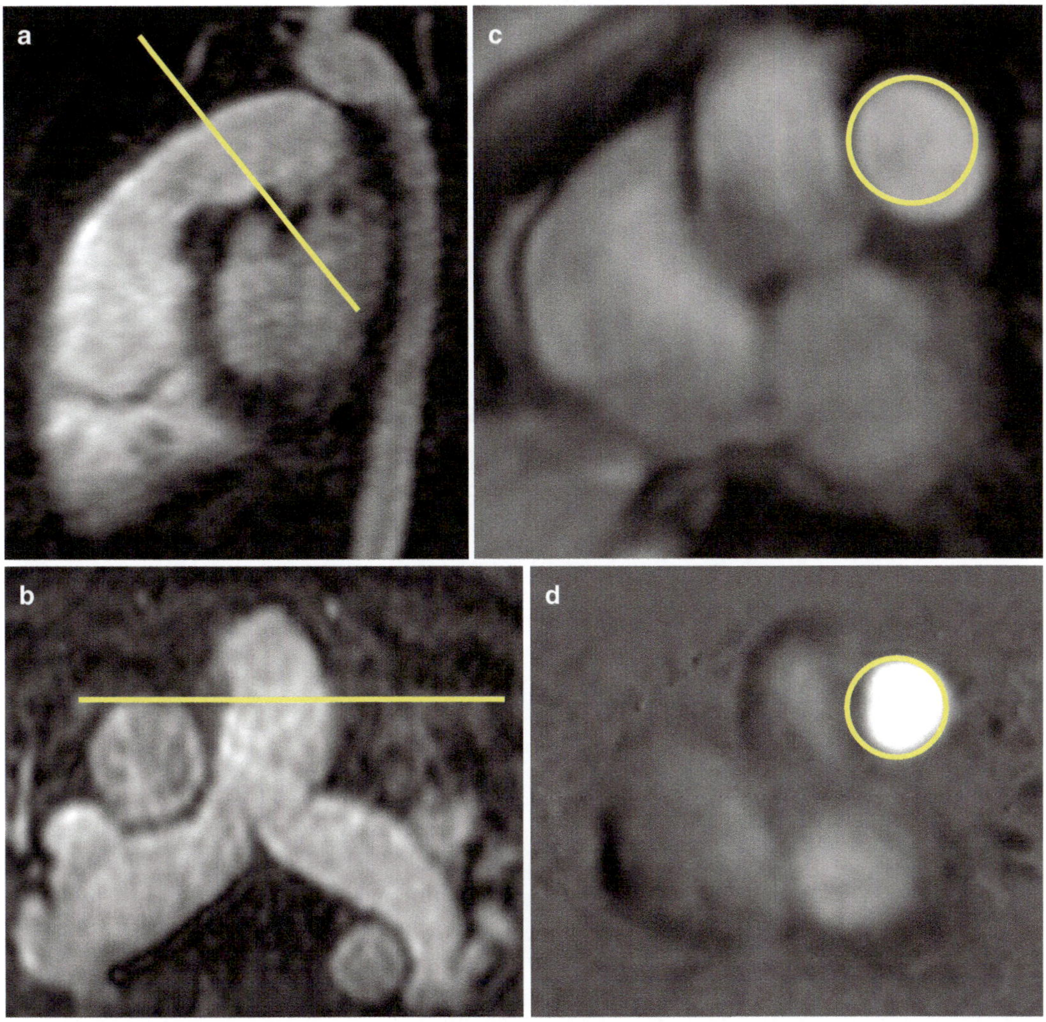

Fig. 20.2 Oblique long axis reconstructed MRA images (**a**, **b**) showing the planning for MPA PC between the pulmonary valve and MPA bifurcation. Magnitude image (**c**) and phase image (**d**) showing the contouring for MPA

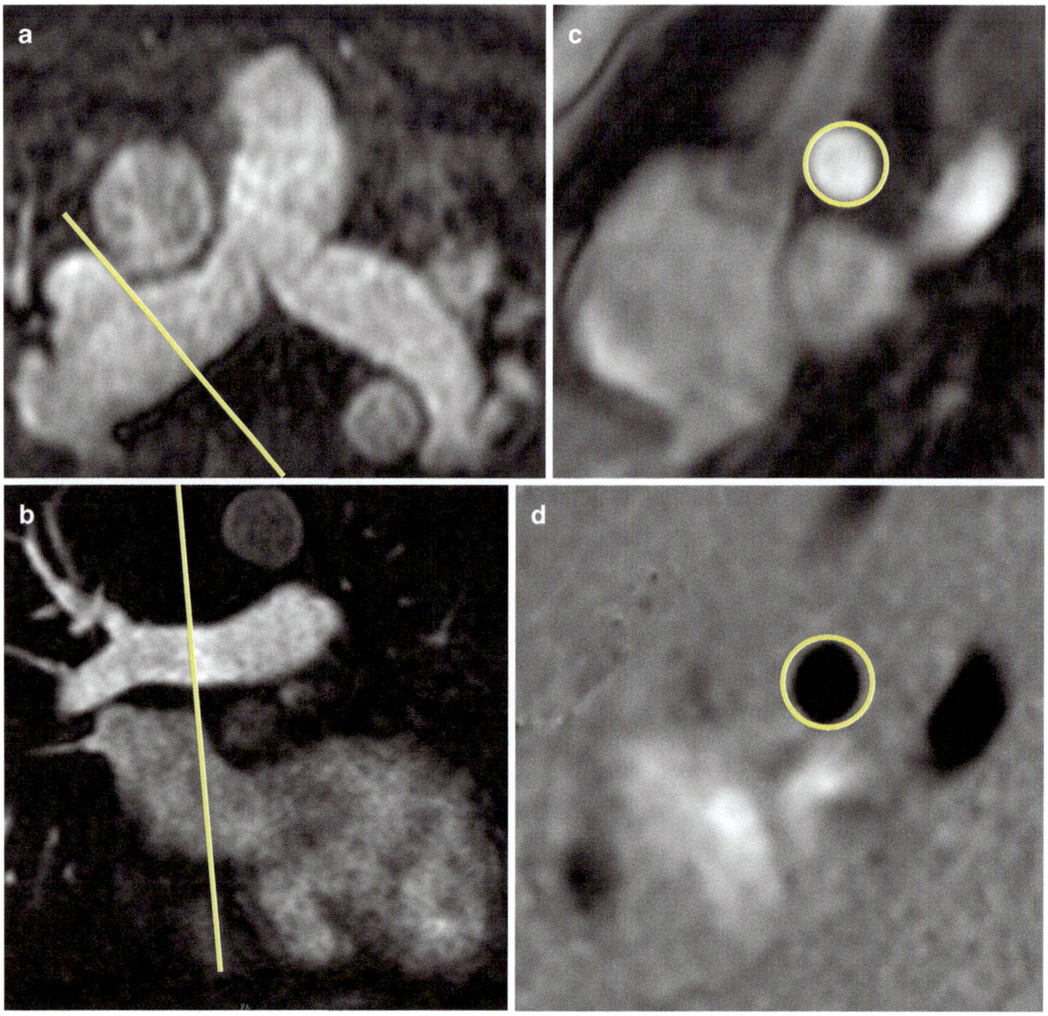

Fig. 20.3 Oblique long axis reconstructed MRA images (**a**, **b**) showing the planning for RPA PC before the upper lobe branch. Magnitude image (**c**) and phase image (**d**) showing the contouring for RPA

20.4.4 Superior Vena Cava

True cross-section view of the SVC is taken just below the azygos vein insertion and the VENC is set at about 100–120 cm/s (Fig. 20.5). Due to the lower VENC used for SVC flow, aliasing at aorta is acceptable.

20.4.5 Descending Aorta

True cross-section of the descending aorta is taken at the level of diaphragm (Fig. 20.6). By selecting the plane at the diaphragmatic level it may also get IVC. VENC is set at 120–150 cm/s.

20.4.6 Pulmonary Veins

Pulmonary venous PC studies are planned from contrast MRA data set (Figs. 20.7, 20.8, 20.9, and 20.10). Both side superior and inferior pulmonary veins are taken just proximal to their insertion with LA. If there are any sizeable middle pulmonary veins, they are taken separately. VENC is set at about 60–90 cm/s

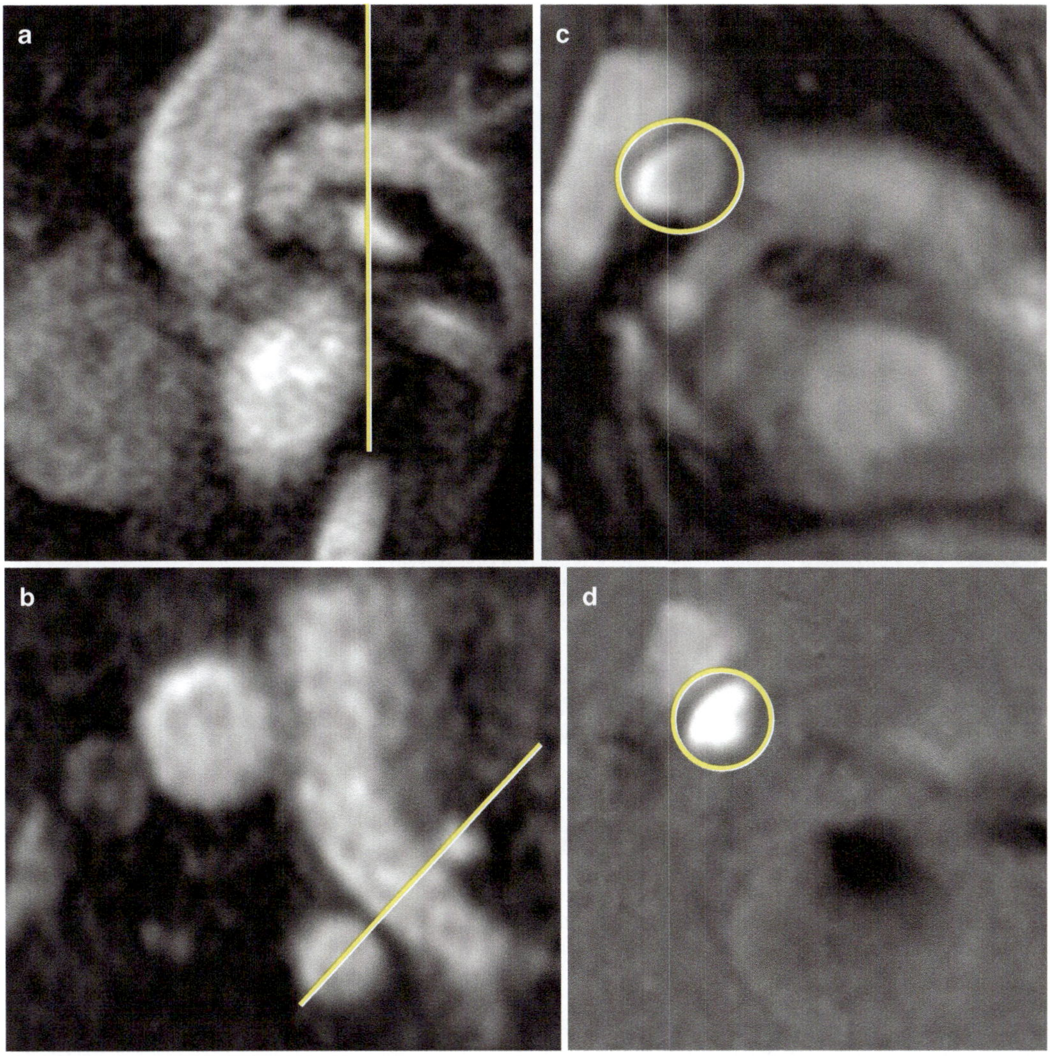

Fig. 20.4 Oblique long axis reconstructed MRA images (**a**, **b**) showing the planning for LPA PC before the upper lobe branch. Magnitude image (**c**) and phase image (**d**) showing the contouring for LPA

20.4.7 Atrio Ventricular Valve

To ensure that this plane remains apical to the valve throughout the cardiac cycle, it should be positioned at the annular level on an end-systolic image. The imaging plane is planned using 2ch and 4ch cine images (Fig. 20.11). The hinge points of the TV and MV leaflets are used as reference points for slice prescription. If the hinge points are not clearly defined, the right and circumflex coronary arteries seen at the atrioventricular junction can be used as alternative landmarks.

Using PC-MRI, both the tricuspid and mitral valves can be assessed simultaneously in the same imaging plane, which cannot be achieved by echocardiography, uniquely allowing assessment of inter-ventricular synchrony. Using this plane, right and left ventricular outflows can also be contoured allowing us to examine the timing of ejection flows in the ventricular outflow tracts.

MRI allows us to accurately quantify the volume of flow over the entire valve area, which is in marked contrast to pulse wave Doppler echocardiography which can only assess flow and flow velocity in a small area.

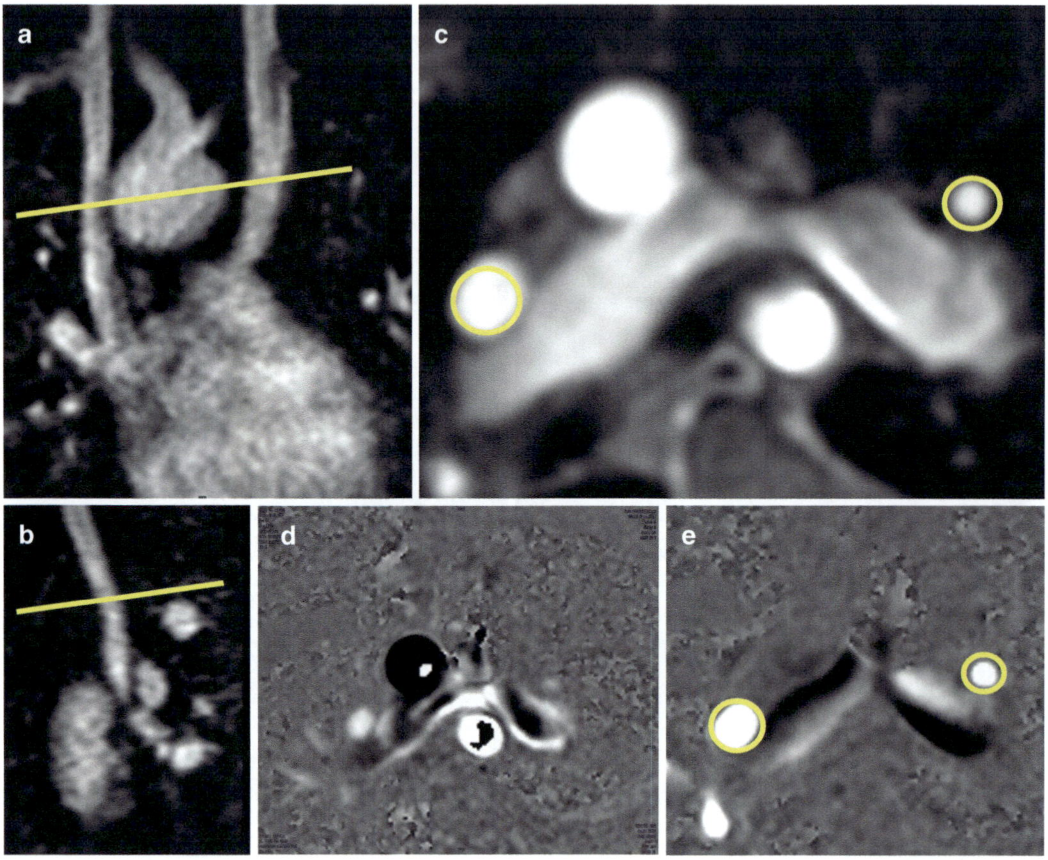

Fig. 20.5 Oblique long axis reconstructed MRA images (**a**, **b**) showing the planning for double SVC PC at the level of MPA bifurcation. Magnitude image (**c**) and phase image (**d**, **e**) showing the contouring for both side SVC. Note the aliasing artifact at ascending and descending aorta due to lower VENC used for SVC flow

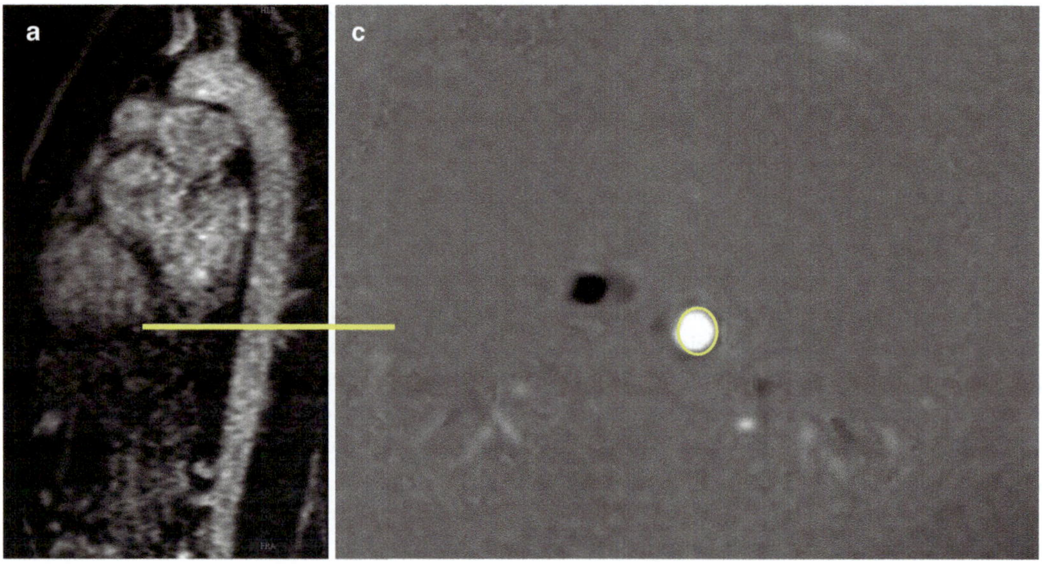

Fig. 20.6 The plane for the descending aorta at the level of the diaphragm includes the suprahepatic IVC

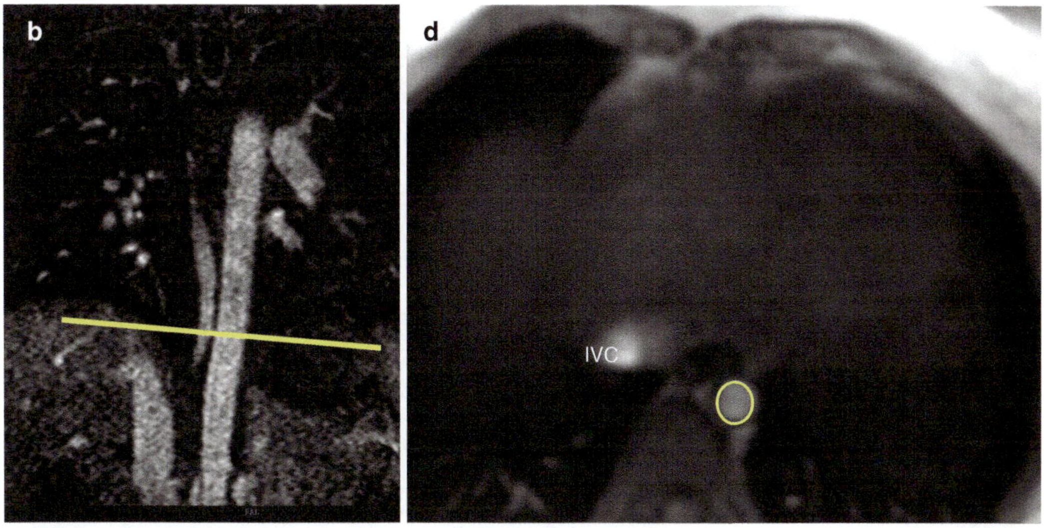

Fig. 20.6 (continued)

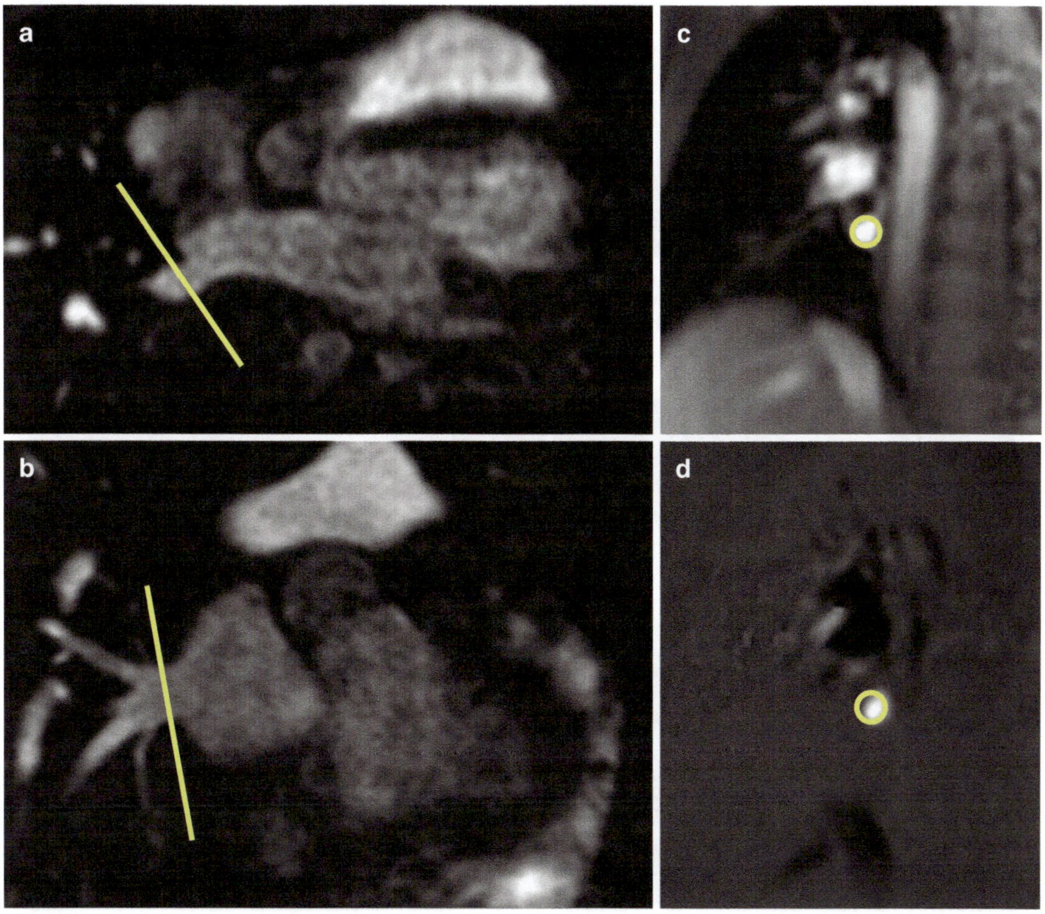

Fig. 20.7 Oblique long axis reconstructed MRA images (**a**, **b**) showing the planning for right inferior pulmonary vein PC close to LA. Magnitude image (**c**) and phase image (**d**) showing the contouring for right inferior pulmonary vein

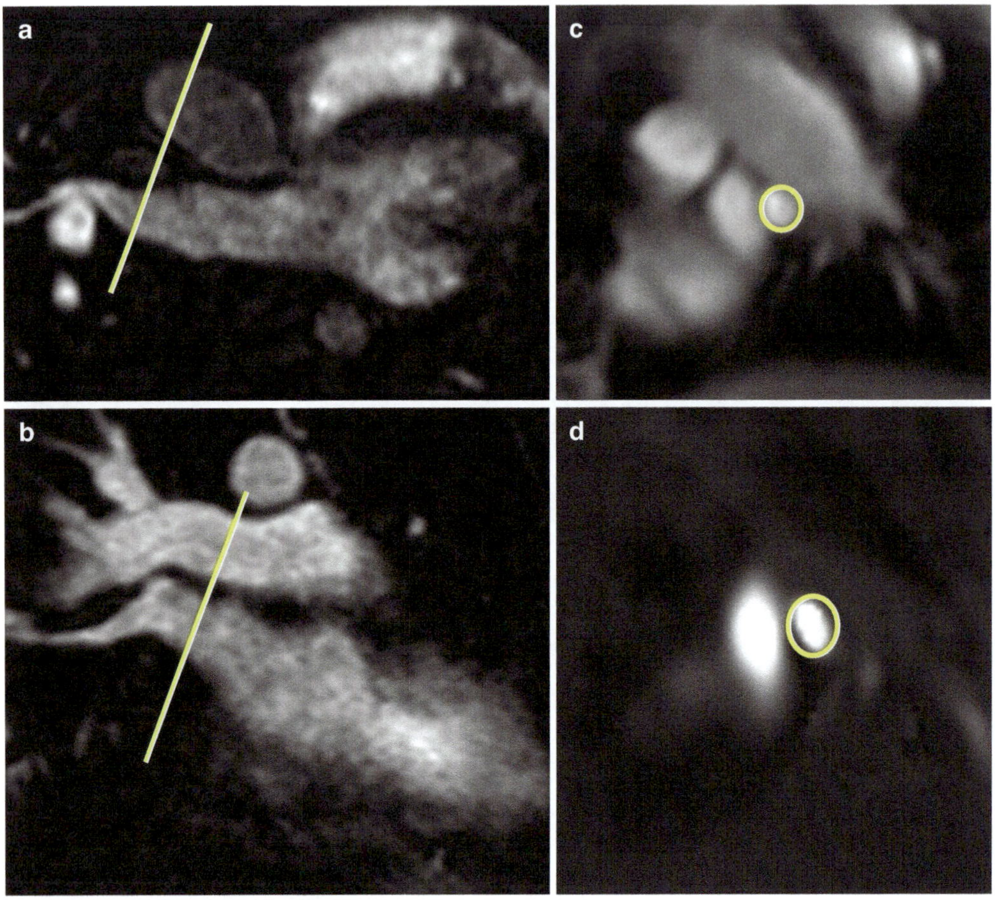

Fig. 20.8 Oblique long axis reconstructed MRA images (**a**, **b**) showing the planning for right superior pulmonary vein PC close to LA. Magnitude image (**c**) and phase image (**d**) showing the contouring for right superior pulmonary vein

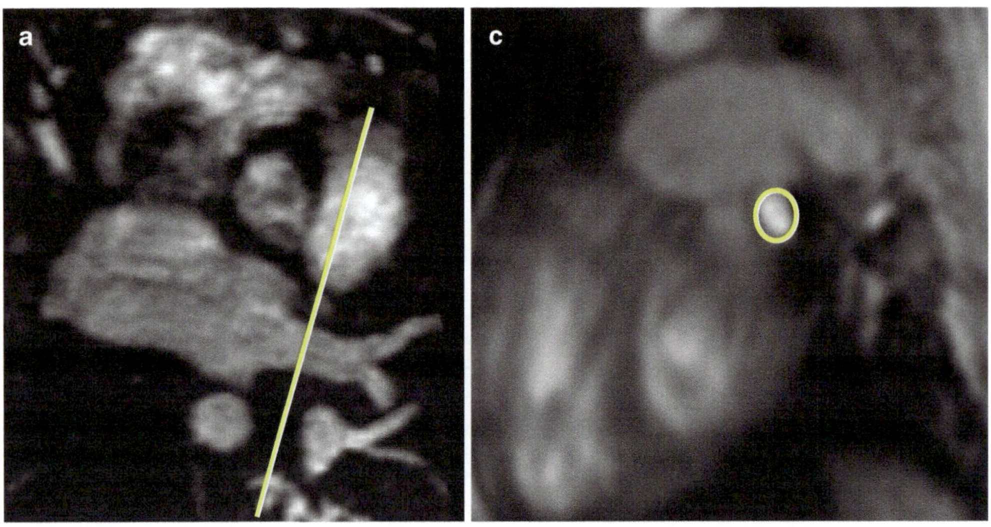

Fig. 20.9 Oblique long axis reconstructed MRA images (**a**, **b**) showing the planning for left upper pulmonary vein PC close to LA. Magnitude image (**c**) and phase image (**d**) showing the contouring for left superior pulmonary vein

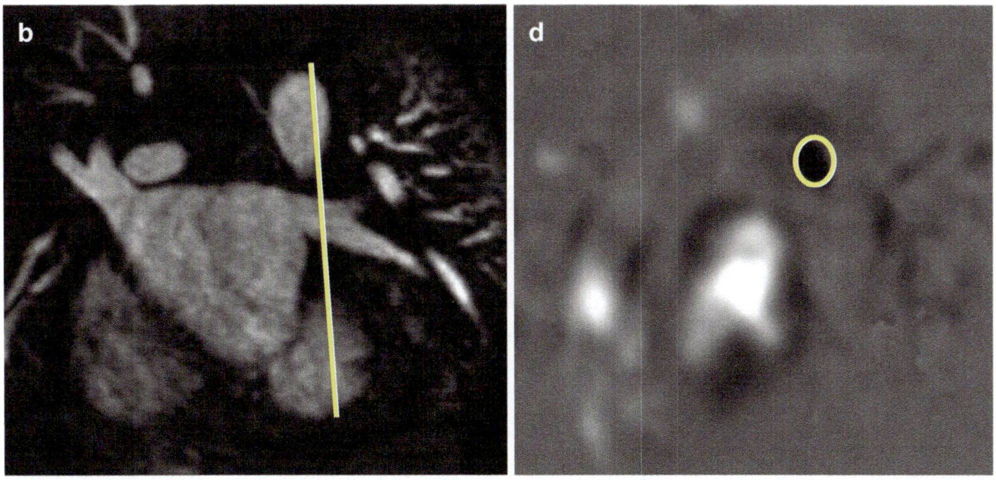

Fig. 20.7 (continued)

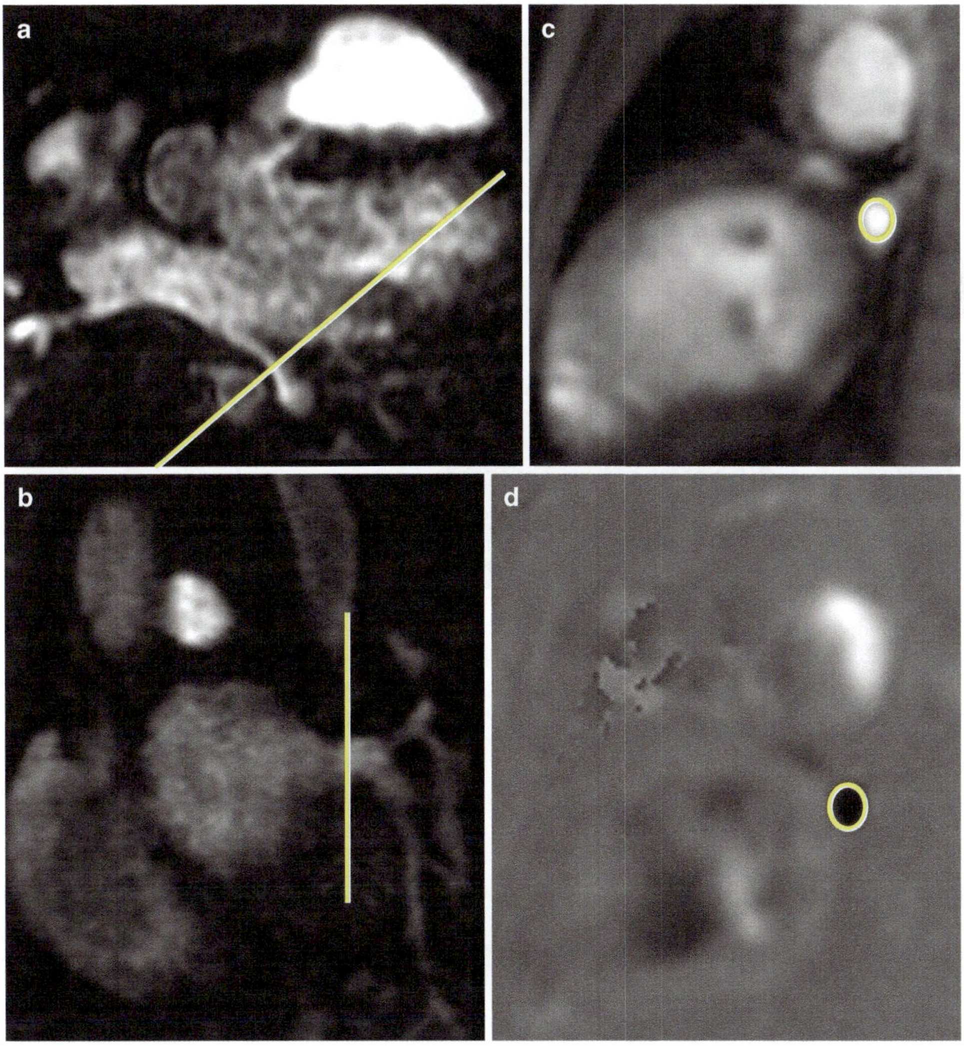

Fig. 20.10 Oblique long axis reconstructed MRA images (**a**, **b**) showing the planning for left inferior pulmonary vein PC close to LA. Magnitude image (**c**) and phase image (**d**) showing the contouring for left inferior pulmonary vein

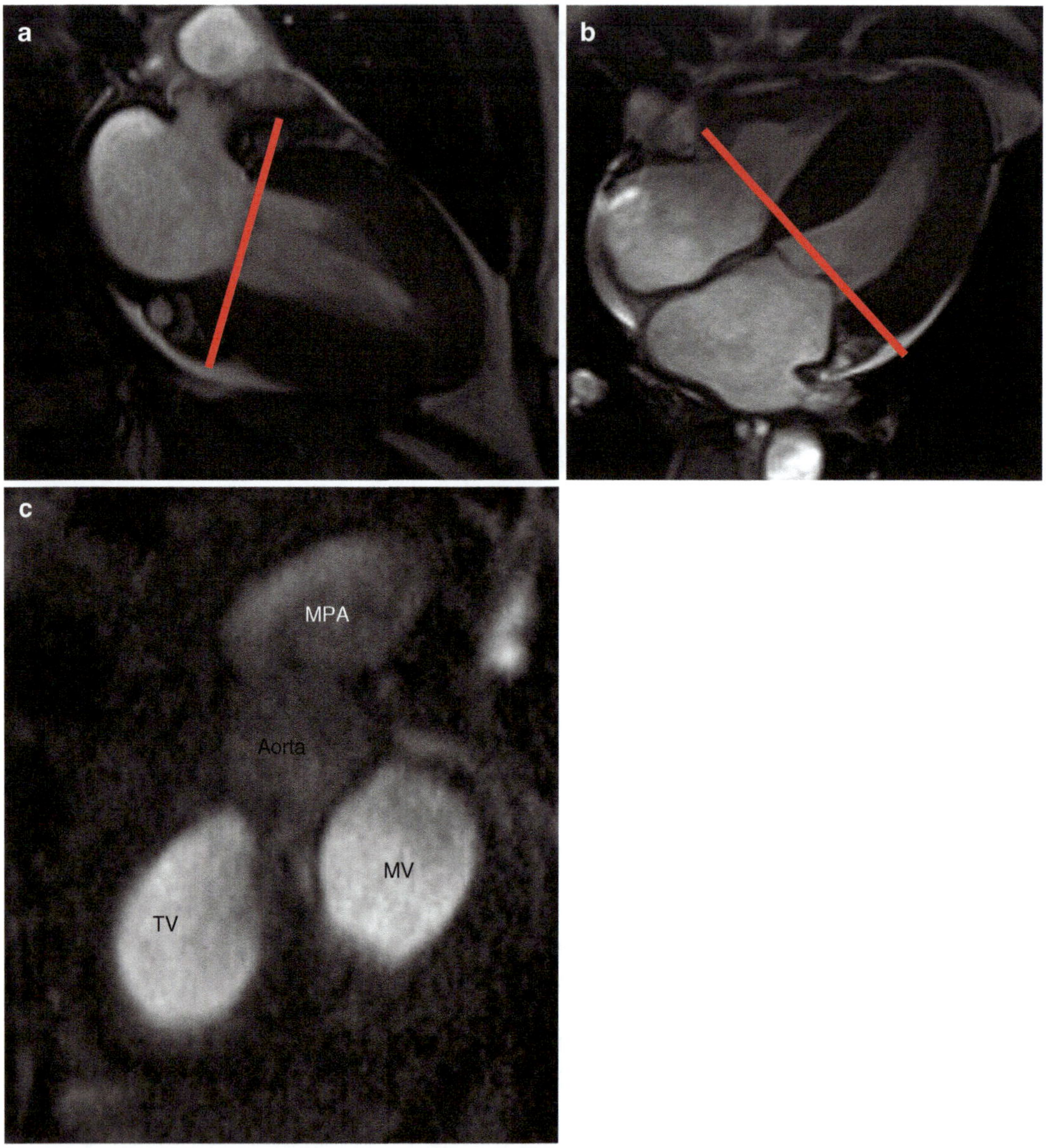

Fig. 20.11 End-systolic 2Ch (**a**) and 4Ch (**b**) cine frame shows the planning for AV valves. Both side AV valves and outflow tracts can be assessed simultaneously from this plane. *TV* Tricuspid valve, *MV* Mitral valve

20.5 Image Post-processing

Velocity and flow are measured with commercial software that allows users to define regions of interest around a vessel lumen or intracardiac region sampled throughout the cardiac cycle [17].

Contours are drawn around the vessel of interest and automatically copied from magnitude to velocity images and vice versa. The automatic contour detection works reasonably well with large vessels like the aorta or pulmonary vessels. But we need to check all ROI (Region of Interest) shape and position in each phase of the cardiac cycle because the vessel moves and changes size during the cardiac cycle. Extra care is usually taken to trace boundaries near the edges of the vessel to eliminate contamination from other vessels and to eliminate errors in the integration due to the inclusion of excess static tissue [18].

Define contours in the magnitude images and always cross-check them in the velocity images. Generally, it is recommended to draw the contours of systolic phases in the velocity images. It is difficult to discern the edges of the vessel on end-diastolic images, on which the edges have the same gray appearance as the surrounding stationary tissue. In the diastolic frames, magnitude images seem to be more suitable for the definition of vessel boundaries.

Abnormal signal, such as susceptibility artifact from the air in the lungs, should be carefully excluded from the region of interest.

To estimate the peak velocity, a small ROI within the high signal intensity area in the velocity image may give a better result than contouring the entire vessel, since arbitrary phase values in the tissue adjacent to the vessel are avoided.

In some cases, flow-related aliased images can be salvaged with a post-processing technique called phase unwrapping [19–22].

Parameters directly calculated from the PC-MRI data include antegrade volume (average positive flow), retrograde volume (average negative flow), peak velocity, and mean velocity. Following parameters are derived from the basic parameters:

(a) Net volume (Average flow) (ml) = Average positive flow − Average negative flow
(b) Regurgitant fraction [%] = (Average negative flow/Average positive flow) × 100
(c) Cardiac output (liters/min) = (Average flow [ml] × heart rate [beats/minute])/1000)
(d) Cardiac index = (Cardiac output/BSA)

20.5.1 Practical Pearls for PC Flow study Post Processing

- Check contour in all slices in both magnitude and velocity images.
- Draw the systolic phase in velocity image and diastolic phase in the magnitude image.
- Draw just outside the vessel wall.
- Background compensation: large area, no vessel/air inside, closer to ROI.

20.5.2 Internal Checking

When the PC-MRI sequences are acquired and post-processed correctly, there should be good agreement between the flows of major vasculature. As a general rule in normal people, ascending aortic flow (stroke volume) will be equal to combined SVC plus descending aortic flow as well as to combined SVC plus IVC flow. Similarly, MPA flow should be equal to combined branch pulmonary arterial flow as well as to all four pulmonary venous flow.

It is to be noted that the LV and RV stroke volume measured by volumetry is equal to ascending aortic and MPA stroke volume measured by PC-MRI, respectively. Any deviation from this agreement needs careful search for valvular regurgitation or shunt lesions.

20.6 Comparison with Doppler USG

The velocity and volume of blood flow may be underestimated using PC-MRI if the vessel of interest is not imaged in a plane exactly perpendicular to the direction of flow. Compared to echocardiography, PC-MRI flow measurements tend to show lower peak velocities, but studies have shown that at Doppler sonography, peak velocities can be overestimated as much as 25% [6].

MRI allows us to accurately quantify the volume of flow over the entire vessel area which is in marked contrast to pulse wave Doppler echocardiography which can only assess flow and flow velocity in a small area. PC-MRI, therefore, has been found superior to Doppler sonography for evaluation of mean flow.

Though PC-MRI has a poorer temporal resolution than echocardiography, it has a number of advantages. Simultaneous assessment of multiple vessels in the same imaging plane is possible in MRI, whereas only one structure can be assessed using pulse wave doppler (Table 20.4).

20.7 Pitfalls of PC-MRI and the Remedies

20.7.1 Improper Selection of VENC

A VENC setting below the peak velocity results in an aliasing or velocity wraparound. It can be well seen in the velocity images, in which the voxels of assumed peak velocities have an inverted signal intensity compared with that of surrounding voxels (Fig. 20.12). However, a VENC that is too high results in less accurate measurements because noise increases with larger VENCs, and flow becomes compressed to a narrow range. The flow jet may not be visualized if the VENC is set too high.

Table 20.4 Comparison between phase-contrast MRI and Doppler USG

	PC-MRI	Doppler echo
Principle	Phase shift	Doppler shift
Flow direction color	Black and white	Red and blue
Flow information	Full cross-section area	Single point
Aliasing	Spectrum overlap	Color mix
Correction for aliasing	Increase VENC	Increase PRF
Temporal resolution	50 ms	<10 ms
	Retrospective gating	Realtime
Imaging during free-breathing	Yes	Limited
Imaging during free arrhythmia	Limited	Yes
Angle dependence	Yes (20°)	Yes (20°)
Flow quantification	In-plane	En face

Large deviations of VENC from ideal VENC affect peak velocity more than flow because the noise is averaged over a number of voxels for flow measurements.

If the VENC is set at no more than three times the ideal VENC, the chance or error in the peak velocity measurement is less than 10%. VENC scout can be used to identify the correct velocity of a stenotic vessel.

20.7.2 Improper Vessel Alignment

Imaging plane can be selected from two orthogonal long axis of the vessel of interest so that it gets true cross-section of the vessel of interest. Accurate cross-section plane of a small curved vessel can be planned from MRA (MR Angiography) data. Deviation of 15° from the orthogonal imaging plane is tolerable for estimation of flow. For small angles, the error is small; a misalignment of 20° produces an error of about 6%.

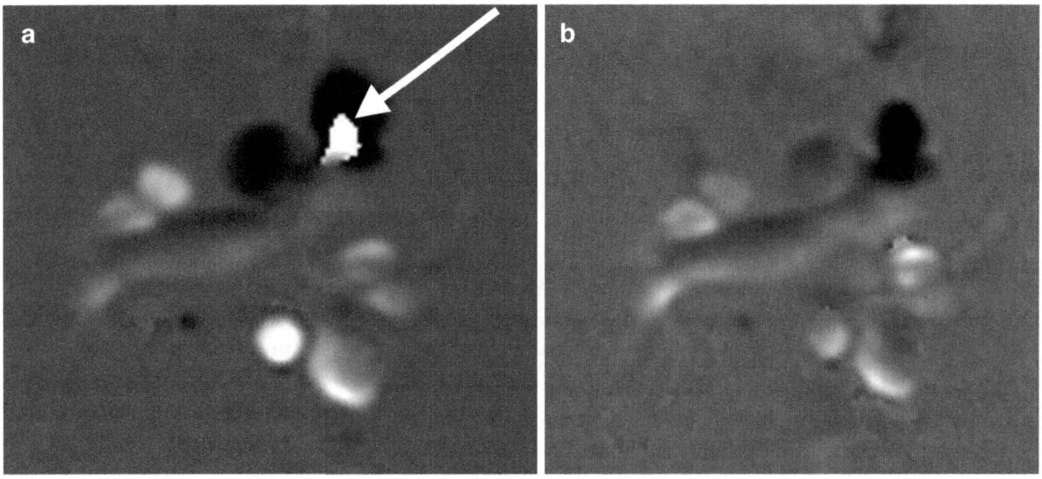

Fig. 20.12 Aliasing artifact within the MPA (arrow in **a**) is removed by increasing the VENC in (**b**)

An ovoid shape of an arterial vessel usually signifies a gross deviation from the ideal orthogonal imaging plane. During data acquisition due to cardiac or respiratory motion, the imaging plane may be changed. Through-plane motion of the heart and blood vessels may impact the accuracy of flow measurements [23, 24]. 3D PC-CMR sequences along with specialized post-processing analysis software can compensate for this motion.

20.7.3 Inadequate Temporal Resolution

Temporal resolution is affected by both views per segment and the number of phases to reconstruct per cardiac cycle. When a low temporal resolution is used, the peak velocity and flow in the great arteries are underestimated. PC-MRI should be acquired with an appropriate temporal resolution because under-sampling will smooth a pulsatile flow curve and cause inaccuracies. The number of reconstructed images should be at least 24–30 to cover all phases of the cardiac cycle. When the heart rate is higher, the number of views per segment should be decreased to maintain adequate temporal resolution as recommended in Table 20.1. The lower the views per segment value, the greater the number of frames to be reconstructed to achieve optimal accuracy.

20.7.4 Inadequate Spatial Resolution

Ideally, there should be at least four true pixel available across the vessel diameter or cardiac valve of interest in both directions. With decreasing spatial resolution, partial volume effects cause underestimation of the flow and peak velocity [14]. The accuracy of flow measurements may suffer while measuring small diameter vessels like coronary arteries [25].

20.7.5 Magnetic Field Inhomogeneity

Susceptibility artifact from metallic implants may affect the estimation of blood flow. So it is recommended to avoid the vessel sampling close to metallic implants [26].

20.7.6 Flow-Related Signal Loss

It can be due to loss of coherence within a voxel, resulting in the inability to detect the phase of the flow signal above that of noise; to inappropriate selection of the velocity range, which in turn leads to poor detection of small vessels with slow flow; and to turbulence, which occurs in valvular stenosis and regurgitation. The latter can be overcome by using short-TE sequences.

20.7.7 Pulsation Artifacts

Pulsation artifacts of the ascending or descending aorta in the phase-encoding direction may overlap with the vessel of interest resulting in a false estimate of blood flow. It can be eliminated by repeating the measurement after changing the orientations of the phase and frequency encoding.

20.7.8 Phase Offset Error

It is a systematic phase error of stationary as well as moving spins. It is largely dependent on local magnetic field inhomogeneities or gradient imbalance. It can be compensated by using background subtraction (Fig. 20.13) or by using phantom correction [27–30].

If the background subtraction is used, the background ROI should be as large as possible. It should be in close vicinity to the ROI so that it can compensate for local phase errors and must not include blood vessels or air.

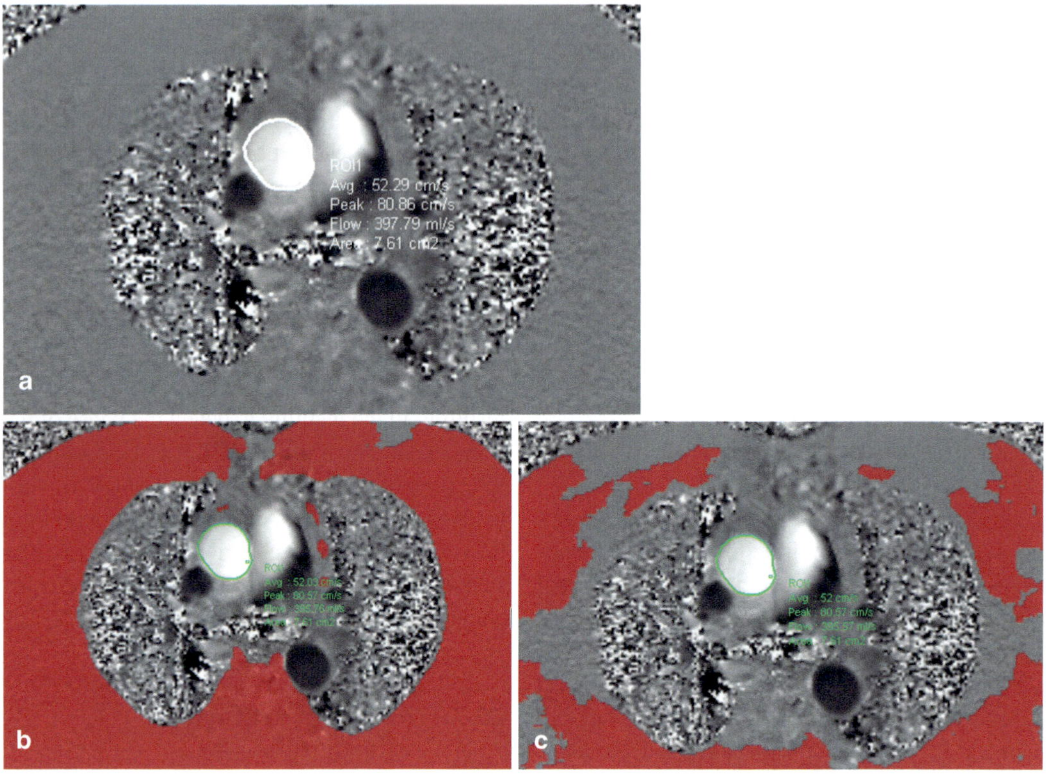

Fig. 20.13 Background correction technique used in Siemens Syngovia software. (**a**) is without background correction, (**b**) with higher threshold and (**c**) with lower threshold background correction

Phase offset error can also be corrected by repeating identical velocity acquisitions on a static phantom and subtracting the corresponding apparent phantom velocities from those of the clinical acquisition. If the phantom is not kept at the correct place while acquiring the data, it will give erroneous results (Fig. 20.14).

20.7.9 Prospective Gating

The use of retrospective gating, as opposed to prospective (triggered) gating, is important for the evaluation of diastolic events (e.g., diastolic function, semilunar valve regurgitation) to ensure capture of complete diastole.

20.8 Clinical Applications of PC-MRI

20.8.1 Presence of Flow

PC-MRI can be used to demonstrate blood flow within the vessel of interest ex. to differentiate cyst from an aneurysm.

It can identify small septal defect by selecting the imaging plane perpendicular to the atrial/ventricular septum (Fig. 20.15). Through-plane velocity images can be used to assess the cross-sectional area of a flow, such as an atrial septal defect or valve opening area.

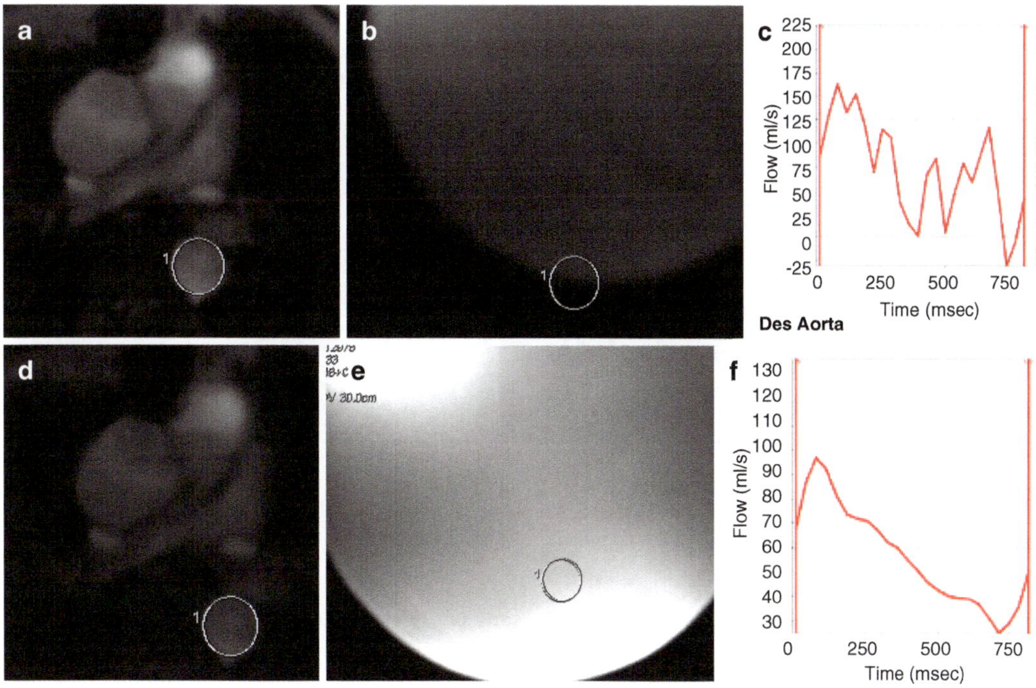

Fig. 20.14 Background correction technique with phantom used in GE Reportcard software. Improper placement of phantom ROI (**b**) leads to an erroneous graph (**c**). After changing the phantom's position (**e**), it got corrected (**f**)

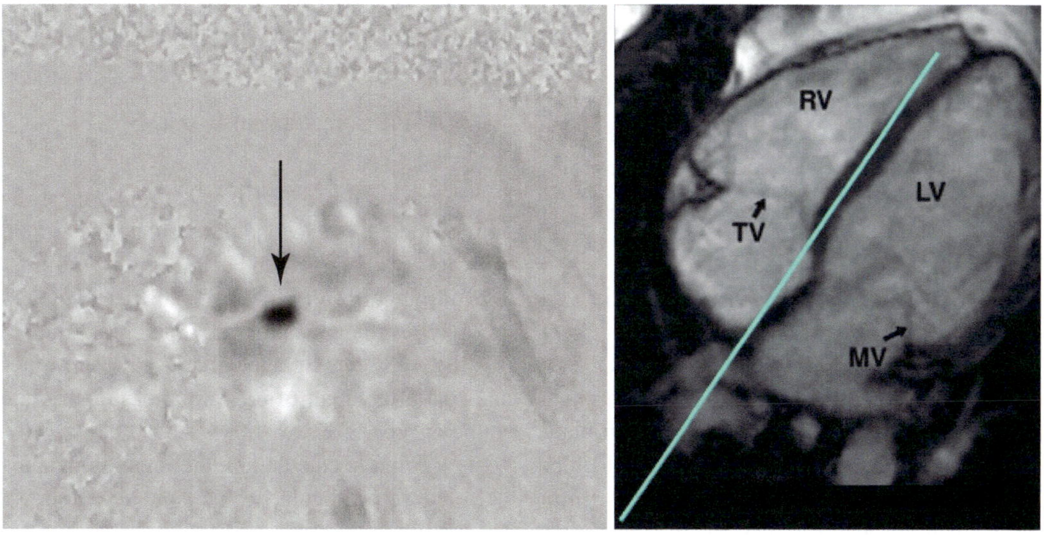

Fig. 20.15 PC-MRI Planning to identify ASD (arrow)

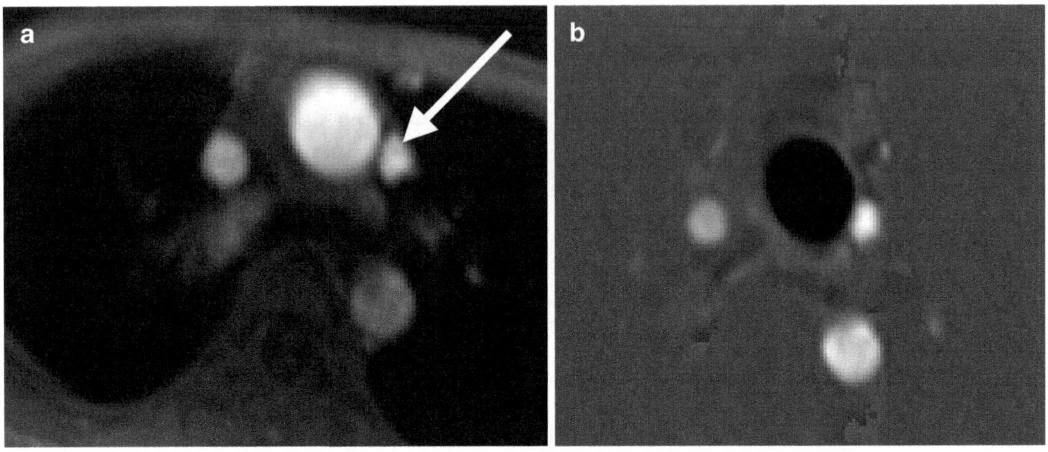

Fig. 20.16 (**a**) Axial MRI just below the level of arch of aorta shows an abnormal vessel (arrow) lateral to ascending aorta. This can be either a double SVC or an anomalous pulmonary vein. (**b**) PC-MRI at the same level shows the abnormal vessel having flow direction similar to RSVC, confirming it as LSVC

20.8.2 To Know the Direction of Blood Flow

It is possible to identify the direction of blood flow in an unknown vessel compared to the direction of the known vessel (Fig. 20.16). Phase-contrast provides image contrast by differing flow patterns and timings, e.g., the true and false lumen in aortic dissection [31, 32].

In aortic dissection peak and mean velocities are lower in the false lumen and bidirectional flow with greater retrograde flow volume in the false than in the true lumen.

20.8.3 Gradient Across the Stenosis

Peak velocity within the stenotic jet can be determined in planes either perpendicular (through-plane velocity measurement) or parallel (in-plane velocity measurement) to the direction of blood flow. In-plane imaging usually provides sufficient pixels for analysis of velocity because the entire length of the abnormal jet is seen well. With through-plane imaging, only a section of the jet is displayed; as a result, depending on the position of this section, through-plane imaging may lead to miscalculation of the true maximum velocity if the plane is too far from the stenotic site or due to signal loss caused by turbulence and eddy currents if the plane is too close to the stenosis. Thus, it is preferable to obtain scan both perpendicular and parallel to the direction of flow.

Determination of the peak velocity within the stenotic vessel or valve can help estimate the pressure gradient across the stenosis according to the modified Bernoulli theorem (Fig. 20.17):

$$\text{Pressure gradient} = 4 \times \left(V_{max}\right)^2$$

It is to be noted that the V_{max} must have the unit of meters per second to calculate the correct pressure gradient, which has the unit of millimeters of mercury (mm Hg). So if the peak velocity is 300 cm/s, then the pressure gradient is equal to 4 × (3)2 = 36 mmHg. Note that CMR determines the spatial gradient of pressure, not the absolute value of pressure.

For accurate calculation, the imaging plane is selected perpendicular to the stenotic jet shown by long axis PC images. This works well when there is one predominant stenotic jet, but fares less well in the setting of multiple jets.

As mentioned earlier in the post processing section, a small ROI within the high signal intensity area in the velocity image may give a better peak velocity measurement. There are a number

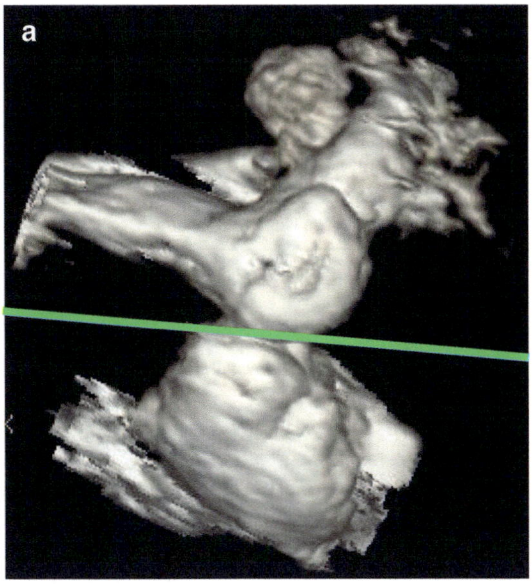

b

Peak Positive Velocity(cm/s)	504.1
Peak Negative Velocity(cm/s)	–459.3
Average flow(ml/min)	1309.1
Average Positive Flow(ml/...	1377
Average Negative Flow(ml/..	–68.1

Summary:Flow 1–PA

Fig. 20.17 Calculation of gradient across the PA band [along the plane of the green line in (**a**)] using the formula $\Delta P = 4\ V^2$. In this case, the summary of the PA flow (**b**) shows the V is about 5 m/s and the gradient across the stenosis is about 100 mmHg

of factors that may lead to erroneous velocity measurements (typically an underestimate) including difficulty in aligning with complex flow jets, partial volume effects, insufficient temporal resolution, signal loss, and misregistration artifacts. So the peak velocity measured with PC-MRI should be used cautiously.

Also, most current clinical systems use segmented techniques that yield average velocities over multiple cardiac cycles. Newer approaches to real-time velocity-encoded cine imaging are preferred when available to capture beat-to-beat variation [33, 34]. Stenosis severity by PC-CMR has shown good agreement with Doppler measurements in the case of aortic and mitral stenosis [35–37].

20.8.4 Calculation of Valve Regurgitation

The technique allows the differentiation of anterograde and retrograde flow so that "negative" (retrograde) flow can be calculated by measuring the area bounded by the curve below the baseline (regurgitant volume). For calculating valve regurgitation the imaging plane should not be taken at the site of the incompetent valve due to artifacts, eddy currents, and the complex motion of the valve through the imaging plane; rather, they must be obtained proximal or distal to the valve annulus [38].

PC-CMR holds particular utility when precise, serial assessment of regurgitant volume as well as ventricular response to volume overload is needed to guide the timing of intervention.

Ascending aortic and MPA velocity maps themselves provide relatively direct data for calculations of the regurgitant volume of the outflow valves. Most phase-contrast analysis software packages calculate forward and reversed flow volumes, and from them, the regurgitant fraction.

Regurgitant volume is equal to the diastolic reversed flow volume (Fig. 20.18).

$$\text{Regurgitant fraction} = (\text{Reverse flow volume} / \text{Forward flow volume}) \times 100$$

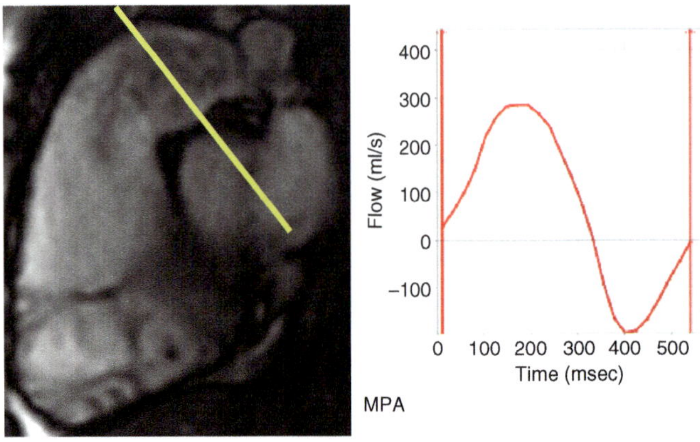

Peak Positive Velocity(cm/s)	97
Peak Negative Velocity(cm/s)	–91
Average flow(ml/min)	3709.7
Average Positive Flow(ml/m...	6874
Average Negative Flow(ml/..	–3164.3

Summary:Flow 2–MPA

Fig. 20.18 Follow-up case intracardiac repair for TOF shows free pulmonary regurgitation (PR). PR fraction is calculated as (3164/6874) × 100 = 46%

Li and colleagues showed reasonable agreement between echo-Doppler and PC-CMR estimates of regurgitation severity in patients with repaired tetralogy of Fallot (TOF) [39]. It is found that with increasing slice distance from the aortic valve, a decrease in measured regurgitant volume occurs due to an aortic compliance effect [40].

Aortic regurgitant volume may be underestimated due to the upward movement of the aortic root in diastole at the time when the regurgitant jet is flowing back into the ventricle. A solution to this source of inaccuracy is the implementation of motion tracking and heart motion adapted flow measurements as described by Kozerke and colleagues [41].

Measuring regurgitant volume across atrioventricular valves may require alternate means of estimation given the non-planar geometry of the regurgitant orifice, the often-eccentric jet directions and motion of the annulus during the cardiac cycle. Mitral regurgitation volume can be calculated from the subtraction of the forward aortic volume by PC-CMR from the LV stroke volume by cine CMR [42].

$$\text{Mitral regurgitant fraction} = \left[\left(\text{LV stroke volume} - \text{aortic forward flow}\right) / \text{LV stroke volume}\right] \times 100\%.$$

Alternatively, the regurgitant volume can be calculated by measuring stroke volume difference between the LV and RV with volumetry. This works well for single valve pathology.

20.8.4.1 Methods to Calculate Isolated Pulmonary Regurgitant Volume

1. RV SV – LV SV
2. QMPA backward flow
3. QMPA forward flow – QAortic forward flow

(SV = stroke volume by volumetric method, *Q* = by PC-MRI flow method, 1 and 3 are Not applicable for multi-valve disease or shunt lesions)

20.8.4.2 Methods to Calculate Isolated Tricuspid Regurgitant Volume

1. RV SV – LV SV
2. RV SV – QMPA forward flow
3. QTV forward flow – QTV backward flow

(SV = stroke volume by volumetric method, *Q* = by PC-MRI flow method, 1 is Not applicable for multivalve disease and associated shunt lesions, 3 is very difficult to draw)

20.8.5 Calculation of Shunts

Phase-contrast MR imaging can potentially provide the most accurate in vivo measurements available of cardiac output and shunt flow [38]. Using CMR cardiovascular shunts can be calculated by direct or indirect method.

Indirect quantification can be performed by measurement of flow in the pulmonary trunk and aorta and calculation of the pulmonary to systemic blood flow ratio (*Q*p/*Q*s). In the absence of a shunt, pulmonary and systemic flow rates are approximately equal, with a ratio of 1.0. In left-to-right shunts, as in atrial septal defect, flow in the pulmonary artery is greater than flow in the aorta (Fig. 20.19). In patent ductus arteriosus, ascending aortic blood flow is greater than the main pulmonary arterial flow, and shunt volume can be calculated by subtraction of the two flows. Lower *Q*p/*Q*s in the older child with large septal defect indicates the development of pulmonary vascular resistance (Fig. 20.20).

Depending on the level of the shunt *Q*p and *Q*s can be calculated using PC-MRI. Generally, combined SVC and descending aortic flow is used to estimate *Q*s. Similarly combined right and left pulmonary arterial flow is taken as *Q*p. Other methods of calculating the *Q*p and *Q*s are given in the table (Table 20.5).

The indirect shunt quantification technique using *Q*p/*Q*s is not accurate when the shunt fraction is low or when there are significant valvular regurgitations. PC flow imaging can be applied directly to the shunt, to find the total volume flow, study its velocity–time waveform or simply to find its direction (Fig. 20.21). For example, by doing the flow study across the PDA gives direct quantification of the shunt volume. Direct measurement of the shunt flow requires careful slice positioning if it moves during the cardiac cycle.

Hundley et al. validated *Q*p:*Q*s by PC-CMR against invasive oximetry and indicator dilution, showing good agreement in shunt fraction [43]. Thomson et al. were able to calculate the shunt

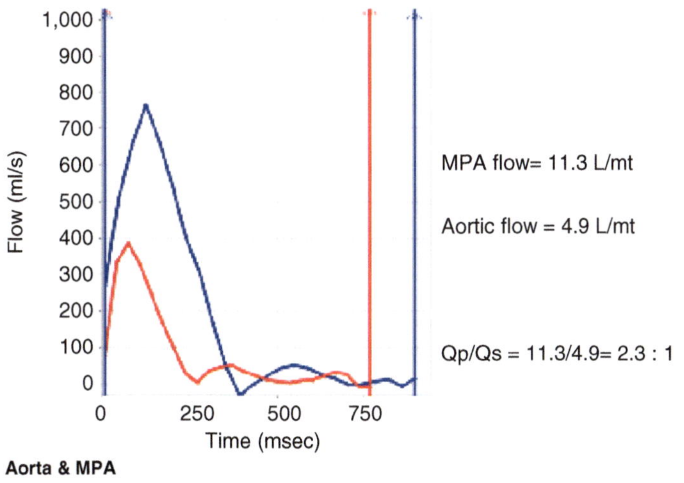

Peak Positive Velocity(cm/s)	78.8
Peak Negative Velocity(cm/s)	–31.9
Average flow(ml/min)	4898.8
Average Positive Flow(ml/m...	5284.1
Average Negative Flow(ml/..	–385.3

Summary:Flow 1–Aorta

Peak Positive Velocity(cm/s)	124.5
Peak Negative Velocity(cm/s)	–114.5
Average flow(ml/min)	11261.9
Average Positive Flow(ml/m...	11999.9
Average Negative Flow(ml/..	–737.9

Summary:Flow 1–MPA

Fig. 20.19 Calculation of *Q*p/*Q*s using MPA and ascending aortic flow in a case of ASD

Fig. 20.20 Large VSD in the adult patient. Both ascending aortic and MPA flows are about 3.3 L/mt with *Q*p: *Q*s ratio of 1:1, suggesting higher pulmonary vascular resistance leading to reduced shunt

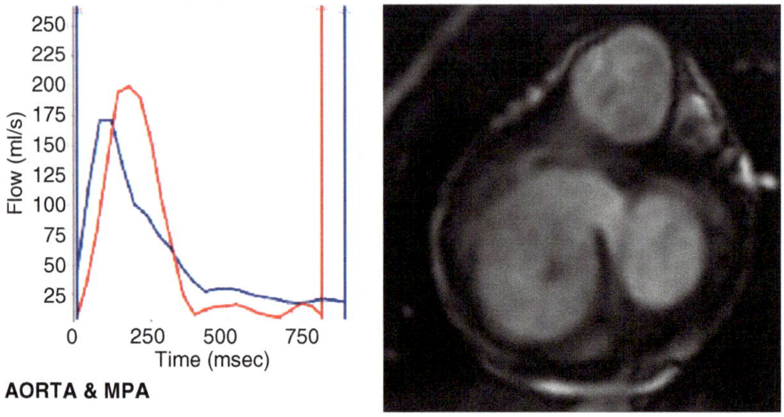

Peak Positive Velocity(cm/s)	102.3
Peak Negative Velocity(cm/s)	–17.5
Average flow(ml/min)	3319.1
Average Positive Flow(ml/m...	3487.5
Average Negative Flow(ml/..	–168.4

Summary:Flow 1–AORTA

Peak Positive Velocity(cm/s)	49.7
Peak Negative Velocity(cm/s)	–19.9
Average flow(ml/min)	3339.8
Average Positive Flow(ml/m...	3584.6
Average Negative Flow(ml/..	–244.8

Summary:Flow 1–MPA

Table 20.5 Methods of calculation of *Q*p and *Q*s

Type of shunt	*Q*p	*Q*s
Intracardiac (ASD, VSD, APVC)	PVs RPA+LPA MPA RV stroke volume (ASD, APVC)	SVC+IVC SVC+DA AA LV stroke volume (ASD, APVC)
Extracardiac (PDA, APW, APC)	PVs RPA+LPA (APW) LV stroke volume (PDA, APW, APC) AA	SVC+IVC SVC+DA RV stroke volume (PDA, APW, APC) MPA

Abbreviations: *ASD* atrial septal defect, *VSD* ventricular septal defect, *APVC* anomalous pulmonary venous connection, *PVs* pulmonary veins, *RPA* right pulmonary artery, *LPA* left pulmonary artery, *MPA* main pulmonary artery, *SVC* superior vena cava, *IVC* inferior vena cava, *DA* descending aorta, *AA* ascending aorta, *PDA* patent ductus arteriosus, *APW* aortopulmonary window, *APC* aortopulmonary collaterals

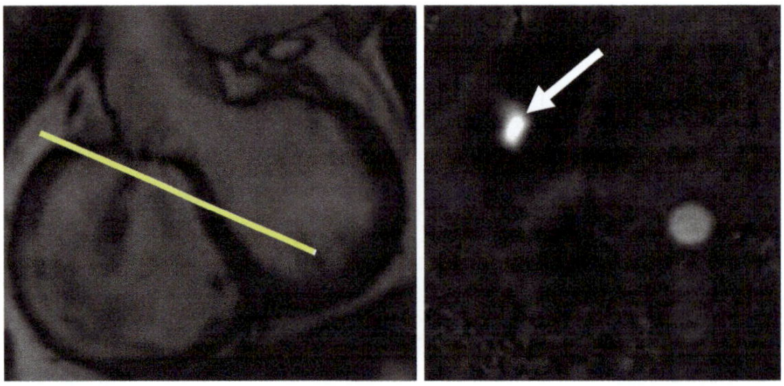

Peak Positive Velocity(cm/s)	264.9
Peak Negative Velocity(cm/s)	–22.8
Average flow(ml/min)	1105.6
Average Positive Flow(ml/m...	1170.6
Average Negative Flow(ml/..	–66.2

Summary:Flow 6–Curve 1

Fig. 20.21 Direct calculation of shunt in a case of post-intracardiac repair for TOF with residual VSD. PC flow study was done perpendicular to the VSD jet (arrow). About 1.1 L/mt is the shunt volume across the VSD with meticulous, sequential acquisitions to obtain the ideal plane for en face ASD flow measurement [44].

In patients with right heart dysfunction of unknown etiology, screening for intra- or extracardiac shunt with through-plane aortic and pulmonic flow quantifications allows for estimation of *Qp*:*Qs*.

20.8.6 Evaluation of Collateral Flow Circulation

The severity of coarctation of the aorta can be assessed by evaluating the collateral flow circulation by PC-MRI. Normally flow volume in the proximal descending aorta is approximately 7% higher than in the distal thoracic aorta, but in patients with coarctation, there may be greater blood flow distally due to retrograde collateral blood flow into the aorta from the intercostal arteries and other aortic branches. The amount of flow in descending aorta at the level of diaphragm minus flow volume just distal to the coarctation segment gives the exact volume of collateral flow. The presence of collateral flow indicates a hemodynamically significant coarctation [45] (Fig. 20.22).

Total APC (aortopulmonary collateral) flow can be calculated by subtracting the sum of right and left pulmonary arterial flows from the sum of the individual pulmonary vein flows (*Q*pv − *Q*pa). It can also be calculated by subtracting the sum of SVC and defending aortic flow from ascending aortic flow.

20.8.7 Assessment of Differential Lung Perfusion

With PC-MRI, differential pulmonary blood flow is quantified by measurement of flow separately in the left and right pulmonary arteries [46]. This is very useful in patients with branch pulmonary artery stenosis with resultant hypoperfusion of the affected lungs to decide on the interventional strategies. It is also helpful to understand the complex flow in Fontan circulation [47].

20.8.8 Velocity Waveforms and Flow Patterns

With good temporal resolution, PC velocity map can be used to detect abnormal blood velocity waveforms during the cardiac cycle.

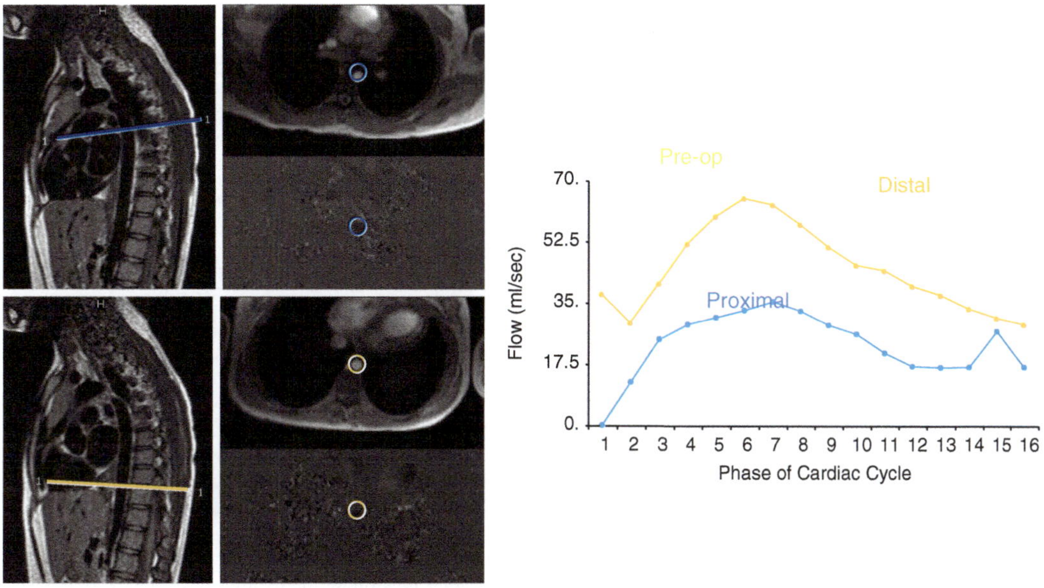

Fig. 20.22 Calculation of collateral flow in the case of coarctation of the aorta. PC flow study at the lower descending aorta (yellow line and graph) show higher flow than upper section (blue line and graph) indicative of collateral circulation suggesting hemodynamically significant coarctation

20.8.8.1 Diastolic Function Assessment by Transmitral Flow

Atrio-ventricular valve inflow velocities are an instantaneous marker of the filling gradient between the atrium and ventricle. AV valve flow is routinely recorded with transthoracic echo (TTE), with diastolic function being inferred from the filling pattern. Previous studies have demonstrated a good correlation between cardiac MR imaging and TTE for the measurement of flow velocities [48–50].

The AV valve flow velocity curve is composed of two waves: E and A (Fig. 20.5). The E wave corresponds to rapid LV filling at early diastole; it is influenced by the pressure gradient between the LA and LV. This gradient depends on LA and LV pressures, LV relaxation and stiffness, and mitral valve inertness. The A wave corresponds to late LV filling at end-diastole after LA contraction; it is influenced by LV stiffness and LA contractility. Normally E wave is taller than A wave. In diastolic dysfunction E/A ratio is altered.

Simultaneous assessment of both side AV valves and both outflows uniquely allows us to assess interventricular synchrony. In patients with post intracardiac repair for TOF (Tetralogy of Fallot), there will be a prolonged ejection time with delayed cessation of forward flow in the pulmonary artery. There is also a delay between cessation of forward flow and tricuspid valve inflow indicating an increased IVRT, the additional finding of diastolic antegrade flow in the pulmonary artery suggests right ventricular diastolic dysfunction (Fig. 20.23).

20.8.8.2 Pulmonary Venous PC

The pulmonary venous flow (PVF) is composed of three waves: S, D, and A. The systolic S wave depends on LA relaxation as well as LV systolic function. The D wave occurs at early diastole and depends on LV relaxation and LA–LV stiffness. The A wave occurs at end-diastole and depends on LA contraction and LV stiffness. In cases of impaired relaxation due to diastolic dysfunction, the amplitude of the pulmonary D wave decreases, with consequent elevation of the S/D ratio.

Loss of normal phasic variation in the pulmonary vein is a feature of significant pulmonary venous stenosis.

20.8.8.3 Assessment of Pulmonary Hypertension

Pulmonary arterial PC-MRI shows a characteristic flow pattern in patients with pulmonary hypertension. This includes an early systolic peak with

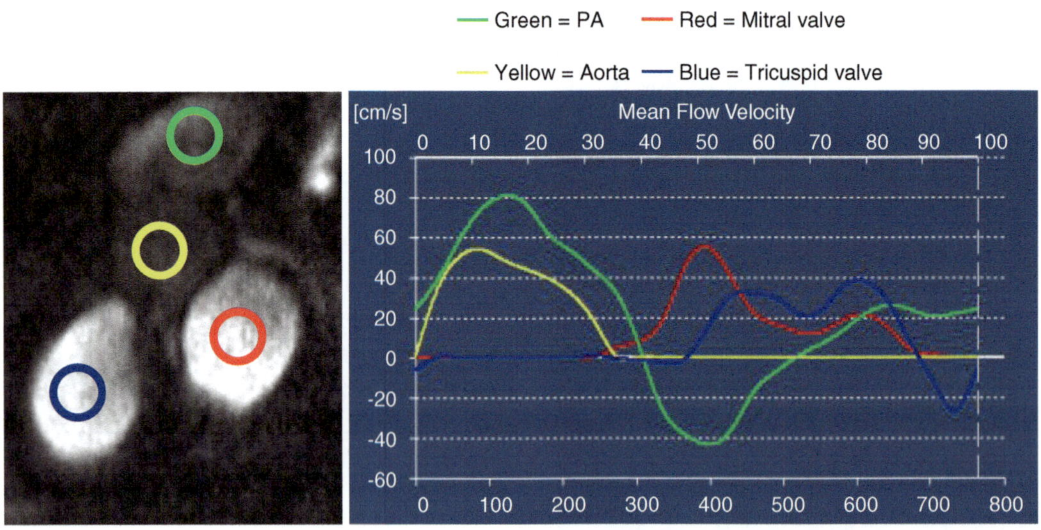

Fig. 20.23 Simultaneous flow assessment at mitral valve (red), tricuspid valve (blue), aorta (yellow), and MPA (green) in a case of post-intracardiac repair for TOF. Due to severe pulmonary regurgitation, there is a prolonged ejection time with delayed cessation of forward flow in the pulmonary artery (green). There is also a delay between cessation of pulmonary forward flow and tricuspid valve inflow (blue) indicating an increased isovolumetric relaxation time, the additional finding of diastolic antegrade flow in the pulmonary artery suggests right ventricular diastolic dysfunction

decreased peak systolic velocity, a rapid deceleration with multiple peaks at late systolic phase, a pronounced flow reversal in early diastole, and irregular oscillations of flow throughout diastole (Fig. 20.24). The average velocity of pulmonary arterial flow measured by PC-MRI is the most useful single parameter in the assessment of pulmonary hypertension [51, 52]. Changes in pulmonary arterial flow patterns after administration of pulmonary vasodilators like 100% oxygen or nitric oxide can be useful in assessing the reversible pulmonary vascular resistance [53] (Fig. 20.25).

20.8.9 Practical Pearls

Different components of PC-MRI interpretation

- Presence of flow: ex. inside shunt, septal defect
- Flow direction—compare with known flow
- Pattern of graph: ex. E/A wave at AV valve
- Peak velocity—for gradient across stenosis
- Total flow (stroke volume)
- Forward and reverse flow—to asses regurgitation fraction

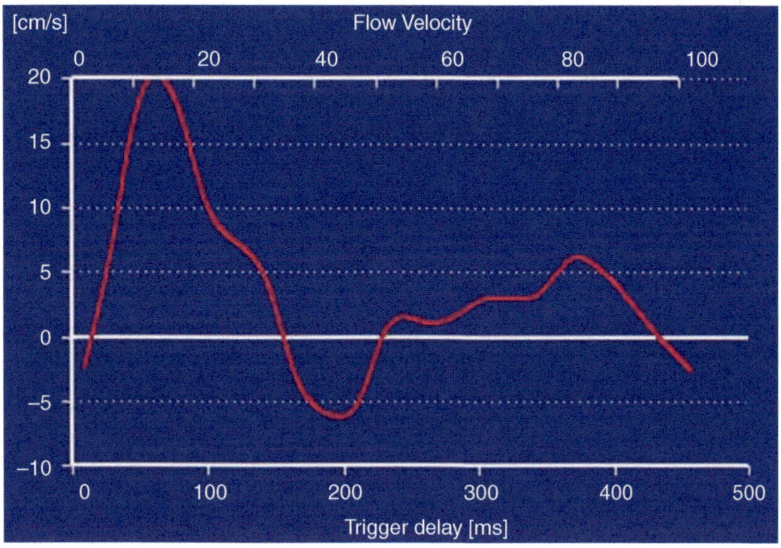

Fig. 20.24 PC flow tracing at the level of the pulmonary artery in a case of severe pulmonary hypertension show an early systolic peak with decreased peak systolic velocity, a rapid deceleration with multiple peaks at late systolic phase, a pronounced flow reversal in early diastole and irregular oscillations of flow throughout diastole

a

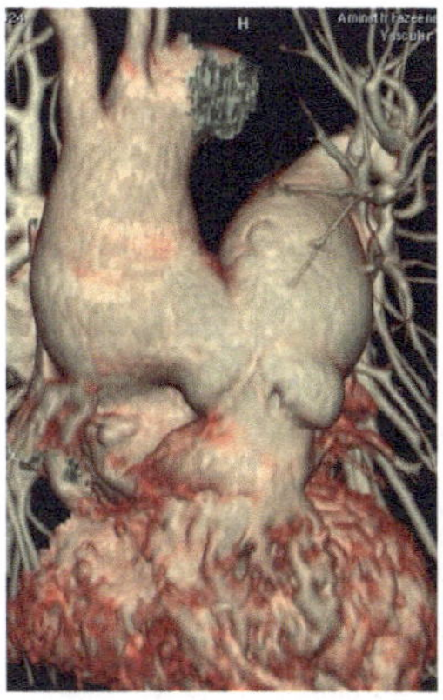

b

FLOWS & FUNCTIONS AT BASELINE (ROOM AIR) :
QS = SVC + ABD AO flows = 1.7 + 2 = 3.7 L/min.
QP = RUPV + RLPV + LUPV + LLPV
2.2 + 1.5 + 1.5 + 1.3 = 6.5 L/min.
Qp:Qs = 1.8:1.
SO2 = 85%-92%.

AFTER ADMINISTERING 100% OXYGEN FOR 10 MINUTES :
QS = 1.2 + 1.8 = 3 L/min.
QP = 2.6 + 1.7 + 1.8 + 1.6 = 7.7 L/min.
Qp:Qs = 2.6:1.
SO2 = 100%.

Fig. 20.25 Pulmonary vasoreactivity testing using PC-MRI. PC flow study in an adult patient with AP window shows an increase in shunt fraction after administering 100% oxygen compared to room air (Ref. to Videos 20.1, 20.2, and 20.3)

20.9 Newer Applications

20.9.1 "Real-Time" Flow Imaging

Even though real-time imaging has coarser spatial and temporal resolutions than conventional PC-MRI methods, it has few unique applications. A range of new clinical applications in short-term flow variations are possible, e.g., exercise testing [54], and in pediatric congenital shunt flow [55] enabling maneuvers as used during ultrasound velocity measurements.

20.9.2 Coronary Artery Blood Flow (CBF)

Resting coronary artery flow rates are typically 90 ml/min and in normal subjects, which may increase by a factor of 4–5 with pharmacological stress. Peak flow velocity is typically <25 cm/s. Examinations under rest and adenosine stress enable the determination of flow reserves and thus the detection of hemodynamically significant stenosis [56, 57].

20.9.3 3D and 4D Flow

ECG synchronized time-resolved 3D (4D) PC-MRI using three-directional velocity encoding offers the possibility of isotropic high spatial resolution and thus the ability to measure and visualize the temporal evolution of complex flow and motion patterns in a 3D volume, without any restrictions to predefined imaging planes [58, 59]. This method has also been used in the evaluation of Fontan pathway dynamics [60].

20.10 Conclusions

PC-CMR currently offers a wide range of clinical applications that show distinct advantages in the evaluation of children with CHD, where invasive studies and X-ray exposure are to be avoided.

Using the recommendations and protocols provided in this chapter, phase-contrast MRI is easy to perform and yields reliable results. In contrast to the results of other techniques, the results of phase-contrast flow measurement can be reevaluated with the same reliability at any time. This is an important prerequisite for standardized and long-term quality assurance of quantitative measurements. With careful planning and post-processing, the error rate of quantification can be kept to less than 10%.

References

1. O'Donnell M. NMR blood flow using multiecho, phase contrast sequences. Med Phys. 1985;12:59–64.
2. Nayler GL, Firmin DN, Longmore DB. Blood flow imaging by cine magnetic resonance. J Comput Assist Tomogr. 1986;10:715–22.
3. Nayak KS, Nielsen J-F, Bernstein MA, et al. Cardiovascular magnetic resonance phase contrast imaging. J Cardiovasc Magn Reson. 2015;17:71. https://doi.org/10.1186/s12968-015-0172-7.
4. Varaprasathan GA, Araoz PA, Higgins CB, Reddy GP. Quantification of flow dynamics in congenital heart disease: applications of velocity-encoded cine MR imaging. Radiographics. 2002;22:895–905.
5. Pelc NJ. Flow quantification and analysis methods. Magn Reson Imaging Clin N Am. 1995;3:413–24.
6. Lee VS, Spritzer CE, Carroll BA, et al. Flow quantification using fast cine phase-contrast MR imaging, conventional cine phase-contrast MR imaging, and Doppler sonography: in vitro and in vivo validation. AJR. 1997;169:1125–31.
7. Lotz J, Meier C, Leppert A, Galanski M. Cardiovascular flow measurement with phase-contrast MR imaging: basic facts and implementation. Radiographics. 2002;22:651–71.
8. Vasanawala SS, Hanneman K, Alley MT, Hsiao A. Congenital heart disease assessment with 4D flow MRI. J Magn Reson Imaging. 2015;42:870–86.
9. Greil G, Geva T, Maier SE, Powell AJ. Effect of acquisition parameters on the accuracy of velocity encoded cine magnetic resonance imaging blood flow measurements. J Magn Reson Imaging. 2002;15:47–54.
10. Ley S, Ley-Zaporozhan J, Kreitner K-F, Iliyushenko S, Puderbach M, Hosch W, et al. MR flow measurements for assessment of the pulmonary, systemic and broncho systemic circulation: impact of different ECG gating methods and breathing schema. Eur J Radiol. 2007;61:124–9.
11. Sakuma H, Kawada N, Kubo H, Nishide Y, Takano K, Kato N, Takeda K. Effect of breath holding on blood flow measurement using fast velocity encoded cine MRI. Magn Reson Med. 2001;45:346–8.
12. Johansson B, Babu-Narayan SV, Kilner PJ. The effects of breath-holding on pulmonary regurgitation mea-

sured by cardiovascular magnetic resonance velocity mapping. J Cardiovasc Magn Reson. 2009;11:1.
13. Ley S, Fink C, Puderbach M, Zaporozhan J, Plathow C, Eichinger M, Hosch W, Kreitner KF, Kauczor HU. MRI Measurement of the hemodynamics of the pulmonary and systemic arterial circulation: influence of breathing maneuvers. AJR Am J Roentgenol. 2006;187:439–44.
14. Tang C, Blatter DD, Parker DL. Accuracy of phase-contrast flow measurements in the presence of partial volume effects. J Magn Reson Imaging. 1993;3:377–85.
15. Kilner PJ, Gatehouse PD, Firmin DN. Flow measurement by magnetic resonance: a unique asset worth optimising. J Cardiovasc Magn Reson. 2007;9:723–8.
16. Miller TA, Landes AB, Moran AM. Improved accuracy in flow mapping of congenital heart disease using stationary phantom technique. J Cardiovasc Magn Reson. 2009;11:52.
17. Kozerke S, Botnar R, Oyre S, Scheidegger MB, Pedersen EM, Boesiger P. Automatic vessel segmentation using active contours in cine phase contrast flow measurements. J Magn Reson Imaging. 1999;10:41–51.
18. Hamilton CA, Moran PR, Santago P 2nd, Rajala SA. Effects of intravoxel velocity distributions on the accuracy of the phase mapping method in phase-contrast MR angiography. J Magn Reson Imaging. 1994;4:752–5.
19. Ghiglia DC, Pritt MD. Two-dimensional phase unwrapping: theory, algorithms, and software. New York: Wiley; 1998.
20. Yang GZ, Kilner PJ, Wood NB, Underwood SR, Firmin DN. Computation of low pressure fields from magnetic resonance velocity mapping. Magn Reson Med. 1996;36:520–6.
21. Xiang QS. Temporal phase unwrapping for CINE velocity imaging. J Magn Reson Imaging. 1995;5:529–34.
22. Firmin DN, Nayler GL, Kilner PJ, et al. The applications of phase shifts in NMR for flow measurements. Magn Reson Med. 1990;14:230–41.
23. Kozerke S, Schwitter J, Pedersen EM, Boesiger P. Aortic and mitral regurgitation: quantification using moving slice velocity mapping. J Magn Reson Imaging. 2001;14:106–12.
24. Kayser HW, Stoel BC, van der Wall EE, van der Geest RJ, de Roos A. MR velocity mapping of tricuspid flow: correction for through-plane motion. J Magn Reson Imaging. 1997;7:669–73.
25. Hundley WG, Lange RA, Clarke GD, et al. Assessment of coronary arterial flow and flow reserve in humans with magnetic resonance imaging. Circulation. 1996;93:1502–8.
26. Wolf RL, Ehman RL, Riederer SJ, Rossman PJ. Analysis of systematic and random error in MR volumetric flow measurements. Magn Reson Med. 1993;30:82–91.
27. Gatehouse PD, Rolf MP, Graves MJ, Hofman MB, Totman J, Werner B, Quest RA, Liu Y, von Spiczak J, Dieringer M, et al. Flow measurement by cardiovascular magnetic resonance: a multi-centre multi-vendor study of background phase offset errors that can compromise the accuracy of derived regurgitant or shunt flow measurements. J Cardiovasc Magn Reson. 2010;12:5.
28. Holland BJ, Printz BF, Lai WW. Baseline correction of phase-contrast images in congenital cardiovascular magnetic resonance. J Cardiovasc Magn Reson. 2010;12:11.
29. Chernobelsky A, Shubayev O, Comeau CR, Wolff SD. Baseline correction of phase contrast images improves quantification of blood flow in the great vessels. J Cardiovasc Magn Reson. 2007;9:681–5.
30. Lankhaar JW, Hofman MB, Marcus JT, Zwanenburg JJ, Faes TJ, Vonk-Noordegraaf A. Correction of phase offset errors in main pulmonary artery flow quantification. J Magn Reson Imaging. 2005;22:73–9.
31. Silverman JM, Raissi S, Tyszka JM, Trento A, Herfkens RJ. Phase-contrast cine MR angiography detection of thoracic aortic dissection. Int J Card Imaging. 2000;16:461–70.
32. Kunz RP, Oberholzer K, Kuroczynski W, et al. Assessment of chronic aortic dissection: contribution of different ECG-gated breath-hold MRI techniques. AJR. 2004;182:1319–26.
33. Nezafat R, Kellman P, Derbyshire JA, McVeigh ER. Real-time blood flow imaging using autocalibrated spiral sensitivity encoding. Magn Reson Med. 2005;54:1557–61.
34. Nayak KS, Pauly JM, Kerr AB, Hu BS, Nishimura DG. Real-time color flow MRI. Magn Reson Med. 2000;43:251–8.157.
35. Caruthers SD, Lin SJ, Brown P, Watkins MP, Williams TA, Lehr KA, et al. Practical value of cardiac magnetic resonance imaging for clinical quantification of aortic valve stenosis: comparison with echocardiography. Circulation. 2003;108:2236–43.
36. Søndergaard L, Hildebrandt P, Lindvig K, Thomsen C, Ståhlberg F, Kassis E, et al. Valve area and cardiac output in aortic stenosis: quantification by magnetic resonance velocity mapping. Am Heart J. 1993;126:1156–64.
37. Lin SJ, Brown PA, Watkins MP, Williams TA, Lehr KA, Liu W, et al. Quantification of stenotic mitral valve area with magnetic resonance imaging and comparison with Doppler ultrasound. J Am Coll Cardiol. 2004;44:133–7.
38. Davos D, Kilner PJ. Calculations of cardiovascular shunts and regurgitation using magnetic resonance ventricular volume and aortic and pulmonary flow measurements. Eur Radiol. 2010;20:410–21. https://doi.org/10.1007/s00330-009-1568-2.
39. Li W, Davlouros PA, Kilner PJ, Pennell DJ, Gibson D, Henein MY, et al. Doppler-echocardiographic assessment of pulmonary regurgitation in adults with repaired tetralogy of Fallot: comparison with cardiovascular magnetic resonance imaging. Am Heart J. 2004;147:165–72.
40. Chatzimavroudis GP, Walker PG, Oshinski JN, Franch RH, Pettigrew RI, Yoganathan AP. Slice loca-

tion dependence of aortic regurgitation measurements with MR phase velocity mapping. Magn Reson Med. 1997;37:545–51.
41. Sebastian K, Juerg Schwitter E. Aortic and mitral regurgitation: quantification using moving slice velocity mapping. J Magn Reson Imaging. 2001;14:106–12.
42. Hundley WG, Li HF, Willard JE, Landau C, Lange RA, Meshack BM, et al. Magnetic resonance imaging assessment of the severity of mitral regurgitation. Comparison with invasive techniques. Circulation. 1995;92:1151–8.
43. Hundley WG, Li HF, Lange RA, Pfeifer DP, Meshack BM, Willard JE, et al. Assessment of left-to-right intracardiac shunting by velocity-encoded, phase-difference magnetic resonance imaging. A comparison with oximetric and indicator dilution techniques. Circulation. 1995;91:2955–60.
44. Thomson LEJ, Crowley AL, Heitner JF, Cawley PJ, Weinsaft JW, Kim HW, et al. Direct en face imaging of secundum atrial septal defects by velocity-encoded cardiovascular magnetic resonance in patients evaluated for possible transcatheter closure. Circ Cardiovasc Imaging. 2008;1:31–40.
45. Steffens JC, Bourne MW, Sakuma H, et al. Quantitation of collateral blood flow in coarctation of the aorta by velocity encoded cine magnetic resonance imaging. Circulation. 1994;90:937–43.
46. Roman KS, Kellenberger CJ, Farooq S, MacGowan CK, Gilday DL, Yoo SJ. Comparative imaging of differential pulmonary blood flow in patients with congenital heart disease: magnetic resonance imaging versus lung perfusion scintigraphy. Pediatr Radiol. 2005;35:295–301.
47. Fratz S, Hess J, Schwaiger M, Martinoff S, Stern HC. More accurate quantification of pulmonary blood flow by magnetic resonance imaging than by lung perfusion scintigraphy in patients with fontan circulation. Circulation. 2002;106:1510–3.
48. Rathi VK, Doyle M, Yamrozik J, et al. Routine evaluation of left ventricular diastolic function by cardiovascular magnetic resonance: a practical approach. J Cardiovasc Magn Reson. 2008;10:36.
49. Paelinck BP, de Roos A, Bax JJ, et al. Feasibility of tissue magnetic resonance imaging: a pilot study in comparison with tissue Doppler imaging and invasive measurement. J Am Coll Cardiol. 2005;45(7):1109–16.
50. Mohiaddin RH, Gatehouse PD, Henien M, Firmin DN. Cine MR Fourier velocimetry of blood flow through cardiac valves: comparison with Doppler echocardiography. J Magn Reson Imaging. 1997;7(4):657–63.
51. Sanz J, Kuschnir P, Rius T, Salguero R, Sulica R, Einstein AJ, Dellegrottaglie S, Fuster V, Rajagopalan S, Poon M. Pulmonary Arterial Hypertension: Noninvasive Detection with Phase-Contrast MR Imaging. Radiology. 2007;243:70–9.
52. Kondo C, Caputo GR, Masui T, et al. Pulmonary hypertension: pulmonary flow quantification and flow profile analysis with velocity-encoded cine MR imaging. Radiology. 1992;183:751–8.
53. Nagendran J, Michelakis E. MRI: one-stop shop for the comprehensive assessment of pulmonary arterial hypertension? Chest. 2007;132:2–5.
54. Hjortdal VE, Emmertsen K, Stenbog E, Frund T, Schmidt MR, Kromann O, Sorensen K, Pedersen EM. Effects of exercise and respiration on blood flow in total cavopulmonary connection: a real-time magnetic resonance flow study. Circulation. 2003;108:1227–31.
55. Korperich H, Gieseke J, Barth P, Hoogeveen R, Esdorn H, Peterschroder A, Meyer H, Beerbaum P. Flow volume and shunt quantification in pediatric congenital heart disease by real-time magnetic resonance velocity mapping: a validation study. Circulation. 2004;109:1987–93.
56. Nagel E, Thouet T, Klein C, Schalla S, Bornstedt A, Schnackenburg B, et al. Noninvasive determination of coronary blood flow velocity with cardiovascular magnetic resonance in patients after stent deployment. Circulation. 2003;107:1738–43.
57. Hundley WG, Hamilton CA, Clarke GD, Hillis LD, Herrington DM, Lange RA, et al. Visualization and functional assessment of proximal and middle left anterior descending coronary stenoses in humans with magnetic resonance imaging. Circulation. 1999;99:3248–54.
58. Wigström L, Sjöqvist L, Wranne B. Temporally resolved 3D phase-contrast imaging. Magn Reson Med. 1996;36:800–3.
59. Markl M, Kilner PJ, Ebbers T. Comprehensive 4D velocity mapping of the heart and great vessels by cardiovascular magnetic resonance. J Cardiovasc Magn Reson. 2011;13:7.
60. Whitehead KK, Sundareswaran KS, Parks WJ, Harris MA, Yoganathan AP, Fogel MA. Blood flow distribution in a large series of patients having the Fontan operation: a cardiac magnetic resonance velocity mapping study. J Thorac Cardiovasc Surg. 2009;138:96–102.

Imaging of Pulmonary Hypertension in Congenital Heart Disease

21

Onkar B. Auti, Ashirwad Pasumarthy, and Vimal Raj

Pulmonary hypertension (PH) is characterized by raised pulmonary artery pressures caused by numerous etiologies and interplay of complex pathological mechanisms. Congenital heart disease (CHD) is the predominant cause of childhood pulmonary hypertension and is seen in a plethora of congenital conditions. Neglected or undiagnosed CHD is an important cause of PH in adults. Although the invasive procedure of right heart catheterization is the gold standard for the diagnosis, multiple noninvasive imaging techniques play a major role in the detection of PH and the underlying cause.

Electronic Supplementary Material The online version of this chapter (https://doi.org/10.1007/978-981-15-6755-1_21) contains supplementary material, which is available to authorized users.

O. B. Auti
Ruby Hall Clinic, Pune, Maharashtra, India

A. Pasumarthy
AIG Hospitals, Hyderabad, Telangana, India

V. Raj (✉)
Department of Cardiothoracic Imaging, Narayana Hrudayalaya, Bangalore, Karnataka, India

21.1 What Is Pulmonary Hypertension?

Since first World Symposium on Pulmonary Hypertension (WSPH) in 1973 till fifth WSPH in 2013, PH has been defined as mean pulmonary artery pressure (mPAP) ≥ 25 mmHg at rest, measured by right heart catheterization [1–3]. However, recent data suggest that normal subjects showed normal mPAP of 14.0 ± 3.3 mmHg [4]. So mean value > 20 mmHg (above the 97.5th percentile) is abnormal. However only abnormal mPAP value is insufficient to define pulmonary vascular resistance. Therefore, sixth WSPH Task Force first revisited the definition of PH, suggesting a new pressure level to define an abnormal elevation in the mPAP > 20 mmHg and the need for PVR ≥ 3 WU to define the presence of precapillary PH [5, 6].

21.2 Classification of PH

Second WSPH in 1998 divided the different categories of PH sharing similar pathological findings, hemodynamic characteristics, and management [2]. Sixth WSPH Task Force also made some modifications in PH classification where it is divided into five main groups (Table 21.1) according to their common pathophysiology. [5, 6]

R. Rajeshkannan et al. (eds.), *CT and MRI in Congenital Heart Diseases*,
https://doi.org/10.1007/978-981-15-6755-1_21

Table 21.1 Updated clinical classification of PH

Updated classification of pulmonary hypertension
1. Pulmonary arterial hypertension • Idiopathic PAH and heritable PAH • Associated with portal hypertension, connective tissue disorders, HIV • Associated with congenital heart diseases and schistosomiasis • PAH long-term responders to calcium channel blockers • PAH with features of pulmonary veno-occlusive disease (PVOD) and/or pulmonary capillary hemangiomatosis (PCH) • Persistent pulmonary hypertension of the newborn (PPHN)
2. Pulmonary hypertension due to left heart disease
3. Pulmonary hypertension due to lung diseases and/or hypoxia • Chronic obstructive pulmonary disease • Interstitial lung disease • High altitude
4. Chronic thromboembolic pulmonary hypertension (CTEPH)
5. Pulmonary hypertension with unclear multifactorial mechanisms • Hematologic disorders • Systemic and metabolic disorders • Complex congenital heart disease (CHD)

Group 1 is referred to as pulmonary arterial hypertension (PAH). PAH is defined by a mean pulmonary arterial pressure of > 20 mmHg at rest in the presence of normal pulmonary capillary wedge pressure ($\leq$15 mm of Hg) and increased pulmonary vascular resistance $\geq$ 3 wood units [7].

PAH was further classified into primary (idiopathic) and secondary PAH. Idiopathic PAH remains a diagnosis of exclusion in the absence of other etiological factors. Secondary PAH is further divided into PAH due to congenital heart diseases (CHD) and PAH associated with portal hypertension, connective tissue disorders, or HIV.

The scope of this chapter is limited to the PAH associated with congenital heart disease; therefore, PH associated with other groups is not discussed further.

CHD is further classified clinically into four major groups according to their physiology (Table 21.2).

Table 21.2 Updated clinical classification of PAH associated with Congenital heart disease

Updated clinical classification of PAH associated with CHD	
1. Eisenmenger syndrome	
2. Left-to-right shunts	
– Correctable	– Non-correctable
3. Pulmonary arterial hypertension (PAH) with coincidental congenital heart disease	
4. Postoperative PAH	

- Group 1 includes any intra- or extracardiac systemic to pulmonary shunt, which over a period of time increases pulmonary vascular resistance (PVR) with a reversal of flow through the shunt (Eisenmenger syndrome).
- Group 2 is moderate to large left-to-right shunt which causes PAH due to volume overload in which cyanosis is not a feature. Left-to-right shunt includes atrial septal defect (ASD), ventricular septal defect (VSD), patent ductus arteriosus (PDA), aorta-pulmonary (AP) window, total and partial anomalous pulmonary venous connection (TAPVC and PAPVC). Complex CHD includes complete atrioventricular defect (AVSD), truncus arterioles, single ventricular physiology with unobstructed pulmonary flow, and transposition of great arteries (TGA) with VSD.
- Group 3 comprises small cardiac defects, regarded as coincidental/idiopathic PAH. Marked elevation in PVR observed in these cases of small cardiac defects, which themselves do not account for the development of elevated PVR.
- Persistent postoperative PAH forms group 4 and has clinically poor prognosis.

21.3 Pathophysiology of PH

Pulmonary vascular bed is a low-pressure, low-resistance system in normal individuals. In patients with pulmonary hypertension, PAP and pulmonary vascular resistance (PVR) are elevated.

Diagram 21.1 Pathophysiology of pulmonary hypertension

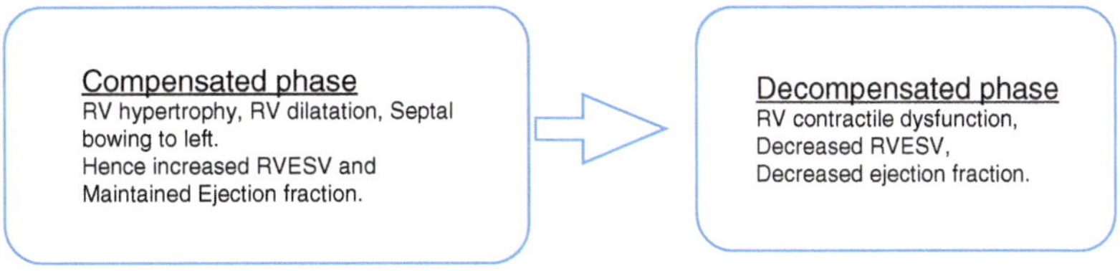

The clinical course of PH is divided into three phases: asymptomatic compensated, symptomatic decompensating, and advanced decompensated.

Right ventricle (RV) is a crescent-shaped thin-walled cavity which pumps blood into pulmonary circulation [8]. RV hypertrophy, RV dilatation, and right atrial enlargement are seen in PH [9].

As PAP increases, there is compensatory hypertrophy of the RV wall with an increase in size to accommodate more blood and in turn increase in end-diastolic volume (EDV). These initial changes are compensatory mechanisms that allow the right ventricle to produce a larger stroke volume and maintain cardiac output. In the advanced decompensated phase, there is RV and RA dilatation with a decrease in ejection fraction. RV changes its shape from crescent to spherical which has a greater cross-sectional area compared to the left ventricle (LV). This results in abnormal septal motion to the left side that impairs LV function [10, 11]. Eventually, the demand for RV for oxygen exceeds the available supply, causing chamber dilatation that leads to tricuspid regurgitation. These processes eventually result in decreased cardiac output and right-sided heart failure. The ability of RV to sustain with pressure and volume overload is the principle determinant of patients' survival and functional capacity [12, 13]. Therefore, morphologic and functional assessment of RV is of utmost importance in the management of PH (Diagram 21.1).

21.4 Pathophysiology of PAH in CHD

In left-to-right shunt, there is a progressive increase in PAP due to an increase in pulmonary blood flow which results in an increase in pressure in the pulmonary arteries leading to abnormal shear stress, circumferential wall stretch, and endothelial dysfunction. Altered expression of vasoactive mediators, such as endothelin-1, prostacyclin, and nitric oxide, results in vasoconstriction, while aberrant expression of vascular endothelial and fibroblast growth factors promotes vascular remodeling (including smooth muscle hypertrophy and proliferation) and increased intracellular matrix deposition [14]. These changes will increase PVR and increase RV and RA pressure. If the pressure in right side of the heart exceeds left heart pressure, then the shunt reverses its direction from left to right which results in cyanosis. This is known as Eisenmenger's syndrome. Interestingly, the development of right-to-left shunt decreases RV pressure and preserves RV ejection fraction, however at the cost of cyanosis and associated complications [15, 16].

Early changes in pulmonary beds are reversible if the heart defect is surgically repaired. Patients with left-to-right shunts usually have normal pulmonary vascular resistance in early age [17]. When surgery is done in later childhood, PVR may fall after the surgery but normal levels not necessarily achieved. And corrective surgery in patients with established PAH may accentuate disease progression and RV failure. This suggests the irreversible nature of PAH where corrective surgery further worsens the outcome [18]. Therefore, the timing of corrective surgery early in life is important.

The development of PAH is much earlier and more frequent in shunts distal to tricuspid valve (post-tricuspid) than shunts proximal to tricuspid valve (pre-tricuspid) as pre-tricuspid shunt causes volume overload whereas post-tricuspid shunt causes volume and pressure overload. Hence, VSDs require early surgical repair compared to ASD and PAPVC [19].

21.5 Prevalence of PAH in CHD

The prevalence of PAH in CHD has fallen in recent years and the number of patients surviving into adulthood has increased markedly due to an increase in detection of underlying causes and prompt cardiac repair [20].

Presently, the majority of PAH in CHD patients seen in clinical practice are adults with neglected heart defects, postoperative residual defects, and inoperable complex CHD [20].

Prevalence PAH in CHD is rare with estimated prevalence of 1.6 to 12.5 cases per million adults. This has a large impact on mortality and morbidity leading to increasing requirements for lifelong care [19].

21.6 Cross-Sectional Imaging

Cross-sectional imaging including CT and MRI play a crucial role in diagnosis of PAH and more importantly identifying the underlying etiology for PAH [21]. Cardiac CT and MRI are useful in the diagnosis and act as complementary modality to echocardiography for diagnosis and management of children with PAH.

21.6.1 CT Protocols

CT protocols primarily depend on the type of scanner (speed of rotation and the width of coverage by the detectors) and the availability of power injectors. The principal aim of CT is to achieve optimal enhancement of right heart chambers and pulmonary arteries. Peripheral intravenous access can be difficult in the pediatric age group. Catheter selection is dependent on the age of the patient and the availability of peripheral venous access. Usually, catheter ≥ 22G can be used in children older than 5 years while catheter < 22G can be used in children younger than 5 years. The rate of dose injection varies according to the size of the IV catheter. Flow rate of 1 ml/s can be used for 24G catheter while 1.5–2.5 ml/s for 22G catheter, 2–4 ml/s for 20G catheter, and 3–5 ml/s for 18–16G catheter are recommended [22]. Dose of contrast is 1–1.5 ml/kg of patient weight followed by saline chase. A bolus-tracking technique is used with the region of interest set in the main pulmonary artery (MPA) and triggering of scan acquisition at a predefined threshold of 150 HU. However, in some cases with severe cardiac dysfunction, hemodilution states in congenital heart disease, the time delay between the threshold being achieved and the scan starting may be different. In such cases, a test bolus technique may be preferred.

21.6.2 MRI Protocols

MRI protocols for assessment of PAH are recommended on 1.5/3 tesla MRI scanner. Four electrode ECG gating is used. Balanced Steady-State Free Precession (bSSFP) stack cine images are taken of uniform thickness without any gaps in at least two planes and in short axis to quantify ventricular function. Phase-contrast imaging is obtained in through-plane in aorta, MPA, RPA, and LPA. Dynamic contrast MR angiography is also obtained using cardiac gating with respiratory compensation.

21.7 Diagnosis and Detection of PAH

21.7.1 CT Assessment

MDCT parameters often used to diagnose PAH is the maximum diameter of the main pulmonary artery (MPA). A diameter > 29 mm is considered as suggestive of PAH in adults [7, 23]. However, this threshold is not very specific, especially in patients with advanced interstitial lung disease (ILD) where dilatation of the pulmonary artery is common due to traction. Threshold of 32 mm is found to be more specific in ILD in adults [24]. Also, normal MPA dimensions cannot exclude the diagnosis of PAH [24].

MPA diameter: ascending aorta diameter ratio is also useful in determining the presence of PAH. MPA diameter should not be greater than ascending aorta diameter in normal circumstances. MPA: aorta ratio of >1 suggests underlying PAH [25]. Segmental pulmonary artery to bronchus ratio of >1:1 in three out of four lobes along with dilated MPV has almost 100% specificity for PAH [26]. Levels at which MPA and aorta to be measured are mentioned in Table 21.3 and depicted Fig. 21.1.

Other features suggestive of PAH are enlargement of the segmental pulmonary arteries greater than 1.25 times the caliber of the adjacent bronchus. Abrupt narrowing or tapering of peripheral pulmonary vessels, right ventricular hypertrophy, right ventricular and atrial enlargement, prominent bronchial artery (greater than 1.5 mm) and reflux of contrast into hepatic veins are other supporting evidence for PAH [24, 27].

A combination of multiple positive findings increases the diagnostic confidence. Combination of segmental artery enlargement and MPA dilatation (>29 mm) has been estimated as 100% specific for the diagnosis of PAH in adults [25].

Egg and banana sign [28] is a specific sign for severe pulmonary hypertension where the pulmonary artery is enlarged to the extent it reaches up to the aortic arch. It is identified by the presence of the pulmonary artery lateral to the aortic arch with the aortic arch being described as the banana and the pulmonary artery as the egg (Fig. 21.2).

Cardiac findings are due to constant raised outflow pressures and subsequent failure. In PAH, RV is dilated with RV:LV ratio of >1 in the axial plane, and RV wall shows hypertrophy (Fig. 21.3). A strong correlation exists between

Table 21.3 Various measurements taken in both CT and MRI

Measurements	
Diameter of MPA	Level of pulmonary bifurcation (Fig. 21.1a)
Diameter of ascending aorta	Level of right PA in axial plane (Fig. 21.1b)
Diameters of right and left PA	Just before branching of lobar arteries
RV measurement	Maximum transverse cavity diameter at the level of tricuspid valve (Fig. 21.3a)
LV measurement	Maximum transverse cavity diameter at the level of mitral valve (Fig. 21.3b)

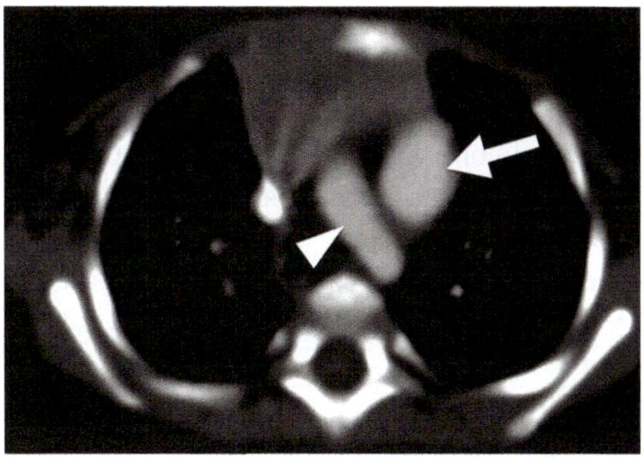

Fig. 21.2 Axial CT images at the level of aortic arch depicting Egg and Banana sign. Note the presence of pulmonary artery (block arrow) lateral to the aortic arch (arrowhead) which is a sign of severe PAH

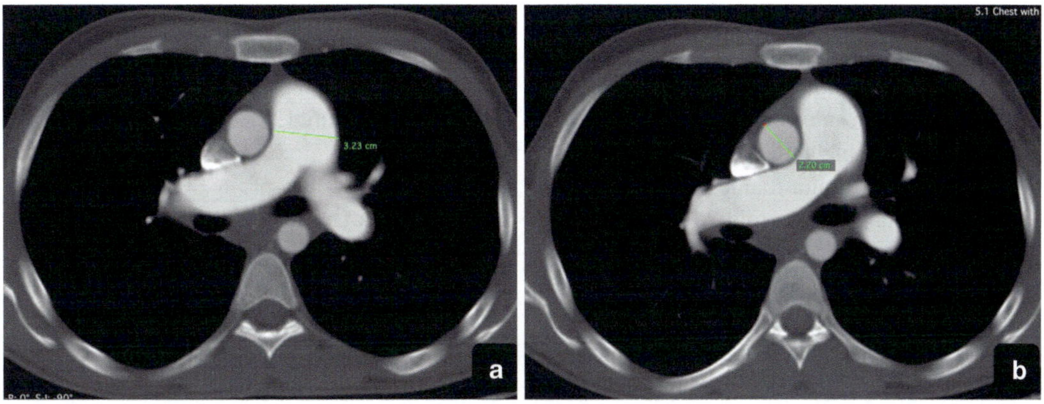

Fig.21.1 Axial CT images at the level of MPA bifurcation showing measurement of MPA (**a**). (**b**) shows an axial CT image at the level of the right pulmonary artery depicting the measurement of ascending aorta. MPA: aorta ratio is more than 1

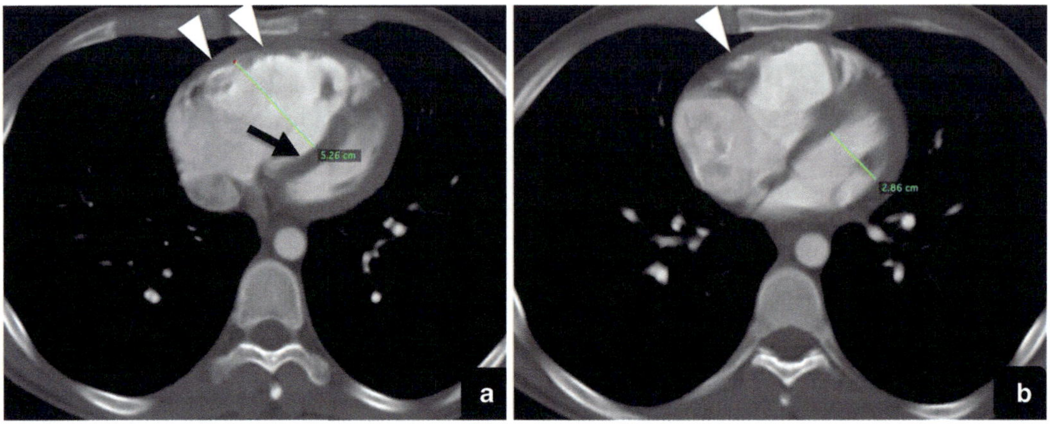

Fig. 21.3 Axial CT images at the level of the tricuspid valve (**a**) and mitral valve (**b**) showing measurements of RV and LV cavity, respectively. RV:LV ratio is more than 1. Note RV hypertrophy (arrowheads) and leftward septal bowing (black arrow)

septal bowing and systolic PAP > 67mm of Hg [29]. Increased septal angle also correlates with raised pulmonary vascular resistance [30]. Other cardiac predictors are RV wall thickness > 6mm, RV/LV wall ratio > 0.32, RV/LV lumen ratio > 1.28, dilatation and reflux of contrast into IVC [31].

21.7.2 MRI Assessment

MRI has advantages of good spatial and temporal resolution, multiplanar imaging capabilities and in addition to CT has better tissue characterization. MRI is useful for diagnosis, establishing etiology, quantification, prognosis, and treatment follow-up.

MRI follows similar anatomical diagnostic criteria as CT scan and shows dilated central pulmonary arteries which are best evaluated in cine SSFP images maximum diameter of great arteries can be calculated in systole. MPA diameter of >29 mm in adults and ratio of MPA:ascending aortic diameter > 1 is used for diagnosis of PAH.

An indirect marker of increased pulmonary arterial pressure (PAP) >70 mm of Hg and high pulmonary vascular resistance (PVR) is the presence of intraluminal hyperintensity on black blood images which is due to slow flow artifact. Presence of turbulent flow artifact in the central pulmonary artery is a qualitative indicator of elevated mPAP [31].

Secondary cardiac changes include RV dilatation and hypertrophy diagnosed by RV: LV ratio of >0.6 and RV wall thickness > 4 mm, respectively [32, 33].

Late gadolinium enhancement is noted at RV insertion sites due to pressure overload indicates mechanical strain. Corresponding elevated T1 values are seen at these sites in T1 mapping sequences. With the time-resolved MR angiography, increased pulmonary transit time is also noted. On functional images, there is increased RV mass, decreased RV function (<35%) which indicates RV failure [31]. On time-resolved three-dimensional phase-contrast imaging prolonged vortical flow in main pulmonary artery indicates RV failure [34].

21.8 Functional Assessment

Several noninvasive parameters are available to reflect the hemodynamics of the pulmonary arterial system which show varying degree of collation with values obtained from right heart catheterization (RHC). Various sequences can be used to assess the ventricular function.

21.8.1 Cine Imaging

MRI is the gold standard for ventricular volume quantification and ejection fraction. While echocardiography has a limited role in the evaluation of RV especially its volumes and function due to its complex shape, MRI is the gold standard in such conditions.

Calculating the RV end-diastolic volume (RVEDV), RV end-systolic volume (RVESV), and RV ejection fraction (RVEF) are key parameters in diagnosing RV failure and severity of PAH. Volume assessment is also important in the follow-up of patients with PAH in monitoring treatment efficacy. Progressive increase in RVEDV and RVESV with decrease in RVEF are strong independent predictors of mortality and treatment failure [18, 35–38].

Various MRI parameters including a decrease in the RV mass, a decrease in RV end-systolic and end-diastolic volumes, and an increase in ejection fraction indicate a good response to therapy.

MRI is also used as a tool for prognostic and risk stratification. The volume of late gadolinium enhancement correlates positively with the RV mass, RV volume, RV dysfunction, and amount of remodeling in the RV wall [31].

Systolic flattening or left-sided bowing of the septum can be very well observed on SSFP images due to high myocardium to blood contrast ratio. The presence of flattering or leftward septal bowing is indicative of PAH. A strong correlation exists with the measurement of the paradoxical curvature of the septum with the severity of PAH. As a result, LV becomes D-shaped and RV becomes progressively concentric [39]. The curvature and bowing of the ventricular septum shows a strong correlation between RV–LV pressure gradient and shows a linear comparison with RV systolic pressure in RHC [40, 41].

21.8.2 Phase-Contrast Imaging

Phase-contrast imaging also known as Q flow imaging is an MRI sequence that detects blood flow and velocity in any vessel. On phase-contrast imaging, low velocity in MPA (<11.7 cm/s) and early retrograde flow are suggestive of PAH [42]. Decreased cardiac output in phase-contrast MRI is an independent adverse prognostic factors. Also, a negative correlation between average velocity in MPA and PAP is noted [42]. Presence of slow flow in the main pulmonary artery correlates with poor prognosis [36]. Elevated PA stiffness results in greater RV afterload.

Pulmonary arterial PC MRI shows a characteristic flow pattern in patients with pulmonary hypertension. This includes an early systolic peak with decreased peak systolic velocity, a rapid deceleration with multiple peaks at late systolic phase, a pronounced flow reversal in early diastole, and irregular oscillations of flow throughout diastole. The average velocity of pulmonary arterial flow measured by PC MRI is the most useful single parameter in the assessment of pulmonary hypertension [43, 44]. Changes in pulmonary arterial flow pattern after administration of pulmonary vasodilators like 100% oxygen or nitric oxide can be useful in assessing the reversible pulmonary vascular resistance [45].

21.8.3 Other Functional Parameters

Other functional parameters include a decrease in the rate of change of area in the pulmonary artery, increased Vmax, increased time to Vmax, increased shear range index, increased trans pulmonary gradient, myocardial tissue velocity, left atrial volume and flow.

PA stiffness can be measured noninvasively using phase-contrast and cine imaging on CMR. Changes in proximal PA stiffness are especially relevant to the progression of PH, as PA stiffness is a good predictor of mortality from right ventricular failure [46–49]. Maximum and minimum PA areas and velocity profiles were measured from cross-sectional CMR images such that PA stiffness indices including pulsatility, distensibility, compliance, and elastic modulus can be calculated [46–49]. Phase-contrast images are acquired through cross-section plane of MPA before bifurcation using the biplane method (Fig. 21.4a, b). Phase-contrast image

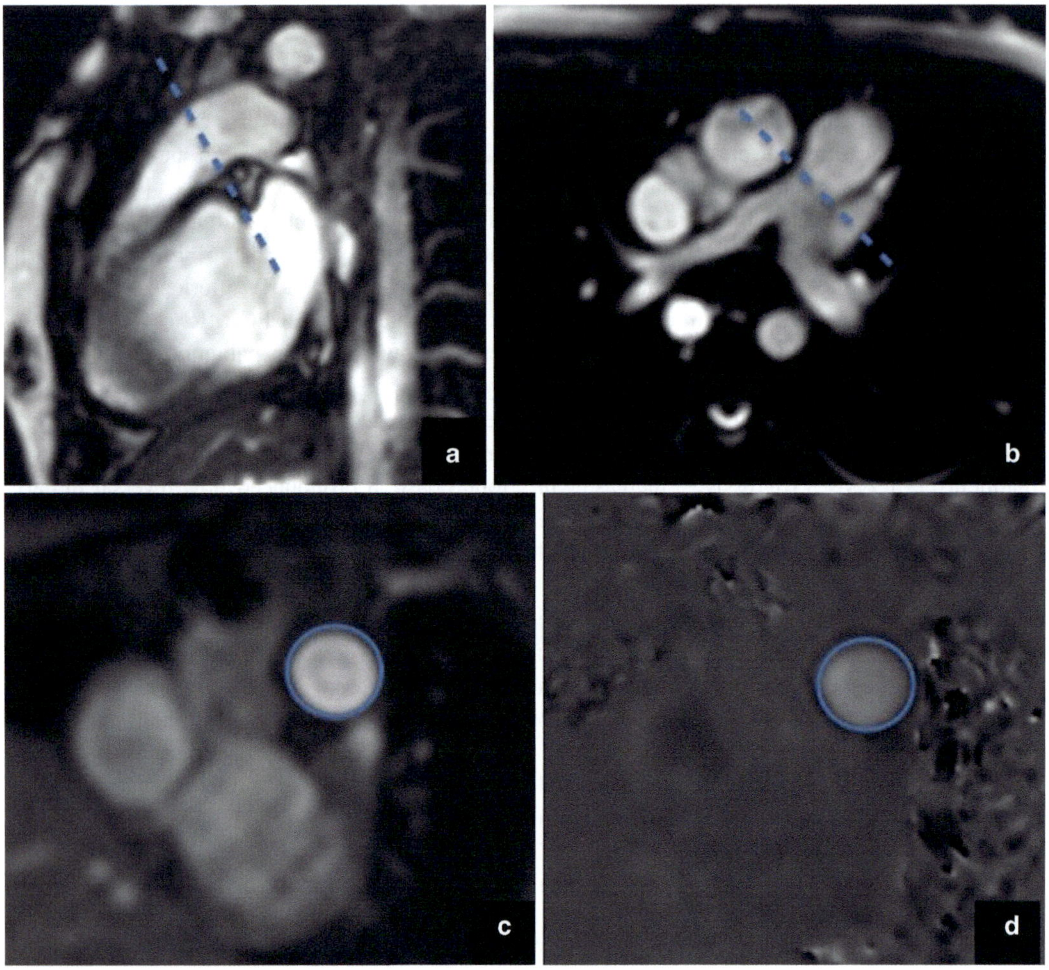

Fig. 21.4 Sagittal SSFP image passing through the long axis of MPA (**a**) and axial CMR images showing the main pulmonary artery with bifurcation (**b**). Dashed line denotes imaging planes for through-plane phase-contrast imaging for MPA. Magnitude image (**c**) and phase image (**d**) of MPA. Circle denotes the region of interest (ROI) for the calculation of PA stiffness indices

appears in magnitude and phase images (Fig. 21.4c, d). Further information like maximum and minimum area of MPA during the cardiac cycle, maximum and minimum velocities, and pressures through MPA can be calculated. PA stiffness assessment by CMR seems to be promising in terms of early identification of pulmonary vascular disease, which may result in earlier diagnosis and treatment.

Attempts to calculate PVR using CMR has also been done and compared with right heart catheterization (RHC) data. Using CMR, PVR can be estimated in WU as 19.38—[4.62 × Ln PA average velocity (in cm/s)] − [0.08 × RVEF (in %)] [50]. Another method to calculate PVR using CMR-derived measurements, and is defined as: (CMR predicted mPAP − CMR predicted PCWP)/CMR phase-contrast CO. CMR predicted PCWP and CO were estimated by left atrial volumetry and pulmonary arterial phase-contrast imaging, respectively. CMR-predicted mPAP = −4.6 + (interventricular septal angle × 0.23) + (ventricular mass index × 16.3). Interventricular septal angle was measured by determining the angle between the mid-point of the interventricular septum and the two hinge points [51]. Noninvasive assessment of PVR using CMR techniques can be as accurate as compared to RHC data and it is a very promising tool in early PH diagnosis, treatment, and follow-up [42, 49–53].

Distensibility of the pulmonary artery, the difference between the cross-sectional area between the end-diastolic and end-systole, of more than 10% indicates a good response to vasodilators therapy [54].

21.9 Role of CT/MRI in PAH Associated with CHD

In the management of PAH related to CHD, identification of the cause is utmost necessary. MRI shows 72% sensitivity and 84% specificity in pediatric pulmonary hypertension when pulmonary artery diameter ≥ 25 mm [55]. CT is very useful in the detection of underlying cause. ASD, VSD, PDA, AP window can be efficiently diagnosed on CT. Figure 21.5 shows CT images of the atrial septal defect with various findings of PAH. VSD and PDA are depicted in Fig. 21.6 as separate cases.

It has shown greater efficacy in detecting sinus venous defects, PAPVC and TAPVC which are difficult to be evaluated on echocardiography [56]. CT is an excellent modality in detecting intra- and extracardiac shunts with greater anatomical detail due to its high spatial resolution, multiplanar and 3D reconstructions as depicted in Fig. 21.7.

CT is also helpful in preoperative evaluation of congenital heart diseases to look for the size of the defect, relations of great arteries, the status of coronary arteries, and atrial and ventricle connections.

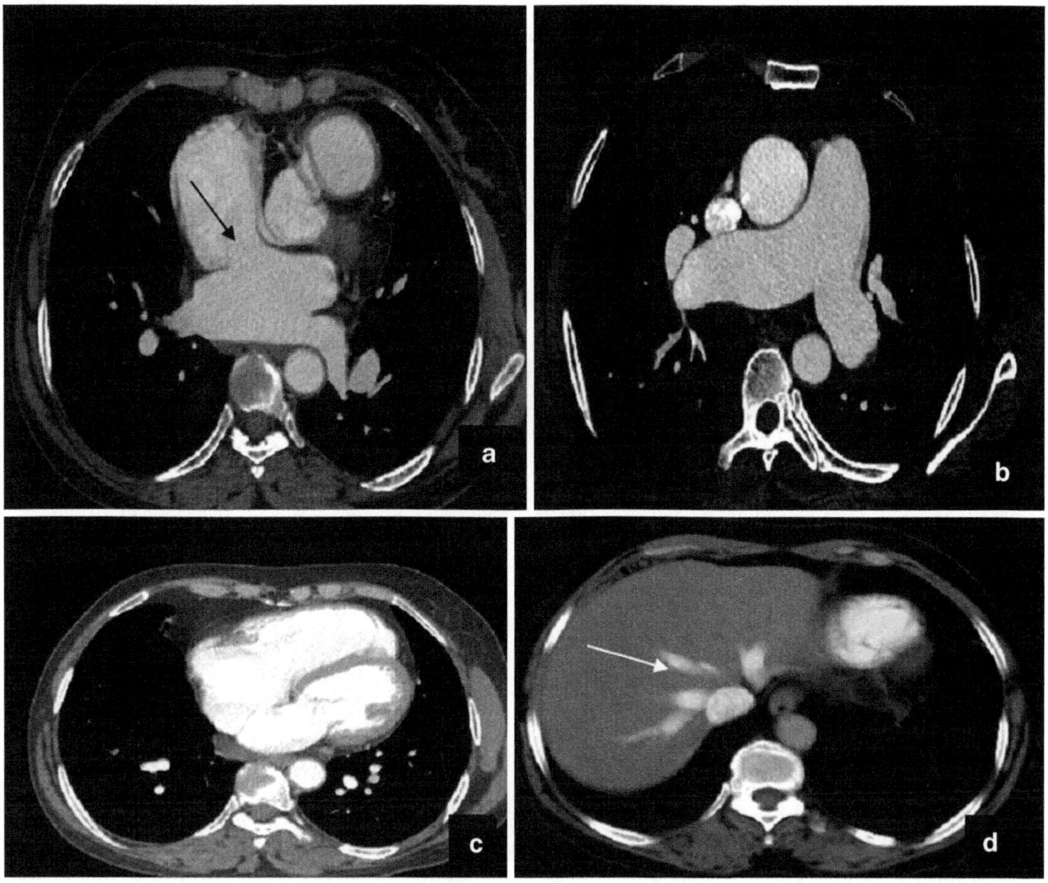

Fig. 21.5 Axial CT images (**a**) showing a large atrial septal defect (black arrow). Features of PAH are seen as dilatation of main and branch pulmonary arteries (**b**), dilated right heart chambers (**c**), and reflux of contrast into hepatic veins (white arrow) (**d**) suggesting tricuspid regurgitation

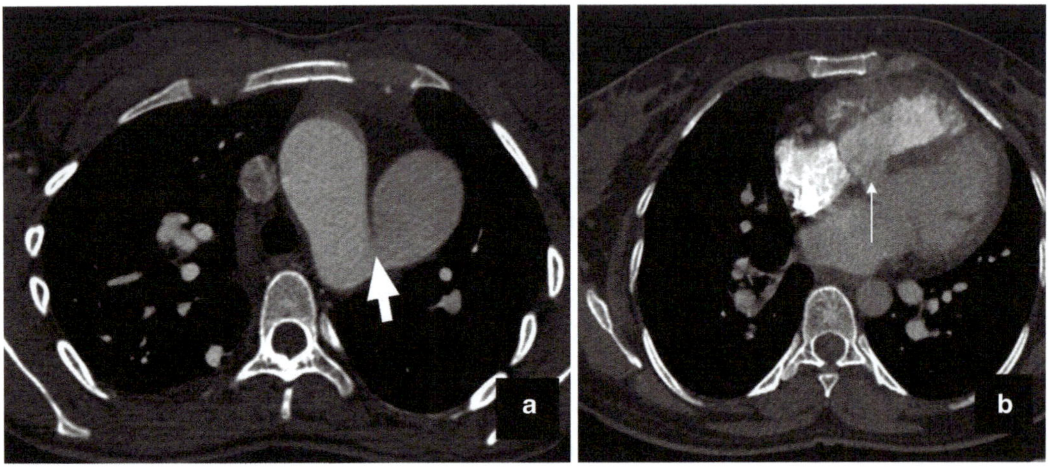

Fig. 21.6 Axial CT image showing large and short PDA (block arrow) communicating aorta and MPA (**a**). Separate CT case demonstrating subaortic VSD (thin white arrow) with overriding of the aorta (**b**)

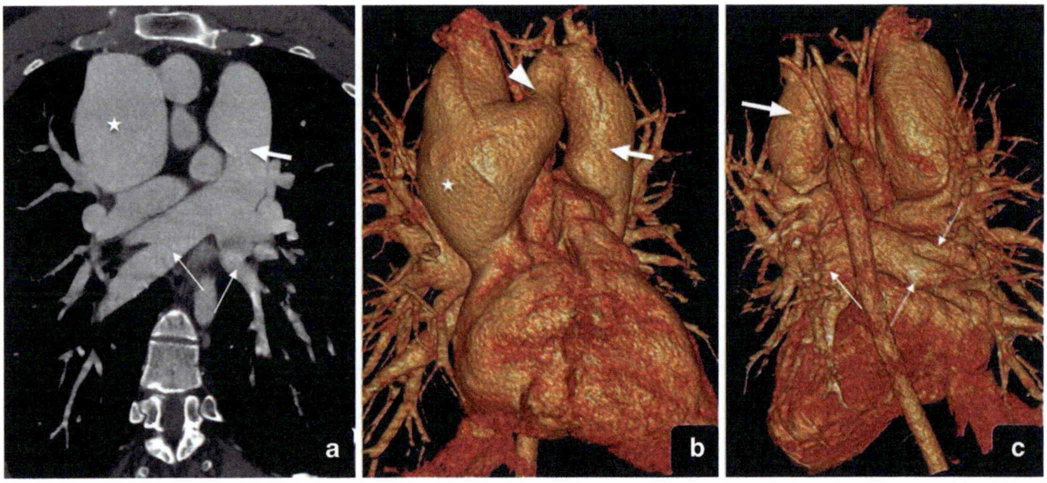

Fig. 21.7 Reconstructed CT image (**a**) and 3D reconstructions (**b** and **c**) showing all pulmonary veins (arrows) joining together to form ascending vertical vein (block arrow) which further drains into an innominate vein (arrowhead) and further into superior vena cava (star). Features are suggestive of supracardiac type of total anomalous pulmonary venous connection (TAPVC)

Both CT and MRI provide greater anatomical details in complex CHDs like transposition of great arteries (TGA), truncus arteriosus, single ventricular physiology, and large AVSD which are important in the decision of surgical correction or palliation.

Abernathy syndrome is a rare vascular malformation known as congenital extrahepatic portosystemic shunt wherein, the portal venous system drains directly into systemic vein bypassing the liver completely or partially. Abernathy malformation is a rare cause of PAH [57]. So, it is important to include the upper abdomen covering the entire portal venous system in the venous phase of CT in every patient who undergoes imaging.

MRI is better than CT in determining the routability of aorta/MPA to ventricles due to high myocardial to blood contrast ratio of SSFP images and multiplanar imaging. It is crucial in

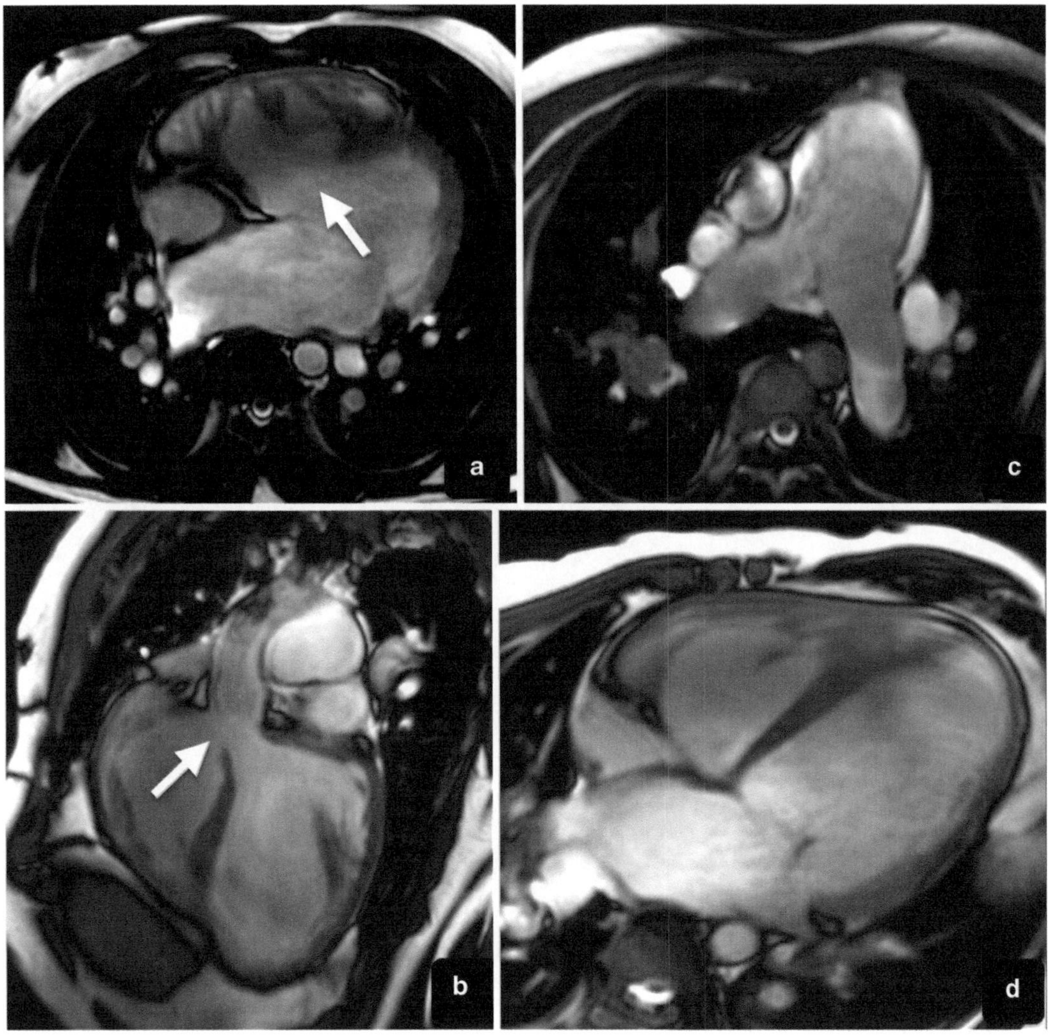

Fig. 21.8 SSFP images show subaortic VSD (arrows) in the axial plane (**a**) and in LVOT view (**b**). LVOT view also demonstrates the feasible routability of aorta to LV. Changes of PAH can be seen as dilated main and branch pulmonary arteries (**c**) and dilatation of RV and LV (**d**)

preoperative assessment in complex CHD (Fig. 21.8).

MRI is helpful in anatomical as well as functional assessment of congenital heart diseases. Anatomical details are better visualized in SSFP images in multiple planes. Phase-contrast imaging is an MRI sequence that detects blood flow and velocity of any vessel. It is the most useful modality in detecting pulmonary blood flow (*Q*p) and systemic blood flow (*Q*s), thereby calculating pulmonary to systemic flow ratio (*Q*p/*Q*s). In the absence of any shunt, *Q*p:*Q*s ratio is equal to 1. If the ratio is more than 1, it indicates the left-to-right shunt and ratio of less than 1 indicates the right-to-left shunt [31]. *Q*p:*Q*s ratio of ≥1.7–2 is used for determining the need for surgical interventions [31, 58].

The pulmonary flow is measured at the level of the main pulmonary artery while the systemic flow is measured at the level of ascending aorta. Both these values are measured perpendicular to the plane of the respective levels. Alternatively, *Q*p can be determined by combined flow in the right and left pulmonary arteries or combined

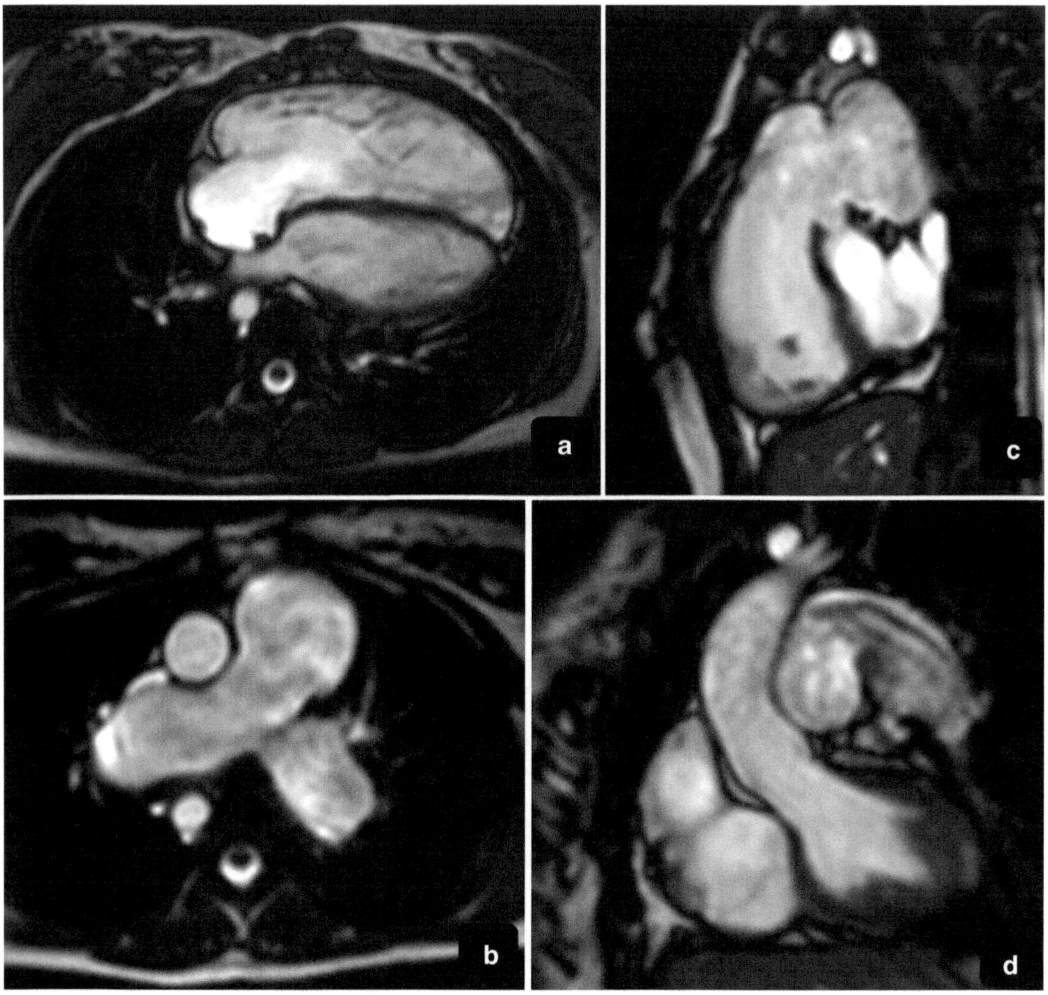

Fig. 21.9 Patient with intracardiac repair for tetralogy of Fallot has been followed up with cardiac MRI for assessment of RV function before pulmonary valve placement. There is an interval development of PAH in the form of dilated RV (**a**) and dilated main and branch pulmonary arteries (**b**). Dilated RVOT is noted with the absence of a pulmonary valve (**c**). VSD patch is noted in the LVOT view (**d**) with no residual VSD

flow in all pulmonary veins. Similarly, *Q*s can be calculated by adding flows of SVC and suprahepatic IVC or adding flows of descending thoracic aorta and SVC.

In postoperative cases, MRI is the most important investigation to follow up on the RV function and ejection fraction. Patients with TOF who underwent intracardiac repair are followed up with MRI and to look for signs of RV dysfunction and PAH for placement of pulmonary valve on appropriate time (Fig. 21.9).

In long-standing PH, due to primary left-to-right shunts, the pulmonary artery pressure eventually rises more than systemic pressure. This leads to a change in the direction of the shunt either from right to left or it becomes bidirectional, a condition called as Eisenmenger's syndrome (ES). Hemodynamically, ES is defined as an elevation of the pulmonary vascular resistance to 12 Wood units (WU) or to a pulmonary-to-systemic resistance ratio equal to or greater than 1.0 [59].

Shunts at the arterial level like PDA and aortopulmonary windows are prone to develop Eisenmenger phenomenon earlier in life as compared to ventricular level shunts and atrial level shunts. Below a certain size, the exact diameter of the defect plays an important role in the development of ES. The threshold is 2–3 cm at the atrial level, 1–1.5 cm at the ventricular level, and 0.5–0.7 cm at the arterial level [60]. ES can also develop postoperatively if communication between systemic and pulmonary circulation persists.

CT is useful in determining the size of defect particularly in shunts at arterial level. Patients with ES are prone to develop in situ thrombosis due to long-standing PAH. CT is an excellent modality to assess pulmonary vasculature which can show, in situ thrombosis in pulmonary arteries in the form of dilatation, eccentric thrombosis, and mural calcifications [61]. There may be devolvement of multiple aortopulmonary collaterals at hilar and intercostal levels.

MR is helpful in anatomic as well as functional assessment of shunts and their follow-up. Phase-contrast images help in the diagnosis of ES as *Q*p:*Q*s becomes equal to 1 (bidirectional shunt) or less than 1 (right to left shunt) [62].

In complex CHD with single ventricle physiology such as hypoplastic left heart syndrome or tricuspid atresia surgical correction with Glenn shunt and then Fontan completion is preferred. The pulmonary vasculature is exposed to nonpulsatile continuous flow from the upper and lower parts of the body. Survival of these patients improved since Fontan procedure was introduced [63, 64]. However, in the long term, there can be gradual attrition of Fontan circulation which results in Fontan circulation failure. PVR is a key factor in the pathogenesis of Fontan failure and even a mild increase in PVR causes a significant decrease in cardiac output [65–67]. CT provides information regarding the patency of Fontan shunt. MRI is more useful in the assessment of pulmonary flows in addition to the ventricular functional assessment. Total pulmonary flow and split flows into RPA and LPA can be calculated from phase-contrast imaging [68]. Using phase-contrast imaging, aortopulmonary collateral burden also can be calculated by calculating the difference between flow across ascending aorta and systemic venous flow. If the collateral burden is high, coiling the collaterals can improve outcomes [69]. Moreover, new techniques like ECG synchronized 3D flow mapping using 3D velocity encoding helps to visualize and assess global and local flows [70].

21.10 Newer Advances in MRI

T1 mapping values have been associated with indices of RV dysfunction [71]. RV T1 mapping is useful to detect diffuse myocardial pathology in RV dysfunction and is an important aspect of PAH prognosis.

Estimation of RV strain rate on cardiac MRI is developing modality in early detection of RV dysfunction. It is one of the important predictors of right heart failure and mortality [72].

21.11 Practical Tips

1. Consider all causes of pulmonary hypertension with reference to the classification of pulmonary hypertension.
2. During CT pulmonary angiography, test bolus technique is better than bolus tracking technique in complicated anatomy and physiology.
3. Consider the combination of multiple positive findings on CT and MRI to diagnose pulmonary hypertension.
4. Functional assessment with MRI can be used in risk stratification and prognosis of PH.
5. Pulmonary artery stiffness and pulmonary vascular resistance can be calculated using phase-contrast MRI images.
6. CT is excellent in the detection of the cause of PH and anatomical assessment in CHD while MRI is useful in functional assessment in CHD and assessing the prognosis of PH.

21.12 Summary

Various imaging techniques help us in diagnosing pulmonary hypertension in underlying congenital heart disease and understanding the underlying pathophysiology. They help in understanding the etiology, classifying the disease, treatment planning, prognosis, and finally in monitoring the treatment. Echocardiography is first-line investigation while CT/MRI play complementary role. CT is predominantly helpful to identify the etiology and anatomical details in CHD. Whereas MRI with its various robust imaging techniques acts as a single stop shop for anatomical information, functional assessment, preoperative assessment, and also postoperative follow-up of patients of CHD-PAH. MRI is becoming increasingly important and may become a standard of care in the near future. Noninvasive assessment of PA stiffness and PVR using CMR techniques are promising tools in early detection of PH, treatment, and follow-up.

Finally, the importance of structured reporting cannot be undermined in such conditions to reduce the incidence of errors, standardizing the reporting format, and encourages the use of lexicon in reporting. Disease-specific report templates can improve report clarity and quality.

Acknowledgment We thank Dr. Ramiah Rajeshkannan, Amrita Institute of Medical Sciences, Kochi, India, for providing Videos 21.4,21.5, 21.6, 21.7, 21.8, 21.9, 21.10, 21.11, 21.12, 21.13, 21.14, 21.15, 21.16, 21.17, 21.18, 21.19, 21.20, 21.21, 21.22.

References

1. Hatano S, Strasser T, editors. Primary pulmonary hypertension. Report on a WHO meeting. Geneva: World Health Organization; 1975.
2. Simonneau G, Galiè N, Rubin LJ, et al. Clinical classification of pulmonary hypertension. J Am Coll Cardiol. 2004;43(Suppl):5S–12S.
3. Simonneau G, Gatzoulis MA, Adatia I, Celermajer D, et al. Updated clinical classification of pulmonary hypertension. J Am Coll Cardiol. 2013;62(25 Suppl):D34–41. https://doi.org/10.1016/j.jacc.2013.10.029. Review. Erratum in: J Am Coll Cardiol. 2014;63(7):746.
4. Kovacs G, Berghold A, Scheidl S, et al. Pulmonary arterial pressure during rest and exercise in healthy subjects: a systematic review. Eur Respir J. 2009;34:888–94.
5. PHA. Hemodynamic definitions and updated classification—impact on clinical practice: a conversation with Erika Berman Rosenzweig and Nicholas Hill. Adv Pulm Hypertens. 2019;18(3):80–3.
6. Simonneau G, Montani D, Celermajer D, Denton C, Gatzoulis M, Krowka M, et al. Haemodynamic definitions and updated clinical classification of pulmonary hypertension. Eur Respir J. 2019;53(1):1801913.
7. Frazier AA, Galvin JR, Franks TJ, Rosado-de-Christenson ML. Pulmonary vasculature: hypertension and infarction. Radiographics. 2000;20(2):491–524.
8. Dell'Italia LJ, Santamore WP. Can indices of left ventricular function be applied to the right ventricle? Prog Cardiovasc Dis. 1998;40(4):309–24.
9. McGoon M, Gutterman D, Steen V, et al. Screening, early detection, and diagnosis of pulmonary arterial hypertension: ACCP evidence-based clinical practice guidelines. Chest. 2004;126(1 suppl):14S–34S.
10. Nauser TD, Stites SW. Diagnosis and treatment of pulmonary hypertension. Am Fam Physician. 2001;63(9):1789–98.
11. Bristow MR, Zisman LS, Lowes BD, et al. The pressure-overloaded right ventricle in pulmonary hypertension. Chest. 1998;114(1 suppl):101S–6S.
12. D'Alonzo GE, Barst RJ, Ayres SM, et al. Survival in patients with primary pulmonary hypertension: results from a national prospective registry. Ann Intern Med. 1991;115(5):343–9.
13. McLaughlin VV, Sitbon O, Badesch DB, et al. Survival with first-line bosentan in patients with primary pulmonary hypertension. Eur Respir J. 2005;25(2):244–9.
14. Adatia I, Kothari SS, Feinstein JA. Pulmonary hypertension associated with congenital heart disease: pulmonary vascular disease: the global perspective. Chest. 2010;137(Suppl 6):52S–61S.
15. Hopkins WE. The remarkable right ventricle of patients with Eisenmenger syndrome. Coron Artery Dis. 2005;16:19–25.
16. Hopkins WE, Waggoner AD. Severe pulmonary hypertension without right ventricular failure: the unique hearts of patients with Eisenmenger syndrome. Am J Cardiol. 2002;89:34–8.
17. Haworth SG. Pulmonary hypertension in the young. Heart. 2002;88:658–64.
18. Balint OH, Samman A, Haberer K, et al. Outcomes in patients with pulmonary hypertension undergoing percutaneous atrial septal defect closure. Heart. 2008;94:1189–93.
19. Galiè N, Manes A, Palazzini M, et al. Management of pulmonary arterial hypertension associated with congenital systemic-to-pulmonary shunts and Eisenmenger's syndrome. Drugs. 2008;68:1049–66.
20. D'Alto M, Mahadevan V. Pulmonary arterial hypertension associated with congenital heart disease. Eur Respir Rev. 2012;21(126):328–37.
21. Devaraj A, Hansell DM. Computed tomography signs of pulmonary hypertension: old and new observations. ClinRadiol. 2009;64:751–60.
22. Tang C, Schoepf U, Chowdhury S, Fox M, Zhang L, Lu G. Multidetector computed tomography pulmonary angiography in childhood acute pulmonary embolism. Pediatr Radiol. 2015;45(10):1431–9.

23. Peña E, Dennie C, Veinot J, Muñiz SH. Pulmonary hypertension: how the radiologist can help. Radiographics. 2012;32:9–32.
24. Alhamad EH, Al-Boukai AA, Al-Kassimi FA, Alfaleh HF, Alshamiri MQ, Alzeer AH, Al-Otair HA, Ibrahim GF, Shaik SA. Prediction of pulmonary hypertension in patients with or without interstitial lung disease: reliability of CT findings. Radiology. 2011;260:875–83.
25. Tan RT, Kuzo R, Goodman LR, et al. Utility of CT scan evaluation for predicting pulmonary hypertension in patients with parenchymal lung disease. Chest. 1998;113:1250–6.
26. Frazier AA, Burke AP. The imaging of pulmonary hypertension. Semin Ultrasound CT MR. 2012;33:535–51.
27. Grosse C, Grosse A. CT findings in diseases associated with pulmonary hypertension: a current review. Radiographics. 2010;30(7):1753–77.
28. Sánchez Nistal MA. Pulmonary hypertension: the contribution of MDCT to the diagnosis of its different types. Radiologia. 2010;52:500–12.
29. Roeleveld RJ, Marcus JT, Faes TJ, et al. Interventricular septal configuration at mr imaging and pulmonary arterial pressure in pulmonary hypertension. Radiology. 2005;234:710–7.
30. Liu M, Ma ZH, Guo XJ, et al. A septal angle measured on computed tomographic pulmonary angiography can non-invasively estimate pulmonary vascular resistance in patients with chronic thromboembolic pulmonary hypertension. J Thorac Imaging. 2012;27:325–30.
31. Goerne H, Batra K, Rajiah P. Imaging of pulmonary hypertension: an update. Cardiovasc Diagn Ther. 2018;8(3):279–96.
32. Ascha M, Renapurkar RD, Tonelli AR. A review of imaging modalities in pulmonary hypertension. Ann Thorac Med. 2017;12:61–73.
33. Giordano J, Khung S, Duhamel A, et al. Lung perfusion characteristics in pulmonary arterial hypertension (PAH) and peripheral forms of chronic thromboembolic pulmonary hypertension (pCTEPH): dual-energy CT experience in 31 patients. Eur Radiol. 2017;27:1631–9.
34. Reiter G, Reiter U, Kovacs G, et al. Blood flow vortices 296 Goerne et al. pulmonary hypertension © cardiovascular diagnosis and therapy. Cardiovasc Diagn Ther 2018;8(3):279–296. cdt.amegroups.com along the main pulmonary artery measured with MR imaging for diagnosis of pulmonary.
35. Katz J, Whang J, Boxt LM, Barst RJ. Estimation of right ventricular mass in normal subjects and in patients with primary pulmonary hypertension by nuclear magnetic resonance imaging. J Am Coll Cardiol. 1993;21(6):1475–81.
36. Hoeper MM, Tongers J, Leppert A, Baus S, Maier R, Lotz J. Evaluation of right ventricular performance with a right ventricular ejection fraction thermodilution catheter and MRI in patients with pulmonary hypertension. Chest. 2001;120(2):502–7.
37. Van Wolferen SA, Marcus JT, Boonstra A, et al. Prognostic value of right ventricular mass, volume, and function in idiopathic pulmonary arterial hypertension. Eur Heart J. 2007;28(10):1250–7.
38. Saba TS, Foster J, Cockburn M, Cowan M, Peacock AJ. Ventricular mass index using magnetic resonance imaging accurately estimates pulmonary artery pressure. Eur Respir J. 2002;20(6):1519–24.
39. Brady D, Lavelle LP, McEvoy SH, et al. Assessing fibrosis in pulmonary sarcoidosis: late-enhanced MRI compared to anatomic HRCT imaging. QJM. 2016;109:257–64.
40. Swift AJ, Wild JM, Nagle SK, et al. Quantitative magnetic resonance imaging of pulmonary hypertension: A practical approach to the current state of the art. J Thorac Imaging. 2014;29:68–79.
41. Dellegrottaglie S, Sanz J, Poon M, et al. Pulmonary hypertension: accuracy of detection with left ventricular septal-to-free wall curvature ratio measured at cardiac MR. Radiology. 2007;243:63–9.
42. Sanz J, Kuschnir P, Rius T, et al. Pulmonary arterial hypertension: noninvasive detection with phase-contrast MR imaging. Radiology. 2007;243:70–9.
43. Sanz J, Kuschnir P, Rius T, Salguero R, Sulica R, Einstein AJ, Dellegrottaglie S, Fuster V, Rajagopalan S, Poon M. Pulmonary arterial hypertension: noninvasive detection with phase-contrast MR imaging. Radiology. 2007;243:70–9.
44. Kondo C, Caputo GR, Masui T, et al. Pulmonary hypertension: pulmonary flow quantification and flow profile analysis with velocity-encoded cine MR imaging. Radiology. 1992;183:751–8.
45. Nagendran J, Michelakis E. MRI: one-stop shop for the comprehensive assessment of pulmonary arterial hypertension? Chest. 2007;132:2–5.
46. Agoston-Coldea L, Lupu S, Mocan T. Pulmonary artery stiffness by cardiac magnetic resonance imaging predicts major adverse cardiovascular events in patients with chronic obstructive pulmonary disease. Sci Rep. 2018;8(1):14447.
47. Ray J, Burger C, Mergo P, Safford R, Blackshear J, Austin C, et al. Pulmonary arterial stiffness assessed by cardiovascular magnetic resonance imaging is a predictor of mild pulmonary arterial hypertension. Int J Cardiovasc Imaging. 2018;35(10):1881–92.
48. Ibrahim E-SH, Bajwa AA, White RD. Assessment of Pulmonary Arterial Hypertension by Magnetic Resonance Imaging. Tomography. 2015;1(1):23–9.
49. Forouzan O, Warczytowa J, Wieben O, François C, Chesler N. Non-invasive measurement using cardiovascular magnetic resonance of changes in pulmonary artery stiffness with exercise. J Cardiovasc Magn Reson. 2015;17(1):109.
50. Garcia-Alvarez A, Fernandez-Friera L, Mirelis J, Sawit S, Nair A, Kallman J, et al. Non-invasive estimation of pulmonary vascular resistance with cardiac magnetic resonance. Eur Heart J. 2011;32(19):2438–45.
51. Swift A, Rajaram S, Hurdman J, Hill C, Davies C, Sproson T, et al. Noninvasive estimation of PA pres-

sure, flow, and resistance With CMR imaging. JACC Cardiovascu Imaging. 2013;6(10):1036–47.
52. Abolmaali N, Seitz U, Esmaeili A, Kock M, Radeloff D, Ackermann H, et al. Evaluation of a resistance-based model for the quantification of pulmonary arterial hypertension using MR flow measurements. J Magn Reson Imaging. 2007;26(3):646–53.
53. Bell A, Beerbaum P, Greil G, Hegde S, Toschke A, Schaeffter T, et al. Noninvasive assessment of pulmonary artery flow and resistance by cardiac magnetic resonance in congenital heart diseases with unrestricted left-to-right shunt. JACC Cardiovascu Imaging. 2009;2(11):1285–91.
54. Kurzyna M, Dabrowski M, Blelecki D, et al. Atrial septostomy in treatment of end-stage right heart failure in patients with pulmonary hypertension. Chest. 2007;131:977–83.
55. Ayhan P, Rana O, et al. Magnetic resonance imaging in pediatric pulmonary hypertension. Tex Heart Int J. 2015;42(3):209–15.
56. Lewis G, Hoey ET, Reynolds JH, et al. Multi-detector CT assessment in pulmonary hypertension: techniques, systematic approach to interpretation and key findings. Quant Imaging Med Surg. 2015;5:423–32.
57. Osorio M, Bonow A, Bond G, Rivera M, Vaughan K, Shah A, et al. Abernethy malformation complicated by hepatopulmonary syndrome and a liver mass successfully treated by liver transplantation. Pediatr Transplant. 2010;15(7):E149–51.
58. Marín Rodríguez C, Sánchez Alegre ML, Lancharro Zapataa Á, Alarcón Rodríguez J. What radiologists need to know about the pulmonary—systemic flow ratio (Qp/Qs): what it is, how to calculate it, and what it is for. Radiología. 2015;57(5):369–79.
59. Wood P. The Eisenmenger syndrome or pulmonary hypertension with reversed central shunt I. Br Med J. 1958;2(5098):701–9.
60. Galie N, Manes A, Palazzini M, et al. Management of pulmonary arterial hypertension associated with congenital systemic-to-pulmonary shunts and Eisenmenger's syndrome. Drugs. 2008;68(8):1049–66.
61. Silversides CK, Granton JT, Konen E, Hart MA, Webb GD, Therrien J. Pulmonary thrombosis in adults with Eisenmenger syndrome. J Am Coll Cardiol. 2003;42(11):1982–7.
62. Kaemmerer H, Mebus S, Schulze-Neick I, Eicken A, Trindade TP, Hager A, et al. The adult patient with eisenmenger syndrome: a medical update after dana point part I: epidemiology, clinical Aspects and diagnostic options. Curr Cardiol Rev. 2010;6(4):343–55.
63. Fontan F, Baudet E. Surgical repair of tricuspid atresia. Thorax. 1971;26:240–8.
64. Wolff D, van Melle JP, Ebels T, et al. Trends in mortality (1975-2011) after one- and two-stage Fontan surgery, including bidirectional Glenn through Fontan completion. Eur J Cardiothorac Surg. 2014;45:602–9.
65. Egbe A, Connolly H, Miranda W, Ammash N, Hagler D, Veldtman G, et al. Hemodynamics of Fontan failure. Circ Heart Fail. 2017;10(12):e004515.
66. Hosein RBM, Clarke AJB, McGuirk SP, et al. Factors influencing early and late outcome following the Fontan procedure in the current era. The "Two Commandments". Eur J Cardiothorac Surg. 2007;31:344–53.
67. Dasi LP, Krishnankuttyrema R, Kitajima HD, et al. Fontan hemodynamics: importance of pulmonary artery diameter. J Thorac Cardiovasc Surg. 2009;137:560–4.
68. Davos C. Global impairment of cardiac autonomic nervous activity late after the Fontan operation. Circulation. 2003;108(90101):II-180–5.
69. Whitehead KK, Gillespie MJ, Harris MA, Fogel MA, Rome JJ. Noninvasive quantification of systemic-to-pulmonary Collateral flow. A major source of inefficiency in patients with superior Cavopulmonary connections. Circ Cardiovasc Imaging. 2009;2:405–11.
70. Markl M, Frydrychowicz A, Kozerke S, Hope M, Wieben O. 4D flow MRI. J Magn Reson Imaging. 2012;36(5):1015–36.
71. Garcia-Alvarez A, Garcia-Lunar I, Pereda D, et al. Association of myocardial T1-mapping CMR with hemodynamics and RV performance in pulmonary hypertension. JACC Cardiovasc Imaging. 2015;8:76–82.
72. Sachdev A, Villarraga HR, Frantz RP, et al. Right ventricular strain for prediction of survival in patients with pulmonary arterial hypertension. Chest. 2011;139:1299–309.

CT Versus MRI in Congenital Heart Disease

22

Shaik Ismail, D. Prashanth Reddy, Bhavana Nagabhushana Reddy, and Sanjaya Viswamitra

22.1 Introduction

The incidence of Congenital Heart Disease (CHD) is 8 per 1000 live births in India [1] and 9.4 per 1000 in the world [2]. In neonates, the incidence of CHD is 6–8 per 1000 neonates. With the advancement in treatment techniques, the survival in CHD patients has increased in the last half-century, particularly with the advent of cardiopulmonary bypass in 1953. We are already seeing this effect with more adults with treated CHD presenting in clinics than children born with CHD [3]. Imaging with CT and MRI will play an important role in detecting complications related to surgery as well as providing prognostic information in this new patient population. In the USA, the annual caseload of adult CHD is 1.4 million with a 5% increase per year and an estimated prevalence of 2.2 million by 2020 [4].

Taussig first used radiography and fluoroscopy to characterize the radiographic appearance of various CHDs. Angiography with cardiac catheterization was the mainstay of CHD imaging until the late 1970s and early 1980s. The emergence of echocardiography in the late 1980s nearly replaced angiography as a primary imaging modality. Echocardiography's ability to provide morphologic, hemodynamic, and functional assessment in a safe and noninvasive manner was the primary reason for this transition [5].

Complex CHD patients often require multidisciplinary imaging techniques for effective diagnosis and treatment planning. The commonly used modalities are echocardiography, CT, MRI, and catheter angiography. These are considered complementary to each other. Transthoracic echocardiography (TTE) is the most commonly used modality as it is cheap, easily available, and does not use ionizing radiation. However, its shortcomings include operator dependence, a limited acoustic window particularly in adult congenital heart disease cases, and its limited capability in the evaluation of extracardiac abnormalities. CT is superior to TTE in the evaluation of pulmonary and systemic venous abnormalities, extracardiac pathology, coronary vessels, and permits visualization of complex anatomy with high spatial and temporal resolution. There is a shift in trend with the increasing use of CT and MRI for imaging in congenital heart disease [3, 6].

22.2 CT Imaging in CHD

Children diagnosed with CHD have an annual exposure from <3 mSv (millisieverts)/year to > 20 mSv/year of radiation resulting from chest

S. Ismail (✉) · D. P. Reddy · B. N. Reddy
S. Viswamitra
Department of Radiology, Sri Sathya Sai Institute of Higher Medical Sciences, Whitefield, Bengaluru, Karnataka, India
e-mail: shaik.i@sssihms.org.in; Prashanth.d@sssihms.org.in; bhavana.n@sssihms.org.in

R. Rajeshkannan et al. (eds.), *CT and MRI in Congenital Heart Diseases*,
https://doi.org/10.1007/978-981-15-6755-1_22

radiography, CT, and cardiac catheterization, depending upon the lesion [7]. Developments such as iterative reconstruction, automated tube current modulation, ECG dose modulation have resulted in a significant reduction in radiation dose, leading to the wider clinical acceptance of this modality. CT has become an important imaging modality, especially in pediatric congenital CHD patients, due to the short procedure time and the need for minimal or no sedation [8].

22.2.1 Technical and Equipment Requirements for Cardiac CT

Recent advances in CT scanner technology have led to a significant improvement in the temporal resolution which was the main factor limiting the widespread use of CT in cardiac imaging. This includes the advent of dual-energy dual-source MDCT which improves temporal resolution by a factor of two, improvements in gantry design permitting a faster gantry rotation time, and increase detector rows with concomitant Z-axis detector coverage.

The increasing utilization of CT for the evaluation of CHD is in part due to the wider availability of cardiac capable multidetector scanners.

22.2.1.1 Spatial Resolution

Spatial resolution is defined as the measurements of the smallest voxel that comprises an image. The standard voxel for all CT scans in the axis of the gantry is 512 × 512. There are new algorithms that offer high resolution 1024 × 1024 matrix. The smaller field of view of around 25 cm for a cardiac scan gives an X–Y resolution of about 0.5 × 0.5 mm. The Z-axis resolution is dependent on the size of the detector and the interpolation techniques, such as "wobble" used while scanning. The detector thickness is between 0.5 and 0.625 mm depending on the scanner. This gives an overall near isotropic data voxel set allowing for preserved image quality in MPRs, vital for CHD evaluation [9, 10].

Coverage in the Z-axis is dependent on the number of detector rows, the speed of gantry rotation, and the pitch that is used. Since the pitch is small for cardiac gated exams, the coverage is mainly depended on the former factors. A 64-slice detector can acquire close to 4 cm of Z-axis coverage in one rotation and is the minimum that is required for consistent quality of cardiac CT imaging. The 256 and 320 slice CT scanners, with Z-axis coverage of 16 cm, are capable of covering the entire heart in a single gantry rotation. The faster the acquisition, the better the compliance of patients, shorter the breath-hold duration, and fewer motion artifacts.

22.2.1.2 Temporal Resolution

Assessment of cardiac structures requires a temporal resolution that is high enough to freeze cardiac motion and is based on the speed of gantry rotation. Modern CT scanners can rotate the gantry through one rotation in as low as 280 ms. The minimum data required for image reconstruction on CT is based on the acquisition of a sufficient number of projections and views of an area of interest. This is typically acquired from at least 180° of gantry rotation and is the time taken for half a gantry rotation. Dual-source scanners can combine 90° of data acquisition from each source which are aligned at right angles to each other to give the best temporal resolution.

With single-source scanners, 180° of data can be acquired either from a single (half) rotation or segmented from multiple rotations. These are "monosegment half scan reconstruction" and "multisegmented multi rotation reconstruction," respectively. For example, a scanner that can rotate the gantry through one full rotation in 300 ms achieves a mono-segment half scan reconstruction temporal resolution of 150 ms. Multisegmented reconstructions can potentially use 60° of information from three successive heartbeats to give a temporal resolution of 100 ms for the same study. The disadvantage is that combining information from three heartbeats may result in misregistration and blurring. In reality, the choice of the reconstruction method is complicated. It is dependent on the heart rate and programmed algorithms of the scanner and is not under manual control. The most reproducible and best quality scans are with dual-

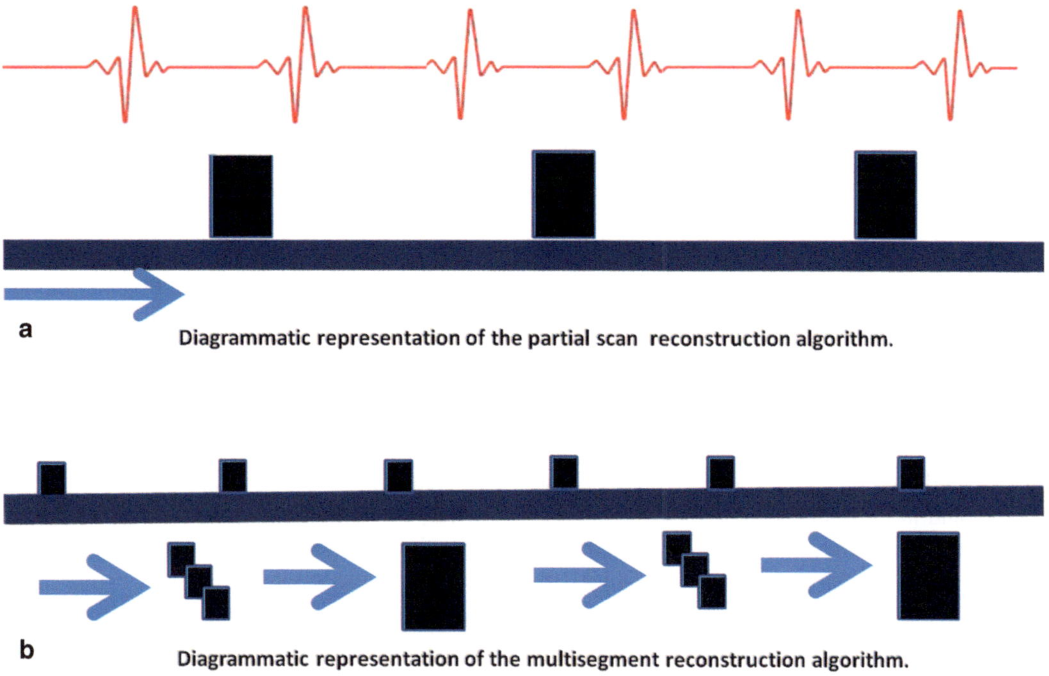

Fig. 22.1 (**a**) "Partial scan algorithm" Data acquisition occurs over 180° of gantry rotation plus the fan angle of the X-ray beam. This can be performed in both prospectively triggered and retrospectively gated acquisitions. In a prospectively triggered acquisition, data acquisition (black boxes) occurs in alternate RR intervals to permit for table move time and gantry rotation time. For example, the top image depicts half scan acquisition per heartbeat over six heartbeats and results in three images. (**b**) "Multisegment algorithm"—In this type of acquisition, data is acquired in a predetermined phase of the cardiac cycle, over multiple heartbeats (small black boxes). In each cardiac cycle, less than 180° of projection data is acquired. The data is then combined to get sufficient data to allow image reconstruction. In the example above, 60° of projection data is acquired in each cardiac phase. The bottom image depicts that for the same six heartbeats result in only two images and require a longer breath-hold with potential for misregistration between the partial acquisition. In practice, the degrees of data acquired depend on the scanner configuration and patient heart rate and is not under manual control. Considering the above algorithm, data from three cardiac cycles is added together to generate the 180° needed for image reconstruction. This effectively reduces the temporal resolution by a factor of 3 (Temporal resolution = Gantry rotation time/2× (number of segments in adjacent heartbeats from which the projection data is acquired)). Variations in the duration of the RR interval will result in misregistration artifacts as such a regular heart rate is a prerequisite. This technique can only be performed in a retrospectively gated scan

source imaging and with mono-segment half scans. Hence, stable and low heart rates, are prerequisites for good quality exams [9, 10] (Fig. 22.1).

22.2.1.3 Pitch

Pitch defines the ratio of table movement to gantry rotation [9]. Cardiac scans require oversampling of data in retrospective ECG-gated scans and thus have a low pitch. This increases radiation dose when compared to prospective ECG gated scans performed in a step and shoot mode. The step and shoot prospective mode is one where there is no table movement during gantry rotation. The table moves between gantry rotations between alternate heartbeats. The acquisition is only during the diastolic phase of the heart and is centered around a 70% R–R window. The advantages are improved image quality with decreased blur at the edges of the coronary vessels and reduced radiation dose while forgoing the information from cardiac motion. This, however, requires good heart rate control. Retrospective gating acquires attenuation data during the entire cardiac cycle. Table movement at a very low pitch is tied to spiral acquisition. This has the advantage of giving additional information regarding cardiac motion at the cost of increased dose [11].

22.2.1.4 High-Pitch CT Scan

A novel method to get around radiation dose and breath-hold times is high pitch scans on dual-source scanners. High-pitch dual-source CT scans use pitch values upto 3.4 as compared to routine retrospective scans which have pitch values of 0.2–0.4. This method can achieve sub mSv exams through the heart with a breath-hold time of close to or less than 1 s [12]. In addition, lowering the voltage to 80 kV can further increase the attenuation of iodine (80 kV is closer to the K edge of Iodine) and increase the contrast of iodine on the images. Children between 1 and 12 years of life are ten times more sensitive to radiation dose and will benefit from low dose high-pitch CT scans [13].

22.2.1.5 ECG Gated Versus Non-gated Study

An important aspect of CT imaging in CHD is whether to use a gated or a non-gated study and, if gated, whether retrospective or prospective.

The advantages of a non-gated study are lower radiation dose, short scan time and thus fewer artifacts due to respiratory motion, and a larger scan coverage. The disadvantage is increased artifacts due to cardiac motion.

Thus, for most CHD, an ECG-gated study is performed. Retrospectively gated study is the most common acquisition mode due to the high heart rate in pediatric CHD patients and the potential added information from cardiac motion. Adults with CHD and without contraindications to beta-blockers may be scanned using prospective ECG triggering provided the heart rate is adequately controlled before the scan [14, 15]. The holy grail of cardiac imaging is to reduce dose while getting the best possible information. Faster scanners, dual source, prospective gating, have the potential to reduce radiation to less than 1.0 mSv in young children [16]. However, the typical dose with prospective gating is around 3 mSv in most institutions with a 64 detector (128 slice scanner) and increases to 10–15 mSv with retrospective gating. It is, thus, recommended that each center follow the ALARA principles and be cognizant of radiation dose and imaging gently while protocoling pediatric CHD exams.

22.2.2 Protocoling a CT CHD Study

The imager needs to review the clinical history and all previous exams prior to protocoling the study. The echo information is critical in understanding what additional information is needed from the CT scan. Common to all is the need to get thin collimation for high-quality MPR images, ECG gating when required to assess chamber and great vessel morphology, isomerism, and coronary arteries. Coverage can vary depending on the nature of the CHD. At a minimum, most CHD requires coverage from above the aortic arch to the diaphragm. Extended coverage may be considered in partial or total anomalous pulmonary venous return, aortic abnormalities, and postoperative patients. While ECG gating is preferred, evaluation for large structures such as the aorta may be performed without gating to reduce the dose and speed up the acquisition [17].

Also critical in protocoling is contrast administration. Dose in a pediatric individual ranges from 1.5 to 2 mL per kg body weight up to a maximum volume of 100 mL at an infusion rate of 1–2 mL/s depending on the iodine concentration in the contrast agent [18]. In pediatric congenital heart disease patients, placement of the IV line can be in either arm. We recommend placing the IV cannula in the left arm as this provides more consistent opacification and detection of the left superior vena cava. Contrast via the right antecubital vein can be considered when evaluating the arch of the aorta and branch vessels as this prevents streak artifacts across this area of anatomy.

The timing of the contrast bolus is performed using the bolus tracking technique or the test bolus technique and is a matter of institutional protocol. Unlike adult coronary evaluation, CHD benefits from uniform opacification of the right and left chambers. Understanding the pathophysiology of CHD is important in achieving this. Streak artifact from the contrast bolus can be reduced by a saline flush.

22.3 MR in Congenital Heart Disease

Cardiac MRI (CMR) consists of multiple sequences that perform a comprehensive morphological and functional analysis of the heart. MRI has the advantage of not using ionizing radiation. It does need multiple sequences in a more constrained MR environment, has a longer acquisition, and typically requires better patient compliance or sedation. Intravenous contrast is not required for all cases in CMR. A typical CMR protocol for congenital heart disease consists of the following components:

1. Morphologic analysis
2. Cine imaging
3. Phase-contrast imaging
4. 3D MR angiography
5. Delayed enhancement imaging
6. Additional sequences

22.3.1 Morphological Imaging

This includes dark blood and bright blood sequences. The high contrast difference between the blood pool and surrounding structures in these sequences is ideal for identifying situs, anomalous systemic and pulmonary anatomy, cardiac chamber identification, aorta and pulmonary artery anatomy in brief. Black blood imaging uses fast spin-echo (FSE or TSE), spin-echo (SE), and HASTE sequences. All black blood images are ECG gated and are acquired during a breath-hold. Multi-slice balanced field echo or steady-state free precession—bSSFP (various vendor-specific abbreviations include TruFISP, FIESTA, BFFE) is used for bright blood imaging [19, 20].

3D bSSFP non-contrast MRA: Since bSSFP has the advantage of inherently high signal and good blood tissue differentiation, this property can be exploited for the generation of images with 3D datasets of the heart. These are usually acquired in any systolic or diastolic rest phase and are acquired with respiratory gating using navigator sequences. The duration of the sequence becomes subject- and sequence-specific [21].

22.3.2 Cine Imaging

CHD results in distinctive types of ventricular load or dilatation. Hence, quantification is essential in the management of patients and is important for the evaluation of postoperative patients such as post Tetralogy of Fallot (TOF) repair cases.

Two main sequences used in cine imaging are spoiled gradient echo (GRE) and bSSFP sequences. Cine sequences are the workhorse of cardiac MR imaging and are used to assess for wall motion abnormalities, ventricular volume quantification, and mass quantification. Cine images can be acquired in any plane without any geometrical assumptions which are the biggest advantage compared to echo and CT. Regions of high-velocity flow and turbulence result in artifacts due to dephasing, phase misregistration, and loss of signal in cine sequences. These artifacts can be greatly reduced with the use of flow compensation in balanced gradients of the bSSFP sequences. Although regurgitant/stenotic jets and shunts can be visualized on these sequences, they are not suited for quantification [19, 20].

22.3.3 Phase-Contrast Imaging (PC)

Phase-contrast (PC) sequences encode phase shifts due to velocity in the MR image and can be used to quantify flow velocity, the direction of flow and volume. PC MR is commonly used in flow quantification of the aorta and pulmonary artery. This quantification permits us to calculate aortic and pulmonary regurgitant volumes directly. Mitral and tricuspid regurgitant volumes can be calculated by subtracting the PC forward flow from the ventricular stroke volumes derived from the analysis of the cine images. PC MRI also provides a means to cross-check volumetric information. In the absence of shunts and regurgitant lesions, the ventricular stroke volume calculated from cine images should be equal to the aortic or pulmonary forward volume measured by PC MRI [22] (Fig. 22.2).

CHD can have both intra- and extracardiac shunting comprising left to right, right to left, or sometimes mixed shunts. Cine phase-contrast MR imaging of the pulmonary artery and aorta blood

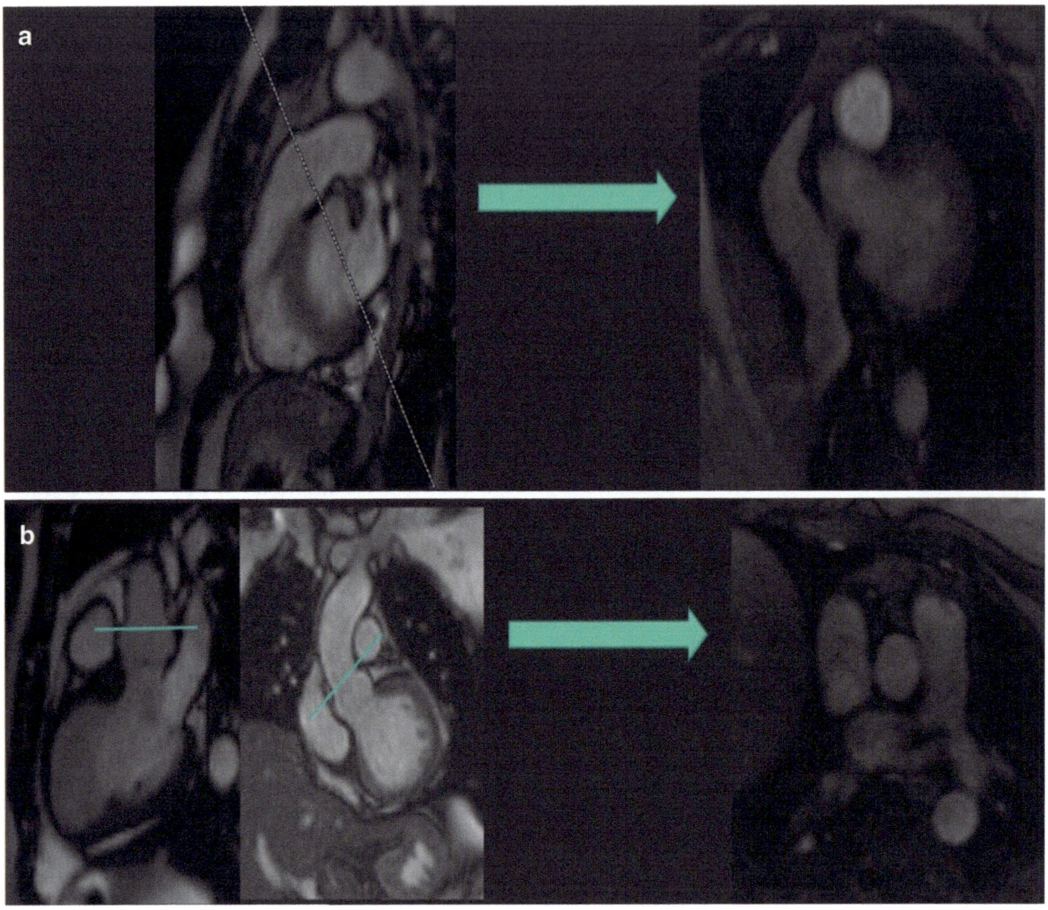

Fig. 22.2 Pulmonary short-axis plane for PC MRI (upper row) is planned from the RVOT view perpendicular to the main pulmonary artery and distal to valve leaflets. The aortic short axis for PC MRI (lower row) is planned from the three-chamber and LVOT views perpendicular to ascending aorta just distal to tips of the valve leaflets at the sinotubular junction level

flow can be used to quantify *Qp*/*Qs*. *Qp* is measured at the level of the main pulmonary artery or pulmonary valve. *Qs* is calculated at the level of ascending aorta or aortic valve. The ideal *Qp*/*Qs* ratio is 1. A ratio of >1.5 represents a significant left to right shunt, whereas a value <1 represents a right to left shunt. The planning for calculation of *Qp*/*Qs* varies depending on the location of the shunt. For example, a PDA would require the calculation of flows in the right and left pulmonary arteries separately.

22.3.4 Delayed Enhancement Imaging

Enhancing areas after gadolinium administration in this sequence represent increased extracellular space which is seen in scar tissue, myocyte injury, and inflammation. This sequence has a limited role in the evaluation of CHD and is usually limited to postoperative evaluation. The presence of a scar is associated with an increased risk of arrhythmia [23].

22.3.5 Contrast-Enhanced Magnetic Resonance Angiography (CE-MRA)

22.3.5.1 3D CE-MRA

It is increasingly being used as the first-line imaging for blood vessels and consists of injecting contrast bolus followed by a saline flush in a very short

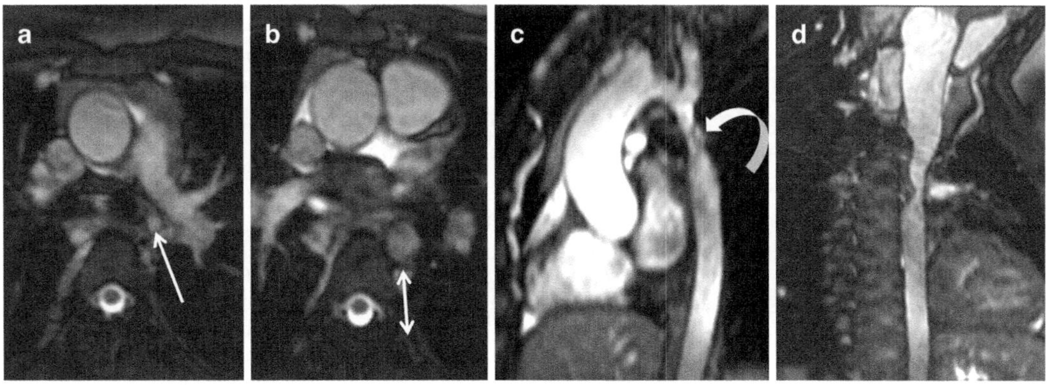

Fig. 22.3 Images (**a**–**d**) for a navigator gated free-breathing 3D bSSFP noncontrast MRA showing coarctation of the aorta, (**c**) Curved multiplanar reformatted images of the aorta can be created to better visualize the anatomical relationship between the aortic arch branches and the coarctation. (**d**) Curved MPR images layout the aorta along a center line trace and are useful for the evaluation of stenoses in tortuous vessels

duration, after achieving peak enhancement in the region of interest, CE-MRA acquisition begins. This is a GRE-based sequence and can be used as a single-phase MRA where entire acquisition time is for one data set of 3D images or time-resolved MRA where the region of interest is imaged over a time interval depicting various stages of enhancement [24, 25]. Most 3D sequences do not pair with ECG gating (Fig. 22.3).

Disease-Specific CMRI Protocol for Common CHD done in our institute based on SCMR guidelines [26].

The basic congenital heart disease protocol consists of:

- Dark blood imaging: FSE/TSE or STIR
- Cine sequences (bSSFP and GRE):
  - Left ventricular short axis, two-chamber and three-chamber, four-chamber views
  - Optional right ventricular three-chamber view, two-chamber view
  - Enface view for shunt quantification
  - Axial stack images axial stack from the diaphragm to the top of the aortic arch
- Phase-contrast imaging (PC)
  - At the level of the aorta (Ao) and pulmonary artery (PA)
- Whole heart angiography using 3D contrast MRA or navigator gated bSSFP sequences

22.4 Protocols for Common Conditions (Table 22.1)

22.5 CT Versus CMR for Congenital Heart Disease

The advantages of CT over MRI

- Short scan duration—reduced need for sedation. A particular concern in the pediatric population.
- Isotropic data set—Thin slices without inter-slice gaps reduce volume averaging, permit MPRs without significant loss of image quality.
- MPRs and 3D VRTs—anatomy can be evaluated in multiple planes which helps assessment of the relation of lesions to surrounding structures and in surgical planning.
- High spatial resolution—Permits coronary evaluation.
- Wide field of view—extracardiac pathologies such as lung findings and upper abdominal findings are better assessed with CT.
- Artifacts due to metallic hardware as less of an issue than in MR imaging.
- Calcium is easily visualized on CT scans. Cardiac relationship to bony structures and

Table 22.1 CMR protocols for common CHD

Indication	Sequences	Important assessment parameters
Shunt evaluation Atrial septal defect, ventricular septal defect, atrioventricular septal defect (ASD/VSD/AVSD) Partial anomalous pulmonary venous return (PAPVC)	• Basic CHD protocol • Whole heart angiography using 3D contrast MRA or navigator-gated bSSFP sequences	Position of defect Ventricular volume and function Shunt quantification Pulmonary vein morphology
Tetralogy of Fallot (TOF)	Basic CHD protocol • Additional—PC CMR: branch PAs	RVOT morphology Pulmonary valve and artery morphology Ventricular volume and quantification Valvular function and flow assessment
Transposition of great arteries (TGA) (pre- and postoperative)	Basic CHD protocol Additional sequences • Cine bSSFP oblique planes to image the SVC and IVC pathways in long axis • CE-MRA or 3D SSFP to image the thoracic vasculature, and systemic and pulmonary venous baffles • PC CMR: AAo, MPA, branch PAs, tricuspid and mitral valves	RVOT Pulmonary artery morphology Aortic arch anatomy Ventricular volume and quantification Valvular function and assessment Coronary artery anatomy assessment
Ebstein anomaly	Basic CHD protocol Additional sequences • Cine bSSFP multiple contiguous slices in the right ventricular three-chamber view and in the four-chamber view • Cine bSSFP contiguous stack-oriented parallel to the functional tricuspid valve plane to visualize the valve en face • PC CMR: AAo, MPA • CE-MRA or 3D SSFP to image the thoracic vasculature	Tricuspid valve morphology, tricuspid regurgitation, and stenosis, pulmonary stenosis, ventricular parameters, presence of an atrial septal defect, *Qp*/*Qs* based on flow measurements
Coarctation of the aorta, before or after repair	Left ventricular short-axis, two-chamber, and three-chamber, four-chamber views Candy view CE-MRA or 3D SSFP to image the thoracic Vasculature PC CMR: Proximal and distal aorta to quantify collaterals	Level of coarctation Presence and extent of collaterals Coarctation gradient Recurrent coarctation in post-op cases LV function and mass

sternotomy wires are better seen in the case of redo sternotomy.

- Coronary artery imaging with CT is well validated and in routine use, whereas MR coronary angiography is not commonly used due to the lower spatial resolution. MR coronary angiography is indicated when the anomalous coronary artery is suspected.
- Easy to perform and understand with a short learning curve

Disadvantages of CT compared with MRI

- Limited functional information—Cardiac function can be quantified from retrospectively gated CT scans. However, this results in a higher radiation dose and is not as accurate as MRI due to the lower temporal resolution. Right ventricular volumetry is not possible. No information about valve function, shunt quantification, and myocardial scar.

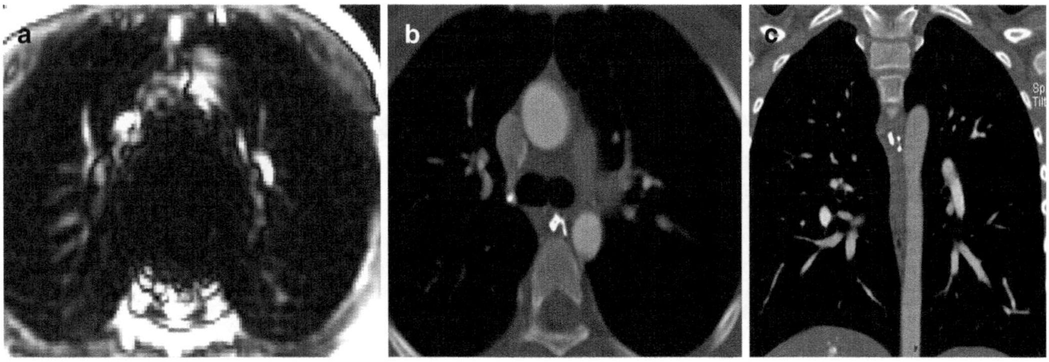

Fig. 22.4 (**a**) Axial SSFP MR image showing severe susceptibility artifact obscuring most of the mediastinal vasculature. (**b**, **c**) Axial and coronal chest CTA shows an embolization coil. Metallic hardware tends to affect MR images more than CT and CT may be preferred in such cases

- Intracardiac anatomy is blurred in non-gated CT.
- Radiation dose.
- Contrast reactions.
- Artifacts due to high heart rate: Beta-blocker may be needed for coronary artery imaging.
- MR sequences can be performed with navigator gating in patients with poor breath-hold capacity whereas there is no compensatory mechanism for respiratory motion on CT.

Advantages of MRI over CT

- No ionizing radiation.
- The higher temporal resolution provides a more accurate assessment of ventricular function.
- Evaluation of ventricular function, volumes, flows is possible.
- True multiplanar acquisition.
- Evaluation of fibrosis with LGE sequence help in determining prognosis.
- Newer techniques—T1, T2 mapping, ECV, DWI, strain. Initial studies have shown them to be promising imaging biomarkers for determining patient prognosis.
- Non-contrast MRA imaging is possible.
- Fewer contrast reactions. Gadolinium is relatively safer than iodine contrast in patients with renal dysfunction.

The disadvantage of MRI compared to CT

- The complexity of performing the scan with a long learning curve to perform and understand. Requires trained technologists.
- Can be time-intensive.
- Need for prolonged sedation. Requires monitored anesthesia care and MR compatible anesthesia equipment.
- Cardiac MRI is contraindicated patients with pacemakers, some types of epicardial leads, and claustrophobia.
- Embolization coils and other metallic implants cause severe distortion of adjacent structures (In-stent stenosis cannot be assessed due to metallic artifacts).
- Lung findings are not well assessed on MRI.
- Small tortuous structures like coronaries and MAPCAs are difficult to assess compared to CT angio (Fig. 22.4).

22.6 3D Printing

3D printing was first developed in the 1980s. The recent explosion in the use of 3D printing technologies brought about by improvement in computing powers and the development of more affordable 3D printers has led to the utilization of this modality for several medical applications including uses in congenital heart disease.

The process of 3D printing involves the generation of a segmented image from a CT or MR data set by highlighting the anatomy of interest. 3D printing for congenital heart disease requires careful segmentation by a trained radiologist. These segmented software models are then sent for printing. Printing time varies depending on the complexity of the model and the printer tech-

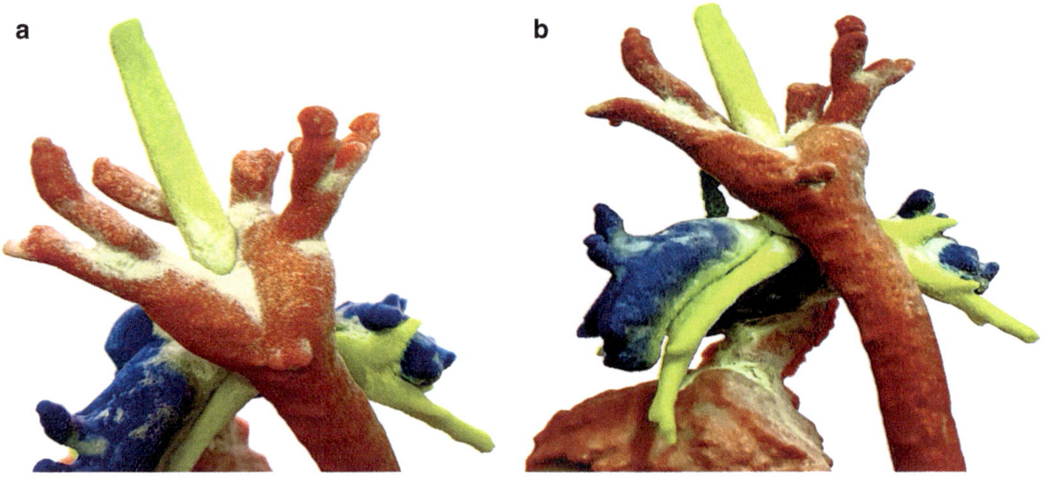

Fig. 22.5 3D printed models demonstrating a double aortic arch. Cardiac structure is segmented using different colors for easy identification (Image courtesy: Dr. Deepa Prasad, Banner Medical Center, Arizona.)

nology varying from 6 to 24 h for CHD cases [27] (Fig. 22.5).

The major benefits of using 3D printed models include:

- Facilitate communication between physicians and patients [28].
- Provide a valuable educational tool for surgeons in training and medical students.
- Improve patient understanding of their disease and may improve adherence to medication and compliance with follow-up recommendations [29].
- They are a useful addition to lectures and improve the audience's understanding of cases such as vascular rings [30].
- 3D models have shown utility in clinical decision making and interventional planning. The complex spatial relationship between structures is more easily understood using a 3D model as compared with 2D images.
- It helps in determining the size of devices used for interventional transcatheter procedures. Applications include atrial septal closure device placement, angioplasty of a pulmonary venous baffle, and device closure of mitral valve leaflet perforation in infective endocarditis [31].

The limitations of current 3D printing technology are:

- Lack of a systematic method for the segmentation of CT or MR datasets.
- Segmentation is complex, operator dependent, and time-consuming [32].
- Materials used for 3D printing do not accurately simulate cardiac structures and cannot show dynamic changes throughout the cardiac cycle [33].
- The model is not sterile and cannot be used by surgeons during a procedure.
- The start-up cost, material, and maintenance costs are quite high.

3D printing is a novel technology with various clinical applications that are only now making inroads into the field of congenital heart disease imaging. The industry has taken note of the potential for this technology and is working to develop cheaper materials, faster printers, and automation of the segmentation procedure which will undoubtedly lead to more widespread use and acceptance in the medical community [34–37].

ECG-gated CT images provide a better dataset than MRI for 3D printing models.

22.7 Imaging in Cardiac Shunts

CT and MRI are increasingly being used in the evaluation of cardiac shunts. CT helps in accurate defect size measurement, vascular assessment, and adjacent lung evaluation.

22.7.1 MRI

Simple shunts are generally evaluated with echocardiography and it is usually the only imaging modality that is required. When echocardiography is suboptimal due to poor windows or complex shunts, MRI can be performed.

MRI has the advantage of shunt quantification with the use of in-plane and through-plane PC imaging. Indirect shunt quantification is performed with the use of flow assessment in the aorta and pulmonary artery for the *Qp*/*Qs* ratio. A ratio of > 1.5–1.75 is considered to be the threshold above which surgery is frequently considered. Direct shunt quantification at the level of the defect through in-plane PC imaging is relatively difficult and technical expertise is a must to perform it accurately [38].

ASD, VSD, PDA, and AVSD are common congenital heart defects diagnosed both in children and adults. The examination begins with TTE which provides a defined morphologic classification, size and can also evaluate flow parameters. CT provides high-resolution images, can accurately classify shunts, and can also assess extra cardiac anatomy. CMR provides both anatomic and functional evaluation of the shunt.

22.7.2 Atrial Septal Defects

22.7.2.1 Types of ASD

- Ostium primum defect
- Ostium secundum defect
- Sinus venosus defect
- Coronary sinus defect

22.7.2.2 Ostium Primum ASD

Ostium primum defect is a partial AV septal defect resulting from the failure of fusion of the septum primum with the endocardial cushions. It is the second most common type of ASD (15–30%) and is located in the anterobasal part of the atrial septum, adjacent to the AV valves [39].

22.7.2.3 Ostium Secundum ASD

They are the most common type accounting for 75% of all cases and are located in the fossa ovalis. The shunt flow is perpendicular to the septum and this differentiates it from PFO where the flow is oblique [39, 40] and various studies have shown that the presence of PFO alone is not associated with increased risk of stroke or death [41].

22.7.2.4 Sinus Venosus ASD

SV ASD is rare accounting for 5–10% of the cases; it is not a true septal defect and results from abnormal resorption of the embryonic venous sinus into the right atrium, therefore resulting in overriding of SVC/IVC into the right atrium with an intact interatrial septum (septum secundum). This condition is more commonly associated with partial anomalous pulmonary venous connections (PAPVC) [39, 40].

22.7.2.5 Coronary Sinus (CS) Defect

This accounts for less than 1% of cases where there is a lack of intervening septum between the coronary sinus and LA is unroofed partially or completely. Structurally, these are classified into four types: type I, CS is completely unroofed with a persistent left SVC; type II, completely unroofed CS with no persistent left SVC; type III, CS is partially unroofed in its mid portion; and type IV, partially unroofed terminal portion [39, 40, 42] (Figs. 22.6 and 22.7).

22.7.2.6 CT and MRI: When and Why

Although echocardiography still is the gold standard for ASD evaluation, CT helps in the assessment of associated anomalies such as PAPVC. Sinus venous ASDs are better visualized on CT than on echocardiography. MRI may be performed when the radiation dose is a concern.

Transcatheter ASD closure is currently being practiced as a safe and successful alternative to open surgical repair and it becomes essential to have information regarding the septal defect, its location, and rim margins before the intervention. Contraindications to transcatheter ASD

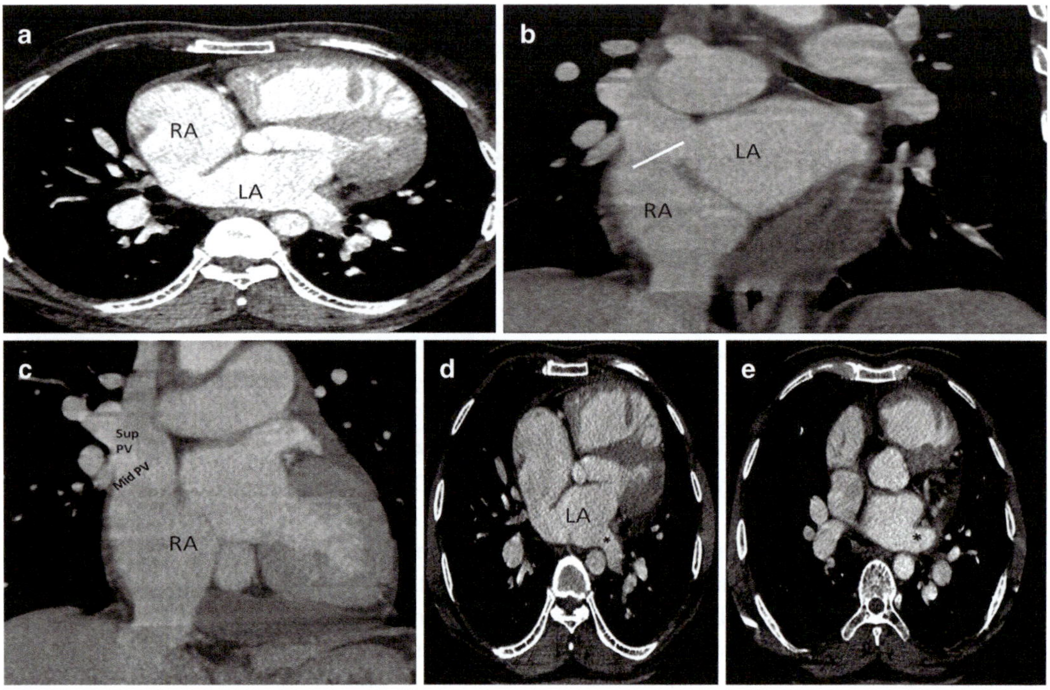

Fig. 22.6 A 25-year-old male with an ostium secundum and sinus venosus ASD (solid white line) and anomalous pulmonary venous drainage of the right upper and middle pulmonary veins into the SVC The left pulmonary veins (asterisk) drain into the LA. The upper lobe pulmonary vein ostium was not visualized on transthoracic echocardiography. CT was done to evaluate for pulmonary vein anatomy

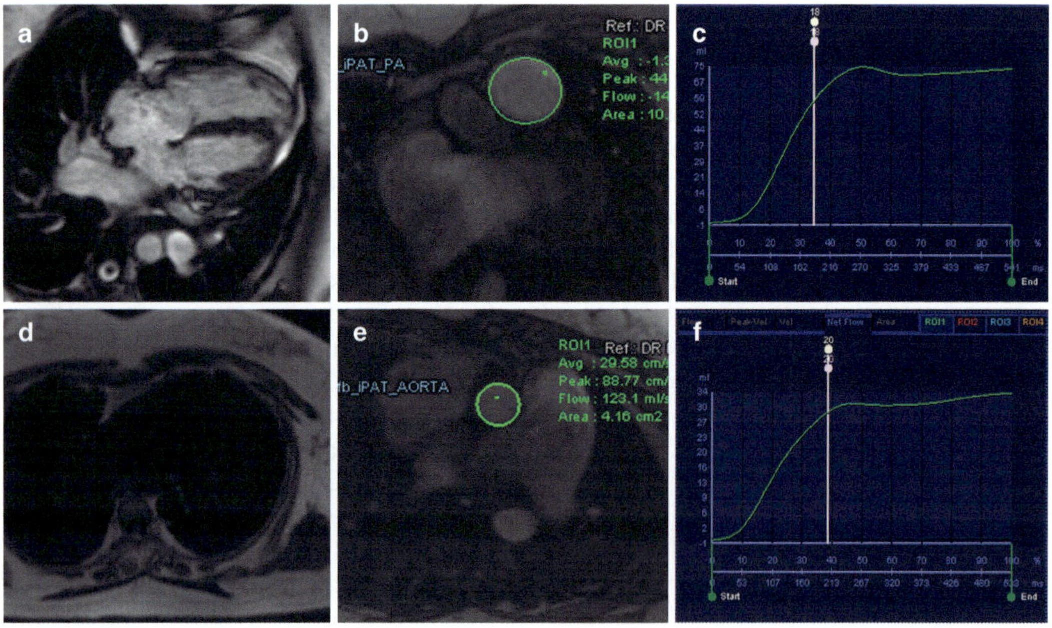

Fig. 22.7 (**a**) bSSFP MRI in a 30-year-old female shows a large ostium secundum ASD. (**b–c**) Show flow analysis of the pulmonary artery. (**d**) Dark blood TSE images show dilated pulmonary arteries. (**e–f**) Show flow analysis of aorta. The *Qp*/*QS* ratio was 2 indicating a physiologically significant shunt

closure are a defect larger than 36–40 mm in maximal diameter, the proximity of the ASD to the atrioventricular valve, venacava, or the coronary sinus. Good device deployment requires a 5-mm minimum rim of atrial tissue surrounding the defect [43, 44]. MRI is done when the radiation dose is a concern and is as accurate as CT in detecting ASDs and associated PAPVC.

22.7.2.7 Practical Pearl

A small ASD may be missed if only a single cardiac phase is evaluated. Visibility of the ASD increases in the cardiac phase where there is shunting through the defect. This is usually in the ventricular end-systole which corresponds to the 30–45% phase. Cardiac motion artifacts also vary depending on the phase and are minimal in the end-diastolic and end-systolic phases. Hence, careful evaluation of the atrial septum on multiple phases is essential. PC MRI oriented along the interatrial septum can identify small ASD. ECG-gated CT is essential to assess small ASD (Fig. 22.8).

22.7.2.8 Atrioventricular Cushion/Septal Defects (AVCD/AVSD)

Embryologically, at day 35–40, the endocardial cushions grow and meet, dividing the atrioventricular canal into right and left openings. The mesenchyme around each orifice proliferates to form the tricuspid and mitral valves.

The existence of a single common fibrous annulus results in a common atrioventricular valve or two separate valves which constitute the basis of the morphological classification.

22.7.2.9 Types of AVSD

The complete AVSD consists of an ostium primum ASD present directly above or at the plane of the atrioventricular valve with a large VSD directly below the atrioventricular valves and a common atrioventricular valve with five to six rudimentary leaflets.

The intermediate form of AVSD consists of an ostium primum ASD and a VSD. There is rudimentary midline tissue dividing the common AV valve into two separate orifices.

The transitional form of AVSD is relatively similar to complete AVSD. The leaflets of the common atrioventricular valve are fixed to the crest of the interventricular septum, resulting in a small VSD.

The partial form consists of a simple OS ASD with a cleft in the mitral valve. There is no associated VSD.

In addition to the above, the alignment of the common AV valve to that of the ventricles results in direction of the flow of blood either equal to the two ventricles resulting in a balanced AVCD or preferentially to one ventricle resulting in an unbalanced AVCD. An unbalanced AVCD can be either right or left dominant based on the larger ventricle [45–47].

22.7.2.10 CT and MRI: When and Why

The initial diagnostic modality is echocardiography. CT is performed for the evaluation of associated anomalies such as PAPCV and pulmonary artery abnormalities. MRI is equally efficient and can be used when the radiation

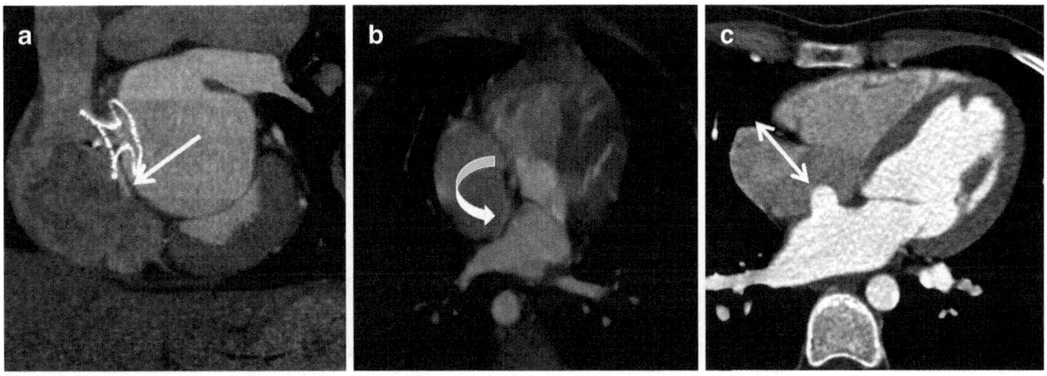

Fig. 22.8 Image (**a**) depicting a residual ASD leak (arrow) after transcatheter defect closure. Image (**b**) showing a patent foramen ovale with oblique direction of flow (curved arrow). Image (**c**) showing bulging of the interatrial septum suggestive of an atrial septal aneurysm

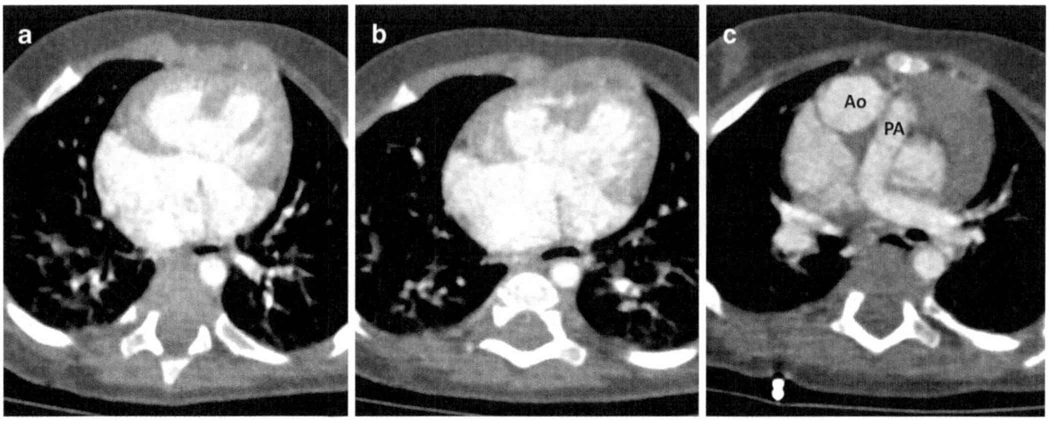

Fig. 22.9 (**a**) CT in a 6-year-old boy demonstrating a single AV valve, ostium primum ASD, the aorta is anterior to the pulmonary artery. These are classical findings of a complete AVCD. (**b**) The ventricles are equal in size indication of a balanced type of ACVD. There was associated pulmonary artery atresia (not shown). (**c**) D type transposition of the great arteries with aorta anterior and to the right of the pulmonary artery

dose is a concern or functional information is required. However, the procedure time for MRI is longer and requires general anesthesia. These are complementary modalities and offer options for troubleshooting in difficult cases (Fig. 22.9).

22.7.2.11 Practical Pearls

Blind spots of echocardiography include the ascending aorta, aortic arch, and the branch pulmonary arteries. CT and MRI provide excellent anatomical detail in this location. AVCD should be suspected when the mitral and tricuspid valve planes are at the same level and there is an elongation of the left ventricular outflow tract.

22.7.3 Ventricular Septal Defects

VSD can be isolated or it can occur in association with other congenital heart diseases (Fig. 22.10).

The unified VSD nomenclature system recognizes four types of VSD [48, 49].

22.7.3.1 Type 1

Type 1 is located just beneath the semilunar valves and above the crista supraventricularis in the conal or outlet septum and consists of the following entities—subarterial, supracristal, conal, infundibular, subpulmonary VSDs. They are commonly associated with prolapse of the anterior aortic leaflet and the defect is bound by the fibrous annulus of the semilunar valves.

22.7.3.2 Type 2

Type 2 VSD involves the membranous septum and further assigned based on the site of involvement as inlet, trabecular, outlet, and confluent (multiple areas of septum involvement). Other synonyms include perimembranous, conotruncal VSD, etc., and these account for up to 80% of VSD.

22.7.3.3 Type 3

Type 3 VSDs are also known as inlet, AV canal type, or endocardial cushion type and are located in the inlet portion of the right ventricular septum, immediately inferior to the septal leaflet of the tricuspid valve. They are commonly associated with AVCD and account for 5% cases of all VSD.

22.7.3.4 Type 4

Type 4 or muscular VSD is entirely bordered by the muscular septum with a rim entirely consisting of septal muscle. Based on its location in the septum, it is classified as inlet, trabecular outlet, or confluent (involves multiple areas of the septum). They account for 20% of all VSDs and they sometimes occur as multiple defects also known as swiss cheese VSD. They are associated with high chances of spontaneous closure (Fig. 22.11).

22.7.3.5 CT and MR: When and Why

Regions that are difficult to visualize on echocardiography such as the apical septum can be better assessed on CT and MRI. CT is useful in the postoperative evaluation and can assess for the morphology of the VSD patch, residual and recurrent VSDs. It can also be used to assess closure devices for residual shunts.

22.7.3.6 Practical Pearl

Multiplanar reformats such as the short-axis and four-chamber views are particularly useful in detecting small VSDs. Small Perimembranous VSDs can be missed if only the axial plane is used for diagnosis. Perimembranous VSDs can be associated with aortic insufficiency. This is due to the disruption of the aortic valve annulus

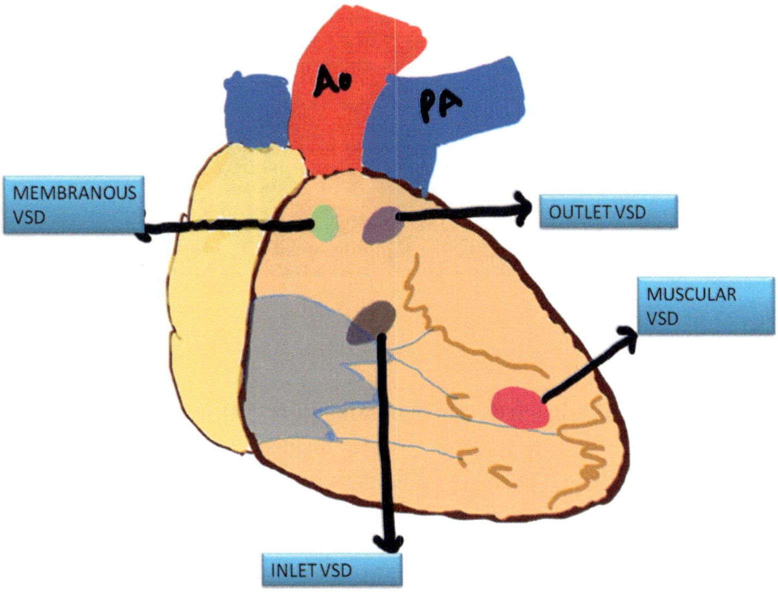

Fig. 22.10 The sites and types of VSD

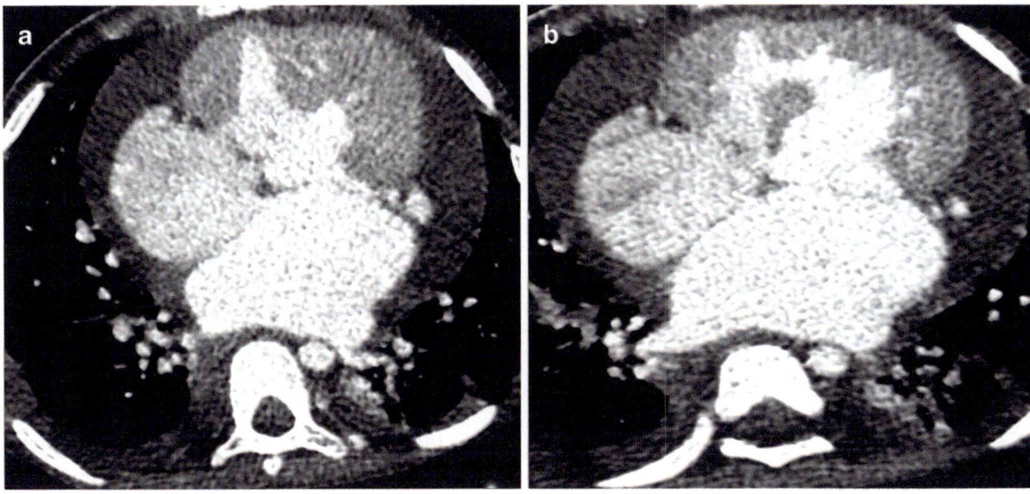

Fig. 22.11 Series of images demonstrating different types of VSDs. Image (**a** and **b**) A 4-year-old girl with incomplete AVCD, perimembranous (double-headed arrow) and muscular VSDs and a small ostium primum ASD. Separate mitral and tricuspid valves are at the same level and are separated by a ridge of tissue that represents fibrous mesenchymal tissue. This is consistent with an incomplete type of AVCD. Images (**c** and **d**) from a different patient demonstrate with small perimembranous type of VSD (asterisk)

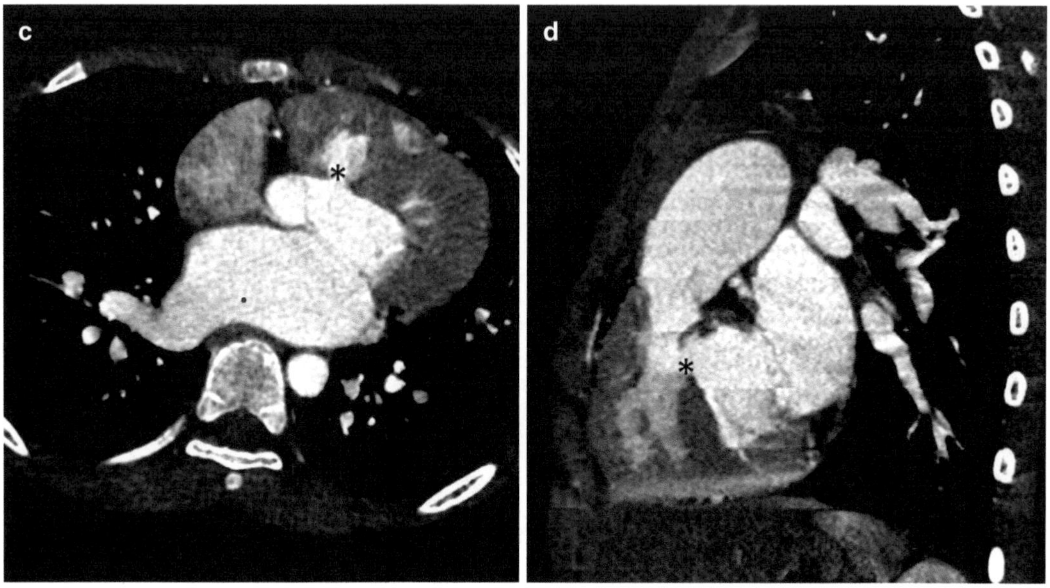

Fig. 22.11 (continued)

and a venturi effect due to the shunt causing prolapse of the semilunar valve cusp. Aortic insufficiency should be assessed if an MRI is done in these cases.

22.8 Venoatrial Anomalies

Pulmonary venous anomalies are characterized by an abnormal number, connection, or drainage of pulmonary veins.

The spectrum consists of:

1. Partial anomalous pulmonary venous connections (PAPVC)
2. Total anomalous pulmonary venous return (TAPVR)
3. Pulmonary vein atresia
4. Pulmonary venous stenosis
5. Pulmonary varix

22.8.1 Partial Anomalous Pulmonary Venous Connection

In PAPVC there is abnormal drainage of the pulmonary veins into the RA or its tributaries. This occurs as a result of persistent fetal pulmonary venous drainage into the RA or systemic veins. This is commonly associated with ASDs and most of the symptomatic patients have PAPVC with ASD rather than isolated PAPVC.

The anomalous right upper lobe (RUL) pulmonary vein drains into the superior vena cava (SVC) or the cavo-atrial junction and in up to 90% of cases, a sinus venosus ASD is also present.

The anomalous right lower lobe pulmonary vein typically drains into the inferior vena cava (IVC) or sometimes into the portal vein or hepatic veins.

If the anomalous drainage is associated with right lung hypoplasia and hypoplastic pulmonary artery it is known as scimitar/venolobar or hypogenic lung syndrome.

The anomalous left upper lobe pulmonary vein commonly drains into the brachiocephalic or innominate vein through a vertical vein. The vertical vein is considered a remnant of the embryologic left cardinal system.

Treatment consists of redirection of the pulmonary veins into the left atrium and closure of any shunt defect if present.

22.8.2 Total Anomalous Pulmonary Venous Return (TAPVC)

In TAPVC all the pulmonary veins fail to connect to the left atrium and drain into RA or its tributaries through primitive fetal connections. Anatomic classification of TAPVC is based on the drainage site. The TAPVC cases have an early presentation with cyanosis and heart failure. Infracardiac type of TAPVC is commonly associated with obstruction [50, 51] (Figs. 22.12, 22.13, and 22.14; Table 22.2).

22.8.3 CT and MR Imaging: Where and Why

In cases of anomalous pulmonary venous drainage, the initial imaging modality is echocardiography. CT helps in the detection of anomalous pulmonary vein courses, site of drainage, and presence of any stenosis. CT accurately helps in their identification which is essential before surgery and it reduces the need for invasive catheter pulmonary angiography [53, 54]. MRI is not frequently used for evaluation of TAPVC in chil-

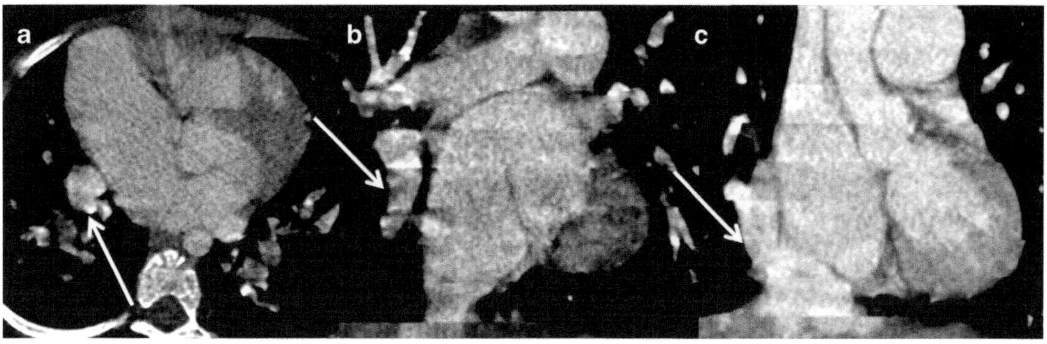

Fig. 22.12 (**a**–**c**) A 9-year-old boy with partial anomalous pulmonary venous drainage. The right-sided veins are forming a common chamber (white arrow) and draining into the RA–IVC junction

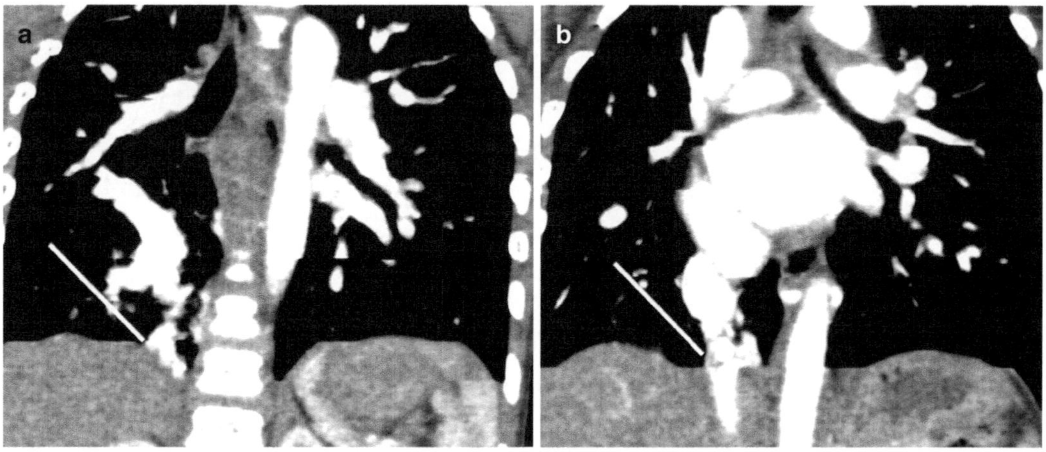

Fig. 22.13 A 3-year-old girl child with CT images (**a**, **b**) demonstrating anomalous Infradiaphragmatic PAPVC or scimitar vein (solid line) drainage into IVC consistent with PAPVC/Scimitar syndrome. (**c**, **d**) hypogenic right lung (arrow) with pulmonary artery hypoplasia (solid arrow) and dextroposition

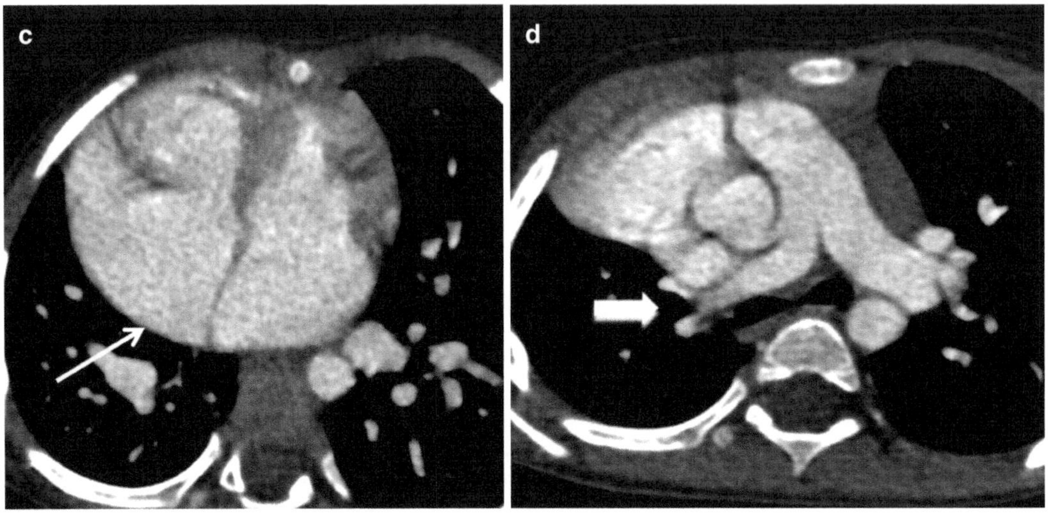

Fig. 22.13 (continued)

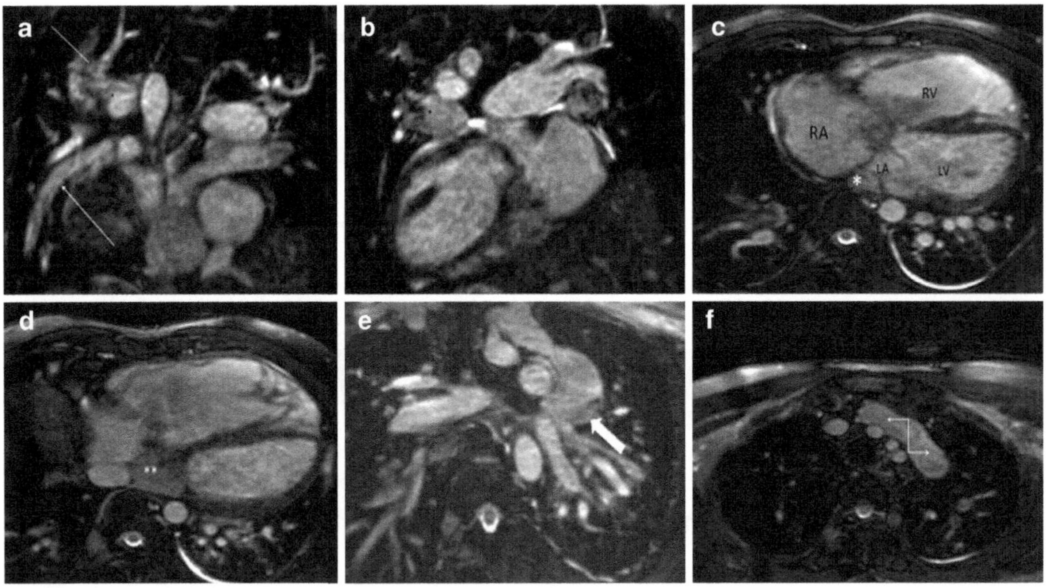

Fig. 22.14 Case demonstrating the utility of MRI for the evaluation of complex pulmonary vein abnormalities. Images (**a–c**) show right-sided pulmonary veins drain into a common chamber (asterisk). Image (**c** and **d**) which drains into the coronary sinus (double asterisk). The LA is small in size as there is no pulmonary vein communicating with the LA. Image (**e** and **f**) left sided pulmonary veins drain into a vertical vein. Solid arrow in Image (**f**) vertical vein draining into the left brachiocephalic vein (wedged double-headed arrow)

dren and neonates as they are adequately evaluated using echocardiography [55]. MRI can be used for PAPVC detection with the use of cine sequences and contrast MRA. The advantages of MRI over CT include functional assessment, flow quantification (*Q*p/*Q*s), and the ability to calculate differential flow to the lungs [56]. The importance of MR imaging is increasing in post-operative cases of PAPVC. Its multiplanar capabilities and SSFP cine images have good blood tissue contrast which helps in the assessment of the dimensions of the pulmonary vein orifice and

Table 22.2 Depicting types of total anomalous pulmonary venous drainage [52]

Type 1—Supra-cardiac—draining into right or left SVC
Type 2—Cardiac—draining into RA or coronary sinus
Type 3—Infra-cardiac—draining into IVC or its tributaries
Type 4—mixed type

to look for the presence of stenosis at the veno-atrial junction, ventricular function, and *Qp*/*Qs* quantification. The abovementioned advantages of CMR also apply to imaging in postoperative anomalous pulmonary vein repair, especially in infradiaphragmatic type which has a high chance of stenosis [56, 57].

22.8.3.1 Practical Pearls

Unexplained findings of pulmonary hypertension such as pulmonary artery dilation or right-sided cardiac chamber enlargement should prompt the radiologist to look for an occult PAPVC.

22.9 Tetralogy of Fallot (TOF)

Tetralogy of Fallot is one of the most common cyanotic congenital heart diseases with an incidence of 1 in 3000. It is associated with genetic abnormalities in about 25% of cases usually 22q1 deletion (DiGeorge Syndrome) or trisomy 21 (Down's syndrome) [58].

22.9.1 Anatomy

TOF results from the anterosuperior deviation of the conal septum. The characteristic anomalies are VSD, overriding aorta, RVOT obstruction (mild to severe obstruction of the RVOT and the pulmonary artery infundibulum with or without pulmonary atresia), and right ventricular hypertrophy.

The RVOT obstruction is in the form of infundibular stenosis (45% cases), isolated pulmonary valve abnormality (10%), a combination of infundibular stenosis and pulmonary valve abnormality (15%), and pulmonary valve atresia (15%). The pulmonary valve is abnormal in TOF cases and its involvement ranges from valve hypoplasia to valvular fusion resulting in stenosis and atresia [59, 60] (Figs. 22.15 and 22.16).

McGoon's ratio is the sum of the diameters of the RPA and LPA just proximal to the first-order bifurcation divided by the diameter of the aorta at the diaphragmatic hiatus. The normal ratio is within 2–2.5. This ratio can be accurately estimated using CT as this region of the pulmonary arteries is better visualized than on echocardiography. McGoon's ratio of greater than 1.5 is a prerequisite for surgical treatment of patients with TOF and pulmonary stenosis.

Nakata index is calculated by dividing the areas of the right and left pulmonary arteries by the BSA. Normal measurement is around 330 ± 30 mm/m^2. A Nakata index of >100–150 mm^2/m^2 is acceptable for complete repair without prior palliative shunt [61] (Fig. 22.17).

22.9.2 Associated Anomalies

Coronary artery anomalies are seen in 5% of cases and can be well assessed on CT [62]. The aortic root shows clockwise rotation in TOF. The LAD arising from the right coronary artery (RCA) is the most common anomaly associated with TOF. It can be confused with a large conus branch on angiography. The single coronary artery is the second most common associated anomaly. The anomalous coronary artery is at risk for injury during transannular repair of the right ventricular outflow tract or pulmonary artery infundibulum.

22.9.3 CT and MRI: When and Why

CT plays an important role in the preoperative imaging of TOF patients. The pulmonary arteries are visualized in excellent detail. Pulmonary artery abnormalities such as infundibular, valvular and supravalvular stenosis, hypoplasia, atresia, and absence are well visualized. The site and size of VSDs and the presence of anomalous coronary artery crossing the RVOT can be assessed.

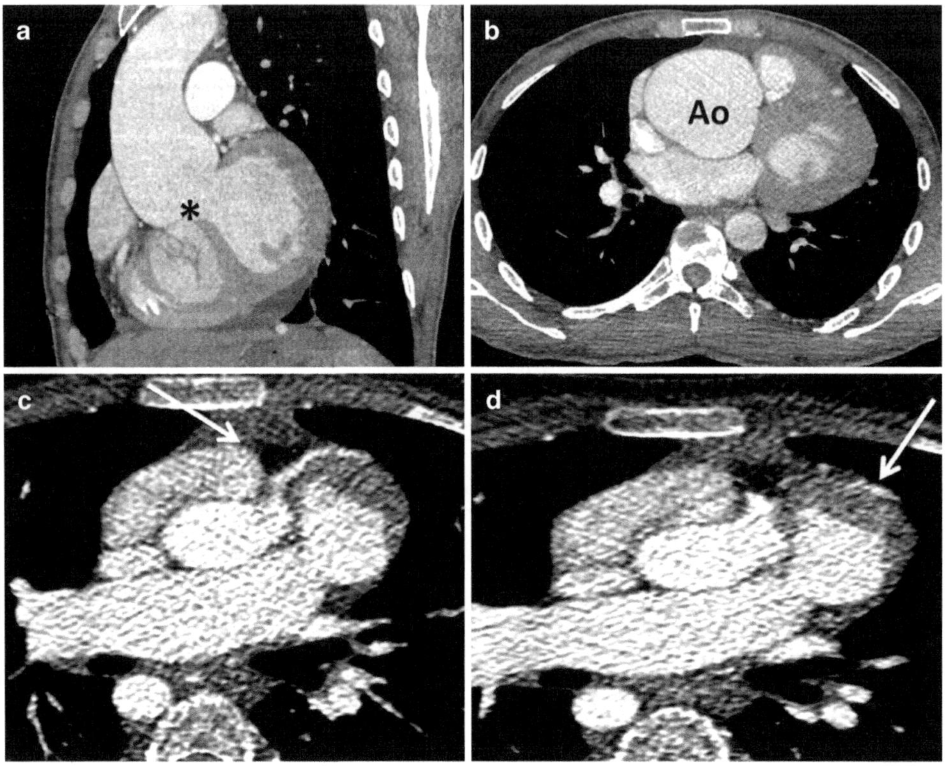

Fig. 22.15 Images demonstrating the utility of CT for the evaluation of the aortic root and coronary artery anatomy in TOF. (**a**, **b**) A 22-year-old male with TOF, perimembranous VSD, aortic override, and aortic root dilation. (**c**) A different case of TOF with an anomalous coronary artery course (arrow). There is an accessory LAD arising from the RCA crossing the RVOT

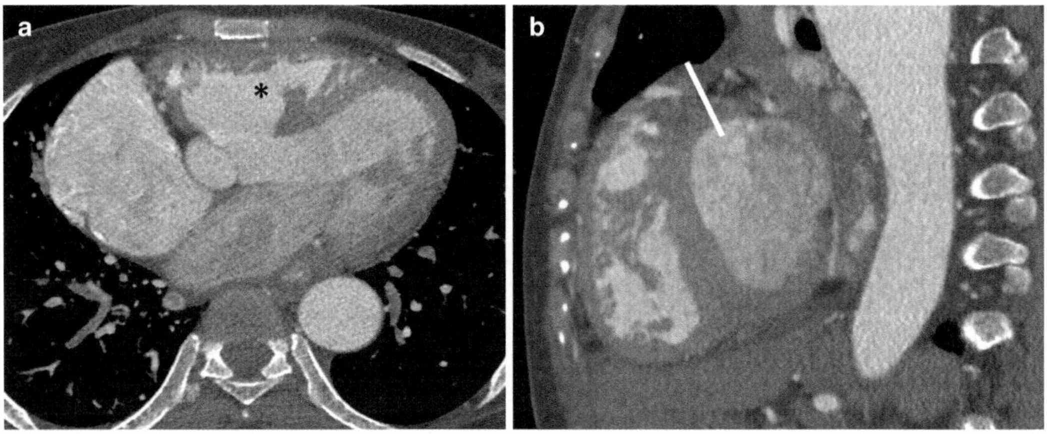

Fig. 22.16 Images demonstrating the utility of CT for the evaluation of pulmonary artery anatomy in TOF with pulmonary atresia. The images show RV hypertrophy (**a**), absent main pulmonary artery with infundibular stenosis and pulmonary atresia (solid white line) (**b**) subaortic perimembranous VSD with aortic override (double-headed arrow) (**c**). The branch pulmonary arteries are severely hypoplastic (**d**, **e**) LPA—arrow, RPA—wedged arrow). There are multiple MAPCAS supplying the lungs

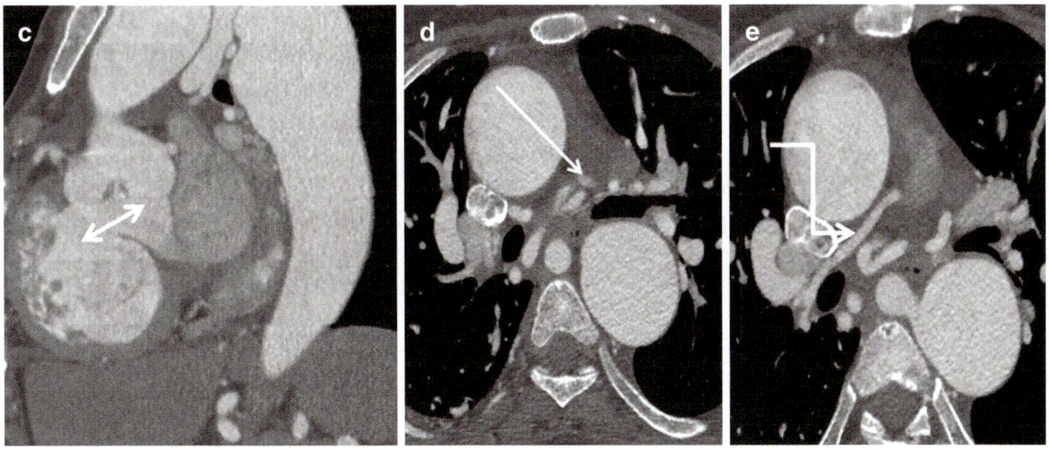

Fig. 22.16 (continued)

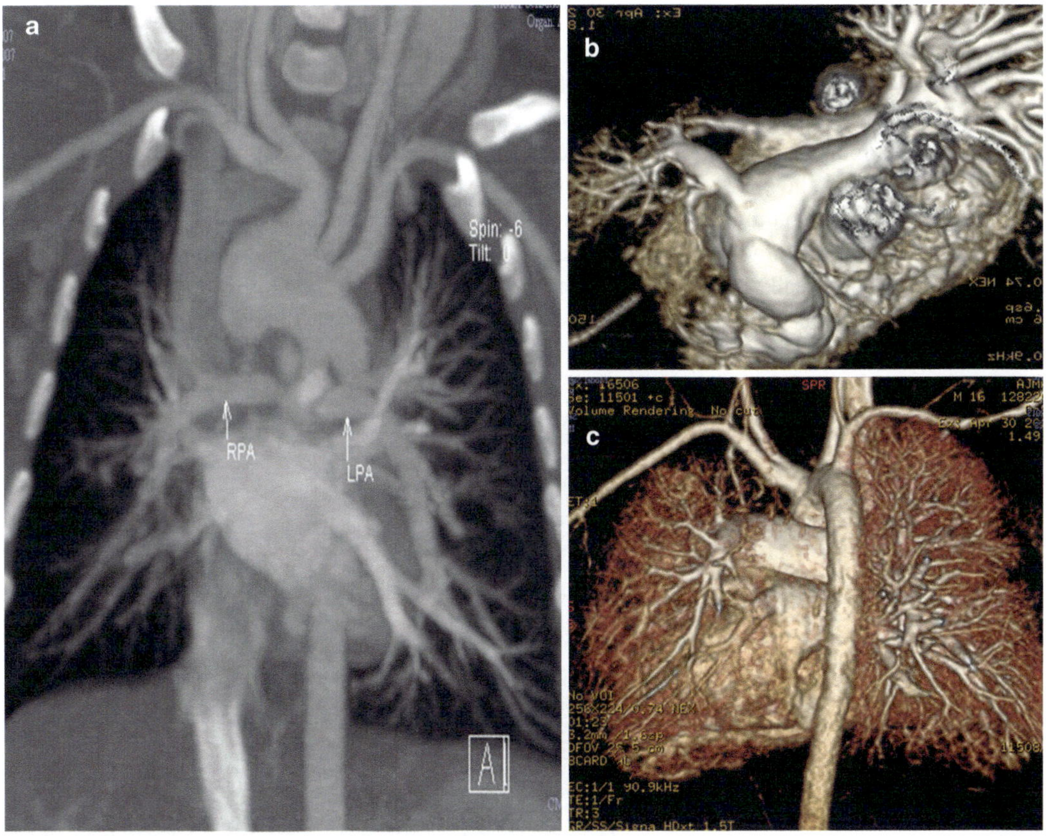

Fig. 22.17 (**a**) Lung arborization on CT versus MRI. (**a**) CTA shows poor arborization in the right lung in a case of pulmonary atresia. The annotated arrows also point to the position where RPA, LPA measurements are to be taken for calculation of McGoon's ratio. (**b**, **c**) MRA of another patient showing poor lung arborization on the left side due to LPA stenosis

CT has the added advantage of identifying major aortopulmonary collaterals (MAPCAs) and can identify their origin and course. This becomes important while planning for a unifocalization surgery. CT is proven to be effective in identifying MAPCA with less radiation compared to conventional catheter angiography [63].

22.9.4 CMR in TOF

The MR evaluation of TOF requires a comprehensive evaluation of the entire heart with a focus on the right ventricle and pulmonary valve. The RVOT is analyzed for stenosis and the pulmonary artery is analyzed for valve-sparing surgery. A perimembranous VSD is obligatory. RV volume quantification and pulmonary artery flow assessment and *Qp*/*Qs* calculation and aortic root assessment.

Echocardiography is the initial modality for the evaluation of postoperative TOF patients. MR screening is recommended starting in the adolescent age group due to the poor acoustic windows for the RV. Chronic pulmonary regurgitation leads to chronic RV volume overload, progressive dilation, and eventually irreversible dysfunction when compensatory mechanisms fail.

The most significant use of CMR in post-TOF repair is in the decision to insert a pulmonary valve which is based on measurements of pulmonary regurgitation, biventricular size, shunt ratio, and the presence of aneurysmal dilation of the RVOT.

Multiple studies have evaluated the RV end-diastolic volume (EDV) and RV end-systolic volume (ESV) in TOF with pulmonary valvular incompetence following complete corrective surgery. Various studies have defined RV volume thresholds which correspond to irreversible RV dysfunction. When these thresholds are exceeded, the RV function is unlikely to improve even after pulmonary valve replacement.

MRI is the current gold standard for RV volumetric measurement. RV volumes are quantified using the disc summation method (area of the RV in each slice multiplied by the slice thickness). This method avoids geometric assumptions and has good inter and intraobserver reliability.

Other complications that are associated with TOF surgery such as conduit stenosis, RVOT aneurysm, and residual VSDs can also be assessed with MRI [64, 65] (Figs. 22.18 and 22.19).

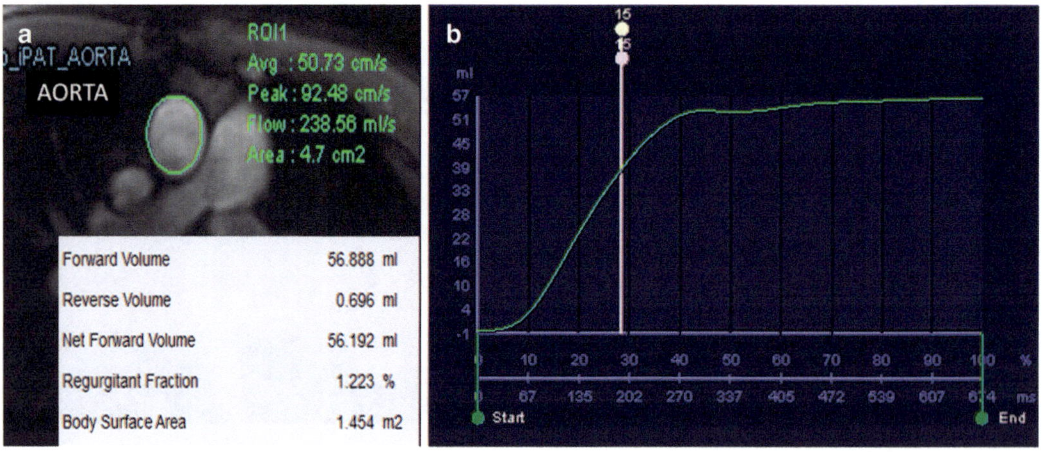

Fig. 22.18 CMR evaluation in post-op TOF. A 30-year-old female with TOF status post complete repair at 12 years of age, CMR with PC flow studies at the aorta and pulmonary artery. (**a**) Aortic flow quantified directly from the PA PC MRI for *Qp*/*Qs* evaluation. (**b**) Pulmonary regurgitation can be quantified directly from the PA PC MRI which demonstrates severe pulmonary regurgitation (regurgitant fraction >40%)

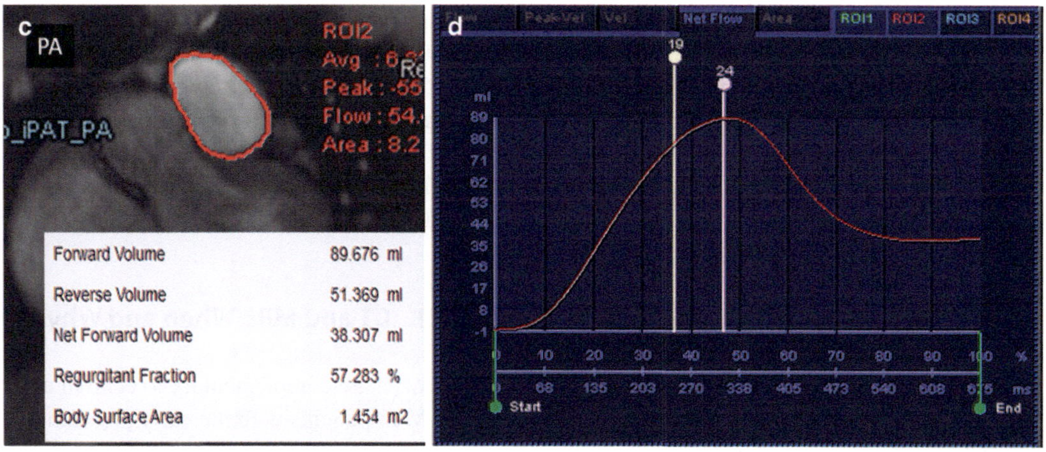

Fig. 22.18 (continued)

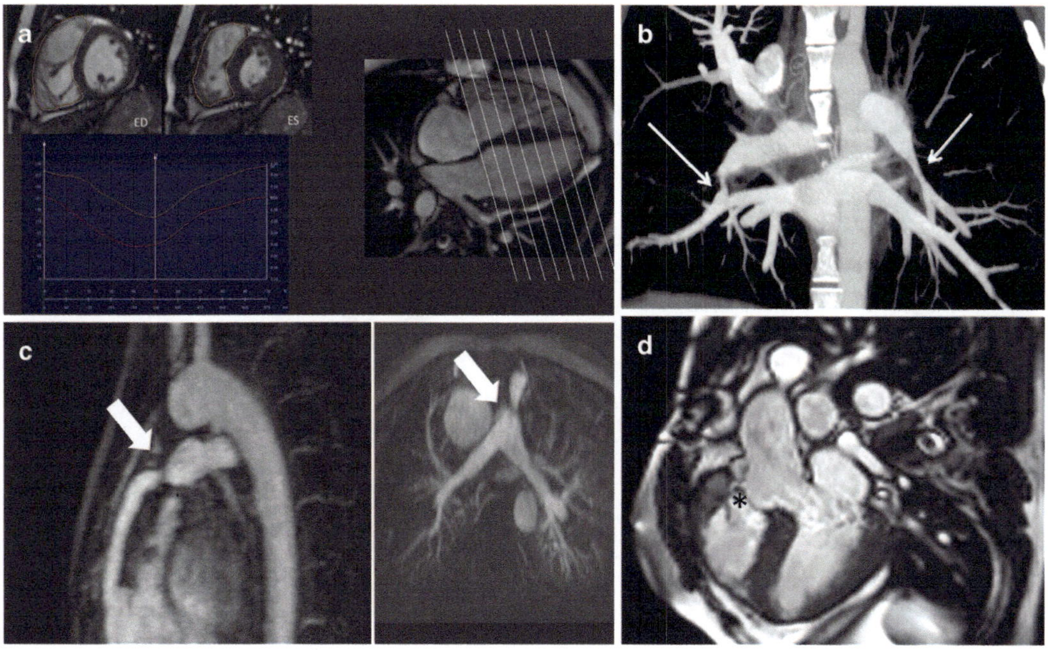

Fig. 22.19 CMR evaluation in post-op TOF. (**a**) demonstrating RV volumetry and contouring using the disc summation technique. (**b**) CT showing branch PA stenosis in an operated TOF patient. (**c**) MRA showing conduit stenosis (solid arrow) in operated TOF cases. (**d**) Turbulent flow across a small defect in a flaccid VSD patch is consistent with a recurrent VSD (asterisk) in operated TOF patients

22.9.5 Practical Pearls

CMR helps guide treatment either by surgical reconstruction of the pulmonary valve or by percutaneous primary pulmonary valve implantation. RVOT diameter can be measured on MRI and diameters ranging from 14 to 22 mm [66] are suitable for valve implantation. RVOT morphology and proximity of proximal coronary arteries to RVOT can also be assessed.

CMR helps in RV volumetry and quantification and helps in guiding treatment and the threshold limit of RVEDVi (end-diastolic volume index) ranges from 150 to 200 mL/m^2 depending on institutional and the surgeon's perspective.

22.10 Double-Outlet Ventricles: DORV

Double-outlet right ventricle (DORV) is a condition in which both the aorta and main pulmonary artery arise from the morphologic right ventricle. DORV is considered present when there is greater than 50% override of the aortic root over the ventricular septal defect (Fig. 22.20).

The pathophysiologic classification of DORV is based on defining the position of the VSD relative to the arrangement of the great arteries. The VSD can be of various types and the position of the VSD relative to the great vessels determines the clinical presentation [67, 68] (Figs. 22.21 and 22.22; Table 22.3).

22.10.1 CT and MRI: When and Why

CT and MRI are complementary to echo in cases of DORV. In patients with the early presentation, echo provides sufficient information. CT helps in

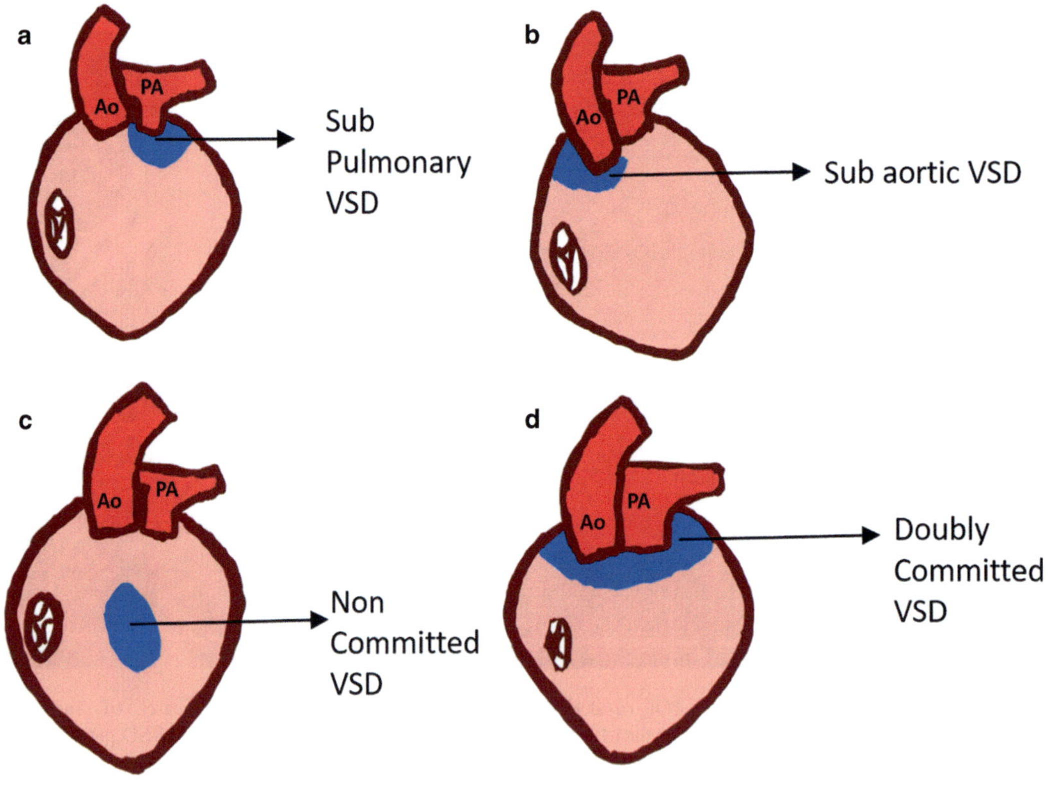

Fig. 22.20 Demonstrating various types of VSD and relative classification of DORV related to VSD. *Ao* Aorta, *PA* pulmonary artery. (**a**) sub-pulmonary, (**b**) sub-aortic, (**c**) noncommitted, (**d**) doubly committed VSD

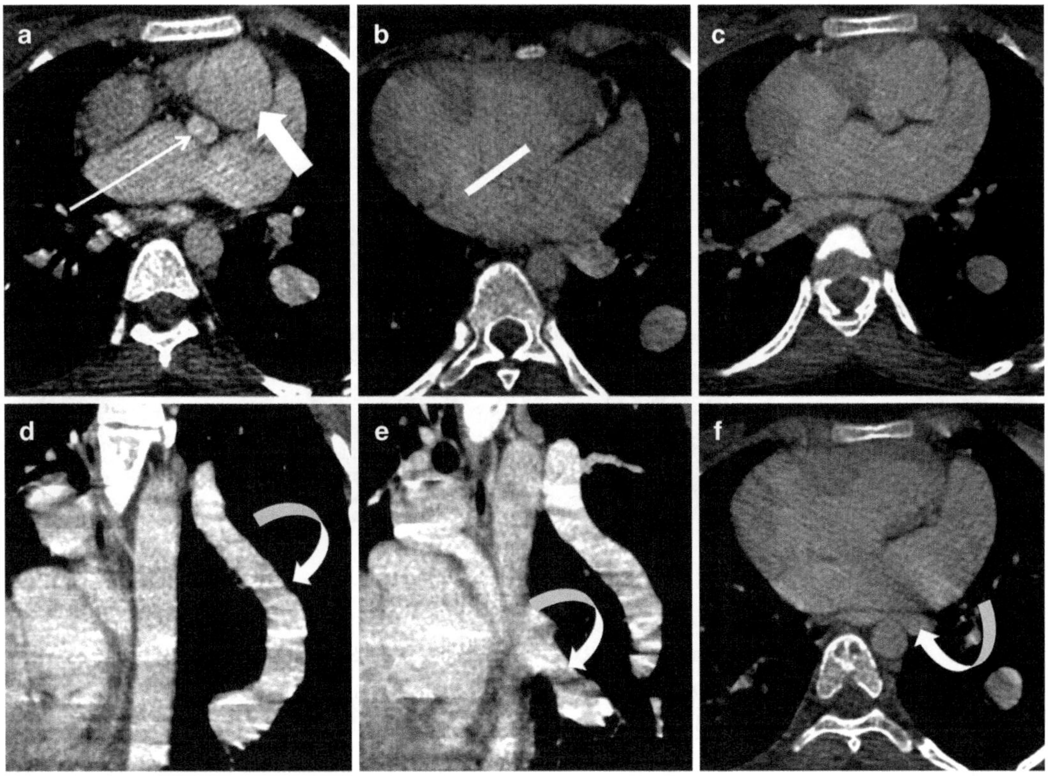

Fig. 22.21 Case of DORV with TAPVC. (**a**, **b**) CT images in a 10-year-old male show dextrocardia, DORV with aorta anterior and to the left of the pulmonary artery (long arrow) in keeping with L malposed aorta (solid arrow), pulmonary atresia (long arrow), and perimembranous VSD (solid line). (**c**–**f**) Supracardiac TAPVC right-sided pulmonary veins (asterisk) form a common chamber and pass posterior to the left atria to drain into the left SVC. The left superior and inferior pulmonary veins drain into the left SVC (asterisk)

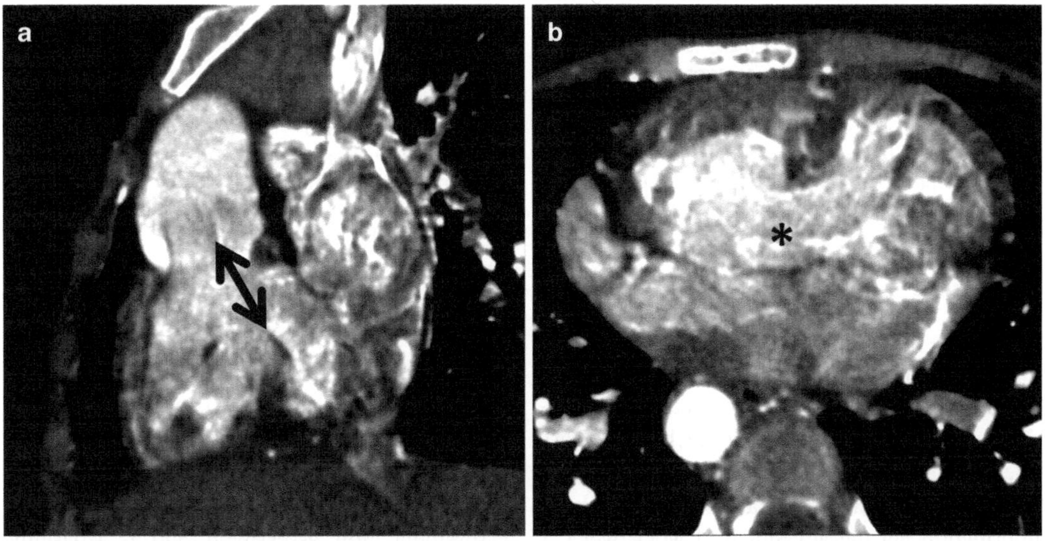

Fig. 22.22 (**a**–**d**) DORV with approximately 80% override (double-headed arrow) with perimembranous VSD (asterisk), OS ASD (solid line), and pulmonary atresia (single-head arrow)

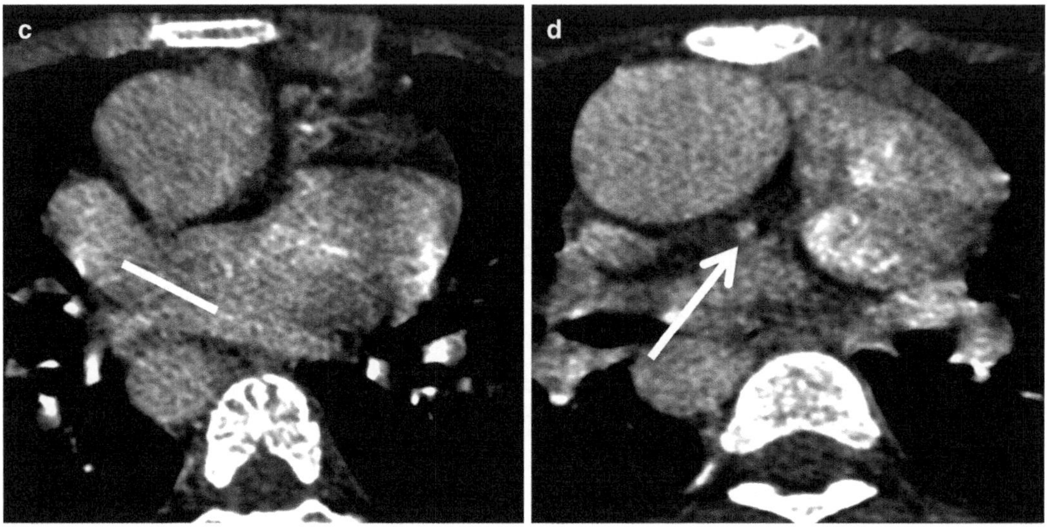

Fig. 22.22 (continued)

Table 22.3 Pathophysiologic classification of DORV—position relative to VSD and great artery relationship

Pathophysiologic classification of DORV—position relative to VSD and great artery relationship			
Subaortic	Subpulmonic	Doubly committed (immediately beneath the semilunar valves)	Noncommitted (remote from both semilunar valves)
Subaortic VSD-type (tetralogy of Fallot-type) DORV accounts for more than half of the DORV cases	Subpulmonary VSD-type DORV—this condition is also known as Taussig–Bing Anomaly and accounts for 30% of patients with DORV	Doubly committed VSD-type DORV occurs in about 10% of cases of DORV	Noncommitted or remote VSD-type DORV occurs in 10% of DORV cases
The great arteries are in normal anatomical relation with the aortic root posterior and to the right of the pulmonary artery origin	The great artery relationship is abnormal in these cases. Aorta is anterior and to right of pulmonary artery	The great arteries are in normal anatomical relationship	The great arteries are normally related
Pulmonary stenosis is present in these patients, and hence this physiology is similar to tetralogy of Fallot, where there is aortic override (more than 50%) into the right ventricle	If pulmonary stenosis is present then physiology represents TOF and if absent its similar to TGA	The LVOT is shared equally between aorta and pulmonary artery and the pathophysiology resembles that of a VSD	The physiology is similar to that of an isolated VSD or atrioventricular canal defect

the assessment of atrial and ventricular morphology, atrioventricular and ventriculoatrial connections, pulmonary artery and its branches, coronary artery anatomy, MAPCAs, and the relationship of the great vessels. MRI can provide the above information but the advantage of MRI over CT is its multiplanar nonconventional imaging plane capabilities where the dynamic relation between the great vessels and VSD can be assessed. In postoperative DORV patients, MR has the advantage of providing accurate ventricular volumetry, shunt quantification and baffle/conduit stenosis assessment, flow assessment, and as a baseline study for follow-up of RV function.

22.11 Transposition of Great Arteries (TGA)

Transposition of great arteries occurs due to embryologic defect involving the conotruncal septum with aorta arising from morphological RV and pulmonary artery arising from morphological LV. Looping of the heart refers to the configuration of the ventricles. D-looping refers to the normal folding of the embryonic heart tube with morphological RV to the right of the LV and L looping is an abnormal configuration where the morphological RV is to the left the LV.

22.11.1 D-TGA (Ventriculoarterial Discordance, Atrioventricular Concordance)

D-TGA occurs due to abnormal conotruncal rotation. The aorta is to the right and anterior to the pulmonary artery. There is D-looping. This results in the aorta arising from morphological RV and the pulmonary artery arising from the morphological LV. The atrioventricular concordance is maintained resulting in a parallel orientation of the systemic and pulmonary circulations. A shunt is necessary for survival.

22.11.2 L-TGA or ccTGA (Atrioventricular and Ventriculoarterial Discordance: Double Discordance)

In L-TGA, the aorta is toward the left and anterior to the PA. There are L-loop configurations of the ventricles. The aorta arises from the RV and the pulmonary artery arises from the LV. The RA is in communication with morphological LV and the LA with the RV. The pulmonary veins drain into the LA. Thus, the end result is ventriculoarterial and atrioventricular discordance.

In simple transposition, there is a small shunt such as a PDA/PFO in more than half of the cases. Complex transposition is associated with other anomalies and consists of a large PDA, ASD, VSD, or coarctation, etc. This becomes important in medical and surgical treatment for the patients with TGA with VSD/ASD/LVOT obstruction and pulmonary atresia [69, 70]. Using a multimodality approach will avoid misdiagnosis.

22.11.3 Surgical Modalities in TGA

Atrial Baffle Procedure It comprises of Senning or Mustard procedure and consists of removal of the interatrial septum and creation of a conduit that directs blood from the SVC and IVC to the left atrium and pulmonary venous return to the right atrium.

Arterial Switch Procedure (ASO/ASP) The main pulmonary artery is anastomosed to the previous aortic root and aorta is anastomosed to the pulmonary artery root following the creation of a neo aorta after the coronary ostia are transected and implanted in the main pulmonary artery root.

Rastelli Procedure A conduit is placed between the LV and aorta through the VSD and between the RV and the pulmonary artery. It is generally done in TGA patients with RVOT obstruction [69, 70].

22.11.4 CT and MRI: When and Why

Morphological evaluation of TGA can be done using either CT or MRI. D-TGA patients present in the neonatal period when echo has a good window and provides accurate information for treatment. CT is used for the morphological analysis of the ventricles, relation of the great vessels, and identifying coronary artery anomalies. CT also has the advantage of identifying other associated abnormalities.

In cases of L-TGA, the majority present in adulthood. The RV supports the systemic circulation for a long time but eventually results in failure when compensatory mechanisms fail. MRI has an important role in quantifying ventricular

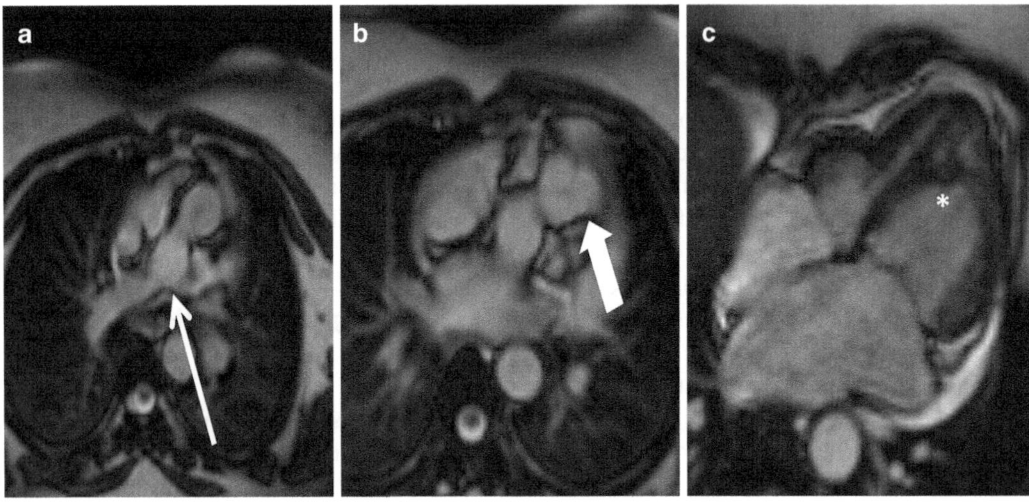

Fig. 22.23 Images (**a–c**) MR Axial HASTE and cine images in a 39-year-old female with atrioventricular and ventriculoarterial discordance, morphological RV (asterisk) is to the left of morphological LV, altered relation of the aorta [thin arrow in (**b**)] and pulmonary artery [thin arrow in (**a**)] with aorta anterior and to left of the pulmonary artery in keeping with corrected TGA (ccTGA)

function, AV valve regurgitation, and in morphological assessment (Fig. 22.23).

22.12 Post-surgical TGA

The main role of CT and MR imaging in postoperative TGA is to first identify the complex anatomy following the surgical procedure as an adjunct to information available on echo.

Following Mustard and Senning procedures, CT and MRI both help in identifying the site of baffle stenosis. Leaks have a risk of paradoxical embolism. MRI has the advantage of quantification of stenosis using PC imaging and also helps in identifying collateral pathways in patients with chronic venous stenosis [69, 70]. The RV supports the systemic circulation in these patients and functional deterioration, hypertrophy, and scarring can occur in the long run [71].

After arterial switch procedure, CT and MRI help in identifying obstruction of the pulmonary arteries and RVOT as they are positioned immediately behind the sternum making echocardiographic evaluation difficult. Dilation of the aortic annulus and neo-aortic root may be seen after surgery and may result in regurgitation [72]. MRI has the added advantage of ventricular volume quantification. Specifically, RV volumetry by MRI is very accurate and can be used as a baseline for follow-up studies (Fig. 22.24).

22.12.1 Ebstein's Anomaly

Ebstein anomaly is defined by the apical displacement of the tricuspid annulus into the right ventricle exceeding 8 mm/m^2 with reference to the mitral valve base plane. The posterior and septal leaflet is hypoplastic and thickened. The anterior leaflet is fenestrated. This apical displacement results in the separation of RV into two parts. The atrialized (aRV) and functional RV (fRV) can be differentiated based on the presence of trabeculations in the functional RV.

22.12.2 CT and MRI: When and Why

The accurate assessment of the morphology of the tricuspid valve, leaflets, chordal attachments, and tricuspid valve is possible on echocardiography [73]. MRI is indicated with the echo window is poor especially in older individuals.

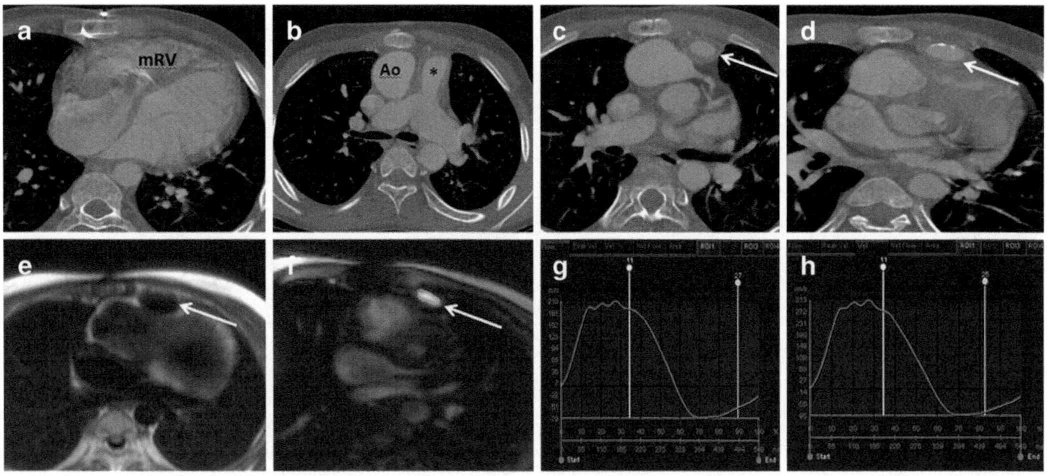

Fig. 22.24 MRI assessment in postoperative TGA. Images (**a**–**d**) demonstrate a 13-year-old male with ventriculoarterial discordance. The aorta to the right of the pulmonary artery (asterisk). CT imaging performed post Rastelli procedure shows mild narrowing of the RV–PA conduit in its mid portion. Images (**e**–**h**) MRI has the added advantage of morphological and functional imaging and revealed an elevated peak systolic velocity (343 cm/s) within conduit confirming the presence of stenosis although the conduit appears wide on CT

The main uses of CMR in Ebstein are the accurate quantification of RV function and volume. The fRV and aRV volumes can be quantified separately. The use of axial stack bSSFP cine images may be preferred over the routine short-axis cine images which are used for LV volumetry as the former has a better interobserver agreement. The axial planes provide a better depiction of tricuspid valve displacement and leaflet coaptation. The role of CMR in Ebstein's is presently not completely defined with very few published studies [74].

CMR has the advantage of providing a morphological, functional evaluation of heart and assessment of tricuspid regurgitation. Shunt quantification can be done in the presence of associated septal defects. CMR helps in determining the Carpentier classification of the type of Ebstein's depending on the atrialized and functional RV volumes as well as tricuspid leaflet morphology.

22.12.3 Carpentier Classification [75]

- Type A: The right ventricular volume is adequate.
- Type B: The atrialized right ventricle is large with a freely moving anterior leaflet of the tricuspid valve.
- Type C: The movement of the anterior leaflet of the tricuspid valve is severely restricted and can cause significant RV obstruction.
- Type D: There is near total atrialization of the right ventricle with a small infundibular component of RV.

The tricuspid regurgitation is quantified by the following formula and can be used when there is no associated shunt [76].

$$\text{TR volume} = \text{RV stroke volume} - \text{Qp}(\text{pulmonary artery forward flow}).$$

CT is used as an adjunct to CMR if there is a contraindication to CMR. The protocoling requires targeted opacification of right-sided chambers with ECG gating and is practically a good method for morphological evaluation of valvular anatomy, ventricular and atrial chambers, and other associated abnormalities (Fig. 22.25).

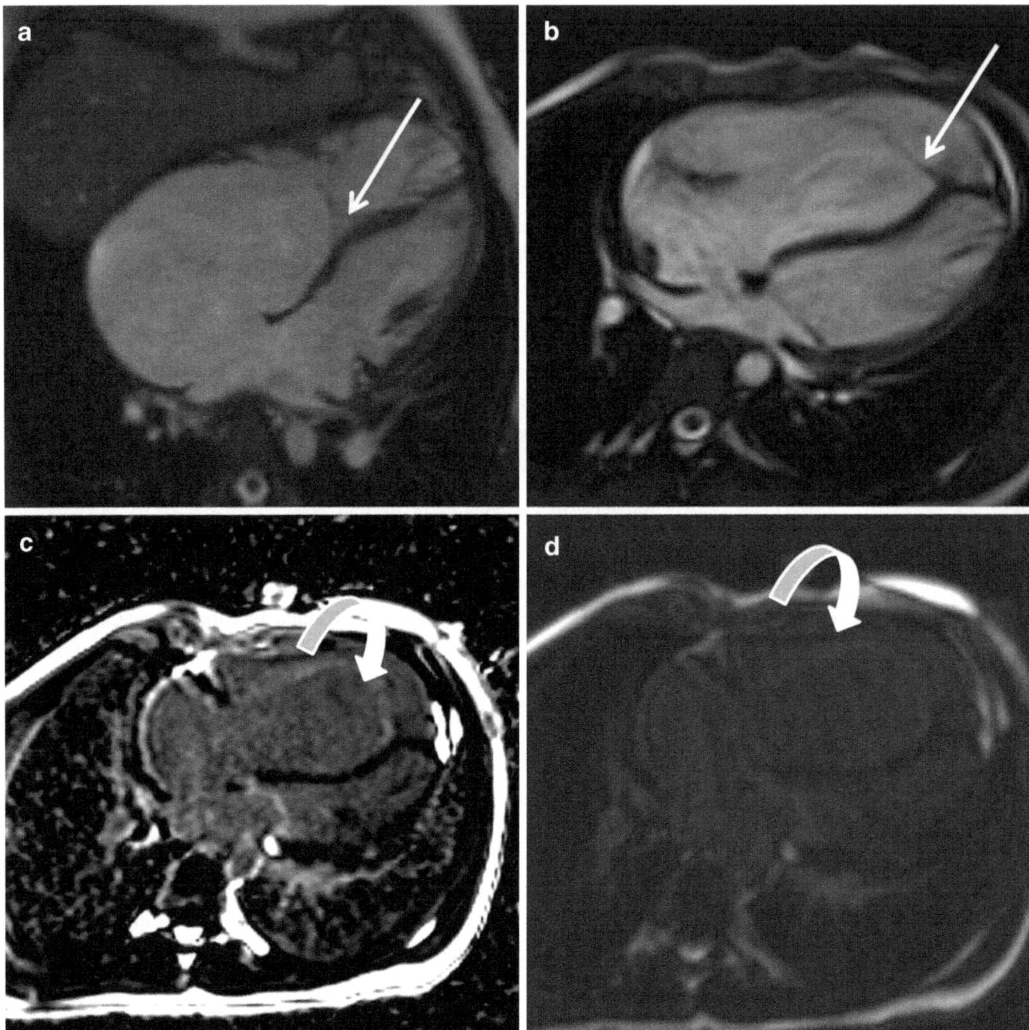

Fig. 22.25 (**a**) Ebstein's anomaly in a 15-year-old male with the apical displacement of the septal leaflet of the tricuspid valve and atrialization of the right ventricle (arrow). The atrialized RV is smooth whereas the functional RV has a trabeculated appearance. (**b**) A 10-year-old with severe Ebstein's anomaly. Phase image (**c**) and magnitude image (**d**) of LGE images showing enhancement (curved arrow) of the dysplastic endocardium in aRV

22.12.4 Practical Pearls

CMR is complimentary to echo and is used for the evaluation of RV quantification and apical displacement of the tricuspid valve. For serial examinations, volumetry should be done in the same plane (axial or short axis) as the previous study.

22.13 Coarctation of Aorta (CoA)

Coarctation of the aorta is a focal discrete narrowing in the aorta just distal to the origin of the left subclavian artery, the previous classification of pre-ductal and post-ductal is not being used currently. The cause of aortic coarctation is unknown but multiple causative factors are implicated ranging from genetic factors, altered fetal hemodynamics, and persistent fetal tissue at the ductus. Most of the cases of aortic coarctation are sporadic; however, a clear genetic predisposition is noted with approximately 4% cases showing associated congenital heart diseases ranging from VSD to hypoplastic heart disease, bicuspid aortic valve being the most common association [77].

The indications for intervention in CoA is the presence of a gradient across the obstruction of more than 20 mmHg and the presence of LV dysfunction even if the gradient is less than 20 mmHg [78] (Figs. 22.26 and 22.27).

22.13.1 CT and MRI: When and Why

MDCT has revolutionized aorta imaging due to the fast imaging times and multiplanar capabilities of modern scanners which provide an accurate anatomical evaluation of the aorta. Bolus tracking techniques helps in proper timing on the contrast bolus to achieve adequate luminal opacification. ECG gating helps in aortic root evaluation which is plagued by artifacts due to cardiac pulsation on non-gated scans. Faster gantry rotation time, wider Z-axis coverage reduce the need for sedation in pediatric cases and provide accurate identification of collaterals. The main concern for use of CT is the radiation dose as multiple examinations may be required; however, with use of high pitch CT and state of the art scanners, the radiation dose may even be lowered to sub-millisievert levels [79].

MRI with the use of black blood, 3D bSSFP non-contrast angiography and cine images can demonstrate the aorta, site of obstruction, and collaterals without the need for contrast agent administration. Contrast-enhanced MRA is the most commonly used technique due to the ease

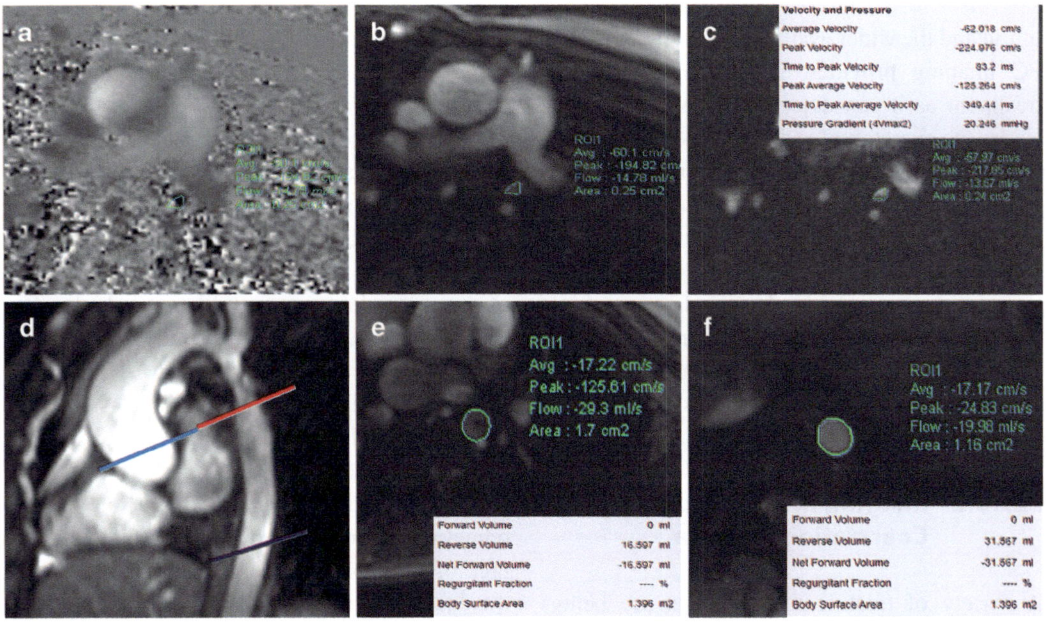

Fig. 22.26 Images demonstrating the utility of MRI in aortic coarctation. (**a–c**) PC images at the level of the coarctation showing measurement of the peak systolic velocity and pressure gradient. In this case, the gradient is 20 mmHg consistent with a hemodynamically significant stenosis. (**d–f**) Collateral flow assessment in a case of CoA is performed by acquiring PC MRI images at levels just below the coarctation and distal to coarctation at the level of the diaphragm. Collateral flow is then calculated by subtracting the flow in the proximal slice just distal to coarctation (red line) from the distal slice (violet line). A cine or phase-contrast image in the short-axis plane of the aortic valve (blue line) is also routinely obtained to assess for bicuspid aortic valve and associated regurgitation or stenosis

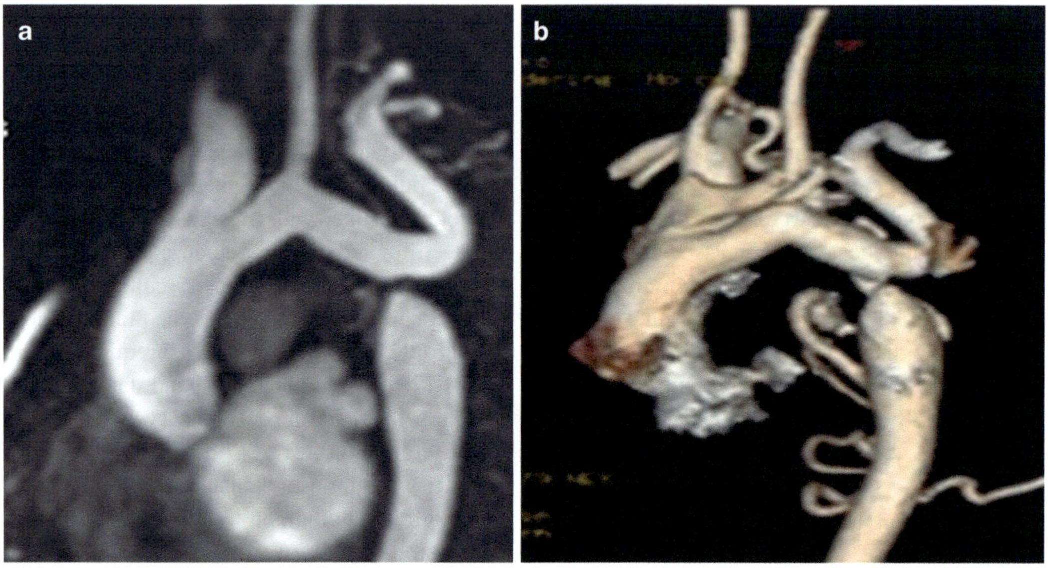

Fig. 22.27 (**a**, **b**) MRA with MPR showing Type A Interrupted aortic arch (IAA) and severe CoA have a similar presentation and hallmark of aortic interruption is a complete absence of continuity between the two segments of the aorta and in IAA the arch is small in caliber and post-stenotic dilation is seen in CoA

of use and the wider availability of this sequence. PC imaging provides information in guiding treatment as it can detect the pressure gradient across the coarctation and can help in calculating the volume of collateral circulation by subtracting the flow in the proximal descending aorta from the distal aorta [80]. Contrast-enhanced MRA is the preferred modality for follow-up because the patients need to undergo multiple studies after treatment where the radiation dose is a concern. But MRI cannot be used to assess the stented segment due to artifacts.

22.13.2 Imaging in Repaired Coarctation of Aorta

A variety of treatment approaches are beings used for coarctation ranging from resection with end to end anastomosis, patch aortoplasty, bypass graft insertion at the site of coarctation, endovascular balloon angioplasty repair, and stenting.

The long-term postoperative complications of CoA are hypertension, recoarctation, aneurysm at the site of intervention, or in the ascending aorta. Associated long-term sequelae are coronary artery disease, or result from bicuspid aortic valve, mitral valve anomalies, infective endocarditis, or cerebral aneurysms.

Recurrent coarctation and aneurysm formation at the postoperative site are the common complications post repair. Aneurysm can result from associated inherent aortic wall abnormality, bicuspid aortic valve, and hypertension. The risk of aneurysmal rupture and dilation is high when the ratio of the caliber of the dilated aorta and diaphragmatic aorta is more than 1.5. There is also a higher risk associated with bicuspid valve and turner syndrome. Hence, there is an increased need for long-term surveillance in these patients. CT and MR both play an important role in periodical evaluation but MR has the added advantage of functional hemodynamic evaluation and the lack of ionizing radiation. The use of 3D MRA has improved the spatial resolution for a detailed evaluation of aorta and its branches [81, 82] (Fig. 22.28).

According to the 2008 AHA/ACC guidelines [83]:

The postoperative coarctation patients need long-term follow-up and need to be monitored for the following:

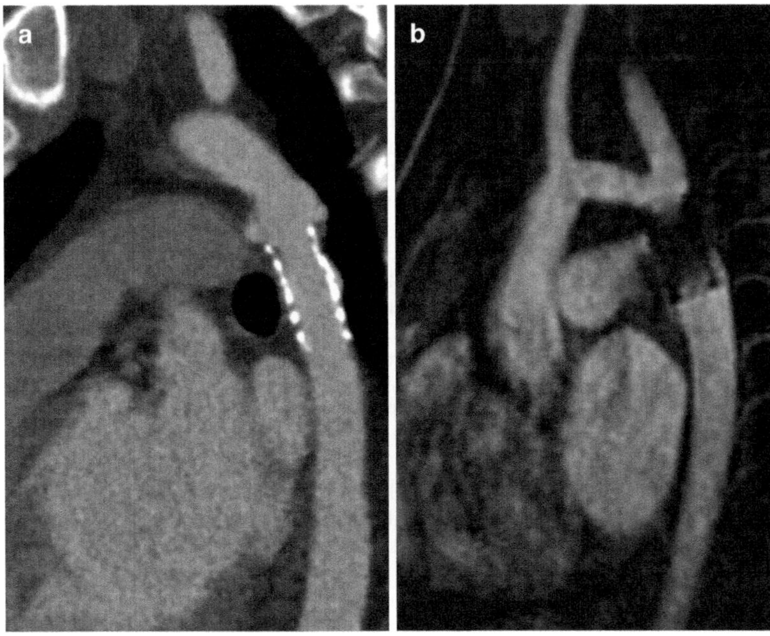

Fig. 22.28 (**a**) CTA shows patent post-coarctation stent very well, but MRA (**b**) shows loss of signal inside the stent due to metal artifact

- Periodical evaluation for systemic hypertension.
- Evaluation of the repair site by Echo, CT, or MR performed within an interval period of less than 5 years.
- Periodical echo evaluation for bicuspid aortic valve, ascending aortic dimensions, and ventricular function.
- Periodical evaluation for berry aneurysms in the brain as there is an increased prevalence of aneurysms in these patients compared to the normal population.
- Endocarditis prophylaxis in patients with a previous history of endocarditis, conduit placement, or for a period of 6 months in cases where prosthetic graft material or stent was used.

22.14 Conclusion

The more widespread availability of CT and MRI has led to increased utilization and acceptance of these modalities among the clinical community. Although echocardiography remains the first-line investigation in most patients, CT and MRI are more often used as a problem-solving modality when there are unanswered questions. For example, echocardiography may pick up a dilated right ventricle raising suspicion for an ASD or PAPVR. This may lead to a TEE, CT, or an MRI which can better delineate pulmonary venous return and sinus venosus defects. In case a shunt is not identified other causes for right ventricular dilation can be well assessed with CT or MRI. These include pulmonary hypertension, organic tricuspid valve disease, and right ventricular cardiomyopathy which are not easily assessed by echocardiography. Echocardiography, CT, and MRI have emerged as complementary and not competitive imaging modalities. A multimodality imaging approach will result in reduced resource cost, avoid unnecessary invasive procedures, and improve patient care.

References

1. Saxena A, Mehta A, Sharma M, Salhan S, Kalaivani M, Ramakrishnan S, Juneja R. Birth prevalence of congenital heart disease: a cross-sectional observational study from North India. Ann Pediatr Card. 2016;9:205–9.
2. Liu Y, Chen S, Liesl Zhan S, Kalaivani M, Ramakrishnan S, Juneja R, Keavney BD. Global birth

prevalence of congenital heart defects 1970–2017: updated systematic review and meta-analysis of 260 studies. Int J Epidemiol. 2019;48(2):455.
3. Ranganath P, Singh S, Abbara S, Agarwal PP, Rajiah P. Computed tomography in adult congenital heart disease. Radiol Clin North Am. 2019;57(1):85.
4. O'Leary JM, Siddiqi OK, de Ferranti S, Landzberg MJ, Opotowsky AR. The changing demographics of congenital heart disease hospitalizations in the United States, 1998 through 2010. JAMA. 2013;309(10):984–6. https://doi.org/10.1001/jama.2013.564.
5. Saremi F. Cardiac CT and MR for adult congenital heart disease. New York: Springer; 2014. p. 23p.
6. Rajiah P, Tandon A, Greil G, Abbara S. Update on the role of cardiac magnetic resonance imaging in congenital heart disease. Curr Treat Options Cardiovasc Med. 2017;19:1. https://doi.org/10.1007/s11936-017-0504-z.
7. Glatz AC, Purrington KS, Klinger A, et al. Cumulative exposure to medical radiation for children requiring surgery for congenital heart disease. J Pediatr. 2014;164:789–794.e10.
8. Machida H, Tanaka I, Fukui R, Shen Y, Ishikawa T, Tate E, Ueno E. Current and novel imaging techniques in coronary CT. Radiographics. 2015;35(4):991–1010.
9. Lin E, Alessio A. What are the basic concepts of temporal, contrast, and spatial resolution in cardiac CT? J Cardiovasc Comput Tomogr. 2009;3(6):40303. https://doi.org/10.1016/j.jcct.2009.07.003.
10. Mahesh M, Cody DD. Physics of cardiac imaging with multiple-row detector CT. Radiographics. 2007;27(5):1495–509. https://doi.org/10.1148/rg.275075045.
11. Raman SP, Mahesh M, Blasko RV, Fishman EK. CT scan parameters and radiation dose: practical advice for radiologists. J Am Coll Radiol. 2013;10:840–6.
12. Goo HW. Image quality and radiation dose of high-pitch dual-source spiral cardiothoracic computed tomography in young children with congenital heart disease: comparison of non-electrocardiography synchronization and prospective electrocardiography triggering. Korean J Radiol. 2018;19(6):1031.
13. Chelliah A, Shah AM, Farooqi KM, et al. Cardiovascular CT in cyanotic congenital heart disease. Curr Cardiovasc Imaging Rep. 2019;12:30. https://doi.org/10.1007/s12410-019-9507-3.
14. Goo HW. State-of-the-art CT imaging techniques for congenital heart disease. Korean J Radiol. 2010;11(1):4.
15. Goo HW, Park IS, Ko JK, Kim YH, Seo DM, Park JJ. Computed tomography for the diagnosis of congenital heart disease in pediatric and adult patients. Int J Cardiovasc Imaging. 2005;21(2-3):347–65.
16. Yang DH, Goo HW, Seo DM, Yun TJ, Park JJ, Park IS, Ko JK, Kim YH. Multislice CT angiography of interrupted aortic arch. Pediatr Radiol. 2008;38(1):89–100. https://doi.org/10.1007/s00247-007-0662-3.
17. Han Y, Kelly B, et al. Computed tomography imaging in patients with congenital heart disease, part 2: technical recommendations. An expert consensus document of the Society of Cardiovascular Computed Tomography (SCCT). J Cardiovasc Comput Tomogr. 2015;9(6):493.
18. Saremi F. Cardiac CT and MR for adult congenital heart disease. New York: Springer; 2014. p. 89p.
19. Bogaert J, Dymarkowski S, Taylor AM, Muthurangu V. Clinical cardiac MRI. Berlin: Springer; 2012. p. 1–29p.
20. Ridgway JP. Cardiovascular magnetic resonance physics for clinicians: part I. J Cardiovasc Magn Reson. 2010;12:71. https://doi.org/10.1186/1532-429X-12-71.
21. Krishnam MS, Tomasian A, Malik S, Singhal A, Sassani A, Laub G, Finn JP, Ruehm S. Three-dimensional imaging of pulmonary veins by a novel steady-state free-precession magnetic resonance angiography technique without the use of intravenous contrast agent: initial experience. Invest Radiol. 2009;44(8):447–53. https://doi.org/10.1097/RLI.0b013e3181a7c6cb.
22. Lotz J, Meier C, Leppert A, Galanski M. Cardiovascular flow measurement with phase-contrast MR imaging: basic facts and implementation. Radiographics. 2002;22:651–71.
23. Babu-Narayan S, Kilner PJ, Li W, Moon JC, Goktekin O, Davlouros PA, Khan M, Ho SY, Pennell DJ, Gatzoulis MA. Ventricular fibrosis suggested by cardiovascular magnetic resonance in adults with repaired tetralogy of fallot and its relationship to adverse markers of clinical outcome. Circulation. 2006;113(3):405–13.
24. Steeden JA, Pandya B, Tann O, et al. Free breathing contrast-enhanced time-resolved magnetic resonance angiography in pediatric and adult congenital heart disease. J Cardiovasc Magn Reson. 2015;17:38. https://doi.org/10.1186/s12968-015-0138-9.
25. Syed M, Raman SV, Simonetti OP. Basic principles of cardiovascular MRI. London: Springer; 2015. 284p. https://doi.org/10.1007/978-3-319-22141-0.
26. Fratz S, Chung T, et al. Guidelines and protocols for cardiovascular magnetic resonance in children and adults with congenital heart disease: SCMR expert consensus group on congenital heart disease. J Cardiovasc Magn Reson. 2013;15:51.
27. Biglino G, Koniordou D, Gasparini M, et al. Piloting the use of patient-specific cardiac models as a novel tool to facilitate communication during clinical consultations. Pediatr Cardiol. 2017;38:813–8.
28. Biglino G, Capelli C, Koniordou D, et al. Use of 3D models of congenital heart disease as an education tool for cardiac nurses. Congenit Heart Dis. 2017;12:113–8.
29. Costello JP, Olivieri LJ, Su L, et al. Incorporating three-dimensional printing into a simulation-based congenital heart disease and critical care training curriculum for resident physicians. Congenit Heart Dis. 2015;10:185–90.
30. Jones TW, Seckeler MD. Use of 3D models of vascular rings and slings to improve resident education. Congenit Heart Dis. 2017;12:578–82.

31. Bhatla P, Tretter JT, Ludomirsky A, et al. Utility and scope of rapid prototyping in patients with complex muscular ventricular septal defects or double-outlet right ventricle: does it alter management decisions? Pediatr Cardiol. 2017;38:103–14.
32. Valverde I, Gomez-Ciriza G, Hussain T, et al. Three-dimensional printed models for surgical planning of complex congenital heart defects: an international multicenter study. Eur J Cardiothorac Surg. 2017;52:1139–48.
33. Zhao L, Zhou S, Fan T, Li B, Liang W, Dong H. Three-dimensional printing enhances preparation for repair of double outlet right ventricular surgery. J Card Surg. 2018;33:24–7.
34. Garekar S, Bharati A, Chokhandre M, et al. Clinical application and multidisciplinary assessment of three dimensional printing in double outlet right ventricle with remote ventricular septal defect. World J Pediatr Congenit Heart Surg. 2016;7:344–50.
35. Cantinotti M, Valverde I, Kutty S. Three-dimensional printed models in congenital heart disease. Int J Cardiovasc Imaging. 2017;33:137–44.
36. Meier LM, Meineri M, Qua Hiasen J, Horlick EM. Structural and congenital heart disease interventions: the role of three-dimensional printing. Neth Heart J. 2017;25:65–75.
37. Huff TJ, Ludwig PE, Zuniga JM. The potential for machine learning algorithms to improve and reduce the cost of 3-dimensional printing for surgical planning. Expert Rev Med Devices. 2018;15:349–56.
38. Debl K, Djavidani B, Buchner S, et al. Quantification of left-to-right shunting in adult congenital heart disease: phase-contrast cine MRI compared with invasive oximetry. Br J Radiol. 2009;82(977):386–91. https://doi.org/10.1259/bjr/18500608.
39. Rajiah P, Kanne JP. Computed tomography of septal defects. J Cardiovasc Comput Tomogr. 2010;4(4):231–45. https://doi.org/10.1016/j.jcct.2010.05.005.
40. Nicolay S, Salgado RA, Shivalkar B, Van Herck PL, Vrints C, Parizel PM. CT imaging features of atrioventricular shunts: what the radiologist must know. Insights Imaging. 2016;7(1):119–29. https://doi.org/10.1007/s13244-015-0452-7.
41. Messe SR, Silverman IE, Kizer JR, Homma S, Zahn C, Gronseth G, Kasner SE. Quality Standards Subcommittee of the American Academy of Neurology.Practice parameter: recurrent stroke with patent foramen ovale and atrial septal aneurysm: report of the Quality Standards Subcommittee of the American Academy of Neurology. Neurology. 2004;62(7):1042–50.
42. Johri AM, Rojas CA, El-Sherief A, et al. Imaging of atrial septal defects: echocardiography and CT correlation. Heart. 2011;97:1441–53. https://doi.org/10.1136/hrt.2010.205732.
43. Geva T, Martins JD, Wald RM. Atrial septal defects. Lancet. 2014;383(9932):1921–32. https://doi.org/10.1016/S0140-6736(13)62145-5.
44. Yasunaga D, Hamon M. MDCT of interatrial septum. Diagn Interv Imaging. 2015;96(9):891–9.
45. Mazur W, Siegel MJ, Miszalski-Jamka T, Pelberg R. CT atlas of adult congenital heart disease. London: Springer; 2013. p. 106–8. https://doi.org/10.1007/978-1-4471-5088-6.
46. Syed MA, Mohiaddin R. Magnetic resonance imaging of congenital heart disease. London: Springer; 2012. p. p55–8. https://doi.org/10.1007/978-1-4471-4267-6.
47. Saremi F, Hassani C, Sánchez-Quintana D, et al. Radiographics. 2016;36(7):1966–86. https://doi.org/10.1148/rg.2016160010.
48. Jacobs JP, Burke RP, Quintessenza JA, Mavroudis C. Congenital heart surgery nomenclature and database project: ventricular septal defect. Ann Thorac Surg. 2000;69:S25–35.
49. Minette MS, Sahn DJ. Congenital heart disease for the adult cardiologist. Circulation. 2006;114:2190–7.
50. Dillman JR, Yarram SG, Hernandez RJ. Imaging of pulmonary venous developmental anomalies. Am J Roentgenol. 2009;192(5):1272–85.
51. Mazur W, Siegel MJ, Miszalski-Jamka T, Pelberg R. CT atlas of adult congenital heart disease. London: Springer; 2013. p. 204–10. https://doi.org/10.1007/978-1-4471-5088-6.
52. Herlong JR, Jaggers JJ, Ungerleider RM. Congenital heart surgery nomenclature and database project: pulmonary venous anomalies. Ann Thorac Surg. 2000;69:S56–69.
53. Himesh V, Vyas SBG, Krishnamurthy R. MR imaging and CT evaluation of congenital pulmonary vein abnormalities in neonates and infants. Radiographics. 2012;32:87–98. https://doi.org/10.1148/rg.321105764.
54. Kim TH, Kim YM, Suh CH, Cho DJ, Park IS, Kim WH, Lee YT. Helical CT angiography and three-dimensional reconstruction of total anomalous pulmonary venous connections in neonates and infants. AJR Am J Roentgenol. 2000 Nov;175(5):1381–6.
55. Oh KH, Choo KS, Lim SJ, et al. Multidetector CT evaluation of total anomalous pulmonary enous connections: comparison with echocardiography. Pediatr Radiol. 2009;39:950–4.
56. Syed MA, Mohiaddin R. Magnetic resonance imaging of congenital heart disease. London: Springer; 2012. p. p76–80. https://doi.org/10.1007/978-1-4471-4267-6.
57. Alsoufi B, Cai S, Van Arsdell GS, Williams WG, Caldarone CA, Coles JG. Outcomes after surgical treatment of children with partial anomalous pulmonary venous connection. Ann Thorac Surg. 2007;84(6):2020–6.
58. Lapierre C, Dubois J, Rypens F, Raboisson MJ, Déry J. Tetralogy of Fallot: preoperative assessment with MR and CT imaging. Diagn Interv Imaging. 2016;97(5):531–41. https://doi.org/10.1016/j.diii.2016.01.009.
59. Yap SC, van Geuns RJ, Meijboom FJ, et al. A simplified continuity equation approach to the quantifi cation of stenotic bicuspid aortic valves using velocity encoded cardiovascular magnetic resonance. J Cardiovasc Magn Reson. 2007;9:899–906.

60. Sagmeister F, Herrmann S, Ritter C, et al. Functional cardiac MRI for assessment of aortic valve disease. Radiologe. 2010;50:541–7.
61. Banderker E, Pretorius E, de Decker R. The role of cardiac CT angiography in the pre- and postoperative evaluation of tetralogy of Fallot. S Afr J Radiol. 2015;19(2):a899. https://doi.org/10.4102/sajr.v19i2.899.
62. Kapur S, Aeron G, Vojta CN. Pictorial review of coronary anomalies in Tetralogy of Fallot. J Cardiovascu Comput Tomogr. 2015;9(6):593–6.
63. Meinel FG, Huda W, Schoepf UJ, Rao AG, Cho YJ, Baker GH, Hlavacek AM. Diagnostic accuracy of CT angiography in infants with tetralogy of Fallot with pulmonary atresia and major aortopulmonary collateral arteries. J Cardiovasc Comput Tomogr. 2013;7(6):367–75. https://doi.org/10.1016/j.jcct.2013.11.001.
64. Ordovas KG, Muzzarelli S, Hope MD, Naeger DM, Karl T, Reddy GP, Marchiori E, Higgins CB. Cardiovascular MR imaging after surgical correction of tetralogy of Fallot: approach based on understanding of surgical procedures. Radiographics. 2013;33:1037–52. https://doi.org/10.1148/rg.334115084.
65. Geva T. Repaired tetralogy of Fallot: the roles of cardiovascular magnetic resonance in evaluating pathophysiology and for pulmonary valve replacement decision support. J Cardiovasc Magn Reson. 2011;13:9. https://doi.org/10.1186/1532-429X-13-9.
66. Oosterhof T, van Straten A, Vliegen HW, Meijboom FJ, van Dijk AP, Spijkerboer AM, et al. Preoperative thresholds for pulmonary valve replacement in patients with corrected tetralogy of Fallot Nusing cardiovascular magnetic resonance. Circulation. 2007;116(5):545–51.
67. Wilkinson JL. Double outlet ventricle. In: Anderson RH, Baker EJ, Macartney FJ, Rigby ML, Shinebourne EA, Tynan M, editors. Paediatric cardiology. 2nd ed. London: Churchill Livingstone; 2002. p. 1353–81.
68. Mazur W, Siegel MJ, Miszalski-Jamka T, Pelberg R. CT atlas of adult congenital heart disease. London: Springer; 2013. p. 233–6. https://doi.org/10.1007/978-1-4471-5088-6.
69. Saremi F. Cardiac CT and MR for adult congenital heart disease. New York: Springer; 2014. p. 230–60.
70. Syed MA, Mohiaddin R. Magnetic resonance imaging of congenital heart disease. London: Springer; 2012. p. p175–88. https://doi.org/10.1007/978-1-4471-4267-6.
71. Hucin B, Voriskova M, Hruda J, Marek J, Janousek J, Reich O, Skovranek J. Late complications and quality of life after atrial correction of transposition of the great arteries in 12 to 18 year follow-up. J Cardiovasc Surg (Torino). 2000;41:233–9.
72. Quaegebeur JM, Rohmer J, Ottenkamp J, et al. The arterial switch operation: an 8-year experience. J Thorac Cardiovasc Surg. 1986;92:361–84.
73. Saremi F. Cardiac CT and MR for adult congenital heart disease. New York: Springer; 2014. p. 364–7.
74. Fratz S, et al. The functional right ventricle and tricuspid regurgitation in Ebstein's anomaly. Int J Cardiol. 2012;167(1):258–61. https://doi.org/10.1016/j.ijcard.2011.12.081.
75. Carpentier A, et al. A new reconstructive operation for Ebstein's anomaly of the tricuspid valve. J Thorac Cardiovasc Surg. 1988;96(1):92–101.
76. Syed MA, Mohiaddin R. Magnetic resonance imaging of congenital heart disease. London: Springer; 2012. p. 133–9. https://doi.org/10.1007/978-1-4471-4267-6.
77. Mazur W, Siegel MJ, Miszalski-Jamka T, Pelberg R. CT atlas of adult congenital heart disease. London: Springer; 2013. p. 154–7.
78. Saxena A, Relan J, Agarwal R, Awasthy N, Azad S, Chakrabarty M, et al. Indian guidelines for indications and timing of intervention for common congenital heart diseases: revised and updated consensus statement of the Working group on management of congenital heart diseases. Ann Pediatr Cardiol. 2019;12(3):254–86. https://doi.org/10.4103/apc.APC_32_19.
79. Karaosmanoglu AD, Khawaja RDA, Onur MR, Kalra MK. CT and MRI of aortic coarctation: pre- and postsurgical findings. Am J of Roentgenol. 2015;204(3):224–33.
80. Hom JJ, Ordovas K, Reddy GP. Velocity-encoded cine MR imaging in aortic coarctation: functional assessment of hemodynamic events. Radiographics. 2008;28(2):407–16.
81. Suradi H, Hijazi ZM. Current management of coarctation of the aorta. Glob Cardiol Sci Pract. 2015;2015(4):44. https://doi.org/10.5339/gcsp.2015.44.
82. Shih M-CP, Tholpady A, Kramer CM, Sydnor MK, Hagspiel KD. Surgical and endovascular repair of aortic coarctation: normal findings and appearance of complications on CT angiography and MR angiography. Am J Roentgenol. 2006;187(3):302–12.
83. Warnes CA, Williams RG, Bashore TM, Child JS, Connolly HM, Dearani JA. ACC/AHA 2008 guidelines for the management of adults with congenital heart disease: executive summary: a report of the American College of Cardiology/American Heart Association Task Force on Practice Guidelines (Writing Committee to Develop Guidelines for the Management of Adults With Congenital Heart Disease). Circulation. 2008;118:2395–451. https://doi.org/10.1161/CIRCULATIONAHA.108.19081.

Echocardiography for Congenital Heart Disease: Fundamental Approach

23

Mahesh Kappanayil and R. Krishna Kumar

23.1 Introduction

Echocardiography is the cornerstone of cardiac imaging and retains its importance even in the current era of advanced imaging modalities. It continues to be the essential primary modality for cardiovascular assessment, by virtue of being an accurate, efficient, and versatile imaging tool that is easily available, affordable, and accessible even at point-of-care. Within the limits of the general limitations of ultrasound (including acoustic windows), echocardiography is a time-proven comprehensive tool for both anatomical and physiological evaluation. The large majority of diagnostic and management decisions with regard to CHD continue to be based on echocardiography, in conjunction with the clinical picture and other basic tools like electrocardiogram (ECG) and X-ray. This is particularly true for neonates, infants, and young children with good acoustic windows. Advanced modalities like invasive catheterization, magnetic resonance imaging (MRI), and computed tomography (CT) are reserved for specific situations and to answer specific study questions.

That said, the choice of one or the other modality, or in many cases, consolidated information gathered from multiple modalities should be dictated by the specific demands of the case. Information obtained from echocardiography is operator-dependent and requires skill and a good understanding of spatial anatomy and physiological correlates. Imparting skills at performing comprehensive echocardiography is an integral part of cardiology training programs. Congenital heart echocardiogram requires a particularly thorough, systematic, and protocol-bound approach in view of the wide range of anatomical complexities and physiological correlates possible in CHD. Techniques and technology are evolving rapidly in tandem with advancements in computational and biomedical engineering sciences.

Modern-day echocardiography is a compendium of multiple instrumentations, techniques, modalities, and applications that include two-dimensional and three-dimensional echocardiograms obtained through transthoracic, transesophageal, or epicardial approaches, and a variety of tools for hemodynamic assessment (color Doppler, spectral Doppler, tissue Doppler, speckle tracking, etc.). Most of these tools and techniques are common for echocardiograms across all ages and indications—pediatric as well as adult, for congenital as well as acquired heart disease. This chapter will focus on the fundamental approach to transthoracic echocardiographic imaging for congenital heart disease.

M. Kappanayil (✉) · R. K. Kumar
Department of Pediatric Cardiology, Amrita School of Medicine, Amrita Institute of Medical Sciences and Research Centre, Amrita Vishwa Vidyapeetham, Kochi, Kerala, India

R. Rajeshkannan et al. (eds.), *CT and MRI in Congenital Heart Diseases*,
https://doi.org/10.1007/978-981-15-6755-1_23

23.2 History of Echocardiography

Beginning with trying to understand how bats navigate in the dark using reflected echos of inaudible sound waves (Lazzaro Spalanzani, 1729–1799), through the discovery of piezoelectricity by the Curies in 1880, "ultrasound" and its applications went through an era of discovery and development to evolve into the "medical ultrasound" as we know it now [1, 2]. The initial applications were in the wartime use of SONAR (Sound Ranging and Navigation System) to detect enemy submarines during World War I and the RADAR (Radio Detection and Ranging) during World War II [2]. Until then, medical applications were quite literally "under the radar"—waiting to be explored. It was in the 1940s that Karl Theo Dussik first demonstrated its application in imaging cerebral ventricles, and Andre Denier proposed using ultrasound to visualize internal viscera [2–4].

The heart—vital, dynamic, and central to life itself has always fascinated scientists, and imaging of the heart became one of the earliest and core challenges in the evolution of ultrasound as a medical imaging tool. Wolfe Dieter Keidel ideated on the possibility of using it to record rhythmic volume variations of the heart [2, 4]. But it was groundbreaking and pioneering work of Inge Edler and Carl Hellmuth Hertz that led to the first real-world application of ultrasound to understand the workings of the human heart [2, 5]. Edler, as cardiologist and director of the Cardiovascular Laboratory at the pioneering cardiac surgical unit at the University of Lund in the 1950s, had the difficult task of evaluating patients with mitral valve disease for surgical mitral valvotomies. With his knowledge of the use of RADAR in World War II, he ideated upon the use of the same principles to "visualize" the heart. His ideas led him to a remarkable association with the brilliant young, physicist Hertz and the ensuing unique collaboration between the two culminated in the birth of "ultrasound cardiography." In October 1953, Edler and Hertz recorded the first moving "pictures" of the heart with an "ultrasound reflectoscope" using a novel technique now known as "time-motion" or "M-mode" [2, 6]. Hertz went on to develop newer techniques of two-dimensional echocardiography and applications of Doppler principles for measuring the rate of blood flow [2]. The initial response of the scientific and medical community to these innovations ranged from disinterest to polite disregard. It was in the subsequent decade of the 1960s that these techniques began to gather traction and momentum. Groundbreaking work by Harvey Fiegenbaum in the United States in the 1960s and his collaboration with Harold Dodge laid the foundations for the first real measurement of ventricular dimensions using M-mode [7]. The term "echocardiography" was coined by Fiegenbaum. Eggleton created the first commercially successful two-dimensional echocardiogram in the 1970s [8]. Refining of Doppler techniques to assess blood flows and combining it with two-dimensional echo to create duplex scanning followed. The power of echocardiography for assessing hemodynamics was unmasked with the ingenious inference by Holen and Hatle that modified Bernoulli's equation which could be used for calculating pressure gradients across stenotic valves [9, 10]. Transesophageal echo techniques were developed in the 1970s [11]. Echocardiography continues to evolve with advancing technology.

23.3 Advantages of Echocardiography

- *Non-invasive* (transthoracic), no radiation.
- *Widely available*—from high-end standalone machines to portable and ultraportable (handheld) devices.
- *Adaptable* to a variety of settings from outpatient clinics, operating rooms, catheterization laboratories, intensive care units to mobile units, rural settings, and bedside situations.
- *Versatile*—provides both anatomical and physiological information; allows for both qualita-

tive and quantitative assessment including responses to drugs, exercises, and maneuvers.
- *Excellent temporal resolution*, therefore very useful in imaging fast-moving structures like cardiac valves and infant hearts.
- *Real-time imaging*, amenable to instant interpretation for rapid decision-making, without dependence on complex post-processing.
- *Reproducible* and suited for multiple, serial evaluations. Normative data allows standardized comparisons of various dimensional and functional parameters.

23.4 Objectives of Echocardiography

Echocardiography has different and distinct roles during the different phases of patient care.

Preoperative assessment (transthoracic, transesophageal): Planning optimal management through:

- Comprehensive morphological diagnosis
- In-depth physiological assessment, correlating it with the anatomy
- Assessing feasibility of surgical or interventional strategies by clearly defining suitability, challenges, and risk factors
- Identifying the need for additional assessment like cardiac catheterization, CT, or MRI

Intraoperative assessment (epicardial, transesophageal):

- Assessment of the effectiveness of repair
- Identify major residual or additional defects

Postoperative assessment (transthoracic):

- Immediate postoperative assessment of the effectiveness of repair, residual lesions, and cardiac functions
- Serial follow-up for lesion-specific or procedure-specific long-term issues including need/timing/suitability for subsequent staged procedures or re-interventions

23.5 General Guidelines for Echocardiography

Dedicated echocardiography rooms in an outpatient clinic setting should have an optimized ambient environment:

- During an examination, the room should preferably be darkened, at best illuminated with a dim, diffuse light, that allows the best appreciation of the details on the backlit screen of the echocardiography machine.
- The patient cot and the echocardiography machine should be suitably arranged to allow both the patient and the echocardiographer to be comfortably positioned throughout the echo study.
- Young children and infants may need sedation to permit comprehensive echo assessment, therefore ensuring provision for administering appropriate sedation and monitoring the patient. Written protocols for type of sedation, dosage, and monitoring should be in place. A darkened prep-room and/or breastfeeding room should preferably be adjoining. Toys, music, parental attention, etc. can also be used as distractions, in place of sedation, in some cases.
- Ensure a comfortable, thermoneutral environment particularly for infants and neonates; this can be done by appropriately swaddling them in blankets/sheets. Ultrasound jelly may be pre-warmed to body temperature.
- Multiparameter vitals monitor, pulse oximeter, oxygen, emergency drugs, and resuscitation equipment should be readily available. Written protocols for emergency management should be established.
- Height and weight recording will allow the indexing of specific parameters.

23.6 Optimal Image Acquisition

23.6.1 Choice of Transducer and Frequency

The vast majority of echocardiograms are transthoracic (TTE), with transesophageal (TEE) and epicardial being restricted to specific situations. CHD patients may vary in age and size from tiny premature neonates to obese teenagers and older individuals. A range of transducers should, therefore, be available, and an appropriate frequency-range transthoracic transducer should be chosen for each patient.

Low frequency (1.5–3 MHz) transducer with greater penetration would be appropriate for older, bigger patients. Higher frequency (≥7.5 MHz) transducers would be required for young children, while 10–12 MHz probes will be optimally suited for imaging neonates. Multi-frequency transducers are also available; imaging parameters should be carefully selected before starting the study. Dedicated Doppler transducer for continuous-wave Doppler is useful.

23.6.2 Standardization and Optimization

- Electrocardiography (ECG) gating during image acquisition is essential to allow accurate interpretation and quantification of the information obtained.
- Height and weight of the subjects should be recorded, allowing indexing of parameters.
- Standard imaging views and protocols should be followed for better comparability and offline interpretation.
- Manual adjustment of specific parameters is necessary—frame rate, depth, sector width, magnification, focus, gain, velocity scales, etc. to optimize images dynamically throughout an exam. Typically one echocardiographic exam may include multiple views and multiple modalities—two-dimensional, M-mode, color Doppler, spectral Doppler, etc., each of them requiring optimization of these settings. Most of the modern-day higher-end echocardiography equipment have "automatic optimization" or "preset" modes, but obtaining perfect images often involves additional manual adjustments.
- One must strive to acquire and archive good quality ("publication quality") images for offline viewing, reporting, or analysis.
- Acquire at least three loops for moving images; longer loops may be recorded where required.
- Reports should be comprehensive, structured, and systematic, preferably on a standard/uniform format.

23.6.3 Imaging Protocols

The comprehensive echocardiographic study involves optimal utilization of multiple modalities in a manner so as to obtain maximal insight into the anatomy and physiology in a given patient. Two-dimensional echo, M-mode, Doppler (Pulse Wave and Continuous Wave) and where available and relevant, tissue-Doppler and three-dimensional echo are the principal imaging modalities used. Transthoracic imaging comprises the vast majority of echocardiographic studies and will be the focus of this chapter.

Why does echocardiography for congenital heart disease require a tailored approach?

- Wide age range of subjects—from neonates to adults.
- Wide range of possible anatomical and structural malformations, requiring a deep understanding of segmental anatomy and three-dimensional spatial relationships.
- Complex interplay between structure and function, requiring hemodynamic understanding and analytical thinking.
- Echocardiographer needs to have an understanding of the management pathways, and the natural and modified history for various types of CHD; the imaging needs to address the pertinent study questions (both anatomic and hemodynamic) to guide management. The wide range and complexity of downstream decision-making adds to the challenges of imaging.

- Requires specific views and a thorough systematic approach.

23.6.4 The Segmental Approach

"Segmental approach" forms the foundation of echocardiography for congenital heart disease, and serves as a guiding principle. It breaks up cardiovascular anatomy and its analysis into three "segments" based on 10 embryological regions [12]:

1. Visceroatrial situs
2. Ventricular looping
3. Great artery relationship

The aim of an echocardiogram is to clearly define each of these elements in a sequential manner. It is standard to use the notational system developed by Van Praagh, using a series of three letters separated by commas, within a parenthesis denoting each of these three elements of anatomy—the first letter denoting situs (S = solitus, I = inversus, A = ambiguous), second letter the ventricular looping (D = dextro loop, L = levo loop), and the third letter great artery relationship (S = solitus, I = inverted, d = dextro-malposition, l = levo-malposition) [13–15].

In simpler terms, during an echocardiogram, the cardiovascular anatomy may be viewed as a jigsaw puzzle with each of the following being a piece of the puzzle—individual systemic and pulmonary veins, the atria, the ventricles, and the great arteries (Fig. 23.1). Add to this the spatial location of the heart and its relationship to other viscera. A comprehensive echocardiogram is directed at locating, characterizing, and then defining the connections of each of these elements. This can be an extremely challenging task given the wide spectrum of abnormalities possible. Following a systematic and logical approach helps address these challenges.

This is achieved by following a specific sequence of scanning views to minimize the

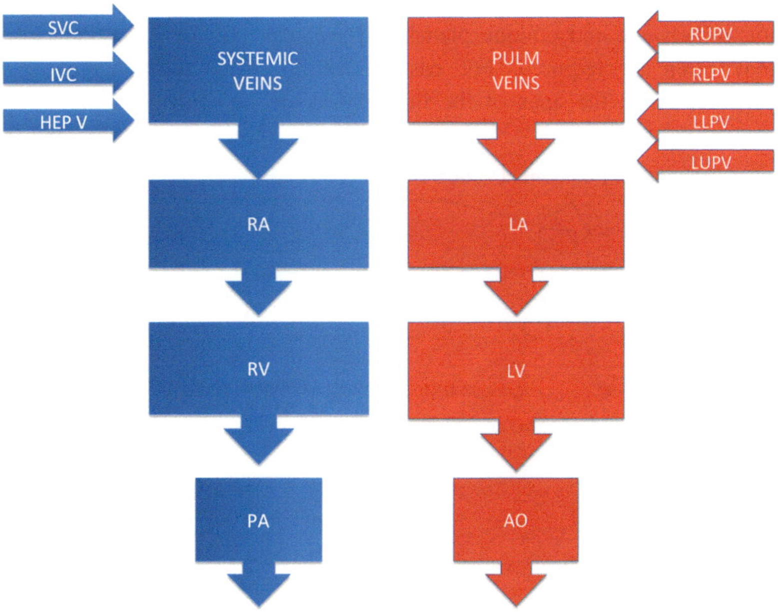

Fig. 23.1 The "jigsaw puzzle" of segmental anatomy. *AO* Aorta, *HEP V* hepatic veins, *IVC* inferior vena cava, *LA* left atrium, *LLPV* left lower pulmonary vein, *LUPV* left upper pulmonary vein, *LV* left ventricle, *PA* pulmonary artery, *PULM VEINS* pulmonary veins, *RA* right atrium, *RV* right ventricle

chances of error. Some of these views are unique to CHD-scans and not routinely used for scanning adults with acquired heart disease. Although it is ideal to follow this sequence for thoroughness and accuracy, exceptions may be made in situations that require expeditious targeted exams or where certain views are limited by poor echo windows. Wherever possible, one must endeavor to adhere to the protocols. The reporting should be just as thorough and must follow a detailed segmental checklist format.

23.7 Views and Scanning Techniques

Five sequential transducer positions are recommended for a systematic scan for congenital heart disease, as shown in Fig. 23.2. The exact probe positions may need to be adjusted in any given patient according to the best available acoustic windows, viscerocardiac positions, and other factors. With the probe in each of the positions, scanning involves "sector sweeps" along specific planes rather than viewing a fixed imaging sector; in-between and oblique planes and sweeps may often be required. For easier anatomical orientation, the apex of the imaging sector should be kept at the bottom of the screen during the subxiphoid and apical views, while it is kept at the top of the screen in other views [16, 17]. Two-dimensional (B-mode) and color flow imaging are both done in each view and sweep. Echocardiographers should be aware of the structures that can be visualized in each view, and interpretation depends upon pattern recognition.

Despite the two-dimensionality of B-mode echo, viewing the heart from multiple positions and sweeping across imaging sectors allow the imager to mentally reconstruct the three-dimensional anatomy and spatial relationships.

23.8 Specific Views

23.8.1 Subxiphoid Views

These views are obtained with the patient lying supine, by positioning the transducer in the epigastrium, just caudal to the xiphisternum. There is no bony interface in these views and the liver can be used to advantage in providing an effective acoustic window to the heart. Children usually have excellent subxiphoid scanning windows and almost the entire segmental anatomy can be elucidated in these views [18–20].

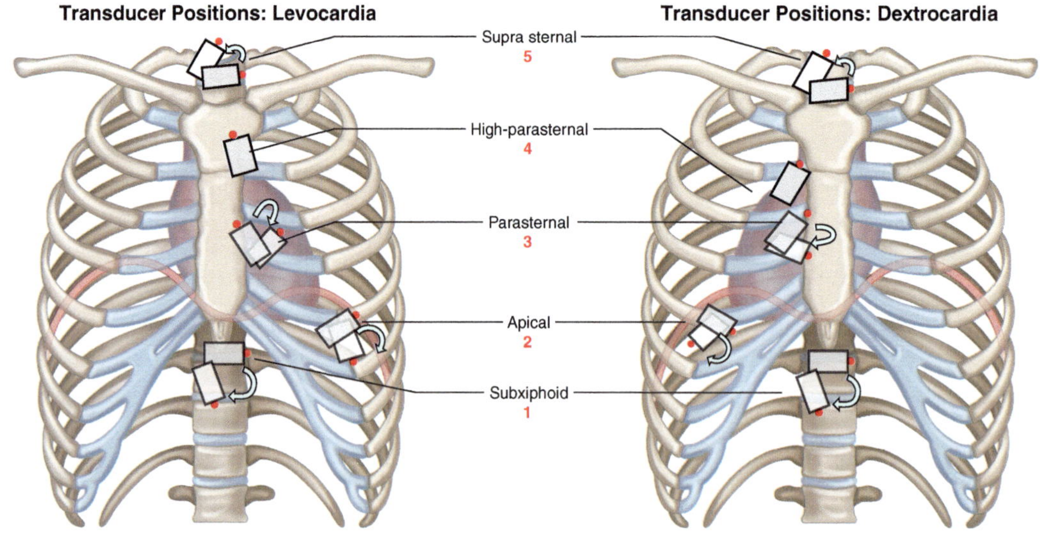

Fig. 23.2 Transducer positions for obtaining various echocardiographic views during assessment for congenital heart disease in levocardia (left) and dextrocardia (right)

Older children or young adults may need to be instructed to volitionally relax their abdominal muscles during a subxiphoid scan; folding the knees with the feet kept flat on the bed may also help keep the anterior abdominal wall relaxed for a good scan.

23.8.2 Subxiphoid Long-Axis Sweep

The transducer is positioned in the subxiphoid area, pointing directly posterior, with the cursor at 3 o'clock position. This serves as a good starting point, by helping to determine the visceral situs. The position/lie of the liver, and the position of inferior vena cava (IVC) and the abdominal aorta in relation to each other and to the spine (Fig. 23.4a) can be clearly seen in this view and would help define visceral situs (solitus, inversus, or ambiguous). Slow, deliberate cranial sweep of the transducer (Fig. 23.3), while keeping the footprint of the transducer anchored, allows visualization of progressively anterior and superior structures:

- Define the relationship of the hepatic veins to IVC (Fig. 23.4b).
- Trace the drainage of IVC into the atrium.
- Note the coronary sinus and posterior aspect of the atrial septum.
- Note the right upper pulmonary vein (Fig. 23.4c).
- Note left atrium (LA) and left ventricle (LV) (Fig. 23.4d).
- Further angulation shows all four cardiac chambers together with atrial septum and part of the ventricular septum (posterior and inlet septum) (Fig. 23.5a).
- Further anterior-superior angulation reveals the great arteries and their connections to the ventricles. In the normal heart, aorta is visualized first, followed by the pulmonary valve and proximal main pulmonary artery (Fig. 23.5b, c).

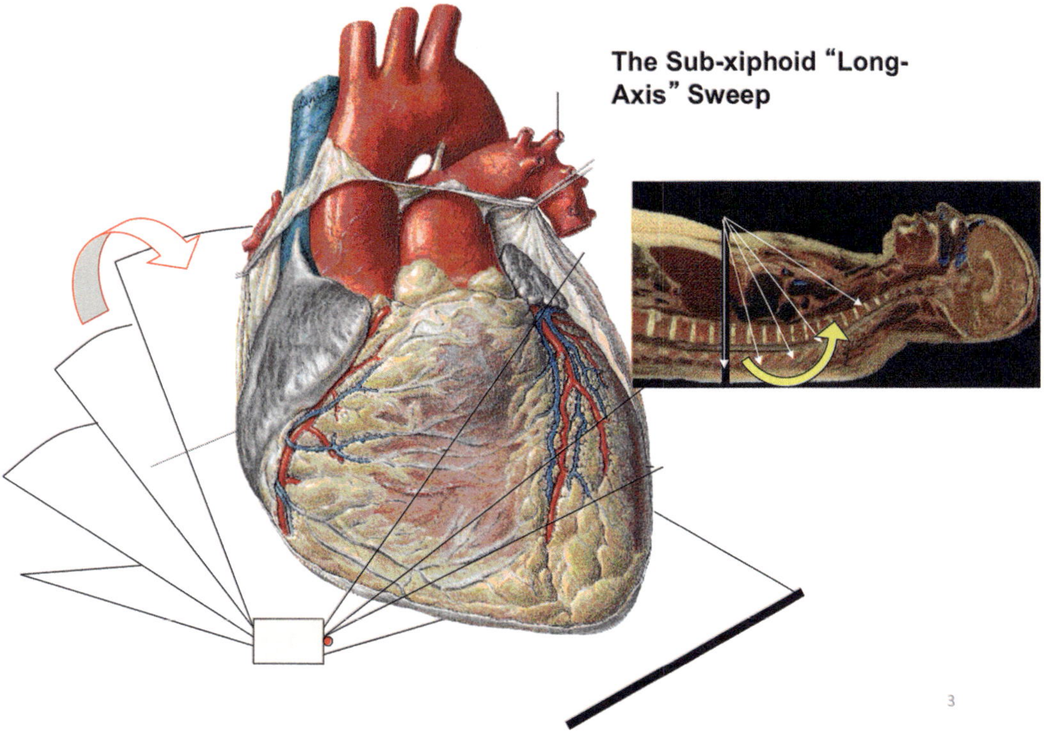

Fig. 23.3 Transducer position and imaging planes for the subxiphoid long-axis views: anterio-superior cuts. The subxiphoid long axis sweep starts in the axial plane in the abdomen and moves superiorly in the direction of the coronal plane

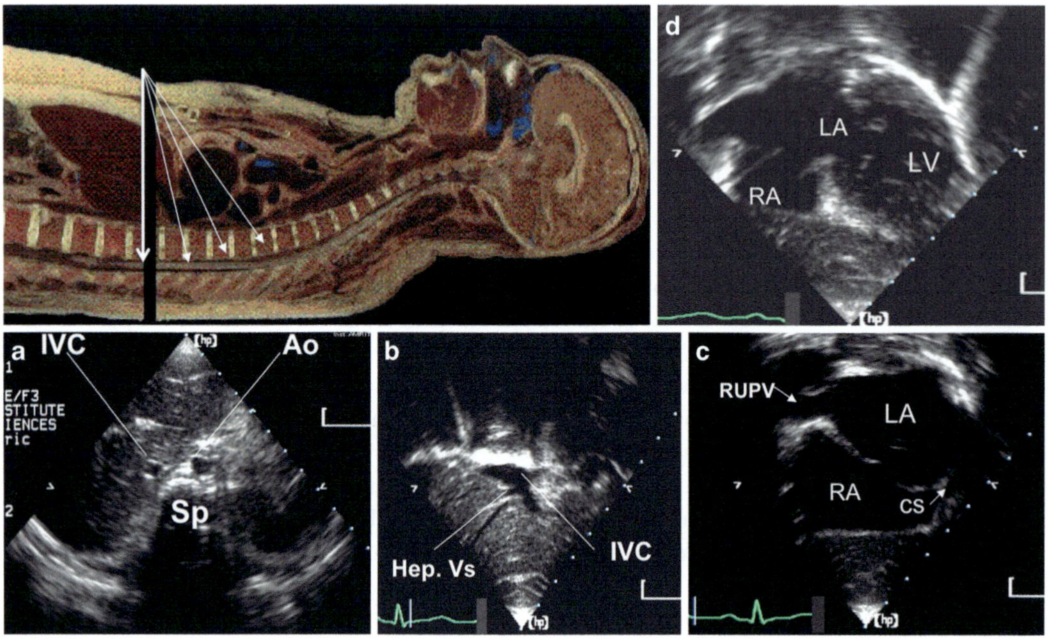

Fig. 23.4 Sequential images obtained during the subxiphoid long axis sweep. (**a**) Posterior cuts for demonstration of situs. This view shows the relationship of the inferior vena cava (IVC) to the aorta (Ao) and the spine (Sp); (**b**) Demonstrating veno-atrial connections: Hepatic veins(HVs), inferior vena cava (IVC) are shown to enter the right atrium (RA); (**c**) Posterior cut of the atrium showing right upper pulmonary vein (RUPV), right atrium (RA), coronary sinus (CS); (**d**) subxiphoid long-axis view showing the left atrium (LA) and the left ventricle (LV)

23.8.3 Subxiphoid Short-Axis Sweep

Rotation of the transducer by 90° from the long axis orientation takes the cursor into a 6 o'clock position (or pointing toward the supine patient's feet) and allows the imaging sectors to cut the heart along its short axis (Figs. 23.2 and 23.6):

- Slide the transducer rightwards along the subxiphoid location to obtain the "bicaval view" where the superior vena cava (SVC), IVC, and the atrial septum can be seen in the long axis (Fig. 23.6a). Using this location as the fulcrum, gradually sweep the probe leftwards (for levocardia, rightwards for dextrocardia) until the sweep covers the entire heart right up to the apex.
- While rightward-most transducer position shows the SVC, IVC, atrial septum, the coronary sinus, and right lower pulmonary vein, slight counterclockwise rotation shows the right upper pulmonary vein entry to the left atrium, and also allows further visualization of the atrial septum [21].
- As the transducer is swept leftwards, the aortic valve, proximal ascending aorta, mitral and tricuspid valves come into view (Fig. 23.6b).
- This is followed by visualization of the right ventricular outflow tract (RVOT), pulmonary valve, and the main pulmonary artery. Defects in the outlet ventricular septum (doubly committed and supracristal) are best seen in this view, as are muscular obstructions of the RVOT (Fig. 23.6c).
- Further leftward sweep shows the ventricular cavities with the intervening muscular ventricular septum. The normal left ventricle (LV) appears rounded and the right ventricle (RV) crescent-shaped (Fig. 23.6d).
- The sweep extending into the apex outlines apical muscular VSDs.
- Slight counterclockwise rotation of probe with the cursor roughly in 5 or 4 o' clock position allows a good visualization of both the

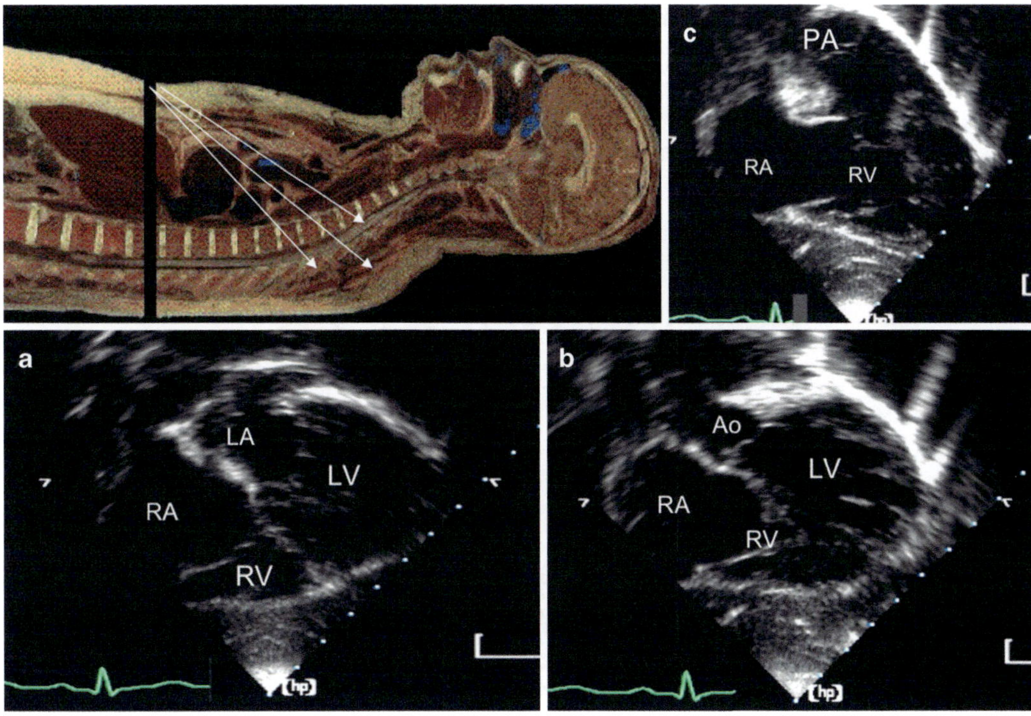

Fig. 23.5 Anterio-superior cuts in the subxiphoid long-axis view. (**a**) The subxiphoid four-chamber view showing the four chambers; right atrium (RA), right ventricle (RV), left atrium (LA), left ventricle (LV). (**b**) Superior angulation from the four-chamber plane shows the origin of the aorta (AO) from the left ventricle (LV). (**c**) on further cranial angulation, from the anterior, most structures are revealed. This plane demonstrates the right ventricle (RV) and the pulmonary artery (PA)

atrioventricular valves en-face and their relationship with the interventricular septum (Fig. 23.7). This can be a particularly useful view while assessing the AV valves in common atrioventricular septal defects (AVSD) and Ebstein's anomaly.

Sweeping back and forth, slowly, with and without color flow mapping allows a thorough assessment. In general, a thorough two-dimensional sweep should precede the use of color flow imaging, to achieve the best frame-rates and resolution to identify structural defects. The "color compare" mode with plain B-mode and color flow imaging arranged side by side allows good visual comprehension. False echo-dropouts can often be identified by the color interface on either side.

An *additional (paracoronal) subxiphoid* view involves keeping the probe in the same location as for the other subxiphoid views, but rotated so that the cursor points toward the patient's left shoulder (about 2 o' clock position), and the transducer angular cranially/anteriorly. This view provides an en-face view of the interventricular septum, with both the inflow and outflows of the RV seen (Fig. 23.8). This view is particularly useful for mapping-out the location of VSDs, and also for characterizing the RVOT anatomy in patients with Tetralogy of Fallot.

In neonates and young children, the subcostal views provide an excellent window to comprehensively assess the anatomy, including a fair visualization of the branch PAs, aortic arch, descending aorta, and patent ductus arteriosus (PDA).

Rather than being dogmatic about "fixed views," an echocardiographer needs to be free and flexible to adjust the scanning views and angulations to trace the structures of interest.

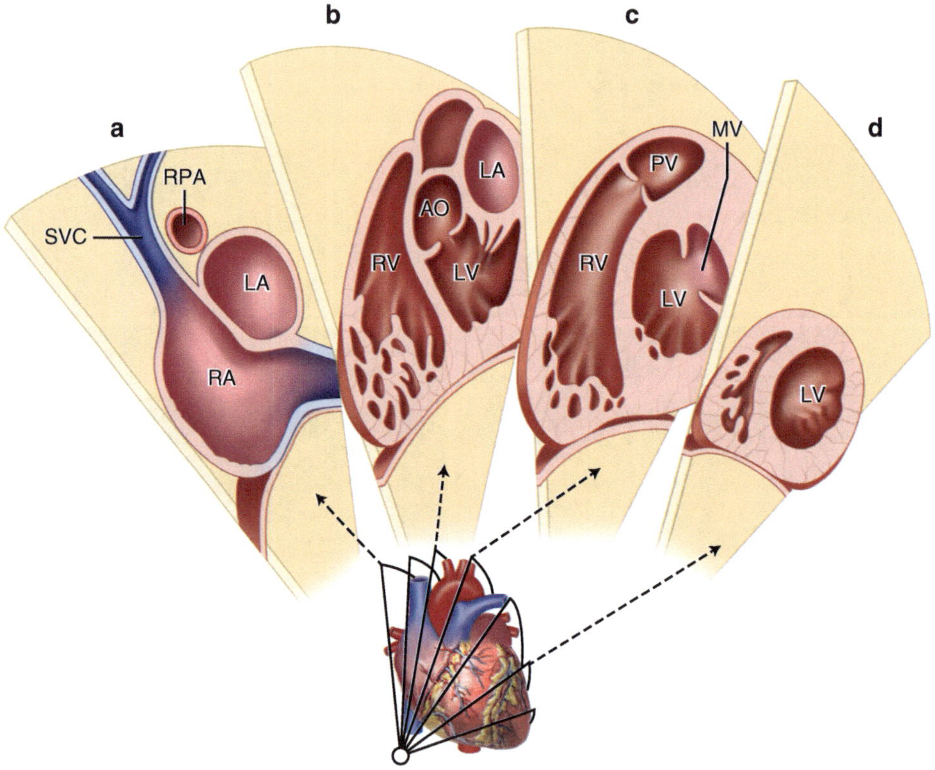

Fig. 23.6 Transducer position and imaging planes for the subxiphoid short-axis (sagittal) views. The sweep should move from right to left. (**a**) The rightward cut is the bicaval view. Both the vena cava (SVC and IVC) are seen. The right pulmonary artery (RPA) is seen behind the SVC. The left atrium (LA) is seen just below the RPA. (**b**) This is at the level of the atrioventricular junction and profiles the membranous septum (MSeptum) just below the aorta (Ao); the inflows of the right ventricle (RV) and left ventricle (LV) are also profiled. (**c**) The next frame is obtained by sweeping to the left and this profiles the right ventricular outflow tract (RVOT) and the pulmonary artery (PA). (**d**) This cut is obtained at the level of the mid-cavity of the left ventricles

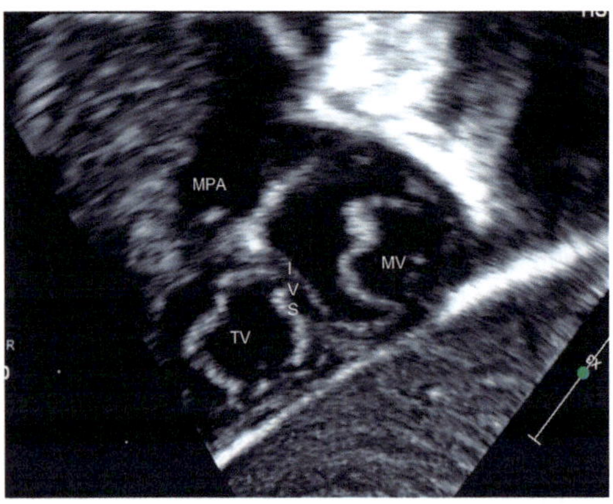

Fig. 23.7 Subxiphoid view obtained by slight counter-clockwise rotation of the transducer from the short-axis view, showing both the atrioventricular valves in cross-section and their relationship to the interventricular septum. *IVS* interventricular septum, *MPA* main pulmonary artery, *MV* mitral valve, *TV* tricuspid valve

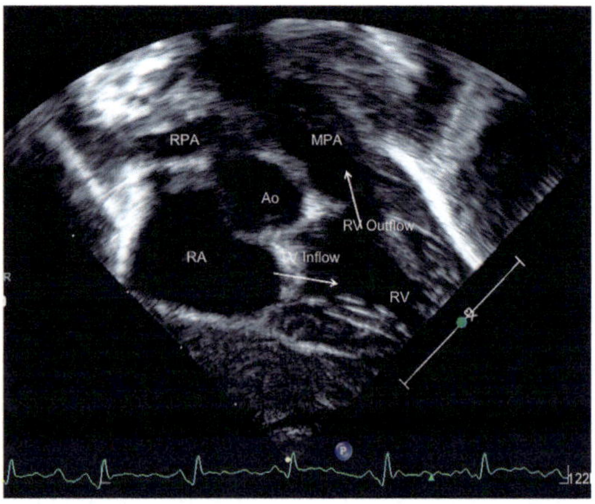

Fig. 23.8 Subxiphoid paracoronal view with the transducer cursor pointing roughly toward 2 o' clock position showing the right ventricular inflow and outflow. The ventricular septum is en-face in this view. *Ao* aorta, *MPA* main pulmonary artery, *RA* right atrium, *RPA* right pulmonary artery, *RV* right ventricle, *TV* tricuspid valve

23.8.4 Apical Views

Apical views are obtained by placing the transducer on the chest wall at the location of the cardiac apex (Figs. 23.2 and 23.9). The ideal location can be determined easily by palpating the chest in most children:

- This view is best obtained by having the patient in a left decubitus position. In smaller children and infants, it may be enough to slightly turn them leftwards using a small pillow or soft support. Satisfactory apical views can be obtained in neonates even in the supine position.
- The transducer should be positioned, usually with the cursor pointing toward the patient's left shoulder, and the imaging sector transecting the heart in an oblique axial plane, until one obtains the "four-chamber" view—showing the two atria, the two AV valves, and the two ventricles (Fig. 23.9b).
- Using this transducer position as the fulcrum, a posterior sweep or angulation will show the posterior aspects of RV and RA along with the coronary sinus (Fig. 23.9a).
- An anterior or cranial sweep from here brings it back to the four-chamber view, and further anterior/cranial angulation shows the left ventricular outflow tract (RVOT)—or the apical "five-chamber" view (Fig. 23.9c).
- Further anterior/cranial angulation reveals the RVOT (Fig. 23.10b).
- Clockwise rotation of the transducer from the four-chamber view gives the apical "two-chamber" view that displays the LV inflow and outflow simultaneously (Fig. 23.10a).

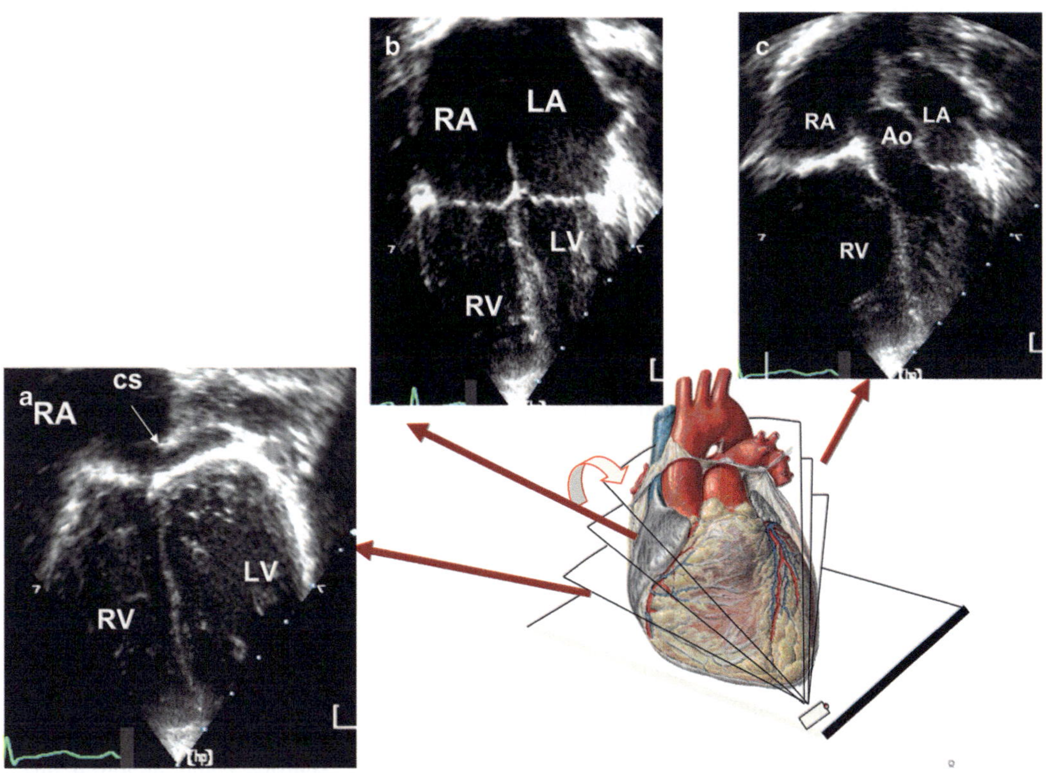

Fig. 23.9 Transducer position and imaging planes for the Apical four- and five-chamber views. Posterior structures such as the coronary sinus and posterior ventricular septum are seen in the inferior cuts (**a**); by sweeping superiorly the mitral and tricuspid valves are profiled (classic apical four-chamber view) (**b**); further sweep superiorly reveals anteriorly located left ventricular outflow tract and aortic valve (**c**). *LA* left atrium, *LV* left ventricle, *RA* right atrium, *RV* right ventricle

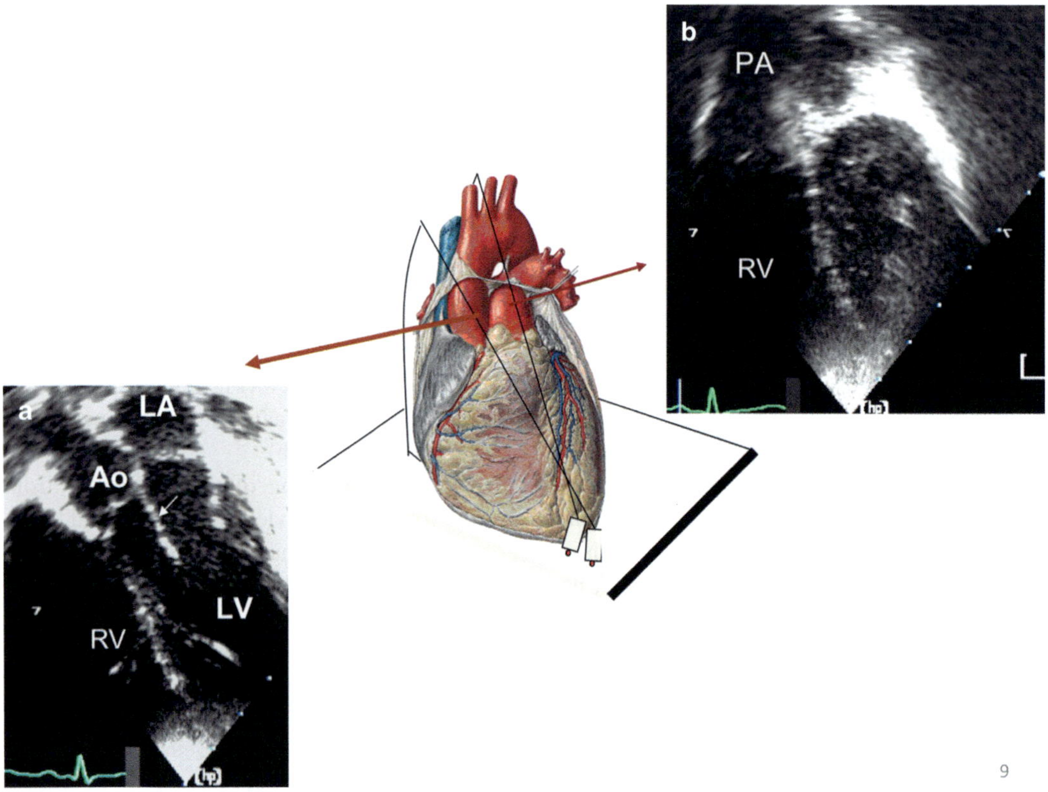

Fig. 23.10 (**a**) The apical long axial view is obtained after clockwise rotation and superior angulations from the apical four-chamber view. This allows an excellent view of the left ventricular outflow. The arrow points to the anterior mitral leaflet. (**b**) Sweeping leftward and further superiorly from the apical long-axial view reveals the right ventricular outflow tract. *Ao* Aorta, *LA* Left atrium, *LV* Left Ventricle, *PA* Pulmonary artery, *RV* Right Ventricle

23.8.5 Parasternal Views

Parasternal Long-Axis (PLAX) view is obtained by keeping the cursor pointing toward the right shoulder (Figs. 23.2 and 23.11):

- This displays the LV in its long axis along with its inflow and outflow. The LA, mitral valve, aortic valve, and the proximal ascending aorta are well visualized in this view (Fig. 23.11b).
- Angling the transducer downwards toward the right hip shows the membranous ventricular septum, and then the tricuspid valve inflow. Sweeping it back brings back the PLAX view (Fig. 23.11a).
- Angulating the transducer back toward the left shoulder brings us back to the classical PLAX view; further angulation in the same direction displays the RVOT, pulmonary valve (Fig. 23.11c).

Parasternal Short-Axis View (PSAX) is obtained by rotating the transducer by 90° from the PLAX position (Fig. 23.12):

- This displays the aortic valve in cross-section, the individual cusps, and the proximal coronary arteries (with a slight adjustment of transducer position). Atrial septum is posterior to the aortic valve, the LA appendage, and the individual pulmonary veins.
- Sweeping toward the apex shows the cross-section of the ventricles, and the mitral valve, the location of the LV papillary muscles, and the ventricular septum.
- Sweeping anterior and sliding up by one or two spaces shows the pulmonary valve (left and

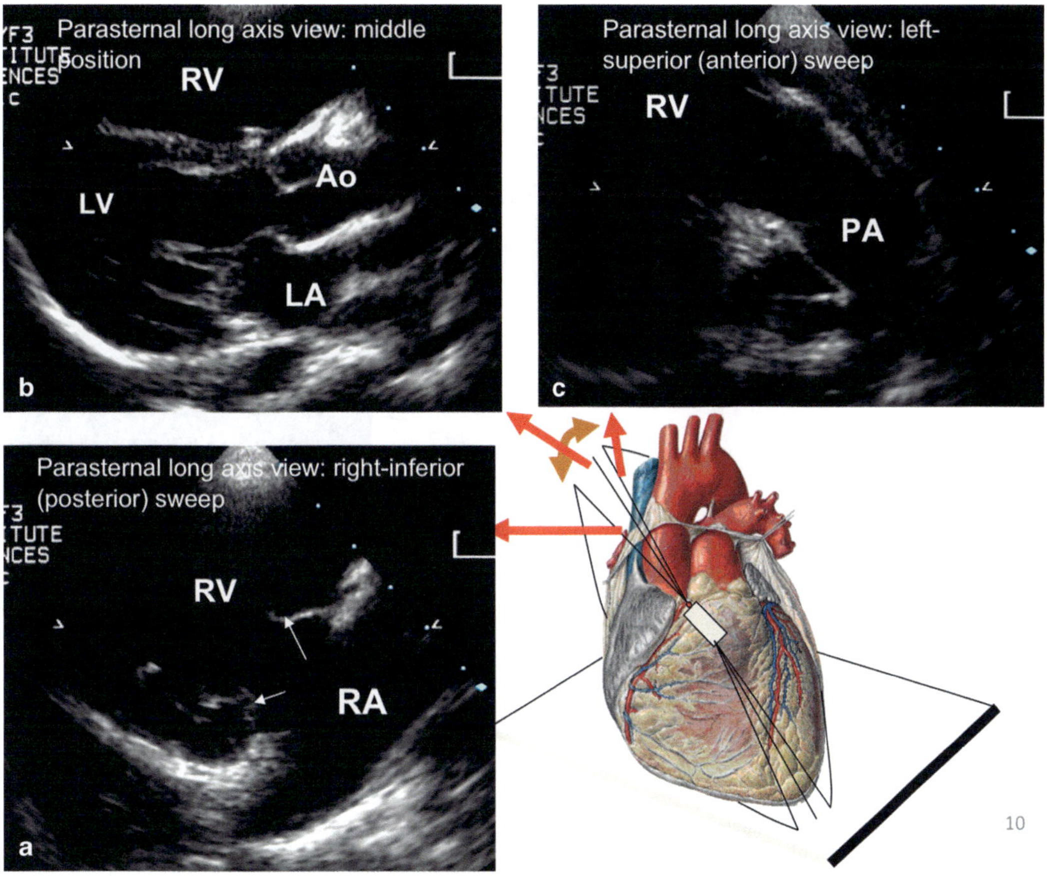

Fig. 23.11 Transducer position and imaging planes for the parasternal long-axis views. The three images are obtained by sweeping rightwards and inferiorly (**a**) and leftwards and superiorly (**c**) from the standard parasternal long-axis view (**b**)

anterior to aortic valve), the main pulmonary artery, and the division of branch pulmonary arteries. The RVOT can be seen wrapping around the aorta in this view. Anterior malalignment of the conal septum and subvalvar RVOT obstructions of TOF can be well appreciated in this view. This view also enables one to distinguish between membranous, intraconal, and subpulmonic VSDs.

23.8.6 High-Parasternal ("Ductal") View

This view is obtained by sliding upward (up to two intercostal spaces) and medially from the transducer location for PSAX view along the left sternal border, rotating it a few degrees counterclockwise and sweeping leftwards—profiling the left pulmonary artery (LPA) and descending aorta in the same view (Figs. 23.2 and 23.13):

- A classical patent ductus arteriosus (PDA) is best visualized in this view, allowing accurate demonstration of its anatomical shape, size, and flows (by applying color flows and Doppler).
- More complex PDA anatomy would require further adjustments to the view to delineate the entire anatomy of the duct and its insertions. Juxta-ductal coarctation of aorta is also well appreciated in this view.
- Sliding the transducer higher into the first/second intercostal space and rotating it clockwise

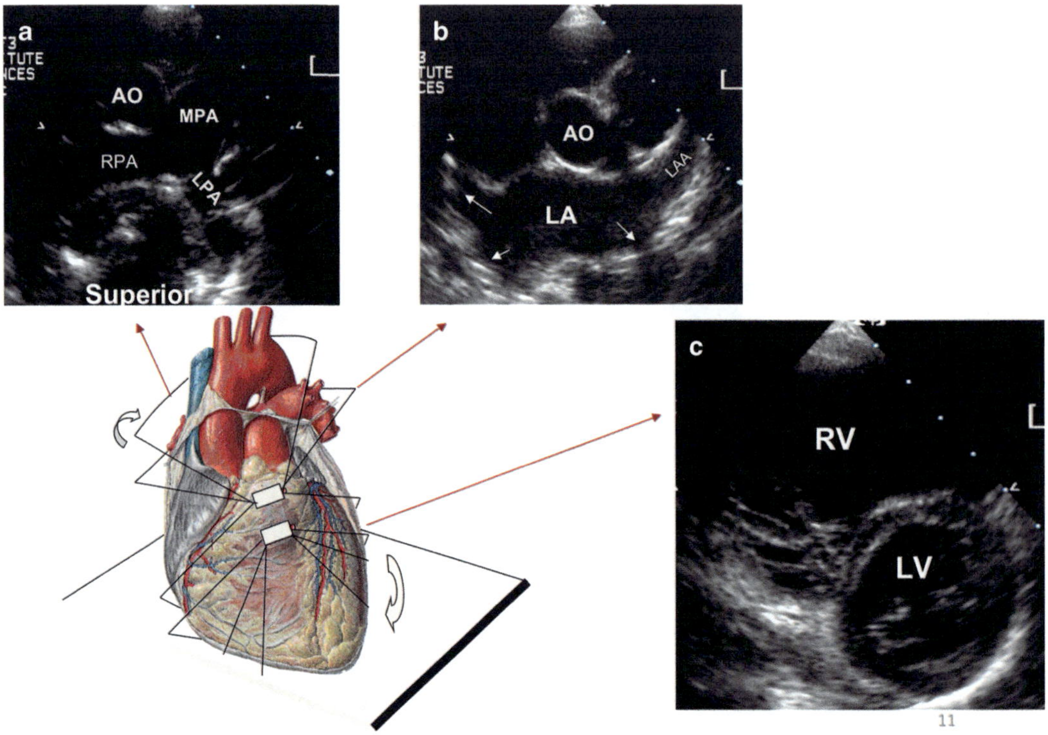

Fig. 23.12 Transducer position and imaging planes for the parasternal short-axis views. Superior sweep (**a**) enables visualization of the branch pulmonary arteries (RPA and LPA), the main pulmonary artery (MPA) is seen to the left of the aorta (Ao). (**b**) Shows images obtained using a slight downward tilt of the transducer in the parasternal short-axis view. This enables visualization of the left atrial appendage (LAA) and the pulmonary veins (arrows). Frame (**c**) is obtained by sliding slightly downwards and pointing the transducer toward the apex. The ventricular cavity cross-section is profiled. *LA* left atrium, *LV* left ventricle, *RA* right atrium, *RV* right ventricle

toward the left shoulder helps demonstrate branch pulmonary arteries especially in pulmonary atresia situations.

High Right Parasternal View is obtained by keeping the transducer along the right sternal border rather than the left with the cursor pointing upwards (12 o' clock position), preferably with the patient in right decubitus position:

- This view profiles the SVC along its long axis, and the sinus venosis part of the atrial septum.
- This view also gives the best orientation of the continuous wave Doppler for assessing the severity of aortic valve stenosis.

23.8.7 Suprasternal Views

This is one of the essential and unique views employed during an echocardiogram for CHD. This requires positioning of the patient with an extension of the neck by using a pillow or roll under the shoulder of the supine patient.

Suprasternal Short-Axis View (Fig. 23.14):

- The transducer is placed in the suprasternal notch with the cursor pointing toward the left shoulder (3 o' clock position) and angled posteriorly by about 45° to show the ascending Aorta in oblique section, the entire length of mediastinal RPA from the PA confluence to the hilum seen below the aorta, and the SVC to the right of aorta.

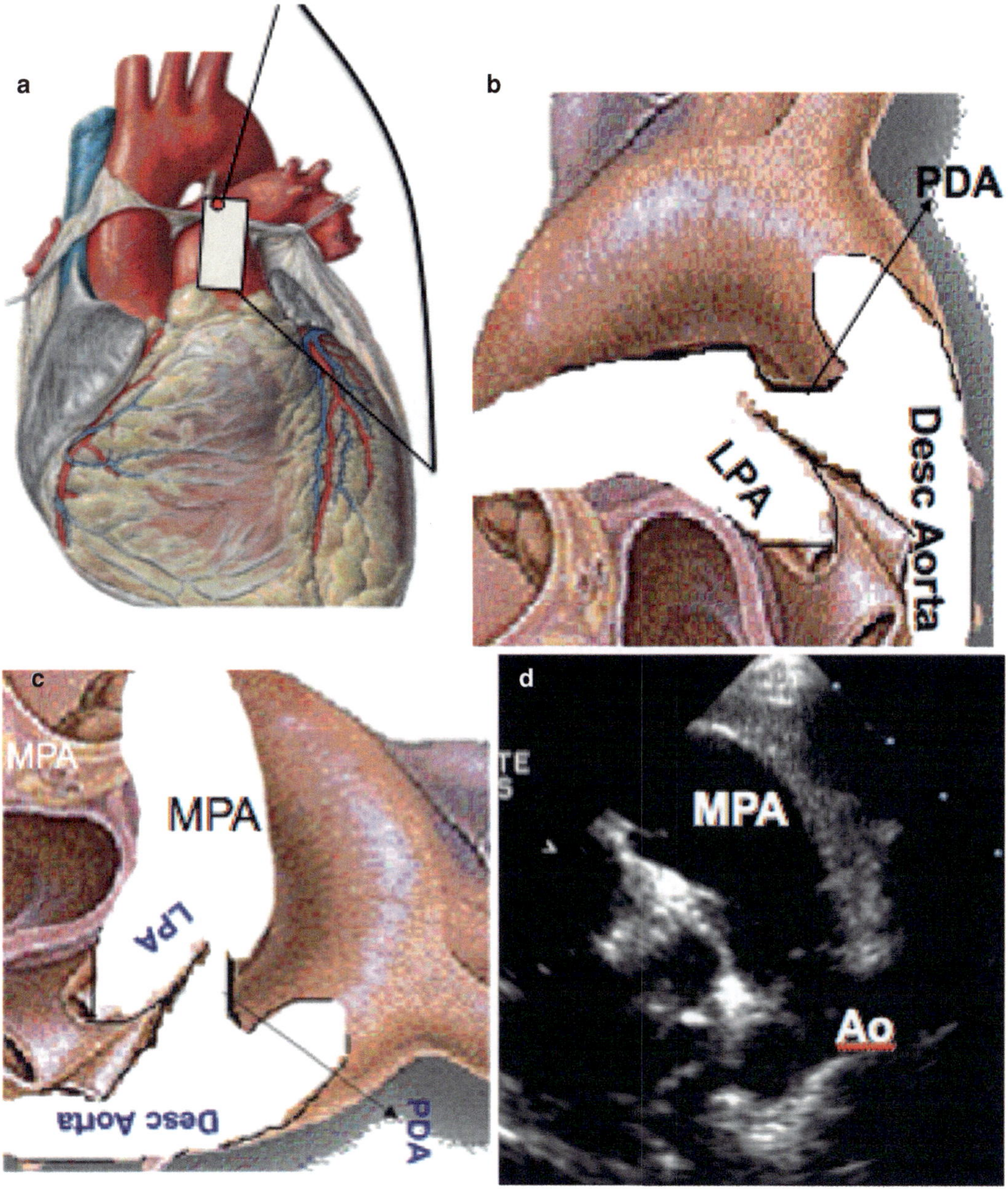

Fig. 23.13 The high parasternal or the ductal view is obtained by placing the transducer high in the precordium, usually in the first intercostal space, (**a**) and obtaining a section of the MPA–LPA and the descending aorta in the parasagittal plane (**b**) To understand the echo image (**d**) the picture in the frame "(**b**)" has been rotated by 90° in a clockwise direction (**c**). The anterior structures are displayed closest to the transducer. *Ao* Aorta, *MPA* Main pulmonary artery, *LPA* left pulmonary artery, *PDA* Patent ductus arteriosus

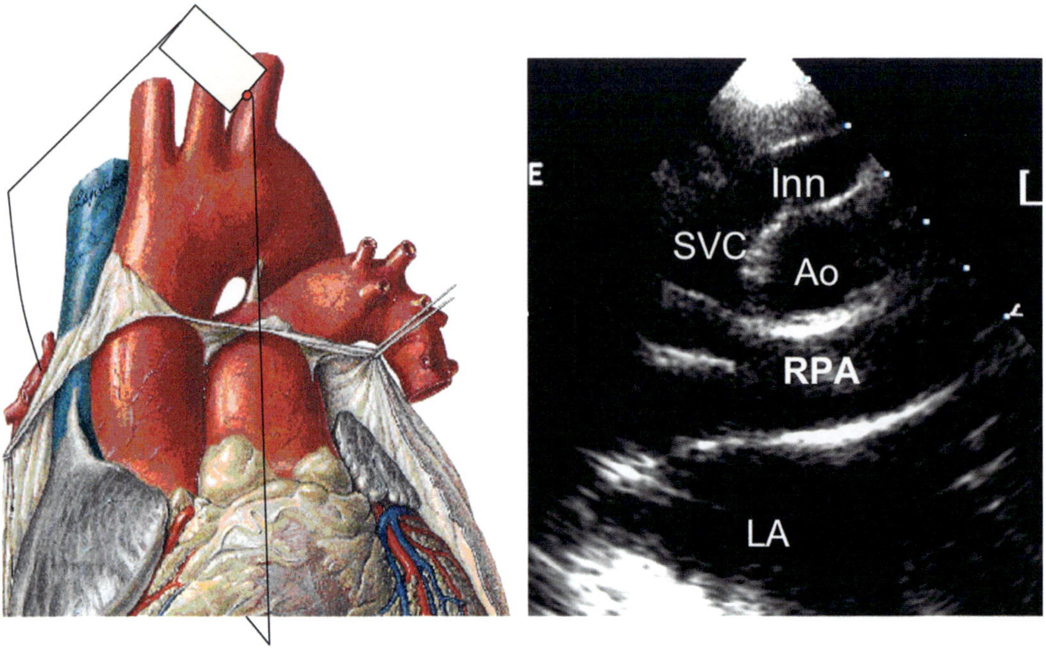

Fig. 23.14 The suprasternal short-axis view cuts the aorta (Ao) in its short-axis (shows up as a circular structure) and cuts the right pulmonary artery (RPA) in its long axis. The innominate vein (Inn) is the closest to the transducer. Other structures seen are superior vena cava (SVC) and left atrium (LA). The frame on the left shows how the imaging plane cuts the structures and the frame on the right shows the echocardiography picture

- Tilting of the transducer enables visualization of the innominate vein and its drainage into the SVC, as well as the drainage of SVC into the RA.
- Cranial tilt of the transducer helps to identify and trace the course of the first aortic branch (usually Innominate Artery) and its bifurcation into the Right Subclavian Artery (RSCA) and the Right Common Carotid Artery (RCCA).
- Absence or hypoplasia of the innominate vein suggests bilateral SVC; left SVC (LSVC) can be imaged by tilting the transducer leftwards of the Aorta, sliding it into the first intercostal space just left of the sternum, and rotating to show the entire course of the LSVC.

Suprasternal Long-Axis View (Fig. 23.15):

- This view is obtained by rotating the transducer counterclockwise (from the short-axis potion) with the cursor pointing toward the patient's left ear (roughly 2 o' clock position such that the aortic arch is profiled along its long axis ("candy cane" view).
- The branches from the aortic arch can be well appreciated. RPA appears in cross-section while a slight leftward tilt profiles the LPA along its long axis.

23.9 Hemodynamic Assessment

Echocardiography can provide a great deal of hemodynamic information, derived from multiple tools that include:

- Two-dimensional visualization of the movements of the cardiac structures (chambers, septae, and valve leaflets)
- Quantification of ventricular fractional shortening (FS) and ejection fraction (EF) using M-mode (Teicholz method), two-dimensional echo (Simpson method), or three-dimensional echo

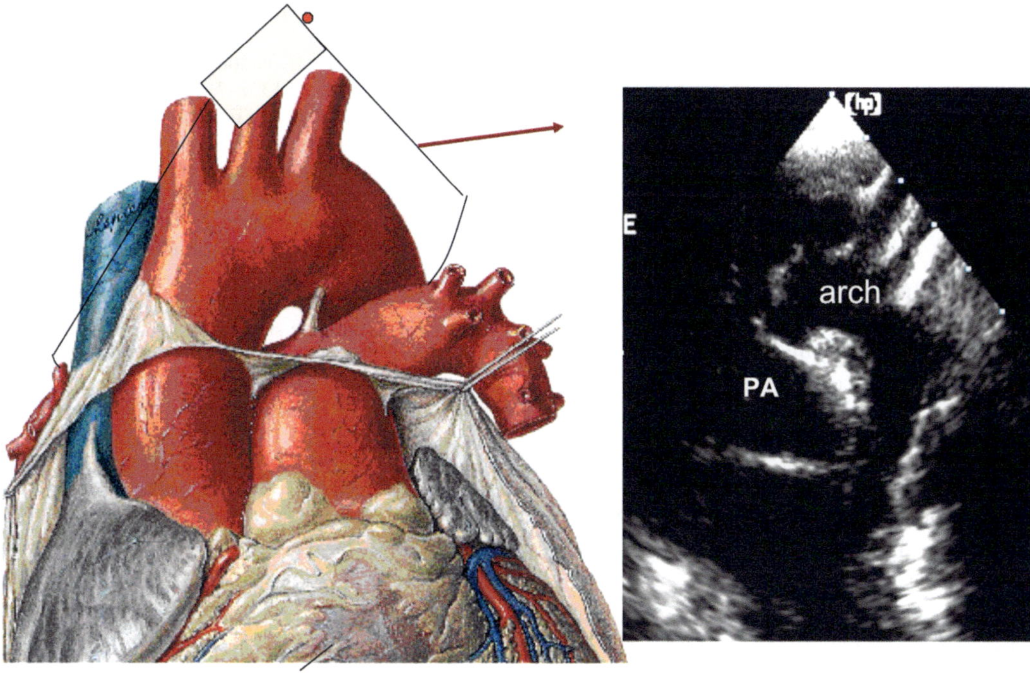

Fig. 23.15 Transducer position and imaging planes for the supra-sternal long-axis views (left). Echocardiogram showing the structures seen in the supra-sternal long-axis view (right). *PA* pulmonary artery, *Arch* Aortic Arch

- Interrogation and interpretation of color Doppler across valves and structural defects
- Spectral Doppler (continuous and pulse wave) to measure blood flow velocities and to derive pressure gradients
- Tissue Doppler indices
- Speckle tracking
- Myocardial strain imaging
- Stress echocardiography

Ventricular volume, systolic function assessment, color Doppler, and spectral Doppler evaluation are essential elements of echocardiography for CHD. Tissue Doppler, speckle tracking, strain imaging, and stress studies usually find greater applications in acquired heart disease and adult echocardiograms. A detailed discussion of hemodynamic assessment is beyond the scope of this chapter. However, it is pertinent to remember that anatomical information must be interpreted and reported in conjunction with the hemodynamic findings in CHD imaging. Management decisions are as reliant on physiological information as on the structural diagnosis.

23.10 Summary

Echocardiography for CHD requires a thorough, sequential, and systematic approach. This is essential for piecing together the disparate parts of the jigsaw puzzle of cardiovascular segmental anatomy and deciphering their three-dimensional spatial inter-relationships. Many views and imaging planes are quite unique to CHD echocardiograms. Almost every view involves dynamic sweeps, tilts, and rotations through the anatomical planes, rather than relying on a fixed image plane. With increasing experience and expertise, the echocardiographer adapts not just to these prescribed views but to infinite in-between viewing planes and views, leading toward understanding and managing CHD.

Final word—"Integrated Imaging Approach".

Diagnosis and management of CHD require the combined and coordinated efforts of personnel, techniques, and technologies across specialties—cardiology, cardiac surgery, radiology, anesthesiology, and intensive care, and so on. No imaging modality can replace good clinical acumen and expertise. All imaging modalities are tools in our armamentarium, with their own strengths and weaknesses, and should be used intelligently either alone or in combination toward understanding and treating CHD. These choices should be dictated by the ability of each modality to answer specific study questions pertinent to each case, balanced with the feasibility and safety. The information thus obtained, as well as the clinical context should be integrated to help guide management.

Acknowledgments Figures 23.2, 23.3, 23.4, 23.5, 23.6, 23.7, 23.8, 23.9, 23.10, 23.11, 23.12, 23.13, 23.14, and 23.15 have been reproduced with permission from Kumar RK. Echocardiography for evaluation of congenital heart disease. In: Prabhakaran D, Kumar RK, Naik N, Kaul U, eds. Tandon's Textbook of Cardiology. Wolters Kluwer, 2019:432–442.

References

1. Curie P, Curie J. Developpement, par pression de l'electricite polaire dans les cristaux hemiedres a faces inclinees. Comptes Rendus. 1880;91:291–5.
2. Singh S, Goyal A. The origin of echocardiography: a tribute to Inge Edler. Tex Heart Inst J. 2007;34(4):431–8.
3. Dussik KT. On the possibility of using ultrasound waves as a diagnostic aid. Neurol Psychiat. 1942;174:153–68.
4. Edler I, Lindstrom K. The history of echocardiography. Ultrasound Med Biol. 2004;30:1565–644.
5. Holmer NG, Lindstrom K, Lundstrom N-R, Marsal K, Olsson B, Pettersson H, Persson HW. In memoriam: Inge Edler—the father of echocardiography. Eur J Ultrasound. 2001;13:179–82.
6. Edler I, Hertz CH. The use of ultrasonic reflectoscope for the continuous recording of the movements of heart walls. 1954. Clin Physiol Funct Imaging. 2004;24:118–36.
7. Feigenbaum H. Evolution of echocardiography. Circulation. 1996;93:1321–7.
8. Wann LS, Weyman AE, Feigenbaum H, Dillon JC, Johnston KW, Eggleton RC. Determination of mitral valve area by cross-sectional echocardiography. Ann Intern Med. 1978;88:337–41.
9. Holen J, Simonsen S. Determination of pressure gradient in mitral stenosis with Doppler echocardiography. Br Heart J. 1980;41:529–35.
10. Hatle L, Angelsen BA, Tromsdal A. Non-invasive assessment of aortic stenosis by Doppler ultrasound. Br Heart J. 1979;43:284–92.
11. Frazin L, Talano JV, Stephanides L, Loeb HS, Kopel L, Gunnar RM. Esophageal echocardiography. Circulation. 1976;54:102–8.
12. Lapierre C, Déry J, Guérin R, Viremouneix L, Dubois J, Garel L. Segmental approach to imaging of congenital heart disease. Radiographics. 2010;30(2):397–411.
13. Van Praagh R. The importance of segmental situs in the diagnosis of congenital heart disease. Semin Roentgenol. 1985;20(3):254–71.
14. Van Praagh R, Vlad P. Dextrocardia, mesocardia, and levocardia: the segmental approach to diagnosis in congenital heart disease. In: Keith JD, Rowe RD, Vlad P, editors. Heart disease in infancy and childhood. 3rd ed. New York, NY: Macmillan; 1978. p. 638–95.
15. Anderson RH, Becker AE, Freedom RM, et al. Sequential segmental analysis of congenital heart disease. Pediatr Cardiol. 1984;5(4):281–7.
16. Henry WL, Demaria A, Gramiak R, et al. Report of the American Society of echocardiography committee on nomenclature and standards in two-dimensional echocardiography. Circulation. 1980;62:212–7.
17. Gutgesell HP. Cardiac imaging with ultrasound: right-side up or upside down? [Editorial]. Am J Cardiol. 1985;56:479–80.
18. Bierman FZ, Williams RG. Prospective diagnosis of d-transposition of great arteries neonates by subxiphoid two-dimensional echocardiography. Circulation. 1980;63:165–73.
19. Bierman FZ, Fellows K, Williams RG. Prospective identification of ventricular septal defects in infancy using two-dimensional echocardiography. Circulation. 1980;62:807–17.
20. Kumar RK. Echocardiography for evaluation of congenital heart disease. In: Prabhakaran D, Kumar RK, Naik N, Kaul U, editors. Tandon's textbook of cardiology. New Delhi: Wolters Kluwer; 2019. p. 432–42.
21. Sanders SP. Echocardiography and related techniques in the diagnosis of congenital heart disease. I. Veins, atria and interatrial septum. Echocardiography. 1984;1:118–217.

3D Prototyping: Technology and Applications for CHD

24

Mahesh Kappanayil

24.1 Introduction

Medical imaging is all about technology. It is that unique space where engineering, medicine, and computer science come together in the most tangible and impactful possible manner. As technology takes quantum leaps, so do its applications in medical imaging. Once we obtain a perfect imaging dataset, it is how we process that information that completes the loop and guides us toward patient management.

The cardiovascular system, and in particular congenital heart disease (CHD) with its wide range of anatomical and positional alterations possible, offers some of the most difficult challenges for medical imaging technology. Both anatomy and physiology, and their mutual correlations need to be deeply internalized. Traditionally, one or more imaging modalities are employed, as per requirements of the case, and all the information thus derived is collated to generate the final mental picture, diagnosis, and a management plan. Comprehending, internalizing, and effectively communicating three-dimensional (3D) spatial anatomy is a crucial element in this process. Even while using two-dimensional planar imaging like 2D echocardiography, the imager constantly attempts to mentally reconstruct the spatial anatomy while sweeping through the planes. 3D echocardiography, computed tomography (CT), and the 3D angiographic sequences in magnetic resonance imaging (MRI) provide 3D volumetric data in the form of stacks or slices of information that can then be viewed slice-by-slice or manipulated and post-processed in various ways to provide a 3D perspective.

Multiplanar viewing and 3D rendering are some of these tools. However, at the end of the day, viewing is still on the 2D screens of workstations and interpretation depends upon the experience, understanding, and spatial intelligence of the viewer [1]. In most units, complex management decisions are taken in multidisciplinary meetings involving cardiologists, surgeons, anesthesiologists, and other members of the team. Communicating the precise anatomical details and getting all the team members on the same page with exactly the same mental picture and understanding of the anatomy is a daunting task, and impacts management decisions and pre-surgical planning.

3D Prototyping or 3D Printing, also known as "additive manufacturing," is an innovative manufacturing process that uses computer-aided processing of three-dimensional image data to create physical "print outs" of virtual objects. Primarily developed for industrial applications, the technology transcends into the space of medicine through its ability to convert volumetric medical imaging

M. Kappanayil (✉)
Department of Pediatric Cardiology, Amrita School of Medicine, Amrita Institute of Medical Sciences and Research Centre, Amrita Vishwa Vidyapeetham, Kochi, Kerala, India

R. Rajeshkannan et al. (eds.), *CT and MRI in Congenital Heart Diseases*,
https://doi.org/10.1007/978-981-15-6755-1_24

data into actual to-scale physical replicas. And since many of the commonly used medical imaging techniques generate 3D datasets—they provide a ready substrate for using the technology in a radical and transformative manner.

24.2 What Is 3D Printing or Additive Manufacturing?

"*Additive manufacturing*" is a fabrication technique that involves the creation of a three-dimensional object from a computer-aided design (CAD) model by successive addition of material layer by layer, under precise computer control. This gives it the unique ability to build extremely complex designs and geometries from a digital 3D model with a very high degree of accuracy in relatively short build-times.

3D printing technology lies at the crossroads of computer science, material science, and fabrication technology. There is a wide range of techniques and materials that can be used, according to the requirements of the object being created. The basic principle of all 3D printing processes is the same—create a digital 3D model, divide it into multiple slices or layers, and then recreate it physically, layer by layer, by adding material through a digitally controlled process using "3D Printers." The different techniques of 3D printing vary in the way the layers are deposited and the type of materials used. Most 3D printing techniques are suitable for printing-out objects derived out of medical imaging data.

24.3 Different Types of 3D Printing Technologies and How They Work

1. *Stereolithography*: Photopolymerization and solidification of a photosensitive resin using digitally guided ultraviolet (UV) light laser. A wide range of such resins are available that can be converted into 3D prints with varying physical and mechanical properties—from flexible to hard, from transparent to opaque. It is a high-precision technique with excellent surface finish, commonly used for printing-out cardiovascular models.
2. *Fused deposition modeling (FDM)*: extrusion and solidification of melted thermoplastic materials. The material is usually fed into the printer in filament form and includes polymers like polylactic acid (PLA), acrylonitrile butadiene styrene (ABS), polycarbonate (PC), high-density polyethylene (HDPE), etc. This is a versatile and robust technique well suited for making hard and durable models with long shelf life.
3. *Selective Laser Melting*: Melting and fusion of powdered hard materials like metal (e.g., titanium), ceramic using a high-powered laser beam.
4. *Selective Laser Sintering*: Sintering of a range of powdered materials like nylon, polyamide (PA), polystyrenes (PS), thermoplastic elastomers, polyaryletherketones (PAEK) and metallic powders using laser.
5. *Polyjet*: Jetting and then solidification of thin layers of photopolymers using UV light. This technology is capable of incorporating multiple materials and multiple colors into one model and is an excellent technique for printing realistic medical models.
6. *Digital Light Processing (DLP)*: similar to stereolithography, except that it uses more conventional light sources like arc lamp with liquid crystal display (LCD) panel to photopolymerize a photosensitive resin material.
7. *Binder Jetting*: binding of the particles of a powdered material (e.g., metal, sand, ceramic) using a liquid-binding agent.

24.4 Brief History of Additive Manufacturing

3D printing as a technology is not new and has been in existence since the 1980s. Hideo Kodama invented a new layer-by-layer approach to manufacturing by polymerizing a photosensitive resin using UV light in 1981 [2]. In 1986, Charles Hull obtained a patent for a stereolithography system, and he subsequently went on to release the world's first commercially available 3D printer, the SLA-1 through his company 3D Systems Corporation [3]. Carl Deckard patented Selective Laser Sintering (SLS) in 1988. Scott Crump is credited with inventing the fusion deposition modeling (FDM) technology, which he patented in 1989. He founded his company Stratasys that released the first commercially available FDM machine in 1992 [4]. The subsequent three decades have seen considerable advances in not just the technology but in the materials used in additive manufacturing.

The turning point was the advent of miniaturized, affordable, desktop versions of these machines with the expiry of the patents governing them in the first decade of the new millennium. Young start-up companies like Makerbot™ with the launch of their desktop FDM 3D printer, and Formlabs™ with their desktop version of an SLA printer, brought the technology into the hands of hobbyists and enthusiasts and captured the popular imagination. These changes, coupled with rapid advances in material science as well as in software spawned a new wave of innovations, and discovery of novel uses for the technology. Medicine, by virtue of an existing need for better ways to visualize imaging data, found a ready application.

24.5 3D Printing in Medicine and in Cardiovascular Sciences

The primary utility for 3D printing technologies in medicine stems from its capability to convert medical volumetric imaging datasets to physical replicas. This has the potential to dramatically simplify the manner in which we view and interact with medical images. Derived from patient-specific imaging data, the 3D printed anatomical models precisely mimic the true anatomy and allow the observers to touch, hold and manipulate imaging data in a uniquely sensory manner, instead of merely viewing it on a 2D screen. The tactile interaction with the model greatly adds to the three-dimensional understanding of complex morphology, and takes away the need to imagine or intellectualize spatial anatomy [5–7].

Tentative exploration of medical applications for 3D printing started as early as the 1990s with its use in bony reconstructive surgeries. In 1999, Wake Forest Institute for Regenerative Medicine used the technology to create a biodegradable scaffold of the urinary bladder of a patient from CT scan, layered it with autologous cells grown from the bladder to create a laboratory-grown bladder for transplantation [8]. Dental, orthopedic, and craniomaxillofacial surgical specialties were among the earliest adopters of the technology, since the early 2000s, since it allowed realistic and relatively simple bony reconstructions for better surgical planning, and subsequently even cutting-guides and implants [9–12].

Utilizing 3D printing in cardiovascular imaging has been a relatively recent development. Modeling cardiovascular anatomy poses unique challenges. The soft tissue characteristics, mobility of the heart, the small size of many of the structures, and breathing and movement artifacts are among the factors that add to technical difficulties in acquiring and then accurately 3D-modeling cardiac imaging data. Also, in the current era when 3D printing is not standard-of-care, has limited accessibility, requires niche expertise, and involves extra costs; it is largely left to the "early adopters" to identify need and implement processes [13–18]. Expectedly, it is in the subset of CHD patients with the most complex anatomies that 3D printing has found its most important early applications. Therefore, it is not surprising that the most common and established use cases have been in complex double outlet right ventricle (DORV) lesions. Understanding of the spatial relationship between the great arteries and their relationship with the ventricles and the ventricular septal defect (VSD) in DORV are critical to planning surgical repair. Multiple studies have shown the significant incremental value of 3D prints in understanding DORV anatomy and planning surgical treatment [15–17, 19, 20]. 3D printing is an effort and expertise intensive process and is, therefore, better reserved for situations that demand its utility. It should address very specific study questions and fulfill specific needs. These questions may pertain to extracardiac or intracardiac anatomical details or both:

- Understanding 3D spatial relationships between various cardiovascular structures, e.g., in complex heterotaxy syndromes, mixed total anomalous pulmonary venous connections (TAPVC), aortopulmonary collaterals, etc.
- Understanding complex intracardiac anatomical details to plan the surgical approach, e.g., in complex double outlet right ventricle (DORV), criss-cross heart, anatomically corrected malposition of great arteries (ACMGA), etc.
- Understanding rare and complex defects for planning the interventional approach, e.g., portosystemic shunt, arteriovenous malformation, aortic aneurysm, etc.
- As a scaffold for designing or customizing patient-specific implants, stents, and valves.
- As teaching, research, and simulation tools [21–23].
- As an effective communication tool [24].
- Creating morphological museums populated by 3D printed models of various pathological entities.
- Biological 3D printing applications.

24.6 Steps in Cardiovascular 3D Printing

24.6.1 Step 1: Imaging

The primary requirement for 3D printing is an optimal volumetric imaging dataset, which could be CT, MRI, or echocardiogram. Anticipating the need for downstream 3D printing can help choose the ideal imaging modality and ensure optimized acquisition.

The choice of modality may depend upon a variety of factors. While 3D echocardiographic datasets would be low-cost, easy to acquire, and free of ionizing radiation and ideal for structures like valve leaflets, ultrasound is prone to artifacts, limited by acoustic windows, and has suboptimal signal/noise ratios. Ultrasound data is, at present, the least optimized for 3D printing. CT scan provides sub-millimeter tissue resolution, can identify bone and calcium, can be safely done even in patients with pacemakers and metal implants, and is ideal for 3D printing. ECG-gated, breath-held, contrast-enhanced CT angiography can provide a spatial resolution of 0.3–0.7 mm. But the trade-off for CT is exposure to ionizing radiation. MRI can provide high-resolution soft tissue and blood pool imaging along with vital functional information, without ionizing radiation or iodinated contrast media. MRI 3D sequences that can be effectively used for 3D printing include contrast-enhanced MR angiography as well as whole heart 3D SSFP sequence with respiratory navigator gating and ECG triggering, with or without contrast. The latter sequence gives excellent imaging of intracardiac details. The disadvantages of MRI are lower spatial resolution than CT, longer scan times, and inability to use it in patients with pacemakers and metal implants. Therefore, the choice of the imaging modality needs to be customized to the requirements, limitations, and the specific study questions of the case. A good quality dataset should have a uniform, good blood to myocardium contrast with no significant artifacts. In case the patient has undergone multiple forms of imaging, the best dataset that answers the study questions should be chosen for further processing. It is also possible to combine data from different imaging modalities into one model using digital co-registration software tools.

CT and MRI data are exported in the DICOM® (Digital Imaging and Communications in Medicine) format. 3D echocardiographic data is exported in the Cartesian DICOM format.

24.6.2 Step 2: Segmentation, Design, and Creation of the Digital 3D Object

Segmentation is the process of registering a region of interest (ROI) from the DICOM images onto a three-dimensional field, and converting the data from slices of pixels into a 3D digital model with proper *X*;*Y*;*Z*-axis coordinates [21] In order to this, the DICOM datasets are imported into specialized software and first subjected to a "pre-segmentation process" that consists of identification and isolation of the ROI and subjecting it to the algorithmic treatment of pixels: thresholding, clustering, edge attraction, and classification

[21]. Segmentation results in the transformation of this data into a 3D model, with the total 3D coordinates being referred to as a "mesh." The segmented mesh is then saved and exported out in 3D file formats such as STL, OBJ, VRML, PLY, and AMF [20] (Fig. 24.1).

A number of commercially available proprietary software as well as open-source software can be used to execute these steps, e.g., Mimics (Materialise, Leuven, Belgium), Simpleware (Synopsis, CA), Seg3D (University of Utah, Salt Lake City, UT), Slicer, Terrarecon (Foster City, CA) and others.

Segmentation is a crucial step in the process of 3D printing, particularly with regard to 3D printing of soft-tissue structures and the cardiovascular system. While segmenting bony structures is usually a quick, thresholding process, cardiovascular image segmentation can be demanding, time-consuming, and heavily dependent upon the expertise of the operator. Differentiation between soft tissue/myocardium/vessels and the blood pool may be difficult and poorly demarcated in some image slices. The individual doing the segmentation should have background knowledge of cardiovascular defects and experience with viewing and interpreting cardiovascular tomographic images. Errors in thresholding can result in errors in the masks generated and thereby in the eventual 3D model. The quality of the imaging dataset, age and size of the patient, breathing and movement artifacts, and inherent complexity of anatomy can all make the segmentation a challenging and expertise-intensive step. Most of the segmenting software have inbuilt digital tools for editing the masks, which allow addition, subtraction, and modification of data that goes into the creation of the masks. The human interface is critical here since it requires skill to correctly interpret the raw DICOM images and to ensure that segmented and edited digital 3D model is an accurate representation of the raw data.

There are several design considerations while segmenting and creating a digital 3D model of a cardiovascular lesion, depending upon the specific intent of the print. Examples are—decisions whether to include the myocardium or only the blood pool, whether to build a solid heart model or a hollow one, whether to build an intact model or a sliced-open one. The model created

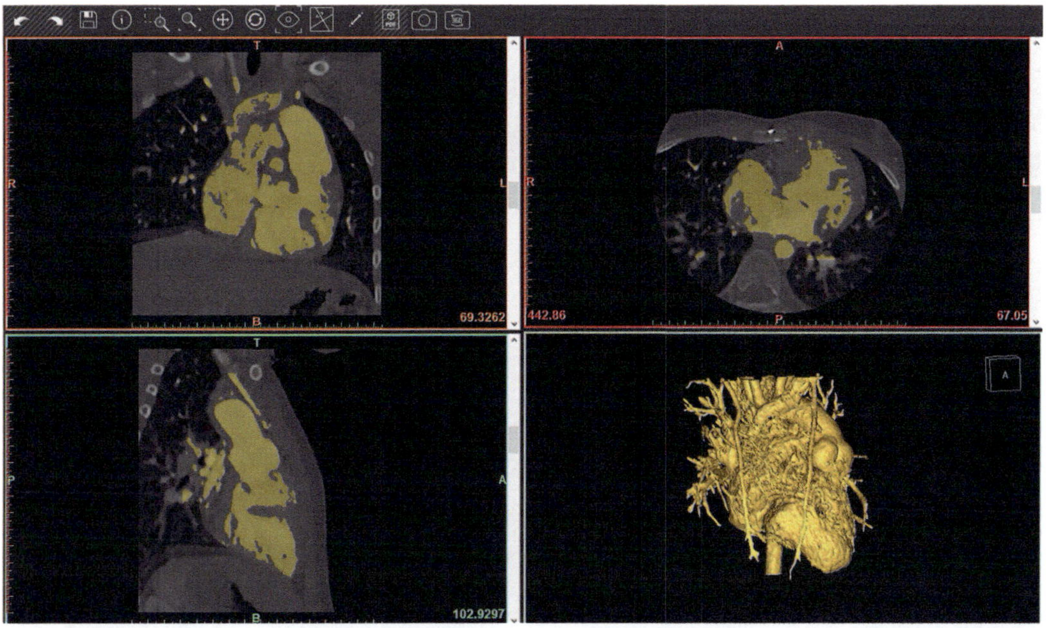

Fig. 24.1 Screenshot showing the isolation of region of interest (ROI) and thresholding of the two-dimensional orthogonal projections to generate an accurate and pertinent three-dimensional image

by segmenting the blood pool out of an angiographic dataset is essentially a voluminogram. Design tools in software allow for the creation of an outer shell or mesh over the voluminogram. Subsequent subtraction of the blood pool while retaining the outer shell results in a hollow heart model that can provide excellent visualization of the intracardiac spaces and the pathways for blood flow. A hollow heart model can be cut open along pre-decided planes at the design stage, using digital cut tools, to allow the best visualization of the intracardiac anatomical challenges, e.g., a sliced-open hollow-heart model would be ideal for understanding the complexity of left ventricle (LV) to aorta pathway in a DORV with remote ventricular septal defect (VSD). For an extracardiac study question like the spatial relationship of aortopulmonary collaterals to descending aorta, or the pattern of pulmonary venous drainage in a case of total anomalous pulmonary venous return (TAPVR), a solid model would suffice (Figs. 24.2, 24.3, and 24.4). Fair knowledge of the potential downstream surgical options is important to add these design elements to the digital 3D file. In case the intent of the model is for a surgical simulation, the decision may be to print a hollow whole-heart model in a material that a surgeon can later cut and inspect the internal details.

The stage of segmentation is an important point of quality check to ensure that the digital 3D model created is accurate and true to the original raw data.

The virtual 3D model can be further edited using digital tools like smoothing and cutting away of unnecessary parts, and labeling, before finally exporting as in a 3D printable file format. Standard tessellation language or STL is one of the most common such file formats. The scale of the object can be accurately customized at the time of export. 1:1 scale is opted for building true-to-life realistic models.

24.6.3 Step 3: Consideration of the Printing Technology and Material to Be Used

The 3D file created in the above steps is ready to be "printed out." The type of printer and the material used is dictated by the purpose and the desired durability, flexibility, complexity, func-

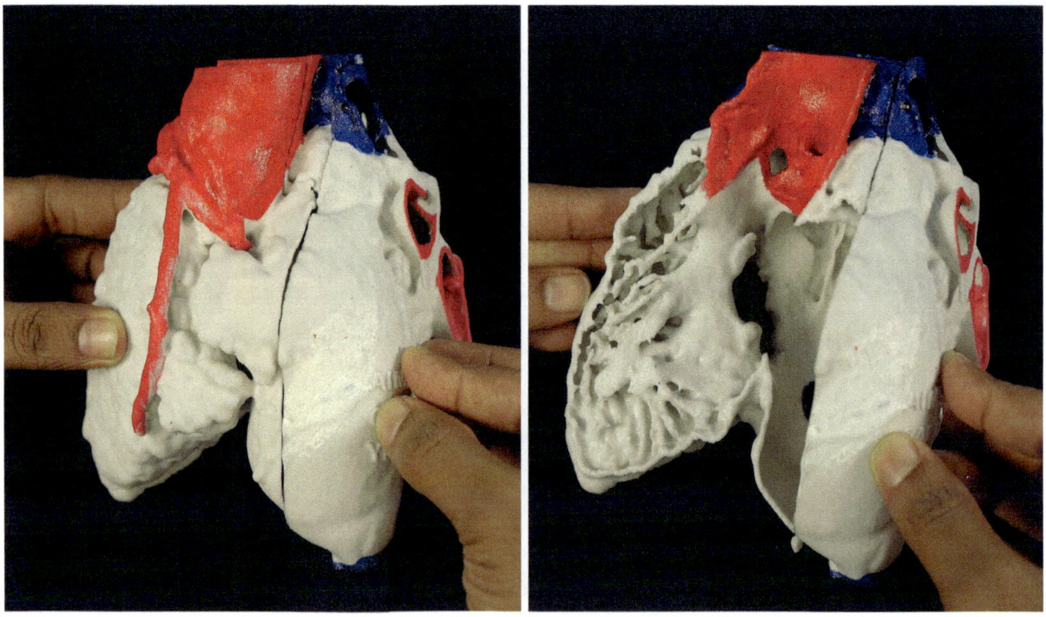

Fig. 24.2 Three-dimensional model of a complex heart with dextrocardia, double outlet right ventricle in the context of heterotaxy syndrome. The "cut-open" design of the model allows a detailed inspection of intracardiac details

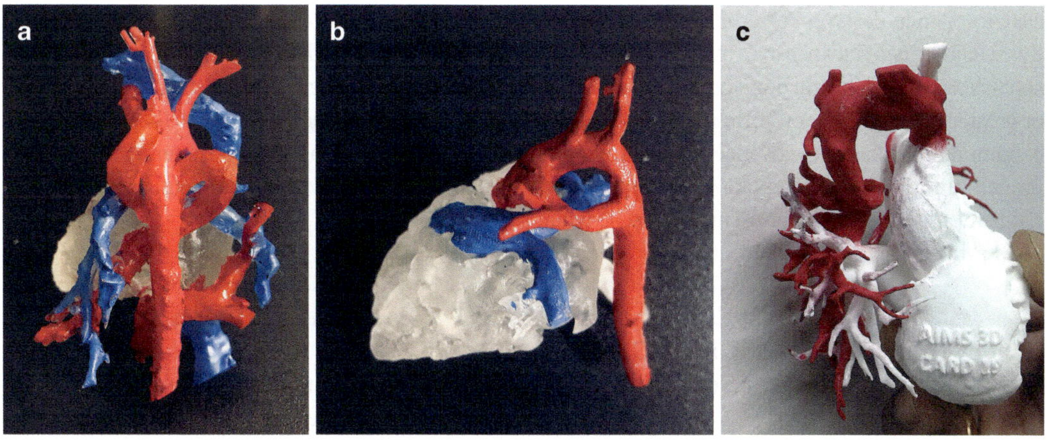

Fig. 24.3 (**a**) shows the pulmonary venous anatomy in a case of a neonate with mixed total anomalous pulmonary venous return. (**b**) Double aortic arch. (**c**) Aortopulmonary collateral from right subclavian artery to right pulmonary artery

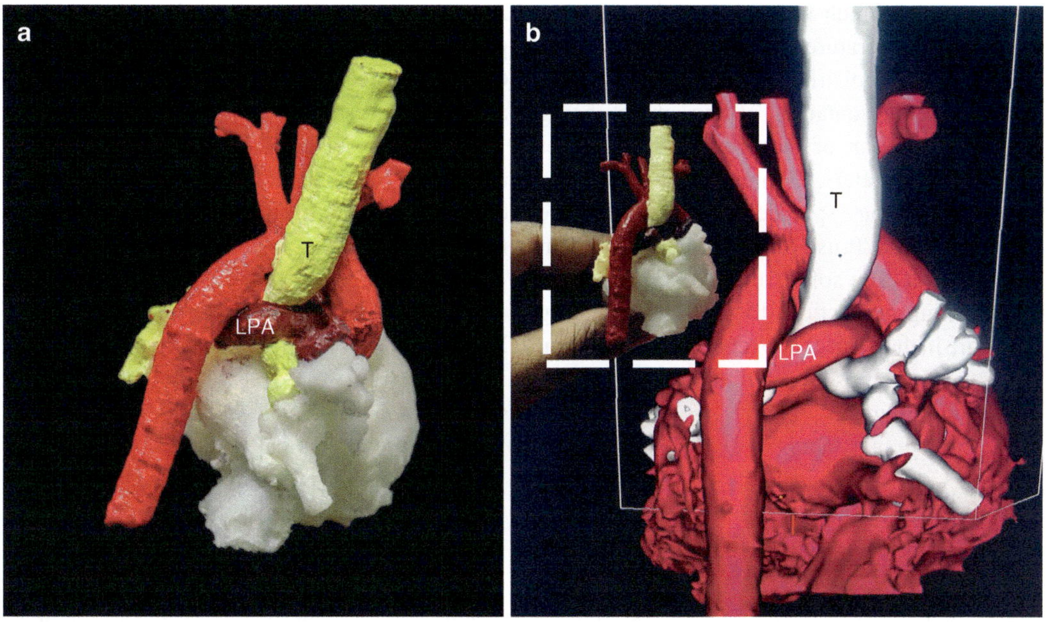

Fig. 24.4 (**a**) Three-dimensional model of LPA-sling showing the trachea (T) and left bronchus compressed by the left pulmonary artery (LPA). (**b**) The 1:1 scale model held in perspective in front of a zoomed up digital image

tionality, surface quality, and esthetics of the model. The choice also depends upon the access to different types of printers and printing materials—which could range from basic desktop FDM and SLA printers, through more advanced and sophisticated polyjet and SLS printers to industrial-grade printers. The cost of the 3D printing process, as well as the turn-around time, can also vary widely accordingly.

An ideal situation for cardiovascular centers would be to have an in-house point-of-care 3D printing facility with good quality, low-maintenance, and easy-to-operate desktop 3D printers that use readily available and inexpensive material. For more sophisticated models utilizing specialized material, or greater capability, the projects can be exported to extramural facilities with advanced printers. Polyjet printers are capable of incorporating multiple materials and multiple colors in a single model, while SLM printers can print titanium.

24.6.4 Step 4: Export of Digital 3D File to 3D Printer Software and Hardware

Digital 3D file is exported to the 3D printer via "slicer software." The slicer software prepares the digital file for printing by converting it into stacks and prescribing the instructions to the printer, which include the printer movements, the temperature of the extruder or printer bed, design and distribution of "support structures," layout/orientation of the object being printed, resolution of the print, and a number of other parameters. Examples of printer or printer technology-specific slicer software are Ultimaker Cura, Prusa Slicer, Slic3r, Voxelizer, and PreForm. The software exports the executable printing instructions to the actual printing hardware in the form of a "g-code." Optimization at this level ensures an accurate print as per the desired requirements.

24.6.5 Step 5: Printing and Post-processing

The digital 3D file is finally converted into a physical 3D model by the printer hardware by adding material to create layer-after-layer in accordance to the slicer. The time taken for this process varies depending upon the type of printer, the type and amount of material required, and the size and complexity of the object. Many of the 3D printing technologies print support structures to support overhangs in the design. These support structures are removed after the print is complete, and the object is further post-processed to give it the final form and finish.

Time, material consumption and cost for 3D printing CHD models depends upon the type of printing technology and material being used, and the complexity and size of the model. With advances in technology and material science, the printing processes are becoming faster and less expensive.

24.7 Caveats of 3D Models

Accuracy and utility of 3D depend upon several variables: (1). The quality of the 3D imaging dataset. (2). Accuracy of interpretation of the raw data by the person involved in pre-segmentation and segmentation processes. (3). Quality and accuracy of the software manipulation (segmentation) of the DICOM images into a digital 3D file. (4). Appropriateness of the design of 3D print to answer specific study questions. (5). Quality and accuracy of the final printing process and post-processing.

3D printing of medical images is not a "plug and play" process. It requires considerable human expertise and effort for an accurate and meaningful application.

24.8 Illustrative Case Examples

- *Patient 1*: an 18-year-old male, hypoxic and polycythemic patient with baseline SO2 75% with complex cyanotic CHD. Despite early diagnosis in infancy, he had been refused cardiac surgery at multiple institutions in the past due to complex anatomy. Multi-modality cardiac imaging that included echocardiography, catheter angiography, and cardiac MRI had led to a morphological diagnosis of situs inversus, dextrocardia, complex DORV, side-by-side great arteries, large conoventricular VSD with inlet extension, severe subvalvar and valvar pulmonary stenosis. Biventricular surgical repair was considered challenging after conventional review of imaging data in multidisciplinary meetings at multiple institutions led to significant ambiguity and disagreement regarding the technical feasibility of biventricular repair. Contrast-enhanced MRA sequence obtained as part of the cardiac MR protocol was extracted and segmented on Materialise Mimics® (Materialise NV, Leuven, Belgium) software, and a "hollow-heart" 3D digital model was created. The model was custom designed with the posterior atrial walls digitally removed, providing a perspective through the atrioventricular (AV) valve annuli, similar to the surgeons' perspective after atriotomy. The model was printed out on a 1:1 scale using polyamide material on an SLS printer. The 3D model provided a dramatically enhanced understanding of the spatial and intracardiac anatomy and aided a clear decision toward biventricular repair. A very clear surgical plan was made on the basis of the 3D print with regard to the tunneling pathway, need and location of right ventriculotomy, and the placement of right-ventricle (RV)-to-pulmonary artery (PA) conduit (Fig. 24.5). The surgical findings correlated well with the 3D printed model. The surgery was successfully executed as per the plan with optimal cardiopulmonary bypass time and postoperative recovery.

- *Case 2*: A 2-month-old infant presented with heart failure, diminished lower limb arterial pulses, and mild desaturation (SO2 90%). The infant had been evaluated previously at other cardiac centers and concerns expressed about complex anatomy. Echocardiogram showed situs solitus, levocardia with criss-cross AV connections, inlet VSD, DORV with coarctation of aorta. Spatial anatomy and the intracardiac anatomy were difficult to comprehend using standard echocardiographic views; custom viewing planes were used to gather anatomical details. Criss-cross hearts with associated defects are among the toughest imaging challenges in CHD imaging and can baffle even experienced and skilled imagers. Conventional review of echocardiographic images suggested the possibility of biventricular repair with intraventricular tunneling of the left ventricle (LV) to aorta via the VSD, along with coarctation repair, through sternotomy approach. In view of the complexity of the anatomy, a 3D print was planned. A cardiac multidetector CT scan was done, and the volumetric data was used to print-out the hollow-heart model in powder-based sandstone material (Fig. 24.6). Two cuts were prescribed during the design stage—a posterior parasagittal cut allowing removal of the atria, and a mid-septal level ventricular short-axis cut.

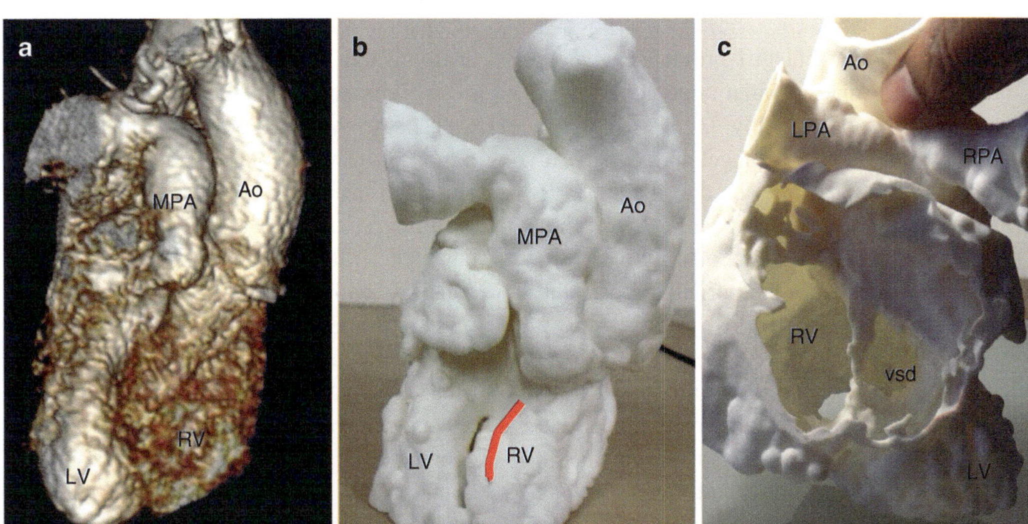

Fig. 24.5 (**a**) Digital 3D reconstruction of Case 1 DORV. (**b**) and (**c**) show the enhanced visual perspective using the 3D model. Red line in (b) marks the planned site of right ventriculotomy. *AO* aorta, *LPA* left pulmonary artery, *LV* left ventricle, *MPA* main pulmonary artery, *RPA* right pulmonary artery, *RV* right ventricle, *vsd* ventricular septal defect

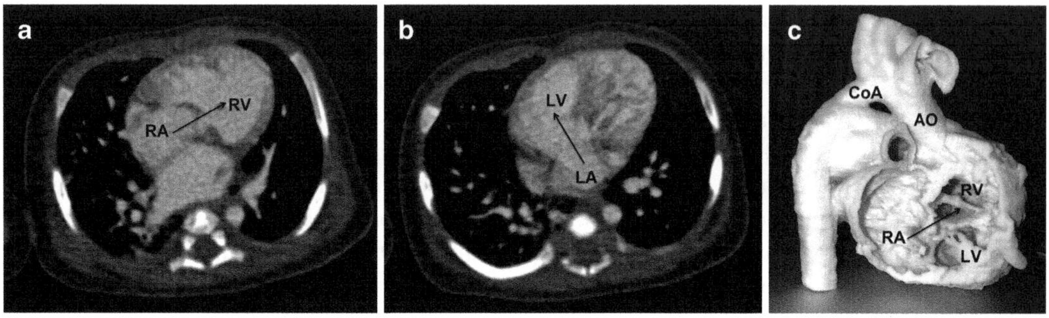

Fig. 24.6 (**a**) and (**b**) show the axial images of criss-cross atrioventricular relationships. (**c**) The three-dimensional model. *AO* Aorta; *CoA* Coarctation of aorta; *LA* left atrium, *LV* left ventricle, *RA* right atrium, *RV* right ventricle

The rare and complex anatomy was well appreciated using the model. It showed the non-feasibility of routing the VSD to the aorta (arising from the superior/leftwards morphological RV). The 3D model led to a drastic change in the surgical plan, with the adoption of a thoracotomy approach for coarctation repair and pulmonary artery band as the first step in single ventricle palliation. Surgery was safely executed. The 3D print helped surgeons avoid a futile sternotomy, cardiotomy, and cardiopulmonary bypass run, thereby minimizing the risk of complications and optimizing the postoperative recovery. Subsequently, the patient was successfully staged through bidirectional Glenn shunt (BDGS) and Fontan operation.

- *Case 3*: A 9-year-old girl presented 3 years after extracardiac Fontan operation with protein-losing enteropathy (PLE). She had been evaluated and managed previously in outside institutions with a cardiac diagnosis of DORV with large, remote VSD, with d-malposed great arteries. Anatomy had been deemed unsuitable for biventricular repair due to the difficult LV-to-aorta routing pathway and borderline smallness of the RV cavity. She had undergone BDGS with pulmonary artery banding (PAB) at 1 year, and extracardiac Fontan completion at 6 years of age. In the context of Fontan failure and PLE, she was reevaluated for the possibility of biventricular conversion or a heart transplant. The complex intracardiac anatomy was resolved using a "hollow heart" 3D model printed using clear resin on an in-house desktop SLA printer. The split-open model was used to make a meticulous plan of the surgical steps for biventricular correction, with Fontan take-down. The surgery was successfully accomplished as per the plan (Fig. 24.7).
- *Case 4*: A 5-day-old female neonate presented with severe cyanosis, tachypnea, and tachycardia. Echocardiogram revealed mixed TAPVR with severe pulmonary artery hypertension. However, standard echocardiographic planes failed to demonstrate the unusually tortuous anatomy of the common pulmonary veins. 3D print created on desktop SLA printer using flexible, transparent resin provided clear anatomical delineation and a roadmap for surgical correction (Fig. 24.3a).
- *Case 5*: A 6-year-old boy with situs inversus, dextrocardia with complex intracardiac anatomy, had been refused corrective surgery on multiple previous occasions at outside hospitals. The interventricular relationship was complex with the left-sided morphological right ventricle wrapping around the leftward, inferior, and posterior morphological left ventricle. The ventricular septal alignment was unusual and difficult to understand through conventional imaging including echocardiogram, MRI, and CT. 3D model allowed detailed understanding, enabling successful corrective surgery (Fig. 24.8).

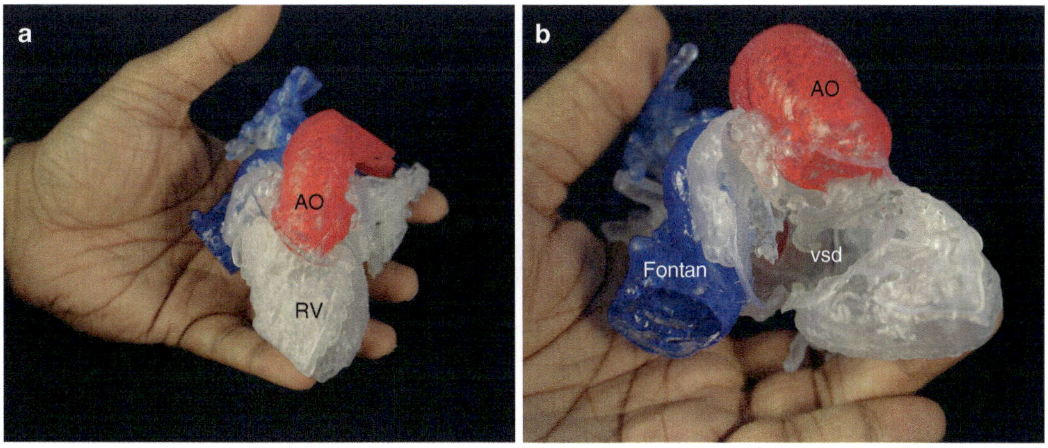

Fig. 24.7 Three-dimensional model of Case 3, clearly showing the relationship of ventricular septal defect (VSD) to aorta (AO). (**a**) shows the external features, while (**b**) reveals the intracardiac features. *AO* aorta, *RV* right ventricle, *vsd* ventricular septal defect

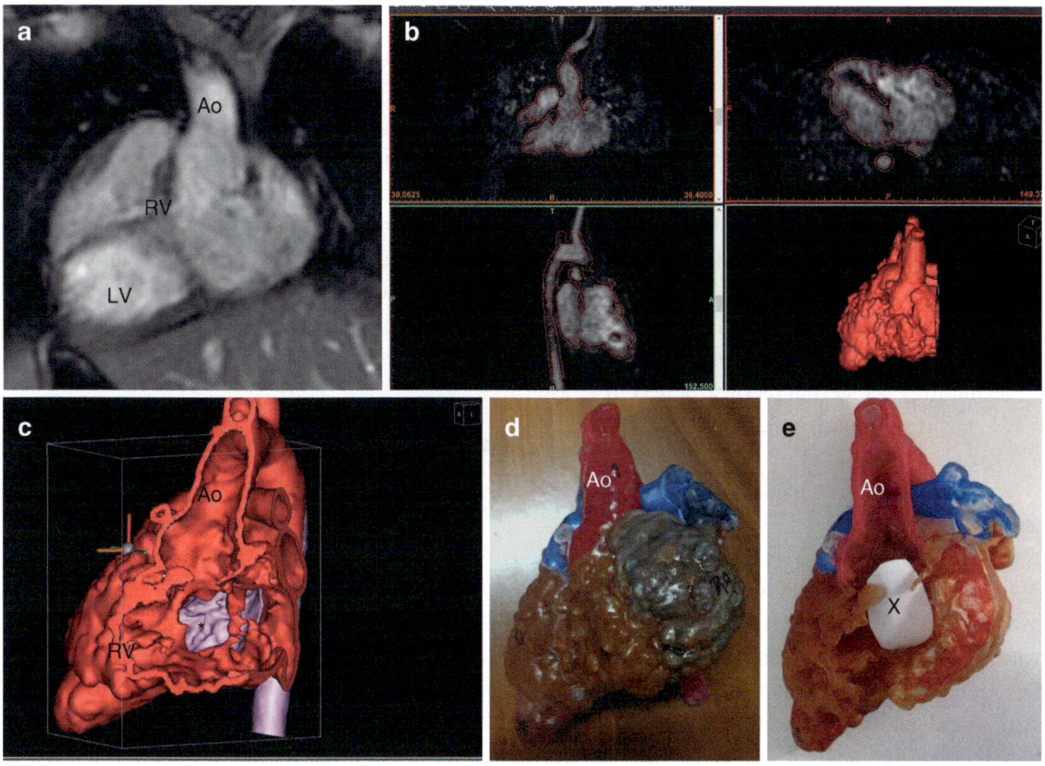

Fig. 24.8 Case 4—(**a**) 2D SSFP coronal image. (**b**) Segmentation process. (**c**) Digital 3D image showing the intracardiac anatomy. (**d**, **e**) Three-dimensional model. *AO* aorta, *RV* right ventricle, *X* simulation of patch-closure and routing of ventricular septal defect

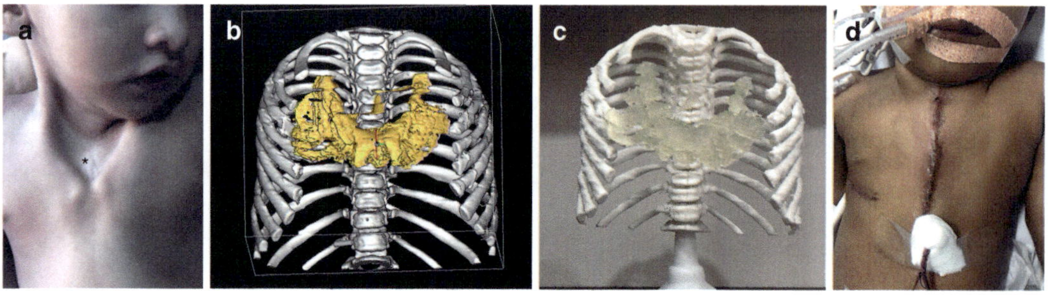

Fig. 24.9 (**a**) Absent sternum in a young infant. (**b**) Digital three-dimensional image of the lesion. (**c**) Three-dimensional model. (**d**) Postoperative image. *marks the region of the sternal cleft on figure (**a**)

- *Case 6:* A 9-month-old child with congenital complete sternal cleft was considered for sternal reconstruction. The thoracic cage of the patient was 3D printed in PLA material using in-house FDM 3D printer and was used to formulate a meticulous surgical plan. The thoracic cage model allowed a clear understanding of the anatomical challenges—the length and shape of the cleft. Surgical reconstruction of the sternum was simulated using a resected length of the right seventh rib from the 3D printed model. The surgery was executed as per the plan with sternal reconstruction using autologous right seventh rib graft laid on a perichondrial bed over the sternal cleft. This was the first such use of 3D printing technology for sternal reconstruction in a case of absent sternum (Fig. 24.9).

24.9 Summary

3D printing is not a novel medical imaging modality, rather it is a novel and more tangible way to interact with medical images. It simplifies spatial understanding and the appreciation of size, shape, and form of actual anatomical parts, thereby enabling accurate surgical planning and range of other applications. Point-of-care (POC) 3D printing laboratories can be easily established within medical institutions, considerably enhancing adoption, reducing turn-around times, reducing costs, and maximizing benefits of medical 3D printing. The digital 3D models generated after segmentation can be preserved in virtual morphology libraries and can be printed out any number of times—providing an infinitesimal repository of all possible pathologies. The virtual 3D files also serve as a substrate to develop the next generation of interactive visualizations in the form of Virtual Reality and Augmented Reality. 3D printing opens up the possibilities for truly personalized medicine with patient-specific surgical guides, implants, devices, and prostheses. Biological 3D printing holds tremendous potential for printing out biological tissues and organs in the future. 3D printing technology has the true potential to be a game-changer in the field of medicine.

References

1. Berney S, Bétrancourt M, Molinari G, et al. How spatial abilities and dynamic visualizations interplay when learning functional anatomy with 3D anatomical models. Anat Sci Educ. 2015;8:452–62.
2. Kodama H. Automatic method for fabricating a three-dimensional plastic model with photo-hardening polymer. Rev Sci Instrum. 1981;52(11):1770–3.
3. History of 3D printing: when was 3D printing invented? All3DP. 10 Dec 2018. Retrieved 22 Nov 2019.
4. 3D printing. Wikipedia contributors. Wikipedia, The Free Encyclopedia. Revised 10 Apr 2020 07:21 UTC. Retrieved 1 Apr 2020 09:16 UTC. https://en.wikipedia.org/w/index.php?title=3D_printing&oldid=950106237.
5. Lunghi C, Alais D. Touch interacts with vision during. Binocular rivalry with a tight orientation tuning. PLoS One. 2013;8:e58754.

6. Hadeed K, Acar P, Dulac Y, Cuttone F, Alacoque X, Karsenty C. Cardiac 3D printing for better understanding of congenital heart disease. Arch Cardiovasc Dis. 2018;111:1–4. https://doi.org/10.1016/j.acvd.2017.10.001.
7. Subat A, Goldberg A, Demaria S, Katz D. The utility of simulation in the management of patients with congenital heart disease: past, present, and future. Semin Cardiothorac Vasc Anesth. 2018;22:81–90. https://doi.org/10.1177/1089253217746243.
8. https://3dprint.com/242602/dr-anthony-atala-explains-the-frontiers-of-bioprinting-for-regenerative-medicine-at-wake-forest. Accessed 11 Apr 2020.
9. Rengier F, Mehndiratta A, von Tengg-Kobligk H, Zechmann CM, Unterhinninghofen R, Kauczor HU, Giesel FL. 3D printing based on imaging data: review of medical applications. Int J Comput Assist Radiol Surg. 2010;5(4):335–41.
10. Webb PA. A review of rapid prototyping (RP) techniques in the medical and biomedical sector. J Med Eng Technol. 2000;24(4):149–53.
11. Torabi K, Farjood E, Hamedani S. Rapid prototyping technologies and their applications in prosthodontics, a review of literature. J Dent (Shiraz). 2015; 16(1):1–9.
12. Winder J, Bibb R. Medical rapid prototyping technologies: state of the art and current limitations for application in oral and maxillofacial surgery. J Oral Maxillofac Surg. 2005;63:1006–15.
13. Cantinotti M, Valverde I, Kutty S. Three-dimensional printed models in congenital heart disease. Int J Cardiovasc Imaging. 2016;33(1):137–44.
14. Hibino N. Three dimensional printing: applications in surgery for congenital heart disease. World J Pediatr Congenit Heart Surg. 2016;7(3):351–2.
15. Garekar S, Bharati A, Chokhandre M, Mali S, Trivedi B, Changela VP, Solanki N, Gaikwad S, Agarwal V. Clinical application and multidisciplinary assessment ofThree dimensional printing in double outlet right ventricle with remote ventricular septal defect. World J Pediatr Congenit Heart Surg. 2016;7(3):344–50.
16. Farooqi KM, Gonzalez-Lengua C, Shenoy R, Sanz J, Nguyen K. Use of a three dimensional printed cardiac model to assess suitability for biventricular repair. World J Pediatr Congenit Heart Surg. 2016;7(3):414–6.
17. Farooqi KM, Uppu SC, Nguyen K, Srivastava S, Ko HH, Choueiter N, Wollstein A, Parness IA, Narula J, Sanz J, Nielsen JC. Application of virtual three-dimensional models for simultaneous visualization of Intracardiac anatomic relationships in double outlet right ventricle. Pediatr Cardiol. 2016;37(1):90–8.
18. Biglino G, Capelli C, Wray J, Schievano S, Leaver LK, Khambadkone S, Giardini A, Derrick G, Jones A, Taylor AM. 3D-manufactured patient-specific models of congenital heart defects for communication in clinical practice: feasibility and acceptability. BMJ Open. 2015;5(4):e007165.
19. Kappanayil M, Koneti NR, Kannan RR, Kottayil BP, Kumar K. Three-dimensional-printed cardiac prototypes aid surgical decision-making and preoperative planning in selected cases of complex congenital heart diseases: early experience and proof of concept in a resource-limited environment. Ann Pediatr Cardiol. 2017;10(2):117–25.
20. Farooqi KM, Mahmood F. Innovations in preoperative planning: insights into another dimension using 3D printing for cardiac disease. J Cardiothorac Vasc Anesth. 2018;32(4):1937–45. https://doi.org/10.1053/j.jvca.2017.11.037.
21. Batteux C, Haidar MA, Bonnet D. 3D-printed models for surgical planning in complex congenital heart diseases: a systematic review. Front Pediatr. 2019;7:23. https://doi.org/10.3389/fped.2019.00023.
22. Jones TW, Seckeler MD. Use of 3D models of vascular rings and sling to improve resident education. Congenit Heart Dis. 2017;12:578–82. https://doi.org/10.1111/chd.12486.
23. Loke YH, Harahsheh AS, Krieger A, Olivieri LJ. Usage of 3D models of tetralogy of Fallot for medical education: impact on learning congenital heart disease. BMC Med Educ. 2017;17:54. https://doi.org/10.1186/s12909-017-0889.
24. Biglino G, Capelli C, Wray J, Schievano S, Leaver LK, Khambadkone S, et al. 3D-manufactured patient specific models of congenital heart defects for communication in clinical practice: feasibility and acceptability. BMJ Open. 2015;5:e007165. https://doi.org/10.1136/bmjopen-2014-007165.

Radiation Issues in Pediatric Cardiac CT Imaging

25

Hemant B. Telkar and Srikanth Moorthy

25.1 Introduction

MDCT uses ionizing radiation, to produce diagnostic information. We as medical professionals should understand the potential advantages and risks of a test and balance them [1, 2].

This is particularly important for diagnostic tests that are performed for congenital heart disease (CHD) on children. It is imperative to have a clear understanding of radiation risk and the measures needed to reduce risk when doing cardiac CT studies in the pediatric population [3].

25.2 Basic Radiation Dosimetry Parameters

MDCT delivers radiation in the form of a narrow, fan-shaped beam of X-rays emitted from the X-ray tube during its rotation around the patient. By using special dosimetry techniques, radiation doses to patients can be calculated. This section describes the basic dosimetry, quantities used to indicate patient doses during CT.

H. B. Telkar (✉)
Infinity Medical Centre, Next to Gandhi (MGM) hospital, Parel, Mumbai, India

S. Moorthy
Amrita School of Medicine, Amrita Institute of Medical Sciences and Research Centre, Amrita Vishwa Vidyapeetham, Kochi, Kerala, India
e-mail: smoorthy@aims.amrita.edu

25.2.1 Absorbed Dose

Absorbed dose (unit-Gray-Gy) is the energy deposited in a small volume of matter (tissue) by the radiation beam passing through the matter divided by the mass of the matter.

CT radiation outputs are described by using the volume CT dose index (CTDIvol, expressed in milligrays) and dose-length product (DLP, expressed in milligray-centimeters). CTDIvol is an estimate of average X-ray tube output from an acquired CT image series, and DLP is the total X-ray tube output integrated throughout the entire scan, which is obtained by multiplying CTDIvol by the scanned length (in centimeters) of the patient. These metrics represent scanner X-ray tube output and not patient dose. For example, at any given CTDIvol value for the same diameter phantom, organ doses are substantially larger for small children than for large adults [4].

25.2.2 Equivalent Dose

The biological effects of an absorbed dose of a given magnitude are dependent on the type of radiation delivering the energy and the amount of radiation absorbed. Biological effect is smaller for X-rays (factor of 1) when compared the heavier alpha particles (factor of 20). The equivalent dose (unit–Sievert-Sv) is calculated as:

R. Rajeshkannan et al. (eds.), *CT and MRI in Congenital Heart Diseases*,
https://doi.org/10.1007/978-981-15-6755-1_25

$$\text{Equivalent dose}(\text{in Sv}) = \text{absorbed dose}(\text{in Gy}) \times \text{radiation weighting factor}$$

For X-rays of the energy encountered in CT, the radiation weighting factor is equal to 1.0. Thus, for CT, the absorbed dose in a tissue, in Gy, is equal to the equivalent dose in Sv.

25.2.3 Effective Dose

It is used to compare the stochastic (chance/probabilistic) risk of non-uniform exposure to radiation. Body tissues react differently to radiation and cancer-induction occurs at a different rate of dose in different tissues. Hence, the effective dose is a measure of the risk of developing fatal cancer in the tissue in question [5]. If the body is uniformly irradiated, the summed effective doses are equal to 1.

Broad estimates of effective dose (E) may be derived from values of Dose Length Product (DLP) for an examination using appropriately normalized coefficients.

$E = E_{DLP} \times DLP$ (mSv). DLP of the whole examination is auto-generated in all modern CT scanners at the end of the exam as part of a "Dose Report."

The DLP can be converted to an Effective dose using the k factor which is specific for body region and age (Table 25.1) [6].

For a cardiac CT, we would then multiply the DLP for chest by the factor as per age to get an effective dose in mSv.

25.3 Radiation Risks from Performing Cardiac CT in Pediatric Age Group

It is generally acknowledged that radiation dose is more concerning for a pediatric than an adult patient due to a relative increase in radiation sensitivity and a longer life span during which an adverse effect may manifest clinically [7].

The probability of absorbed X-rays to induce cancer is thought to be very small for radiation doses of the magnitude that are associated with CT procedures [8, 9]. Such estimates of the cancer risk from X-ray exposure have a broad range of statistical uncertainty and there is some scientific controversy regarding the effects from very low doses and dose rates.

Under prolonged, high-dose exposure, X-rays can cause other adverse health effects, such as skin erythema (reddening), hair loss, skin tissue injury, genetic effects, and birth defects [10].

But at the exposure levels associated with diagnostic cardiac CT, these adverse effects would not occur and have not been documented to date. However, some of these children may have to undergo repeated CT examinations and the cumulative dose can considerable. In appropriate patients, cardiac CT provides invaluable information and it is expected that more and more scans will be performed in the future. The potential for harmful radiation exposure should always

Table 25.1 Normalized effective dose per dose-length product (DLP) for adults (standard physique) and pediatric patients of various ages over various body regions

	k (mSv/Gy^{-1} cm^{-1})				
Region of body	0 year old	1 year old	5 year old	10 year old	Adult
Head and neck	0.013	0.0085	0.0057	0.0042	0.0031
Head	0.011	0.0067	0.0040	0.0032	0.0021
Neck	0.017	0.012	0.011	0.0079	0.0059
Chest	0.039	0.026	0.018	0.013	0.014
Abdomen and pelvis	0.049	0.030	0.020	0.015	0.015
Trunk	0.044	0.028	0.019	0.014	0.015

be kept in mind and the examination should be tailored to minimize risk from radiation.

25.4 Steps for Lowering the Radiation Dose from CT to Pediatric Population

All imaging modalities that utilize radiation must adhere to the "as low as reasonably achievable" (ALARA) concept regarding the delivered dose from the exam.

For cardiac CT, variability in the scanning parameters, size of the child, length of the body imaged, and whether or not ECG triggering was prospective or retrospective can affect the radiation dose [11, 12].

Below is a broad framework of Dos and Don'ts in available resources with imaging specialists.

25.4.1 Appropriate Selection of Patient

Perform a CT scan for congenital heart disease (CHD) only when it will provide required diagnostic information not available with another nonionizing radiation diagnostic tool, e.g., 2D Echo, or the overall patient risk is less than other imaging modalities (vascular access, contrast exposure, anesthesia, and sedation).

- Perform CT only when clinically indicated.

25.4.2 Patient Centering in the Gantry

Patient centering is a key aspect to achieving optimal image quality balanced with radiation dose and should be taught to all concerned staff responsible for patient positioning. Since the distance of the skin from the focal spot of the CT scanner determines the entrance dose to the skin of the patient (inverse-square law), positioning the child in the middle of the CT gantry reduces the radiation dose [13].

- The patient should be in the center of gantry.

25.4.3 Contrast Delivery

Contrast injection should be optimized so that the right quantity is injected with proper synchronization with image acquisition so that only one scan is needed for all information (try and avoid multiple runs) [14]. A plain scan is not needed in almost all CHD cases.

- Limit the number of acquisitions.

25.4.4 Appropriate Coverage

Limit the scan range to the area of interest (decrease *z*-axis coverage). CT radiation dose is directly proportional to the *z*-axis scan length [15]. When all other acquisition parameters are kept constant, the Dose Length Product (DLP) is directly proportional to CTDIvol scan length. It is essential that the scan length be minimized to include only the area of interest to reduce radiation dose.

- Remember 1 cm of extra coverage increases radiation by 20%.

25.4.5 mAs and kVp Settings

Keeping other factors constant, decreasing the kVp from 120 to 80 can result in up to a 65% dose reduction [16, 17].

Adjust scanner output for pediatric patients to 70 or 80 kVp for most children and 90 or 100 kVp for adolescents [18] (Figs. 25.1 and 25.2).

Lower voltage can also help reduce the amount of contrast material required for CT angiography

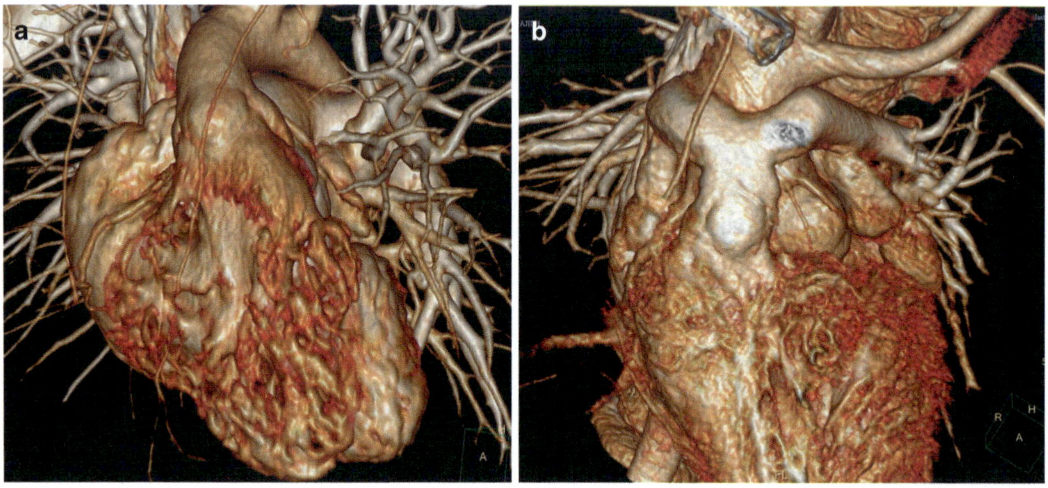

Fig. 25.1 CT scan of a case of transposition of great arteries (TGA) taken using 100Kv shows a smooth VRT image (**a**). But similar scan in a case of post-arterial switch using 80 Kv shows noisy but diagnostic quality image (**b**)

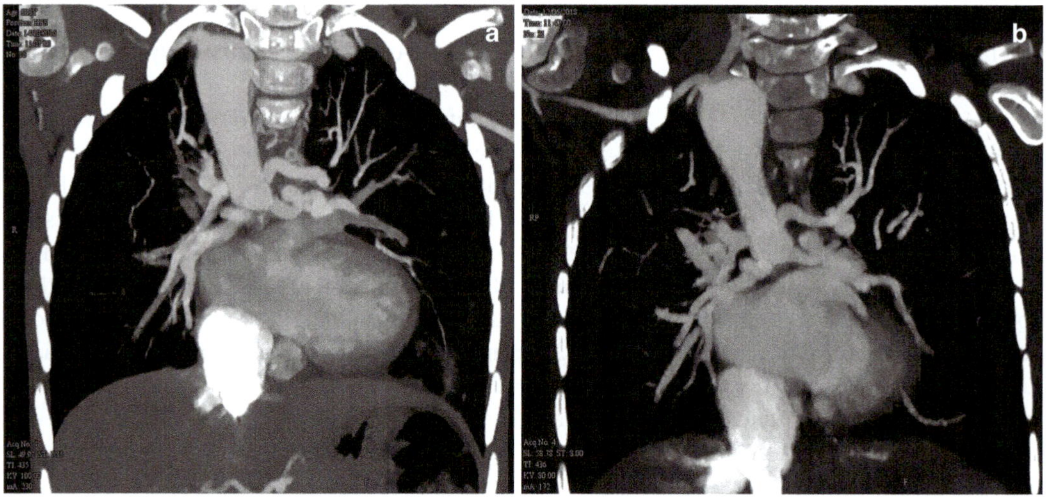

Fig. 25.2 CT MIP of a child with pulmonary atresia showing aorta-pulmonary collaterals. (**a**) was taken with 100 Kv showing smooth image and (**b**) was taken 2 years later using 80 Kv showing relatively noisy but diagnostic quality image

because iodine enhancement increases substantially at lower voltage [19, 20].

Automatic Tube current modulation or Automated Exposure Control [AEC]) modulates mAs based on the topographic (scout) image. It can reduce radiation dose by up to 40–50% over standardized imaging algorithms and works best when the patient is centered in the gantry [21].

All modern scanners have pediatric protocols for all regions, which will optimize all these parameters to the best advantage. The important thing is to ensure that this option is used for children.

- The lowest possible tube current (mAs) for a given tube potential (kVp) should be used in cardiac CT.

25.4.6 Pitch of Scan

Use the highest pitch scan mode or a volumetric scan mode minimizes both image acquisition time and radiation dose [22].

The radiation dose is inversely proportional to pitch when using helical scan mode. The latest generation of dual-source CT technology (in which dose is independent of pitch) permits scanning at a very high pitch (up to 3.4) because of the presence of two X-ray tubes [23].

The highest pitch scan modes decrease the time of image acquisition compared to standard pitch scan modes, and, therefore, can also decrease the need for sedation or anesthesia in young patients.

- Use the highest pitch for pediatric cardiac CT scans.

25.4.7 Thicker Detector Width

Thicker collimation is recommended when imaging larger structures, or for functional imaging, i.e., fine detail is not needed.

Thicker collimation (0.75–1 mm) will reduce radiation dose, improve image signal, and decrease image acquisition time [24]. Spatial resolution and visualization of small structures such as the coronary arteries, however, will be a challenge and appropriate width is set based on what information is needed.

- Use an appropriate scan width to reduce radiation dose.

25.4.8 Iterative Reconstruction

The use of iterative reconstruction results in improved image quality with standard scanner output, or lower radiation doses without loss of image quality if the scanner output is prospectively decreased. Multiple studies using different vendor's equipment have shown iterative reconstruction decreases radiation dose up to 40–50% [25, 26].

- Use iterative reconstruction algorithm.

25.4.9 Prospective/Retrospective ECG Gating and Non-ECG Pulsing

Gated studies deliver higher radiation dose than non-gated studies. Consider scanning without ECG gating when coronary and intracardiac anatomy is not necessary.

The lowest dose of ECG-gated scans will be obtained with a regular and slow heart rate. For coronary artery imaging, consider heart rate lowering medications and coronary vasodilators that allow prospective ECG triggered techniques to be used. This can reduce the radiation dose by at least 30% [27].

Higher heart rates often need a wider acquisition window for detailed coronary imaging increasing radiation dose. The highest doses may be obtained with an irregular heart rate during the scan monitoring phase, as the acquisition window will be automatically widened to capture a diagnostic image [28].

For both retrospectively and prospectively ECG-gated scans, the percentage of the R-R interval with full radiation can be narrowed to a single cardiac phase. The minimum acquisition window that will provide the necessary information based on indication and heart rate should be used. Some scanners offer automatic windowing to optimize the window and reduce the radiation dose to the patient based on patient-specific ECGs.

- Use non-ECG gated study whenever possible and prefer prospective gating to retrospective gating if the scanner allows.

In the end, proper training of all staff involved in cardiac CT of pediatric patients is essential to achieve an ALARA scan, keeping in mind that we need diagnostic information and not very beautiful appearing smooth images of the cardiac structures. It is better to record the dose calculated for each scan at the end of the final report to be self-accountable, to keep a track of cumulative radiation in children undergoing repeat scans and as a benchmark for future improvement.

Key Points

- Perform cardiac CT in children only when clinically indicated.
- Remember 1 cm of extra coverage increases radiation by 20%.
- The lowest possible tube current (mAs) for a given tube potential (kVp) should be used in cardiac CT.

References

1. Brenner DJ, Hall EJ. Computed tomography—an increasing source of radiation exposure. N Engl J Med. 2007;357:2277–84. https://doi.org/10.1056/NEJMra072149.
2. Lee CI, Haims AH, Monico EP, Brink JA, Forman HP. Diagnostic CT scans: assessment of patient, physician, and radiologist awareness of radiation dose and possible risks. Radiology. 2004;231:393–8.
3. Almohiy H. Paediatric computed tomography radiation dose: a review of the global dilemma. World J Radiol. 2014;691:1–6.
4. Huda W, Rowlett WT, Schoepf UJ. Radiation dose at cardiac computed tomography: facts and fiction. J Thorac Imaging. 2010;25(3):204–12.
5. Hausleiter J, Meyer T, Hadamitzky M, et al. Radiation dose estimates from cardiac multislice computed tomography in daily practice: impact of different scanning protocols on effective dose estimates. Circulation. 2006;113(10):1305–10.
6. American Association of Physicists in Medicine. The measurement, reporting, and management of radiation dose in CT. Report no. 96. College Park, MD: American Association of Physicists in Medicine; 2008.
7. Brenner DJ, Elliston CD, Hall EJ, Berdon WE. Estimates of the cancer risks from pediatric CT radiation are not merely theoretical. Med Phys. 2001;28:2387–8.
8. Berrington de Gonzalez A, Darby S. Risk of cancer from diagnostic X-rays: estimates for the UK and 14 other countries. Lancet. 2004;363:345–51.
9. Cohen S, Liu A, Gurvitz M, et al. Exposure to low-dose ionizing radiation from cardiac procedures and malignancy risk in adults with congenital heart disease. Circulation. 2018;137:1334–45.
10. Imanishi Y, Fukui A, Niimi H, Itoh D, Nozaki K, Nakaji S, Ishizuka K, Tabata H, Furuya Y, Uzura M, Takahama H, Hashizume S, Arima S, Nakajima Y. Radiation-induced temporary hair loss as a radiation damage only occurring in patients who had the combination of MDCT and DSA. Eur Radiol. 2005;15:41–6. https://doi.org/10.1007/s00330-004-2459-1.
11. Earls JP, Leipsic J. Cardiac computed tomography technology and dose-reduction strategies. Radiol Clin N Am. 2010;48(4):657–74.
12. Bae KT, Hong C, Whiting BR. Radiation dose in multidetector row computed tomography cardiac imaging. J Magn Reson Imaging. 2004;19(6):859–63.
13. Strauss KJ, Goske MJ, Kaste SC, et al. Image gently: ten steps you can take to optimize image quality and lower CT dose for pediatric patients. AJR. 2010;194:868–73.
14. Lell MM, Jost G, Korporaal JG, et al. Optimizing contrast media injection protocols in state-of-the art computed tomographic angiography. Investig Radiol. 2015;50(3):161–7.
15. Tzedakis A, Damilakis J, Perisinakis K, Karantanas A, Karabekios S, Gourtsoyiannis N. Influence of z overscanning on normalized effective doses calculated for pediatric patients undergoing multidetector CT examinations. Med Phys. 2007;34:1163–75.
16. Lira D, Padole A, Kalra MK, Singh S. Tube potential and CT radiation dose optimization. AJR Am J Roentgenol. 2015;204(1):W4–W10.
17. Sodickson A. Strategies for reducing radiation exposure in multi-detector row CT. Radiol Clin N Am. 2012;50(1):1–14.
18. McCollough CH. Maximizing dose reductions with cardiac CT. Int J Cardiovasc Imaging. 2009;25(6):647.
19. Sodickson A, Weiss M. Effects of patient size on radiation dose reduction and image quality in low-kVp CT pulmonary angiography performed with reduced IV contrast dose. Emerg Radiol. 2012;19(5):437–45.
20. Leschka S, Stolzmann P, Schmid FT, et al. Low kilovoltage cardiac dual-source CT: attenuation, noise, and radiation dose. Eur Radiol. 2008;18(9):1809–17.
21. Yu L, Li H, Fletcher JG, McCollough CH. Automatic selection of tube potential for radiation dose reduction in CT: a general strategy. Med Phys. 2010;37(1):234–43.
22. Primak AN, McCollough CH, Bruesewitz MR, Zhang J, Fletcher JG. Relationship between noise, dose, and pitch in cardiac multi-detector row CT. Radiographics. 2006;26:1785–94.
23. Goetti R, Leschka S, Baumuller S, et al. Low dose high-pitch spiral acquisition 128-slice dual-source computed tomography for the evaluation of coro-

nary artery bypass graft patency. Investig Radiol. 2010;45(6):324–30.
24. Kalra MK, Sodickson AD, Mayo-Smith WW. CT radiation: key concepts for gentle and wise use. Radiographics. 2015;35:1706–21.
25. Singh S, Khawaja RD, Pourjabbar S, Padole A, Lira D, Kalra MK. Iterative image reconstruction and its role in cardiothoracic computed tomography. J Thorac Imaging. 2013;28(6):355–67.
26. Leipsic J, Labounty TM, Heilbron B, et al. Estimated radiation dose reduction using adaptive statistical iterative reconstruction in coronary CT angiography: the ERASIR study. AJR Am J Roentgenol. 2010;195(3):655–60.
27. Shuman WP, Branch KR, May JM, et al. Prospective versus retrospective ECG gating for 64-detector CT of the coronary arteries: comparison of image quality and patient radiation dose. Radiology. 2008;248:431–7.
28. Leschka S, Scheffel H, Desbiolles L, et al. Image quality and reconstruction intervals of dual-source CT coronary angiography: recommendations for ECG pulsing windowing. Investig Radiol. 2007;42(8):543–9.

GPSR Compliance

The European Union's (EU) General Product Safety Regulation (GPSR) is a set of rules that requires consumer products to be safe and our obligations to ensure this.

If you have any concerns about our products, you can contact us on ProductSafety@springernature.com

In case Publisher is established outside the EU, the EU authorized representative is:

Springer Nature Customer Service Center GmbH
Europaplatz 3
69115 Heidelberg, Germany

Batch number: 10731383

Printed by Printforce, the Netherlands